W9-APD-602

BASIC PATHOLOGY

Second Edition

STANLEY L. ROBBINS, M.D.

Professor and Chairman, Department of Pathology,
Boston University School of Medicine

MARCIA ANGELL, M.D.

1976

W. B. SAUNDERS COMPANY • Philadelphia • London • Toronto

W. B. Saunders Company: West Washington Square
Philadelphia, PA   19105

1 St. Anne's Road
Eastbourne, East Sussex BN21 3UN, England

833 Oxford Street
Toronto, Ontario M8Z 5T9 Canada

Library of Congress Cataloging in Publication Data

Robbins, Stanley L

Basic pathology.

1. Pathology.   I. Angell, Marcia, joint author.
   II.   Title.

RB111.R6 1976   616.07   75–19853

ISBN 0-7216-7599-9

Listed here is the latest translated edition of this book
together with the language of the translation and the publisher

Spanish (*1st Edition*) — NEISA, Mexico City, D.F., Mexico

Basic Pathology   ISBN   0-7216-7599-9

© 1976 by W. B. Saunders Company. Copyright 1971 by W. B. Saunders Company.
Copyright under the International Copyright Union. All rights reserved. This book is protected by copyright. No part of it may be reproduced, stored in a retrieval system, or transmitted in any form or by any means, electronic, mechanical, photocopying, recording, or otherwise,
without written permission from the publisher. Made in the United States of America. Press
of W. B. Saunders Company. Library of Congress catalog card number 75-19853.

Last digit is the print number: 9   8   7   6   5   4   3   2   1

To
Sarah Rachael
and to
Lara and Elizabeth

Preface to the Second Edition

The favorable response to the first edition of *Basic Pathology* has made us wary of altering the book's goals and structure. The second edition, then, is also meant to be a "thin" book in which major diseases are discussed rather fully, minor ones more briefly, and very rare ones not at all. Again Part One concerns the general mechanisms of disease, with heavy emphasis on pathogenesis, and Part Two deals with specific diseases of the various organ systems from a strongly clinical perspective.

However, while the basic goals and structure of the book remain largely unchanged, the second edition is in substance a new text. The extensive revision was dictated not by any compulsion of the authors to tamper, but by the significant advances in the understanding of disease processes that have been made over the past few years. Particularly startling have been the changes in our conceptions of carcinogenesis, autoimmune diseases, lymphomas, glomerular diseases and viral hepatitis. Indeed, very few areas of pathology have remained unaffected by the influx of new information. In addition, two new chapters have been added. The discussions of environmental diseases, previously dispersed throughout the text, are brought together and expanded somewhat in a chapter of their own. Neuropathology, which was "freely omitted" in the first edition, is now conceded to be "best covered" in a text such as this.

The incorporation of new knowledge and the addition of two chapters have inevitably meant that, despite our good intentions, a thin book put on some weight. All we can say in our defense is that the added weight is not fat but muscle.

STANLEY L. ROBBINS

MARCIA ANGELL

Acknowledgments

The writing of acknowledgments after completion of a manuscript is a pleasant task for two reasons. It signals the completion of the text, but more importantly, it provides an opportunity to express our indebtedness to those who have contributed so much to us and to this book.

Foremost among those to whom we owe a large debt of gratitude is our editorial assistant, Ms. Kathy Pitcoff. Kathy expertly and enthusiastically participated in every phase of the preparation of this text: the preliminary library research; the typing and editing of manuscript; the maintenance of the voluminous and sometimes labyrinthine files; and the final meticulous screening of the proofs. The many errors that do *not* appear in this text are a testament to her uncompromising standards and to her dedication to this book. Such errors as may persist are the responsibility of the authors. We are also grateful to Mrs. Pam R. Adler for her support and encouragement.

Other colleagues and friends have helped in innumerable ways. Particularly deserving of acknowledgment are Drs. Hugues Ryser, Michael Bennett and Vinay Kumar for their expert and wise suggestions and critiques of sections of the manuscript. Drs. Leonard Gottlieb, Enrique Soto, Robert Terry, Michael Gerber, Remedios Rosales and Thomas Kemper all graciously provided illustrative "treasures" from their collections.

The burdens involved in the preparation of a text fall not only on the authors but also on their families, especially their spouses. This is even more true with a second edition, since any burden grows more oppressive with time. To Elly Robbins, apologies and much, much gratitude for her patient, willing acceptance of the many incursions imposed on her life by this book. The junior author (M. A.) is very grateful, once again, to her husband, Michael Goitein. Through his encouragement and devotion, along with judiciously measured advice, he contributed immeasurably to this book. M. A. also wishes to acknowledge the more brutal encouragement of her 6 year old daughter, Lara, who glanced at a few pages of the first edition, tossed it aside, and suggested, "Next time you write something, make it interesting." We have both tried very hard to do that.

We are also grateful for the cooperation and support of our publishers, the W. B. Saunders Company, in the enormous task of putting our efforts "between covers." While many individuals unknown to us undoubtedly made valuable contributions, a few merit specific citation: Ms. Catherine Fix, for her expert editing of the manuscript; Ms. Lorraine Battista for her skilled assemblage of the book; Mr. Herbert Powell, for his patient processing of the proof; and particularly Mr. Jack Hanley, Vice President and Editor, Health Sciences, for his unfailing courtesy to the authors and his enthusiastic faith in this text.

Finally, each of us would like to pay tribute to the other for endless patience and for resolute dedication to the distant vision. The joint authorship has more than survived these many years; it has thrived, not only because of a shared understanding of the complexities involved in such a cooperative effort, but even more because of our deep respect for each other.

S. L. R.

M. A.

Preface
to the
First Edition

Of books as well as men it may be observed that fat ones contain thin ones struggling to get out. In a sense this book bears such a relationship to its more substantial progenitor, Robbins' *Pathology*. It arose from an appreciation of the modern medical student's dilemma. As the curriculum has become restructured to place greater emphasis on clinical experience, time for reading is correspondingly curtailed. For this reason, we have attempted to extract from the body of knowledge of pathology the basic information necessary not only for the student but also for the busy clinician. However, by no means is *Basic Pathology* a synopsis. The weight loss has not resulted from pruning, but rather signals the emergence of an entirely new book with its own structure and approaches guided by the recent literature.

To produce the "thin" book, we freely omitted such subjects as neuropathology and diseases of the eye and of the skin which we believe are best covered in texts dealing with these specialties. Rare and esoteric lesions are omitted without apology, and infrequent or trivial ones described only briefly. We felt it important, however, to consider rather fully the major disease entities. It is our hope that sensible judgments have been made both in the subject matter included and, perhaps more importantly, in that excluded. In this, we have assumed the task more often left to the hapless student—that of establishing priorities. It represents an act of courage on our part which we are eager to exhibit, mindful that it places us squarely open to justifiable charges of omission.

The book is divided into two parts. The first deals with the general mechanisms and language of disease. Special emphasis is given to the pathogenesis of disease because we believe that an understanding of this is necessary to appreciate the dynamic nature of disease as it evolves from its incipient stage to its full expression. As far as is reasonable, pertinent biochemical and metabolic derangements are correlated with structural (and ultrastructural) alterations. And throughout we have tried to show the wider ramifications of the disease process as it affects other organs and distant parts of the body and, most importantly, the patient as a whole.

The second part of the book treats the pathology of specific diseases. We have chosen to give this section a strongly clinical orientation in the belief that such an approach is not only more interesting, but also of greater value in correlating morphologic changes with their manifestations. Thus, in most chapters the various disorders of an organ or system are divided into groups based on the clinical syndromes evoked in a typical patient. For example, in the chapter dealing with the respiratory system, major headings include "acute cough," "chronic cough," "acute dyspnea" (breathlessness), and "chronic dyspnea." The major respiratory diseases can reasonably be considered to present themselves in one of these four ways. We hope that this approach may make the book useful for nurses and allied health personnel as well as for medical students and clinicians. It should be emphasized that we are not offering an exhaustive differential diagnosis of symptom complexes. Clearly, this would be inappropriate in a text of pathology. Rather, the aim of our approach is to present the material in a relevant and assimilable manner. Pathology is not concerned primarily with cadavers; its genesis is in the living patient, and its greatest usefulness is to him. We hope that we have in some measure succeeded in relating pathology to its origins and to its significance.

STANLEY L. ROBBINS

MARCIA ANGELL

Contents

PART

ONE

CHAPTER 1

Disease at the Cellular Level

Begging the forgiveness of the clergy and the poets let us begin this consideration of pathology with the observation that man is basically a complex aggregation of highly specialized cells. The health of the individual has its origins in healthy cells. Disease, on the other hand, reflects dysfunction of a significant number of cells. It is necessary then to begin our consideration of pathology with an examination of disease at the cellular, and indeed, subcellular levels.

The normal cell is a restless, pulsating microcosm constantly modifying its structure and function in response to changing demands and stresses. Until these stresses become too severe, the cell tends to maintain a relatively constant or narrow range of structure and function, designated as normal. Thus, normal homeostasis is a fluid rather than a static, rigid state. Just as the individual must adapt to the constantly changing demands and stresses of life, so must the cell. Within limits, cellular adaptation achieves an altered but steady state, preserving the health of the cell despite continued stress. However, if the limits of adaptive capability are exceeded, injury or even cell death results. In response to progressive levels of stress, then, the cell may: (1) adapt, (2) be reversibly injured or (3) die. We can draw an analogy to a stately tree exposed to a wind storm. Up to a point the tree bends and yields to the stresses of the wind forces but rapidly resumes its erectness when the stresses abate. The wind-swept conformation of the tree on the shore line is a beautiful example of an adaptive, altered, but steady state permitting continued survival and growth. More severe wind may break branches and strip leaves, but such injury is compatible with recovery and survival. A hurricane, however, may be more than the tree can withstand and leave it an uprooted victim of stresses too great for survival.

The normal cell, the adapted cell, the injured cell and the dead cell are hazily delimited states along a continuum of function and structure. In response to sustained mild to moderate stress the cell might pass through a succession of stages of adaptation and injury, only to die eventually. More severe stress might induce direct injury and, of course, intense injury might kill immediately. One cannot assume that all stressed or injured cells pass through every stage of reaction. Whether a specific form of stress induces adaptation, injury or cell death depends not only on the nature and severity of the stress, but also on many variables relating to the cells themselves, e.g., particular vulnerability, differentiation, blood supply, nutrition and previous state of health. For example, liver cells are peculiarly vulnerable to inhaled or ingested carbon tetrachloride. Moreover, chronic consumption of large amounts of alcohol (itself a hepatotoxin) increases the liver cells' vulnerability to CCl$_4$. On the other hand, ganglion cells and myocardial cells are the first injured by oxygen deprivation (hypoxia), and ischemia (loss of blood supply) of the kidney first damages cells in the proximal convoluted tubules, sometimes not affecting the other tubules at all.

In many instances there are ready explanations for these particular vulnerabilities. Once absorbed, carbon tetrachloride is metabolized in the liver and Cl and CCl$_3$, radicals far more toxic than the parent compound, are released here. Thus, liver cells bear the brunt of this form of injury. Renal tubular cells often are damaged by CCl$_4$, but the reasons are less obvious. Since ganglion cells are dependent entirely upon oxidative phosphorylation, they are extremely vulnerable to oxygen deprivation. Cardiac muscle cells have an extremely high rate of metabolism and thus are almost equally susceptible to hypoxia. Sometimes the site of attack or delivery of the stressful influence determines the particular cells affected. For example, the pulmonary parenchyma is attacked directly by inhaled toxic gases. Despite these obvious explanations there are other instances in which stressful agents induce changes in mysterious sites. We do not know why, for example, the poliomyelitis virus attacks principally anterior horn ganglion cells in the spinal cord or why a toxic level of lead absorbed into the bloodstream exerts its effect principally on the hematopoietic system, the central nervous system and the kidneys. Nonetheless, it is important to know the major targets of the various forms of stress in order to make an educated guess at the etiology of the cellular change from the selective sites of involvement. Thus, the child with an anemia and manifestations of diffuse central nervous system involvement may well be a victim of lead poisoning.

All stresses and noxious influences exert their effects first at the molecular and biochemical levels. Regrettably, such deeply fundamental changes are only rarely detectable, even with sophisticated methods of study. Only when the functional alterations are fairly well advanced is it possible to determine whether the cell has adapted; in turn, functional adaptation must continue for some time before it induces morphologic changes. The structural lesions of reversible injury become evident only after some indeterminate period of stress, and similarly, the structural manifestations of cell death become evident only some time after the cell has died. The biochemical and functional changes always precede and,

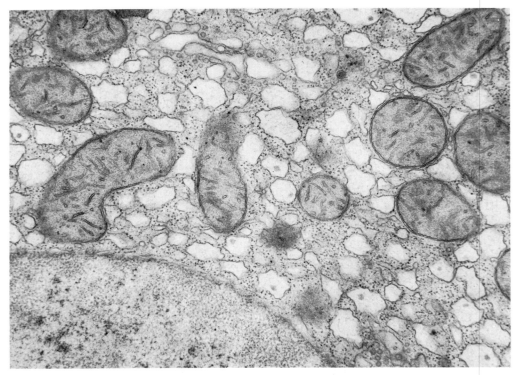

Figure 1–1. Rat liver cell four hours after carbon tetrachloride intoxication, showing well developed swelling of endoplasmic reticulum and shedding of ribosomes. Mitochondria at this stage are unaltered. (From Robbins, S. L.: Pathologic Basis of Disease. Philadelphia, W. B. Saunders Company, 1974. Courtesy of Dr. Iseri.)

indeed, induce the morphologic alterations. The time lag required to produce the recognizable changes of cellular adaptation, injury or death varies with the sophistication of the methods used to detect these changes. With histochemical or ultrastructural techniques changes can be seen in minutes or hours, but it may be much longer before they become evident with the light microscope or on gross inspection (Figs. 1–1 and 1–2). Despite sophisticated methods of morphologic and biochemical investigation, the boundary lines be-

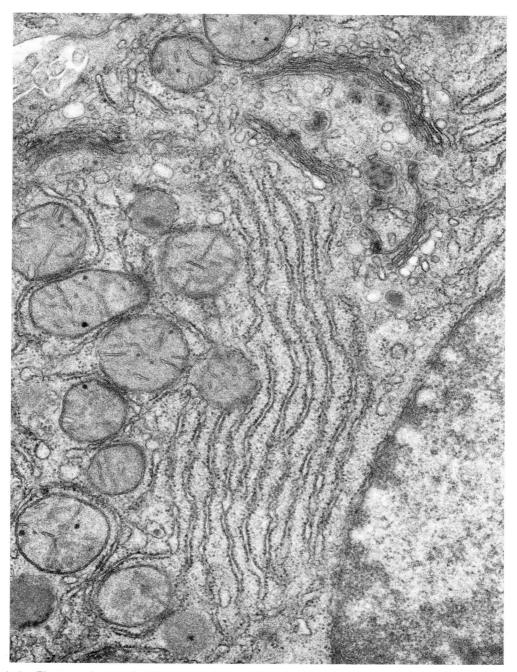

Figure 1–2. Electron micrograph of a portion of a normal rat liver cell (for comparison with Fig. 1–1). The nucleus with its double membrane is at lower right. Golgi complexes are seen in the upper right as parallel arrays of membranes associated with small vesicles. Evident also are the mitochondria and stacks of rough endoplasmic reticulum studded with ribosomes.

tween these stages are still difficult to define, and there are no clear benchmarks by which the severely stressed but still normal cell can be distinguished from the cell that has been taxed to the point of injury. Similarly, there are no certain parameters by which the injured but still viable cell can be differentiated from one that is fatally injured.

The following sections consider first the broad categories of stresses and noxious influences that induce cellular adaptation, injury and death; then the morphology of these three states will be taken up individually.

CAUSES OF CELLULAR ADAPTATION, INJURY AND DEATH

The stresses that induce altered morphologic states in the cell range from the gross physical violence of a crushing blow to the near-physiologic demands of prolonged increased physical activity. The muscled legs of the ballet dancer represent an adaptive response to high levels of functional and metabolic demands—i.e., a significant increase in the size of individual muscle cells. This adaptive alteration creates a new steady state which not only is functionally desirable, but also, like the shore-line tree, is pleasing to the eye. Most forms of stress or noxious influences ultimately affect fundamental cellular mechanisms or components, such as: (1) maintenance of the integrity of the cellular membranes, both that enclosing the cell and those of the internal organelles; (2) maintenance of the ionic and osmotic homeostasis of the cell; (3) production of energy needed for the cell's normal metabolic processes; (4) synthesis of proteins (enzymic and structural); and (5) the cell's genetic apparatus. The broad categories of adverse influences known to affect these basic cellular functions include: (1) hypoxia, (2) increased work demand, (3) chemicals and drugs, (4) physical agents, (5) microbiologic agents, (6) immune mechanisms, (7) genetic defects, (8) nutritional imbalances, and (9) aging.

HYPOXIA

Hypoxia, an extremely important and common cause of cell injury and cell death, impinges on aerobic oxidative respiration. Loss of blood supply, which may occur when the arterial flow or the venous drainage is impeded by vascular disease or luminal clots, is the most common cause of hypoxia. Another frequent cause is inadequate oxygenation of the blood due to cardiorespiratory failure. Loss of the oxygen-carrying *capacity* of the blood, as in anemia or carbon monoxide poi-

soning (producing a stable carbon monoxyhemoglobin that blocks oxygen carriage) is a third, less frequent basis for oxygen deprivation. Cyanide too is a cellular asphyxiant, inactivating cytochrome oxidase within the aerobic respiratory system. Depending on the severity of the hypoxic state, cells may adapt, undergo injury or die. For example, if the femoral artery is narrowed, the muscle cells of the leg may shrink in size (atrophy). This reduction in cell mass achieves a balance between metabolic needs and the available oxygen supply. More severe hypoxia would, of course, induce cell injury or cell death.

WORK OVERLOAD

When persistently stressed by increased metabolic demands, cells may first adapt by increasing the number of organelles, as for example the endoplasmic reticulum, myofilaments or mitochondria, leading to an increase in cell size. Eventually, however, such cells may decrease in size, presumably as a result of "exhaustion atrophy." Extreme work overload may ultimately kill the cell (though it must be admitted that irrefutable documentation of this is lacking). It is contended, for example, that in the form of diabetes mellitus caused by inadequate insulin secretion, prolonged high blood glucose levels may overwork the already taxed beta cells to the point of destruction. An imbalance between the level of metabolic activity and the available blood supply (similar to the injury caused by hypoxia) may be operating here. Alternatively, the increased metabolic activity might induce sufficient depletion of the aerobic energy reserves to force the cell to fall back on anaerobic glycolytic mechanisms. This event could create a sufficient drop in the intracellular pH to cause injury. It is sufficient to say that work overload is a known cause of cellular adaptation and may well be a cause of cell injury or cell death.

CHEMICALS (INCLUDING DRUGS)

Chemicals and drugs are important causes of cell adaptation, injury and death. Virtually any chemical agent or drug may be implicated. Even an innocuous substance such as glucose, if sufficiently concentrated, may so derange the osmotic environment of the cell that it causes injury or cell death. The habitual use of barbiturates evokes adaptive alterations in liver cells. Agents commonly known as poisons may cause severe cell damage and possibly, of course, death of the whole organism. We still know disappointingly little about the pathways by which many of these chemicals and drugs effect their changes, but presumably they all act on some vital function of the cell, such as membrane permeability, osmotic homeostasis or the integrity of some enzyme or cofactor. As mentioned earlier, the individual agent usually has specific targets within the body, affecting some cells and sparing others. In some cases this selectivity reflects the cell populations involved in the absorption, transport and metabolism of the agent. Barbiturates evoke changes in liver cells because it is these cells which are involved in the degradation of such drugs. When mercuric chloride is ingested it is absorbed from the stomach and excreted through the kidneys and colon. Thus it exerts its principal effects on these organs. Here the mercury presumably inactivates enzymes or competes for radicals such as $-SH$. As was pointed out earlier, however, we do not always have such simplistic explanations for the selective points of attack of the many chemicals and drugs which induce cellular changes.

PHYSICAL AGENTS

Trauma, extremes of heat or cold, sudden changes in atmospheric pressure, radiant energy and electrical energy all have wide ranging effects on cells. *Mechanical trauma* may cause subtle but significant dislocations of the intracellular organization of organelles, or at the other extreme, may destroy the cell by completely disrupting it.

Cold and heat are evident causes of stress, cell injury and even cell death. *Low temperature* acts in a number of ways. At first it induces vasoconstriction and impairs the blood supply to cells. Injury to the vasomotor control, with marked vasodilatation, stagnation of blood flow and sometimes intravascular clotting, may follow. When the temperature becomes sufficiently low, intracellular water crystallizes. Damaging *high temperatures* may of course incinerate tissues, but long before this point increased temperature causes injury by inducing hypermetabolism, exceeding the capacity of the available blood supply. Hypermetabolism also leads to the accumulation of acid metabolites, which lowers the pH of the cell to critical levels. Moreover, heat may denature proteins, including vital enzymes.

Sudden changes in atmospheric pressure also may lead to impairment of the blood supply to cells. Deep sea divers or tunnel diggers, when working under increased atmospheric pressure, have higher levels of atmospheric gases dissolved in their blood. If such individuals return to normal pressure too quickly the dissolved gases come out of solution rapidly and form air bubbles within the circulation. Oxygen is readily redissolved, but nitrogen is less soluble and may persist as small bubbles that become trapped in the microcirculation, blocking blood flow and ultimately causing hypoxic injury to cells. This disorder is called "caisson" disease.

The damaging effects of *radiant energy* were all too vividly illustrated by the atomic bombs (p. 233). Less grotesque exposure to radiant energy may also be injurious, either because of direct ionization of chemical compounds contained within the cell or because of ionization of cellular water, producing free "hot" radicals which secondarily interact with intracellular constituents. Radiant energy also induces genetic mutations which may injure or even kill cells (Totter, 1968).

Electrical energy generates heat when it passes through the body and may thus produce burns. More importantly, however, it may interfere with neural conduction pathways and often causes death from cardiac arrhythmias. The extent of damage induced by electrical current depends on its voltage and amperage, the tissue resistance (hence the generation of heat) and the pathway followed by the current from its point of entrance in the body to its point of exit.

MICROBIOLOGIC AGENTS

A host of living agents, ranging in size from the submicroscopic viruses to grossly visible nematodes, may attack man, causing cell injury, cell death, or indeed death of the individual. Here it is possible to discuss only a few generalizations about how these living forms affect cells. *Viruses* and *rickettsias* are obligate intracellular parasites, that is, they can survive only within living cells. The interaction between viruses and host cells takes many forms. Many viruses parasitize cells apparently without affecting them; these have been termed "passenger viruses." Those which induce cellular changes fall into two broad categories: (1) agents capable of causing cell death (cytolytic) and (2) agents which stimulate cell replication and possibly cause tumors (oncogenic).

The cytolytic viruses behave in a remarkably varied fashion. Although we do not understand the mechanisms involved, many have a highly specific cytotropism, and thus damage only specific types of cells. For example, the virus of poliomyelitis (acquired as an enteric infection) destroys only ganglion cells in the central nervous system, particularly anterior horn cells. The virus of viral hepatitis (acquired either as an enteric infection or by contamination of the blood from the use of infected hypodermic needles or blood transfusions) injures only hepatocytes. On the other hand, other viruses, such as the cytomegalovirus, attack cells in a variety of organs. Some viruses, such as that causing herpes simplex, may remain latent in the cells of the body throughout life. However, when the resistance of cells is only slightly reduced, the virus may cause disease. Thus herpes simplex may cause vesicles in the oral cavity or on the lips ("cold sores") when the patient is suffering from a respiratory illness, when his lips have been exposed to intense sunburn or when his general immune status is depressed. Yet the virus can be isolated from many individuals in the absence of such lesions. The cytomegaloviruses, also latent in many healthy individuals, may cause death when the patient is immunodeficient or develops some severe debilitating disease. The term "opportunistic infection" is applied to these disorders produced by microorganisms which generally are not pathogenic (disease producing) unless the individual is predisposed. Some cytolytic viruses cause disease soon after they parasitize the cells of man, as for example the viruses causing influenza, measles, mumps and many other conditions. Recently, it has become apparent that certain viruses, appropriately termed "slow viruses," require months or years to evoke cellular changes and disease. Progressive multifocal encephalopathy and subacute sclerosing panencephalitis, uncommon central nervous system diseases, are examples of slow viral infections (p. 666) (Marx, 1973).

We still do not know how viruses cause cytolysis and cell death. They may subvert the metabolism of the cell to their own growth requirements or compete for substrates essential to the life of the cell. Rapid intracellular replication and accumulation of virions may virtually explode the cell. Viruses may also induce antigenic changes within cells, and the immune response may mediate cell destruction. The mechanism of slow virus infection is, if possible, even more obscure. On the one hand it is proposed that the infectious agent is in some way defective and overproduces the nucleoprotein core but not the capsular envelope (possibly responsible for some of its antigenicity). Alternatively, it is suggested that the host may suffer from some T-cell immunodeficiency, rendering him incapable of mounting an adequate immune response (Editorial, 1974a).

As mentioned earlier, when some viruses (oncogenic viruses) infect the cells of man they do not cause cell death. Instead they not only stimulate cellular replication but also induce changes in the genotype and phenotype of the cell (transformation). This is the basis for the viral induction of cancers, which has been established so well in animals and is suspected in man (p. 93).

Bacteria, although they are extracellular parasites, are almost as unpredictable in their effects as viruses. Some are harmless commensals and some even contribute to man's survival. The *Escherichia coli* flora of the gut, for example, constitute a valuable source of vitamin K. However, even *E. coli* may cause disease in infants, who have little or no immunity to these otherwise innocuous organisms, or in debilitated or immunodeficient adults. Similarly, many individuals harbor potentially pathogenic bacteria in the oropharynx but develop a significant clinical infection only when rendered vulnerable. The administration of broad spectrum antibiotics may destroy the normal coliform flora of the gut and permit swallowed staphylococci to multiply wildly within the intestinal tract. A staphylococcal enteritis then ensues, which can lead to bacteremia and death. These, then, are opportunistic infections. In contrast, other bacteria, such as the agents causing syphilis, gonorrhea or plague, almost always cause disease if the organism gains a portal of entry. To the best of our knowledge there is no counterpart of slow viral infections among the bacterial diseases.

How bacteria evoke cellular injury and disease is still imperfectly understood. Some organisms liberate exotoxins capable of causing cell injury at a distance from the site of implantation of the bacteria. Other agents elaborate endotoxins that are released only on disintegration of the organisms. In addition, some bacteria may damage cells by elaborating a variety of enzymes such as lecithinase (*Clostridium perfringens*), capable of destroying cell membranes, or hemolysins (beta hemolytic streptococci), which lyse red cells. Another potential mechanism of bacterial injury is the development of hypersensitivity to the agent, leading to damaging immunologic reactions.

We know little about how *fungi, protozoa* and *helminths* cause cell damage and disease. Some, such as the histoplasma, coccidioides and the blastomycetes, induce sensitization reactions; but others, such as actinomycoses, do not. How protozoa induce cell injury is sometimes remarkably clear and at other times obscure. Amebiasis is caused by a protozoan which elaborates powerful proteolytic enzymes and so destroys tissues wherever it implants. The plasmodia of malaria invade and eventually destroy red cells by releasing toxic metabolites as well as malarial pigment derived from hemoglobin. The causative agent of toxoplasmosis, however, is an obligate intracellular protozoan which causes considerable tissue damage in its sites of localization by obscure mechanisms. Helminthic infections have their own specific sites of localization and induce cell injury for the most part by obscure means. The agent of trichinosis preferentially invades striated muscle (cardiac and skeletal) and eventually destroys parasitized cells. The trichina worm may usurp the energy supplies of the cell, or possibly its metabolic end-products are toxic, but these explanations are speculative. Filariasis is characterized by intense fibrosis at sites of localization, but we do not understand why such inflammatory fibrosis evolves. In conclusion, it must be admitted that with microbiologic infections, the ultimate mechanism of cell injury and cell death very often remains uncertain.

IMMUNE MECHANISMS

Immune reactions have come to be recognized as not uncommon causes of cell damage and disease. The trigger antigen may be exogenous in origin, as for example the resin of poison ivy, or may be endogenous, e.g., cellular antigens. The latter evoke so-called autoimmune diseases. The effect of immune reactions on cells is discussed in some detail in Chapter 6, page 167.

GENETIC DERANGEMENTS

Critical to the cell's homeostasis is its normal genetic apparatus. Mutations, whatever their origin, may have no recognizable effect, may deprive the cell of a single enzyme (*inborn errors of metabolism*), or may be so severe that they are incompatible with cell survival. The mutation may appear during gametogenesis, in the early zygote or in adult cells (a somatic mutation). Indeed, as you will learn later, somatic mutations may underlie the origins of cancerous transformation of cells. As is well known, some genetic abnormalities are transmitted as familial traits, as for example sickle cell anemia. More is said about genetic derangements in Chapter 5, page 123.

NUTRITIONAL IMBALANCES

It is sad to report that deficiencies in nutrition not only are important causes of cell injury today, but threaten to become devastating problems in the future. Protein-calorie deficiencies (which scourge many of the developing nations) are the most obvious examples. Avitaminoses also are rampant in deprived populations and are not uncommon even in industrialized nations having relatively high standards of living. Ironically, excesses in nutrition, privileged only to upper economic groups, may also become important causes of morbidity and mortality. Excess calories and diets rich in animal fats are now strongly implicated in the development of athero-sclerosis. Obesity alone leads to an increased vulnerability to certain disorders. Indeed, atherosclerosis and obesity, both related to the untoward effects of nutritional excesses, have become virtually epidemic in some countries such as the United States.

AGING

Aging must be mentioned as a cause of cell injury and death. While the changes of aging are considered by some to be merely physiologic consequences of life, their variable rate of development in individuals and among races and ethnic groups strongly suggests that some poorly understood, selective factors may be partially responsible for the cell injury and death in advanced years. In one individual, neuronal function may persist remarkably effectively into the eighth and ninth decades of life, while other less fortunate individuals become living vegetables in the sixth and seventh decades of life. The basis for these differences is still obscure, but factors other than age are under intense scrutiny.

Having discussed the major causes of cellular adaptation, injury and death and their possible mechanisms of action, we can now turn to the morphologic expressions of the changes incurred.

CELLULAR ADAPTATION

Just as animals, including man, have adapted to environmental changes in the evolution of their species, so do cells adapt to changes in their microenvironment. The normal cell does not exist in a rigidly fixed functional and morphologic state. Rather it traverses a fluid range of structure and function reflecting the changing demands of daily life. When stresses or noxious influences impinge upon the cell, it will, to the extent possible, adapt and achieve an altered steady state, permitting it to survive within its changed environment. We have just begun to understand the many facets and manifestations of cellular adaptation. A few of the better defined examples follow.

Induction of enzymes and organelles, such as mitochondria, ribosomes and endoplasmic reticulum, is one manner of adaptation to prolonged stress. The actively metabolizing liver cell has more oxidative enzymes and mitochondria than does the unstressed cell. If the liver cell is called upon to produce large amounts of plasma proteins, or similarly, if the plasma cell is stimulated to synthesize gamma globulins in an immune reaction, an increased number of ribosomes is formed. The liver cell chronically exposed to barbiturates is an excellent example of adaptation (Jones and Fawcett, 1966). Barbiturates are detoxified in the liver by oxidative demethylation, which involves hydroxylating enzymes found in the smooth endoplasmic reticulum (SER). The barbiturates stimulate *(induce)* the synthesis of more hydroxylating enzymes as well as more SER membranes. In this manner, the cell is better able to detoxify the drugs and so adapt to its altered environment. As one might surmise, as the liver cell develops greater capability to detoxify barbiturates so does the individual, and drug tolerance develops.

The induction of SER and its enzyme systems in liver cells by chronic exposure to barbiturates has effects on the metabolism of other compounds which are also degraded by hydroxylating reactions. As we shall see later (p. 21). CCl_4 is one such compound and bilirubin (p. 508) is another. Enzyme induction has recently come to the forefront in terms of the relationship between smoking and cancer of the lung. It has been observed that patients with this form of cancer have increased levels of cellular aryl hydrocarbon hydroxylase. This enzyme is capable of splitting hydrocarbon residues found in tobacco smoke into potentially cancerogenic compounds (Editorial, 1974*b*). Conceivably, patients who develop this form of cancer are those genetically most vulnerable to induction of this hydroxylase by cigarette smoke. Thus the adaptation of cells to their abnormal environment unfortunately sometimes has dire consequences to the host.

*Sequestration of focal injury—autophagy—*is a mechanism by which focal injuries within a cell, or worn out or old organelles, are sequestered and thereby isolated from the vital remainder of the cell. The injured focus (damaged organelles) is wrapped in membranes derived from the endoplasmic reticulum, thus creating an autophagic vacuole (Ericsson, 1969). While such a proposition is seductive and satisfying as a cellular protective mechanism, recent studies raise some puzzling issues. Trump and his co-workers (Arstila et al., 1972) have shown that mitochondria enclosed within autophagic vacuoles are not different from control mitochondria. The degradation of the mitochondria seems to begin after they are enclosed within the autophagic vacuole. Is it possible that autophagy occurs throughout life and is one part of the cycle of constant cell renewal? Alternatively, perhaps sequestered mitochondria are indeed damaged but the changes are too subtle to be detected by presently available means. In any event, cellular structures may be enclosed within membrane-bound sacs known as *auto-phagic vacuoles* or *cytosegresomes*. Thereafter, the autophagic vacuole fuses with lysosomes to produce an *autolysosome*. In this way the cellular structures enclosed in the vacuole are exposed to the degradative action of lysosomal enzymes. When the cellular debris cannot be totally digested it persists as a membrane-bound *residual body*. Most often, the undigested residuum consists of partially degraded, polymerized cellular membranes. With the light microscope these residual bodies appear as yellow-brown *lipofuscin* granules. Since autophagy occurs throughout life, lipofuscin accumulates progressively and these residual bodies are sometimes called *metabolic* or *"wear and tear" pigment.* It is of interest that liver cells and epithelial cells lining the kidney tubules, and possibly other cells, may extrude residual bodies, thereby unburdening the cell. Whether extruded or not, autophagy and the creation of residual bodies is by no means incompatible with normal cell function and represents a protective phenomenon permitting cell survival despite focal intracellular injury.

The cell may also adapt to an unfavorable environment by an increase or decrease in size. *Increase in cell size without an increase in the number of cells in a tissue is hypertrophy.* The cells are enlarged because more ultrastructural components are synthesized. As a consequence, the entire organ or tissue is enlarged. Hypertrophy is best exemplified in striated muscle cells, both those in the heart and those in skeletal muscle. Increased workloads induce hypertrophy of skeletal muscle cells, as is plainly evident in the biceps of the manual laborer and the legs of the athlete and ballet dancer. Elevated blood pressure (hypertension) leads to hypertrophy of the cardiac muscle cells and cardiac enlargement as an adaptive response (Fig. 1–3). *Such adaptive hypertrophy implies synthesis of enzymes, mitochondria, endoplasmic reticulum and myofilaments, achieving an equilibrium which permits a tolerable level of metabolic activity per unit volume of cell.* Hypertrophy is not limited to muscle cells; it may be seen in any cell, such as the liver cell or the renal tubular epithelial cell, which is called upon to increase metabolic activity.

On the other hand, when its level of function is diminished a cell may shrink. *A decrease in cell size and therefore in the size of the organ is designated atrophy.* Atrophy represents an adaptation to decreased workload, disuse, diminished blood supply or loss of endocrine stimulation. Thus atrophy is encountered in the skeletal muscles of a limb which is immobilized in a plaster cast or paralyzed by loss of innervation. Reduction in blood supply, when not sufficient to kill dependent cells, will

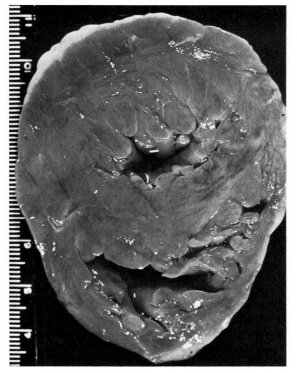

Figure 1–3. A cross section of a heart with marked left ventricular hypertrophy. The left ventricular wall is over 2 cm. in thickness (normal, 1 to 1.5 cm.). On the right side of the interventricular septum, the mottled, dark area is a focus of fresh ischemic necrosis (myocardial infarct).

bodies and lipofuscin granules. Thus, many atrophic, shrunken organs, particularly those composed of muscle cells, develop a brown pigmentation—a condition known as "brown atrophy." The heart in the aged individual, for example, may weigh only 200 to 250 grams (normal 350 to 400) and be dark brown in color, the so-called *brown atrophy of the heart.*

It should be noted in passing that small organ size may not necessarily imply atrophy. *Hypoplasia* (failure to develop fully) also produces an abnormally small organ. *Aplasia* or *agenesis* (total failure of the structure to develop) may also occur. Obviously, aplasia is compatible with life only when nonvital structures are involved, despite a common belief that some automobile drivers have aplasia of the brain.

The limits of cell adaptation are finite, however, and thus the point may be reached at which the vagaries of life not only buffet but actually begin to injure the cell.

CELLULAR INJURY

As mentioned, the cell's ability to adapt to stress or adverse environmental conditions is limited. When the limits are exceeded, cellular injury results, which may of course lead to cell death. There is no sharp line differentiating adaptive morphologic change from cell injury; nor is there sharp delimitation between the morphologic parameters of reversible injury and lethal injury. For example, it may be impossible to differentiate severe atrophic changes in cells due to restriction of blood supply from alterations reflecting ischemic injury. Similarly, if cells are exposed to a chemical poison, such as mercury, the cells may suffer nonlethal injury or be irreversibly damaged, depending on the level of the toxic agent. Despite intensive study, the "point of no return" may be impossible to delineate morphologically. Thus, as mentioned earlier, *adaptive changes, reversible damage and the morphologic manifestations of cell death represent a continuum, with one stage merging imperceptibly with the next.*

The morphologic changes which indicate cell injury become apparent only some time after the critical damaging biochemical event. The biochemical changes first lead to functional derangement, which eventually leads to the morphologic alterations. The time required for observable changes to develop depends on the methods used to detect them. For example, hypoxic injury to the heart muscle cells can be detected biochemically within 5 to 15 minutes by loss of oxidative enzymes, depletion of glycogen and reduction of ATP

cause them to atrophy. It is more than likely that immobilization of an extremity and denervation of muscles act by reducing blood flow. The ovaries, testes and secondary sex organs atrophy in advanced life, presumably as a result of loss of hormonal stimulation. The brain also atrophies in later life (as so many students suspect in their professors), possibly because of progressive atherosclerosis and restriction of blood supply.

Traditionally atrophy was divided into physiologic and pathologic categories, implying that atrophy of the brain, for example, is physiologic in advanced years of life but pathologic when induced by loss of blood supply (Fig. 1–4). Another classification employed special terms such as disuse atrophy, neurogenic atrophy, vascular atrophy and endocrine atrophy. *Ultimately all forms of atrophy imply some adverse environment requiring the cell to regress to a smaller size at which it may still survive but at a lower level of function.* At the ultrastructural level, the decrease in cell mass is seen as the breakdown of cell components accompanied by an increased number of autophagic vacuoles. Many of these autophagic vacuoles ultimately are converted into residual

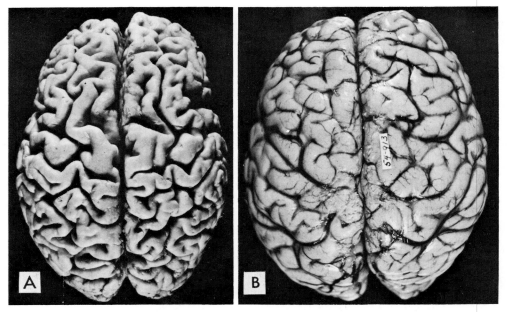

Figure 1–4. *A,* Physiologic atrophy of the brain in an 82 year old male. The meninges have been stripped. *B,* Normal brain of 35 year old male. (From Robbins, S. L.: Pathologic Basis of Disease. Philadelphia, W. B. Saunders Company, 1974.)

stores. Ultrastructural alterations, such as swelling and decrease in the matrix density of mitochondria, become evident very soon thereafter (Jennings et al., 1969). Classical light microscopic changes become evident only after 4 to 12 hours.

As was pointed out earlier, despite the availability of elegant and sophisticated methods of investigation, in the great majority of instances we still do not know the precise loci at which various noxious influences exert their first effect. Ultimately the basic physiologic functions of the cell, such as respiration and the production of ATP, maintenance of normal membrane permeability, osmotic and ionic homeostasis and preservation of the genetic apparatus, become deranged. Fundamental questions remain, however. What specific biochemical function or structural macromolecules does hypoxia affect first? Does irradiation damage DNA polymerase first, preventing synthesis of DNA, or does it instead act on bonds in the double helix, destroying already formed DNA? Considering the cell's complexity, it is not surprising that we do not yet understand the precise targets of cell injury. Complex interactions, such as feedback inhibition, induction and allosteric inhibition, represent delicately balanced mechanisms and damage to any one function leads, in ever-widening circles, to other derangements (Monod et al., 1963). If the cell's oxidative respiration is impaired, for example, synthesis of proteins is soon affected because

of lack of ATP. Loss of protein synthesis in turn leads to inability to maintain the integrity of membranes, and so on. Conversely, damage to protein synthesis means loss of formation of enzymes, which in turn affects aerobic respiration. Since any single function of the cell may involve numerous pathways and organelles, the problem is compounded. For example, oxidation of long-chain fatty acids appears to be carried out principally in mitochondria. Fatty acid synthesis, involving the production of malonyl-CoA and the step-like elongation of fatty acids by the addition of acetyl-CoA, however, occurs in the soluble portion of the cytoplasm. The synthesis of proteins for the formation of lipoproteins takes place in the rough endoplasmic reticulum. But where do they become linked to lipids? Some evidence suggests that this step takes place in the smooth endoplasmic reticulum. Clearly, then, fat metabolism involves numerous pathways and organelles. Furthermore, varying types of injuries may exert similar effects. It is well documented that certain chemical agents, viruses and radiant energy all can attack the chromosome. Thus, the problem of understanding precisely how injuries act on the cell is not a small one.

With this overview of the still unresolved problems relating to an understanding of the pathogenesis of cell injury we can turn to the consideration first of the morphologic manifestations of cell injury at the ultrastructural level, then of the morphologic manifestations at the light microscopic level, and finally attempt to correlate the functional and structural derangements.

MORPHOLOGIC EXPRESSIONS OF CELL INJURY — ULTRASTRUCTURAL

Cells react to injury in a limited number of ways. Damage to one biochemical function may affect one type of organelle first, but like a ripple in a pond, ultimately other functions and organelles are soon involved. Therefore, whatever the primary target, in time all forms of injury extend to involve the entire structure of the cell. For these reasons, it has been difficult to establish for most forms of injury the temporal sequence of morphologic alterations. Two agents, hypoxia and CCl₄, however, have been studied intensively in this respect and will be considered later (p. 20) in the correlation of deranged function with structure. In this presentation, each of the major ultrastructural components of the cell will be considered separately, detailing the pattern of morphologic change evoked by most injuries; the functional correlates will be presented later.

The pathologic changes in organelles compatible with cell recovery cannot be segregated clearly from those indicative of irreversible lethal damage. Obviously, when all mitochondria are destroyed and the entire internal structure of the cell is reduced to a shambles, the changes denote cell death; but even subtle dislocations may denote severe injury or cell death. A moment's reflection reveals that the normal cells examined with the electron microscope (and most examined with the light microscope) are in fact, dead. Death resulted instantaneously by immediate fixation which stopped all enzymic activity and thus preserved the ultrastructural architecture. In other words, organellar alterations only develop in cells which are living, and it is impossible to judge from the severity of these changes if the "point of no return" has been passed. Just recall how difficult it is to tell whether a plant can recover from lack of water by simply examining a drooping, dehydrated leaf.

Injury induces changes in the *conformation and size* of cells. With phase microscopy, the normal living cell in tissue culture is a pulsating microcosm, extending and retracting pseudopods and restlessly modifying its shape. It is probably not as fidgety in organized tissues. There is limited motion (pulsation) of internal organelles, but always within a fairly narrow range. When the cell is injured, the tempo of their motion becomes more feverish. If the injury is lethal, the motions and contortions slowly abate and eventually cease,

as the cell passes through a writhing agony before it dies (Bessis, 1964). When motion has ceased, the cytoplasmic pseudopods are retracted and the cell and nucleus both shrink. Buckley (1972) has documented this sequence in thermally injured cultured cells.

The *plasma membrane* is involved, primarily or secondarily, in virtually every form of injury. Early in the cell's response to adverse influences no morphologic alteration in the cell membrane can be discerned by electron microscopy; but biochemical studies unmistakably disclose increased permeability, permitting increased intake of sodium, water and calcium ions, as well as leakage of intracellular potassium, enzymes and cofactors. As will be discussed on page 20, this phenomenon of leakage of enzymes often provides important diagnostic information to the clinician. Sometimes this increased permeability is associated with paradoxic thickening of the plasma membrane. With progressive injury, breaks and discontinuities may appear. In lower animal forms, these breaks are repaired by a remarkable phenomenon, i.e., extrusion and coagulation of the perimeter of the cytoplasm. This peripheral coagulum effectively reestablishes a continuous enclosing plasma membrane. Conceivably the same phenomenon occurs in man. Membrane blebs, vesicles and elongated tubular projections may also appear in injured cells. In addition, lamellated concentric membranous layers, referred to as *myelin figures*, are sometimes encountered within the cytoplasm of injured cells. The derivation of these structures is still somewhat uncertain; but one proposal suggests that with membrane injury there is release of membranous lipoproteins into the cell. Dissociation of these lipoproteins releases hydrophilic phosphatides which bind water and become arrayed in molecular layers separated by aqueous interfaces. Thus, lamellated figures resembling layered myelin are created (Buckley, 1963).

Mitochondria almost invariably are altered when a cell is injured. One of the most common responses is an increase in size caused either by an increase in intramitochondrial components (very likely an adaptive response) or by mitochondrial swelling. The latter is associated with the cell's increased intake of sodium and water and efflux of potassium and magnesium. Along with swelling, the mitochondrial matrix becomes more translucent, developing sparse, finely divided precipitates and sometimes, in dying cells, flocculated dense granules. Often the dense granules contain calcium, which has leaked into the mitochondria because of the abnormal permeability of their membranes. All manner of mitochondrial pleomorphism (diversity of size and shape) may appear, but it must be appreciated that in the living normal cell the mitochondria undergo continuous convoluted motion — dividing, fusing, branching and changing in size and shape. Hence, some of the pleomorphic forms encountered in injured cells may merely represent fixation of the mitochondria at one instant in their busy lives (Fig. 1–5). In more severe injuries, the

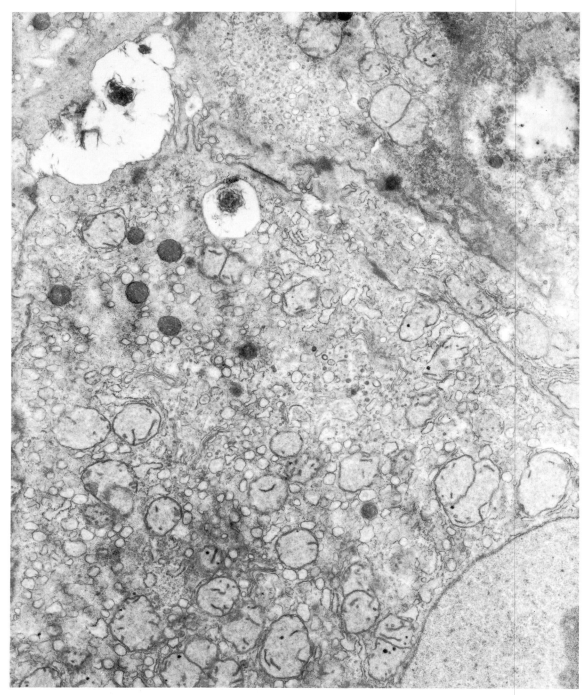

Figure 1–5. A liver cell from a rat exposed to a hepatotoxin for four days. Note the swollen, distorted mitochondria and cisternae of the ER. Bile stasis is evident in the distended canaliculus between cells, at the upper left.

mitochondrial cristae and internal membranes fragment and are disrupted. This, of course, is associated with loss of function of the related electron transport and enzymic systems.

The endoplasmic reticulum (ER), ribosomes and Golgi apparatus share in the general response to injury. The ER is a sensitive indicator of cell injury and has been called the "intracellular sponge." Dilatation of the ER is usually the first manifestation of deranged osmotic homeostasis of the cell. In severe forms of injury, fragmentation and vesiculation, particularly of the smooth ER, develop. Certain injurious agents, such as CCl$_4$, which specifically damage membranes, cause shedding of ribosomes from the rough endoplasmic reticulum and dissociation of polysomes. Sometimes the ribosomes themselves are separated into their 50S and 30S units (Smuckler and Benditt, 1963). Other abnormalities in the endoplasmic reticulum have been described, including the formation of whorled patterns, dense closely packed clumps and, as indicated earlier, autophagic vacuoles (p. 10). Dilatation of the Golgi apparatus has been described during hypoxic and other forms of cell injury.

Lysosomes, with their contained hydrolases, once were thought to play a primary role in cell injury and cell death; thus they were referred to as "suicide bags." It was thought that organellar dislocations and the eventual destruction of the cell were mediated by rupture of the lysosomes and release of their powerful catalytic enzymes. Recent studies indicate quite clearly, however, that lysosomes are relatively stable and remain morphologically intact despite severe cellular injury. They burst only after cell death and so release their enzymes to digest the cell's carcass (Hawkins et al., 1972). These findings do not preclude the possibility, however, that in reversible cell injury lysosomes may become abnormally permeable. As the pH of the cell falls, the leaked catalytic enzymes are activated. In support of this concept, it has been shown that free acid phosphatase and beta glucuronidase are sometimes present within the cell sap despite apparent morphologic preservation of the lysosomes. Indeed, it is possible to protect cells against many forms of injury by the prior administration of such membrane stabilizing agents as adrenal steroids.

As you recall, lysosomes participate in cell injury in other ways. They fuse with autophagic vacuoles to bring about the dissolution of contained biodegradable debris, including worn-out cellular organelles, and thus participate in the formation of residual bodies, including lipofuscin pigment.

A number of other ultrastructural changes appear in injured cells. *Loss of the normal complement of glycogen granules* is an early consequence of injury. It is most evident in damaged liver and striated muscle cells (including those of the heart). In the normal liver cell, glycogen is widely distributed in the cytoplasm in the form of dense particles frequently clumped together into rosettes. In heart muscle cells, the glycogen granules are more widely dispersed. When a myocardial cell is rendered hypoxic by ligation of a coronary artery for 5 to 15 minutes, there is substantial loss of glycogen (Jennings et al., 1969). Presumably deprived of its aerobic respiration, the cell falls back on glycolytic mechanisms and utilizes stored glycogen as the source of energy. It is important to note that in order to evaluate the glycogen content of cells, prompt and appropriate fixation is necessary. Glycogenolysis occurs quickly with inadequate preservation of tissues. Moreover, glycogen is slowly soluble in aqueous solutions and so may be spuriously depleted in tissues preserved in aqueous fixatives, such as formalin. To assay the glycogen content of cells adequately it is necessary to employ frozen sections of fresh tissues or of tissues fixed in absolute alcohol (avoiding paraffin embedding), and then utilize special stains. The periodic acid–Schiff (PAS) stain imparts a rose-violet color to the glycogen and Best's carmine imparts a rose-pink color.

In many forms of cell injury, *lipid droplets* appear within the cytoplasm. The droplets (liposomes) take the form of homogeneous round to oval inclusions of increased density which seem to be surrounded by a membrane-like margin. The rim is probably composed of a monolayer of phospholipids; their hydrophilic ends constitute the interface between lipid droplet and cytoplasm. Fat droplets are most likely to develop in those cells involved in secondary fat metabolism (e.g., liver cells) or in cells utilizing lipids as a source of energy (e.g., cardiac muscle cells). Sufficient lipid may accumulate to be readily visible with the light microscope or even grossly, and so will be discussed in greater detail in a following section (p. 17).

Hyaline inclusions appear in a variety of forms under a variety of circumstances. *The term "hyaline" embraces all material which has a homogeneous pink appearance under the light microscope.* When resolved under the electron microscope the hyalin may be amorphous or have a complex substructure. For example, hyaline inclusions are sometimes found in liver cells of alcoholic patients. Using electron microscopy, it can be seen that the hyalin has a fibrillar substructure and apparently represents a synthetic product of obscure nature, having a large component of protein (Iseri and Gottlieb, 1971). Hyaline droplets may also be seen in the epithelial cells of the proximal convoluted tubules of the kidney in certain forms of renal disease (e.g., mercury poisoning and other diseases associated with heavy proteinuria). There is now substantial evidence that whenever the glomerular filtrate contains large amounts of protein it is reabsorbed in the proximal convoluted tubular epithelial cells and appears as hyaline droplets within the cytoplasm. This alteration, therefore, is not truly a manifestation of cell injury.

Pigments, calcium deposits and a variety of other substances may appear within cells, but these will be the subjects of later considerations.

MORPHOLOGIC EXPRESSIONS OF CELL INJURY—LIGHT MICROSCOPIC

Traditionally the light microscopic morphologic changes indicative of nonlethal injury to cells are called *degenerations.* It is important to understand that *the term degeneration always implies reversible injury.* In this present day of electron microscopy it is evident that degenerative changes detectable with the light microscope occur only some time after more subtle ultrastructural alterations are discernible. The morphologic expressions of cell injury visible with the light microscope involve principally the cytoplasm. The nucleus is remarkably unaffected, save, perhaps, for some clumping of the chromatin against the nuclear membrane. *Three distinctive patterns of degeneration can be recognized: cellular swelling, hydropic degeneration and fatty change.* There is some virtue in differentiating among these three patterns because they offer clues to the nature of the injury. For example, fatty change in the liver is characteristic of alcoholism but is rare in viral hepatitis. Conversely, the acute stages of viral hepatitis typically are marked by striking hydropic degeneration (ballooning) of liver cells. However, it must not be assumed that individual agents always induce specific morphologic alterations; at best the correlations are imperfect. Sometimes an injurious influence first induces cellular swelling, followed by hydropic degeneration, in turn leading to fatty change. Such a sequence is not invariable, however. Sometimes cellular swelling passes directly to fatty change or, alternatively, the manifestations of cell injury may not progress further.

Cellular swelling is virtually the standard primary morphologic response to all forms of reversible injury. In the past this morphologic change was called *"cloudy swelling"* because the cytoplasm of such swollen cells has a clouded, ground glass appearance. It usually implies loss of intracellular reserves of energy or increased permeability of cell membranes leading to an increase of intracellular water.

Certain features of the control of normal cell water should be recalled here. The cationic composition of the intracellular fluid differs markedly from that of the extracellular fluid. The chief intracellular cations are potassium and magnesium; those in the extracellular fluid are sodium and calcium. The electrochemical forces, as expressed by the Gibbs-Donnan equilibrium, tend to draw sodium into the cell. The high intracellular content of protein cannot pass the semipermeable plasma membrane; therefore the cell requires active (energy dependent) transport of sodium out of the cell to maintain its normal osmolality. This active extrusion of sodium is known commonly as the "sodium pump."

If normal cell membrane permeability is impaired or the intracellular sources of energy are depleted, the sodium concentration tends to equalize on both sides of the membrane. Water passively follows the sodium into the cell, resulting in swelling. Thus, impairment of oxidative phosphorylation and depletion of the normal levels of ATP deprive the cell of its sodium pump (Majno et al., 1960). Alternatively, the initial lesion might be increased membrane permeability, which then permits sodium and calcium to leak into the cells. The presence of the latter cation compounds the problem, since it is a potent uncoupler of oxidative phosphorylation. At the same time, potassium diffuses out of the cell. At the ultrastructural level the cellular swelling can be resolved as swelling of the ER and the mitochondria. The mitochondrial swelling is a consequence of both loss of energy sources and increased membrane permeability, rendering the cell unable to maintain its osmotic homeostasis.

Cellular swelling is a difficult morphologic change to appreciate with the microscope, but it can sometimes be inferred from the compression of the microvasculature. It is more easily discerned ultrastructurally and, paradoxically, at the level of the whole organ. When all cells in an organ are involved there is an increase in overall weight and turgor and some pallor (because of the compression of the microvasculature). Remember, this form of cellular alteration represents an early and completely reversible manifestation of injury.

Hydropic degeneration (vacuolar degeneration) is a more severe form of cellular swelling. It represents sufficient accumulation of water within the cell to produce clear vacuoles when observed with the light microscope (Fig. 1–6). In large part the vacuoles represent markedly

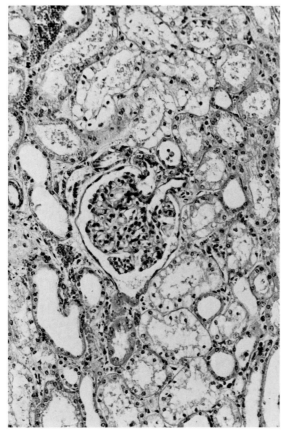

Figure 1–6. Hydropic degeneration of renal tubular epithelial cells seen in the center field above and below the glomerulus. The cleared, vacuolated cells contain dark displaced nuclei, suggesting that the hydropic degeneration has been followed by death of the cells.

distended ER. This type of reversible injury or cellular degeneration is particularly prominent in the epithelial cells of the kidneys in patients suffering from severe hypokalemia (low levels of potassium in the blood). Chloroform and carbon tetrachloride toxicity, as well as viral hepatitis, may cause hydropic degeneration in the liver cells. The gross morphologic changes evoked in hydropic degeneration are identical with those encountered in cellular swelling.

Fatty change is the most ominous of the cellular degenerations. Although reversible, it often implies severe injury and may even forebode cell death. It is characterized microscopically by the accumulation of fat vacuoles within parenchymal cells. Early there are numerous small vacuoles dispersed throughout the cytoplasm, creating a foamy appearance under the light microscope, but the nucleus is not displaced. More intense lipid accumulation leads to coalescence of these small droplets into one or more very large vacuoles,

which frequently distend the cell and displace the nucleus, sometimes compressing it against the plasma membrane (Fig. 1–7). Indeed, in very advanced fatty change, the cell may appear to be transformed to a fat storage cell. Sufficient accumulation may distend the cell until it ruptures the plasma membrane and coalesces with adjacent cells into a so-called fatty cyst. Whatever the size of the vacuoles, with routine tissue stains (e.g., hematoxylin and eosin) they appear as cleared spaces. Standard histologic techniques employ lipid solvents which remove the vacuolar contents. However, with appropriate aqueous fixatives and frozen section techniques, the lipid content can be preserved and stained with Sudan IV or Oil Red O, imparting a red-orange coloration to the lipid globules.

Fatty change is most commonly encountered in the liver, heart and kidneys, because the cells of these organs either are involved in fat metab-

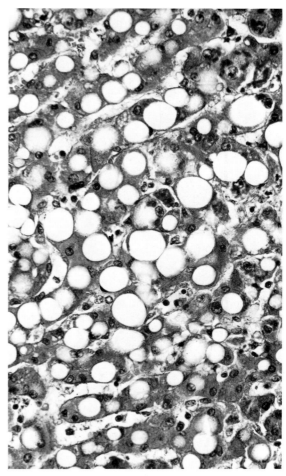

Figure 1–7. High power detail of marked fatty change of liver. The variability in size of vacuoles is evident. In some cells, the well preserved nucleus is squeezed into the displaced rim of cytoplasm about the fat vacuole.

olism or are largely dependent upon lipids for their energy sources. *Marked fatty change within the liver may increase its size two to three times and transform it into a soft, greasy, yellow organ* that readily fractures under slight pressure. Such fatty change is commonly encountered in chronic alcoholism, and it is often followed by the fibrous scarring of alcoholic cirrhosis. Severe protein deficiency states (kwashiorkor) and protein-calorie malnutrition also induce fatty change in the liver. Such extreme degrees of fat accumulation are not common in other forms of cell injury. Lesser degrees of fatty change in the liver are seen in diabetes mellitus, carbon tetrachloride or chloroform poisoning, halothane toxicity, phosphorus and gold poisoning, prolonged hypoxia and, in the experimental animal, in lipotropic deficiencies and following the administration of ethionine.

In the kidneys, fatty change most often involves the epithelial cells of the proximal convoluted tubules. When it is of a sufficiently marked degree, the fat causes the kidney to appear pale, slightly yellow and variably enlarged. This change occurs principally in profound hypoxia or after reabsorption of lipoproteins in renal diseases that induce abnormal excretion of these substances. In the kidneys, the fat manifests itself as small vacuoles within the cytoplasm of the epithelial cells. Sometimes the fat-laden cells bulge into the lumina of the tubules and rupture.

In the heart, fatty change takes the form of minute fat vacuoles in the cytoplasm of the myocardial fibers. It usually follows hypoxia from severe anemia or infections, such as diphtheria, which involve toxins injurious to the heart. In the former circumstance, the fat is distributed in bands, producing a so-called *thrush breast* effect, i.e., alternating bands of pale and normal myocardium. The pale bands of fatty change are thought to represent those areas of the heart most remote from blood vessels and therefore most hypoxic. In the second pattern, the toxin diffuses throughout the entire myocardium and produces a uniform fatty alteration, rendering the myocardium pale and slightly yellow. If these changes are not marked, they are often missed on gross inspection. In fact, it may be necessary to use the special techniques mentioned previously to visualize the fat droplets microscopically.

The pathways by which fat accumulates in injured cells have been studied most intensively in the liver. In essence, *fatty change in hepatocytes results from an imbalance between intracellular synthesis or accumulation of lipids and their oxidation or release.* Fat is normally presented to the liver in two forms: (1) free fatty acids, liberated from the peripheral fat depots by lipoprotein lipase; and (2) chylomicrons, formed by the mucosal cells of the intestinal tract following fat absorption. The chylomicrons, composed mostly of triglycerides combined with small amounts of cholesterol esters, phospholipids and lipoproteins, are first hydrolyzed, liberating free fatty acids and glycerols. Thereafter, the free fatty acids from the peripheral depots and from the chylomicrons are synthesized within the liver cells into triglycerides as well as cholesterol esters and phospholipids. Triglyceride synthesis probably occurs within the endoplasmic reticulum. Some of the synthesized triglycerides are oxidized as a source of energy and some are complexed to proteins to create lipoproteins destined for export out of the cell (Lombardi, 1966; Isselbacher and Greenberger, 1964).

Against this background of normal metabolism we can see how the various clinical disorders lead to fatty change in the liver. *The most common derangements involve (1) excessive synthesis of triglycerides, (2) decreased utilization (oxidation) of fatty acids and (3) impaired exportation of lipoproteins.* Some disorders act at more than one locus within this complex metabolic process. Hypoxia presumably interferes with fatty acid oxidation by mitochondria. Protein-calorie starvation induces increased mobilization of depot fat and excessive transport of fatty acids to the liver. At the same time, protein deficiencies presumably deprive the liver of lipotropic agents (choline and methionine) required for the synthesis of phospholipids and lipoproteins. The mechanisms involved in alcoholism are still somewhat controversial and are discussed in some detail on page 525. Here it is sufficient to say that the dispute centers on the question of whether alcohol itself is a hepatotoxin, injuring liver cells directly and impairing utilization and export of lipids, or whether the chronic alcoholic patient coincidentally lives on a diet deficient in proteins and lipotropes. The weight of evidence favors the view that alcohol is a direct hepatotoxin (Rubin and Lieber, 1967, 1974). DiLuzio (1973) claims that the mechanism of injury is peroxidation of the lipid moiety of membranes. This theory is supported by his observations that alcohol-induced fatty change in the liver can be blocked by the administration of anti-oxidants.

The significance of fatty change for cell function depends on its setting, but *in all circumstances, fatty change, even when quite marked, is reversible and is compatible with survival of the cell if the underlying cause is controlled.* Fatty change in the liver or kidneys may simply imply a metabolic overload of cells not affecting function, at least for a while. Fatty change in the myocardium, however, may impair function sufficiently to lead to cardiac failure. Similarly, extreme fatty change may be a cause of hepatic or renal failure. Of course, if the injury is sustained or severe enough, cell death will ensue. It should be noted that while cell death may follow fatty change, cells may die without undergoing this form of cellular degeneration.

The term "fatty change" now encompasses the older designations "fatty degeneration" and "fatty infiltration." *Fatty degeneration* was applied to the abnormal accumulation of lipids in injured cells rendered unable to metabolize or mobilize lipid—i.e., a true cellular degeneration. In contrast, normal cells might be presented with more lipid than they could metabolize and the accumulation of fat within the cell might in time cause injury. To this phenomenon the term *fatty infiltration* was applied. Nonetheless, large amounts of intracellular lipid, whatever the mechanism involved, ultimately impair cell function, and there seems little virtue, therefore, in continuing to make this distinction.

Fatty change affects parenchymal cells and should not be confused with *stromal infiltration of fat.* The latter refers to the accumulation of increased amounts of fat within the interstitial tissues of certain tissues and organs. This strange phenomenon is of obscure nature. Presumably the multipotential fibroblasts in the interstitium become filled with lipid and in effect are converted to "obese" fat cells. Stromal infiltration by fat tends to be associated with obesity or with atrophy of parenchymal cells, but the correlations are imperfect. The heart and pancreas are most often involved. In the heart, stromal infiltration of fat is seen mainly in the right ventricle, where strands of grossly visible fat extend from the subepicardial fat directly through the ventricular wall and appear as small yellow accumulations beneath the endocardium. Thus, the parenchymal cardiac muscle bundles are separated by the fatty strands, but the muscle cells themselves are unaffected. Similarly, the lobules of the pancreas may be separated by large septa of typical adult fatty tissue. As far as can be determined, the fat does not affect the function of either the heart or pancreas.

In the past the term "degeneration" was also applied to a variety of changes, none of which is a cellular injury. These usages require clarification. The term *hyaline degeneration* has been used to describe any cellular or subcellular structure having a homogeneous, glassy pink appearance in routine tissue stains. As stated earlier, *this tinctorial characteristic is caused by a number of alterations, none of which represents a specific pattern of degeneration.*

For example, old collagenous fibrous tissue appears hyaline, but this is not a sign of cellular degeneration. The term "hyalinized" has also been used to describe blood vessels in long-standing hypertension. In this disease the vessel walls become hyalinized and appear glassy pink, obscuring the underlying cellular detail. The same term has been applied to deposits of amyloid, now known to represent an abnormal synthetic product (partly immunoglobulin) of cells. Pink hyaline cytoplasmic droplets within the damaged liver cells in the chronic alcoholic person were described earlier (p. 15). Similar hyaline deposits are sometimes encountered in primary liver cell cancers, as well as other forms of liver disease. Severe febrile illnesses, such as typhoid fever, diphtheria and Weil's disease, sometimes cause a form of muscle change that has been referred to as Zenker's hyaline degeneration (in all probability a variant of coagulative necrosis, to be described later). Spherical hyaline masses known as "Russell bodies" occur within plasma cells in many forms of chronic inflammatory disease. Studies using immunofluorescence have shown that these represent immunoglobulins, at least in part. You will recall that hyaline droplets may appear within the epithelial cells of the proximal tubules of the kidney in mercury poisoning and in any other form of renal disease producing severe proteinuria (p. 16). It is apparent that the term "hyaline" is purely descriptive and is rather loosely applied to a variety of changes, none of which is a true cellular degeneration.

Mucoid degeneration is another common misnomer. It has been applied to abnormal poolings or accumulations of ground substance rich in mucopolysaccharides. Clearly, this is not a cellular degeneration. "Mucoid degeneration" is equally misapplied to excessive elaboration of mucinous secretions produced by inflammatory or neoplastic states affecting mucus-producing epithelial cells. Like old soldiers, these terms refuse to die.

Fibrinoid degeneration, another inappropriate term, is not a true regressive alteration of cells, but rather refers to a pink, amorphous, sometimes granular deposit resembling fibrin, typically seen in a focus of tissue injury. Often the site of deposition is in vessel walls or in connective tissue. *This pattern of injury is characteristic of immunologic disease,* although it does not always have an immunologic origin. Fibrinoid may also be found in the base of peptic ulcers and indeed in some normal placental villi.

The nature of fibrinoid is a controversial subject. With usual tissue stains, it appears as a deeply eosinophilic, amorphous material which sometimes entraps white cells or other necrotic cells. It is often located within the intima and media of vessel walls. Many substances have been identified in fibrinoid, including protein residues, DNA, fibrin, gamma globulins and complement. Its precise composition varies with the underlying disorder. Presumably, complement serves as the chemotactic influence for the polymorphonuclear leukocytes. The presence of immunoglobulins and complement strongly supports the belief that this material results from an antigen-antibody union that binds complement, and that this immune mechanism is the basic cause of the underlying tissue injury (Dixon, 1961). Whereas the fibrinoid material by itself is not a form of cellular degeneration, the underlying causes which lead to the precipitation of fibrinoid may also induce cellular injury, providing some basis for the otherwise inappropriate term "fibrinoid degeneration."

CORRELATION OF DERANGED FUNCTION WITH ALTERED STRUCTURE

Only a few forms of cellular injury have been studied intensively enough to permit correlation of the derangements in function with the consequent structural changes. Two—hypoxic and carbon tetrachloride injury—are presented here.

Hypoxia is one of the most common causes of cell injury in clinical medicine. Hypoxic damage (cell injury and cell death) of myocardial cells, known as myocardial infarction, causes 20 to 25 per cent of all deaths in industrialized nations. The hypoxia is almost invariably the consequence of ischemia, resulting from atherosclerotic narrowing or occlusion of a coronary artery. In this situation the impaired blood supply to the myocardial cells rapidly leads to lowering of ATP reserves and to a drop in intracellular pH owing to the accumulation of lactic acid (Vogt and Farber, 1968). The precise biochemical target of hypoxia is still not certain. Gallagher and associates (1956) propose that the first alteration induced by hypoxic injury is loss of respiratory cofactors involved in the Krebs cycle. Ozawa and his colleagues (1967) suggest instead that the ischemia activates some extramitochondrial lipolytic enzymes, which damage mitochondrial membranes. On the other hand, Vogt and Farber (1968), studying mitochondria from renal tubular cells, show that while ATP reserves are rapidly depleted, the mitochondria from these cells retain the capacity for oxidative phosphorylation. They speculate that other mechanisms may cause the depletion of ATP reserves. In any event, with loss of the ATP reserves, the sodium pump is slowed and cellular swelling, accompanied by swelling of the mitochondria and the ER, results. Glycolytic pathways are then activated, with lowering of the cellular pH. The shift in intracellular pH imposes a further obstacle to enzyme function. Maintenance of membrane integrity is impaired, throwing a greater burden on the sodium pump, at the same time permitting calcium to diffuse into the cell, where it acts as a potent uncoupler of oxidative phosphorylation, thus compounding the injury. Increased membrane permeability may permit lysosomal enzymes, which are activated within the lowered pH of the cell, to leak.

Besides unhinging the osmotic homeostasis of the cell, increased membrane permeability permits the diffusion of intracellular enzymes into the intercellular fluid and then into the bloodstream. Elevated blood levels of these enzymes thus become important clinical parameters of cell injury and, of course, cell death. For example, the cardiac muscle cells contain glutamic-oxaloacetic transaminase (GOT), pyruvic transaminases, isoenzymes of lactic dehydrogenase (LDH) and creatine phosphokinase (CPK). When the patient sustains hypoxic injury to the heart (myocardial infarction) the serum levels of GOT, LDH and CPK rise (Galen, 1975). Indeed, it is possible to estimate the amount of myocardium damaged by serial quantitative studies of these enzymes. It is worth noting here, and will be discussed in greater detail on p. 300, that the individual enzymes leak out at different rates, reaching peak levels at varying time intervals following a myocardial infarct. Other tissues, such as the lung, liver, pancreas and kidney, are also rich sources of GOT and LDH. Thus, ischemic damage to the lung (pulmonary infarction), which is readily confused clinically with myocardial infarction, also induces elevated serum levels of these enzymes. But CPK is found only in the heart, skeletal muscles and brain. Because disorders of the brain and skeletal muscle usually evoke clinical syndromes totally distinct from myocardial infarction, elevated CPK levels are of great diagnostic value in suspected cases of myocardial infarction.

Following initial biochemical disarray, the intracellular dysfunction and morphologic disorganization progress with ever-increasing rapidity. Shedding of ribosomes from the endoplasmic reticulum, cystic dilatation of the reticulum producing large vesicles, further swelling, distortion and rupture of mitochondria, and formation of plasma membrane vesicles and blebs all follow. Nuclear changes, such as clumping of the euchromatin to the nuclear membrane, also become evident, but such changes are reversible. As the extent of the injury mounts and the cells die, the nucleus undergoes further alterations characteristic of cell death, to be described later. *It is to be noted that the major morphologic hallmarks of reversible cellular injury are found in the cytoplasm. Irreversible cell injury, however, is denoted by nuclear changes.*

Carbon tetrachloride-induced injury is another model of cell injury that has been studied intensively. It has long been known that administration of CCl$_4$ to the experimental animal induces fatty change and eventually cell death, principally in liver and renal tubular epithelial cells. At high dosage levels, CCl$_4$ may act as a direct solvent on membrane lipids, but most of the evidence indicates that carbon tetrachloride derives its toxicity from its two highly active radicals, CCl$_3$ and Cl. Both radicals react with unsaturated lipids, such as are found in membranes, to form unstable organic free radicals, which in turn may interact with oxygen to produce organic peroxides. This sequence is called peroxidation, and it is the key event in the various biochemical and morphologic alterations observed in carbon tetrachloride-induced liver injury (Chopra et al., 1972). The evidence that antioxidants protect the cell against carbon tetrachloride injury supports this view (DiLuzio, 1973). Ultrastructural studies indicate that the endoplasmic reticulum of the hepatocyte is the primary target in CCl$_4$ injury (Rao and Recknagel, 1969). It appears that these organelles possess enzyme systems which are involved in the peroxidation of membrane lipids as well as the oxidative demethylation of drugs such as phenobarbital. As a consequence, pretreatment of animals with phenobarbital induces the synthesis of more enzymes and thereby enhances the toxic action of carbon tetrachloride on the hepatic cell (Reynolds et al., 1972). It is a classic instance in which enzyme and microsomal induction by one agent synergizes the injury-producing potential of another, enhancing the hepatotoxicity of carbon tetrachloride. Shedding of ribosomes from the rough endoplasmic reticulum, loss of the ordered array, dilatation and vesiculation of the cisternae and disruption of polysomes follow these initial alterations. These ultrastructural lesions have been correlated with a decreased capacity for protein synthesis (Smuckler, 1968; Smuckler and Trump, 1968), and inability to synthesize proteins leads to an inadequate maintenance of membranes—not only the plasma membranes but also those of organelles. Thus, cellular permeability, as well as permeability of other membrane-bound organelles such as the mitochondria, increases. Accordingly, there is an influx of sodium, water and calcium. The calcium unhinges mitochondrial oxidative phosphorylation, adding depletion of ATP to the cellular burden. Cellular swelling is followed by the appearance of lipid within the cell. The lipid accumulation is probably related to damage to the protein synthetic apparatus, which impairs production of lipoproteins necessary for the exportation of lipids. In summary, then, carbon tetrachloride is a model of injury in which the precise locus of attack—i.e., the lipid component of membranes—is fairly well delineated. Thereafter, as has already been made clear in the discussion of hypoxic injury, a whole chain of events is set into motion and if the membrane damage is sufficiently severe, the fatty change may progress to cell death.

CELL DEATH

Cell death is a logical but unfortunate extension of cell injury. Neither biochemical nor morphologic studies can predict with certainty which injured cells have passed the "point of no return" and are doomed to die. Cells can be recognized as dead only after they have undergone a sequence of changes referred to as necrosis. *Necrosis may be defined as the morphologic changes caused by the progressive degradative action of enzymes on the lethally injured cell.* The time required for the evolution of unmistakable evidence of necrosis varies with the specific cell type, its metabolic activity, temperature and the extent of cellular injury before the point of irreversibility has passed. Majno and his colleagues (1960), studying the liver cell, showed that it was possible to make light microscopic diagnoses of ischemic rat liver cell necrosis only 7 to 8 hours after the cells had died. Curiously, necrosis was recognizable grossly at 3 to 4 hours because of the abnormally opaque and pale appearance of the tissues. Yet at this point light microscopic examination disclosed cells that appeared possibly viable. Equally curiously, it is more difficult to recognize a dead cell with the electron microscope than with the light microscope. One can get too close to the trees to see the forest.

The morphologic changes of necrosis are effected largely by two concurrent processes: activation of intracellular enzymes *(autolysis)* and denaturation of proteins (possibly a consequence of increasing intracellular acidity). Most of the catalytic enzymes are derived from intracellular lysosomes which rupture after the cell has died. But, in addition, some lytic action is contributed by the lysosomal enzymes of immigrant leukocytes, a phenomenon termed *heterolysis*. The constellation of changes indicative of necrosis is then the result of biochemical reactions which ensue in the living patient after the cells have died. Since such reactions require time (minutes to hours), it is impossible on morphologic grounds to determine the precise instant of cell death. All too often coronary artery insufficiency and myocardial infarction cause sudden death of the patient—the well known story of the individual who drops dead on the street. As expected, examination of the heart in such a patient yields no signs of myocardial necrosis. The only telling evidence which may be available is occlusion of a coronary artery.

Neither is it possible in man to predict how much injury the cell can sustain before it will die. In experimental systems, one can determine the critical level of a certain form of injury requisite to kill a specific form of cell. For example, it can be shown that when the rat kidney is deprived of its blood supply for 20 minutes, after which the blood flow is restored, the renal tubular epithelial cells, although injured, eventually recover. However, 30 minutes of ischemia produces irreparable damage (Vogt and Farber, 1968). In order to determine cell death in these cases, the animal was allowed to live for 24 hours and the renal tubular cells examined for necrosis. Obviously, such experimental data are not available for man.

As far as we know there is no single biochemical or metabolic function which constitutes the cell's "Achilles' heel." Most likely the lethal injury takes the form of destruction of one of many enzyme systems vital to the cell's homeostasis. Once a single enzyme system has been unhinged, the functional derangements fan out in ever-widening circles, as was pointed out in the discussion of reversible cell injury. It is entirely possible that cells may survive the initial insult but succumb to its ramifications. Cells, then, may "die" piecemeal. Certainly this is often true at the level of the entire organism. Clinical practice offers many examples of the ability of the heart and lungs to continue to function for at least some time after cerebral function ceases; and in turn, the heart may continue to beat for a limited period of time after respiration has ceased. Thus, it is probable that certain functions of the cell persist transiently after it has already suffered fatal injury at some specific locus. Indeed, as you recall, focal cytoplasmic injuries or damaged organelles may be sequestered by the process of autophagy, but if the injury is lethal, this adaptive, protective mechanism is overwhelmed. Thus, at the functional as well as the morphologic level, it is impossible to identify the precise target, the specific point in time or the amount of disruption that constitutes irreversible injury incompatible with cell survival.

MORPHOLOGIC EXPRESSIONS OF CELL DEATH—NECROSIS

The ultrastructural changes in cell death need not be presented in great detail, since they are merely a progression and accentuation of those of cell injury described earlier (p. 13) (Trump et al., 1962). As indicated, only when the ultrastructural disorganization becomes extreme can the cell be recognized as dead. Conversely, cell death may occur with little if any ultrastructural disorganization, particularly when the cell is killed abruptly, providing no time for ultrastructural disorganization to evolve (e.g., immersion of healthy cells in a fixative). Usually, however, in the process of dying, some disorganization of the cytoplasmic organelles becomes evident.

Although cytoplasmic changes are the major indicators of reversible injury (degeneration), the hallmarks of cell death are found in the nucleus. You recall that with reversible injury the chromatin often becomes clumped against the nuclear membrane. With death of the cell further nuclear changes appear, in the form of one of three patterns. The basophilia of the chromatin may fade progressively (*karyolysis*), a change which presumably reflects the activation of the RNases and DNases as the pH of the cell drops. A second pattern is *pyknosis*, characterized by nuclear shrinkage and increased basophilia. Here the DNA apparently condenses into a solid, shrunken basophilic mass. In the third possible pattern, known as *karyorrhexis,* the pyknotic or partially pyknotic nucleus undergoes fragmentation. With the passage of time (a day or two), in one way or another the nucleus in the necrotic cell totally disappears. Meanwhile, the cytoplasm has become transformed into an acidophilic, granular opaque mass. This acidophilia represents an affinity for acid dyes (eosinophilia), resulting in part from denaturation of cytoplasmic proteins (which exposes basic groups) and in part from activation of acid ribonuclease, which destroys the normally basophilic cytoplasmic RNA. In this manner, the necrotic cell becomes converted into an acidophilic anucleate carcass. With the exception of the erythrocyte, all anucleate cells in man are dead.

Once the cell has died and has undergone the early alterations described above, one of three distinctive sequences ensues. The necrotic cell may undergo *liquefactive necrosis, coagulative necrosis* or, in special circumstances, *caseous necrosis.* The factors determining which of these pathways will be followed are still poorly understood, but some speculations will be offered later.

Liquefactive necrosis presumably occurs when cells die but when at least some of their catalytic enzymes are not destroyed. The liquefaction is brought about mainly by autolysis involving intracellular enzymes, principally those released from ruptured lysosomes. Heterolysis, mediated by the lysosomal enzymes of white cells that gather at the site of necrosis, is also a contributing factor. Liquefactive necrosis is particularly characteristic of focal bacterial infections, since bacteria constitute powerful stimuli to the accumulation of white cells (Fig. 1–8). For obscure reasons, hypoxic death of cells within the central nervous system evokes liquefactive necrosis, yet hypoxic death of heart muscle cells, liver cells, kidney cells and, in fact, most other cells in the body is followed by coagulative necrosis (discussed next). Whatever the pathogenesis, liquefaction essentially digests the dead carcasses of cells and often leaves a tissue defect filled with immigrant leukocytes, creating an abscess, described on page 47.

Coagulative necrosis implies preservation of the basic outline of the coagulated cell for a span of at least some days. Presumably the injury or the subsequent increasing intracellular acidosis denatures not only structural proteins but also enzymic proteins and so blocks the proteolysis of the cell. For a time, then, the general morphologic shape of the cell is remarkably preserved. Coagulative necrosis, as pointed out, is characteristic of hypoxic death of cells in all tissues save the brain. The

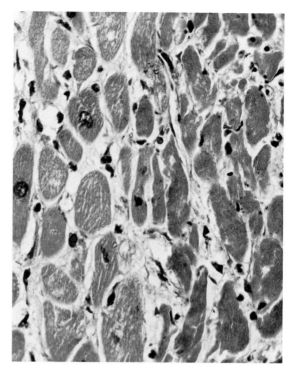

Figure 1–9. Myocardium, with preserved normal fibers on the left. The right half of the figure reveals coagulative necrosis of the fibers, with loss of nuclei and clumping of the cytoplasm, but with preservation of basic outlines of the cells.

myocardial infarct is a prime example. Here acidophilic, coagulated, anucleate cells persist for weeks (Fig. 1–9). Ultimately the necrotic myocardial cells are removed by fragmentation and phagocytosis of the cellular debris by scavenger white cells or by the action of proteolytic lysosomal enzymes brought in by the immigrant white cells. Some diseases, such as yellow fever and viral hepatitis, are characterized by coagulative necrosis of isolated cells. This sequence was once referred to as Zenker's hyaline degeneration, better called *Zenker's hyaline necrosis.* In this setting the coagulated cells are in time converted to rounded hyaline spheres called *Councilman bodies* (Klion and Schaffner, 1966). Coagulative necrosis may also be seen in the centers of rapidly growing cancers which outstrip their blood supply.

Caseous necrosis, a distinctive form of coagulative necrosis, is encountered most often in foci of tuberculous infection. The term "caseous" is derived from the gross appearance (i.e., white and cheesy) of the areas of necrosis. Histologically, the necrotic focus appears as an amorphous granular debris seemingly composed of fragmented, coagulated cells with a distinctive inflammatory enclosing border known as a granulomatous reaction (p.

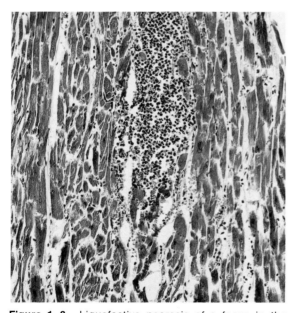

Figure 1–8. Liquefactive necrosis of a focus in the myocardium caused by bacterial seeding. The focus is filled with white cells, creating a myocardial abscess.

49). It is important to be able to recognize this morphologic pattern, because it is evoked by only a limited number of agents. Among these, tuberculosis is preeminent, as is discussed in greater detail on page 399.

Ultimately, in the living patient, most necrotic cells and their debris disappear. Even coagulated cells are eventually removed by a combined process of enzymic digestion and fragmentation, with phagocytosis of the particulate debris by scavenger leukocytes. If necrotic cells and cellular debris are not promptly destroyed and reabsorbed, they tend to attract calcium salts and other minerals and become calcified. This phenomenon, so-called *dystrophic calcification*, may occur despite normal serum levels of calcium and in the absence of systemic derangements of calcium metabolism. Usually it is seen in areas of coagulative necrosis, in foci of enzymic fat necrosis (p. 25), in old scars and in certain forms of tumors (leiomyomas and thyroid adenomas). Such tumors tend to grow slowly, and atrophy and death of central cells leads to foci of collagenization and calcification. Dystrophic calcification also is common in foci of cell destruction caused by certain microbiologic infections (i.e., tuberculosis, histoplasmosis, trichinosis and coccidioidomycosis), and is an almost inevitable accompaniment of advanced atherosclerosis (p. 266). The coronary arteries and the abdominal aorta, for example, are sometimes converted into rigid, calcified pipes. Severely damaged heart valves, particularly in chronic rheumatic heart disease and arteriosclerotic heart disease, are also prone to dystrophic calcification (Fig. 1–10).

Dystrophic calcification is a phenomenon of some clinical importance. The radiographic finding of a calcified lesion in the apex of the lung strongly suggests the presence of an old tuberculous or fungal lesion, which may or may not still be active. Similarly, calcifications in atherosclerosis may be disclosed by x-rays as densities almost invariably implying an advanced stage of this arterial disorder. Thus, the tendency for calcium to be deposited in foci of cell destruction is of more than academic importance.

The biochemical mechanisms resulting in dystrophic calcification are poorly understood and may indeed vary among the various settings. One theory proposes that denaturation of proteins first exposes reactive groups, which then bind phosphates released in the disintegration of the cell. In turn, the phosphates bind calcium (Glimcher and Krane, 1962). The calcification of arterial lesions in atherosclerosis has been attributed to alteration of the ground substance in the region of the atheromas, predisposing to binding of cal-

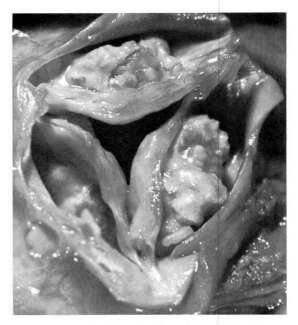

Figure 1–10. A view looking down onto the unopened aortic valve in a heart with healed (old) rheumatic aortic endocarditis. The semilunar cusps are thickened and fibrotic. Behind each leaflet are seen irregular masses of piled up dystrophic calcification.

cium ions. Whatever the pathway, dystrophic calcification usually develops slowly, over months and years. Occasionally it is seen remarkably soon after cell injury, as in some cases of pulmonary tuberculosis or acute toxic destruction of renal tubular epithelium.

Hypercalcemic (metastatic) calcification should be mentioned, if only briefly, to differentiate it from dystrophic calcification. The fundamental derangement here is hypercalcemia, which predisposes to the deposition of calcium salts in normal vital tissues. The major causes of hypercalcemia and the particular sites usually involved in hypercalcemic calcification are presented on page 616.

Wherever calcification occurs, in both the dystrophic and hypercalcemic forms, the calcium appears as a blue-black (in ordinary tissue stains), amorphous to granular deposit, sometimes within the injured cells but more often between cells. Sometimes the accumulation of calcium salts obliterates the underlying native structures. Old foci of calcification may undergo metaplastic bone production, creating hard masses that persist throughout life.

Having discussed the possible outcomes of necrosis, we must turn to some older usages of the term "necrosis" which require clarification. The term *gangrenous necrosis* is generally applied to a limb which has lost its blood supply and has been attacked by bacterial agents. In reality this is not a specific pattern of cellular necrosis but describes the cell and tissue changes produced by a combination of hypoxia and bacterial action. The surgeon is wont to refer to such changes as *wet gangrene*. If the limb is not attacked by bacteria, but has simply undergone loss of blood supply, and if the tissues and cells have suffered hypoxic coagulative necrosis, the condition may be referred to as *dry gangrene*. It is, in reality, ischemic coagulative necrosis.

Enzymic fat necrosis is descriptive of focal areas of destruction of fat resulting from abnormal release of activated pancreatic enzymes into the substance of the pancreas and the intestinal cavity. This occurs in the uncommon but calamitous abdominal emergency known as "acute hemorrhagic pancreatic necrosis." The activated proteases digest the fat cell membranes, and the activated lipases split the triglyceride esters contained within fat cells. The released fatty acids combine with calcium to produce grossly visible chalky white areas of necrosis described more completely in the consideration of the pancreas (p. 538). Enzymic fat necrosis is not a specific form of necrosis; the cellular changes are essentially liquefactive.

Traumatic fat necrosis differs from enzymic fat necrosis and moreover is not truly a distinctive pattern of cell death. Usually it is encountered in superficial adipose tissue, frequently in the female breast. It was once thought to be caused by local trauma. However, in nearly 50 per cent of the cases no history of trauma can be elicited. The designation "traumatic fat necrosis" is therefore somewhat inappropriate. Its causation is unknown but essentially it comprises focal rupture of fat cells with release of neutral and split fats, which evoke a striking leukocytic inflammatory response. This entity is described more completely in the consideration of the breast (p. 585).

In closing this discussion of necrosis it is to be emphasized that the recognition of cell death is of great importance because it implies irreversible loss of vital functioning parenchyma.

INTRACELLULAR ACCUMULATIONS

This section deals with an assortment of intracellular accumulations that may or may not impair the normal function of the cell. In general, intracellular accumulations imply either (1) presentation to the cell of excessive amounts of some normal metabolite, (2) accumulation of some abnormal nonmetabolizable product, or (3) excessive intracellular synthesis of some product. Intracellular accumulation of glycogen in diabetic patients who have prolonged high blood glucose levels is an example of the first mechanism. The second pathway might involve the intracellular accumulation of some abnormal product resulting from an inborn error of metabolism. The third instance is exemplified by excessive synthesis of some pigment, such as melanin, encountered in certain disease states, such as adrenal insufficiency. Some of these intracellular accumulations are apparently without functional effect, but others overload the cell and cause cell injury and dysfunction. All are important, however, because they provide morphologic evidence of the underlying causation or disease.

GLYCOGEN

Glycogen accumulation is a distinctive and relatively uncommon form of cell change. Some designate this cellular alteration as *glycogen infiltration*, but this is merely semantics. The condition is encountered in patients having deranged carbohydrate or glycogen metabolism — more specifically, in diabetes mellitus and a constellation of inborn errors of metabolism known collectively as the glycogen storage diseases.

Diabetics have high blood glucose levels and consequent glycosuria. Increased glucose reabsorption in the renal tubular epithelial cells follows, principally affecting the terminal straight portion of the proximal convoluted tubules and the loop of Henle (p. 137). The glucose is stored in the form of glycogen, which accumulates sufficiently to cause clear vacuolation of the cytoplasm of the cells in these tubules. Often the glycogen vacuoles displace the nuclei to the base of the cell. Glycogen accumulation in the diabetic is also encountered in liver cells where, for reasons that are not clear, it is most visible in the nuclei, which appear swollen and cleared. Although there is also an increase of intracytoplasmic glycogen in the liver cell, it is difficult to discern in ordinary tissue sections by light microscopy. No renal or hepatic functional deficit is associated with the glycogen accumulation.

In the glycogen storage diseases there is a genetic lack of one or more of the enzymes involved in either the mobilization of glycogen or the synthesis of normal glycogen. When an abnormal glycogen is synthesized, it cannot be mobilized and it accumulates. The sites of glycogen deposition in the several forms of the glycogen storage diseases are extremely variable and may affect the cells of the heart, liver, kidneys or other organs, depending upon which particular enzyme system is deficient. For example, the most common pattern, von Gierke's disease (p. 152), is caused by a deficiency of glucose-6-phosphatase which principally affects the liver and kidneys, and these organs bear the brunt of this metabolic overload. Pompe's disease (p. 153), in contrast, is characterized by a lack of a lysosomal glucosidase in striated muscles, including myocardial cells, and consequently normal glycogen cannot be metabolized by these cells and accumulates in skeletal muscles and the heart. In these storage disorders, the glycogen may accumulate to such excessive amounts that it causes cell and organ enlargement, dysfunction and, indeed, death of the patient at an early age. Whatever its setting, intracellular glycogen accumulation requires special stains, such as the PAS, to differentiate the clear vacuolation from intracellular lipids and water.

LIPIDS

As was pointed out in the discussion of fatty change (p. 17), lipid accumulations may be encountered in *injured* cells, which are unable to handle normal amounts of lipid. Here, however, we are concerned with the overload of apparently *normal* cells with lipid. The very common and serious disorder *atherosclerosis* is an example of lipid overload. In this disease the cells within the intima of arteries are laden with lipids, principally cholesterol and cholesterol esters, very likely derived from plasma lipids. The lipids accumulate principally within myointimal cells in the intimal layers of the aorta and large arteries, producing focal plaques (atheromas) which encroach on the vascular lumina and simultaneously injure the underlying media, as is described in detail on page 269. Most severely affected individuals have hyperlipidemia and hypercholesterolemia, which probably play an important causative role in the development of the arterial disease. Intracellular accumulations of cholesterol and cholesterol esters within phagocytic cells are also encountered in other hypercholesterolemic states, some of which are hereditary and others acquired. Usually these intracellular accumulations are located in subepithelial histiocytes and in tendons, where they produce tumorous masses known as *xanthomas*. These individuals are also likely to develop severe atherosclerosis. Scavenger macrophages may accumulate large amounts of lipid debris, particularly in inflammatory foci and in areas of trauma to fat depots. All cells overloaded with lipids appear foamy or develop large vacuoles; these require fat stains for determination of the nature of the intracellular accumulation.

PROTEINS

Protein accumulations may be encountered in cells either because excesses are presented to the cells or because the cells synthesize excessive amounts. Normally, trace amounts of albumin, filtered through the glomerulus, are reabsorbed in the proximal convoluted tubules. Any disorder producing heavy proteinuria leads to excessive reabsorption of protein, which appears in the form of spherical globules within the cytoplasm of these cells. The globules represent overstuffed lysosomes. If the proteinuria abates, the accumulated protein can be lysed. Accumulations of protein, presumably immunoglobulins, in plasma cells may create homogeneous, rounded, acidophilic *Russell bodies* (Gray and Doniach, 1970). Why they appear in some plasma cells is unclear, but it is speculated that they reflect excessive stimulation of antibody production.

COMPLEX LIPIDS AND CARBOHYDRATES

Intracellular accumulations of a variety of abnormal metabolites characterize a growing list of inborn errors of metabolism collectively referred to as the "storage diseases" (p. 151). These abnormal products collect within cells throughout the body, principally those in the reticuloendothelial system. The abnormal products range from complex lipids (in Gaucher's, Tay-Sachs and Niemann-Pick diseases) to complex carbohydrates (in Hurler's and Hunter's syndromes) to other, more exotic products, such as glycolipids and mucolipids. In all of these rare conditions, the precise identification of the stored product requires specific biochemical or enzymic analyses.

PIGMENTS

Pigments, of either exogenous or endogenous origin, may accumulate within cells. While most are relatively innocuous, they often provide valuable clues to the existence and nature of an underlying disorder.

EXOGENOUS PIGMENTS

Accumulations of exogenous carbon dust in the macrophages of the alveoli and the lymphatic channels blacken the tissues of the lungs *(anthracosis)*. It is a universal indication of the air pollution to which the coal miner and the urban dweller are exposed. When these macrophages drain to the regional lymph nodes, they similarly blacken them. However, anthracosis does not interfere with normal respiratory function, nor does it predispose to infection, except in extreme instances, as in coal miners. Those living in iron mining communities may develop a rustlike discoloration of the lung (*siderosis*). Here again, the pigmentation does not seem to be associated with damage but implies heavy air pollution. In some of these mining areas, however, the iron dust is associated with silica dust (*siderosilicosis*), and the silica may produce serious lung disease (page 383). Tattooing, now largely out of style, may cause dermal pigmentation of an innocuous but sometimes embarrassing nature. The tattoo pigment has the distressing property of persisting in situ throughout life in dermal macrophages, creating difficulties if one wishes to marry "Alice" when the adornment is seductively titled "Mary."

ENDOGENOUS PIGMENTS

Four major forms of pigment are of endogenous origin. Hemosiderin and bilirubin are hemoglobin-derived; lipofuscin and melanin are not. Each is considered briefly below.

Hemosiderin is a golden-yellow to brown, granular or crystalline, iron-containing pigment. The substructure of hemosiderin and its special staining characteristics are discussed in more detail on page 327. It appears within and between cells whenever there is a local or systemic excess of iron. Local excesses of iron may be produced by internal hemorrhages (within tissues or closed body cavities) or by long-standing vascular congestion that presumably leads to minute hemorrhages. The common bruise following an injury provides an excellent example of the local formation of hemosiderin. The color changes which occur in the bruise reflect the transformation of the hemoglobin. The bruise begins with the blue-red color of erythrocytes which accumulate at the site of hemorrhage. These are phagocytized by macrophages, which break down the hemoglobin to produce at first biliverdin (yellow-green), then bilirubin (green-brown) and eventually hemosiderin (golden yellow). The lung in long-standing heart failure and particularly in mitral stenosis is a prime example of protracted congestion leading to the appearance of hemosiderin in phagocytic mononuclear cells in the alveoli. These pigmented macrophages thus are often called "heart failure" cells (Fig. 1–11). *Systemic hemosiderosis* is encountered whenever there is iron overload in the body. Depending upon the amount and cause of the iron excess, the pigment may be confined to the reticuloendothelial cells throughout the body or in addition be deposited in parenchymal cells, such as those in the liver, kidneys, endocrine glands, pancreas and other organs. Involvement of

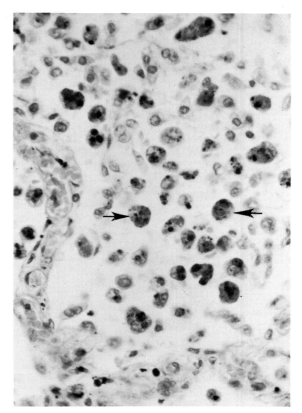

Figure 1–11. An alveolus in the lung of a 63 year old female with heart failure of 3 years' duration. The large macrophages ("heart failure cells") contain clumped hemosiderin pigment within their cytoplasm (arrows).

these organs is characteristic of *hemochromatosis*, the most extreme example of systemic iron overload. Further consideration of this disorder is presented on page 530.

In most instances, the intracellular accumulation of hemosiderin pigment does not damage the cell and so does not impair either cell or organ function. Indeed, the iron contained within this pigment can be mobilized and hemosiderin will therefore disappear in time if the cause for the excess iron abates. As is well known, a black and blue bruise eventually disappears. However, massive accumulations of hemosiderin in phagocytic cells (such as those in lymph nodes and spleen) may cause their destruction, with release of the pigment into extracellular spaces. The heavy accumulations of iron in hemochromatosis are also suspected of impairing liver and pancreatic structure and function, but it is still not certain that the hemosiderin itself is the injurious agent.

Bilirubin, a brown-green pigment, is also derived from hemoglobin, and is normally present in bile. It is largely produced from the breakdown of senescent red cells, which are phagocytized by RE cells, principally in the spleen but also in the liver and bone marrow. The heme pigment (porphyrin) ring is split, iron is released and, by a series of oxidation-reduction reactions in which heme-oxygenase participates, biliverdin and then bilirubin are produced. Most of this degradation probably occurs within lysosomes. A small amount of bilirubin is synthesized directly in the bone marrow as a by-product of hemoglobin formation. More details on the subsequent metabolism of bile pigment are presented on page 508. Here it suffices to say that bilirubin appears within cells only when there is some derangement in its secretion by liver cells or some other disorder such as an obstruction to the biliary tract. These conditions usually lead to an accumulation of bilirubin in the blood and tissues resulting in icterus (jaundice). The bilirubin is visible within cells morphologically only when the jaundice is well marked. It appears as a mucoid, green-brown to black, amorphous, globular, intracytoplasmic deposit. Most often hepatocytes are affected, but in severe jaundice bilirubin also may be observed in renal tubular epithelial cells and dermal macrophages. Although moderate bilirubin accumulation is well tolerated by the hepatocytes, massive accumulation may lead to functional impairment.

Lipofuscin has already been described as metabolic "wear and tear" pigment (p. 10). As far as we know it does not affect cell function.

Melanin, an endogenous dark brown granular pigment, is not derived from hemoglobin. It is normally found in melanocytes, the malpighian layer of the skin and mucous membranes, and in the retina and leptomeninges. Occasionally melanocytes are encountered in the ovaries, adrenal medulla, bladder or substantia nigra of the brain. Melanin is derived from tyrosine through the action of tyrosinase, an enzyme normally present in melanocytes. The tyrosinase catalyzes the formation of dihydroxyphenylalanine (DOPA) which, through a sequence of somewhat obscure steps, is polymerized and then coupled with protein to produce melanin (Fitzpatrick and Lerner, 1953). At the level of the light microscope, the melanin appears as brown to black amorphous intracytoplasmic granules. At the ultrastructural level, the DOPA which is synthesized in the granular endoplasmic reticulum is aggregated or polymerized in the Golgi apparatus and incorporated there into small membrane-bound organelles known as melanosomes (Seiji and Iwashita, 1965).

In the epidermis, melanin usually is found in the basal malpighian layer. The melanocytes which synthesize the pigment are found in the dermis and they, as it were, transfer the pigment to the epidermal cells through dendritic processes which form bridges between the basal cells of the epithelium and the melanocytes. A similar mechanism accounts for the pigmentation of the cells of the hair follicle. Aggregates of these dermal melanocytes create freckles which darken, as is well known, after exposure to sunlight because of the actinic stimulation of melanin synthesis.

In man, melanin synthesis is under adrenal and pituitary control. Adrenal steroids suppress and pituitary ACTH stimulates its synthesis. Animals possess a clearly identified pituitary melanocyte-stimulating hormone (MSH), but the existence of MSH in man is not well established and its role may be performed by ACTH.

Albinos suffer from a hereditary lack of tyrosinase. Thus they are unable to synthesize melanin and are extremely vulnerable to sunlight. They lack the protective pigment mantle in the skin against the actinic activity of sunlight, as well as the light shielding action of the pigment in the eye. Such persons therefore are prone to developing sunburn and skin cancers and have extreme visual sensitivity to light.

Excess melanin synthesis in the skin is encountered in adrenal insufficiency (Addison's disease). In this disorder, the low levels of circulating adrenal steroids lead to compensatory overproduction of pituitary ACTH. Increased amounts of melanin are also found in pigmented nevi and often in malignant melanomas, sometimes transforming these cancers into black masses (Fig. 1–12).

SOMATIC DEATH

Having discussed cell death, it is necessary to define briefly *somatic death,* i.e., the death of the individual. It is not easy to determine the precise moment at which somatic death may be said to have occurred. This difficulty assumes great medical, ethical and legal importance in these days of organ transplantation, when it is necessary to remove an organ from a donor within minutes or, indeed, within seconds of death. The problem has been compounded by the increased sophistication of medical technology, since the heartbeat may now be prolonged artificially by electrical pacemakers, respirations be maintained by respirators and the temperature of the body sustained by electric blankets. All, however, would agree that cessation of all organ function characterizes death. Some are now urging that this definition be limited only to flattening of the electroencephalogram, indicating cessation of brain function, irrespective of

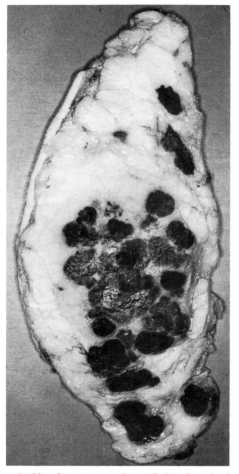

Figure 1–12. A cross section of the female breast from a 48 year old patient with a malignant melanoma arising in the skin of the neck. The deeply pigmented cancer seeded widely throughout the body, giving rise to these intensely black nodules within the breast.

other organ function. Whatever the precise moment of death, once all vital functions have ceased, a sequence of postmortem changes appears. *Algor mortis* applies to the loss of body heat as the temperature of the body gradually equilibrates with its environment. The rate of cooling depends upon the temperature differential between the body and its environment. *Livor mortis* refers to the gradual seepage of blood out of the normal vascular channels, with engorgement of dependent tissues, usually beginning within two to three hours. *Rigor mortis* refers to postmortem rigidity. This usually begins within six to eight hours, depending upon the body temperature at the time of death and on the environmental temperature. It affects the muscles of the upper part of the body first, progressing toward the lower extremities. Rigor usually begins to abate about 16 to 20 hours after death, once again beginning in the cephalad

region of the body. Ultimately, the tissues putrefy or decompose by the action of both intracellular and bacterial catalases.

SUMMARY

This chapter deals with the ultimate basis of all organic disease — namely, the effect of abnormal microenvironments on cells. The elaborate microcosm of the cell responds in varying ways to the slings and arrows that come its way in its daily existence. The nature and extent of the response depend on many factors which relate both to the host and to the injurious agents. Important among these are the cell's specific vulnerabilities, still poorly understood; its degree of differentiation (highly specialized cells are in general more easily injured); and its general environment, including blood supply, nutrition, and so forth. Critical parameters with respect to the injurious influence are its specific nature, duration and intensity. Depending upon these variables the cell may:

1. Undergo adaptation.
2. Be reversibly injured.
3. Be irreversibly injured and die.
4. Accumulate normal or abnormal products.

Cellular adaptation, reversible injury and cell death represent three stages in a continuum of the response of the cell to noxious influences. Adaptation, as you recall, may involve induction (of enzymes, altered metabolic pathways, organelles, myofilaments), autophagy, hypertrophy or atrophy.

When the challenge exceeds the capacity of the cell to adapt, it may become reversibly injured and undergo one of the many biochemical and structural alterations termed degenerations. Three specific patterns were described: cellular swelling, hydropic degeneration and fatty change. The exact pattern of degeneration that eventuates depends on the specific cell involved, its principal metabolic activity and the type, duration and intensity of the injurious agent. *Reversibility is implicit in the concept of cellular degeneration.*

With stronger challenges, the cell may be irreversibly injured and die. The line between reversible and irreversible injury is not sharply delimited. For the recognition of cell death we are dependent on more or less crude indicators of loss of vital metabolic processes or loss of vital structures, manifested by nuclear changes (pyknosis, karyorrhexis or karyolysis). As was pointed out, by the time such morphologic degradation can be recognized, the cell has already been irreversibly injured or dead for some time. Thus the morphologic changes which follow cell death are encompassed within the term necrosis and are the result of the dynamic processes of autolysis, heterolysis and denaturation of proteins. Three distinctive patterns of necrosis were described: liquefactive, coagulative and caseous.

Normal and abnormal cells may accumulate a variety of products. Some are presented to the cell in excess, others are synthesized in excess within the cell and still others accumulate because they are incapable of metabolic degradation. A variety of intracellular accumulations were cited, including glycogen, lipids, proteins and abnormal products resulting from inborn errors of metabolism. Calcium salts and pigments, of both exogenous and endogenous origin, may also accumulate within cells.

This gamut of cellular changes will be encountered over and over again throughout all subsequent considerations of disease states. Just as an individual's state of health is predicated on healthy cells, so does illness arise in altered and damaged cells.

REFERENCES

Arstila, A. V., et al.: Studies on cellular autophagocytosis. A histochemical study on sequential alterations of mitochondria in the vacuoles of rat liver. Lab. Invest., 27:317, 1972.

Bessis, M.: Studies on cell agony and death: An attempt at classification. *In* Ciba Foundation Symposium: Cellular Injury. Boston, Little, Brown & Co., 1964, p. 287.

Buckley, I. K.: Microscopic pathology of injured living tissue. Int. Rev. Exp. Path., 2:241, 1963.

Buckley, I. K.: A light and electron microscopic study of thermally injured cultured cells. Lab. Invest., 26:201, 1972.

Chopra, P., et al.: Mechanism of carbon tetrachloride hepatotoxicity, an in vivo study of its molecular basis in rats and monkeys. Lab. Invest., 26:716, 1972.

DiLuzio, N. R.: Anti-oxidants, lipid peroxidation and chemical induced liver injury. Fed. Proc., 32:1875, 1973.

Dixon, F.: Discussion on composition of fibrinoid. Mechanisms of cell and tissue damage produced by immune reactions. II. International Symposium, Immunopathology. Basel, Benno Schwabe and Co., 1961, p. 90.

Editorial: Measles and multiple sclerosis. Lancet, 1:247, 1974a.

Editorial: Aryl hydrocarbon hydroxylase inducibility and lung cancer. Lancet, 1:910, 1974b.

Ericsson, J. L. E.: Studies on induced cellular autophagy. Characterization of the membranes bordering autophagosomes in the parenchymal liver cells. Exp. Cell. Res., 56:393, 1969.

Fitzpatrick, P. B., and Lerner, A. B.: Terminology of pigment cells. Science, 117:640, 1953.

Galen, R. S.: The enzyme diagnosis of myocardial infarction. Hum. Pathol., 6:141, 1975.

Gallagher, C. H., et al.: Enzyme changes during liver autolysis. J. Path. Bact., 72:247, 1956.

Ginn, F. L., et al.: Disorders of cell volume regulation. I. Effects of inhibition of plasma membrane adenosine triphosphatase with Oubain. Am. J. Cell. Biol. 53:1041, 1968.

Glimcher, M. J., and Krane, S. M.: Studies on the interactions of collagen and phosphate. *In* McLean, F. C. (ed.): Radioisotopes and Bone, A Symposium. Philadelphia, F. A. Davis Co., 1962, p. 393.

Gray, A., and Doniach, I.: Ultrastructure of plasma cells containing Russell bodies in human stomach and thyroid. J. Clin. Path., 23:608, 1970.

Hawkins, H. K., et al.: Lysosome and phagosome stability in lethal cell injury. Am. J. Path., 68:255, 1972.

Iseri, O. A., and Gottlieb, L. S.: Alcoholic hyalin and megamitochondria as separate and distinct entities in liver disease associated with alcoholism. Gastroenterology, 60:1027, 1971.

Isselbacher, K. L., and Greenberger, N. J.: Metabolic effects of alcohol on the liver. New Eng. J. Med., 270:351, 402, 1964.

Jennings, R. B., et al.: Ischemic injury of the myocardium. Ann. N.Y. Acad. Sci., 156:61, 1969.

Jones, A. L., and Fawcett, D. W.: Hypertrophy of the agranular endoplasmic reticulum in hamster liver induced by phenobarbital (with a review on the functions of this organelle in liver). J. Histochem. Cytochem., 14:215, 1966.

Klion, S. M., and Schaffner, F.: The ultrastructure of acidophilic "Councilman-like" bodies in the liver. Am. J. Path., 48:755, 1966.

Lombardi, B.: Considerations on the pathogenesis of fatty liver. Lab. Invest., 15:1, 1966.

Majno, G., et al.: Death and necrosis: Chemical, physical, and morphologic changes in rat liver. Virchows. Arch. Path. Anat., 333:421, 1960.

Marx, J. L.: Slow viruses: role in persistent disease. Science, 180:1351, 1973.

Monod, J., et al.: Allosteric proteins and cellular systems. J. Molec. Biol., 6:306, 1963.

Ozawa, K., et al.: The effect of ischemia on mitochondrial metabolism. J. Biochem., 61:512, 1967.

Rao, K. S., and Recknagel, R. O.: Early incorporation of carbon labelled carbon tetrachloride into rat liver particulate lipids and proteins. Exp. Molec. Path., 10:219, 1969.

Reynolds, E. S., et al.: Lipid parenchymal cell injury. IX. Phenobarbital potentiation of endoplasmic reticulum denaturation following carbon tetrachloride. Lab. Invest., 26:219, 1972.

Rubin, E., and Lieber, C. S.: Alcohol-induced hepatic injury in nonalcoholic volunteers. New Eng. J. Med., 278:869, 1968.

Rubin, E., and Lieber, C. S.: Fatty liver, alcoholic hepatitis and cirrhosis produced by alcohol in primates. New Eng. J. Med., 290:128, 1974.

Seiji, M., and Iwashita, S.: Intracellular localization of tyrosinase and site of melanin formation in melanocytes. J. Invest. Derm., 45:305, 1965.

Smuckler, E. A.: Structural and functional alteration of the endoplasmic reticulum during carbon tetrachloride intoxication. *In* Campbell, P. N., and Gran, F. C. (ed.): Structure and Function of the Endoplasmic Reticulum in Animal Cells. New York, Academic Press, 1968, p. 11.

Smuckler, E. A., and Benditt, E. P.: Carbon tetrachloride poisoning in rats: alteration in ribosomes of the liver. Science, 140:308, 1963.

Smuckler, E. A., and Trump, B. F.: Alterations in the structure and function of the rough-surfaced endoplasmic reticulum during necrosis in vitro. Am. J. Path., 53:315, 1968.

Totter, J. R.: Mechanism of radiation injury. Environ. Health Ser. (Radiol. Health), 33:2, 1968.

Trump, B. F., et al.: An electron microscope study of early cytoplasmic alterations in hepatic parenchymal cells of mouse liver during necrosis in vitro (autolysis). Lab. Invest., 11:986, 1962.

Vogt, M. T., and Farber, E.: On the molecular pathology of ischemic renal cell death. Am. J. Path., 53:1, 1968.

laries, as well as opening of inactive capillary beds. Concomitantly, the postcapillary venules dilate and fill with the rapidly flowing blood. Thus, the microvasculature at the site of injury becomes congested, producing hyperemia in the inflammatory site. With very mild injuries, the vascular alterations may not progress beyond this point, but with more severe tissue injury, the hyperemia is followed by slowing of the blood flow, which may progress to total stasis. Stagnation of flow is the consequence of several events. Concomitant with the development of hyperemia, the venules and capillaries become abnormally permeable, resulting in the escape of plasma water (described in the next section). The viscosity of the blood is thus increased, leading to both packing (sludging) of the red cells and increased frictional resistance to flow. The veins, already overloaded by the increased flow in the area, likewise are affected by hemoconcentration and increased frictional resistance to flow. Thus, the outflow from the local site is impeded, which contributes to the stasis and stagnation. Pressure measurements in the venules and capillaries reveal an increased hydrostatic pressure (important to our later consideration of exudation). The red cell clumps and stasis disorganize the laminar flow pattern of the normally rapidly moving stream, and white cells are displaced to the periphery of the microvessels (margination) (Fig. 2–1). Sometimes, depending on the severity of the injury, the blood may actually clot at this stage of the reaction to form a thrombus (p. 219). Usually, however, this implies direct damage to endothelial cells. Soon after the white cell margination becomes evident, leukocytes escape from their vascular confinement and appear in the perivascular tissues.

The time relationships of these vascular changes depend to some extent on the severity of the injury. Arteriolar dilatation becomes evident within a few minutes of the injury. Slowing and stagnation are apparent within 10 to 30 minutes, and in severe injuries clotting may be seen at this time.

VASCULAR PERMEABILITY CHANGES AND EXUDATION

Increased vascular permeability with the escape of plasma (including plasma proteins) and white cells is known as exudation and is a major feature of all acute inflammatory reactions. It accounts for an increase in the volume of interstitial fluid (edema) and tissue swelling at the local site of injury. *The increased permeability first affects venules but rapidly extends to capillaries.* The mechanisms leading to this increase in permeability in acute inflammation

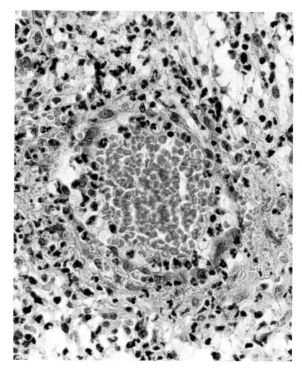

Figure 2–1. A dilated congested venule with peripheral orientation (margination) of neutrophils. Many neutrophils have emigrated into the perivascular edematous tissue.

are still incompletely understood. Indeed, even normal microvascular permeability is still something of an enigma. Let us first consider the normal state.

Permeability, in the biologic sense, refers to the rate of penetration of a substance through a barrier. It is equally applicable to water and to electrolytes, but in the context of the inflammatory reaction, greatest interest centers on the escape of much larger particles, the plasma protein molecules. Omitting much detail, we may state that the microcirculation consists essentially of continuous channels of branching and anastomosing endothelium-lined tubes. In the arterioles, the wall includes muscular elements, whereas in the capillaries there are only scattered pericytes. The venules differ little from the capillaries but they have a poorly developed muscular layer. The endothelial cell layer is enclosed within a continuous basement membrane. Although lacking in liver sinusoids and very thin in the lungs, in most tissues, the basement membrane is sufficiently well developed to be visualized by electron microscopy. Often it splits to enfold pericytes. The endothelial cell itself has been likened to a fried egg in appearance, with the central thick portion enclosing the nucleus, from which a thin attenuated sheet extends out in all directions. Its surface is pitted and scalloped by numerous invaginations (*caveolae intracellulares*). Many times, small intracellular vesicles formed by the pinching off of invaginations are attached to the plasma membrane. These vesicles are interpreted as evidence of micropinocytosis, which, as we shall see later, may represent a mechanism of fluid transfer across the endothelial cell.

The endothelial lining of all venules and of most capillaries in the body is of the so-called *continuous* type, i.e., an unbroken cytoplasmic layer with complicated interlocking interendothelial junctions (Karnovsky, 1967). *Fenestrated* patterns are found in the endocrine and exocrine glands, where the endothelial cytoplasm is perforated by pores. Similar pores are present in the endothelial cells of the glomeruli, but here the pores may be closed by diaphragms (Luft, 1964). A discontinuous pattern, with wide intercellular junctions and possibly large fenestrations, is present in the bone marrow, spleen and liver. With these notable exceptions, however, the microvasculature is characterized by interlocking endothelial junctions. How then does fluid escape from the capillaries and venules in the normal interchange of interstitial fluid? Although the endothelial cells in capillaries and venules with continuous lining may come close to each other, they do not fuse, and a space of about 4 to 6 nanometers (nm.) separates contiguous cells. Normally this scant space is filled by an amorphous substance described as "fuzz" or "extraneous substance" (Luft, 1966). The nature of this substance is uncertain but it is presumed to be a secretory product of the endothelial cell, probably acid mucopolysaccharide in nature. It appears to be analogous to the extraneous coat or glycocalyx found in many other cells, such as those lining the intestinal tract.

The precise nature of the interendothelial cell junctions is of considerable interest. For years, physiologists have postulated the existence of pores through which protein-poor fluid might pass in the normal state, but electron microscopy has failed to reveal pores in capillaries and venules save for the specialized capillary patterns already mentioned. However, the small fuzz-filled spaces between endothelial cells correspond quite well to the hypothetical pores sought by the physiologist. The magnitude of these spaces is appropriate for the passage of plasma water and small molecules such as the inorganic electrolytes and glucose. The constant interchange of plasma water between the vascular and extravascular compartments must occur through these small crevices and, as proposed by Starling, be controlled by hydrostatic and osmotic pressures within and without the vascular compartment.

The normal interendothelial cell junctions in capillaries and venules are too narrow to permit even the passage of albumin, the smallest of the plasma proteins. Therefore, an active, energy dependent transport mechanism is postulated to explain the passage of the small amounts of plasma proteins characteristic of normal interstitial fluid. The caveolae intracellulares may fill with plasma and form small endocytic vesicles. Movement of these vesicles across the endothelial cell cytoplasm and discharge of their contents at the basal surface might well provide the mechanism for the escape of the larger molecules. In support of this proposal, Karnovsky (1967) has shown considerable vesicle transport of horseradish peroxidase, which approximates the albumin molecule in size. Energy dependent vesicular transport may thus constitute the pathway of passage of the trace amounts of protein macromolecules normally found in interstitial fluid.

As we shall see, the basement membrane on which endothelial cells abut in capillaries also constitutes a filtration barrier. It is composed of a feltwork of fibers and filaments, creating a layer varying in thickness from less than a hundred to approximately 150 nm.

With this brief overview of the normal fluid exchange, it is now possible to consider the development of inflammatory exudation and edema at sites of acute inflammation. *Inflammatory exudates have a high specific gravity, about 1.020,* and often contain 2 to 4 grams per cent of protein as well as white cells which have emigrated. They may even have as much protein as whole plasma (6 to 7 gm. per cent). In contrast, *non-inflammatory transudates generally have a specific gravity below 1.012,* because essentially they comprise ultrafiltrates of plasma. Thus, in mild injuries, only a thin albuminous fluid escapes, while more marked damage allows the passage of the much larger globulins and even fibrinogen. Of course, severe injuries might rupture vessels, allowing the escape of all the constituents of blood. The correlation between severity of injury and the size of the molecule that is able to escape is referred to as *molecular sieving. Two events occurring in the inflammatory response are responsible for molecular sieving: a rise in hydrostatic pressure within the microcirculation and unlocking of endothelial cell junctions.* Direct measurements have demonstrated that arteriolar vasodilatation is followed by a rise in pressure within capillaries and venules. This increased intravascular pressure might well explain the passive transport of larger volumes of fluid and small molecules across the filtration barrier. However, the pressure rise is not sufficient to explain the escape of the larger protein macromolecules. Widening of endothelial cell junctions, beautifully documented in electron micrographs by Majno and Palade (1961), comes into play to explain the passage of large molecules (Fig. 2–2). Myofibrils identified in endothelial cells permit contraction of these cells, providing an explanation for the widening of the interendothelial junctions (Majno and Leventhal, 1967). When tracer particles such as carbon black are introduced into the circulation of an animal and then some substance such as histamine or serotonin (which increases vascular permeability) is injected, the large tracer molecules pass through the widened intercellular junctions. They then are trapped against the basement membrane and later somehow manage to squeeze through. Here, then, is the mechanism by which macromolecules may escape, to produce the protein-rich exudates of inflammatory reactions. Mild injuries may induce little widening of the junctions and result in only protein-poor exudates having a specific gravity not much higher than that of transudates. As the severity of the injury increases, so does the widening of the interendothelial cell space, permitting the formation of ever more protein-rich exudates.

The basement membrane constitutes a second filtration barrier. The method by which large protein molecules and white cells traverse it remains a mystery. However, it can be shown in sequential studies that after a transient period of entrapment, these larger particles, as well as white cells, eventually penetrate to enter the surrounding tissues. High resolution electron micrographs disclose no defects or visible channels.

The timing and rate of development of exudation and edema at the site of acute inflammation also vary with the severity of the injury. The use of carbon tracer particles and vital dyes (such as trypan blue), which complex to albumin and thus provide tagged macromolecules, has permitted detailed exploration of the phenomenon of exudation. These findings, derived from experimental models in animals, are believed to be completely relevant to man. When the skin of the guinea pig is exposed to graded severities of thermal injury, three temporal patterns of exudation can be identified (Sevitt, 1958, 1964).

Mild injuries induce an *immediate permeability response*, which begins within 1 to 2 minutes following the application of heat and phases

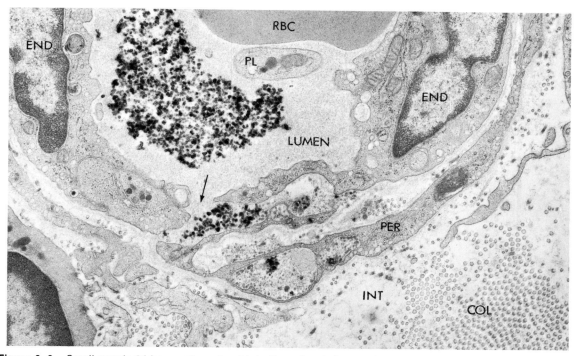

Figure 2–2. Small venule 24 hours after a local injection of an inflammation-provoking toxin. The arrow points to a gap between endothelial cells (END) through which some of the small, particulate, dark carbon particles have escaped and now lie trapped between the endothelial cells and an enclosing pericyte (PER). INT, interstitium; COL, collagen fibers; RBC, erythrocyte; PL, platelet. (Courtesy of Dr. R. Cotran.)

out within 15 to 30 minutes. Rarely this reaction may persist for as long as an hour. As we shall see, this immediate response appears to be mediated largely by histamine, because it can be blocked by antihistamines. Electron micrographs of the inflammatory site indicate that the venules are the principal site of leakage; the capillaries appear relatively unaffected. This pattern of inflammatory exudation is encountered in very mild clinical inflammatory reactions.

Slightly more severe injuries induce a so-called *delayed response*. Here the increase in permeability is delayed for a period ranging from 30 minutes to 10 hours and reaches a peak, depending on the time of onset, between 4 to 24 hours after the injury (Wilhelm, 1973). It appears that the delayed wave of increased permeability involves leakage from both venules and capillaries. Why the development of exudation is delayed in moderate forms of injury is not yet well understood. One might speculate that the injury damages endothelial cells, which only become necrotic and leaky after some time lag.

Severe levels of injury induce an *immediate (early) sustained reaction*. Here the increase in permeability rises to an early peak, as in the immediate response, but remains at a high plateau at least as long as the delayed pattern. Presumably here the more intense levels of heat have caused not only the death of endothelial cells but their immediate disruption, causing abnormal leakage in both capillaries and venules. It should be emphasized that although these three patterns of permeability response can be identified clearly in the experimental model, and may also occur in man, in all likelihood *clinically significant injuries produce the immediate sustained reaction*. Mention should be made again that even in severe injuries no morphologic alteration of the basement membrane can be identified by electron microscopy. Unquestionably biophysical changes are present which are beyond the range of detection.

MEDIATORS OF THE VASCULAR RESPONSE

What mechanisms bring about the vascular events (vasodilatation and increased permeability) characteristic of the inflammatory response? Mediators have long been suspected for the following reasons: (1) whatever the nature of the injury, the initial inflammatory reaction is virtually stereotyped, (2) there is a latent period between injury and the development of the full-blown reaction, and (3) certain aspects of the reaction can be suppressed, at least partially, by drugs.

NEUROGENIC MECHANISMS

In the very early phases of the reaction to injury, neurogenic mechanisms participate. Recall that following injury there is a very fleeting phase of arteriolar vasoconstriction, followed soon by dilatation of the arterioles leading into the inflammatory focus. Insights into these events are provided by the "triple response of Lewis" (Lewis, 1927). When the skin is heavily stroked by a dull instrument, such as the tip of a pencil or a ruler edge, a *dull red line* corresponding to the line of pressure appears in approximately 1 minute. Soon a *bright red halo* or *flare* surrounds the stroke mark. Thereafter, the third component appears — the *edematous wheal (swelling)* along the line of the original stroke mark. Lewis showed that the second component of this triple response — the flare — could be blocked by prior anesthesia or interruption of the nervous pathways into the area. He concluded that this event was mediated by neurogenic vasodilatation of arterioles. Presumably this occurs through an antidromic axon reflex arc involving the vasomotor innervation of the arterioles. The first and third components of the triple response were not affected by blocking of the nervous pathways, and Lewis attributed these to the release in injured tissues of an "H substance" which he later designated as histamine. The transient phase of vasoconstriction in the usual injury is, then, neurogenic in origin, but soon the antidromic reflex inhibits the vasoconstrictive impulses and contributes to the vasodilatation. Even without neural connections, however, the major aspects of the acute inflammatory response would take place, because, as we shall see, the principal mediators are chemical.

CHEMICAL MEDIATORS

So many chemical mediators have been identified that we are confronted with an embarrassment of riches. Which are significant in man and what their specific roles may be are still poorly understood and highly contentious. Those reasonably well characterized can be divided into three large groups:

1. Amines — histamine and 5-hydroxytryptamine (serotonin), coupled perhaps with the inactivation of epinephrine and norepinephrine.

2. Plasma proteases (esterases) and polypeptides — kallikrein, plasmin, lysosomal esterases, kinins and fractions of complement.

3. Miscellaneous — slow reacting substance (SRS), lymph node permeability factor (LNPF), neutrophil lysosomal basic proteins, prostaglandin E and lysolecithin.

Many other mediators have also been described in the literature but their participation in the inflammatory response in man has not yet been sufficiently clarified to merit mention here.

Histamine is generally acknowledged to be a major mediator of the first wave of vascular adjustments in the acute inflammatory response. It is widely distributed in the body in three forms—free, labile and bound (in platelets, basophils and mast cells). The free and labile forms probably contribute little to the inflammatory reaction, since they are present only in small amounts in most tissues. The richest source of histamine is the mast cells, normally present in the connective tissue adjacent to blood vessels. The histamine is contained within membrane-bound granules. Release of active histamine involves degranulation of the mast cell, cleavage of ionic bonds binding histamine to protein and alterations of the granule membrane, rendering it permeable or vulnerable to rupture. In man, histamine causes dilatation of arterioles and increased permeability in capillaries and venules, principally in the latter. It can be isolated from inflammatory sites soon after injury, but the amounts rapidly dwindle within the first 60 minutes, so it participates largely in the early phase of the response. Histamine, then, cannot be the mediator of the wave of increased permeability in the delayed response, nor can it explain the continued high level of permeability in the sustained response (Miller and Melmon, 1970).

5-Hydroxytryptamine (serotonin) induces dilatation and increased permeability in the microcirculation of rodents. In fact, in some animal species it may be more potent than histamine in effecting these changes. In such animals, it is released from platelets, mast cells and basophils, but it is not as abundant in analogous cells in man. Moreover, it has been impossible to prove that serotonin significantly affects capillary permeability in man (Page, 1958). While the possibility that serotonin is involved in the acute inflammatory response in man cannot be ruled out, it is doubtful that it is a major chemical mediator.

Inactivation of epinephrine and norepinephrine may be important phenomena in the development of the inflammatory vascular reaction. Both agents have a vasoconstrictive and antipermeability effect. Spector and Willoughby (1964) have proposed that activation of enzymes such as monoamine oxidase may occur at the site of injury and lead to inactivation of the catecholamines, thus potentiating the vascular dilatation and increased permeability of the inflammatory response.

Plasma proteases and polypeptides comprise a group of agents believed to play an important role in the inflammatory reaction. Three complex systems are found within this group: (1) the kinins, (2) the fibrinolytic system and (3) the complement system. As will be seen, there are many interrelationships. The *kinin* system effects the ultimate release of the vasoactive agents bradykinin (9 amino acids) and lysyl-bradykinin (10 amino acids) from their inactive precursors, the kininogens (alpha globulins), normally present in the plasma. The mode of release has long been controversial but undoubtedly involves activated proteases. As best understood at present, the initial event involves the activation of factor XII (Hageman factor) in the clotting system by contact with "surface-active agents" such as glass, kaolin, collagen and antigen-antibody complexes. Conceivably, injury alters the endothelium, in some way rendering it surface active, or exposes collagen in damaged walls of venules or capillaries. A fragment of factor XII has been recently identified as pre-kallikrein activator or PKA (Wuepper and Cochrane, 1972; Movat, 1972). Activated PKA is then able to convert pre-kallikrein into its active proteolytic form, i.e., the enzyme kallikrein. In turn, kallikrein acts on the kininogens in the plasma to release the vasoactive compounds bradykinin and lysyl-bradykinin, as is schematized in Figure 2–3. Other pro-

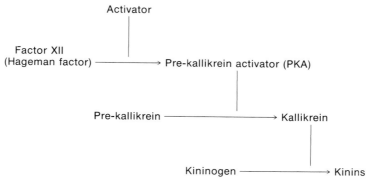

Figure 2–3. Formation of kinins. [Modified from Cochrane, C. G., and Wuepper, K. D.: The first component of the kinin-forming system in human and rabbit plasma. Its relationship to clotting factor XII (Hageman factor). J. Exp. Med., *134*:986, 1971.]

teases may also release the kinins, as is discussed in the next section. In passing, it might be noted that PKA may well have been present in the mediator known as globulin-permeability factor, accounting for its vasoactivity.

The kinins are the most potent inflammatory agents known. They induce arteriolar dilatation, increase capillary and venular permeability, enhance the migration of leukocytes to sites of injury in some animals and when applied to a blister base cause pain. It is evident that the kinins evoke many of the changes encountered in the inflammatory response. They are, however, almost as transient as histamine and therefore must exert their major effect during the early phases of the acute reaction. They probably are not involved in the later occurring events (Willoughby, 1972).

The *fibrinolytic system* contributes to the vascular phenomena of inflammation via the kinin system. Plasminogen activated to plasmin may play a role in the inflammatory response in three possible ways: (1) by direct action on the kininogens, liberating kinins (a slow action relative to the speed and potency of plasma kallikrein); (2) by releasing PKA from activated factor XII, which will in turn liberate kinins; and (3) by cleaving the third component of complement, as will now be described.

The *complement system* may be involved in all inflammatory reactions but most certainly plays a role in those related to immune reactions. Cleavage products of activated C'3 and C'5 fractions increase capillary and venular permeability. These fragments have now been demonstrated to play a major role in the vascular phenomena of the immune disorder known as anaphylaxis (p. 173) and so the fragments are called anaphylatoxins. Whether fractions of complement play a role in non-immunologic injuries is still a vexatious issue. Willoughby (1973) contends that complement fractions launch all inflammatory reactions. It is proposed that breakdown products of proteins activate the complement system, leading to release of vasoactive fractions, which in turn release other chemical mediators. However, a recent study suggests that complement depletion has little effect on the evolution of the nonspecific acute inflammatory response (Wahl et al., 1974), so we must leave this issue as still unsettled.

The *miscellaneous group of mediators* includes a number of factors whose role in man has not been established with certainty. Many are of fairly recent isolation and possibly more study will confirm their importance. *Slow reacting substances (SRS)* are defined as agents which slowly contract the guinea pig ileum and are released from tissues or cells by any injury. Two forms have been identified: SRS-C and SRS-A. The evidence today suggests that SRS-C is in fact one of the prostaglandins (described below). SRS-A, first encountered in anaphylactic reactions, may also play a role in non-immunologic inflammatory responses. In immune responses, SRS-A is released together with histamine, and so it probably contributes to the early phase of the inflammatory response, but it may also be a mediator of the later events. *Lymph node permeability factor (LNPF)* is a relatively membrane-free extract of lymph node cells. It has been implicated in certain immune reactions, principally of the delayed hypersensitivity type (p. 176). Whether it contributes to non-immunologic inflammatory responses is uncertain (Willoughby and Spector, 1964). LNPF probably represents a mixture of substances, and to date the specific vasoactive fraction has not been characterized chemically. *Lysosomal products from neutrophils* may participate in the inflammatory response in a number of ways. Lysosomal enzymes are capable of liberating kinins from their inactive precursors. In addition, the lysosomes contain cationic or basic proteins which enhance vascular permeability. They may well have this effect by acting on mast cells to release histamine (Ranadive and Cochrane, 1968). Lysosomes also contain proteases that digest elastin, collagen and basement membrane and may thereby enhance vascular permeability. In any event, the contents of lysosomes derived from neutrophils may well be important in inflammatory reactions, since these leukocytes escape from the blood and accumulate very early at sites of inflammation. Conceivably lysosomal products contribute to the full evolution of the reaction. *Prostaglandin E (PGE)*, a member of a family of fatty acids, is a new addition to the list of potential mediators. It has been proposed that PGE is synthesized at the inflammatory focus by a PG synthetase. PGE causes increased vascular permeability in many species. Its potency (on a weight basis) is somewhat higher than that of histamine and approximately equal to that of the kinins. Moreover, PGE appears to weakly attract white cells to inflammatory sites and to sensitize the pain receptors to mechanical and chemical stimulation. In experimentally produced inflammatory models, the action of PGE subsides within 15 to 20 minutes and is thus unlikely to be involved in the sustained and delayed responses. It has also been proposed that PGE may intensify the effects of other chemical mediators (Moncada et al., 1973). It is apparent that PGE evokes many of the effects associated with the inflammatory response and currently this substance is receiving much attention as an important mediator of the inflammatory response (Kaley and Weiner, 1971). *Lysolecithin* may be another mediator of the delayed response to injury (Cotran and Majno, 1964). Injection of dilute solutions of lysolecithin induces increased permeability in the venules and capillaries, closely simulating the delayed phase of the inflammatory reaction. This agent is of interest since it may be released by complement, which is often present at inflammatory sites.

In the presence of so many possible mediators, it has been exceedingly difficult to determine which are involved in the various phases of the evolution of the reaction to injury. It seems reasonable to conclude that histamine, perhaps soon followed by the kinins, initiates the early vascular phenomena, but as pointed out earlier, some contend that complement fractions are the triggers which release these mediators. The liberation of kinins must involve other agents, such as PKA, plasmin and possibly enzymes derived from neutrophil lysosomes. What can be said of the later appearing wave of increased permeability in the delayed response and of the immediate but sustained response? Conceivably LNPF, SRS and lysolecithin contribute to these events. There is, however, a strong suspicion that direct damage to endothelial cells induced by clinically significant injuries underlies the later increased permeability seen in the more severe forms of injury. The time required for the biochemical degradation of such damaged cells could account for the delayed phase of increased permeability. Of course, even more severe injuries might kill the endothelial cells outright and simultaneously destroy their mechanical and filtration integrity. This may explain the sustained response which begins soon after the onset of the inflammatory reaction. Indeed, very intense damage might rupture entire vessels, leading to hemorrhagic exudation. Nevertheless, in less dramatic injuries it must be clear that despite the plethora of possible mediators, we still do not understand fully the genesis of the vascular phenomena of the inflammatory response.

WHITE CELL EVENTS

The massing of white cells, principally neutrophils and macrophages, at a site of injury may well constitute the most important aspect of the inflammatory reaction. White cells are capable of engulfing foreign particulate matter, including bacteria and the debris of necrotic cells, and their lysosomal enzymes contribute in a number of ways to the defensive response. The lymphocyte plays very little, if any, role in the acute phases of inflammation, but principally contributes to the reactions in chronic long-standing inflammatory processes and in those of immunologic origin. Lymphocytes will be considered later in the discussion of chronic inflammation (p. 44). We can consider the sequence by which white cells aggregate and act at the inflammatory site under the following headings: (1) margination and pavementing, (2) emigration, (3) chemotaxis, (4) aggregation and (5) phagocytosis. Each of these topics will now be discussed briefly; for more detail reference can be made to the excellent review by Hersh and Bodey (1970).

MARGINATION AND PAVEMENTING

In the inflammatory focus, the onset of stagnation in the microcirculation induces red cell clumping to form aggregates larger than individual leukocytes. According to physical flow laws, these red cell masses assume a central location within the axial stream and the white cells are displaced to the periphery *(margination)*. Thus they come to occupy positions in contact with the endothelial surfaces. At first they slowly tumble or roll along the endothelial surface in the sluggish margins of the stream, but soon the cells appear to stick and *pavement* the endothelial surfaces. Platelets and red cells may also adhere, but when this occurs a clot usually forms to produce complete occlusion of the vessel. The question of why leukocytes stick to the endothelium is still unanswered. Three possibilities must be entertained: (1) the leukocyte is altered and becomes abnormally sticky, (2) the endothelium is altered in some way, rendering it sticky, or (3) some substance having adhesive properties is elaborated or precipitated. Conceivably each of these alterations is involved, and indeed, there are observations in support of all three. Injury of leukocytes by micropuncture renders them more adhesive. Moreover, following injury, white cells lose their essentially spherical shape and develop pseudopods. Normally the white cell and the endothelial cell repel each other by electrochemical negative charges. The pseudopods, carrying only relatively few charges, might contact and adhere to the endothelial surface. In this way, a point of anchorage results that might lead to firm adherence. Calcium may play some role in this adherence, serving as a bridge between the negative charges on the endothelial cell and those on the white cell. Chelation of calcium by EDTA has been shown to block the massing of white cells at sites of injury (Thompson et al., 1967). In support of changes in endothelial cells is the observation that white cells tend to stick to the side of the vessel nearest the site of injury (Allison et al., 1955). Finally, the possibility that some substance may serve as an adhesive directs attention to the alterations in the extraneous coat of endothelial cells. This substance might undergo chemical alteration, rendering it sticky. Whatever the cause, it is clear that at the inflammatory focus margination and pavementing of white cells accompany circulatory stasis. It is of interest, however, that the administration of large doses of adrenal steroids reduces or totally blocks the phenomenon of pavementing. Steroids are known to stabilize cell membranes, but how this action can be extrapolated to its deterrent effect on leukocytic pavementing is still unclear. It is possible, however, that this action of steroids may in some measure account for the well known inhibitory effect of steroids on the inflammatory response. The patient on long-term adrenal steroid therapy is especially susceptible to uncontrolled bacterial infections.

EMIGRATION

As the term implies, emigration refers to the process by which motile white cells migrate out of blood vessels. Although all leukocytes are more or less motile, the most active are the neutrophils and monocytes, the most sluggish are the lymphocytes. Many elegant studies have confirmed that the principal sites of emigration of white cells are the loosened intercellular junctions (Florey, 1962; Marchesi, 1961) (Fig. 2–4). Emigration is an active ameboid process and indeed once outside the vessel, the neutrophils can continue to move as fast as 20 micrometers (μm.) per minute. A second phenomenon has also been noted; on occasion a spurt of red cells may burst through the vessel wall behind an exiting white cell. This red cell movement, called *diapedesis* ("to walk between"), is believed to be passive and to result from hydrostatic pressure squeezing the thin envelope through a small defect. Thus, red cell diapedesis is a passive phenomenon, whereas white cell emigration is an active, energy dependent process.

Detailed study of emigration has disclosed a number of interesting points. First, the peak of the wave of leukocytic emigration does not coincide with that of increased vascular permeability. Indeed, white cells may in some manner extrude themselves through unaltered, apparently closed interendothelial cell junctions. In general, however, just as venules become leaky before capillaries in most inflammatory responses, white cell emigration in like manner first becomes evident in the venules and only later involves the capillaries. The first cells to appear in perivascular spaces

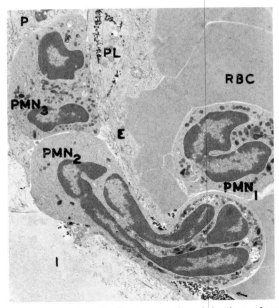

Figure 2–4. Venule 10 hours after injection of an inflammation provoking toxin. A neutrophil (PMN$_2$) is seen squeezing through (emigrating from) the lumen into the perivascular tissue. PMN$_3$ has already emigrated and is trapped between the endothelium (E) and the pericyte (P). Carbon particles (see arrow at lower right corner) will undoubtedly follow PMN$_2$. I, interstitium; PL, platelet. (Courtesy of Dr. R. Cotran.)

are the neutrophils, usually followed by monocytes (once outside the vascular compartment, monocytes are referred to as macrophages or histiocytes). This sequence is attributed to the greater number of neutrophils in the circulation and to the fact that neutrophils are more motile than monocytes. Moreover, as will be seen, factors which facilitate emigration of monocytes may be produced by or potentiated by neutrophils. In the animal rendered neutropenic, monocyte emigration is blocked.

CHEMOTAXIS (LEUKOTAXIS)

Long ago it was suggested that the direction of migrating white cells might be determined by chemical substances which create a gradient along which cells would migrate toward the focus of highest concentration. Such chemotactic factors may be released at sites of injury. One view of chemotaxis proposes that the factors induce directed linear migration of leukocytes. However, chemotaxis may take other forms (Keller, 1972). The factor(s) may lead to trapping of randomly wandering cells at the locus of highest concentration, or chemotactic factors might enhance random migration.

Although a host of factors can be demonstrated to be chemotactic in vitro, it is still not certain that they are effective in vivo. Chemotaxis can be graphically documented in vitro in the Boyden chamber. A micropore membrane permeable to migrating cells separates an upper compartment containing the cell suspension from the lower compartment containing the test chemotactic solution. The number of cells which have migrated through the filter is a measure of the chemotactic effectiveness of the solution in the lower compartment. Using this experimental system, it can be shown that certain agents isolated from inflamed tissues operate only on neutrophils, others only on monocytes, while a few affect both (Ward, 1974). In addition, agents have been identified for eosinophils and basophils.

Chemotactic factors for neutrophils include substances released from various types of viruses and bacteria, a protease split fraction of the third and fifth components of complement, a trimolecular complex of complement ($C'5$, $C'6$, $C'7$), collagen degradation products, components of the kinin system, including the enzyme kallikrein and plasminogen activator, and a fibrinopeptide released from fibrinogen

by the action of thrombin (Keller, 1972; Gamow et al., 1971; Houck and Chang, 1971; Kay et al., 1973; Zigmond and Hirsch, 1973). Table 2–1 reveals additional chemotactic agents. In this bewildering array, some probably act in all inflammations, others may act principally in immune reactions. For example, it is likely that the complement fractions have their principal role in immune injuries, but whether they are also operative in other inflammations is uncertain (Wahl et al., 1974). It is not unreasonable to propose that in a particular inflammatory reaction one factor or a small group of factors may be most abundant and operative, while in another instance other agents come into play. The primary effective agent may vary from one inflammatory reaction to another.

Chemotactic agents acting on monocytes and macrophages include: fragments of $C'3$ and $C'5$, bacterial factors, L-forms (protoplasts), kallikrein and plasminogen activator, and fractions from neutrophils and lymphocytes. It is worth noticing that neutrophils, possibly

TABLE 2–1. SUMMARY OF THE INFLAMMATORY RESPONSE

Events		Site	Morphologic Alteration	Mediator or Mechanism
Hemodynamic Alterations		Arterioles	Vasodilatation	Neurogenic Chemical: histamine, serotonin (?)
		Venules	Vasodilatation	Chemical: histamine, kinins, complement fractions, lysosomal products, prostaglandin E (?), serotonin (?)
		Capillaries	Vasodilatation and opening of inactive channels	
Permeability Changes	Early	Venules	Dilatation, congestion and widening of endothelial junctions	Physical: increased hydrostatic pressure Chemical: histamine, kinins, complement fractions, lysosomal products, prostaglandin E (?), serotonin (?)
	Late	Capillaries	Dilatation, congestion and widening of endothelial junctions	Physical: increased hydrostatic pressure, direct endothelial injury (?) Chemical: lysolecithin (?), LNPF (?), SRS (?)
White Cell Events	Margination and Pavementing	Venules and capillaries	Peripheral orientation and adherence to endothelial surfaces	Interruption of laminar flow
	Emigration	Venules and capillaries	Escape from vessels	?
	Aggregation	—	Accumulation at site of injury	Chemotactic agents: For neutrophils: complement fractions, fibrin fractions, lymphocyte factors, fractions of red cell membranes, collagen degradation products, components of kinin system. For macrophages: bacteria, L-products, neutrophil fractions, lymphocyte factors
	Phagocytosis	—	Engulfment of bacteria and debris	Doing their thing!

the basic peptides in their lysosomal granules, play an important role in the formation of chemotactic agents for macrophages. Herein may lie the explanation for the fact that neutrophils constitute the first wave of leukocytic emigration, followed only later by monocytes. Chemotactic agents for macrophages are also released from sensitized lymphocytes following contact with antigen. This last factor appears to be different from *migration inhibition factor (MIF)* but it could explain the aggregation of macrophages in cell-mediated immune reactions.

Chemotactic factors must also exist for lymphocytes, because these cells accumulate in *allergic* (immunologic) inflammatory reactions and also predominate in *non-allergic* chronic inflammations. To date, however, no agents chemotactic for lymphocytes have been identified which are effective in the Boyden chamber.

Although the evidence that chemotactic factors are effective clinically is still fragmentary, some very recent provocative observations suggest that they do indeed function in vivo. Reports are now appearing in the literature describing patients whose impaired defense against microbiologic infection is attributed to defective neutrophil or mononuclear leukocyte chemotaxis (Clark et al., 1973; Snyderman et al., 1973). Such intriguing hereditary entities as the Chediak-Higashi syndrome and the "lazy leukocyte syndrome" (Miller et al., 1971) have been identified and are apparently characterized by deficient chemotactic mechanisms. Acquired leukocytic defects have also been identified in diabetics and in patients with tumors and bacterial and viral infections, as well as other disorders (Ward, 1974). Therefore, defects in chemotaxis may well impair the inflammatory response by retarding the aggregation of white cells at the site of injury.

AGGREGATION OF LEUKOCYTES

The massing of leukocytes at a site of injury constitutes a major histologic hallmark of acute inflammation. The accumulation of these cells follows a fairly predictable sequence. *In most acute reactions (such as those caused by common pathogenic bacteria, thermal and chemical injury) the first cells to appear, as mentioned previously, are neutrophils. Later monocytes (or macrophages) outnumber the neutrophils.* In the Boyden chamber, neutrophils respond to chemotactic stimuli within 90 minutes, whereas monocytes require 5 or more hours. Still later, lymphocytes and plasma cells may appear, but these cells almost always imply chronicity of the inflammation and so will be discussed in greater detail later. As we shall see, there are exceptions to this general

sequence. Certain organisms, such as the tubercle and typhoid bacilli, evoke a predominantly mononuclear reaction from the outset. Similarly, viral infections and many other immune reactions are characterized principally by the accumulation of lymphocytes. Despite these exceptions, most acute inflammations are marked by large numbers of neutrophils.

Several influences act to determine the sequence of appearance of the various white cell types in the inflammatory focus. Although both neutrophils and monocytes begin to emigrate at about the same time, the neutrophils appear first, as we have seen, owing in large part to their greater mobility and to the fact that they are present in greater number in the circulation. Moreover, the inflammatory state may cause a systemic reaction in which the marrow participates with increased production of leukocytes, particularly neutrophils. Menkin (1940) described an alpha globulin fraction of inflammatory exudate which he called "leukocyte-promoting factor," but the effect of this agent has not been clearly established. Many other poorly defined protein derivatives of necrotic cells and bacteria, two of which have been termed "neutropoietin" and "leukopoietin G," have a similar stimulant effect on the marrow production of leukocytes, particularly the neutrophils. The white cell count of the peripheral blood may rise to 20,000 to 30,000 cells per mm.^{3} or more, and the great preponderance (80 to 90 per cent) are neutrophils. However, even under normal circumstances neutrophils have a very short life span (from hours to 4 days), and in addition they are known to be particularly vulnerable to the accumulation of lactic acid. Thus, in an inflammatory focus their life span may be even more abbreviated, and maintenance of the neutrophil population in the inflammatory focus therefore requires constant recruitment from the blood. In the course of days, as the chemotactic factors dwindle—an occurrence to be expected—the emigration of neutrophils begins to slow.

For mysterious reasons, the recruitment of macrophages is far more sustained than that of neutrophils. In experimental injuries, it can be shown that neutrophils emigrate in far greater numbers in the first few days, but with the passage of time monocytes (macrophages) begin to enter an inflammatory focus in greater number than neutrophils (Ryan and Spector, 1970). Thus, after two or three days, macrophages outnumber the neutrophils in most inflammations. Once present, they persist because they are relatively resistant to the falling pH usually found in the inflammatory site. In addition, their normal life span ranges from many months to years, considerably longer than that of neutrophils. It has been proposed that macrophages proliferate at inflammatory sites (Spector and Willoughby, 1971), but a recent study suggests that during an inflammatory reaction, proliferation of these cells begins while they are still in the circulation (Van Furth et al., 1973). Whatever the mechanisms involved, it is possible to approximate the age of an acute inflammatory response by noting whether macrophages outnumber the neutrophils. If they do, the lesion is probably at least several days old.

PHAGOCYTOSIS

Phagocytosis of bacteria and unwanted debris and the release of powerful catalytic enzymes from the lysosomes of both neutrophils and macrophages constitute two of the dominant benefits to be derived from the inflammatory reaction in most forms of injury (Zucker-Franklin, 1968). The term "phagocytosis" literally means "cell-eating." A great many cells in the body are capable of phagocytosis, but of principal interest now are the neutrophils and macrophages. Eosinophils, too, are phagocytic, but lymphocytes and plasma cells are not. Although reticuloendothelial cells are also actively phagocytic, these cells are principally effective in removing foreign particulate matter from the circulation. Thus, they come into play when in proximity to injury or when the invading agents become blood-borne.

The precise details of phagocytosis have been well studied by electron microscopy (Brewer, 1963). The first step in phagocytosis is attachment of the leukocyte to the particle. The cell then appears to flow partially around the particle, to create, in effect, a deep pocket. The mouth of the pocket eventually closes to entrap the "victim" in a sac bound by a membrane derived from the plasma membrane of the phagocyte. Lysosomes subsequently attach to this sac and by fusion with it bring their enzymes to bear directly on the destruction and removal of the offending particle. The energy consumed in phagocytosis is derived from glycolytic pathways (Douglas, 1970). Whereas both neutrophils and macrophages are actively phagocytic, the macrophage is less fastidious and is capable of engulfing material eschewed by the neutrophil. The macrophage is of prime importance, then, in removing debris at the inflammatory site.

The phagocytic activity of leukocytes is modified by many influences. Most important is the presence of antibodies or fractions of complement, collectively known as opsonins. Opsonins are normally present in the serum but are increased in amount in specific immune reactions. The opsonins coat bacteria and render them more vulnerable to phagocytosis. They are of particular importance in the phagocytosis of certain virulent organisms. For example, neutrophils cannot engulf virulent pneumococci in the absence of immune serum (Wood et al., 1946). How opsonins work is still not clear. They may alter the surface of bacteria, inactivate toxic substances or simply serve as colloid, facilitating the adherence of the phagocyte to the foreign body. Surfaces against which the bacteria or foreign bodies can be cornered, as it were, also facilitate phagocytosis. Accordingly, fibrin strands provide effective aids. This phenomenon is particularly important in the lungs, where the alveolar spaces would permit bacteria to float around unless they became enmeshed in fibrin. In addition, phagocytosis is favored by higher body temperatures, and thus febrile reactions and the local increased heat in inflammatory sites enhance the phenomenon.

The importance of phagocytosis in defense against bacterial infections is dramatically demonstrated in patients who have some disorder leading to deficient marshalling of white cells at inflammatory foci. Patients with granulocytopenia (a deficiency of circulating neutrophils) often die of uncontrolled bacterial infections. Similarly, mention has already been made of the "lazy leukocyte syndrome" also characterized by recurrent and uncontrolled microbiologic infections. The use of powerful immunosuppressant drugs in transplant patients often depresses the bone marrow, accounting for the fact that infections are the major cause of death in these patients.

Once a microorganism has been engulfed, what is its fate? Most are readily destroyed by the phagocyte. But some, particularly virulent organisms, may destroy the leukocyte. On the other hand, certain organisms, such as the acid-fast bacilli causing tuberculosis and leprosy, are able to survive within phagocytes. Thus, drainage of the white cells through the lymphatics to the lymph nodes results in spread of the infection. The factors that determine whether engulfed bacteria will be killed within their membrane-bound prisons or will survive are poorly understood. Following phagocytosis, neutrophils undergo a marked increase of metabolic activity, characterized by increased oxygen uptake, increased glycolysis, and increased production of lactic acid, resulting in lowering of the ambient pH (Rossi and Zatti, 1964). The acidity favors activation of the lysosomal enzymes of the neutrophil. These include lysozyme (an enzyme capable of degrading bacterial cell walls), which is present in large amounts in neutrophils. Phagocytes also produce hydrogen peroxide, which has an antibacterial action. Another antibacterial substance called phagocytin has been described (Hirsch and Cohn, 1960). Very low concentrations of phagocytin promptly kill a wide range of organisms. Among the variety of potential bactericidal agents possessed by phagocytes, the lysosomal enzymes are probably of greatest importance, since they are known to be capable of digesting proteins, nucleic acids and complex lipids, and bacteria basically represent a composite of these substances.

Before closing the discussion of phagocytosis, it should be emphasized that this leukocytic activity is not directed only against bacteria. Inert exogenous debris, such as small fragments of wood or steel, as well as endogenous cellular debris may be phagocyted and thus be removed from the inflammatory focus. If the unwanted intruder is too large to be incorporated within a phagocyte, large multinucleate foreign body giant cells may be produced. These are of sufficient size to enclose remarkably large particles and are described in greater detail on page 49. Thus, the phenomenon of phagocytosis contributes significantly to the "clean up" at sites of injury.

It must now be clear, as observed early in this chapter, that the inflammatory response is a highly integrated and complex process. An effort to summarize it was presented in Table 2–1, but it should be remembered that the attempt to assign mediators to specific phases of the response is somewhat arbitrary, as indicated in the previous discussion.

DIFFERENTIATION OF ACUTE, CHRONIC AND SUBACUTE INFLAMMATION

To this point, the inflammatory process has been described in terms of the immediate reaction to injury. This immediate reaction gives rise to acute inflammation. Acute reactions are seen when the stimulus to inflammation is transient, as for example with physical trauma, burns (whether caused by excess heat or by chemicals) and microbiologic infections which are rapidly eradicated by the defensive forces of the body. In contrast, some inflammatory stimuli persist for weeks and even years, as in the instance of a large foreign body which is not removed. Similarly, the inhalation of silica dust may lead to a chronic protracted inflammation within the lung known as silicosis. Silica particles are relatively insoluble and persist as a continuing inflammatory stimulus. Rarely, some responses merit the intermediate designation "subacute." Inflammatory reactions may thus be acute, chronic or subacute, with consequent modification of the morphologic pattern.

ACUTE INFLAMMATION

The *acute inflammatory response* to an injurious influence of brief duration is characterized principally by *vascular and exudative changes.* Trivial injuries may elicit only few changes and be confined largely to transient local hyperemia, which subsides in the course of 24 to 36 hours. More intense injuries of brief duration evoke not only the hemodynamic vascular changes described earlier but also full-blown exudative changes. Therefore, they are accompanied by local tissue swelling, which represents the accumulation of extravascular exudate. As will be seen when we discuss the intensity of injury, the nature of the exudate will vary according to the extent of widening of the interendothelial junctions. The white cells which participate in the acute reaction are almost entirely neutrophils and macrophages.

CHRONIC INFLAMMATION

Chronic inflammation results whenever the injurious agent persists. Such reactions are characterized by a *proliferative (fibroblastic) rather than an exudative reaction.* The proliferative component represents the onset of fibroplasia in the margins of the injury. The exudation of the acute phase has largely subsided, although sometimes it persists from the earlier acute phase, and the white cell population has slowly evolved from one predominantly of neutrophils and macrophages to one of macrophages and lymphocytes, possibly admixed with plasma cells (Fig. 2–5). Thus, the leukocytic exudation in chronic inflammation is often referred to as mononuclear, to distinguish it from polymorphonuclear. It should be noted that with active chronic inflammation, with an as yet uncontrolled inflammatory stimulus, the center of the inflammatory focus may be rich in neutrophils surrounded by an inflammatory reaction of mononuclear cells and fibroblasts. The neutrophils will persist until the injurious influence has been completely neutralized. A good example of an active chronic inflammatory process is the peptic ulcer of the duodenum or stomach. *An ulcer is a local excavation of the surface of an organ or tissue resulting from the sloughing of inflammatory necrotic tissue* (Fig. 2–6). Peptic ulcers may persist for years. The base of the ulcer is often covered by a layer of acute exudate composed of fibrin and enmeshed neutrophils. Deep to this layer large numbers of lymphocytes, macrophages and some plasma cells are found. Deeper yet there may be dense fibrosis indicative of the chronicity of the ulcer crater. Thus, in the same lesion we see an acute neutrophilic exudate as well as unmistakable evidence of chronic inflammation.

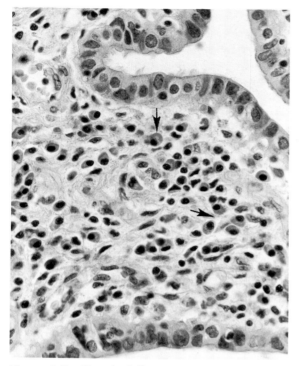

Figure 2–5. Chronic inflammation of the fallopian tube. The subepithelial connective tissue is infiltrated with mononuclear white cells, principally plasma cells marked by eccentric nuclei (see arrows).

Some inflammations are difficult to categorize as either acute or chronic, because indeed there is no sharp line either clinically or morphologically which divides them. Arbitrarily it is often said that when an inflammation lasts longer than 4 to 6 weeks, it is chronic. However, since much depends on the effectiveness of the host response and the nature of the injury, time limits are without meaning. Some agents evoke low grade, smoldering responses which never have a significant acute phase. Conceivably, a very transient acute reaction may have been present, perhaps lasting only a few days, but very soon the morphologic pattern assumes the characteristics of chronic inflammation. The reaction in the lungs to inhaled silica particles, mentioned before, is a good example. There is, indeed, a very transient neutrophilic exudation within the pulmonary tissues soon after lodgment of the silica particles. However, within days the inflammatory reaction changes to one marked by macrophages, lymphocytes and a few plasma cells, accompanied by a fibroblastic response. Other agents evoke a *granulomatous inflammation*, which also is of a chronic nature virtually from its onset. More details on this special pattern of reaction will be given subsequently. Thus, no time limit clearly separates acute from chronic inflammation.

Rather, *the differentiation rests on the morphologic pattern of the inflammatory reaction.*

Why lymphocytes and plasma cells aggregate at non-immunologic chronic inflammatory sites, and the role these cells play, remain mysterious. Circulating lymphocytes are motile, but much less so than neutrophils and monocytes. They emigrate between endothelial cells as do the neutrophils and macrophages. Little is known about chemotactic influences for lymphocytes. In the circulating blood, there are two populations of these cells, one short-lived (the B-cells, p. 168) and the other extremely long-lived (the T-cells, p. 167), having a life span measured in terms of years. Plasma cells are of course not present in the circulation normally and presumably are formed at the site of injury by the differentiation of B-lymphocytes. Since lymphocytes and plasma cells are the agents of humoral and cell-mediated immunity, they understandably accumulate at sites of immunologic injury. Conceivably, within inflammations of long duration, there is release of cellular antigens, which in effect provide an immunologic component to the inflammatory response.

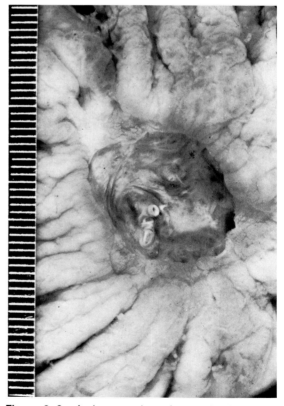

Figure 2–6. A close-up view of a peptic ulcer of the stomach. The crater is surrounded by the rugal folds of the gastric mucosa. An eroded artery, which caused the fatal hemorrhage, protrudes from the floor of the ulcer.

SUBACUTE INFLAMMATION

Subacute inflammation can be dealt with briefly, since it not only is poorly defined but also is of doubtful validity as a specific form of inflammation. Such validity as it may possess relates to its being an intergrade between acute and chronic inflammation. When the term "subacute inflammation" is applied, it generally indicates a response which has some exudative component but also some of the fibroplastic and mononuclear features of the chronic reaction. Often the term "subacute" is misapplied to remitting or subsiding acute inflammations when neutrophils have largely disappeared and the leukocytic reaction is primarily composed of macrophages, a few lymphocytes and, for some unknown reason, a scattering of eosinophils.

MORPHOLOGIC PATTERNS OF ACUTE AND CHRONIC INFLAMMATION

The immediate response to all forms of injury is virtually stereotyped, as described earlier. Within the first few days, however, several influences relating to the injurious agent begin to condition and modify the course and morphologic expression of the inflammatory response. These influences can be best categorized as: (1) intensity of the injury and consequent nature of the exudate and (2) pathogenicity of the specific causative agent. At the conclusion of this chapter, the various *host* factors which modify the quality and adequacy of the response will be considered.

MORPHOLOGIC PATTERNS BASED ON INTENSITY OF INJURY AND CHARACTER OF EXUDATE

Exudation and consequent edema or swelling is one of the characteristic features of the inflammatory response. It is virtually always present in the acute inflammatory reaction but may also persist into the chronic stages. In very mild injuries, it may be so slight as to escape detection.

The nature and amount of exudate depend in general on the intensity of the injury. This generalization is not always valid since, as will become apparent later, the specific injurious agent also influences the nature of the exudate. Nonetheless, it is permissible to say that mild injuries tend to evoke a watery exudate low in protein. Such an inflammatory process is designated a *serous inflammatory reaction.* A good example of a serous reaction is the skin blister that follows a mild burn. In the course of a few days, the serous exudate is slowly resorbed and the inflammatory state subsides.

With more severe injuries and the resulting greater vascular permeability, larger molecules pass the vascular barrier. A *fibrinous inflammatory exudate* develops when the vascular leaks are large enough to permit the passage of fibrinogen molecules. Acute rheumatic carditis classically evokes a fibrinous pericarditis (Fig. 2–7). In the same way, ischemic necrosis of a portion of the myocardium (myocardial infarct) often causes a fibrinous pericarditis in the overlying epicardium. Fibrinous exudates may be removed by fibrinolysis. However, when the fibrin is not removed, it may stimulate the ingrowth of fibroblasts and blood vessels and thus lead to scarring. Conversion of the fibrinous exudate to scar tissue (termed *organization*) within the pericardial sac will lead either to opaque fibrous thickening of the pericardium and epicardium in the area of exudation or, more often, to the development of fibrous strands which bridge the pericardial space. In this way the pericardial sac may be partially or totally obliterated; the latter is designated obliterative pericarditis. Similarly, organization of fibrinous exudate in the pulmonary alveoli results in filling of the air spaces by a fibroblastic connective tissue, irre-

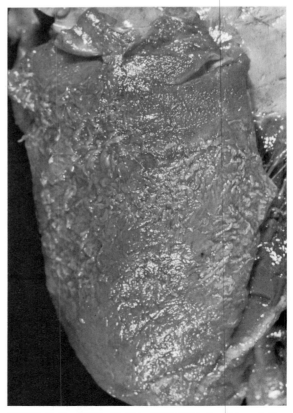

Figure 2–7. View of the epicardial surface of the heart, heavily layered with a shaggy fibrinous exudate—the so-called "bread and butter" pericarditis.

vocably impairing the respiratory function of the organized lung parenchyma. It is evident then that fibrinous exudation may have more serious consequences than serous exudation.

More severe inflammatory responses, particularly those caused by microbiologic agents, are characterized by the emigration of large numbers of leukocytes to produce a *purulent or suppurative inflammatory reaction*. A classic example of such a response is acute suppurative appendicitis. The lumen of the appendix may be filled with suppuration, better known as "pus." Large amounts of exudate may permeate the appendiceal wall and layer the serosal covering of the organ. A suppurative exudate may be resolved by proteolytic enzymes largely derived from leukocytic lysosomes and thus be removed. Alternatively, the exudate may become organized and sometimes calcified. Indeed, suppurative reactions are even more apt to undergo organization than fibrinous reactions. For this reason, an acute bacterial suppurative pericarditis is much more likely to result in fibrous obliteration of the pericardial cavity than is a fibrinous pericarditis. The obliteration may be associated with dense interadherence of pericardium and epicardium. Indeed, sometimes the enclosing fibrous tissue seriously hampers cardiac function by restricting diastolic expansion of the heart, a condition known as constrictive pericarditis. Calcification of such connective tissue adds a further impediment to cardiac function, creating a calcified rigid encasement of the heart *(concretio cordis)*. The calcified fibrous scar constitutes a gravestone that permanently marks the site of prior suppurative inflammation.

Hemorrhagic inflammatory reactions are encountered in intense injuries which cause necrosis and rupture of vessel walls. This pattern is particularly common in certain meningococcal and rickettsial infections in which the organisms cause inflammatory necrosis of small blood vessels. Hemorrhagic exudates, too, may become organized and calcified, but this occurs less often than in suppurative reactions. It is apparent then that the various patterns of inflammatory exudate conditioned by the intensity of the injury have greatly differing potentials to the patient.

Some inflammatory reactions are characterized by mixed patterns of exudation — for example, serofibrinous or fibrinosuppurative. An injury may evoke a serous reaction at the outset, with subsequent transformation to the fibrinous or suppurative patterns as the inflammation develops to its full intensity. Whatever the mixture, the presence of large amounts of fibrin or suppuration within an inflammatory focus constitutes an invitation to the ingrowth of fibroblasts and blood vessels,

with organization of the exudate. We know very little about the influences that determine whether resolution or organization will occur, but the outcome may be related to the length of time that such exudates persist at the inflammatory site.

MORPHOLOGIC PATTERNS BASED ON CAUSATIVE AGENT

Most injuries, such as physical trauma, excess heat, chemical burns and exposure to excess radiant energy, evoke fairly nonspecific patterns of inflammation. In contrast, infections with microbiologic agents tend to evolve into somewhat distinctive patterns of inflammatory reaction. Although it is not always possible to identify the specific causative agent by the morphology, an educated guess can be made as to the possible etiology, permitting institution of appropriate cultural and serologic diagnostic procedures. Even in this era of "wonder drugs" the limited range of effectiveness of each against the myriad microorganisms makes it critically important to establish the precise etiology of an infectious disease so that the most appropriate antibacterial treatment can be employed. The following remarks will be limited to some of the more distinctive inflammatory reactions evoked by certain microorganisms.

Localized suppurative infections are caused by a great variety of bacteria that collectively are referred to as pyogens (pus producers). *Pus may be defined as an inflammatory exudate rich in proteins which contains viable leukocytes admixed with cell debris derived from necrotic native and immigrant white cells.* Included among the pyogens are staphylococci, many gram-negative bacilli (*Escherichia coli, Klebsiella pneumoniae, Proteus* strains and *Pseudomonas aeruginosa*), the meningococci, gonococci and pneumococci. Infections with these agents induce local collections of pus at the site of implantation. Staphylococci are perhaps the most frequent cause of localized suppurative or pyogenic infections. When implanted beneath the skin or in a solid organ, the pyogens produce an *abscess* — a localized collection of pus. Pyogenic infections of the skin range from the simple hair follicle infection *(folliculitis)* to the *furuncle* (more popularly known as a "boil") to the multiple deep-seated abscesses known as *carbuncles*. The gram-negative rods, on the other hand, are more often the cause of suppurative urinary tract infections, such as those that involve the urinary bladder *(cystitis)* or the kidney *(pyelonephritis)*. The favorite site of attack of the gonococcus is the genital tract (male or female), while the meningococcus implants on the oronasopharyngeal mucosa, whence it spreads to the meninges (*suppurative meningitis*). All the pyogens, wherever they become implanted, are capable of invading blood vessels to produce bacteremia, with the potential seeding of any or all of the other organs and tissues in the body. In this fashion, a neglected staphylococcal or gonococcal infection, for example, may give rise to bacterial implantation on the heart valves (*bacterial endocarditis*), or to meningitis or a brain abscess. In the course of progression of any infection, the regional lymph nodes or the entire lymphoid system of the body may become involved, as will be discussed more fully later.

A subgroup of suppurative infections is the *spreading suppurative infection* classically caused by the streptococci, particularly those of the beta hemolytic Lancefield group A. Infections with these organisms tend to trek rapidly through large areas of tissue, such as an entire forearm, one side of the face or even large tracts of the abdominal wall. Characteristic of such spreading infection is brawny edema and fiery red hyperemia of the inflammatory area known as *cellulitis* (also referred to as a *phlegmon*). Instead of producing focal abscesses filled with thick purulent exudate, the streptococci tend to evoke a watery suppurative reaction distributed throughout the cleavage planes and tissue spaces. This morphologic pattern reflects the bacterial elaboration of large amounts of hyaluronidases that break down polysaccharide ground substance, fibrinolysins that digest fibrin barriers and lecithinases that destroy cell membranes. As might be anticipated, in this type of spreading infection, the lymphatics are particularly prone to secondary involvement (*lymphangitis*). In these infections one can sometimes observe subcutaneous red streaks extending proximally from areas of injury toward the regional lymph nodes. The regional nodes undergo striking inflammatory reactive hyperplasia, and too often the organisms invade the bloodstream, producing bacteremia. Sometimes a streptococcal infection remains fairly superficial and affects only the skin, superficial subcutaneous tissues and skin lymphatics in a pattern known as *erysipelas*.

The other, less virulent Lancefield groups of streptococci tend to produce focal suppurative reactions in the pattern of the pyogens already mentioned. It should be noted that the immunologic reactions to the streptococcal infections may themselves be responsible for very serious poststreptococcal systemic diseases, such as rheumatic fever (p. 313) and glomerulonephritis (p. 436).

Membranous (sometimes called *pseudomembranous*) *inflammation* is the term given to those inflammatory reactions on the surface of an organ or tissue that are characterized by the formation of a superficial membranous layer of exudate containing the causative agents, precipitated fibrin, necrotic native cells and inflammatory white cells. This pattern is most frequently encountered in the oropharynx, trachea, bronchi and gastrointestinal tract. *Diphtheria and moniliasis are classic examples of membranous inflammations of the pharyngeal and respiratory regions.* In diphtheria, the causative organism, *Corynebacterium diphtheriae*, establishes itself superficially on the surface of the mucous membranes of the pharyngeal region or the trachea and major bronchi, and here it evokes an inflammatory exudation of fibrin and white cells admixed with necrotic cells. A gray-white, tough membrane is produced. Should it become loosened and be inhaled, it may cause asphyxiation, particularly in the young child. Diphtheritic infections, however, have other serious implications, resulting from the absorption into the bloodstream of a very powerful exotoxin elaborated by the organism, which often causes severe injury to the myocardial cells (*cardiomyopathy*). Monilial infection of the oral cavity, commonly referred to as *thrush*, produces patches of gray-white membrane. In this infection, the membrane is made up largely of the fungal mycelia, with only scant amounts of inflammatory exudate. The membranous inflammation of the intestinal tract, termed *membranous enterocolitis*, is of uncertain etiology. It is most frequently found in the colon but may also involve the lower small intestine. Superficial but severe staphylococcal infection of the bowel mucosa has been postulated as one cause. Staphylococci ordinarily cannot compete with the abundant normal flora of the gut. Overgrowth of staphylococci therefore is usually encountered in patients receiving broad spectrum antibiotics which wipe out the coliforms and thus permit the antibiotic resistant staphylococci to overgrow. Debilitation, or perhaps impairment of the vascular supply in the gut, may also predispose to the overgrowth of staphylococci. Membranous inflammatory reactions at this site are usually found to comprise massive amounts of staphylococci along with white cell and mucosal cell debris bound up in fibrinous precipitate. Although other agents produce membranous inflammation in the gut, the recognition of this pattern of reaction provides at least one clue to the etiology of the process.

Diffuse involvement of the RE system and focal histiocytic aggregations are characteristics of the Salmonella infections. Within this group, typhoid fever, produced by *Salmonella typhi*, is the most serious disorder. The other organisms tend to produce less threatening febrile illness, often with gastrointestinal manifestations. In these diseases, there is widespread involvement of the lymph nodes, as well as of the spleen and liver. In all sites, the RE cells are hypertrophied. These often undergo proliferation to produce focal aggregations of RE cells or histiocytes. In the gastrointestinal tract, typhoid fever induces hyperplasia and enlargement of Peyer's patches, often with ulceration of the overlying mucosa.

Perivascular accumulations (cuffing) and interstitial infiltrations of mononuclear leukocytes are characteristic of most viral and rickettsial infections. Lymphocytes and macrophages—and, to a lesser extent, plasma cells—are involved principally. Rarely, in extremely acute viral infections, there may be a polymorphonuclear leukocytic reaction. Thus, the various viral agents that cause encephalitis (p. 665) tend to evoke mononuclear cuffing about the small vessels of the brain substance. Poliomyelitis is similarly characterized by mononuclear interstitial and perivascular infiltrates. In addition, viral myocarditis is characterized by intercellular edema and infiltrations of mononuclear white cells (Fig. 2–8). The response to rickettsial infections is virtually the same except that there is often proliferation of the endothelial cells as well as a perivascular reaction. Actual parasitization of the endothelial cells by the rickettsial organisms appears to lead to the proliferative reaction in these cells. There is often necrosis and

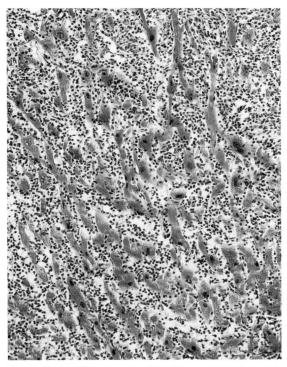

Figure 2–8. Viral myocarditis. The myocardial cells are widely separated by edema and an infiltration of mononuclear white cells.

rupture of the walls of the small blood vessels as a result of this involvement. *Typhus fever,* for example, produces striking vascular and perivascular reactions in the brain and any other tissue affected. *Rocky Mountain spotted fever* causes a similar reaction, not only in the brain but also in the small vessels of the skin, hence the skin rash.

We still do not understand such a predictable mononuclear infiltrate. There is some suspicion that immunologic mechanisms are involved, thus evoking a response principally from immunologically competent cells, i.e., lymphocytes, plasma cells and macrophages.

Granulomatous inflammation is a distinctive morphologic pattern of inflammatory reaction encountered in relatively few diseases. *Tuberculosis is the archetype of the granulomatous diseases, but syphilis, sarcoidosis, cat-scratch fever, lymphogranuloma inguinale, leprosy, brucellosis, some of the mycotic infections, berylliosis and reactions to irritant lipids* are also included. Recognition of the granulomatous pattern, for example, in a lymph node biopsy is of great importance because of the limited number of possible etiologies, some of which are extremely threatening. *A granuloma consists of a microscopic aggregation of plump fibroblasts or histiocytes (macrophages) that have been transformed into epithelial-like cells, and are therefore designated epithelioid cells, surrounded by a collar of mononuclear leukocytes, principally lymphocytes and occasionally plasma cells.* Older granulomas develop an enclosing rim of fibroblasts and connective tissue. Frequently, but not invariably, *large giant cells* are found in the periphery or sometimes in the center of granulomas. These giant cells may achieve diameters of 40 to 50 μm. (micrometers). They comprise a large mass of cytoplasm containing numerous (20 or more) small nuclei. Two types of giant cells are encountered. The *Langhans type* is said to be characteristic of tuberculosis, but in reality it may be found in any of the granulomatous reactions. The nuclei in this form tend to be arranged about the periphery of the cell, sometimes encircling the cytoplasm, and at other times producing horseshoe patterns. The individual nuclei are quite small and have a diameter of only a very small fraction of the diameter of the entire cell. *The foreign body type giant cell* differs in that the numerous nuclei are scattered throughout the cytoplasm in no distinctive pattern. Both forms of giant cells are believed to arise from fusion of histiocytes or from division of the nuclei without separation of cells. Although some investigators rely heavily on the finding of giant cells, *the identification of a granulomatous reaction actually rests with the recognition of the conversion of macrophages into epithelioid cells.*

The formation of granulomas is a reflection

of the buildup of cell-mediated immunity to the causative agent. The following sequence is postulated. The etiologic agent—for example, the tubercle bacillus—is implanted in the lung. At the very outset, neutrophils and macrophages aggregate at the site. The macrophages engulf the bacilli. During the ensuing 10 to 14 days, cell-mediated immunity to the bacilli develops, leading to the generation of specifically sensitized lymphocytes. These cells then accumulate at the site of infection and liberate several soluble factors (lymphokines), some of which attract, immobilize and activate more macrophages (Mackanass, 1972). Simultaneously, the macrophages undergo epithelioid cell transformation. This transformation is believed to represent a reaction on the part of the macrophage to the absorption or ingestion of some substance which causes enlargement of the cell, with the production of an abundant granular cytoplasm. In some of these epithelioid cells, phagocytized bacilli or fragments of bacilli can be found within the cell cytoplasm. In other cells, however, no recognizable bacterial fragments can be seen. It has been proposed, and in fact has been reasonably well documented, that the lipids in the wall of the tubercle bacillus evoke such transformation. Waxes that contain macromolecular lipids of quite unusual chemical structure, containing about 40 to 50 per cent mycolic acid and 40 to 50 per cent polysaccharides, as well as amino acids, have been extracted from *Mycobacterium tuberculosis* (White, 1966). Injection of such extracts into guinea pigs evokes a characteristic local granuloma formation, complete with giant cells. It is not certain that the same fraction is responsible for all the granulomatous reactions in the many diseases and circumstances mentioned above. However, it is of interest that lipids such as those used as solvents for certain drugs often induce a granulomatous inflammatory response to a subcutaneous or intramuscular injection.

Although all the disorders previously mentioned are characterized by granuloma formation, certain variations in the granulomatous pattern are encountered among the various diseases. *The granuloma of tuberculosis classically has central caseous necrosis* (described on p. 23) (Fig. 2–9). The fusion of many caseating granulomas may give rise to extensive macroscopic lesions of caseous necrosis involving large areas of the lung. These are readily detectable on x-ray. The same caseating lesion is produced in all tissues affected. In contrast, *sarcoidosis almost never produces central necrosis, and so the sarcoid granuloma is often called a "hard tubercle,"* while the tuberculous granuloma is often referred to as a "soft tubercle." Syphilis produces gummatous necrosis in the center of its granuloma. Gummatous necrosis tends to have a rub-

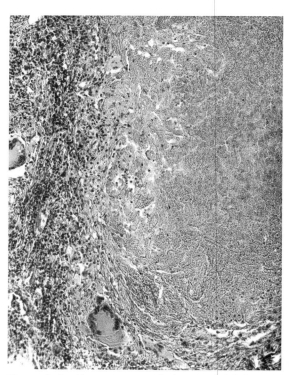

Figure 2–9. Caseous necrosis (upper right) in a tuberculous granuloma (a caseating tubercle). In the necrotic focus, all cell detail is obliterated by granular debris. The enclosing wall contains several large multinucleate giant cells of the Langhans type, with peripheral orientation of the nuclei.

bery consistency, firmer than the soft, cheesy texture of the tuberculous reaction. Berylliosis may cause central necrosis, but classically polymorphonuclear leukocytes are present in the necrotic center, a distinctly unusual finding in tuberculosis. Some of the differential features are outlined in Table 2–2.

Fibrinous exudations and *fibrinoid deposits* are characteristic of most immunologic injuries. On this basis, for example, rheumatic fever and systemic lupus erythematosus (SLE) are marked by fibrinous pericarditis or fibrinous pleuritis. *Even more characteristic of immunologic injury are necrotizing lesions in the walls of small vessels accompanied by deposits of fibrinoid material and leukocytic infiltrates* within the necrotic vessel walls. Further details are given in the complete discussion of diseases of immune origin in Chapter 6.

It has been the purpose of this section to point out that some injuries and etiologic agents produce more or less characteristic patterns of inflammation. Often one sees a diagnosis such as "inflammatory reaction with mononuclear perivascular cuffing." The tendency for specific agents to create predictable lesions in certain tissues provides some guidance in determining the precise etiology. In addition, the morphologic inflammatory reac-

TABLE 2–2. MAJOR GRANULOMATOUS INFLAMMATIONS*

DISEASE	CAUSE	TISSUE REACTION
Tuberculosis	Mycobacterium tuberculosis	Noncaseating tubercle (granuloma prototype): A focus of epithelioid cells, rimmed by fibroblasts, lymphocytes, histiocytes, occasional Langhans' giant cell. Caseating tubercle: Central amorphous granular debris, loss of all cellular detail.
Sarcoidosis	Unknown	Noncaseating granuloma: Giant cells (Langhans' and foreign body types); asteroids in giant cells; occasional Schaumann's body (concentric calcific concretion).
Certain fungal infections		Granuloma usually larger than single tubercle with central granular debris; often contains causal organism and recognizable neutrophils.
	Histoplasma capsulatum	Organism is yeast-like, round to oval, budding, 2 to 4 μm.; usually intracellular.
	Cryptococcus neoformans	Organism is yeast-like, sometimes budding; 5 to 10 μm.; large, clear capsule.
	Blastomyces dermatitidis	Organism is yeast-like, budding; 5 to 15 μm.; thick, doubly refractile capsule.
	Coccidioides immitis	Organism appears as spherical (30–80 μm.) cyst containing endospores of 3 to 5 μm. each.
Syphilis	Treponema pallidum	Gumma: Microscopic to grossly visible lesion, enclosing wall of histiocytes, fibroblasts and lymphocytes; plasma cell infiltrate; center cells are necrotic without loss of cellular outline.
Cat-scratch fever	Virus ? Chlamydiae?	Rounded or stellate granuloma containing central granular debris and recognizable neutrophils; giant cells uncommon.
Berylliosis (chronic)	Beryllium	Fibrosing granuloma resembling noncaseating lesions of sarcoidosis. Asteroids and Schaumann's bodies may be present.
Lymphogranuloma inguinale (venereum)	Chlamydiae?	Granulomatous enclosing rim composed mostly of macrophages and reticuloendothelial cells about a microabscess containing viable and necrotic neutrophils.

*Modified from Robbins, S. L.: Pathologic Basis of Disease. Philadelphia, W. B. Saunders Co., 1974.

tion can be characterized in terms of the duration and intensity of an injury and the character of the exudate. Thus, it is possible to speak, for example, of an acute, suppurative staphylococcal pericarditis.

ROLE OF LYMPHATICS, LYMPHOID TISSUE AND RE SYSTEM

As major components of the body's defense mechanism, the lymphatics and lymphoid tissues become involved in any significant inflammatory reaction. *Lymphatics* are almost as omnipresent as capillaries. They are lined with continuous epithelium having loose cell junctions and basement membranes in the larger channels. In an inflammatory response, there is increased regional lymphatic flow of a fluid having a higher than usual protein content and containing increased numbers of leukocytes. These vessels drain off the fluid and cellular exudate from the area of reaction. It has always been somewhat puzzling that the delicate channels do not become compressed or obliterated by the pressure of the inflammatory transudation or exudation. On the contrary, they are often dilated. Delicate fibrils have been identified extending at right angles from the walls of lymphatics into the adjacent tissues (Leak and Burke, 1968). As the tissue pressure mounts, traction is exerted on these fibrils to maintain the patency of the lymphatics. This traction might also increase the dimensions of the loose intercellular junctions and thus provide ready pathways for the entrance of fluid, proteins and cells.

Lymphatic drainage, regrettably, also provides channels for the dissemination of the injurious agent. Inflammatory involvement of lymphatic channels (*lymphangitis*) and the regional filtering lymph nodes (*reactive lymphadenitis*) may develop. Reactive lymphadenitis is characterized by increased numbers of the lymphoblasts and histiocytes in the cortical follicles. Often there is phagocytosis of cell debris by the RE cells of the sinuses and follicles. Occasionally polymorphonuclear cells and particulate debris can be identified in the sinuses. If significant numbers of viable bacteria drain to the node, they may set up secondary sites of necrosis, leading to the destruction of the lymph node, with accumulation of exudate in these sites.

Nevertheless, the regional lymph nodes constitute important secondary lines of defense, which, in general, tend to screen off the infection from the remainder of the body. As would be expected, if these secondary lines of defense are overwhelmed, the inflammatory reaction may extend throughout the body and produce generalized involvement of all lymphoid tissues and reticuloendothelial organs, such as the spleen and liver. This dissemination is encountered only in severe inflammatory reactions and usually implies drainage of the infection through the blood as well as through the entire lymphatic system. Lymphadenopathy may be produced by primary or secondary neoplastic involvement of these structures, but in these disorders the enlargement is not accompanied by tenderness nor, usually, by overt lymphangitis. With microbiologic infections that involve the bloodstream, generalized tender lymphadenopathy appears, accompanied by hepatomegaly and splenomegaly. For this reason, the astute clinician always palpates for enlargement of the lymph nodes, liver and spleen in febrile patients suspected of having a disseminated microbiologic infection.

The reticuloendothelial (RE) system may be viewed as another line of defense which polices the bloodstream. It is composed of widely dispersed cells having as a common denominator the capacity to take up vital dyes, such as trypan blue, and to phagocytize particulate matter circulating in the blood. The constituent cells include the fixed littoral cells lining the lymphatic channels, the lymphoid, marrow and the splenic tissues; the Kupffer cells of the liver; scattered endothelial cells of the blood vessels; and tissue histiocytes or macrophages. Monocytes can also be considered a part of the RE system. All of these cells participate in the defense of the body by removing particulate matter, such as circulating bacteria or other macromolecular debris. In malaria, for example, the RE cells are loaded not only with plasmodia but also with malarial pigment derived from hemoglobin released by the lysis of parasitized erythrocytes. Thus, generalized lymphadenopathy, hepatomegaly and particularly splenomegaly are seen in this infection. In the course of such phagocytic activity, the RE system can become overloaded, producing what is referred to as *reticuloendothelial blockade.* When such occurs, it has the serious implication of removing the body's last line of defense, thus exposing all of the tissues of the body to the offending agent.

CLINICAL MANIFESTATIONS OF ACUTE AND CHRONIC INFLAMMATION

From what has already been said, and indeed as everyone knows from personal experience, inflammations are painful and cause other local manifestations. Some (streptococcal tonsillitis is a good example) also evoke systemic signs and symptoms, such as fever, malaise and loss of appetite. It is our purpose here to correlate the inflammatory changes already described with the resultant clinical findings.

The local manifestations of acute inflammation and active chronic inflammation have long been known as the *cardinal signs of inflammation* — i.e., *rubor* (redness), *calor* (heat), *tumor* (swelling), *dolor* (pain) and *functio laesa* (loss of function). The pathophysiology of some of these cardinal signs is readily evident. The local heat and redness result from the increased blood flow in the microcirculation at the site of injury. The swelling is obviously the consequence of exudation, with its increase of interstitial fluid. Pain is less easily explained. It has been attributed simplistically to pressure on nerve endings resulting from exudation. Although this explanation may be valid, there is a suspicion that chemical mediators may be involved. Recall that when applied to a blister base, the kinins evoke pain. Similarly, prostaglandins may in some way increase neural sensitivity. Not unreasonably, any one or indeed all of these mechanisms may be operative. The causes of loss of function are equally obscure. One could propose on mechanistic grounds that a painful infection in or about the elbow joint might lead to voluntary immobilization of the joint; but such an explanation would hardly suffice for the loss of liver function seen in diffuse hepatitis. Conceivably, the hyperemia of inflammation raises the temperature in the microenvironment of the cells, impairing enzyme function; or the increased metabolic activity of an inflammatory focus might lower the pH and interfere with function in that way. These suggestions are, however, hypothetical. We simply do not understand functio laesa.

The cardinal signs classically are evoked by all significant acute inflammations. They may also be present with active chronic inflammations, i.e., those in which cellular necrosis is still present in the chronic inflammatory focus. As the flame of the inflammatory focus burns out, the cardinal signs fade and disappear. The redness and local heat abate first, then the pain, but the swelling and loss of function may persist for some time, even in those chronic inflammatory responses which smolder for months. Eventually all the cardinal signs disappear, leaving perhaps only some induration (increased consistency) as a sign of the proliferative fibroplasia of chronic inflammation.

Systemic manifestations, all too familiar to anyone who has suffered from a severe sore throat or a respiratory infection, may be evoked by acute or chronic inflammation. Fever is one of the most prominent systemic manifestations, particularly in inflammatory states associated with spread of organisms into the bloodstream. Bacteremia usually induces a high fever (102° to 104° F.), characterized by dramatic swings in the temperature, producing so-called spikes on the temperature chart. Usually these patients have violent shaking chills, which may indeed rattle the bed. It is postulated that bacteria release pyrogens, possibly in the nature of endotoxins. Endogenous pyrogens are also proposed; these may be released from neutrophils and monocytes when these cells are exposed to bacterial endotoxins, to antigen-antibody complexes or to the products of necrotic cells (Atkins et al., 1967). The precise nature of the endogenous pyrogen has not been well established but it is thought to be a lipoprotein derived from cell membranes. There is evidence from experimental animals that pyrogens act on the thermoregulatory mechanisms in the hypothalamus that control the production and dissipation of body heat. The phenomenon has been likened to "setting the hypothalamic thermostat at a higher level" (Atkins, 1960).

Leukocytosis (increase in the number of circulating white cells) is another characteristic of significant acute and chronic inflammations. In acute appendicitis, for example, the white cell count may well rise to 18,000 to 25,000 leukocytes per mm.³ of blood. Indeed, some inflammatory states evoke extreme elevations of the white count to levels above 50,000 mm.³ of blood. Such extreme elevations are sometimes called *leukemoid reactions* because they approach the white cell count encountered in leukemia. In most nonspecific inflammations, the leukocytosis is due to an absolute as well as relative increase in the number of circulating neutrophils. Some mechanisms involved in the production of this neutrophilia have already been mentioned (p. 42).

Not all inflammatory states evoke a neutrophilic leukocytosis. Infectious mononucleosis, whooping cough, mumps, German measles and undulant fever characteristically produce a lymphocytosis instead. Allergic inflammatory reactions (hay fever, bronchial asthma and systemic angiitides) and parasitic infections typically elicit an eosinophilia. Moreover, the white cell count in the circulating blood actually drops in certain inflammatory states. Infections caused by viruses, rickettsiae and protozoa, and the salmonelloses, as well as overwhelming bacterial infections, may be marked by leukopenia rather than leukocytosis.

Mention has already been made of the response of the lymphoid and reticuloendothelial systems to inflammations; thus, local or generalized lymphadenopathy, sometimes accompanied by splenomegaly and hepatomegaly, may be present.

A number of other ill-defined and inconstant systemic manifestations may appear in patients with febrile inflammatory states—e.g., headache, listlessness, malaise, loss of appetite and general disability. One would suspect the formation of humoral substances as the underlying basis for these nonspecific complaints, but none has been identified. Despite our lack of understanding of their origins, malaise, debility and the other manifestations of general ill health are clinically significant, since they are responsible for much of the suffering of the patient with inflammatory disease.

REPAIR

In the inflammatory-reparative reaction, repair begins soon after the injury, while the acute inflammatory reaction is still in full swing. But it cannot be completed until the injurious agent has been destroyed or neutralized. *Repair consists of the replacement of dead cells by viable cells.* These new cells may be derived either from the parenchyma or from the connective tissue stroma of the injured tissue. It is hardly necessary to point out that in the evolutionary process mammals have lost the capacity to regenerate total structures, such as a limb, as so many of the simpler aquatic and amphibious animals do. Indeed, the regenerative capacity of man is quite limited. Only some of his cells are capable of regeneration and then only under specific conditions. Repair of destroyed cells therefore usually involves some connective tissue proliferation with the formation of a fibrous scar. Although the anatomic continuity of the tissue may be restored thereby, such repair is obviously imperfect since it replaces functioning parenchymal cells with nonspecialized connective tissue. Scarring thus diminishes the reserve of the organ or tissue involved.

Morphologic descriptions of parenchymal regeneration will be presented first, then connective tissue scarring will be described, followed by a discussion of our present understanding of the mechanisms and forces that govern repair.

PARENCHYMAL REGENERATION

Replacement of destroyed parenchymal cells by proliferation of reserve cells can occur only in those tissues in which the cells retain the capacity to replicate (McMinn, 1967). Other factors also influence the regenerative process, but first let us consider the ability of cells to divide. *The cells of the body have been divided into three groups, based on their regenerative capacity: labile, stable and permanent.* The first two groups are able to proliferate throughout life, while permanent cells cannot reproduce themselves. Obviously, injury which destroys permanent cells can never be repaired by proliferation of the preserved parenchymal elements.

Labile cells continue to multiply throughout life to replace those shed or destroyed by normal physiologic processes. These include the cells of all epithelial surfaces, as well as lymphoid and hematopoietic cells. Included among the epithelial surfaces are the epidermis, the linings of the oral cavity, gastrointestinal tract, respiratory tract, the male and female genital tracts and the linings of ducts. In all these sites the surface cells exfoliate throughout life and are replaced by continued proliferation of reserve elements. Indeed, the lining of the small intestine is totally replaced every few days. The regenerative capacity of such cells obviously is enormous. The cells of the bone marrow and the lymphoid structures, including the spleen, are also labile cells. In these tissues, there is constant replacement of cells that have a life span ranging from a few days to possibly years.

Stable cells retain the latent capacity to regenerate, but under normal circumstances do not actively replicate because they have a sur-

vival time measured in terms of years and possibly equal to the life of the organism. The parenchymal cells of all glands in the body, including the liver, pancreas, salivary and endocrine glands, kidney tubular cells and glands of the skin, are stable cells. For example, mitotic figures are rare to the point of being virtually nonexistent in normal adult liver, yet the liver has the capacity to regenerate large excised portions. It is possible to remove 80 per cent of the liver in an experimental animal and find, in about a week, a liver of essentially normal weight. Within an hour after partial hepatectomy, changes can be identified in parenchymal cells throughout the residual liver substance. By 24 hours the cells, nuclei and nucleoli more than double in size, and soon thereafter mitoses appear (Bucher, 1967). Restoration of the normal liver weight is accomplished largely by an increase in the size of the residual lobules. Such regenerated tissue is completely functional. There may be in addition some disorderly proliferation of hepatocytes and blood vessels along the lines of surgical excision, creating disorderly liver lobules. This marginal regeneration can participate in most of the metabolic functions of the liver, but because the hepatocytes are not arrayed regularly along bile canaliculi, their function in the excretion of bile is impaired or lost. Man too has a remarkable capacity to regenerate excised liver, as has been documented in patients who have had hepatectomies for primary liver cell carcinoma.

The mesenchymal cells of the body and their derivatives also fall into the category of stable cells. It is well known that fibroblasts and the more primitive mesenchymal cells retain great regenerative capacity. Moreover, many of these mesenchymal cells have the further ability to differentiate along a number of lines, thus making possible the replacement of specialized mesenchymal elements. Injuries involving bone are often accompanied by differentiation of mesenchymal cells into chondroblasts or osteoblasts. In adipose tissue, these same mesenchymal cells may become repositories for the storage of lipids and in this way be transformed into fat cells.

Muscle cells have been held by some workers to be stable cells and by others to be permanent cells. The evidence that skeletal, cardiac and smooth muscle cells are capable of regenerating is at best scanty and uncertain. Most of this evidence is derived from studies of lower animals (Reznick, 1969; Hay, 1971). It will suffice to say here that if muscle cells do have some regenerative capacity, it is extremely limited. Certainly scarring almost inevitably follows myocardial infarction and one does not encounter, in the margins of the in-

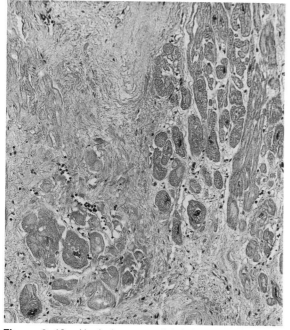

Figure 2–10. Healed myocardial infarct. Dense collagenous scar has replaced most of the myocardial fibers in the area of ischemic necrosis.

farct, replicative activity in the still vital myocardial cells (Fig. 2–10). Similarly, scarring follows injuries to the smooth muscle of the wall of the intestines and uterus. Yet enlargement of the uterus during pregnancy is thought to be accomplished by both hypertrophy and hyperplasia of smooth muscle cells. Whether muscle cells should be considered as stable or permanent cells remains an unsettled issue.

Permanent cells comprise only neurons and, as mentioned above, possibly muscle cells. Destruction of a neuron, whether it is in the central nervous system or in one of the ganglia, represents a permanent loss. However, this statement does not refer to the ability of the nerve cell to replace its severed axon process. If the cell body of the neuron is not destroyed, the cell may regrow any of its extended processes. New axons grow at the rate of 3 to 4 mm. per day, but in such regrowth, they must follow the preexisting pathway of the degenerating axon, or the regrowth becomes tangled and disoriented and, therefore, nonfunctional. The disoriented, growing axon process may give rise to a mass of tangled fibers, sometimes termed an *amputation* or *traumatic neuroma*. It is for this reason that coaptation of severed nerves is of importance in surgical repair; it provides an appropriate "road map" for the regenerating axon fibers.

The perfection of parenchymal repair of an injury depends on more than the ability of cells to regenerate. Preservation of the stromal architecture or framework of the injured tissue is also necessary. In the regeneration of the liver mentioned earlier, it was pointed out that some restoration of size is accomplished by replication of cells within residual lobules. Such cells, which have normal orientation to the liver framework and to the vascular sinusoids and biliary canaliculi, may achieve perfect function. At the line of surgical excision the regeneration is disorderly and complete function (such as secretion of bilirubin into the bile) cannot be assumed by these masses of cells. Similarly, if the kidney is exposed to a toxic agent which destroys renal tubular cells but does not affect the tubular basement membranes or the underlying stroma, regeneration of tubular cells may completely restore normal structure and function. If, on the other hand, the stromal framework of the tubules is lost, as with a renal infarct, perfect reconstruction is not possible, and scarring ensues. Thus the perfection of repair depends to a considerable extent on the survival of the basic framework of the tissue. When this is lost, regeneration may restore mass but not complete function.

A further conditioning influence on regeneration is the obvious necessity for preservation of some portion of the original structure. Total destruction of a kidney cannot be followed by regeneration. The remaining kidney may undergo some compensatory enlargement, but the totally destroyed kidney is irrevocably lost. Similarly, total destruction of hair follicles, sweat glands or sebaceous glands cannot be followed by replacement of these lost adnexal structures. Thus, deep burns or loss of large amounts of skin may be followed by regeneration of an epidermis devoid of adnexal structures.

REPAIR BY CONNECTIVE TISSUE

Proliferation of fibroblasts and capillary buds and the subsequent laying down of collagen to produce a scar is the usual consequence of most tissue damage. The only exceptions have already been cited. Connective tissue scarring is a ubiquitous and efficient method of repair but, as has been indicated, it necessitates a loss of specialized parenchymal function (Fig. 2–11). *Connective tissue repair is traditionally considered as either primary union, e.g., that which takes place when surgical wound margins are nicely coapted by sutures, or as secondary union, e.g., that which occurs when the loss of tissue prevents such coaptation.* In the former instance, there is little or no loss of substance; exudate and necrotic debris are minimal and the repair occurs quite promptly. When there has been a significant loss of tissue, as in an open wound, and there is a considerable amount of exudate or necrotic

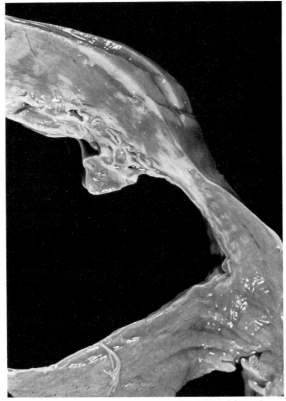

Figure 2–11. The pale areas within the thinned out cross section of the heart are fibrous scar resulting from the replacement of myocardial fibers by scar tissue.

debris to be removed, the healing takes place more slowly. The defect must be filled by the slow buildup of newly formed, highly vascularized connective tissue. This tissue, which is rich in young fibroblasts and capillaries and often contains leukocytes, is termed *granulation tissue*. Only after all the debris is removed and the defect has been filled is the healing completed by the reepithelialization of the wound.

Healing by primary union ("first intention") may be described as follows:

Within the *first postoperative day* after the wound has been coapted by sutures, the line of incision promptly fills with blood clot. The surface of this clot dries, creating a crust or scab, and thereby seals the wound. The usual acute inflammatory reaction ensues in the margins of the wound, and a significant polymorphonuclear infiltrate is present.

During the *second day*, two separate activities begin concurrently: reepithelialization of the surface and fibrous bridging of the subepithelial cleft. Both depend heavily on the fibrin meshwork in the blood clot, since it provides a structural scaffold along which the epithelial cells, fibroblasts and capillary buds migrate. Small tongue-like processes of cells protrude toward the midline from the epithelial

margins. Within 48 hours these spurs connect to complete the epithelial covering of the wound. At first, the surface epithelium is quite thin and may consist of only a single layer of cells in the mid-portion of the incision. Soon thereafter, progressive proliferation gives rise to the many layered differentiated squamous epithelium characteristic of the normal epidermis. Damaged hair follicles, sweat glands and sebaceous glands may similarly regenerate. However, as was previously mentioned, adnexal structures which have been totally destroyed cannot be replaced. During the second day, the fibroblasts at the margin of the incision hypertrophy and develop increased basophilia of their cytoplasm.

By the *third postoperative day* the acute inflammatory response begins to subside, and the neutrophils are largely replaced by macrophages which debride the wound margins of destroyed cells as well as bits and pieces of fibrin. Concurrently, mitotic activity appears within fibroblasts and vascular sprouts grow (at the remarkable rate of 0.1 to 0.2 mm. per day) into the subepithelial cleft to begin the process of organization of the exudate.

By *day 5* the incisional space is usually filled with a highly vascularized, loose, fibroblastic connective tissue rich in ground substance. Scattered collagen fibrils may now be present.

By the *end of the first week*, then, the wound is covered with an epidermis of approximately normal thickness, and the subepithelial cleft is bridged by a vascularized connective tissue beginning to lay down collagen fibrils.

During the *second week* there is continued proliferation of fibroblasts and vessels and the progressive accumulation of collagen. By now the fibrin scaffold has entirely disappeared. The scar is still bright red owing to the increased vascularization and, as will be seen (p. 60), it has not yet attained significant tensile strength. Indeed, most of the tensile strength of a recent wound is attributable to the coapting surgical sutures and to the epithelial bridge. However, the inflammatory reaction has now almost completely abated, leaving only a few scattered macrophages and perhaps a sparse infiltrate of lymphocytes.

By the end of the second week the basic structure of the scar is already established and a long process, which will achieve blanching of the scar by compression of the vascular channels, accumulation of collagen and steady increase in the tensile strength of the wound, is under way. As will be discussed later, however, even well healed surgical scars may never regain the tensile strength, extensibility and elasticity of normal unwounded skin (Dunphy, 1967).

Healing by secondary union ("second intention healing") is a more prolonged process because of the need to remove all dead tissue and necrotic debris and to fill in the tissue defect with vital cells. Some parenchymal regeneration is possible at the margins, but within the wound itself all architectural framework is lost, and so most of the repair is accomplished by connective tissue scarring. The base and margins of the defect are first layered with granulation tissue. Fibroblastic proliferation and capillary budding begin while the acute and sometimes chronic inflammatory reaction is still active in the center of the wound. As the leukocytes remove the exudate and debris the wound "granulates" in from its margins. At the same time, in surface wounds the epithelial margins migrate and proliferate but only insofar as the underlying granulation tissue provides a base upon which they may grow. To some extent, the advancing epithelial cells grow downward over the edges and indeed a small mass of buried epithelium may be found in the newly formed granulation tissue.

A second remarkable phenomenon—*wound contraction*—aids in the repair of large defects, at least those on the surface of the body. It has been shown that a defect of about 40 cm.² in the skin of a rabbit becomes reduced over the course of six weeks to 5 to 10 per cent of its original size, largely by contraction. Remarkably, *all wounds halve their size at about the same rate.* Similar contraction may occur in deep wounds, but it has been less well studied. The mechanism of wound contraction is still somewhat uncertain but appears to involve contraction of fibroblasts within the granulation tissue (Majno and Leventhal, 1967). Indeed, myofilaments have been identified within these cells, justifying their designation as *myofibroblasts* (Gabbiani et al., 1972). By shortening, these multipotential mesenchymal cells are able to reduce significantly the size of the defect which must be filled eventually by granulation tissue and covered with epithelium.

While wound contraction greatly speeds and facilitates the repair of surface wounds, it has undesirable aspects. Contractures may result, which can block full extension of joints or lead to disfiguring deforming scars, particularly in the face and neck region. Intensive efforts are now being directed toward control of wound contracture when it may yield these undesirable consequences (Peacock, 1973).

In review, then, healing by second intention differs in important ways from healing by first intention. Invariably large tissue defects have more necrotic cells and exudate which must be cleared. Ingrowth of granulation tissue plays a far more prominent role in second intention healing. Moreover, this granulation tissue almost always has a more intense suffusion with neutrophils and macrophages because of the stronger inflammatory reaction elicited by the larger lesion. And, finally, wound contraction occurs only when there are large defects, since there is no significant loss of tissue in wounds which heal by first intention. As a consequence of these features, healing by second intention almost invariably results in the production of more scar and greater loss of specialized function. Thus, in large skin wounds there may be permanent loss of skin appendages (hair, sweat and sebaceous glands) in the scarred area. Obviously first intention healing proceeds to completion more rapidly than the more complicated healing by second intention.

Two aberrations may occur in wound healing, whether the process is by first or second intention. The accumulation of excessive amounts of collagen may give rise to a protruding, tumorous scar known as a *keloid*. Recent evidence indicates that collagen accumulation in wound healing reflects a balance between synthesis and lysis of this fibrous protein. As is discussed in greater detail on page 62, keloid formation is now attributed to an inadequate rate of lysis (Forrester, 1973). Keloid formation appears to be an individual predisposition and, for reasons unknown, this aberration is somewhat more common in blacks. The other deviation in wound healing is the formation of excessive amounts of granulation tissue which protrudes above the level of the surrounding skin and in fact blocks reepithelialization. This has been called *exuberant granulation* or, with more literary fervor, *"proud flesh."* Excessive granulations must be removed by cautery or surgical excision to permit restoration of the continuity of the epithelium.

Although the focus of much of the preceding discussion has been repair of skin wounds, the same basic characteristics of repair apply to the healing of defects in other organs and tissues of the body. Thus, repair of an abscess in the lung or an infarct in the kidney pursues the same course as that of an open wound on the surface of the body. The necrotic tissue and inflammatory debris must be removed. Similarly, the cell loss must be replaced, to the extent possible, by marginal regeneration of parenchymal cells, followed by ingrowth of vascularized connective tissue which, over the course of months, becomes progressively more collagenous. Thus, as was emphasized earlier, healing of most wounds represents a combination of parenchymal regeneration and connective tissue scarring, although in the individual instance one phenomenon may be predominant.

BONE REPAIR

Repair of a bone injury is essentially another instance of connective tissue healing. It differs from soft tissue repair insofar as formation of the specialized calcified tissue of bone involves the activity of osteoblasts and osteoclasts. These pivotal cells are derived from the periosteum and endosteum in the area of injury or, possibly, from the metaplastic transformation of primitive mesenchymal cells or fibroblasts in the adjacent connective tissues. Repair of a bone may be so perfect that it cannot be visualized at a later date by x-rays or even histologic examination.

Repair of a fracture may be taken as a model of the processes of bone healing. Bone, with its contained marrow, is a highly vascularized tissue. When fractured, there is considerable hemorrhage into the site. A clot fills the region between the two fractured ends, as well as any space created by tearing of adjacent tissues, such as the periosteum and endosteum. Cellular proliferation and neovascularization along the meshwork of the blood clot ensues just as has been described in the healing of a soft wound. By day 2 or 3, rapidly proliferating chondroblasts and osteoblasts looking very much like plump fibroblasts appear in the areas proximate to the injured periosteum and endosteum. Immobilization of the bone is critical because continued movement interferes with deposition of such rigid tissues as cartilage and calcified matrix that are so necessary for bony union. Toward the end of the first week, in the appropriately immobilized fracture, islands of cartilage appear in the highly vascularized connective tissue which has replaced the clot (Udupa and Prasad, 1963). The combination of fibroblastic tissue and islands of cartilage forms a fairly firm but still yielding fusiform sleeve that bridges the fracture site. This bridging tissue is known as a *soft tissue* or *provisional callus (procallus)*. By the end of the first week some calcium is deposited in the cartilaginous matrix, further hardening the provisional callus and splinting the fractured ends of the bone. About this time, the osteoblasts of periosteal and endosteal origin begin to secrete osseomucin, creating trabeculae of osteoid. Eventually the procallus becomes traversed by a maze of osteoid trabeculae laid down in a haphazard pattern. Progressive calcification of the osteoid bony callus ensues. In this manner, the provisional callus is replaced ultimately by *bony callus.* The fracture is now rigidly united, but there is excess bone within the marrow space and encircling the external aspect of the fracture site. This stage of repair might be reached in four to six weeks, depending upon a number of conditions, which will be mentioned later in this chapter. Total healing of the fracture might be extended for many weeks or months and involves the combined action of osteoblasts and osteoclasts. The excess bone within the marrow space, as well as around the fracture, is slowly remodeled

(i.e., resorbed by osteoclasts), while at the same time neo-osteogenesis and increased calcification within the normal bone contours further strengthen and reinforce the trabeculae. Ultimately, the marrow cavity is restored to its original dimensions, and the bone marrow regrows to its prefracture stage of development. Stress—or more precisely, direction of thrust of weight bearing—appears to guide the pattern of remodeling. If a fractured long bone is anatomically aligned, only the new bone directly sealing the fracture site persists. With malalignment or bowing, neo-osteogenesis will occur along the concave aspect to bring about appropriate thrust lines for weight bearing, while the convex aspect is resorbed. The periosteum is reformed by the combined action of the fibroblasts and osteoblasts, and only some connective tissue scarring in the adjacent muscles may be left as a sign of the former injury. Additional details of this remarkable reconstitution of original structure may be found in the excellent discussion by Ham and Harris (1956).

Many factors are important in this healing process in bone. Primary among them is adequate immobilization. It should be apparent that if the fractured ends are not firmly immobilized, *hard* tissue, such as the calcified osteoid trabeculae, cannot be formed. Instead, collagenized fibrous tissue may replace the soft tissue callus, which will block all possibility of later bony repair. In the same way, interposition of nearby soft tissues between the fractured ends will likewise block the formation of the new bone bridges between the two fractured ends.

If hemorrhage is excessive, a large provisional callus is formed, which requires more time to be replaced. At the same time, the excess hemorrhage leads to the formation of a larger bony callus that must eventually be remodeled and removed.

Infection of a fracture site is a serious complication. Bacteria introduced into the fresh blood clot literally run amok. The infection not only causes secondary tissue damage but also inhibits callus formation.

Proper reduction of the fracture greatly speeds repair. If the ends have not been fragmented, realignment reduces the distance between the fractured ends and permits rapid union. It is remarkable to observe at a much later date a fracture that could not be realigned—the repair may be slowed but, as long as other complications do not exist, it proceeds nonetheless. The bony union will in time be sufficiently strong to bear weight, and the remodeling may eventually create a straight shaft, although it may be shortened owing to the loss in length created by the initial bowing. Obviously, miracles do not happen and if the malalignment is marked, deformity or non-union may result. An additional consideration in bone repair is the metabolic environment. Involved here are an adequate blood supply, nutrition (particularly vitamin C and calcium) and normal levels of hormones (particularly estrogens), which appear to influence osteoblastic activity. Of these factors, the blood supply is most critical. A fracture that destroys the arterial supply, or multiple fractures that create devascularized bone fragments, greatly retard and sometimes block bone healing for months or years. Despite all these limiting qualifications, the repair of bone injury is one of the most remarkable demonstrations of the reparative capacity of the body.

MECHANISMS INVOLVED IN REPAIR

As mentioned earlier, several features of the reparative process deserve closer study: (1) factors that govern epithelialization of a wound, (2) the stimuli to proliferation and (3) events involved in scarring and development of wound strength.

EPITHELIALIZATION

Epithelialization of an injury on any surface of the body begins within hours. It should be reemphasized that such epithelial regrowth requires a foundation of vital cells upon which the epithelial margins may advance. Three separate features of epithelial activity have been identified: migration, proliferation and differentiation. This division is somewhat artificial because the three activities overlap to a considerable extent (Johnson, 1964).

Epithelial *migration* can be identified in wounds of the skin within 12 hours of injury. Small pseudopod-like processes composed of cells from the basal layer of the epidermis protrude toward the center of the wound. The forces actuating such migration are poorly understood. The phenomenon is best exemplified in the mucosal lining of the small intestine where the entire epithelial surface is totally replaced every 3 to 4 days (Leblond and Stevens, 1948). In such renewal, the cells deep within the crypts of Lieberkühn are the focus of active proliferation. The new cells migrate along the sides of the villus and are extruded at the tip. There is virtually no mitotic activity of cells once they have advanced halfway up the individual villus, and from here on the process is entirely one of migration. It might be argued that such movement results from the pressure of newly formed cells deep in the crypts pushing the nondividing cells ahead of them. There is, however, evidence from the study of corneal healing

and the repair of wounds in young embryos that migration may occur in the absence of proliferation (Weiss and Matoltsy, 1959). How can cells seemingly rooted to a basement membrane migrate? While considerable attention has been focused on possible changes in cement substance or in desmosomes, no alterations that would facilitate such mobility have been detected. Alternatively, it is postulated that cells are normally migratory, and injury merely releases pressure constraints to permit cells to break their basal attachments. To date, we do not know whether the primary change is in the moorings of the cell or in the constraints upon its normal migratory tendencies (Abercrombie and Ambrose, 1962).

Cellular proliferation becomes evident in the epithelial margins within 24 hours. The mechanisms that initiate such mitotic activity will be discussed later in our consideration of growth stimuli. During migration and proliferation, the cells are quite undifferentiated. Epidermal cells, for example, show no evidence of keratinization and in the intestinal tract there is little evidence of such specializations as the formation of secretory granules or enzymes. Once the wound is covered, however, *differentiation* begins and along with the proliferation of the epidermal cells the surface layers assume their characteristic flattening and keratinization, and the cells in the intestinal mucosa assume their usual tall columnar appearance, punctuated by vacuoles of mucous secretion. For further details of this interesting phenomenon of epithelialization and for characterization of the cellular changes at the level of the electron microscope, reference should be made to the excellent review by Johnson (1966).

STIMULI TO CELL PROLIFERATION

An enormous body of data has accumulated on the stimuli to cell proliferation in wounds. The widely varying proposals, all speculative, can be divided into those supporting the elaboration of some factor or substance which stimulates cells to grow and those supporting the concept that loss of inhibitory influences underlies cellular proliferation. *The weight of evidence at the present time favors release of growth restraints in the immediate environment of the wound.* This concept is based on the proposition that all cells are genetically programmed for mitotic division. This ability is permanently repressed in some cells, as in those already described as permanent cells; it is continuously operative in labile cells, and can be derepressed (activated) in stable cells. Such a concept is basic to the genetic model proposed by Jacob and Monod (1963).

Loss of inhibitory influences as the stimulus to cell proliferation in wounds is supported by a considerable body of evidence. Perhaps the most widely accepted hypothesis in this regard is that of *contact inhibition* (Abercrombie, 1966, 1967). According to this view, cells are inhibited from proliferation by the interchange of signals or substances at contact points. When contact is lost, as in the margins of a wound, replication begins. Contact inhibition is best documented in vitro. If two small explants of fibroblasts are introduced into a culture flask separated by some distance, radial strands of cells grow out in all directions. When strands of cells from these explants come into contact, cell division stops in those cells but continues in cells which have not established contact with their neighbors. The nature of the signal which passes between the cells in contact is still uncertain, but the explanations of Loewenstein (1969) offer a possible mechanism. He suggests that electrochemical charges normally flow between stable cells, passing through specialized regions of the cell membrane known as *nexuses*. This electrical flux in some way inhibits cell replication. The cells in the margin of a wound no longer receive signals from their neighbors and so begin to replicate. Could the wound injury alter the nexus junctions and impair the passage of cell to cell signals?

Another explanation for loss of inhibitory influences postulates reduced levels in the wound margin of diffusable substances which normally restrain cell proliferation. Bullough (1966) calls the repressor substances *chalones* (Greek for "to reef the sails") and proposes that with tissue injury there is a loss of chalones by diffusion from epidermal cells into the wound. The reduced concentration of chalones in the local site turns off specialized cell function and diverts cellular activity to mitotic division. Interestingly, in tissue culture chalones from epidermal cells suppress the mitotic division of only epidermal cells and not that of other cell types, such as fibroblasts or liver cells (Iversen, 1968). Of even more interest is the fact that chalones derived from the epidermal cells of man, for example, appear to act on the epidermal cells of all species. It should be noted that the proliferative reaction in the epidermis is sharply localized to the area of the wound, extends only about 1 mm. from the wound margin and is without effect on the fibroblasts and blood vessels within the dermis.

Weiss (1955) offers another model. He views restraint on cellular growth as dependent on a balance between "*templates*" which initiate cell replication and "*antitemplates*," both found within cells. In this hypothesis, the antitemplates are more freely diffusable and with

wounding diffuse out of cells, permitting the templates to initiate cell replication by default. As cells regrow into the wound, the increased cellular population produces sufficient antitemplates to counteract the templates.

Another view of the stimuli to cell proliferation in wounds proposes the elaboration of *stimulatory factors*. Ancient writings contain references to various plant products, ointments and potions which favor wound healing. More contemporary studies allude to wound hormones (*trephones*), growth promoting factors and possible increased levels of pituitary growth hormone as stimuli to cell proliferation in the wound. Most of the evidence derives from studies of the regeneration of the liver following hepatectomy. In one experimental system, a hepatectomized rat is linked in parabiotic union to a normal rat. Increased mitotic activity in the liver of the normal parabiont is offered as evidence of a circulating growth stimulator (Hurowitz and Studer, 1960). However, in a virtually identical experimental model, the existence of a humoral stimulatory factor was denied (Heimann et al., 1963). Without belaboring this issue further, it can be summarized by stating that to date there is no conclusive proof of the existence of stimulators of cell replication in wounds.

Most of the preceding observations relate to parenchymal cells. The stimuli to replication of fibroblasts and endothelial cells are, if possible, even less well understood. One suggestion offers lowering of oxygen tensions within the center of wounds as the stimulus to the growth of these mesenchymal cells (Remensnyder and Majno, 1968). Interesting as all these observations may be, they are still hypotheses. The entire problem of what turns cellular replication on and off is a fertile and important field requiring further study. Conceivably here lies also the key that will unlock the mystery of cancer.

COLLAGENIZATION AND WOUND STRENGTH

Scarring is an inevitable consequence of all repair save for the ideal situation in which an entirely parenchymal injury permits perfect regeneration and reconstitution of the original architecture. Fibroblasts are the workhorses of scar formation, aided by the newly formed blood vessels, which bear the needed supplies of oxygen and nutrients (Van Winkle, 1967). The kinetics of the ingrowth of fibroblasts and newly formed blood vessels into an area of injury have been intensively studied by Cliff (1965) and Schoefl (1963). By time lapse cinemicroscopy, they have shown that reparative tissue advances into a model injury at the remarkable rate of 0.1 to 0.2 mm. per day. They also noted that endothelial cell proliferation in the newly formed blood vessels occurs just behind an advancing tip of nonproliferating cells. The endothelial cells then migrate along the luminal surface of the blood vessels to achieve their position in the advancing end of the new sprout. It has been observed that frequently two newly formed capillary buds will fuse to produce an arcade from which new buds will arise. The lymphatic vessels demonstrate this same phenomenon. Miraculously, blood vessels only join other blood vessels, while lymphatics show the same snobbishness, and the twain never fuse!

Collagen is the essential product of the fibroblast which ultimately provides the tensile strength necessary in wound healing. As is well known, collagen fibers are formed by the precise alignment and precipitation of monomer collagen molecules. The monomer molecule (approximately 300 nm. in length and 1.5 nm. in diameter) is made up of three polypeptide (alpha) chains, each containing slightly more than 1000 amino acids. The alpha chains run colinearly throughout the length of the molecule and are entwined together in the form of a left-handed helix. The alpha chains are synthesized within the fibroblasts, probably on the ribosomes attached to the endoplasmic reticulum, but possibly on free polyribosomes. Hydroxylation of the proline (representing approximately 10 per cent of the amino acid residues in a collagen alpha chain) and lysine occurs after the formation of the polypeptide chain. The newly synthesized polypeptides pass through the endoplasmic reticulum, are modified en route, and are extruded from the cell as procollagen. The precise fashion by which the procollagen monomers are secreted from the fibroblast remains uncertain, but many details on this process are provided in the excellent review by Miller and Matukas (1974). It is believed that hydroxylation is a necessary step for the transport of the monomers across the cell membrane (Kivirikko and Prockop, 1972). Once outside the cell, the soluble monomers are converted to the relatively insoluble mature collagen by formation of both intramolecular and intermolecular cross links involving aldehyde groups, aldol condensations and Schiff bases (Forrester, 1973). The cross linking occurs within the ground substance secreted by the fibroblasts. Indeed, it has been shown that mature insoluble collagen can be formed in vitro from soluble procollagen in the absence of cells (Gross, 1965). Thus, the role of the fibroblast is the elaboration of procollagen (soluble collagen) and appropriate ground substance. Clearly, the seemingly banal fibroblast is a most educated cell.

There is striking coordination between the secretion of the collagen monomers and the elaboration of components of the ground substance to produce the many forms of connective tissue found in the body. Consider for a moment the differences among cartilage, bone, tendon and dermal connective tissue. The extracellular ground substance is rich in mucopolysaccharides, such as chondroitin and hyaluronic acid and their derivatives, as well as glycosoaminoglycans. The contribution of this ground substance to collagenization is best brought out in the healing of second wounds. Not uncommonly in clinical practice, an abdominal wound ruptures or reopens within the first two postoperative weeks. Such wound dehiscence, as it is known, implies failure of the primary wound to undergo normal healing. Most often it is a consequence of infection in the primary wound, but excessive hemorrhage, inadequate alignment and coaptation of tissue layers and a host of other factors may be involved, as will be discussed later. Of principal interest here is the fact that the healing of such second wounds occurs much faster than primary wound healing if the underlying obstacles to healing are removed and the wound is resutured. It has been reported that in 5 to 7 days a resutured wound has a tensile strength two times that which primary wounds would achieve in a similar time span (Peacock, 1962). This remarkably accelerated healing is attributed to higher concentrations of procollagen and mucopolysaccharides already present at the site.

The biosynthesis of collagen is dependent on an adequate supply of nutrients to the fibroblast. The requisite amino acids and vitamin C (ascorbic acid) are critical (Gould, 1966). In the vitamin C deficient individual there is apparent disorganization of the ribosomes and polyribosomes within fibroblasts; this morphologic change is accompanied by faulty incorporation of hydroxyproline and hydroxylysine in the collagen chains. The best evidence to date suggests that ascorbic acid is needed to catalyze the action of the hydroxylases involved in the hydroxylation of proline and lysine within the alpha chains. When hydroxylation fails to occur, there is inadequate secretion of the monomers and soluble collagen cannot be converted into mature fibrillar collagen. Thus, wounds in the scorbutic patient heal poorly and have little tensile strength. Hemorrhages are likely to occur in such wounds because avitaminosis C also leads to inadequate formation of cement substance between endothelial cells, which results in excessive friability of small blood vessels. Lack of vitamin C is therefore a serious handicap to repair.

The strength of a healed wound is largely a func-

tion of its collagen content. While most studies of wound healing have focused on the breaking strength of the wound, i.e., its tensile strength, Forrester (1973) rightly points out that extensibility (force required to produce extension) and other parameters are equally important. Here, however, we shall confine our attention to tensile strength. Surprisingly, in an age of space exploration, it has proven impossible to obtain any consensus on the rate of increase of tensile strength in skin wounds and the level of strength ultimately acquired by well healed wounds. As a reasonable synthesis of the many conflicting and varying reports, it can be said that *healed skin wounds ultimately achieve 70 to 90 per cent of the strength of unwounded skin, never regaining full strength* (Douglas, 1963, 1969; Dingman, 1973; Forrester, 1973). It must be admitted, however, that other experts such as Adamsons and his co-workers (1964) contend that healed wounds may achieve greater strength than normal unwounded skin. These reported differences, of great clinical importance, can neither be resolved nor rationalized.

The acquisition of tensile strength follows a sigmoid curve. The first phase has been described as the catabolic period when there may actually be destruction of collagen. The second (anabolic, proliferative or collagen) phase generally begins on day 5. Thereafter there is a progressive increase in tensile strength up to day 100, followed by a virtual plateau which is maintained for years and perhaps for the life of the patient. When the plateau phase is more closely investigated we find that the total collagen content of a wound stabilizes while collagen is still being actively synthesized. Clearly, collagen is being removed from the wound at the same time that it is being added (Riley and Peacock, 1966, 1967). This dynamic state is achieved by collagenase, which breaks down mature collagen into its soluble procolla-

gen form. Thus, lysis of collagen is an important controlling factor. As mentioned earlier, keloid production is probably the consequence of inadequate lysis. Another interesting observation emerges from the study of the collagen content of wounds. On biochemical grounds, the collagen content of wounds returns to normal levels far more rapidly than recovery of wound strength. Indeed, Forrester (1973) points out that the collagen content of the wound reaches normal levels by 60 to 70 days, at a time when the wound has recovered only 25 to 35 per cent of its strength. Thus, strength in wounds is not simply a function of the amount of collagen but also relates to the extent of collagen cross linking and possibly to some sort of interaction between collagen fibers and connective tissue ground substance.

Since wounds require 100 days to regain 70 to 90 per cent of the tensile strength of unwounded skin, how it is possible to discharge patients from the hospital within the first postoperative week? The answer lies in the art and skill of the surgeon and his use of sutures. Carefully sutured wounds have approximately 70 per cent of the strength of unwounded skin immediately following surgery (Lichtenstein et al., 1970). If sutures are removed at the end of the first week, wound strength is only at approximately the 5 to 10 per cent level. But sutures are not unalloyed blessings. As foreign bodies, they themselves constitute an inflammatory stimulus and thus to some extent impede repair. Indeed, there is good evidence that tape-closed wounds heal more rapidly and more effectively than sutured wounds. For this reason some suture material now used is slowly soluble, presumably timed to degrade along with the progressive increase in the collagenous strength of the wound. It should be amply evident now that the study of wound repair has wide-ranging ramifications, particularly for the postoperative patient.

OVERVIEW OF THE INFLAMMATORY—REPARATIVE RESPONSE

At this point, a backward look may help to interrelate the multitude of changes occurring simultaneously or sequentially in the inflammatory-reparative response. Figure 2–12 offers an overview of the possible pathways. This schema reemphasizes certain important concepts. Not all injuries result in permanent

damage; some are resolved with almost perfect repair. More often, the injury and inflammatory response result in residual scarring. While it is functionally imperfect, the scarring provides a permanent patch that permits the residual parenchyma more or less to continue functioning. Sometimes, however, the scar it-

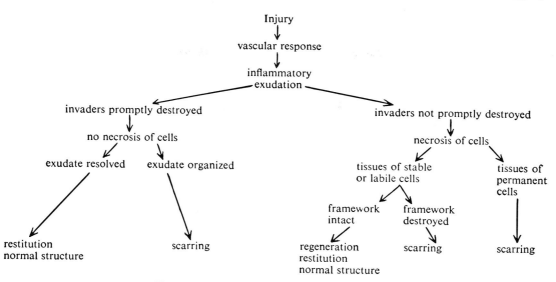

Figure 2–12. Pathways of reparative response.

self is so large or so situated that it may cause permanent dysfunction, as for example in a healed myocardial infarct. In this case, the fibrous tissue not only represents a loss of preexisting contractile muscle, but also constitutes a permanent burden to the overworked residual muscle.

FACTORS MODIFYING THE QUALITY AND ADEQUACY OF THE INFLAMMATORY—REPARATIVE RESPONSE

The quality and adequacy of the inflammatory reaction and reparative response are determined by factors relating to both the injurious agent and to the host. The outcome of an injury is determined by the balance achieved between the defensive, healing capability of the host and the destructive influence of the injurious agent. Much has already been said about the impact of the intensity, duration and nature of the injury. Here we are primarily concerned with the host factors, which are equally important in this equation. Only the more important ones will be discussed, under the headings of systemic and local influences.

SYSTEMIC INFLUENCES

The role of *age* in modifying the quality and adequacy of the inflammatory-reparative re-

sponse is surprisingly controversial. The "prevailing wisdom" holds that the elderly heal more slowly and less adequately than the young (Dingman, 1973). This has been attributed to a decrease in the rate of fibroplasia, a decrease in the rate of parenchymal cell proliferation and an increased susceptibility to infection of "clean wounds." Yet there is little valid documentation of this view. A recent study points out that there was no difference between *tensile strength* values of the healing wounds of two age groups of rats, one young (8 months old) and the other old (20 months of age). However, the thickness of the scar was greater in the younger animals (Sussman, 1973). In another study no significant differences were found in the adequacy of repair among various age groups of rats (Abt and von Schuching, 1963). Moreover, it is extremely difficult in man to segregate the influence of age from the effects of the virtually omnipresent atherosclerosis in the aged, which reduces the blood supply to sites of injury and thereby impairs wound healing.

The *nutrition* of the patient is of unchallenged importance. Both experimental and clinical observations indicate that severe protein depletion impairs wound healing (Levenson et al., 1950). Although the protein deficient patient can derive most of the tissue building blocks for wound repair by mobilization of body tissues, methionine and cystine may be in inadequate supply for the *sulfation* of the mucopolysaccharides of the ground substance. Accordingly, there is inadequate synthesis of collagen. Indeed, it has been held that supplementation of even normal diets with methionine and cystine has a beneficial effect on the healing process (Rosenberg and Caldwell, 1965). The important role played by vitamin C in the normal formation of collagen has already been cited. Deficiencies of ascorbic acid block hydroxylation of proline and lysine and thus result in defective collagen production (Ross and Benditt, 1962). Administration of vitamin C to the deficient animal is followed within 24 hours by a striking return to normal collagen production. Zinc may be another substance required for adequate wound healing (Pories et al., 1967). It has been said that in the United States levels of this metal in the normal diet are marginal. In the wound, zinc is largely concentrated in the margins, where there is most active parenchymal regeneration and fibroplasia. Possibly, this element acts as an enzymic cofactor.

Derangements in the blood may have a profound effect on the inflammatory-reparative response. No one would deny that a deficiency of circulating granulocytes (*granulocytopenia*), whatever its cause, predisposes to bacterial infections and renders the leukocytic exudation inadequate to control bacterial invasion. The loss of neutrophils also impairs lysosomal proteolysis of dead cells and exudate, hampering repair. Similarly, there is no controversy over the role of *bleeding abnormalities (hemorrhagic diatheses)* in expanding the inflammatory reaction and thus slowing repair. The breakdown products of excessive hemorrhage in an area of injury represent further stimuli to the inflammatory response, and the clotted blood provides a rich substrate for the growth of itinerant bacteria. Moreover, the clot with its hemoglobin must be removed before repair can be completed. On the other hand, there is disagreement over the role of *anemia* in the impairment of wound healing. It has been reported that in experimental animals anemia does not significantly hamper the inflammatory response nor slow repair (Levenson et al., 1950, 1965). Nonetheless, a definite beneficial effect in lowering the incidence

of wound complications was reportedly achieved by deferring operation upon infants until their anemia had been corrected (Musgrave and Brenner, 1960). Although it is entirely possible that anemia may hamper the inflammatory-reparative response, there is no unequivocal evidence in support of this notion. It must be recognized that the anemic patient often has nutritional deficiencies or concomitant disease, which makes it extremely difficult to segregate the effect of the individual variables.

Immunity requires only brief mention here since it is obviously an important influence in microbiologic disease and will be discussed fully in Chapter 6. When immunity is not present from the outset of an infection, the development of humoral and cell-mediated responses to the invading agent may be crucial in eventually bringing the infection under control.

Diabetes mellitus is a particularly important predisposing factor in microbiologic infections. Diabetics tend to develop significant clinical infections more frequently than controls. They are particularly likely to develop tuberculosis, skin infections, infections of the urinary tract and mycotic infections. It is not that they are more vulnerable to bacterial invasion but rather that they are less able to control the invasion once established. The nature of this susceptibility to infection is still incompletely understood. Diabetics are prone to develop generalized arterial disease and so may suffer from inadequate blood supply to the area of injury. Sometimes they are dehydrated and have serious electrolyte disturbances. Because the skin of diabetic patients contains high levels of glucose, survival of implanted bacteria is favored. A low level of lactic acid in the skin removes one of the major inhibitory influences to bacterial growth. The neutrophils of diabetic patients have decreased phagocytic capacity. All of these abnormalities hamper the inflammatory response and render the diabetic patient vulnerable to serious infections.

Hormones, particularly the adrenal steroids, have a depressant effect on the inflammatory and reparative reactions. Cortisol is most active in this regard, but other glucocorticoids behave similarly. The precise site of action of the steroids is still uncertain. In experimental animals, high levels of cortisol prevent the increased vascular permeability of the acute inflammatory response (Ebert and Barclay, 1952). Corticosteroids also appear to interfere with the pavementing of leukocytes, thereby diminishing emigration. In addition, the membrane stabilizing action of steroids may hamper release of vital lysosomal enzymes (Weissman and Thomas, 1963). Steroids also significantly hamper repair. In the experimental animal pretreated with cortisol, fibroplasia is inhibited, new collagen formation is retarded, and neovascularization is slowed (Bhussry and Rao, 1968). Again, the mechanisms are not established. There is a hint that the steroids may impair formation of the mucopolysaccharide ground substance so important in the formation of mature collagen (Dunphy and Udupa, 1955). It has also been suggested that steroids block the synthesis of nucleic acids and impair the uptake of amino acids by fibroblasts, both of these effects resulting from hormonal action on the plasma membrane of the fibroblast. Although there is thus considerable evidence that the glucocorticoids have profound inhibitory effects on all phases of the inflammatory-reparative response in the experimental animal, it should be cautioned that these results have been achieved by pretreatment of the animals with high levels of steroids. It is uncertain that the usual therapeutic doses employed in clinical medicine have a significant effect in man. However, because it is impossible to know the precise threshold level or duration of treatment which might have an effect on the inflammatory-reparative response in the individual, it is generally considered unwise to administer glucocorticoids to patients with infections or wounds unless other disorders are present which demand their use.

LOCAL INFLUENCES

Adequacy of local blood supply may well be the single most important influence in determining the quality and adequacy of the inflammatory-reparative response. Arterial disease which reduces blood flow and venous disorders which retard drainage seriously hamper the response to injury. For this reason, even a trivial injury to the toe in an aged individual with advanced atherosclerosis of the arteries in the lower leg may culminate weeks or months later in an amputation of the leg. Varicose veins of the leg result in hampered venous efflux, cause chronic edema of the lower leg and restrict adequate arterial inflow. Secondarily infected ulcerations (well recognized by the designation "varicose ulcers") are common following injuries to the legs of these patients.

Infection of "clean wounds," whatever their cause, is a serious hindrance to repair. The more intense inflammatory reaction and copious exudation tend to separate tissue edges, build up pressure within the inflammatory site and contribute to destruction of both native and immigrant white cells, thus enlarging the initial tissue injury. Healing by first intention may perforce be transformed into healing by second intention, with its more protracted course.

Foreign bodies are fairly obvious stimuli to inflammation and impediments to healing. Indeed, they must be removed by enzymic action (if they are biodegradable), by sequestration within multinucleate giant cells or by extrusion from the wound, either spontaneously or with the aid of surgery. Repair cannot be completed until one of these resolutions has been achieved. It must be remembered that sutures represent foreign bodies. Meticulous coaptation of wound margins permits primary union and not only reduces the amount of inflammation but also greatly facilitates and speeds repair. On the other hand, as we have seen, sutures constitute stimuli to inflammation and, when on the skin surface, invite bacterial contamination of the suture tracts. The use of just enough and not too many sutures is not only a surgical science but also an art.

Immobilization of wounds is of primary importance in fractures. It may also be beneficial in large soft tissue injuries in which movement may induce secondary hemorrhages and dislocation of tissue approximation.

Location of the injury may significantly alter the end result. It is apparent that perfect reconstruction of tissues is possible only when the site of injury involves stable and labile cells. All destruction of permanent cells must result in irrevocable loss of specialized function. The functional loss may be unimportant when there is a large reserve, although to some extent the reserve is thereby diminished. Thus the location of an injury impinges on the adequacy and quality of the end result. The location of the response also has other implications. Inflammations may arise within natural body cavities or tissue spaces, such as the peritoneal, pleural and pericardial spaces, or in loose connective tissue. Although inflammatory exudate may readily fill the spaces, if resolution follows, virtually normal structure and function are restored. Similarly, resolution of inflammatory exudate within the pulmonary alveoli may leave no permanent damage if the pulmonary parenchyma has not been destroyed. At some later date, the lungs might appear entirely normal. By contrast, bacterial invasion of the liver or kidney with the production of an abscess might be repaired by marginal parenchymal regeneration but almost inevitably involves some scarring.

In closing, it is hardly necessary to point out that an understanding of the basic mechanisms and principles of inflammation and repair is fundamental to the proper treatment of the innumerable injuries encountered in everyday medicine. Stated in another way, clinical treatment of tissue injury consists, in essence, of the attempt to modify favorably by judicious interventions the physiologic and pathologic processes of the inflammatory and reparative response. A century ago "laudable pus" was a common expression, which implied recognition of the important role of the inflammatory reaction in the body's defense. Often the pus is indeed laudable.

REFERENCES

Abercrombie, M.: Contact inhibition and its biological implications. Nat. Cancer Inst. Monog., *26*:249, 1966.

Abercrombie, M.: Localized formation of new tissue in an adult mammal. Symp. Soc. Exp. Biol., *11*:235, 1967.

Abercrombie, M., and Ambrose, E. J.: The surface properties of cancer cells. A review. Cancer Res., *22*:252, 1962.

Abt, A. F., and von Schuching, S.: Aging as a factor in wound healing. Arch. Surg., *86*:627, 1963.

Adamsons, R. J., et al.: The relationship of collagen content in wound strength in normal and scorbutic animals. Surg. Gynec. Obstet., *119*:323, 1964.

Allison, F., Jr., et al.: Studies of the pathogenesis of acute inflammation. I. The inflammatory reaction to thermal injury as observed in the rabbit ear chamber. J. Exp. Med., *102*:655, 1955.

Atkins, E.: Pathogenesis of fever. Physiol. Rev., *40*:580, 1960.

Atkins, E., et al.: Release of an endogenous pyrogen *in vitro* from rabbit mononuclear cells. J. Exp. Med., *126*:357, 1967.

Bhussry, B. E., and Rao, S.: Histochemical response to experimental skin injury in rats. Biochem. Pharm. (Suppl.). Oxford, England, Pergammon Press, 1968, p. 51.

Brewer, D. B.: Electron microscopy of phagocytosis of staphylococci. J. Path. Bact., *86*:299, 1963.

Bucher, N. L. R.: Experimental aspects of hepatic regeneration. New Eng. J. Med., *277*:686, 738, 1967.

Bullough, W. S.: Cell replacement after tissue damage. *In* Illingworth, C. (ed.): Wound Healing. Boston, Little, Brown & Co., 1966, p. 43.

Clark, R. A., et al.: Defective neutrophil chemotaxis and cellular immunity in a child with recurrent infections. Ann. Int. Med., *78*:515, 1973.

Cliff, W. J.: Kinetics of wound healing in rabbit ear chambers, a time lapse cinemicroscopic study. Quart. J. Exp. Physiol., *50*:79, 1965.

Cotran, R. S., and Majno, G.: A light and electron microscopic analysis of vascular injury. Ann. N.Y. Acad. Sci., *116*:750, 1964.

Dingman, R. O.: Factors of clinical significance affecting wound healing. Laryngoscope, *83*:1540, 1973.

Douglas, D. M.: Wound Healing and Management. Baltimore, Williams & Wilkins Co., 1963.

Douglas, D. M.: Wound healing. Proc. Roy. Soc. Med., *62*:513, 1969.

Douglas, S. D.: Analytic review: disorders of phagocyte function. Blood, *35*:851, 1970.

Dunphy, J. E.: The healing of wounds. Canad. J. Surg., *10*:281, 1967.

Dunphy, J. E., and Udupa, K. N.: Chemical and histochemical sequences in normal healing of wounds. New Eng. J. Med., *253*:857, 1955.

Ebert, R. H., and Barclay, W. R.: Changes in connective tissue reaction induced by cortisone. Ann. Int. Med., *37*:506, 1952.

Florey, H. W.: General Pathology, 3rd edition. Philadelphia, W. B. Saunders Co., 1962.

Forrester, J. C.: Mechanical, biochemical and architectural features of surgical repair. Adv. Biol. Med. Phys., *14*:1, 1973.

Gabbiani, G., et al.: Granulation tissue as a contractile organ: a study of structure and function. J. Exp. Med., *135*:719, 1972.

Gamow, R. I., et al.: Analysis of chemotaxis in white blood cells. Biophys. J., *11*:860, 1971.

Gould, B. S.: Collagen biosynthesis. *In* National Academy of Sciences: Wound Healing, Proceedings of a Workshop. Washington, D.C., National Research Council, 1966, p. 99.

Gross, J.: The behavior of collagen units as a model in morphogenesis. J. Biophys. Biochem. Cytol., Suppl. *2*:261, 1965.

Ham, A. W., and Harris, W. R.: Repair and transplantation of bone. *In* Bourne, G. H. (ed.): The Biochemistry and Physiology of Bone. New York, Academic Press, 1956, p. 475.

Hay, E. D.: Skeletal muscle regeneration. New Eng. J. Med., *284*:1033, 1971.

Heimann, R., et al.: Liver cell proliferation due to biliary obstruction. Studies in parabiotic rats. Exp. Molec. Path., *2*:442, 1963.

Hersh, E. M., and Bodey, G. P.: Leukocytic mechanisms in inflammations. Ann. Rev. Med., *21*:105, 1970.

Hirsch, J. G., and Cohn, Z. A.: Degranulation of polymorphonuclear leukocytes following phagocytosis of microorganisms. J. Exp. Med., *112*:1005, 1960.

Houck, J., and Chang, C.: The chemotactic properties of the products of collagenolysis. Proc. Soc. Exp. Biol. Med., *138*:69, 1971.

Hurowitz, R. B., and Studer, A.: Effect of partial hepatectomy on mitosis rate in CCl4-induced liver damage of parabiotic rats. Arch. Path., *69*:511, 1960.

Iversen, O. H.: Effect of epidermal chalone on human epidermal mitotic activity in vitro. Nature (London), *219*:75, 1968.

Jacob, F., and Monod, J.: Elements of regulatory circuits in bacteria. *In* Harris, R. J. C. (ed.): Biological Organization at the Cellular and Super-Cellular Level. London, Academic Press, 1963, pp. 1–24.

Johnson, F. R.: The reaction of epithelium to injury. *In* Annual Reviews, Brit. Postgrad. Med. Fed.: The Scientific Basis of Medicine. New York, Oxford University Press, 1964, p. 279.

Johnson, F. R.: Wound epithelialization. *In* National Academy of Sciences: Wound Healing, Proceedings of a Workshop. National Research Council, Washington, D.C., 1966, p. 48.

Kaley, G., and Weiner, R.: Prostaglandin E: A potential mediator. Ann. N.Y. Acad. Sci., *180*:338, 1971.

Karnovsky, M. J.: The ultrastructural basis of capillary permeability studied with peroxidase as a tracer. J. Cell. Biol., *35*:213, 1967.

Kay, A. B., et al.: Generation of chemotactic activity for leukocytes by the action of thrombin on human fibrinogen. Nature (London), *243*:56, 1973.

Keller, H. U.: Chemotaxis and its significance for leukocyte accumulation. Agents and Actions, *2*:161, 1972.

Kivirikko, K. I., and Prockop, D. J.: Partial purification and characterization of protocollagen, lysine hydroxylase from chick embryos. Biochim. Biophys. Acta, *258*:366, 1972.

Leak, L. V., and Burke, J. F.: Ultrastructural studies on the lymphatic anchoring filaments. J. Cell. Biol., *36*:129, 1968.

Leblond, C. P., and Stevens, C. E.: Constant renewal of intestinal epithelium in albino rats. Anat. Rec., *100*:357, 1948.

Levenson, S. M., et al.: The healing of soft tissue wounds: the effects of nutrition, anemia and age. Surgery, *28*:905, 1950.

Levenson, S. M., et al.: The healing of rat skin wounds. Ann. Surg., *161*:293, 1965.

Lewis, T.: The Blood Vessels of the Human Skin and Their Responses. London, Shaw, 1927.

Lichtenstein, I. L., et al.: The dynamics of wound healing. Surg. Gynec. Obstet., *130*:685, 1970.

Loewenstein, W. R.: Transfer of information through cell junctions and growth control. Canad. Cancer Conf., *8*:162, 1969.

Luft, J. H.: Fine structure of the diaphragm across capillary "pores" in mouse intestine. Anat. Rec., *148*:307, 1964.

Luft, J. H.: Structure of capillary and endocapillary layer as revealed by ruthenium red. Fed. Proc., *25*:1773, 1966.

Mackaness, G. B.: Lymphocyte-macrophage contraction. *In* Lepow, I. H., and Ward, P. A. (eds.): Inflammation: Mechanisms and Control. New York, Academic Press, 1972, p. 163.

Majno, G., and Leventhal, M.: Pathogenesis of histamine type vascular leakage. Lancet, *2*:99, 1967.

Majno, G., and Palade, G. E.: Studies on inflammation. I. The effect of histamine and serotonin on vascular permeability: an electron microscopic study. J. Biophys. Biochem. Cytol., *11*:571, 1961.

Marchesi, V. T.: The site of leucocyte emigration during inflammation. Quart. J. Exp. Physiol., *46*:115, 1961.

McMinn, R. M. H.: The cellular morphology of tissue repair. Int. Rev. Cytol., *22*:63, 1967.

Menkin, V.: The Dynamics of Inflammation. Experimental Biology Monographs. New York, Macmillan Co., 1940, pp. 64, 180.

Miller, E. J., and Matukas, V. J.: Biosynthesis of collagen, the biochemist's view. Fed. Proc., *33*:1197, 1974.

Miller, M. E., et al.: Lazy leukocyte syndrome. A new disorder of neutrophil function. Lancet, *1*:665, 1971.

Miller, R. L., and Melmon, K. L.: The related roles of histamine, serotonin and bradykinin in the pathogenesis of inflammation. Ser. Haematol., *3*:5, 1970.

Moncada, F., et al.: Prostaglandins, aspirin-like drugs and the oedema of inflammation. Nature (London), *246*:217, 1973.

Movat, H. C.: Chemical mediators of the vascular phenomenon of the acute inflammatory reaction and of immediate hypersensitivity. Med. Clin. N. Amer., *56*:541, 1972.

Musgrave, R. H., and Brenner, J. C.: Complications of cleft palate surgery. J. Plast. Reconst. Surg., *26*:180, 1960.

Page, I. H.: Serotonin (5-hydroxytryptamine); the last 4 years. Phys. Rev., *38*:277, 1958.

Peacock, E. E., Jr.: Some aspects of fibrogenesis during the healing of primary and secondary wounds. Surg. Gynec. Obstet., *115*:408, 1962.

Peacock, E. E., Jr.: Biologic frontiers in the control of healing. Am. J. Surg., *126*:708, 1973.

Pories, W. J., et al.: Acceleration of wound healing in man with zinc sulphate given by mouth. Lancet, *1*:121, 1967.

Ranadive, N. S., and Cochrane, C. G.: Isolation and characterization of permeability factors from rabbit neutrophils. J. Exp. Med., *128*:605, 1968.

Remensnyder, J. P., and Majno, G.: Oxygen gradients in healing wounds. Amer. J. Path., *52*:301, 1968.

Reznick, M.: Origins of myoblasts during skeletal muscle regeneration. Lab. Invest., *20*:353, 1969.

Riley, W. B., and Peacock, E. E., Jr.: Collagenolytic enzyme in human tissues. Surg. Forum, *17*:90, 1966.

Riley, W. B., and Peacock, E. E., Jr.: Identification, distribution and significance of a collagenolytic enzyme in human tissues. Proc. Soc. Exp. Biol. Med., *124*:207, 1967.

Rosenberg, B. F., and Caldwell, F. T., Jr.: Effect of single amino acid supplementation upon the rate of wound contraction and wound morphology in protein-depleted rats. Surg. Gynec. Obstet., *121*:1021, 1965.

Ross, R., and Benditt, E. P.: Wound healing and collagen formation. II. Fine structures in experimental scurvy. J. Cell. Biol., *12*:533, 1962.

Rossi, F., and Zatti, M.: Changes in the metabolic pattern of polymorphonuclear leukocytes during phagocytosis. Brit. J. Exp. Path., *45*:58, 1964.

Ryan, G. B., and Spector, W. G.: Macrophage turnover in inflamed connective tissue. Proc. Royal Soc. Lond., *175*:269, 1970.

Schoefl, G. L.: Studies on inflammation. III. Growing capillaries: their structure and permeability. Virchows. Arch. Path. Anat., *337*:97, 1963.

Sevitt, S.: Early and delayed edema and increase in capillary permeability after burns of the skin. J. Path. Bact., *75*:27, 1958.

Sevitt, S.: Inflammatory changes in burned skin, reversible and irreversible effects and their pathogeneses. *In* Thomas, L., Uhr, J. W., and Grant, L. (eds.): Injury, Inflammation and Immunity. Baltimore, Williams & Wilkins Co., 1964, p. 183.

Snyderman, R., et al.: Defective mononuclear leukocyte chemotaxis: a previously unrecognized immune dysfunction. Studies in a patient with chronic mucocutaneous candidiasis. Ann. Int. Med., *78*:509, 1973.

Spector, W. G., and Willoughby, D. A.: Vasoactive amines in acute inflammation. Ann. N.Y. Acad. Sci., *116*:839, 1964.

Spector, W. G., and Willoughby, D. A.: Vascular and cellular aspects of inflammation of the skin. Adv. Biol. Skin, *11*:29, 1971.

Sussman, M. D.: Aging of connective tissue: physical properties of healing wounds in young and old rats. Am. J. Physiol., *224*:1167, 1973.

Thompson, P. L., et al.: Suppression of leucocytic sticking and emigration by chelation of calcium. J. Path. Bact., *94*:389, 1967.

Udupa, K. N., and Prasad, G. C.: Chemical and histochemical studies on the organic constituents in repair in rats. J. Bone Joint Surg., *45B*:770, 1963.

VanFurth, R., et al.: Quantitative study on the production and kinetics of mononuclear phagocytes during an acute inflammatory reaction. J. Exp. Med., *138*:1314, 1973.

Van Winkle, W., Jr.: The fibroblast in wound healing. Surg. Gynec. Obstet., *124*:369, 1967.

Wahl, S. M., et al.: The effect of complement depletion on wound healing. Am. J. Path., *75*:73, 1974.

Ward, P. A.: Leukotaxis and leukotactic disorders. Am. J. Path., *77*:519, 1974.

Weiss, P.: Biological Specificity and Growth. Princeton, N.J., Princeton University Press, 1955.

Weiss, P., and Matoltsy, A. G.: Wound healing in chick embryos in vivo and in vitro. Develop. Biol., *1*:302, 1959.

Weissman, G., and Thomas, L.: Studies of lysosomes. II. The effect of cortisone on the release of acid hydrolases from a large granule fraction of rabbit liver induced by an excess of vitamin A. J. Clin. Invest., *42*:661, 1963.

White, R. G.: The effect of mycobacteria on macrophage mobilization and granuloma formation. *In* Illingworth, C. (ed.): Wound Healing. Boston, Little, Brown & Co., 1966, p. 27.

Wilhelm, D. L.: Chemical mediators. *In* Zweifach, B. W., Grant, L., and McCluskey, R. T. (eds.): The Inflammatory Process, Vol. II. New York, Academic Press, 1973, p. 303.

Willoughby, D. A.: The inflammatory response. J. Dent. Res., *51*:226, 1972.

Willoughby, D. A.: Mediation of increased permeability. *In* Zweifach, B. W., Grant, L., and McCluskey, R. T. (eds.): The Inflammatory Process, Vol. II. New York, Academic Press, 1973, p. 251.

Willoughby, D. A., and Spector, W. G.: The lymph node permeability factor: a possible mediator of the delayed hypersensitivity response. Ann. N.Y. Acad. Sci., *116*:874, 1964.

Wood, W. B., et al.: Studies of the mechanisms of recovery in pneumococcal pneumonia. J. Exp. Med., *84*:387, 1946.

Wuepper, K. D., and Cochrane, C. G.: Plasma prekallikrein: isolation, characterization and mechanism of activation. J. Exp. Med., *135*:1, 1972.

Zigmond, S. H., and Hirsch, J. G.: Leukocyte locomotion and chemotaxis. New methods for evaluation and demonstration of a cell-derived chemotactic factor. J. Exp. Med., *137*:387, 1973.

Zucker-Franklin, D.: Electron microscopic studies of human granulocytes: structural variations related to function. Sem. Hemat., *5*:109, 1968.

CHAPTER 3

Neoplasia and Other Disturbances of Cell Growth

Neoplasia literally means new growth, and the mass of cells that composes the new growth is known as a neoplasm. Perhaps the best definition of a neoplasm was offered by Willis (1952)—"A neoplasm is an abnormal mass of tissue, the growth of which exceeds and is uncoordinated with that of the normal tissues, and persists in the same excessive manner after the cessation of the stimuli which evoked the change." Generally, neoplasms have two other characteristics. They seem to behave as parasites and compete with normal cells and tissues for their metabolic needs. Thus, neoplasms may flourish in patients who are otherwise wasting. Neoplasms also enjoy a certain degree of autonomy, and more or less steadily increase in size regardless of their local environment and the nutritional status of the host. To an extent, then, they are uncontrolled growths. Their autonomy, however, is by no means complete. Some neoplasms require endocrine support, and, indeed, such dependencies can sometimes be exploited to the disadvantage of the neoplasm. Moreover, all are critically dependent on an adequate blood supply derived from the host. Despite these dependencies *a neoplasm is best considered as a parasitic, abnormal mass of cells which grows more or less progressively unless excised or controlled by therapeutic intervention.*

All cells in the body possess the inherent capacity to undergo mitosis since all have the same genome as the zygote. Under certain pathologic conditions even the so-called permanent cells retain the ability to proliferate (Hay, 1971; Kiviat et al., 1973). The spectrum of cellular proliferations, in order of progressively severe growth derangement, can be divided into: (1) regeneration, (2) hyperplasia, (3) metaplasia, (4) dysplasia and (5) neoplasia. Regeneration has already been considered in the section on healing of wounds. Hyperplasia, metaplasia and dysplasia, although characterized by abnormal cellular proliferation, also represent controlled forms of cell growth which are reversible when the inciting stimulus abates. So far as we know, neoplasia, the most extreme form of abnormal cell growth, is almost always irreversible unless, of course, the neoplastic cells are removed or destroyed by therapeutic intervention. The cells within a neoplasm may be virtually normal in appearance or they may be strikingly abnormal, as encountered in some cancers. Neoplasms composed of virtually normal cells are, by and large, benign and have low growth potential. In contrast, cancer cells display a wide range not only of morphologic appearance but also of cellular growth activity. To some degree they are undifferentiated and anarchic, an appearance referred to as anaplasia (described in more detail on p. 74). To place neoplastic proliferation in perspective, the controlled disturbances of cell growth, i.e., hyperplasia, metaplasia and dysplasia, will be considered first, followed by a discussion of the basic aspects of neoplasia. In Chapter 4 the clinical aspects of neoplasia will be considered.

NON-NEOPLASTIC CELL GROWTH

The three distinctive patterns of controlled non-neoplastic cell growth considered here—hyperplasia, metaplasia and dysplasia—must not be viewed merely as graded levels of cellular proliferation. There are important qualitative as well as quantitative differences among these three patterns. However, there is also much overlap among the patterns. Thus one may find hyperplastic cells which have simultaneously undergone metaplasia and, similarly, dysplasia may coexist with metaplasia. Nonetheless, each of these entities may exist in pure form and be readily differentiated from the others.

HYPERPLASIA

The term hyperplasia is applied to a form of controlled cell proliferation characterized by an absolute increase in the number of cells in a tissue or organ. The individual cells are essentially normal in appearance, but may have somewhat larger and slightly hyperchromatic nuclei, as well as abnormally prominent nucleoli. There may also be some increase in the number of organelles, such as mitochondria and free ribosomes, in the individual cell. *The fundamental characteristic of hyperplasia, however, is a quantitative increase in the number of cells without significant alteration in their structure or function.* As a consequence of the increased number of cells, the affected tissues or organs usually increase in volume.

Hyperplasia may represent either a physiologic or pathologic process. *Physiologic hyperplasia* is best exemplified by the glandular proliferation of the female breast at puberty and during pregnancy and lactation. Physiologic hyperplasia of the smooth muscle cells also occurs in the gravid uterus, and here it is accompanied by striking hypertrophy of preexisting smooth muscle cells. The enlargement of one kidney in response to the destruction or removal of the other is another form of physiologic hyperplasia, sometimes specified

as *compensatory hyperplasia.* The remaining kidney is enlarged because of an increase in the size of the individual nephrons, which in turn is produced largely by hyperplasia of tubular epithelial cells, perhaps accompanied by some hypertrophy of the individual cells. New nephrons or glomeruli are not formed, but the capillary tuft of the glomerulus may become enlarged by proliferation of endothelial cells forming more complex capillary loops. The stimuli to such compensatory hyperplasia are poorly understood and have been the subject of intense investigation. Circulating humoral factors, work overload and a variety of enzyme imbalances have been proposed but not established (Malt, 1969).

Pathologic hyperplasia may be induced by a variety of abnormal stimuli. In most instances it is the result of the excessive hormonal stimulation of target cells. For example, various forms of abnormal endometrial hyperplasia are produced by excessive estrogen stimulation, such as may be encountered in patients with certain ovarian tumors (granulosal-luteal cell tumors) which elaborate estrogens. This type of endometrial hyperplasia remains within control, and while it may cause abnormal uterine bleeding, it is not a neoplastic change. However, it is important to note that a *significant number of women with endometrial hyperplasia later develop endometrial cancer. Here is one instance, and there are others, in which controlled cell proliferation may lead to uncontrolled neoplastic proliferation.* We do not understand why this sometimes happens, but some speculation will be presented later. Pathologic hyperplasia is also seen in a variety of forms of thyroid disease known as goiter. Such hyperplasia (considered in more detail on p. 600) may be caused by prolonged or excessive secretion of pituitary thyrotropic hormone or by the presence of abnormal serum immunoglobulins. It will suffice to say here that in a small percentage of cases, thyroid hyperplasia may provide the soil for the later development of a thyroid cancer, another example of the transition from hyperplasia to neoplasia.

The hyperplastic process represents cell proliferation which remains under control and is reversible. For example, if the source of excess estrogen (such as a granulosal cell tumor) can be controlled or removed, the endometrial hyperplasia spontaneously disappears. Hyperplasia of the glands in the breast regresses almost completely after pregnancy and lactation. Physiologic and compensatory hyperplasia obviously serve a useful purpose; the *pathologic hyperplasias, however, are not only intrinsically diseases but also constitute soils for the development of neoplasia, as was pointed out.* This well-known phenomenon provides grounds for the widely held belief that prolonged stimulation of mitotic activity is potentially dangerous, since it produces an environment in which cells may escape from normal homeostatic control.

METAPLASIA

Metaplasia is another form of controlled, abnormal cell growth. It is essentially characterized by an *adaptive substitution by one type of adult or fully differentiated cell for another type of adult cell.* For example, under conditions of chronic irritation or inflammation the more delicate and vulnerable ciliated, pseudostratified columnar epithelium of the bronchi and bronchioles may be replaced by more rugged stratified squamous epithelium. The pseudostratified columnar cells probably do not themselves undergo conversion to squamous cells, but rather the evidence points toward stimulation of growth of the reserve cells within the respiratory epithelium along new pathways of differentiation.

Metaplasia may occur in both epithelial and connective tissue cells. In the epithelia it usually takes the form of substitution for a columnar mucus secreting surface by a stratified squamous epithelial surface. This pattern of metaplasia is seen in the gallbladder, trachea, bronchi or bronchioles, endocervical glands and excretory ducts of any gland of the body, whenever these sites are chronically inflamed or irritated (Fig. 3–1). Vitamin A deficiency, for obscure reasons, is an important cause of epithelial metaplasia leading to keratinizing stratified squamous epithelium in the respiratory passages and the renal calyces and pelves.

Connective tissue metaplasia may be encountered after injury to soft tissue. Scarring is sometimes followed by metaplasia of fibroblasts to osteoblasts, and bone may thus be formed in the area of injury. Similar osseous metaplasia may be seen in traumatic injury to muscle, producing a lesion known as "myositis ossificans." Epithelial metaplasia is almost always reversible, but the connective tissue metaplasias that form bone are usually irreversible and leave permanent markers at the site of old injury.

Teleologically, metaplasia most often represents an adaptive or protective response insofar as the squamous metaplastic epithelium is better able to survive in its adverse environment than was the preceding columnar or pseudostratified epithelium. However, the change is not without drawbacks since it usually implies some loss of specialized function. For example, in the respiratory tract there is loss of ciliary and mucous protective functions of the normal columnar epithelium.

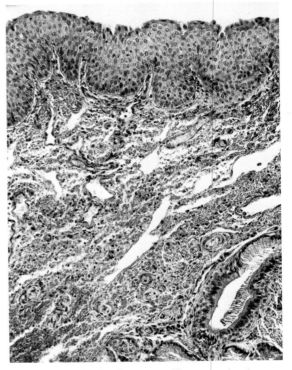

Figure 3–1. Tracheal mucosa. The normal columnar, mucus secreting lining epithelium (similar to that seen in the gland at lower right) has been totally replaced by stratified squamous cells.

Often the metaplastic transformation is quite orderly and, in fact, may faithfully reproduce an epithelial architecture that exactly resembles normal squamous epithelium. At times, however, particularly when there is persistent chronic irritation or inflammation, the metaplastic epithelium is somewhat disorderly—i.e., the cells vary slightly in size and shape, do not have the usual orientation to each other and may have slight variations in nuclear size and chromaticity. Such changes are called "*atypical metaplasia*"; they represent a transition between the orderly pattern of metaplasia and the disorderly pattern of dysplasia.

DYSPLASIA

In the spectrum of non-neoplastic (i.e., controlled) proliferations, dysplasia is the most disorderly. Frequently it is the forerunner of a cancer, although the causes for this very important transition are by no means clear. Dysplasia is encountered principally in the epithelia. *It comprises a loss in the uniformity of the individual cells, as well as a loss in their architectural orientation.* Dysplastic cells exhibit considerable pleomorphism (variation in size and shape) and often possess deeply stained (hyperchromatic) nuclei, which are abnormally

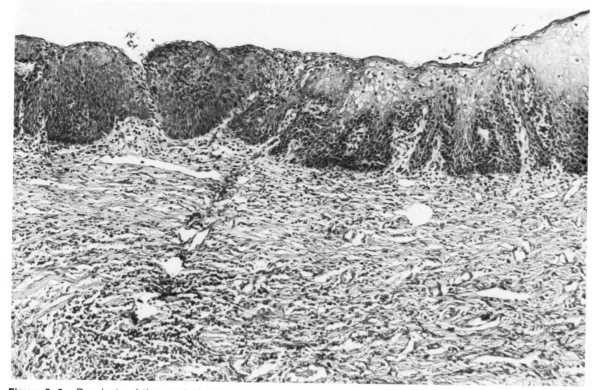

Figure 3–2. Dysplasia of the cervical mucosa. The normal epithelium is seen at the right. Note the gradual conversion into the dysplastic epithelium at the left. The dysplastic cells are smaller, more crowded together, and there is loss of the orderly maturation of the surface layers.

large for the size of the cell. Mitotic figures are more abundant than usual, although almost invariably they conform to normal patterns. Frequently the mitoses appear in abnormal locations within the epithelium. Thus, in dysplastic stratified squamous epithelium, mitoses are not confined to the basal layers and may appear at all levels and even in surface cells. There is considerable architectural anarchy. For example, the usual progressive maturation of tall cells in the basal layer to flattened squames on the surface may be lost and replaced by a disordered scrambling of dark basal-appearing cells throughout the entire thickness of the epithelium (Fig. 3–2).

Dysplasia is characteristically associated with protracted chronic irritation or inflammation. Classically it is encountered in the cervix, respiratory passages, oral cavity and gallbladder. Chronic cervicitis is the antecedent of cervical dysplasia. Dysplasia in the respiratory passages is encountered in chronic bronchitis or bronchiectasis and is notably present in the airways of habitual cigarette smokers. In the gallbladder, gallstones and chronic inflammation of the gallbladder wall frequently precede dysplastic change.

Dysplasia is a reversible, and therefore presumably a controlled, cellular proliferation. When the underlying, inciting stimulus is removed, the dysplastic alterations revert to normal. However, this is an extremely important type of cell change since malignant transformation sometimes supervenes. Why this occurs is still unknown. In the more extreme forms of dysplasia, the cellular abnormalities begin to approach those seen in cancerous growths. It appears that some mysterious line is crossed, whereby dysplastic cells escape the normal homeostatic controls and assume the autonomy encountered in tumorous growths. It is entirely possible that within the dysplastic epithelium, the more frequent mitoses provide a higher chance of mutation, with the production of aberrant cells freed from regulation. There are other speculations, but more is said about these in the consideration of carcinogenesis.

NEOPLASIA

In common medical usage a neoplasm is often referred to as a "tumor" and the study of tumors is called "oncology" (from *oncos,* tumor, and *logos,* study of). Strictly speaking, a tumor is merely a swelling that could be produced by, among other things, edema or hemorrhage into a tissue. However, the term "tumor" has now come to be applied almost solely to neoplastic masses which may cause swellings on the body surface; use of the term for non-neoplastic lesions has virtually disappeared. In oncology the division of neoplasms into benign and malignant categories is most important. This categorization is based on a judgment of a neoplasm's potential clinical behavior. A tumor is said to be benign when its cytologic and gross characteristics are considered relatively innocent, implying that it will remain localized, cannot spread to other sites and is, therefore, generally amenable to local surgical removal and survival of the patient. It should be noted, however, that benign tumors can produce more than localized lumps, and sometimes they are responsible for serious disease. A benign tumor that occludes a vital artery by its expansile pressure or obstructs the common bile duct, for example, may in fact be of more consequence to the patient than a malignant tumor of the skin that is readily excised. *Malignant tumors are collectively referred to as cancers.* The derivation of the word cancer is somewhat lost in antiquity. Hippocrates referred to solid malignant masses as carcinoma, a word derived from the Greek term for crab. Later the Latin term for crab, "cancrum," was applied to these malignant growths; and presumably it is from this origin that we find the term cancer first used in the seventh century as follows: "But some say that it is so called because it adheres to any part that it seizes upon in an obstinate manner, like the crab." "Malignant," as applied to a neoplasm, implies that it can invade and destroy adjacent structures and spread to distant sites to cause death. Obviously, not all cancers pursue so malignant a course. Some are discovered early and are successfully treated. But the designation "malignant" constitutes a red flag, which denotes that in the mind of the pathologist, immediate therapy must be instituted, or progressive spread will follow that may preclude later eradication of the lesion.

NOMENCLATURE

All tumors, benign and malignant, have two basic components: (1) the parenchyma, made up of proliferating neoplastic cells and (2) the supporting stroma, made up of connective tissue, blood vessels and possibly lymphatics. As will be seen, *it is the parenchyma of the neoplasm which largely determines its biological behavior and is the component from which the tumor derives its name.* The stroma, however, provides support for the growth of parenchymal cells and is therefore of considerable importance.

Most benign tumors are composed of parenchymal cells which closely resemble the tissue of origin. Thus they can be classified according to their histogenesis. They are designated by attaching the suffix "-oma" to the cell type from which the tumor arises. A benign tumor arising in fibrous tissue composed of fibrocytes is termed a fibroma; a benign cartilaginous tumor is a chondroma. Benign tumors of epithelial origin defy such easy classification since there are insufficient distinctive names for the great variety of epithelia in the body. Many organs or sites have similar epithelia—i.e., columnar cells line ducts of all glands of the body. Accordingly, among benign epithelial neoplasms some are classified on the basis of their microscopic and some on the basis of their macroscopic patterns. Others are classified by their cells of origin. *Adenoma is the term applied to benign epithelial neoplasms producing gland patterns, as well as to those derived from glands but not necessarily reproducing gland patterns.* A benign epithelial neoplasm growing in gland-like patterns arising from the columnar lining of the gallbladder would be termed an adenoma, as would a mass of benign epithelial cells producing no glandular patterns but having its origin in the adrenal cortex. Benign epithelial neoplasms growing on any surface, which produce distinctive finger-like warty growths or microscopic projections, are designated papillomas or polyps. Some benign tumors form large cystic masses as in the ovary and are referred to as cystomas or cystadenomas. If papillary projections are formed on the epithelial linings of these cystic tumors, they may be further qualified as papillary cystadenomas.

The nomenclature of malignant tumors essentially follows that of benign tumors, with certain additions. *Malignant neoplasms arising in mesenchymal tissue or its derivatives are called sarcomas.* A cancer of fibrous tissue origin is a fibrosarcoma and a malignant neoplasm composed of lymphocytes is a lymphosarcoma. An osteogenic sarcoma would be expected to contain osteoblasts forming bone. But, as we shall see, while this usage is quite appropriate, some writers also consider all sarcomas arising in bone as osteogenic sarcomas even though, for example, they might be made up entirely of malignant appearing fibrocytes having a periosteal origin. Here we shall adopt the generally acceptable practice of designating sarcomas by their histogenesis—i.e., the cell type of which they are composed. *Malignant neoplasms of epithelial cell origin are called carcinomas.* It must be remembered that the epithelia of the body are derived from all three germ layers; thus, a malignant neoplasm arising in the renal tubular epithelium (mesoderm) is a carcinoma, as are the cancers arising in the skin (ectoderm) and lining epithelium of the gut (endoderm). Carcinomas may be further qualified. *Squamous cell carcinoma* would denote a cancer originating in any of the stratified squamous epithelia of the body, and *adenocarcinoma*, a lesion in which the neoplastic epithelial cells grow in gland patterns. Sometimes the tissue or organ of origin can be identified, as for instance in the designation of renal cell adenocarcinoma, or cholangiocarcinoma, which implies an origin from bile ducts. Sometimes the tumor grows in a very embryonic or undifferentiated pattern and must be called poorly differentiated carcinoma.

Classification and terminology are important because they represent the language by which physicians convey the specific clinical significance of a given neoplasm. When the pathologist reports a seminoma of the testis to the surgeon, the precise significance of that term must be recognized. "Seminoma" implies a carcinoma of the testis having a propensity for metastasis to lymph nodes along the iliac arteries and aorta. This condition nonetheless has a fairly good prognosis, since the lesion in its primary site is usually resectable, and the lymphatic metastases are remarkably radiosensitive. A high cure rate may be expected; fewer than 10 per cent of patients with this condition die as a result of their cancer. By contrast, the term "embryonal carcinoma of the testis" indicates a much more grave disease. This form of cancer, virtually indistinguishable grossly from the seminoma in its primary site, has a tendency to metastasize to the lung, liver, bone marrow and brain, and moreover, it is usually radioresistant. A 50 per cent mortality rate within two years of surgical resection may be expected. Terminology therefore often conveys clinical significance.

The specific names of the more common forms of neoplasia are presented in Table 3–1. It should be noted that *most neoplasms are composed of one neoplastic cell type.* A few have more than one neoplastic cell type, but if all are derived from one germ layer these neoplasms are called *mixed.* Neoplasms having cells derived from more than one germ layer are referred to as *teratomas.* Presumably the teratoma arises from toti- or multipotential cells which have the ability to differentiate along several germinal lines. In such neoplasms, cells and organoid structures are found which resemble the derivatives of two or three of the basic germ lines. Although all of these cellular lines may be benign, experience teaches that teratomas, however innocent appearing, tend to manifest malignant behavior.

Table 3–1 also reveals, as may be noted, many inappropriate usages. Under tumors of

mesenchymal origin one finds the synovioma and mesothelioma listed as malignant tumors. Benign counterparts are not listed since all tumors arising from such tissues and cells are considered to be potentially cancerous, however well differentiated they may appear to be. It would be more consistent to designate these lesions as synoviosarcoma and mesotheliosarcoma, but the inappropriate usage is firmly fixed in all medical writing. In the same way, one should note that the seminoma is a form of testicular carcinoma, the melanoma is more appropriately called a melanocarcinoma and the hepatoma is a carcinoma of hepatic cell origin (hepatocellular carcinoma).

There are additional instances of inappropriate terminology. The *hamartoma* is a localized overgrowth of mature cells normally found in an organ. The cells in the hamartoma, while mature and normal, do not recreate the normal organization of the tissue in which they are found. Thus one may see a mass of disorganized hepatic cells, blood vessels and possibly bile ducts within the liver, or there may be a disorganized accumulation of cells indigenous to the spleen, creating an apparent tumor within the spleen. The designation hamartoma is appropriate inasmuch as the aggregation of cells may create a small tumor but the lesion is not a true neoplasm; rather, it is a form of congenital anomaly. Another misnomer is the term *choristoma.* This congenital anomaly is better described as a *heterotopic rest* of cells. For example, a small nodule of very well developed and normally organized pancreatic substance may be found in the submucosa of the stomach, duodenum or even small intestine. This heterotopic rest may be replete with islets of Langerhans, as well as exocrine glands. The term choristoma, connoting a neoplasm, imparts to the heterotopic rest a gravity far beyond its usual trivial significance. In all probability the rest merely reflects an embryogenic defect. Regrettably, neither life nor the terminology of neoplasms is simple.

DIFFERENTIAL CHARACTERISTICS OF BENIGN AND MALIGNANT NEOPLASMS

Nothing is more important to the patient with a tumor than being told "it is benign." Many criteria are used by the clinician and pathologist to make such a judgment, and the following discussion presents the characteristics of neoplasms used to differentiate the benign from the malignant. At the conclusion of this presentation Table 3–3 summarizes these points (p. 84). At the outset, however, it should be stressed that although the great majority of neoplasms can be judged either benign or malignant, some fall in the interme-

TABLE 3-1. CLASSIFICATION OF TUMORS*

TISSUE OF ORIGIN	BENIGN	MALIGNANT
I. Simple (composed of one single neoplastic cell type)		
A. Tumors of Mesenchymal Origin		*sarcomas*
(1) Connective Tissue and Derivatives		
fibrous tissue	fibroma	fibrosarcoma
myxomatous tissue	myxoma	myxosarcoma
fatty tissue	lipoma	liposarcoma
cartilage	chondroma	chondrosarcoma
bone	osteoma	osteogenic sarcoma
notochordal tissue	chordoma	chordoma (or better, chordo-sarcoma)
(2) Endothelial and Related Tissues		
blood vessels	hemangioma:	angiosarcoma
	capillary	
	cavernous	
	sclerosing	
	hemangioendothelioma	endotheliosarcoma (multiple sarcoma—Kaposi's sarcoma)
lymph vessels	lymphangioma	lymphangiosarcoma
	lymphangioendothelioma	lymphangioendotheliosarcoma
synovia		synovioma (synoviosarcoma)
mesothelium (lining cells of body cavities)		mesothelioma (mesothelio-sarcoma)
brain coverings	meningioma	
glomus	glomus tumor	
? blood vessels of bone marrow		? Ewing's tumor (endotheliosarcoma)
(3) Blood Cells and Related Cells		
hematopoietic cells		granulocytic leukemia
		monocytic leukemia
lymphoid tissue		malignant lymphomas
		lymphocytic leukemia
		plasmacytoma (multiple myeloma)
reticuloendothelial system		reticulum cell sarcoma (malignant lymphoma, histiocytic type)
		? Hodgkin's disease
(4) Muscle		
smooth muscle	leiomyoma	leiomyosarcoma
striated muscle	rhabdomyoma	rhabdomyosarcoma

diate gray zone and cannot be assigned to either category with certainty. All neoplasms, from the most innocuous and unmistakably benign to the most anaplastic and certainly malignant, constitute a spectrum of abnormal cellular growth. The line which demarcates the innocent from the treacherous is not sharply defined. Some growths possess certain features which indicate a benign nature, whereas other features suggest malignant potential. Moreover, there is not always perfect concordance between the morphology of a neoplasm and its biologic behavior. Thus, some innocent appearing lesions are sometimes quite aggressive. Occasionally the reverse is true. Only the ultimate course of the tumor clearly demonstrates its true nature, and when the pathologist is called upon to predict this behavior he must rely to some extent upon subjective interpretation. Happily, morphology and the differential character-

istics to be discussed are generally good predictors of behavior for most neoplasms.

DIFFERENTIATION AND ANAPLASIA

Differentiation and anaplasia refer only to the parenchymal cells. The stroma, as mentioned, plays a supporting role. *The differentiation of parenchymal cells refers to the extent to which these cells resemble their normal forebears and thus achieve their fully mature, specialized, functional and morphologic characteristics.* Thus, a well differentiated, striated muscle cell in a tumor would closely resemble its normal counterpart. These cells might also retain their normal function, as has been shown by tissue culture of well differentiated tumor cells. In contrast, a poorly differentiated cell in a neoplasm has achieved no specialized characteristics and thus resembles an embryonic, primitive stem cell. The well differentiated parenchymal cell achieves a high level

TABLE 3–1. CLASSIFICATION OF TUMORS *(Continued)*

TISSUE OF ORIGIN	BENIGN	MALIGNANT
B. Tumors of Epithelial Origin		*carcinomas*
stratified squamous	squamous cell papilloma	squamous cell or epidermoid carcinoma
skin adnexal glands:		
hair follicles		basal cell carcinoma
sweat glands	sweat gland adenoma	sweat gland carcinoma
sebaceous glands	sebaceous gland adenoma	sebaceous gland carcinoma
epithelium lining:		
glands or ducts—well differentiated group	adenoma	adenocarcinoma
	papilloma	papillary carcinoma
	papillary adenoma	papillary adenocarcinoma
	cystadenoma	cystadenocarcinoma
poorly differentiated group		medullary carcinoma
		undifferentiated carcinoma (simplex)
respiratory tract		bronchogenic carcinoma
		bronchial "adenoma"
neuroectoderm	nevus	melanoma (melanocarcinoma)
renal epithelium	renal tubular adenoma	renal cell carcinoma (hypernephroid)
liver cells	liver cell adenoma	hepatoma or liver cell carcinoma
bile duct	bile duct adenoma	bile duct carcinoma (cholangiocarcinoma)
urinary tract epithelium (transitional)	transitional cell papilloma	papillary carcinoma
		transitional cell carcinoma
		squamous cell carcinoma
placental epithelium	hydatid mole	choriocarcinoma
testicular epithelium		seminoma
		embryonal carcinoma
II. Mixed (more than one neoplastic cell type, usually derived from one germ layer)		
salivary glands	mixed tumor of salivary gland origin	malignant mixed tumor of salivary gland origin
renal anlage		Wilms' tumor
III. Compound (more than one neoplastic cell type derived from more than one germ layer)		
totipotential cells in gonads or in embryonic rests	teratoma, dermoid	One or more elements become malignant, e.g., squamous cell carcinoma arising in a teratoma (teratocarcinoma)

*From Robbins, S. L.: Pathologic Basis of Disease. Philadelphia, W. B. Saunders Company, 1974.

of specialization while at the same time retaining its proliferative capability. This highlights an important aspect of neoplasia: Under normal circumstances only primitive cells retain the unlimited capacity to divide and replicate; *in neoplasia, specialization may occur without loss of replicative capability.*

We may now turn to the parenchymal differences between benign and malignant neoplasms. In general, *benign neoplasms are extremely well differentiated.* The cells resemble very closely the normal counterparts from which the tumor took origin. Thus, in a lipoma, one finds mature fat cells with clear, vacuolated cytoplasm loaded with lipids. The leiomyoma is made up of mature, smooth muscle cells. Indeed, if one examines only a few of these cells under high power without appreciating their location within a discrete nodule, it may

be impossible to recognize the well differentiated cells in the leiomyoma as belonging to a tumor. *In well differentiated parenchymal cells of benign tumors, mitoses are extremely scant in number and those present are of normal type.* Frequently, one has difficulty in finding a mitotic figure and is left wondering how the tumor achieved its size.

Malignant tumors display a wide range in parenchymal cell differentiation, from those deceptively well differentiated to those completely undifferentiated. *But, in general, all types of malignant neoplasia display some degree of anaplasia. Indeed, anaplasia is one of the most reliable hallmarks of malignancy.* Literally, anaplasia means "to form backward." It implies "dedifferentiation" or loss of the structural and functional differentiation of normal cells. There is objection to the use of the term

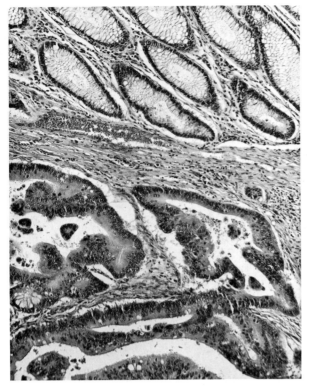

Figure 3–3. Well differentiated adenocarcinoma of the colon. The normal colonic mucosa is shown at the top. The invasive cancerous glands, showing preservation of the columnar palisade of cells and occasional vacuoles of mucus secretion, can be seen at bottom.

"dedifferentiation" since it now appears that anaplasia represents a failure of differentiation of reserve or stem cells rather than a regression of existing adult cells. All highly differentiated cells develop from primitive precursors. Presumably, when a cancer arises division and proliferation of the cells is not accompanied by differentiation and specialization, thus yielding a mass of more or less anaplastic, undifferentiated cells (Figs. 3–3, and 3–4).

Anaplastic cells display marked pleomorphism, i.e., marked variation in size and shape. This pleomorphism exceeds that found in dysplastic cells. Characteristically the nuclei are extremely hyperchromatic and large. The nuclear-cytoplasmic ratio may approach 1:1 instead of the normal 1:4 or 1:6. Giant cells may be formed which are considerably larger than their neighbors, possessing either one enormous nucleus or several nuclei. Anaplastic nuclei are variable and bizarre in size and shape. The chromatin is coarse and clumped, and nucleoli may be of astounding size. More important, the mitoses are often numerous and distinctly atypical; anarchic multiple spindles may be seen that sometimes can be resolved as

tripolar or quadripolar forms, often with one spindle enormously large and the others puny and abortive (Fig. 3–5). In addition, anaplastic cells fail to develop recognizable patterns of orientation to each other. They grow in sheets or masses, with total loss of communal structures, such as gland formations or stratified squamous architecture. Thus anaplasia is the most extreme disturbance in cell growth encountered in the spectrum of cellular proliferations. It is placed in some perspective in Table 3–2.

Studies of the anaplastic cell by electron microscopy have yielded no features that would not be anticipated from light microscopy. As the cells become more anaplastic or undifferentiated, organellar abnormalities become more prominent. Nuclei tend to be misshapen and contain increased amounts of chromatin and unusually large nucleoli. The mitochondria vary more in size and shape than in their normal forebears, and these changes are accompanied by disorganization of the endoplasmic reticulum. In some actively growing neoplastic cells there is an increase of ribosomes and polyribosomes.

Anaplasia is a hallmark of cancer. It does not ap-

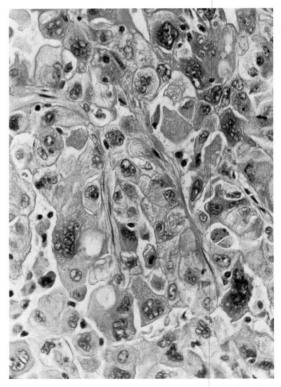

Figure 3–4. An anaplastic carcinoma of the liver. There is great variability in size and shape of the cells. The nuclei are highly pleomorphic, and several hyperchromatic tumor giant cells are readily evident—some with multiple nuclei.

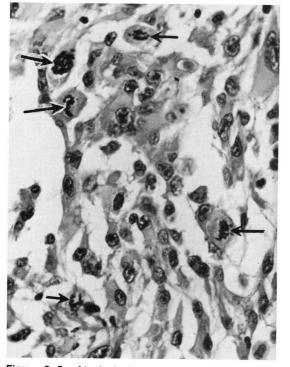

Figure 3–5. Atypical mitoses in a rapidly growing carcinoma of the pancreas. The disorganized mitotic figures (see arrows) reflect the anarchic reproduction of anaplastic tumor cells.

pear in benign neoplasms. It is almost always an irreversible change. Although there are rare instances of anaplastic cancer cells which have undergone maturation and differentiation accompanied by reversion of the original neoplasm to a more benign form, such happy occurrences are rare exceptions. They raise the interesting issue of what provoked such maturation of the anaplastic cells to more differentiated and controlled forms.

The cytologic abnormalities of anaplasia provide the basis for the Papanicolaou smear test for cancer. In essence, Papanicolaou demonstrated that when cancers are present in organs or tissues, examination of secretions of fluids in contact with the tumor may disclose the presence of individual anaplastic cells. Because they often lack cohesiveness, tumor cells are readily shed and thus become available for examination. This method is of great clinical use with bronchial, vaginal and gastric secretions, prostatic fluid, ascitic fluid, nipple discharge and urine. The procedure and its clinical applications are described more fully on page 114.

Occasionally, a malignant neoplasm will be extremely well differentiated and may not be recognizable as malignant by morphologic evaluation of its parenchyma. For example, virtually normal thyroid parenchyma may appear in a lymph node in the neck, where it obviously does not belong and where it must represent dissemination of a very well differentiated cancer. Such a phenomenon is, however, the exception, and the generalization obtains that most cancers have some degree of undifferentiation and anaplasia; and, conversely, anaplasia when present implies cancer. *Anaplasia and evidence of invasion of normal tissues are the two principal criteria by which a diagnosis of cancer is made in a primary lesion.* Obviously, if the tumor has spread, there is no doubt.

Well differentiated parenchymal cells may retain the specialized function of the parent cells from which the neoplasm arose, such as hormone production or mucin secretion (p. 108). Such function is correlated with the level of morphologic differentiation and so is more characteristic of benign than of malignant neoplasms. Pituitary, thyroid, parathyroid, adrenal, pancreatic and gonadal tumors may all elaborate hormones characteristic of their site of origin. Most often, these functioning neoplasms are benign, yet they may have

TABLE 3–2. SPECTRUM OF DISTURBANCES OF CELL GROWTH

ENTITY	EPITHELIAL CHANGE	REVERSIBILITY
Hyperplasia	An increase in the number of essentially normal cells. *Example:* breast epithelium in pregnancy.	Yes
Metaplasia	Substitution by one type of adult or fully differentiated cell for another type of adult cell. *Example:* replacement of columnar mucus-secreting cells in respiratory passages by squamous cells.	Yes
Dysplasia	Variation in the size and shape of cells (pleomorphism), accompanied by a loss of normal orientation and by an increase in the number of cells; mitotic figures, if present, are normal. *Example:* the disorganization and thickening of the cervical epithelium in long-standing chronic cervicitis.	Yes
Anaplasia	Greater pleomorphism than dysplasia—sometimes complete loss of differentiation of cells accompanied by hyperchromasia and by an increased number of mitotic figures, some of which may be abnormal. *Example:* seen only in cancers and when present is indicative of malignancy.	No

great and sometimes even lethal significance to the patient. A parathyroid adenoma only a few millimeters in diameter may produce sufficient parathormone to cause life-threatening hyperparathyroidism. An adenoma of the islet cells of Langerhans no larger than 1 cm. in diameter may cause serious hyperinsulinism and even death from hypoglycemia.

Cancers, too, may retain specialized function. Well differentiated carcinomas of the colon often secrete mucin. There may even be hypersecretion of mucin, which explodes out of cells to create great lakes that literally dissect through the cleavage planes of the colonic wall and greatly facilitate the spread of the tumor. The highly specialized function of tumors may take the form of production of characteristic secretions, hormones or enzymes. Well differentiated squamous cell carcinomas of the epidermis elaborate keratin. Well differentiated hepatocellular carcinomas elaborate bile, providing the most reliable morphologic indicator of the hepatic origin of the tumor. Osteogenic sarcomas elaborate osseomucin and thus form bone. Choriocarcinomas elaborate gonadotropin-like hormones and indeed produce levels very much higher than are encountered in pregnancy. The appearance of this hormone in the serum or urine of a male is virtually pathognomonic of a choriocarcinoma. Similarly, disappearance of the hormone following therapy implies successful eradication of the lesion. Functioning endocrine neoplasms produce some of the most bizarre and interesting endocrinopathies encountered in medicine.

Tumors may also produce enzymes and other humoral factors, and indeed, when enzyme profiles are obtained on well differentiated tumor cells, few differences are noted from their normal counterparts (Bennett et al., 1959). The elaboration of enzymes by well differentiated tumors sometimes provides a valuable diagnostic test. Carcinoma of the prostate, especially when it is metastatic, may elaborate sufficient acid phosphatase to produce detectable levels in the serum.

In addition to enzymes, many tumors elaborate a variety of factors of obscure nature that have well defined clinical effects. For example, renal cell carcinoma may be a source of erythropoietin, which induces polycythemia (abnormally high red cell counts in the peripheral blood). When the primary renal neoplasm is removed, the red cell count returns to normal.

In the more anaplastic and undifferentiated tumors, functional activity appears to be centered on proliferation. Failure of the cell to differentiate morphologically is associated with a failure to develop the enzyme systems and organelles required for specialized function (Paul, 1966). Thus an anaplastic carcinoma arising in the columnar epithelium of the colon may not be capable of secreting mucin. Similarly, poorly differentiated cancers arising from the adrenal cortex are rarely able to elaborate corticosteroids. This observation was best documented in a series of experimentally induced hepatomas (liver cell carcinomas) in rats. The tumors ranged from extremely well differentiated—so-called minimal deviation hepatomas—to poorly differentiated and, in general, rapidly growing neoplasms. The many enzymes involved in liver function were produced by the slowly growing, well differentiated hepatomas but were reduced or not elaborated in the case of the more undifferentiated neoplasms (Farina et al., 1968).

One of the most fascinating aspects of functional neoplasms is the elaboration by certain tumors of substances apparently foreign to the normal tissue of origin. Such activity must represent derepression of genetic coding in the tumor cells that is totally repressed in normal counterparts. For example, certain undifferentiated carcinomas, such as those of the lung, have been found to secrete adrenocorticotropic hormone (ACTH). Other tumors may elaborate antidiuretic hormone (ADH). Peritoneal fibrosarcomas may elaborate insulin (Omenn, 1973; Lipsett et al., 1964). Cancers of several organs (colon, pancreas, lung and stomach) may produce carcinoembryonic antigen which is characteristic of normal embryonic tissues but not found in adult tissues (Zamcheck et al., 1972). Some hepatocellular carcinomas elaborate alpha fetal globulin (Abelev, 1968). Such globulins normally are produced in the liver in fetal life and disappear from the circulating blood soon after birth. Apparently the coding for such synthetic activity becomes repressed at or soon after birth, never to emerge again except when neoplastic transformation occurs. In the case of ACTH and nonpituitary tumors, we can only hypothesize that the code for such synthetic activity resides in all cells in the body since all have the same genome. Normally the code for ACTH is repressed in all cells save the few found in the anterior pituitary. In neoplasia, this codon, for entirely mysterious reasons, erupts into synthetic activity.

In closing this discussion of function, we may state that it is apparent that *well differentiated cells, such as are found in benign neoplasms and in some cancers, resemble their cells of origin not only morphologically but also functionally. In anaplastic tumors the cells' function is directed towards proliferation and other synthetic activities are lost. Therefore, the more rapidly growing and the more anaplastic a tumor, the less likely is functional activity.*

The stroma is vital to the survival and growth of a neoplasm since it provides structural support for the parenchyma and carries with it the nutrient blood supply. Folkman (1971) has ingeniously shown that when individual tumor cells are grown in vitro the expansion of the cell cluster or clone reaches a critical size (2 to 3 mm.) and then stops. Analogously, when tumor cells are inoculated into an animal they cannot grow into a large tumor mass until a blood supply is developed from the adjacent tissues. Folkman proposes that the growing parenchymal cells elaborate an "angiogenesis factor" which stimulates neovascularization of the incipient neoplasm. Further evidence of the critical dependence of the parenchyma on its stromal blood supply is provided by the frequency with which the central region of a rapidly expanding cancer undergoes ischemic necrosis as the neoplasm outgrows its blood supply. This may account for some shrinkage in tumor mass, but regrettably the vital cells ultimately continue to proliferate and recoup losses. Thus the capacity of the parenchyma to survive and multiply is dependent on the adequacy of the blood supply and stromal support. This dependency is presently receiving attention as a possible "Achilles' heel" by which cancer might be destroyed in the patient. Currently a compound known as ICRF-159 has been shown, by angiography and other techniques, to impair vascularization of tumors (Editorial, 1974). Use of this compound in the treatment of human cancer is still in the exploratory stage, but its consideration verifies the critical importance of the blood supply in neoplastic growth.

The amount of connective tissue stroma determines the texture of the tumor. Some neoplasms have very little fibrous stroma and are soft and fleshy. This is particularly true of rapidly growing sarcomas and, indeed, the term sarcoma means "fleshy tumor." Certain other neoplasms evoke a very strong stromal proliferative reaction, known as *desmoplasia,* and thus develop a gritty hardness. These tumors are referred to as scirrhous (e.g., scirrhous carcinoma of the breast). Infrequently, islands of metaplastic cartilage or bone are found in the stroma. Occasionally, the stroma contains a mononuclear infiltrate of lymphocytes, plasma cells and histiocytes. This is of interest since it is interpreted as an immunologic reaction by the host against the tumor. More will be said about tumor immunology later, but here we should point out that such a stromal infiltrate is particularly characteristic of certain cancers of the testis and female breast.

MODE AND RATE OF GROWTH OF NEOPLASMS

The manner and the rate of growth differ somewhat in benign and malignant neoplasms. All tumors begin in a single cell or in a field or cluster of cells. The assumption is often made that the mode of growth is progressive division of the tumor nidus and that the time required for cell division conditions the rate of growth. A further assumption is that all neoplastic cells divide more rapidly than normal cells. While this may be true for certain neoplasms, it may come as a surprise to learn that in some tumors the cell cycle is much longer than in many normal tissue cells (Baserga, 1965). The time required for certain cancer cells to divide has been reported to be as long as three months. For smooth muscle cells in tumors it may be five to six months (Johnson et al., 1960). *The growth of tumors, then, is not due exclusively to an acceleration of the proliferative process, but involves such considerations as the fraction of cells participating in the proliferative pool, the life span of the cells and, even more important, the extent of cell loss through death or exfoliation.* The concept that neoplasms may increase in size because of prolongation of the life cycle of the cells is of more than theoretical interest. It raises the possibility that a fundamental attribute of cancer may be some defect in the differentiation and maturation of cells. The concept of cancer as a disease of disordered cell differentiation and maturation has received its strongest support from the study of leukemia—a malignant process affecting the white cells of the blood and bone marrow. To quote Gallo (1973), "The mechanism of leukemogenesis in man appears to involve a block or an aberration in the normal process of bone marrow leukocyte differentiation rather than a primary proliferative disorder."

Yet another possibility must be considered, particularly in the case of malignant neoplasia. Could growth occur by progressive recruitment of contiguous normal cells? There is experimental evidence that when a culture of normal cells is exposed to cancerogenic influences, such as certain chemicals (to be discussed later) or viruses, some cells are transformed into cancer cells earlier than others. If this observation is applied to the in vivo process in man it may suggest that cancerogenic influences expand the size of a cancer by the progressive transformation of additional normal cells. On the other hand, the originally transformed cells alone may exert a recruiting influence on their normal neighbors.

Whatever the mode of tumor growth *the rate of growth of a neoplasm generally correlates inversely with the level of parenchymal differentiation, and it might also be added that the aggressiveness of a neoplasm correlates to a considerable extent with its rate of growth.* Benign tumors, which are almost always well differentiated, typically increase in size slowly and steadily over a span of years or perhaps decades. Relative to benign neoplasms cancers enlarge rapidly and must either be controlled or eradicated or they will cause the death of the host within months to years. However, it should be noted that exceptions to these generalizations abound. Many benign tumors appear to plateau in size, never to resume progressive enlargement. As will be seen, benign tumors tend to become enclosed within a fibrous capsule. Perhaps expansile growth against the capsule eventually impairs the blood supply to the neoplasm, reducing the vitality of some of the cells and so decreases the proliferating pool. Hormone dependence, and in all probability other influences still unknown, may also contribute to this apparent cessation of growth. It is certainly a well documented fact that in almost all benign neoplasms it is extremely difficult to find mitotic figures. Unquestionably some must be present, but they are exceedingly few in number.

The uterine leiomyoma is a good prototype of the growth behavior of a benign tumor. These tumors may slowly increase in size over the span of years. During pregnancy, perhaps because of hormone stimulation, the rate of enlargement may increase. As the patient gets older the tumor enlargement may slow or even stop. Not infrequently leiomyomas of the uterus are discovered in 30 to 40 year old women on abdominopelvic examination. If the tumors are not removed, because of the patients' unwillingness to have surgery, they may not increase appreciably in size over subsequent years. Indeed, following the menopause they sometimes shrink and many postmenopausal women are found to have leiomyomas largely replaced by collagenous fibrous tissue, sometimes with calcification. Presumably the tumors underwent fibrocalcific atrophy following loss of the requisite levels of ovarian hormones.

Despite the fact that cancers increase in size more rapidly than benign neoplasms, it must not be assumed that cancers kill within months or a few years of their inception. A great deal has been learned about their life histories from longitudinal studies of patients

bearing cancers. This brings us to the concept of *carcinoma-in-situ (ca-in-situ).* Best studied is the cancer of the covering epithelium of the uterine cervix which is readily accessible to observation and biopsy. The Papanicolaou cytologic test, described more completely later in this book (p. 114), has provided a means whereby shed tumor cells in the vaginal secretion permit the identification of cervical carcinomas at an early stage when they have not yet evoked visible alterations in the cervix. At this stage the cancers are in-situ, i.e., *they are confined to transformation of cells within their original location and have not spread across the basement membrane into the adjacent tissue* (Fig. 3–6). The peak incidence of in-situ cervical carcinoma is found in women about 25 to 30 years of age. The average age of patients with visible alterations in the cervix indicating overt cancer is 40 to 45 years of age. This lag period indicates that these neoplasms require years to evolve from the in-situ stage to clinically apparent masses (Johnson et al., 1968). We know less about the life history of other visceral cancers mainly because they are less accessible to observation. It is clear, however, that most carcinomas begin as in-situ lesions which are present for years before the tumors produce symptoms or can be detected by radi-

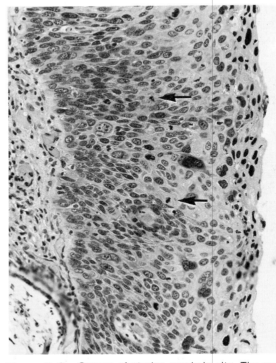

Figure 3–6. Cancer of uterine cervix in situ. The anaplastic mucosa is thickened, but there is no evidence of invasion of the underlying stroma. Note the disorderliness of the cells, the numerous tumor giant cells, pleomorphism and mitotic figures (arrows) well above the basal zone.

ographic or other clinical studies. Thus it is evident that the increase in size of tumors from small but clinically apparent masses to larger masses constitutes only the tip of the iceberg. Much has transpired below the surface during the years following the origin of the lesion as an inapparent in-situ process.

Despite these generalizations cancers are not always predictable in their biology. Although most enlarge progressively, some may suddenly shrink in size, presumably because they outgrow their blood supply and undergo ischemic necrosis. Certain cancers appear to enter periods of dormancy while others may suddenly enlarge explosively. Host factors undoubtedly contribute to this behavior. For example, hormone-dependent carcinoma of the female breast may grow wildly during pregnancy. Many cancers of the prostate can be forced into long periods of dormancy by orchiectomy, which deprives them of required androgenic support. Immune reactions generated by the host against the neoplasm may also play some role in modifying the growth rate of the cancer. More will be said about this later, but it must be emphasized here that *cancers and benign neoplasms are not totally autonomous; their life history is subject to host influences.*

SPREAD OF TUMORS—INVASION AND METASTASIS

A benign neoplasm stays localized at its site of origin. It does not have the capacity to spread to distant sites, as do cancers. Fibromas, lipomas or leiomyomas, for example, slowly increase in size by expansile growth, compressing and possibly distorting the surrounding normal tissues. As they slowly expand, *most develop an enclosing fibrous capsule that separates them from the host tissue.* This capsule is probably derived from the stroma of the native tissue as the tissue cells atrophy under the pressure of the expanding tumor. The stroma of the tumor itself may also contribute to the capsule. However, it should be emphasized that *not all benign neoplasms are encapsulated.* The leiomyoma of the uterus, for example, is quite discretely demarcated from the surrounding smooth muscle by a zone of compressed and attenuated normal myometrium, but there is no well developed capsule. Nonetheless, a well defined cleavage plane exists around these lesions. A few benign tumors are neither encapsulated nor discretely defined. This is particularly true of some of the fibroblastic and vascular benign neoplasms of the dermis. These exceptions are pointed out only to emphasize that *while encapsulation is the rule in benign tumors, the lack of a capsule does not imply that a tumor is malignant.* Occasionally, benign tumors may rupture through their capsule to extend pseudopods into the surrounding tissue. The pseudopods are usually clearly attached to the main mass, grow along a broad front, and are not easily confused with the infiltrative growth of malignant neoplasms.

Cancers grow by progressive infiltration, invasion, destruction and penetration of the surrounding tissue (Fig. 3–7). They do not develop capsules. There are, however, occasional instances in which a slowly growing malignant tumor deceptively appears to be encased by the stroma of the surrounding native tissue, but usually microscopic examination will reveal tiny, crablike feet penetrating the margin and infiltrating adjacent structures. This invasion tends to occur along anatomic planes of cleavage. The infiltrative mode of growth makes it necessary to remove a wide margin of surrounding normal tissue when surgical excision of a malignant tumor is attempted. Hence, cancer surgery is known as radical surgery. The surgeon must have knowledge of the invasive potential of the various forms of cancer since there are striking differences among them.

Cancers have the ability to disseminate to distant

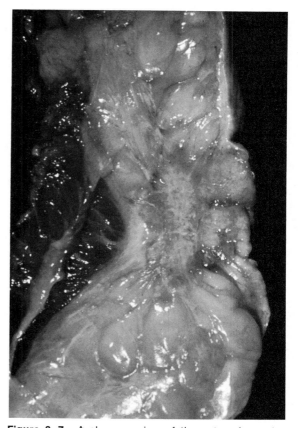

Figure 3–7. A close-up view of the cut surface of a cancer of the female breast. The infiltrative tumor has eroded through the skin (right) and its finger-like extensions pull on the adjacent fat and dark pectoral muscles (left).

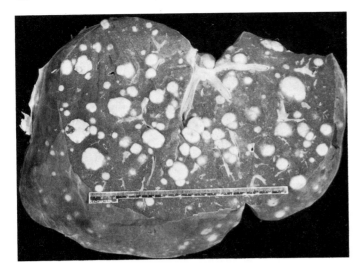

Figure 3–8. A liver studded with metastatic cancer.

sites. This tumor seeding of remote tissues and organs is known as metastasis, and the discontinuous implants are known as metastases. Metastasis unequivocally identifies a neoplasm as malignant, since benign neoplasms do not have this capacity. With rare exceptions, all cancers have the ability to metastasize (Fig. 3–8). The exceptions include malignant neoplasms originating in glial cells (gliomas — note the historically sanctioned paradoxic term for a form of cancer) and basal cell carcinoma of the skin. Both forms are perfectly able to infiltrate locally. Indeed, the basal cell carcinoma is a particularly invasive lesion, but only rarely does it metastasize.

Malignant neoplasms disseminate by one of four pathways: (1) seeding throughout the body cavities, (2) direct transplantation, (3) lymphatic permeation, and (4) transport through blood vessels.

Seeding of cancers occurs when, for example, a carcinoma in the mucosa of the colon, having penetrated the wall of the gut and the visceral peritoneum, reimplants at distant sites throughout the peritoneal cavity. Neoplastic seeding may also be encountered in the other body cavities, i.e., the pleural, pericardial and subarachnoid spaces. One wonders whether malignant tumors may similarly reimplant along an intact epithelium. For example, might a gastric carcinoma reimplant at lower levels of the gastrointestinal tract, or a renal cancer seed the bladder? If such occurs, it is indeed rare.

Transplantation refers to the transport of tumor cell fragments by surgical instruments or the surgeon's gloved hands to sites away from the origin of the cancer. There are actual recorded instances in which this form of transplantation has occurred, and the possibility is certainly well documented by the use of this method in the experimental laboratory. It is, fortunately, an extremely rare pathway of dissemination in clinical practice, perhaps a tribute to the awareness of all surgeons of this possibility. The rarity may also be due to immune mechanisms or the tumor's inability to find suitable conditions for its survival and growth when introduced into viable tissues by this artificial means.

Lymphatic drainage provides the most common pathway for metastatic spread of carcinomas. While it is said that sarcomas rarely spread through lymphatics but instead tend to use the blood vessel route, both forms of cancer use either or both routes. Lymphatic involvement tends to follow the natural drainage paths of the site of tumorous involvement. Thus, bronchogenic carcinomas arising in the respiratory passages disseminate first to the tracheobronchial and mediastinal nodes (Fig. 3–9). Carcinoma of the breast drains first to the axillary nodes, but in time, other local groups of nodes along the internal mammary artery and supra- and infraclavicular regions might be seeded. When the tumor completely replaces the node, it may block the usual drainage paths and produce bizarre retrograde spread along secondary lymphatic channels. Thus, with mediastinal node involvement, one may find progressive extension retrogressively from there to the para-aortic nodes below the diaphragm. Once the tumor has become established in a lymph node, further dissemination may occur from this site.

Some oncologists do not consider regional lymph node spread as a form of metastasis. They view such spread as lymphatic drainage. The problem is not one of semantics alone, since in their view the lymph nodes provide a

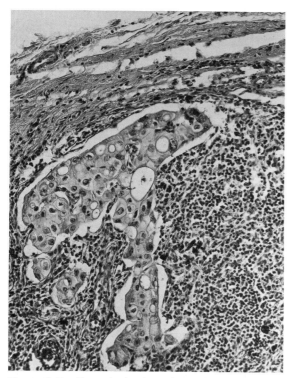

Figure 3–9. Spread of a bronchogenic carcinoma to a mediastinal lymph node. The tumor cells lie within a lymphatic channel.

primary line of defense against further dissemination. Thus, they argue that surgical removal of lymph nodes when not unmistakably involved by metastatic disease is not only unnecessary, but is also unwise since it destroys a defense line. This issue is one of the more vexed in the surgical treatment of cancer and has not yet been resolved.

Blood vessel invasion is the most important pathway of dissemination of tumor seedings to sites other than lymph nodes. Arteries are rarely penetrated, perhaps because of their thick muscular walls. However, they are not completely immune, and on occasion may be eroded, leading to massive, sometimes fatal hemorrhage. Veins and capillaries, with their thinner walls, are much more vulnerable. Certain cancers are notable for their ability to penetrate veins. The renal cell carcinoma can sometimes be found growing along the renal vein in a solid column of cells that occasionally extends up the inferior vena cava to enter the right side of the heart in a long, unbroken, snakelike cord. Hepatocellular carcinomas have the same propensity for invasion of the portal and hepatic veins. Blood vessel spread follows patterns dictated by the vessel involved and its usual pattern of flow. A carcinoma arising within the stomach or else-where in the gastrointestinal tract would first invade the tributaries of the portal vein and thus metastasize to the liver. Carcinomas in organs draining through the inferior and superior vena cavae are most often metastatic to the lung since the small tumor fragments (emboli) are filtered out in the pulmonary vascular bed. Cancers arising in the midline and in close proximity to the vertebral column, such as those of the prostate and thyroid, tend to embolize through the paravertebral plexus, and thus seed the vertebral column. It must be emphasized that in the microscopic study of a surgically removed cancer, invasion and penetration of blood vessels, lymphatics, and perineurial spaces are highly important observations in making a prognosis. They do not, however, necessarily indicate remote dissemination, since implantation may not have occurred and, as we shall see, many factors influence the ability of cancer cells to survive in their metastatic sites.

In a later section (p. 89) the mechanisms involved in the ability of malignant tumors to invade and metastasize will be considered. Although they remain for the most part mysterious, within them may lie the key to methods of controlling and conceivably eradicating cancer. Here we end our consideration of the features which serve to differentiate benign from malignant neoplasms with a recapitulation of the major points of comparison (Table 3–3).

GRADING AND STAGING OF CANCER

There is a great need for methods to quantify the probable clinical aggressiveness of a given neoplasm and, further, to express its apparent extent and spread in the individual patient. Comparisons of end results of various therapeutic modalities are meaningless unless the patients are comparable with respect to the nature, degree of malignancy and extent of their cancers. The end results of treating extremely small, highly differentiated thyroid adenocarcinomas which are localized to the thyroid gland will be very different from those obtained from treatment of highly anaplastic thyroid cancers which have invaded the neck organs.

The grading of a cancer attempts to establish some estimate of its aggressiveness or degree of malignancy based on the cytologic differentiation of tumor cells and the number of mitoses within the tumor. The cancer may be classified as grade I, II, III or IV with increasing anaplasia. Criteria for the individual grades vary with each form of neoplasia and so will not be detailed here. One of the most widely used grading systems is the so-called Broder's classification of squamous cell carcinomas of the skin. Unfortunately, histologic grading is not often a

TABLE 3–3. COMPARISONS BETWEEN BENIGN AND MALIGNANT TUMORS

CHARACTERISTICS	BENIGN TUMOR	MALIGNANT TUMOR
Differentiation and anaplasia	Resembles tissue of origin, absence of anaplasia	Less differentiated cells, often atypical, anaplasia often present
Mode and rate of growth	Usually progressive enlargement, slow growing	May enlarge progressively or erratically, fast growing
Spread of tumors	Expansile, localized, encapsulated	Unencapsulated, invasive, metastatic

helpful prognostic aid because often the correlation between the level of anaplasia of a neoplasm and its biologic behavior is not perfect.

The staging of cancers is based on the size of the primary lesion, its extent of spread to regional lymph nodes and the presence or absence of metastases. The two major agencies concerned with the staging of malignant disease are The International Union Against Cancer (UICC) and The American Joint Committee on Cancer Staging (AJCS). The UICC has evolved a so-called *TNM system*—T for primary tumor, N for regional lymph node involvement and M for metastases. This method of staging is applicable to all forms of neoplasia (Commission on Clinical Oncology, 1968). A specific neoplasm would be characterized using this system as T1, T2, T3 or T4, with increasing size of the primary lesion; N0, N1, N2 or N3, to indicate progressively advancing nodal disease; and M0 or M1 according to whether there are distant metastases. As will be seen in the consideration of certain forms of visceral cancer, the stage T1 is often further subdivided to indicate those lesions which are in-situ and those with minimal local invasion. Unfortunately, the American Joint Committee on Cancer Staging has adopted a different nomenclature and divides all cancers into stages 0 to IV, incorporating within such staging the size of primary lesions as well as the presence of nodal spread and of distant metastases (Copeland, 1965). It is not necessary here to attempt to reconcile these two systems of staging since examples will be cited in later chapters dealing with specific forms of cancer. There are still other classifications for specific forms of cancer, as for example Duke's classification of rectal carcinoma. It is obvious that the accuracy of cancer staging depends entirely on clinical appraisal of the extent of invasion and metastasis of the neoplasm. Errors must necessarily occur, since in one patient metastases may be obvious, whereas they remain occult in other patients. Nonetheless, these attempts at characterizing the extent of the neoplasm provide the basis of a common language in comparing the end results of various modalities of therapy. One hopes the endless controversies in the literature arising from claims and counterclaims about whose patients were "sicker" and therefore less amenable to cure will eventually disappear.

CARCINOGENESIS

It is widely known that the cause or causes of cancer still elude us, but sometimes the many inroads that have been made toward the resolution of this monumental problem are unappreciated. Many agents which produce cancer in animals and in man have been identified, and promising leads have been gained as to their mode of action. At the risk of evoking some alarm we must concede that the subject of carcinogenesis is only slightly less monumental than the disease itself. Here we will attempt to present only sufficient detail to provide a coherent story. We will discuss first some of the fundamental attributes of the cancer cell, then the agents known to be carcinogenic which impose some of these attributes, followed by theories on the mechanism or mechanisms by which such attributes are acquired.

ATTRIBUTES ACQUIRED BY CANCER CELLS

Fully evolved cancer cells differ in many respects from normal cells, and these differences are summed up in the term "*transformation.*" Such transformation may be *defined as an inheritable change in the characteristics and attributes of cells manifested by: loss of control of growth potential; loss of contact inhibition in culture; changes in morphology, antigenic structure, biochemistry and usually karyotype; as well as other poorly understood attributes involving the ability to invade and metastasize.* Transformation described in these terms relates to cells that have undergone total metamorphosis from the normal cell to the fully evolved cancer cell. There are many reasons for believing that a preneoplastic sequence of more subtle intracellular alterations, at levels not discernible by present techniques, precedes such complete transformation. There is also considerable evidence that the evolution from a normal cell population to a clinically overt cancer involves a number of discrete cell populations, each of which has more of the attributes of cancer cells than the preceding generation. Foulds (1969) terms this "tumor progression." A corollary of this concept proposes that up to a certain stage transformation may be reversible. Depending on the cell population, potency of the carcinogen, replicative activity of the cells and a number of other variables it can be shown in tissue culture that some clones of transformed cells will revert to normal (Rabinowitz and Sachs, 1968). Spontaneous regression of cancer in man has also been reported (Everson and Cole, 1966), but unfortunately as far as we know it is extremely rare. While transformation is not always irrevocable, in all likelihood reversion can occur only early in the process.

Some of the attributes of neoplastic transformation, particularly those relating to changes in cellular morphology, have already been mentioned in the discussion of anaplasia. Other attributes will be considered under the following headings: (1) loss of controls, (2) changes in antigens, (3) karyotypic changes, (4) biochemical changes, (5) membrane changes and (6) ability to invade and metastasize. Many biologic features are involved, some of which may be highly important to the fundamental nature of the cancerous process. *It is most important to stress at the outset that while one may suspect that neoplastic transformation has taken place in cells displaying some or all of these attributes, the ultimate and only reliable criterion is the ability of the transformed cell to give rise to a malignant tumor when implanted in an appropriate host.*

Loss of Control.

A dominant attribute of the transformed cancerous cell is its apparent escape from regulatory mechanisms which control the growth of normal cells. Such loss of control is most clearly demonstrable in cell culture. When normal cells capable of being cloned in an appropriate culture medium replicate, small colonies characterized by radial cords of cells migrating out from the center of the colony are created. The colonies tend to be flat, forming a monolayer of cells. When neighboring colonies impinge on each other the cells in contact with each other stop proliferating. This event is referred to as *contact inhibition.* In contrast, when cells are exposed to some oncogenic influence such as a virus or chemical carcinogen, those cells undergoing neoplastic transformation create colonies composed of tangled masses of cells piled up on each other in multiple layers. Proliferation is not inhibited by contact. Similarly, when cells derived from a cancer in man or animals are cloned in culture media, the colonies exhibit the same tangled, haphazard conformation, and contact inhibition is lost. Such behavior is attributed to loss of control mechanisms, but the precise nature of these controls is poorly understood (Abercrombie and Heaysman, 1954).

The controls may lie in the tissues; they may be systemic or even intracellular. In an earlier chapter mention was made of *chalones* (p. 60). You recall that these are tissue extracts which are capable of inhibiting mitosis in cultures of normal as well as tumor cells derived from the specific tissue yielding the extract. Thus chalones derived from normal epidermis are effective against cell cultures of epidermal cells derived from cancers (Editorial, 1973c). A systemic control might be "*immunologic surveillance.*" As will be seen, in the course of neoplastic transformation, cells develop specific antigenic profiles which differentiate these cells from all normal cells. In theory, the normal immune system should immediately destroy these antigenic deviants. Conceivably some breakdown in the immune mechanism or some change rendering the cells immunologically unrecognizable might permit the emergence of a cancer (Burnet, 1970). Indeed, defects in the immune system lower host resistance to carcinogenesis and increase the incidence of cancers (p. 108).

Despite these possibilities, *more credence is given at present to breakdown or loss of control mechanisms at the level of the cell.* Membrane alterations impairing cell to cell communication have been identified in cancer cells. A decreased number of specialized regions of contact (nexuses) in cancer cells has been demonstrated ultrastructurally (McNutt and Weinstein, 1969). Intercellular electrical connections, via ionic exchange, which occur among normal cells of various epithelia (Loewenstein, 1966) were not found among several forms of cells derived from human cancers (Kanno and Matsui, 1968). Gene mutations, affecting metabolic circuits involved in DNA, RNA and protein synthesis, and epigenetic alterations, involving gene expression and mRNA template stability, have all been described and provide plausible explanations for loss of intracellular regulatory controls (Green, 1970b; Harington, 1970; Mazia, 1970). More will be said about some of these changes in the following discussion.

Changes in Antigens.

As mentioned, the transformed or cancerous cell acquires a new antigenic profile which makes it immunologically distinct from all normal cells, including its normal forebears (Klein, 1968). All the known methods for producing tumors in animals (oncogenic viruses, carcinogenic chemicals and irradiation) evoke these tumor-specific antigens (TSA) in transformed cells, and TSA have been identified in many, if not all, cancers in humans.

Experimental tumors induced by oncogenic viruses, whether they are DNA or RNA viruses, have TSA specified by the virus. *Virtually all tumors induced by a common virus, whether in the same animal, in different animals of the same species or in different species, have identical tumor antigens.* While the antigens are virus-specific they are different from the antigens of the virion itself. Presumably these new antigens are coded for by the virus, although the precise mechanisms of DNA agents differ from those of RNA viruses. In contrast, *chemical- or radiation-induced tumors possess TSA which are different for each tumor and are not related to the carcinogen.* Thus even if several tumors were induced in the same animal by methylcholanthrene, each tumor would be antigenically different (Klein, 1969). It appears that most "spontaneous" cancers in man also possess TSA. There are striking differences in the antigenic potency of human tumor cells; although some possess relatively strong antigenic determinants, most are only weakly antigenic.

It has been shown in animals that TSA, apparently located within the cell membranes, can evoke an immune response in the host. They behave like normal histocompatibility antigens in transplant rejections. An experimental animal may thus develop an immune reaction against an induced cancer, but the response is weak. Immunity to the TSA can be better demonstrated by repeated injections of macerates of tumor cells or by a procedure which involves the induction of a neoplasm followed after an interval of time by excision of the tumor. Subsequent efforts to induce a neoplasm by inoculation of the same tumor cells will result in rejection of the tumor by the immune response of the host. Hence, these membrane-bound TSA are also referred to as tumor-specific transplantation antigens (TSTA).

In addition to these membrane-bound antigens, oncogenic DNA viruses also induce virus-specific *nuclear* antigens, referred to as T-antigens. Experimental cancers induced by RNA viruses, chemicals and radiation do not produce T-antigens. Located within the nuclei, these T-antigens are of interest because of the suspicion that they may be responsible for the oncogenic potential of DNA viruses. You recall that some forms of cancer produce fetal antigens (p. 115). These too represent neoantigens differentiating the tumor cells from their non-tumorous forebears.

It is clear that immune responses to tumors do develop in animals and humans bearing tumors (Hellstrom et al., 1969). *Tumor immunity takes the form of both humoral and cell-mediated responses.* The latter is undoubtedly the more important, as it is in the case of transplant rejection. Under appropriate in vitro conditions, it is possible to demonstrate destruction of cultured tumor cells by specific sensitized "killer" cells. Several key questions arise. Is the new antigenic profile "fundamental to the conversion of a normal cell to a neoplastic cell or is it merely a consequence of the change?" (Law, 1969). Moreover, why doesn't the host's immune response immediately reject the tumor once it has acquired its foreign antigenic profile? Finally, can these antigenic differences be exploited to the benefit of the patient? This last query will be addressed later in the discussion of clinical aspects of neoplasia (p. 109). With regard to the first question, it is as yet unclear whether neo-antigenicity is fundamental to the acquisition of cancerous attributes. On the one hand there is the fact that when cells are first transformed by certain viruses (the polyoma virus) they do not always have detectable TSA, suggesting that the antigenic changes are not essential to transformation (Hare, 1967). On the other hand, neo-antigenicity has been revealed in hyperplastic premalignant lesions and skin papillomas induced in experimental animals by chemical carcinogens (Lappé, 1969; Slemmer, 1972). These new antigenic profiles appeared in preneoplastic lesions and persisted in unchanged form until malignant neoplasms subsequently developed. Conceivably they might be important in the acquisition of the cancerous behavior.

Why the host's immunologic response fails to destroy a tumor bearing "foreign antigens" is still a mystery, although several possible explanations have been offered. (1) Tumor cells might proliferate so rapidly that by the time the immunologic response has been mounted the tumor has become so large it insulates its own centrally located cells from the immune reaction. (2) Prolonged exposure of the host to the antigens may induce immunologic paralysis or tolerance. (3) The immune response might not be cytotoxic. As will be discussed later, serum factors, possibly antibodies or free tumor antigens or antigen-antibody complexes, function in some way to block the destructive activity of sensitized lymphocytes (p. 109) (Baldwin et al., 1974; Hellstrom and Hellstrom, 1974). (4) Carcinogenesis itself may imply some defect in the immunologic responsiveness of the host. Indeed, there are many indications of reduced immunologic competence in patients with cancer (p. 108)

(Eilber and Morton, 1970; Liebowitz and Schwartz, 1973). The immune reaction is not always powerless, however, and there are instances in which immunity does aid in the control and possibly the regression of some neoplasms. Perhaps, in the last analysis, the normal individual develops many "incipient" cancers which fortunately are struck down in most of us by an effective immune response.

Karyotypic Changes. Chromosomal abnormalities characterize nearly all forms of human cancer except for many cases of acute leukemia and childhood cancers. These karyotypic abnormalities are very inconstant from case to case but they are very similar among the cells within one tumor (Atkin, 1970). The abnormalities take the form of changes in chromosome morphology or number or both. The weight of evidence favors the view that these changes in karyotype are acquired after the cancer cell has completely evolved, and do not underlie the transformation. As mentioned, in most cases of acute leukemia and in childhood cancers, the karyotypes may be normal. Occasional solid tissue cancers in adults also have completely normal karyotypes. In the experimental animal "minimal deviation" hepatocarcinomas are euploid (Nowell and Morris, 1969). There is, therefore, considerable evidence that *abnormalities in the karyotype are not requisite for transformation but are acquired during the evolution of cancer cells.* This in no way precludes the possibility that far more subtle alterations, such as point mutation, frame shift mutation, and deletion, duplication and rearrangement of genes, underlie the initiation of neoplastic transformation. Such alterations, of course, would not be visible in the karyotype. Indeed, it will become clear in the later presentation of the mechanisms of carcinogenesis (p. 100) that a considerable amount of evidence points toward some subtle, invisible mutation as the critical event in cancerous transformation of all cells.

Granting that visible karyotypic changes are probably late events in cancerous transformation, what are the acquired patterns of chromosomal abnormality and is there a specific marker for cancer? With respect to the first question, the range of karyotypic abnormality is almost limitless, extending from all manner of aneuploidy to all forms of individual chromosomal morphologic aberrations (Sandberg and Hossfeld, 1970). There is still a great deal of disagreement as to whether all the cells of a tumor exhibit the same karyotype. The weight of evidence suggests that the abnormalities, whatever their nature, tend to be rather constant within a tumor. It appears that all the cells arise from a single deviant cell. Despite this, some of the cells in a tumor differ from the others, at least to some extent. Knudson and his collaborators (1974) contend that such differences can be accounted for by sequential mutations in successive generations of cells. But some cancers clearly yield a bimodal distribution of karyotypes, indicating that more than one stem line is present. More will be said about the controversy surrounding the monoclonal or polyclonal origin of cancer later (p. 99).

Only one chromosomal marker identifying a specific form of neoplasia has been identified in nearly all patients. The abnormality is an abbreviated G-22 autosome known as the Philadelphia (Ph) chromosome, which is characteristic of chronic myelogenous leukemia. This abnormality is present in the normoblastic, megakaryocytic and granulocytic cells in all but a few patients having this form of leukemia (Nowell and Hungerford, 1960). At one time the Philadelphia chromosome was thought to be the consequence of a partial deletion of autosome 22, but recent reports indicate that the abnormality is due to a translocation of one of the long arms of autosome 22 to autosome 9 (Borgaonkar, 1973). It will be pointed out later that a few cases of chronic myelogenous leukemia do not have the Ph chromosome and these may represent a distinct disease variant (p. 354).

Biochemical Changes. The subject of the biochemical attributes acquired by cancer cells is both large and immensely complex. Several generalizations can be made. (1) None of the observed biochemical aberrations in cancer cells can be construed as hallmarks of cancer. (2) The better the differentiation of the cancer cell, the more nearly its enzyme profile resembles that of its normal forebears. (3) The more anaplastic and undifferentiated the tumor cell, the greater the deviation from the enzyme system of the normal cell. (4) *Ultimately all primitive anaplastic cells converge on a common simplified metabolic and enzyme pattern* sometimes referred to as "the biochemical uniformity of tumors." As always the question arises—is the observed aberration fundamental to the carcinogenic process or is it a secondary attribute acquired as a consequence of neoplastic transformation? Regrettably, at the present time this question cannot be answered with certainty.

Warburg observed that in cancer cells there is a return to a primitive pattern of anaerobic metabolism even in the presence of oxygen—so-called aerobic glycolysis—which is now recognized as a characteristic of all rapidly growing cells, neoplastic and non-neoplastic (Friedkin, 1973). Similarly, "the biochemical uniformity of tumors" reveals no profound insights into the nature of cancer. Weinhouse (1960) has aptly stated, "The highly neoplastic cell which has been transplanted many generations is like a stripped down racing car in which other metabolic activities have been subordinated to the overwhelming compulsion to divide." Support for this view comes from the study in rats of experimental hepatomas which range from "minimal deviation lesions" to rapidly growing anaplastic cancers (Morris, 1965). A slowly growing, highly differentiated "minimal deviation" hepatoma has virtually the same enzyme profile as the normal liver cell. The rapidly growing, poorly differentiated lesions show many biochemical deviations from the normal liver cell. The levels of some enzymes, such as phosphotransferases, aldolases, pyruvate kinases and phosphorylases, may be depleted or disappear in very undifferentiated tumors, whereas other enzymes, which are minimal or absent in the normal cell of origin, appear (Weinhouse, 1973). Indeed, the poorly differentiated cell in the very rapidly growing hepatocarcinoma comes to resemble the fetal liver cell and may even elaborate alpha fetal globulin. It has been proposed, but without proof, that shifts in enzymes are fundamental phenotypic alterations, stemming from altered gene expression, which enable the cancer cell to utilize metabolic "fuel" more efficiently for uncontrolled proliferation. Most investigators believe, however, that the biochemical changes in cancer cells are probably only incidental expressions of the aberrations of cell maturation or of the mutations involved in the process of neoplastic transformation.

Quite recently, *one biochemical attribute has been identified which appears to be common to all tumor cells—namely, the activation of fibrinolysins.* Indeed, fibrinolysis appears to be necessary for growth of tumor cells (Ossowski et al., 1973). Fibrinolytic activity is seen when cells are transformed in vitro by oncogenic viruses and chemical carcinogens, and it has also been found in a variety of human and animal tumor cell lines. The mechanism by which the neoplastic cells initiate fibrinolysis has been shown to depend on two protein factors. One is present in all vertebrate sera, the other is released by cells following transformation. The serum factor has been identified as plasminogen. The cell factor is an arginine-specific protease which activates plasminogen. These observations help to explain why cells transformed by oncogenic agents do not grow in the absence of serum (Temin et al., 1972). Moreover, although the active fibrinolysin, plasmin, has particularly high affinity for fibrinogen and fibrin, it is also a highly potent trypsin-like enzyme that is capable of degrading a wide variety of peptides. Could such activity favor the invasiveness and spread of cancer? The full significance of this fibrinolytic activity has not yet been fully explored but deserves close attention.

Membrane Changes. A host of alterations appear in the cellular membranes of cancerous cells, raising the possibility that *the fundamental nature of cancer might be loss of cell control as a consequence of membrane changes.* The membrane alterations take many forms. Loss of contact inhibition, discussed earlier (p. 60), might well be the consequence of membrane changes. Decreased adhesiveness of cancer cells, demonstrated by Coman (1944), has been explained by a number of observations which are not necessarily mutually exclusive. Normal epithelial cells, for example, have well established desmosomes which anchor one cell to another. The cells in tumors arising in such epithelia often fail to develop desmosomes. It has been reported that tumor cells have a higher negative surface charge than normal cells. This high negative charge tends to repel contiguous cells. There is reduction in the amount of calcium within tumor tissue, and this may be associated with decreased cell to cell anionic bonding (DeLong et al., 1950). Any one or all of these alterations would help to explain the decreased adhesiveness of cancer cells as a result of alterations in cellular membranes.

Another approach to the study of membrane changes in neoplastically transformed cells concerns the binding of certain phytoagglutinins (lectins). In general, cells which have been neoplastically converted in cell culture are more agglutinable by diverse lectins than are their normal forebears and presumably have more agglutinin receptors (Burger, 1970). Conceivably, bound agglutinin may contribute to the disordered clumped patterns of growth seen in malignant clones in cell culture. Normal growth can be restored by covering the agglutinin receptors with a monovalent agglutinin. However, it should be emphasized that similar agglutinability has been found in some non-tumor cells, and so the significance of these receptor sites as an attribute of neoplastic transformation is still doubtful (Hozumi et al., 1972).

It has also been reported that the membranes of cells in malignant growths are more permeable than are normal cellular membranes (Holley, 1972). It is proposed that cancer cells thus receive increased internal concentrations of nutrients that stimulate cell growth. It must not be forgotten that membrane changes may affect not only the plasma membrane but also those of the nucleus, mitochondria and endoplasmic reticulum, possibly leading to widespread metabolic and behavioral alterations. The significance of all these membrane alterations is still unclear, but Wallach (1968) proposes that *in the last analysis, cancer is a membrane disease.*

Capacity to Invade and Metastasize. It has already been pointed out that cancers in man usually have the capacity to erode, destroy and metastasize. These attributes are not necessarily present from the outset of neoplastic transformation. It may be that each of these attributes is acquired separately, possibly in a variable sequence. For example, the basal cell carcinoma of the skin is known to be a highly infiltrative, erosive form of cancer, once called a "rodent ulcer," yet it almost never metastasizes. In contrast, there are rare reported instances of in-situ carcinomas of the uterine cervical epithelium which have metastasized at a stage when the primary lesion was not yet grossly visible. Ordinarily in-situ cancers are thought to be incipient and, indeed, by definition have not invaded through the basement membrane. Thus invasiveness, destructiveness and the ability to metastasize may constitute separable attributes acquired sooner or later by most cancer cells, unfortunately acquired only too often by most clinically significant cancers of man.

The alterations which confer the capacity to invade on cancer cells are not well understood. At one time invasiveness was attributed to the expansile pressure of the growing mass. But pressure cannot explain the observation that when small fragments of normal and tumor tissue are placed in contact with each other in a culture flask, with ample room about them, the tumor cells preferentially invade the normal tissue (Easty and Easty, 1963). A number of changes may be relevant to invasiveness. Decreased adhesiveness might lead to a rapidly spreading form of growth. Loss of contact inhibition would appear to permit continued replication of cancer cells despite the constraints of the normal surrounding tissue. Elaboration of enzymes, such as fibrinolysins, which are also capable of degrading peptides probably contributes to invasiveness. The high metabolic activity of tumor cells might release increased amounts of lactic acid and other metabolites into their microenvironment, which could injure surrounding normal cells and pave the way for invasion. An immunologic reaction with consequent inflammatory edema might open tissue planes. As has been pointed out in the review of this subject by Easty (1966), however, all of these speculations remain unproved, and so the precise basis for invasiveness is still poorly understood.

Metastatic dissemination of a cancer is obviously its most feared consequence. There has been, therefore, considerable study of the factors involved in the ability of cancer cells to disseminate through the pathways already described. It is reasonably well established that the mere dissemination of cancer cells through the bloodstream or via the lymphatics cannot be equated with the appearance of metastases. Even when 250,000 cancer cells were injected into the bloodstream of experimental animals, approximately 20 per cent of the animals failed to develop metastases (Fisher and Fisher, 1959a). That immunity may play a role in protection against metastasis can be shown in the experimental animal, but the evidence for this in man is still scant.

Obviously the ability of isolated cancer cells or small clusters of cells to remain viable in transport through the blood vessels, lymphatics or natural body cavities is involved in metastatic spread. This attribute might relate to their increased growth vigor. Decreased adhesiveness of cancer cells, which permits their separation from the local primary growth, is also involved in metastasis. But the necessity for the cell or clump of cells (tumor emboli) to lodge in some site where it can develop its own blood supply is probably most important. The elaboration of an *"angiogenesis factor"* has been postulated (p. 79). Metastases are not common in the spleen. It has been argued that the narrow but thick-walled penicilliary arterioles of this organ trap emboli before they reach the thin-walled sinusoids of the spleen, which might permit penetration and implantation of tumor cells. This explanation may be simplistic, however, because it is well documented that melanocarcinoma frequently metastasizes to the spleen. Moreover, although the richness of the blood supply would seem to affect the probability of blood-borne dissemination to an organ, we find that striated muscle, one of the most richly supplied tissues of the body, is a rare site of metastasis. Could the contractile motions of muscle block the lodgment of tumor emboli? Again, why does the bronchogenic carcinoma, after it spreads to the regional lymph nodes, have such a predilection for the adrenal glands that the lymph nodes and the adrenals may be the only sites of metastatic dissemination (Fig. 3–10)? Much remains to be learned.

Other influences may be important. In experimental animals surgical trauma or the administration of cortisone or pituitary extracts increases the number of metastases and, contrariwise, hypophysectomy inhibits the formation and growth of certain forms of metas-

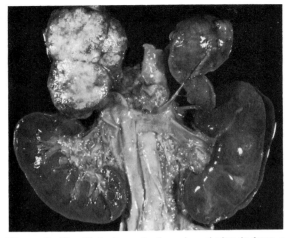

Figure 3–10. Metastases to the adrenal glands from a bronchogenic carcinoma. The gland at the left has been hemisected to reveal the extent of the cancer (note that the kidneys are unaffected).

tases (Fisher and Fisher, 1959b, 1961). These observations underscore the endocrine dependence of certain forms of cancer. Similarly, some cancers in man are more or less hormone dependent (pp. 554 and 588). Metastatic carcinomas of the female breast and endometrium may be arrested in their growth by ovariectomy. In general, however, ablation of endocrine glands yields only temporary remissions rather than dramatic cures.

In closing, it should be pointed out that, as a rule, *the more undifferentiated or anaplastic a cancer, the greater is its potential for invasion and metastasis.* However, there are many exceptions to this rule; many well differentiated lesions metastasize widely and many poorly differentiated lesions do not metastasize. It follows, therefore, that frequently there is a great discrepancy between the "deceptively bland look" (differentiation) of a malignant tumor and its vicious behavior; the converse is also possible. This often repeated observation has given rise to a concept of *biological predeterminism* (MacDonald, 1951). It is postulated that the growth rate and aggressiveness of cancer are genetic characteristics of the individual tumor. As we have said, the qualities of differentiation, proliferation, invasiveness and dissemination are separate attributes of the cancer cell, which may be acquired independently. Thus, some differentiated tumors may have an inherent capacity to metastasize, whereas others may have a different genotype and phenotype. While we may generalize about cancer as a biological phenomenon, the individual patient may be an exception. Many a cancer patient who might reasonably have been expected to die within a year has outlived his doctor!

CARCINOGENIC AGENTS AND THEIR CELLULAR INTERACTIONS

A wide variety of agents capable of inducing cancer in experimental animals has been identified, including: (1) chemical carcinogens, (2) oncogenic viruses and (3) radiation. Moreover, certain chemicals and radiation have likewise been shown to be responsible for some cancers in man and the evidence implicating viruses grows stronger daily. While it is impossible to present the entire catalogue of carcinogens here, some of the more important follow.

Chemical Carcinogens. The first carcinogens discovered were chemicals. They are of great interest for several reasons. First, one would like to discover a common denominator for the many carcinogenic chemicals, and indeed hints have begun to emerge. Second, some investigators estimate that as many as 80 to 90 per cent of all human cancers are attributable to chemicals (Higginson, 1972). It is now 200 years since the London surgeon Sir Percival Pott related scrotal skin cancer in British chimney sweeps to exposure to soot. Three years later, inspired by this observation, the Danish Chimney Sweeps Guild ruled that its members must bathe daily. No public health measure since that time has achieved so much in the control of a form of cancer! It was not until 1915 that Yamagiwa and Ichikawa reawakened interest in Pott's observation by inducing cancer in a rabbit's ear by repeated applications of coal tar. Subsequently Kennaway and Cook isolated from crude coal tars the much more potent, pure polycyclic hydrocarbons. Since then hundreds of chemicals have been shown to cause cancer. Contemporary studies have suggested that many of these agents are actually precarcinogens, which must be metabolically converted to proximate carcinogens and then perhaps further activated to ultimate carcinogens (Heidelberger, 1973; Miller and Miller, 1966). Some of the major classes of chemical agents will be discussed briefly, followed by a consideration of common properties which may be of significance in their carcinogenicity (Miller, 1970a).

Polycyclic aromatic hydrocarbons are among the strongest chemical carcinogens. Best studied are 7,12-dimethyl benz(a)anthracene; dibenz(a,i)anthracene; benzo(a)pyrene; and 3-methylcholanthrene. All induce in vitro neoplastic transformation of a variety of cell types derived from many animal species as well as cancers in vivo in most laboratory animals. They evoke neoplasms when painted on the skin or when introduced subcutaneously or into specific organs. Such universality is a characteristic of very strong carcinogens. It is now established that these *hydrocarbons must be metabolically converted to proximate or ultimate carcinogens.* A series of studies undertaken by Boyland and by Sims and co-workers have documented that microsomal enzymes of cellular origin, such as those in liver cells, oxidize benzo(a)pyrene and dibenz(a,i)anthracene to form epoxides (Boyland, 1950; Grover and Sims, 1970). The epoxides bind covalently to cell proteins and preferentially to the guanine residues of the polynucleotides, RNA and DNA (Hoffman et al., 1970). Binding to DNA appears to correlate most closely with the carcinogenicity of the hydrocarbon metabolite (Duncan and Brookes, 1972). It therefore appears that *hydrocarbons exert their effect via reactive epoxides which, by binding with DNA, cause a point mutation or other permanent alteration in the template.* However, the possibility of altering the expression of DNA by, for example, the binding to repressor proteins cannot be ruled out.

Man, like other species, is vulnerable to the effects of polycyclic hydrocarbons. Reference has already been made to the scrotal cancer of chimney sweeps. Very likely the lung cancers of cigarette smokers are additional lamentable examples. It has been observed recently that an enzyme which can be isolated from lung tissue—aryl hydrocarbon hydroxylase—may be responsible for transforming certain of the polycyclic hydrocarbons in smoke residues into an ultimate carcinogen, i.e., an epoxide (Kellerman et al., 1974).

Several *azo dyes* and *aromatic amines*, such as N-dimethyl-4-aminoazobenzene (DMAB) or "butter yellow"; N-methyl-4-aminoazobenzene (MAB); 2-acetyl aminofluorene (AAF); and 2-naphthylamine are potent carcinogens. Studies of these agents led to our first understanding of the phenomenon of metabolic conversion to proximate or ultimate carcinogens (Miller and Miller, 1966). It had long been known that feeding MAB to rats induced tumors in the liver but not in the gastrointestinal tract. It is now clear that MAB is metabolized in the liver. The proximate carcinogens of both MAB and AAF are their N—OH— esters, and for AAF the major carcinogenic metabolite has been identified as the sulfuric acid ester (DeBaun et al., 1970). *Whereas the ultimate metabolites bind covalently to proteins and to RNA, it appears that their carcinogenicity relates principally to their ability to bind preferentially to the eighth carbon of guanine in DNA* (Matsushima and Weisburger, 1969). Metabolites of DMAB and 2-naphthylamine also form strong bonds to liver DNA. Thus it appears that, like polycyclic hydrocarbons, the aromatic amines require conversion to ultimate carcinogens which ultimately bind to cellular macromolecules, particularly to DNA, and so alter cell structure and function.

Man, too, is susceptible to the effects of aromatic amines. Workers in aniline dye and rubber industries have a strikingly increased incidence of bladder cancer related to their exposure to 2-naphthylamine. This volatile agent, absorbed through the skin and lungs, induces its effects in the bladder, suggesting that some metabolite present in the urine is the ultimate carcinogen. It is sobering to realize that DMAB was once used as a food coloring agent in margarine and that AAF was developed as a potential insecticide. The contribution these may have made to neoplasia in man has not been established.

Alkylating agents are important carcinogens, and they probably provide the clearest insight into the basic mechanism of action of all chemical carcinogens. Alkylating agents such as nitrosamines and betapropiolactones are known mutagens. *The nitrosamines are transformed, either enzymatically or nonenzymatically, into agents that donate methyl and ethyl groups to RNA and DNA.* Both the N–7 of guanine and the O–6 of guanosine are the specific receptor sites for the methyl and ethyl groups (Loveless, 1969). Guanines so alkylated pair with thymine rather than with cytosine, thus creating a mutation. It appears that here, too, binding to DNA, rather than to RNA or proteins, is the critical event in the carcinogenic action of the alkylating agents (Colburn and Boutwell, 1966, 1968a, 1968b). The *nitrosamines* have evoked considerable interest recently because of the possibility that they might be formed in the body from various amine precursors and nitrites (Editorial, 1973b). Nitrites are added to food as preservatives. Many amines are normally present in food. Sander (1971) established that a number of secondary amines are nitrosated under the conditions of temperature and acidity found in the mammalian stomach. Whether such nitrosation occurs in man is difficult to judge, but is obviously worrisome. In any event it is clear that tumors can be induced in a wide range of animal species by nitrosamines, and man is probably not immune.

A host of *other chemicals* have been identified as carcinogens (Miller, 1970a). Some are inorganic and some are naturally occurring compounds found in the foodstuffs of animals and man. A wide variety of inorganic chemicals has been shown to be carcinogenic in animals, and some are implicated in the causation of human cancer. Beryllium, cadmium, chromium, cobalt, iron, lead, nickel, selenium, zinc and titanium have all been shown to be carcinogenic following administration to experimental animals. Arsenic has been implicated in the causation of cancer in man. Similarly, nickel is suspected of being carcinogenic for man (Sunderman, 1971). An increased number of cases of lung cancer and nasal sinus cancer has been reported among nickel workers. While these workers were also exposed to the inhalation of other metals, most of the evidence points to nickel as the primary carcinogen.

As mentioned, carcinogens have been identified in a variety of naturally occurring substances (Miller, 1973), including our food (Crosby et al, 1972). Food may also contain substances that alter metabolism and enhance the response to carcinogens (Sabine et al., 1973). Reference has already been made to nitroso-compounds in foods. Particularly interesting among the possible carcinogens found in food are the *aflatoxins produced by many strains of Aspergillus flavus*. These molds can grow on almost any vegetable in warm, moist conditions. In particular, large amounts of aflatoxins may contaminate badly stored and harvested peanuts (ground nuts), corn or cotton seed. Aflatoxin B_1 has been shown to be a potent hepatocarcinogen for many species of animals, including trout, ferrets and rats. Aflatoxins have been identified in market samples of food for man, especially in tropical countries such as India and Africa (Editorial, 1973a). Peers and Linsell (1973), in a large survey, documented that the incidence of liver cancer in a district of Kenya correlated directly with the level of aflatoxin intake in the daily diet. The total cancer incidence in this district was 19.9 per 100,000 per year. Liver cancer alone contributed 10.8 and 3.8 cases per 100,000 per year in men and women respectively. Indirect evidence exists that aflatoxin B_1 is activated by liver enzymes and binds to DNA (Goldblatt, 1969). Another mold-derived carcinogen for animals is *actinomycin D*. This antibiotic binds to DNA through hydrogen bonds (Svoboda, 1970). One wonders whether man may be at risk through his sometimes indiscriminate use of antibiotics.

A long list of other chemical carcinogens might be detailed. Ethionine, which is strongly carcinogenic to rat liver, is an analogue of the amino acid methionine. It appears to donate an ethyl group to various macromolecules. Stilbestrol has evoked some concern. Recent reports state that adolescent girls whose mothers received stilbestrol for threatened abortion have an increased risk of carcinoma of the vagina (Herbst et al., 1971, 1975) (p. 563). It still is not clear whether the carcinogenic action is related directly to the estrogenic effect of the synthetic hormone or instead is related to one of its metabolites. The

hormone may act merely as a stimulator of cell proliferation, rendering the vaginal cells susceptible to other carcinogenic influences. More will be said about this in the later discussion of the mechanism of action of carcinogens. The implied passage of the hormone or some metabolite across the placenta is also of interest. A doleful roster of the agents demonstrated to be carcinogenic in man is cited in Table 3–4, which is drawn from the report of Heidelberger (1973). It is safe to say that we have only begun to probe the depths of the "sea of carcinogens in which we swim."

The study of chemical carcinogens and their cellular interactions has contributed significantly to the understanding of a number of fundamental principles involved in carcinogenesis. As Ryser (1971) has recently pointed out, the following are basic to the biology of chemical carcinogenesis: (1) the effects of carcinogens are dose dependent, additive and irreversible, (2) carcinogenesis does not occur immediately but requires a period of time, (3) whatever the cellular changes involved, they are transmitted to daughter cells, (4) carcinogenesis can be influenced by factors that are not themselves truly carcinogenic and (5) carcinogenesis requires cell proliferation. These points will now be briefly discussed.

A specific threshold amount of a carcinogen is required to induce cancers in vivo and to transform cells in vitro. Above this amount, a dose dependency has been shown in a number of careful quantitative studies. The number of cells transformed in vitro is proportional to the amount of carcinogen above the basal minimal level. Moreover, the sequential addition of small doses has the same potency as a single administration of a comparable total dose. This observation indicates that whatever the effect, it is additive. Thus, cancers might emerge from the summation of a number of small "hits." Moreover, it indicates that *the critical event inflicted by the carcinogen is fixed in the cell and is apparently not subject to significant repair.*

TABLE 3–4. CHEMICALS RECOGNIZED AS CARCINOGENS IN HUMANS*

AGENT	AFFECTED ORGAN
Soots, tars, oils	Skin, lungs
Cigarette smoke	Lungs
2-Naphthylamine, benzidine, 4-aminobiphenyl, 4-nitrobiphenyl	Urinary bladder
N, N-bis (2-chloroethyl)-2-naphthylamine	Urinary bladder
bis (2-chloroethyl)-sulfide	Lungs
Nickel compounds	Lungs, nasal sinuses
Chromium compounds	Lungs
Asbestos	Lungs, pleura

*From Heidelberger, C.: Current trends in chemical carcinogenesis. Reprinted from FEDERATION PROCEEDINGS, *32*: 2154, 1973.

A time lag exists between the administration of a chemical carcinogen and the induction of cancerous transformation. The duration of the lag or latent period depends upon a number of factors, including the susceptibility of the cell and the dose and potency of the carcinogenic agent. In cell cultures morphologic changes can be seen within hours or days, but when such transformed cells are inoculated into appropriate hosts they almost always fail to produce tumors. Only after an absolute minimum period of latency, generally of the order of 50 or more days, will tumor growth in isologous hosts be evoked by the transferred cells. During this latent period the cells are dividing and may, in fact, have passed through up to 30 generations. Over this time a number of behavioral and karyotypic changes may appear (Sivak and Van Duuren, 1968). It is evident, then, that *true malignant transformation, capable of evoking tumors in appropriate hosts, must be preceded by some finite period of premalignant change.*

The cellular change evoked by a carcinogen is transmitted to daughter cells. This phenomenon can be demonstrated in a variety of experimental systems. For example, in vivo it may take as long as a year for a skin cancer to be produced in the mouse following a single application of an appropriate dose of carcinogen. We know that the generation cycle for mouse skin cells is approximately six days; therefore, many generations of cells must have developed from the original treated cells. *Obviously the critical cancerous change is heritable from one generation of cells to the next.* The events of this period of latency, however, are still not completely understood. Some speculations will be offered when we discuss current theories on the ultimate mechanisms involved in carcinogenesis.

That carcinogens can be influenced by factors not themselves truly carcinogenic is an important aspect of the biologic process, as was brilliantly shown by Berenblum in 1941. He demonstrated that non-tumorigenic doses of a carcinogen might be coupled with the action of other agents such as croton oil or phenol (themselves virtually non-carcinogenic) to evoke a cancer. He referred to the carcinogenic agent as the *initiator* and the croton oil as the *promoter.* This observation was important because it documented the facts that more than one step may be involved in the transformation of a normal cell to a cancer cell, and that sequential modifications can bring about the transformation process. Since this pioneer work it has been shown that the active constituents of croton oil are phorbol esters. When used alone in high concentrations, these esters may themselves lead to a low tumor incidence. However, even in low dosages they have a promoting effect which will lower the "threshold" of response to carcinogenic initiators. *The principal action of promoters appears to be stimulation of cell replication* (Hennings and Boutwell, 1970). It can be shown in skin cells that proliferative activity increases markedly following a single application of croton oil, reaches a maximum within 24 hours and returns to normal within 72 hours. Even when the promoter is applied long after the initiator its effect is not diminished, but if the promoter is applied first and the initiator follows at some later time (more than 72 hours later), the result is essentially that which would be obtained by the initiator alone. *Thus the stimulatory effect of the promoter is limited or reversible, while that of the initiator is probably irreversible.*

The fact that cellular proliferation enhances the carcinogenicity of initiators helps to explain a number of clinical observations. It has long been known that patients with cirrhosis of the liver are particularly vulnerable to the development of hepatocarcinomas. Presumably the regenerative activity in such damaged livers potentiates the emergence of the cancer. Chronic cervicitis is a frequent antecedent to cellular dysplasia, which in turn is ultimately transformed to carcinoma of the cervix in a significant number of patients. It has long been known that hormones may influence cancer production in animals, and it has long been suspected that, particularly when hormones are present in excess, they may have the same effect in humans. For example, high levels of estrogen may contribute to breast cancer in women (Noble, 1964) (p. 587). Whether hormones exert their effect by acting as initiators or as promoters is not known. The role of cellular proliferation in the process of carcinogenesis is still uncertain. Conceivably, it may permit the most deviant cells to outgrow the more normal cells. More likely, cell proliferation (mitotic division) in some way amplifies or fixes an early critical carcinogenic event.

In brief review, the study of chemical carcinogenesis has yielded the following facts about the emergence of a cancer. Initiating agents evoke dose-dependent, additive and irreversible changes that are transmitted to all the progeny of the affected cells. Some latent (?pre-neoplastic) period must follow between initiation and the emergence of a demonstrable tumor, during which time repeated cell divisions occur. The implication is strong that sequential steps, possibly involving multiple mutations or other events, may be taking place during the replication of "initiated" cells.

Oncogenic Viruses. Few topics have produced sharper polarization of experimental

TABLE 3–5. ONCOGENIC VIRUSES*

A. DNA Viruses (about 50)
  1. Papilloma (Shope) Virus Group
      papilloma viruses of rabbit, man, dog, cows, and others
  2. Polyoma Virus Group
      polyoma (Py) virus (murine)
      simian virus (SV 40)
  3. Adenoviruses
      human adenoviruses (31 strains, at least 12 of which induce tumors in newborn animals and/or transform cells in vitro)
      simian adenoviruses (6 viruses)
      avian adenoviruses
      bovine adenoviruses
  4. Herpes Viruses
      ? Burkitt's lymphoma (man) — Epstein-Barr virus (EBV)
      ? Nasopharyngeal carcinoma (man) — Epstein-Barr virus (EBV)
      ? Cervical cancer in women — Herpes virus II
      Lucke's carcinoma (frog)
      Marek's disease (chicken)
      Lymphoreticular disease (owl monkey and marmosets) — herpes saimiri
B. RNA Viruses (about 100)
  1. Avian Leukemia-Sarcoma (Rous) Viruses (20 or more)
  2. Murine Leukemia-Sarcoma Viruses
  3. Murine Mammary Tumor Virus (3 types)
  4. Leukemia-Sarcoma Viruses of Cat, Hamster, Rat and Guinea Pig

*Modified from Dr. M. Green. Reproduced with permission from "Oncogenic viruses," Annual Review of Biochemistry, Volume 39, p. 701. Copyright © 1970 by Annual Reviews, Inc. All rights reserved.

oncologists than the issue of viruses as possible carcinogens in man. One group believes that proof that viruses cause certain neoplasms in man is almost at hand, while others contend that the evidence for viral oncogenesis in man is at best fragmentary, and at worst, greatly overblown. All agree, however, that some viruses are incontrovertibly oncogenic in animals. A list of some of the known oncogenic viruses and those highly suspect is offered in Table 3–5. A few details follow about some of the more significant of these viruses.

The *DNA viruses* are able to induce tumors in certain animals and to transform susceptible cells in vitro. *The introduction of DNA viruses, such as SV 40 and Py, into cell cultures leads to one of two results: (1) productive infection, i.e., replication of the virus accompanied by destruction and lysis of permissive cells (those derived from natural hosts) or (2) abortive infection with neoplastic transformation of up to 40 per cent of nonpermissive cells (those derived from non-natural hosts).* The species specificity of viruses is singularly rigid. The SV 40 virus, for example, lyses monkey cells, but is oncogenic in hamsters and multimammate mice. In culture it transforms cells from rats, mice, guinea pigs or rabbits, but it does not cause tumors when introduced in vivo into these animals. It is important to note that once transformation has occurred, no infectious DNA virions are released, nor can the virus be isolated directly from transformed cells. The evidence now suggests that the viral DNA is incorporated into the host cell DNA, analogous to the lysogenized state of bacteria infected with bacteriophage. The viral agent can be identified in such transformed cells by "rescue techniques," i.e., fusion of the transformed cells with permissive cells, causing cell lysis and release of mature infectious virions. The significance of these findings will be discussed presently.

The *papilloma, polyoma* and simian *vacuolating viruses* (SV 40) are grouped together as the *papova viruses.* Within this group the papilloma virus, in addition to inducing lesions in lower animals, is responsible for *the common wart and mucosal papilloma in man. These two lesions are the only proven viral tumors in man, and it should be noted that both of the lesions are benign.* The Py (polyoma) virus was isolated from adult mice, in which species it produces no apparent ill effect. When injected into newborn rodents, however, it is capable of producing several types of tumors (parotid, kidney, breast and connective tissue), hence its designation "polyoma." The SV 40 and Py viruses are extremely small and possess only enough genetic information to code for about 5 to 10 proteins of 20,000 molecular weight. This fact is of interest in terms of the number of viral genes needed to induce cancerous transformation.

The adenoviruses, of medium size, include 50 or more strains, 31 of which have been isolated from humans. The adenoviruses cause acute respiratory and ocular disease in man but have not been shown to cause cancer. Green (1970a) assayed 130 human tumors for adenovirus mRNA and found none. However, when introduced into a cell culture of nonpermissive cells, adenoviruses are able to induce transformation.

"Question: *do herpesviruses cause cancer in man?* Answer: of course they do" — so reads the title of a recent editorial by Rapp (1973). Not everyone would agree with this bluntly stated point of view, but the evidence supporting it, particularly in the case of Burkitt's lymphoma, is interesting and provocative. *Following are some of the basic observations relating the herpes-like Epstein-Barr virus (EBV) to Burkitt's lymphoma.* To begin with, it is known that a herpes virus is the cause of a lymphoid tumor of chickens known as Marek's disease. Another herpes virus (Herpes saimiri) is responsible for a rapidly growing fatal lymphoreticular tumor in the owl monkey and marmoset. Both of these disorders of lower animals closely resemble Burkitt's lymphoma in man. Viral genome has been identified in lymphoblasts cultured from Burkitt's lymphoma of man (zurHausen et al., 1972). The viral DNA is known to be associated with host cell DNA, although the nature of the molecular connection remains unclear. Exposure of normal human lymphoid cells of fetal origin to the EBV induces in these cells the following changes: (1) the morphology of the cell is changed to a blastoid form, (2) continuous proliferation is induced, (3) the cells may be carried in long term culture, a characteristic not ordinarily found in the absence of a transforming virus and (4) other alterations characteristic of fully evolved cancer cells are present (Epstein and Achong, 1973). All patients with Burkitt's lymphoma have high titers of antibodies to the virus, contrasting with much lower antibody titers in approximately 50 per cent of normal controls (Klein, 1972). In sum, cells derived from the Burkitt's lymphoma appear to possess the viral genome. The EBV brings about apparent malignant transformation of lymphoid cells in vitro with continuous proliferation of these cells, and patients with this lymphoma have immunologic evidence of exposure to the EBV (Henle and Henle, 1974). However, it should be pointed out that the virus has not been isolated directly from neoplastic tissue, nor can it be "rescued." Thus, the evidence is still circumstantial.

It is of interest in this regard that the EBV is established as the cause of infectious mononucleosis, a disorder characterized by striking inflammatory proliferation of the lymphoid tissue throughout the body (Allen and Cole, 1972). It is hypothesized that the EBV is a widely prevalent agent to which a great many individuals are exposed early in life. Most have only a subclinical infection and develop an effective immunity to this agent without ever having demonstrated the classic manifestations of infectious mononucleosis. Some, however, develop overt infectious mononucleosis. According to this hypothesis there is a third group of individuals who, on exposure, develop levels of immunity sufficient to prevent infectious mononucleosis but not to eradicate the virus. Such individuals are at risk of developing Burkitt's lymphoma. Conceivably, a cofactor, such as concurrent infection which stimulates the reticuloendothelial system (?malaria), or some immunodepressant influence, potentiates the oncogenic activity of the virus and the development of Burkitt's lymphoma. More will be said about this causal relationship later (p. 348) but for now it is sufficient to say that the EBV is strongly suspected of being the cause of Burkitt's lymphoma. In closing this discussion, it should be mentioned that the EBV is also implicated in

the causation of carcinoma of the nasopharynx (Allen and Cole, 1972).

A herpes simplex virus (type 2 or genital herpes virus) has recently been implicated in the causation of cancer of the uterine cervix, but the evidence is not as strong as that regarding Burkitt's lymphoma (Melnick et al., 1974). Significant findings include: (1) The epidemiology of cervical cancer and genital herpes virus infection are remarkably similar. (2) Neutralizing antibodies to the virus are more often present in cervical cancer patients than in controls. (3) Women with genital herpes virus infections have a higher incidence of cervical epithelial abnormalities. (4) Viral antigens have been visualized by immunofluorescence in cervical cancer cells. These provocative findings are considered in greater detail on page 566.

Some *RNA viruses* called "leukoviruses" or "oncornaviruses" are also oncogenic. In contrast to the oncogenic DNA viruses, the oncornaviruses cause cancer in their natural hosts, which include a wide variety of vertebrates, including mammals. The first oncogenic viruses discovered, by Ellerman and Bang in 1908, proved to be RNA viruses after it had been shown that they caused chicken leukemia. They were also identified as the cause of pigeon sarcoma by Rous in 1911, of mammary tumors in mice by Bittner in 1936, of mouse leukemia by Gross in 1951 and of mouse sarcoma by Harvey in 1965 and by Moloney in 1966 (Allen and Cole, 1972). *Unlike the DNA viruses, the oncornaviruses not only transform the cells of their natural host but also replicate in them simultaneously.* Thus even in transformed cells a steady state is reached in which some nearly constant number of virions is produced in each cell every hour. Despite the release of infectious virions by transformed cells, transmission of the infectious agent horizontally (from one infected animal to another susceptible host) is generally not possible, although transmission may occur vertically (congenitally).

RNA viral particles usually can be seen with the electron microscope in infected cells. These particles take one of several forms. Those associated with leukemia and sarcoma in animals, "C-particles," consist of a dense central spherical nucleoid, 40 nanometers (nm) in diameter, symmetrically separated from its outer spiked envelope by a narrow electron-lucent space. The RNA mammary tumor viruses, described as "B-particles," have a nucleoid of similar size, which is quite frequently eccentric rather than centrally placed within its outer envelope. Often these particles appear to be formed by budding from the host cell membrane. "A-particles" are dense ring or doughnut-shaped forms which are thought to be precursors of both the C- and B-particles.

For a long time, the manner by which RNA viruses produce heritable changes in successive generations of transformed cells challenged the imagination. It was speculated that in some way the RNA viral genome altered the DNA of the host cell. The first breakthrough came with the observation that actinomycin D, which inhibits RNA transcription from DNA templates, blocked viral production. It was then shown that no virus would be produced by transformed cells if cellular DNA synthesis was blocked. Moreover, homology between RNA from Rous sarcoma virus and portions of DNA from virus infected cells was demonstrated. All this evidence suggests that cell replication is necessary for viral synthesis and that the DNA of transformed cells somehow contains the information for synthesis of the viral RNA. Temin and Baltimore then independently documented the existence of an RNA-directed DNA polymerase associated with oncornaviruses (Temin and Mizutani, 1970; Baltimore, 1970). *The RNA-directed DNA polymerase, better known as "reverse transcriptase," synthesizes DNA using the viral RNA as a template.* Then recombination of this viral DNA with the cellular DNA alters the genome of the host cell, inducing neoplastic transformation. With replication of the transformed cell the viral-coded DNA is simultaneously replicated and so the information for synthesis of viral RNA is incorporated into all transformed cells. The DNA incorporated into the genome of the host cell is thus referred to as "provirus."

It has now been shown that *the RNA-dependent DNA polymerase is a universal attribute of RNA tumor viruses* (Spiegelman et al., 1970a). By molecular hybridization the DNA incorporated into transformed cells has been shown to be complementary to the viral RNA. The single stranded viral RNA functions as a template for a single strand of DNA. For integration into the genome of mammalian cells, the single stranded DNA must be converted into double stranded DNA. Such conversion might require a DNA-directed DNA polymerase and, indeed, Spiegelman and his associates (1970b), among others, have demonstrated DNA-directed DNA polymerase in virions of several of the RNA oncogenic viruses. Whether the DNA-directed DNA polymerase is a separate enzyme from the reverse transcriptase or instead represents two activities of the same enzyme is unclear. Recently reverse transcriptase was identified in several viruses which induce respiratory diseases in sheep. This evidence appeared to contradict the dogma that RNA-dependent DNA polymerase implied oncogenicity. Subsequently it was proved that these "slow viruses" (so-called because the incubation periods of the diseases span months to years) are capable of inducing transformation of mouse embryo cells (Takemoto and Stone, 1971). More surprising was the isolation of "reverse transcriptase" from normal cells (Mizutani, 1973). However, as we shall soon see, this finding is compatible with some of the newer theories of RNA viral oncogenesis which follow.

Studies of RNA viral oncogenesis have led to some surprise findings and much speculation. Apparently uninfected chick cells can be made to yield oncornaviruses (Hanafusa et al., 1970), and it can be shown that these presumably normal cells contain DNA homologous to the RNA of the oncornaviruses (Baluda and Nayak, 1970). To explain these observations two intriguing theories have been offered. One, promulgated by Todaro and Huebner (1972), proposes that the genome of many and perhaps all vertebrate species contains information for the synthesis of RNA tumor viruses. It is transmitted from cell to cell and from animal to animal as a repressed gene (*"virogene"*). Chemical or other carcinogenic influences may derepress only the information in the virogene necessary for oncogenic transformation. This specific information within the virogene is referred to as the *"oncogene."* According to this theory, then, a repressed capability for oncogenicity is present in all cells. Provocative as the theory may be, it has been impossible to identify such repressed malignant genetic information in normal human cells, and the oncogene theory has been seriously challenged (Temin, 1974; Spiegelman et al., 1974).

The *"protovirus"* theory of Temin (1971), on the other hand, postulates that particles with virus-like properties are involved in intercellular communications in normal cells. These particles, which probably contain RNA, pass between all cells. Once in the recipient cell the RNA may be inscribed in the DNA by "reverse transcriptase." Modification of the normal protovirus by radiation or chemicals might yield an oncogenic RNA virus (Temin, 1972). The protovirus concept, in addition to its oncogenic implications, has another interesting ramification. It implies that the DNA of normal cells is not necessarily stable and may be altered at any time by protovirus. Conceivably, normal cell differentiation might involve changes in cellular genome induced by protovirus.

We should note that both the oncogene and protovirus concepts imply that all other carcinogenic agents, including DNA viruses, serve only to derepress or alter viral information normally present in all vertebrate cells, thus leading to the release of active oncornaviruses. It has further been proposed that activation of transforming virus from either the virogene or the protovirus occurs frequently, and that these deviant cells are destroyed by the normal immune system. Patients with a defective immune system, either hereditary or acquired, might then have an increased risk of cancer. Such an increased risk has been documented by many investigators (Hoover and Fraumeni, 1973; Fudenberg, 1971). However, as will become clear, the increased frequency of cancer in immunodeficient individuals may have other explanations (p. 109).

In addition to causing tumors in lower animals RNA viruses are suspected of being involved in certain forms of human cancer: mammary adenocarcinoma and leukemia. With respect to human breast cancer the evidence is voluminous but regrettably confusing (p. 586). Type B-like virus particles have been reported in milk samples from women who have familial histories of breast cancer (Moore et al., 1971). More recent reports, however, deny such findings (Henderson, 1974). Immunologic studies have revealed that the sera of patients with mammary cancer neutralize the infectivity of mouse mammary tumor virus (MMTV) more often than do the sera of control patients (Charney and Moore, 1971). Moreover, Schlom, Spiegelman and co-workers recently demonstrated by hybridization experiments that the cells in approximately two thirds of 29 malignant mammary tumors from women contained DNA specifically homologous to the RNA of the murine mammary tumor virus (Axel et al., 1972). To quote these investigators, "... human mammary tumors contain particles that have both 70S RNA and RNA-instructed DNA polymerase. Furthermore, the DNA synthesized hybridizes to the RNA of the mouse mammary tumor virus." The question arises: if milk from predisposed mothers does contain viral particles, do breast-fed female offspring show a higher incidence of breast cancer than their formula-fed sisters? In the single available detailed study, no such association could be found (Tokuhata, 1969). The studies summarized here do not provide compelling evidence implicating a viral agent in human breast cancer. They do, however, raise many suspicions of a viral etiology (Schlom and Spiegelman, 1973).

An RNA viral causation of leukemia in humans is also suspected. Gallo and his colleagues (1974) have isolated from acute leukemia cells a reverse transcriptase having the physical and biochemical properties of a viral reverse transcriptase. This enzyme is closely related immunologically to reverse transcriptase isolated from type C primate tumor virus. Drawing ever closer to the ultimate goal, type C viral particles were isolated recently from cultured human leukemic cells (Gallagher and Gallo, 1975). Leukemic cells derived from man also possess DNA and RNA having sequences related to the DNA and RNA of murine and primate leukemogenic agents (Hehlman et al., 1973; Spiegelman et al., 1974). In addition, type C particles have been visualized in human acute lymphocytic leukemia and lymphosarcoma cells (Dmochowski, 1973). However, type C particles are often present in the embryos of normal animals and man. Therefore, it must be appreciated that these particles, if they are indeed viral, may be mere passengers and not causative agents. In conclusion, many "footprints" of RNA viruses have been found in certain forms of neoplasia in man, but absolute proof of their role in the etiology of malignancy is still lacking.

Radiation Carcinogenesis. *Radiation is a known carcinogen for both animals and man.* Its oncogenicity is most likely related to its mutagenic effect (Cole and Nowell, 1965). It has been shown that ultraviolet irradiation may impose errors, such as thymine-thymine dimers, in the structure of DNA. Such errors, however, can be repaired, and it is necessary for cell replication to occur soon after exposure for permanent fixation of the radiation-induced injury (Borek and Sachs, 1966). The role of radiation injury in tumor formation is still not known. Five possibilities exist: (1) it may impose genetic changes, leading to loss of controls of cell replication, (2) it may merely accelerate cellular aging associated with an increased incidence of spontaneous mutations and cancer, (3) it may activate oncogenic viruses in a manner compatible with the protovirus and oncogene theories cited earlier, (4) it may exert its effect by alteration of the microenvironment of cells, thus affecting gene expression, or (5) it might stimulate cells to proliferate, leading to the selection of mutants with the most vigorous growth (Warren, 1970).

The history of radiation-induced cancers in man goes back to the early radiologists. These pioneers sometimes placed their hands in the x-ray beam to ascertain the function of their instruments. Many developed skin cancers, as indeed did Roentgen himself. Miners of radium in middle Europe and of uranium in the United States have a significantly increased incidence of bronchogenic carcinoma, presumably induced by the chronic inhalation of radon and its daughter products (United States Congress Joint Committee on Atomic

Energy, 1968). Bone tumors occurred among those workers engaged in radium painting of watch dials who pointed their fine brushes by wetting them with their lips. Additional evidence of the oncogenicity of radiation comes from the study of survivors of the atomic blasts at Hiroshima and Nagasaki. After a time lag of 5 to 10 years the incidence of leukemia (usually acute myelogenous) in exposed individuals was approximately 15 times higher than that of controls (Bizzozero et al., 1966). In addition there is tragic evidence that even the *therapeutic* use of radiation has led to cancers in man. Radiation of the head and neck region for the treatment of a now recognized innocent condition known as "persistence of the thymus" was followed many years later by an increased rate of thyroid cancer in those exposed (Duffy and Fitzgerald, 1950; Refetoff et al., 1975). Similarly, radiation of the scalp in children for tinea capitis, a fungal infection, was followed by a significantly increased incidence of both malignant and benign head and neck tumors, especially those of the brain, the parotid gland and the thyroid (Modan et al., 1974). Thus it is abundantly clear that radiation may induce tumors, a fact that justifies the old maxim "Be sure the treatment is not worse than the disease."

Other Carcinogens. Other agents, particularly *hormones*, have been implicated in the causation of tumors. Whether these agents act as initiators or as promoters is still not clear. They may merely contribute to some underlying initiating influence. There has long been clinical concern that an absolute or relative excess of hormones might induce cancer in endocrine-responsive organs. The experimental work with rats of Biskind and Biskind (1944) is pertinent to this question. They demonstrated that when the ovaries are transplanted into the spleen, tumors develop in the ovaries. Presumably in this experimental model ovarian hormones are drained directly through the liver and inactivated. Thus feedback inhibition of the pituitary is lost. The resultant excessive levels of pituitary gonadotropins first induce proliferation and then neoplasia of the ovaries. The possible role of hyperestrinism in the induction of human endometrial hyperplasia and endometrial carcinoma is mentioned on page 572. The fact that breast cancer is significantly more common in the United States than in Japan has been explained on the basis of a relative hyperestrinism in American women (Segi, 1969). We do not know why, but it cannot be ascribed solely to greater numbers of pregnancies and, thus, relief from cyclic hormones. Environmental factors may be involved. Other instances can be cited in which hormones apparently have caused tumors in experimental animals. Cancer of the thyroid has been induced in experimental animals by excessive levels of pituitary thyroid stimulating hormone. Breast cancers have been induced by excessive exposure to either gonadotropin or prolactin hormone. In most of these experiments the neoplasm initially is somewhat hormone dependent; thus its growth can be inhibited and sometimes reversed by reduction or total withdrawal of the tropic hormones. Clinical experience has also taught that ovariectomy and adrenalectomy may slow or sometimes completely inhibit the growth of breast cancer in women; orchiectomy may similarly affect prostatic cancer. However, in all of these forms of hormone-related neoplasia it is possible that the causative influence is not the hormone stimulation but rather some underlying initiating influence promoted by the hormones which themselves merely stimulate replication and so favor the ultimate emergence of the neoplasm.

Cancers have also been induced in experimental animals by plastic films, methyl cellulose, metal foils and chronic irritation (Brand et al., 1967). Presumably plastic films serve as physical barriers between cells which reduce the area of cell to cell contact and thus in some way diminish normal intercellular controls (Loewenstein, 1969). Might plastic prostheses such as heart valves or vascular grafts be oncogenic in man?

The role of chronic irritation or injury in oncogenesis may be that of promotion via cell replication, already cited as important in the process of carcinogenesis. On the other hand, it is highly doubtful whether a single physical blow could lead to cancer. Repeatedly the courts of law hear of an individual who is discovered to have a neoplasm for example in a subcutaneous location or in the breast, following an injury. There is no evidence derived from animal studies in support of such a sequence of events. It is much more likely that the trauma focused attention on a preexisting occult neoplasm.

In concluding this presentation of carcinogenic agents we should point out that *there is almost certainly no single cause of cancer. Indeed, it is far more attractive to postulate that several influences act in concert or sequentially to bring about the final transformation of the affected cell or cells.* Strong advocates of the role of viruses in oncogenesis, however, contend that all cells possess viral information in the form of either RNA or DNA which is capable of being activated and initiating carcinogenesis. According to this view all other influences serve only to activate or derepress this latent genetic information. For now, however, it is prudent to consider cancer as a group of diseases not all necessarily caused by a single agent but more likely the result of a multiplicity of oncogenic influences.

MECHANISMS OF CARCINOGENESIS

Having discussed the attributes that differentiate normal cells from neoplastic cells and some of the known carcinogens, we must now address the following important questions: (1) What cells and tissues in man are at risk of developing cancer? (2) What are the critical molecular events involved in the carcinogenic process, and do these events involve the genome of the cell (somatic mutation) or are they epigenetic (affecting only gene expression)? (3) Does neoplastic transformation occur as a single event or does it involve a sequence of events, resulting ultimately in a cancer cell? In considering the answers to these questions it should be remembered that cancer may not be a single disease, but rather a group of closely related diseases. Moreover, it is highly likely that more than one pathway may lead to cancer. Nonetheless, the many possible pathways have sufficient commonality to permit discussion of cancer as an entity.

What cells and tissues are at risk of developing cancer? The best answer might be, any cell in the body. Benign tumors probably arise from normal, mature somatic cells. Cancers, too, may arise in normal, differentiated cells. But, as has been pointed out, *cancers are more likely to develop either in cells whose homeostasis has already been disturbed or in those which are actively replicating.* The historic concept that cancers originate in sequestered rests of embryonic cells is no longer thought to be correct, although rarely a tumor is found which strongly suggests such a sequence, e.g., a teratoma located in the mediastinum. Teratomas usually arise from the totipotential germ cells in the gonads. When found in the mediastinum they can only be explained by the sequestration of embryonic totipotential cells. Save for this rarity, there is little to support the view that sequestered embryonic rests are important in the etiology of cancers.

Regenerative, hyperplastic, metaplastic and dysplastic proliferations are fertile soils for the origin of a cancer. Mention has already been made of the development of endometrial carcinoma in patients having certain forms of endometrial hyperplasia (p. 69). The association of cervical carcinoma with long-standing chronic cervicitis and dysplasia of the cervical epithelium is well known. Carcinomas arising in the lungs of habitual cigarette smokers are almost invariably preceded by metaplastic and dysplastic changes within the columnar epithelial lining of the respiratory airways. Liver cell carcinomas (approximately 70 per cent) arise in cirrhotic livers undergoing regeneration following some extensive injury. Cancers also have been known to arise in scarred areas within the lung; these are descriptively referred to as scar cancers. Osteogenic sarcomas typically are tumors of adolescents, arising during the time of maximum skeletal growth. When encountered in adults, they are usually superimposed on preexisting Paget's disease, a disorder characterized by increased osteoclastic and osteoblastic activity. Undifferentiated carcinomas, wherever they arise, probably take origin from the reserve cells which continually divide and differentiate to replace shed or lost specialized cells. Such a turnover occurs constantly, as for example in the lining of the intestinal tract. It is important to recognize, however, that in the great majority of situations these proliferations do not give rise to a tumor.

Certain cellular abnormalities and pathologic states progress to cancer with sufficient frequency to be known as *"precancerous lesions."* The term is a poor one, since in individual cases it can never be certain whether a patient will or will not develop a cancer. Nonetheless, in a large series of patients suffering from the same disorder, the association is unmistakable, and therefore the term "precancerous" is well entrenched. Some of these *precancerous conditions include chronic atrophic gastritis; solar keratosis of the skin; leukoplakia of the oral cavity, vulva and penis; and certain genetic disorders, including xeroderma pigmentosum, Fanconi's anemia, Bloom's syndrome and familial polyposis of the colon.* If a patient has had chronic atrophic gastritis for several decades, for example, he has about a 10 to 15 per cent chance of developing a gastric carcinoma, a much greater likelihood than in normal controls (Zamcheck et al., 1955). Even so in most so-called precancerous conditions, the percentage of cases undergoing cancerous transformation is fairly low.

It is still not possible to determine with certainty whether cancers arise in a single cell *(the clone theory)* or in a field of simultaneously affected cells *(the field theory)*. Both theories may be valid. Some cancers may be monoclonal, others polyclonal. The best evidence for the derivation of a cancer from a single aberrant cell derives from the study of plasma cell (B-cell) neoplasias. Each plasma cell neoplasm produces a single specific pattern of gamma globulin that is constant throughout the life of the particular patient, as though a single cell were synthesizing all the protein. Thus these plasma cell neoplasias have been referred to as *monoclonal gammopathies*. Other evidence for the monoclonal origin of cancers has been presented by Fialkow (1974). There is also some evidence, however, that some cancers are polyclonal, as was also pointed out in the earlier discussion of the karyotypes (p. 87). The issue is more than academic. The field theory implies that many cells may simultaneously undergo neoplastic transformation or, alternatively, that some cells may be affected before others, giving rise to the sequential appearance of several cancers in a given locus. Multicentric and multiple cancers in a specific tissue are well documented clinical occurrences. For example, a patient with a bladder cancer is at increased risk of developing a second malignant neoplasm at another site within the bladder, perhaps months to years after the appearance of the first. Similarly, multicentric foci of cancer may appear in the stomach of a patient with chronic atrophic gastritis. The appearance of bilateral breast carcinomas also supports the field theory of cancer evolution. Clearly, if oncogenic influences such as chemicals, viruses or radiation are at work, one cell or a cluster of cells might be transformed before the others, but with sufficient time and exposure, many or perhaps all may eventually become transformed. We must conclude then that some cancers are believed to be monoclonal, while others may be polyclonal.

Does the critical molecular event leading to carcinogenesis constitute a genetic alteration in the involved cells (a somatic mutation) or some epigenetic change resulting in failure of differentiation or maturation (Prehn, 1971)? It has been emphasized repeatedly that neoplastic transformation involves heritable changes, passed from one cell to its progeny. It is natural to assume that heritable changes must be inscribed into the genome of the cell. However, as Farber (1968) points out,

We must not forget that our current concept of cell differentiation allows an alternate hypothesis—no change in information content of the DNA but rather a change in the 'packaging' of the DNA which somehow controls the functional expression of a selected part of the information content of the DNA. If essentially all diploid cells in a single multicellular organism with the exception of mosaics possess the same genomic information then one can have a large number of potential heritable cellular phenotypes without any change in the information content of DNA. Since differentiated cells almost always breed true—liver makes liver makes liver, etc.—then an heritable alteration in the cell can result from some change in the environment in which the DNA functions. Conceivably, some examples of neoplastic cells may represent such an alteration. Could a change in tRNA or other RNA or in one or more of the cellular proteins be responsible for such a phenomenon?

A host of observations can be cited supporting the view that cancer is fundamentally a failure of differentiation or maturation of cells. As was pointed out earlier (p. 79), cancers may increase in size because the cells have a longer life cycle. Such "immortality" might well be the consequence of metabolic, epigenetic alterations which slow the rate of cellular maturation and differentiation. Pierce (1967) offers evidence that normal cells may arise from malignant cells. Initiation of cells in vitro may be reversible. Highly malignant neuroblastomas have undergone conversion to relatively benign ganglioneuromas involving maturation and differentiation of neuroblasts into ganglion cells. The genetic programs in such cancerous cells thus appear to be intact. Other arguments pointing towards carcinogenesis as a *non*-genetic alteration have been marshalled by Dustin (1972). The epigenetic view of cancerous transformation can not be dismissed.

On balance, *the weight of evidence favors the view that carcinogenesis involves some alteration in cellular DNA, i.e., a somatic mutation.* It was pointed out that while chemical carcinogens interact with a variety of cellular macromolecules, such as proteins and RNA, most of the evidence points toward their interaction with DNA as the critical event. Ames and his co-workers (1973) ingeniously documented that many of the chemical carcinogens are mutagens. They exposed bacterial mutants (having deranged enzyme systems) to chemical carcinogens which had previously been activated by liver cell homogenates, with release of the proximate or ultimate carcinogenic principles. The carcinogens in this model caused frame shift mutations and reversion of the bacterial mutants. Moreover, simple alkylating agents caused base pair substitutions. There is therefore abundant evidence documenting the interaction of chemical carcinogens with DNA. Oncogenic DNA viruses, as you recall, are in some manner incorporated into the genome of the cell, and RNA viruses, by virtue of their "reverse transcriptase," alter the genome of the host cell (Temin, 1974). In effect, then, all the oncogenic viruses induce somatic mutations in transformed cells. Ionizing radiation is a well-known mutagen. Experimental data, therefore, strongly support the mutational theory of carcinogenesis.

In addition, support for cancerous transformation as a somatic mutation can be derived from studies of so-called "spontaneous" tumors of man. These studies also underscore the fact that host factors are important in the evolution of a cancer. Most cancers have their peak incidence in the advanced years of life, when spontaneous mutations are more frequent in replicating cells. A variety of genetic conditions associated with abnormalities in the karyotype predispose to neoplastic transformations, some in early life. Cells already having some mutation are at increased risk of further mutations (Zimmerman, 1971). Down's syndrome, usually an aneuploid state, is associated with a ten- to twenty-fold increase in the incidence of myelogenous leukemia (Miller, 1970b). Patients with recessively inherited chromosomal breakage syndromes, such as Fanconi's anemia and Bloom's syndrome, also have a high incidence of leukemia (German, 1972). In vitro studies have also shown that cells from patients with gross chromosomal aberrations or with an increased rate of spontaneous chromosomal breakage have a greater susceptibility to neoplastic transformation. Thus lymphocytes and fibroblasts from patients with Fanconi's anemia have an abnormal sensitivity to x-rays, as measured by chromosomal breaks per cell per rad (Higuraski and Conen, 1971). Fibroblasts from patients with Down's syndrome or Fanconi's anemia are especially vulnerable to viral transformation (Miller and Todaro, 1969). A highly interesting documentation of the role of chromosomal instability in carcinogenesis is found in the recessively inherited disorder xeroderma pigmentosum. When exposed to sunlight, patients with this disorder are likely to develop multiple cutaneous cancers. The primary defect in this disease is in the genetically determined enzyme system necessary for repair of DNA damage due to ultraviolet light (Cleaver, 1969). Sunlight induces the formation of dimers in the DNA of exposed epithelial cells (a mutation), and these patients cannot repair the mutation since they lack the enzyme necessary for excising the dimer. Presumably the sunlight-induced mutation favors the development of additional mutations, thus leading to cancerous transformation.

A great deal of evidence has been marshalled in support of the concept that *sequential mutations are involved in carcinogenesis.* Knudson (1974) has proposed a "two mutations" theory. The first may be inherited, rendering the individual especially vulnerable to the development of some form of cancer. Such tumors tend to occur earlier in life than other cancers and are often termed "hereditary" cancers. Alternatively, the first mutation may be acquired later in life. The second mutation is presumably always acquired. According to this theory, then, patients with retinoblastoma, neuroblastoma, Wilms' tumor and other "childhood" cancers have hereditary mutations which permit the development of a cancer at a very early age. The two mutations theory may also apply to the cancers of young adults. For example, the risk of breast cancer

developing in relatives of a patient is higher when the patient has bilateral, premenopausal breast cancer than when the cancer is unilateral and occurs after the menopause (Anderson, 1972). Presumably the premenopausal cancer patient has a germ cell mutation and the mutation is also borne by relatives. Not all members of the family need be equally predisposed because of incomplete gene penetrance or a second mutational event negating the first. Many other instances are encountered of cancers in adults which are bimodal in distribution and in which there are strong hints of a genetic predisposition to explain the early peak. When the two mutations are both acquired, we have the situation which obtains with most forms of sporadic cancer, encountered usually in the later years of life. Thus, the accumulated data suggest that the initial mutation is only pre-neoplastic and additional mutations must occur for complete neoplastic transformation. Much, of course, depends on the potency of the carcinogenic influence and on the host. In vitro, with susceptible cells, a single treatment with a very strong carcinogen, such as methylcholanthrene, may induce transformation of 100 per cent of the cells (Mondal and Heidelberger, 1970). Similarly, advanced age with its increased incidence of mitotic errors; active cell replication for whatever reason; and genetic disorders associated with chromosomal mutations or instability all render cells more vulnerable to rapid and complete transformation. Such conditions might in a sense be considered pre-neoplastic. Some animal models of carcinogenesis first exhibit nodular hyperplasia, then benign neoplasia and ultimately malignant neoplasia (Farber, 1973). Presumably the cells in such situations first acquire increased growth vigor, then some cellular controls are lost, which results in the growth of a benign neoplasm, and ultimately total transformation occurs, producing a cancer. Therefore, it would appear that carcinogenesis is an evolutionary rather than a revolutionary process.

Based on these concepts, *a summarizing hypothesis for the evolution of a cancer in man might take the following form. A carcinogenic influence induces some genetic injury in one or more cells as the initiating event. Promoting influences, if present, favor mitosis and so provide the opportunity for the introduction of further mutations in actively replicating cells. Concomitantly or sequentially, the same or other carcinogenic influences continue to impinge on the field, inducing additional mutations in cells already having undergone some alteration of their DNA.* Indeed, it has been amply documented that many forms of carcinogens may collaborate in effecting neoplastic transformation. The action of viruses is enhanced by chemical carcinogens, and the reverse is equally true (Salaman et al., 1963). Thus in man the effects of chemical carcinogens, for example, might be followed after a period of time by exposure to oncogenic viruses. One wonders about the co-carcinogenic effect of the hydrocarbons in cigarette smoke and such agents as the adenoviruses in the induction of lung cancer. Analogously one could posit that chemical carcinogens and ultraviolet irradiation have a role in the induction of skin cancer. Sequential multiple hits on the cell would impose greater and greater mutational errors. In this manner neoplastic transformation and malignancy might evolve.

There are, however, defense mechanisms against the evolution of a cancer cell. It is well known that certain mutations in DNA can be repaired. The emergence of neo-antigens (tumor specific antigens) and the consequent immune response might destroy deviant cells before they have gained a foothold. The primary event might not be adequate to confer on the cells a growth advantage sufficient for tumor induction; without further promotion or additional influences, the initiated cells might revert to normal or be destroyed. We have no way of knowing how often deviant cells are destroyed, but just as man has evolved defenses against infections and can repair injuries, he has undoubtedly evolved some defenses against the emergence of cancer.

If we grant the above hypothesis of cancer induction and assume that transformed cells escape destruction, what is the fundamental nature of the cancer phenotype? The question persists although speculations abound. Perhaps membrane changes allow easier passage of nutrients, conferring on the cancer cell a greater ability to grow. Alternatively, the membrane changes might result in decreased sensitivity to contact inhibition and loss of cell controls. Perhaps altered enzyme systems impair the maturation or differentiation of cells and confer extraordinary longevity, so that accumulating cells form a tumorous mass. Conceivably loss of the ability to synthesize intracellular repressors or loss of regulatory genes might underlie the cancerous change. A long list of other speculations might be offered. But, in the final analysis, how the genetic mutation or epigenetic alteration brings about such a profound phenotypic event remains an enigma shrouded in mystery.

REFERENCES

Abelev, G. I.: Production of embryonal serum alphaglobulin by hepatomas: review of experimental and clinical data. Cancer Res., 28:1344, 1968.

Abercrombie, M., and Heaysman, J. E. M.: Observations on the social behavior of cells in tissue culture. II.

"Monolayering" of fibroblasts. Exp. Cell Res., 6:293, 1954.

Allen, D. W., and Cole, P.: Viruses and human cancer. New Eng. J. Med., 286:70, 1972.

Ames, B. N., et al.: Carcinogens are mutagens: a simple test system combining liver homogenates for activation and bacteria for detection. Proc. Nat. Acad. Sci. U.S.A., 70:2281, 1973.

Anderson, D. E.: A genetic study of human breast cancer. J. Nat. Cancer Inst., 48:1029, 1972.

Atkin, M. B.: Cytogenetic studies on human tumors and premalignant lesions: the emergence of aneuploid cell lines and their relationship to the process of malignant transformation in man. In Genetic Concepts and Neoplasia, (University of Texas M.D. Anderson Hospital and Tumor Institute), p. 36. Baltimore, Williams & Wilkins, 1970.

Axel, R., et al.: Presence in human breast cancer of RNA homologous to most mammary tumor virus RNA. Nature (London), 235:32, 1972.

Baldwin, R. W., et al.: Immunity in the tumor-bearing host and its modification by serum factors. Cancer, 34(Suppl.):1452, 1974.

Baltimore, G.: RNA-dependent DNA polymerase in virions of RNA tumor viruses. Nature (London), 226:1209, 1970.

Baluda, N. A., and Nayak, D. P.: DNA complementary to viral RNA in leukemic cells induced by avian myeloblastosis virus. Proc. Nat. Acad. Sci. U.S.A., 66:329, 1970.

Baserga, R.: The relationship of the cell cycle to tumor growth and control of cell division: a review. Cancer Res., 25:581, 1965.

Bennett, L. L., Jr., et al.: Searches for exploitable biochemical differences between normal and cancer cells. IV. Utilization of nucleosides and nucleotides. Cancer Res., 19:217, 1959.

Berenblum, I.: The co-carcinogenic action of croton resin. Cancer Res., 1:44, 1941.

Biskind, M. S., and Biskind, G. R.: The development of tumors in the rat ovary after transplantation into the spleen. Proc. Soc. Exp. Biol. Med., 55:176, 1944.

Bizzozero, O. J., Jr., et al.: Radiation related leukemia in Hiroshima and Nagasaki, 1946–1964. I. Distribution, incidence and appearance time. New Eng. J. Med., 274:1095, 1966.

Borek, C., and Sachs, L.: In vitro cell transformation by X-radiation. Nature (London), 210:276, 1966.

Borgaonkar, D. S.: Philadelphia chromosome, translocation and chronic myeloid leukaemia. Lancet, 1:1250, 1973.

Boyland, E.: Biological significance of metabolism of polycyclic compounds. In Williams, R. T. (ed.): Biological Oxidation of Aromatic Rings. Symposia, Biochemical Society, No. 4, 1950, p. 40.

Brand, K. G., et al.: Carcinogenesis from polymer implants: new aspects from chromosomal and transplantation studies during premalignancy. J. Nat. Cancer Inst., 39:663, 1967.

Burger, M. M.: Proteolytic enzymes initiating cell division and escape from contact inhibition of growth. Nature (London), 227:170, 1970.

Burnet, F. M.: The concept of immunological surveillance. Progr. Exp. Tumor Res., 13:1, 1970.

Charney, J., and Moore, D. H.: Neutralization of murine mammary tumor virus by sera of women with breast cancer. Nature (London), 229:627, 1971.

Cleaver, J. E.: Xeroderma pigmentosum: a human disease in which an initial stage of DNA is defective. Proc. Nat. Acad. Sci., U.S.A., 63:248, 1969.

Colburn, N. H., and Boutwell, R. K.: I. The binding of beta propiolactone to mouse skin DNA in vivo. Its correlation with tumor initiating activity. Cancer Res., 26:1701, 1966.

Colburn, N. H., and Boutwell, R. K.: II. The in vivo binding of beta propiolactone to mouse skin DNA, RNA and protein. Cancer Res., 28:642, 1968a.

Colburn, N. H., and Boutwell, R. K.: III. The binding of

propiolactone and some related alkylating agents to DNA, RNA and protein of mouse skin. Relation between tumor initiating power of alkylating agents and their binding to DNA. Cancer Res., *28*:653, 1968*b*.

Cole, L. J., and Nowell, T. C.: Radiation carcinogenesis. The sequence of events. Science, *150*:1782, 1965.

Coman, D. R.: Decreased mutual adhesiveness. A property of cells from squamous cell carcinomas. Cancer Res., *4*:625, 1944.

Commission on Clinical Oncology of the Union Internationale Contre le Cancer (International Union Against Cancer): TNM Classification of Malignant Tumors. Geneva, International Union Against Cancer, 1968.

Copeland, M. M.: American Joint Committee on Cancer Staging and End Results reporting. Objectives and progress. Cancer, *18*:1637, 1965.

Crosby, N. T.: Estimation of steam-volatile N-nitrosamines in foods at the 1 μg/kg level. Nature (London), *238*:342, 1972.

DeBaun, J. R., et al.: N-hydroxy-2-acetylaminofluorene sulfotransferase: its probable role in carcinogenesis and in protein-(methion-S-yl) binding in rat liver. Cancer Res., *30*:577, 1970.

DeLong, R. P., et al.: The significance of low calcium and high potassium content in neoplastic tissue. Cancer, *3*:718, 1950.

Dmochowski, L.: Molecular mechanisms in viral neoplasia of animals and their implications in the origin of cancer in man. Am. J. Clin. Path., *60*:3, 1973.

Duffy, B. J., Jr., and Fitzgerald, P. J.: Thyroid cancer in childhood and adolescence, a report on 28 cases. Cancer, *3*:1018, 1950.

Duncan, M. E., and Brookes, P.: Metabolism and macromolecular binding of dibenz(a,c)anthracene and dibenz(a,h)anthracene by mouse embryo cells in culture. Int. J. Cancer, *9*:349, 1972.

Dustin, P. E., Jr.: Cell differentiation and carcinogenesis: a critical review. Cell Tissue Kinet., *5*:519, 1972.

Easty, G. C.: Invasion by cancer cells. *In* Ambrose, E. J., and Roe, F. J. C. (eds.): The Biology of Cancer. London, D. van Nostrand, 1966, p. 78.

Easty, G. C., and Easty, D. M.: An organ culture system for the examination of tumor invasion. Nature (London), *199*:1104, 1963.

Editorial: Cancer and food. Lancet, *2*:1133, 1973*a*.

Editorial: Environmental nitrosamines. Lancet, *2*:1243, 1973*b*.

Editorial: Chalones: possibly an horse. Lancet, *2*:1248, 1973*c*.

Editorial: ICRF-159. Lancet, *1*:344, 1974.

Eilber, R. F., and Morton, D. L.: Impaired immunologic reactivity and recurrence following cancer surgery. Cancer, *25*:362, 1970.

Epstein, M. A., and Achong, B. G.: Various forms of Epstein-Barr virus infection in man: established facts and a general concept. Lancet, *2*:836, 1973.

Everson, T. Z., and Cole, W. H.: Spontaneous Regression of Cancer. Philadelphia, W. B. Saunders Co., 1966.

Farber, E.: Biochemistry of carcinogenesis. Cancer Res., *28*:1859, 1968.

Farber, E.: Carcinogenesis—cellular evolution as a unifying thread: presidential address. Cancer Res., *33*:2537, 1973.

Farina, F. A., et al.: Metabolic regulation and enzyme alterations in the Morris hepatomas. Cancer Res., *28*:1897, 1968.

Fialkow, P. J.: The origin and development of human tumors studied with cell markers. New Eng. J. Med., *291*:26, 1974.

Fisher, B., and Fisher, E. R.: Experimental studies of factors influencing hepatic metastases. III. Effect of surgical trauma with special reference to liver injury. Ann. Surg., *150*:731, 1959*b*.

Fisher, B., and Fisher, E. R.: Experimental studies of factors influencing hepatic metastases. IX. The pituitary gland. Ann. Surg., *154*:347, 1961.

Fisher, E. R., and Fisher, B.: Experimental studies of factors influencing hepatic metastases. I. The effect of number of tumor cells injected and time of growth. Cancer, *12*:926, 1959*a*.

Folkman, J.: Tumor angiogenesis: therapeutic implications. New Eng. J. Med., *285*:1182, 1971.

Foulds, L.: Neoplastic Development. Vol. I. London, Academic Press, Inc., 1969.

Friedkin, M.: The biochemist's outlook on cancer research. Fed. Proc., *32*:2148, 1973.

Fudenberg, H. H.: Genetically determined immune deficiency as the predisposing cause of "autoimmunity" and lymphoid neoplasia. Am. J. Med., *51*:295, 1971.

Gallagher, R. E., and Gallo, R. C.: Type C RNA tumor virus isolated from cultured human acute myelogenous leukemia cells. Science, *187*:350, 1975.

Gallo, R. C.: Summary of recent observations on the molecular biology of RNA tumor viruses and attempts at application to human leukemia. Am. J. Clin. Path., *60*:80, 1973.

Gallo, R. C., et al.: The evidence for involvement of Type C RNA tumor viruses in human leukemia. Cancer, *34*(Suppl.):1398, 1974.

German, J.: Genes which increase chromosomal instability in somatic cells and predispose to cancer. Progr. Med. Genet., *8*:61, 1972.

Goldblatt, L. A.: Aflatoxin: Scientific Background, Control and Implications. New York, Academic Press, 1969.

Green, M.: Oncogenic viruses. Ann. Rev. Biochem., *39*:701, 1970*a*.

Green, M.: Effect of oncogenic DNA viruses on regulatory mechanisms of cells. Fed. Proc., *29*:1265, 1970*b*.

Grover, P. L., and Sims, P.: Interactions of the K-region epoxides of phenanthrene and dibenz(a,h)anthracene with nucleic acids and histone. Biochem. Pharmacol., *19*:2251, 1970.

Hanafusa, T., et al.: Recovery of a new virus from apparently normal chick cells by infection with avian tumor viruses. Proc. Nat. Acad. Sci. U.S.A., *67*:1797, 1970.

Hare, J. D.: Transplant immunity to polyoma virus-induced tumor cells. IV. A polyoma strain defective in transplant antigen induction. Virology, *31*:625, 1967.

Harington, J. S.: Adaptation of cellular control processes in relation to cancer and its therapy. J. Theor. Biol., *28*:31, 1970.

Hay, E. D.: Skeletal-muscle regeneration. New Eng. J. Med., *284*:1033, 1971.

Hehlman, R., et al.: Molecular evidence for a viral etiology of human leukemias, lymphomas and sarcomas. Am. J. Clin. Path., *60*:65, 1973.

Heidelberger, C.: Current trends in chemical carcinogenesis. Fed. Proc., *32*:2154, 1973.

Hellstrom, I., et al.: Studies on immunity to autochthonous tumors. Proc. Trans. Soc., *1*:90, 1969.

Hellstrom, K. E., and Hellstrom, I.: Lymphocyte mediated cytotoxicity and blocking serum activity to tumor antigens. Adv. Immunol., *18*:209, 1974.

Henderson, B. E.: Type B virus and human breast cancer. Cancer, *34* (Suppl.):1386, 1974.

Henle, W., and Henle, G.: Epstein-Barr virus and human malignancies. Cancer, *34*:(Suppl.):1368, 1974.

Hennings, H., and Boutwell, R. K.: Studies on the mechanisms of skin tumor promotion. Cancer Res., *30*:312, 1970.

Herbst, A. L., et al.: Adenocarcinoma of the vagina. New Eng. J. Med., *284*:878, 1971.

Herbst, A. L., et al.: Prenatal exposure to stilbestrol. A prospective comparison of exposed female offspring with unexposed controls. New Eng. J. Med., *292*:334, 1975.

Higginson, J.: *In* Environment and Cancer. 24th Symposium, Fundamental Cancer Research. Baltimore, Williams & Wilkins, 1972, p. 69.

Higuraski, M., and Conen, P. E.: In vitro chromosomal radiosensitivity in Fanconi's anemia. Blood, *38*:336, 1971.

Hoffman, H. D., et al.: Chemical linkage of polycyclic hydrocarbons to deoxyribonucleic acids and polynucleotides in aqueous solution and in a buffer-ethanol solvent system. Biochemistry, 9:2594, 1970.

Holley, R. W.: A unifying hypothesis concerning the nature of malignant growth. Proc. Nat. Acad. Sci. U.S.A., 69:2840, 1972.

Hoover, R., and Fraumeni, J. F.: Risk of cancer in renal-transplant recipients. Lancet, 2:55, 1973.

Hozumi, M., et al.: Surface properties of non-tumorigenic variants of mouse mammary carcinoma cells in culture. Brit. J. Cancer, 9:393, 1972.

Johnson, H. A., et al.: Labeling of human tumor cells in vivo by tritiated thymidine. Lab. Invest., 9:460. 1960.

Johnson, L. D., et al.: Epidemiologic evidence for the spectrum of change from dysplasia through carcinoma-in-situ to invasive cancer. Cancer, 22:901, 1968.

Kanno, Y., and Matsui, Y.: Cellular uncoupling in cancerous stomach epithelium. Nature (London), 218:775, 1968.

Kellerman, G., et al.: Aryl hydrocarbon hydroxylase inducibility and bronchogenic carcinoma. New Eng. J. Med., 289:934, 1974.

Kiviat, M. D., et al.: Smooth muscle regeneration in the ureter. Electron microscopic and autoradiographic observations. Am. J. Path., 72:403, 1973.

Klein, G.: Tumor specific transplantation antigens. G.H.A. Clowes Memorial Lecture. Cancer Res., 28:625, 1968.

Klein, G.: Experimental studies in tumor immunology. Fed. Proc., 28:1739, 1969.

Klein, G. E.: Herpesviruses and oncogenesis. Proc. Nat. Acad. Sci. U.S.A., 69:1056, 1972.

Knudson, A. G.: Heredity and human cancer. Am. J. Path., 77:77, 1974.

Lappé, M. A.: Tumor specific transplantation antigens: possible origin in premalignant lesions. Nature (London), 223:82, 1969.

Law, L. W.: Studies of the significance of tumor antigens in induction and repression of neoplastic disease. Cancer Res., 29:1, 1969.

Liebowitz, S., and Schwartz, R. S.: Malignancy as a complication of immunosuppressive therapy. Adv. Int. Med., 17:95, 1973.

Lipsett, M. B., et al.: Humoral syndromes associated with nonendocrine tumors. Ann. Int. Med., 61:733, 1964.

Loewenstein, W. R.: Permeability of membrane junctions. Ann. N.Y. Acad. Sci., 137:441, 1966.

Loewenstein, W. R.: Transfer of information through cell junctions and growth control. Canadian Cancer Conf., 8:162, 1969.

Loveless, A.: Possible relevance of O–6 alkylation of deoxyguanosine to the mutagenicity and carcinogenicity of nitrosamines and nitrosamides. Nature (London), 223:206, 1969.

MacDonald, I.: Biological predeterminism in human cancer. Surg. Gynec. Obstet., 92:443, 1951.

Malt, R. A.: Compensatory growth of the kidney. New Eng. J. Med., 280:1446, 1969.

Matsushima, T., and Weisburger, J. H.: Inhibitors of chemical carcinogens as probes for molecular targets: ANA as decisive receptor for metabolite from N-hydroxy-N-2-fluorenyl acetomide. Chem. Biol. Interactions, 1:211, 1969.

Mazia, D.: Regulatory mechanisms of cell division. Fed. Proc., 29:1245, 1970.

McNutt, N. S., and Weinstein, R. S.: Carcinoma of the cervix: deficiency of nexus intercellular junctions. Science, 165:597, 1969.

Melnick, J. L., et al.: The causative role of herpesvirus Type 2 in cervical cancer. Cancer, 34(Suppl.):1375, 1974.

Miller, E. C., and Miller, J. A.: Mechanisms of chemical carcinogenesis: nature of proximate carcinogens and interactions with macromolecules. Pharm. Rev., 18:805, 1966.

Miller, J. A.: Carcinogenesis by chemicals. An overview. G.H.A. Clowes Memorial Lecture. Cancer Res., 30:559, 1970a.

Miller, J. A.: Naturally occurring substances that can induce tumors. In Toxicants Occurring Naturally in Foods, 2nd ed. Food and Nutrition Board. New York, National Acad. of Sciences, 1973, p. 508.

Miller, R. W.: Neoplasia in Down's syndrome. Ann. N.Y. Acad. Sci., 171:637, 1970b.

Miller, R. W., and Todaro, G. J.: Viral transformation of cells from persons at high risk of cancer. Lancet, 1:81, 1969.

Mizutani, S.: DNA polymerases in RNA tumor viruses and possible "protoviruses." Am. J. Clin. Path., 60:19, 1973.

Modan, D., et al.: Radiation induced head and neck tumors. Lancet, 1:277, 1974.

Mondal, S., and Heidelberger, C.: In vitro malignant transformation of the progeny of single cells derived from C_3H mouse prostate. Proc. Nat. Acad. Sci. U.S.A., 65:219, 1970.

Moore, D. H., et al.: Search for human breast cancer virus. Nature (London), 229:611, 1971.

Morris, H. P.: Studies on the development, biochemistry and biology of experimental hepatomas. Adv. Cancer Res., 9:227, 1965.

Noble, R. L.: Tumors and hormones. In Pincus, G., Thimann, K. Z., and Astwood, E. B. (eds.): Hormones: Physiology, Chemistry and Applications. Vol. 5. New York, Academic Press, 1964, p. 559.

Nowell, P. C., and Hungerford, D. A.: A minute chromosome in human chronic granulocytic leukemia. Science, 132:1497, 1960.

Nowell, P. C., and Morris, H. P.: Chromosomes of "minimal deviation" hepatoma: a further report on diploid tumors. Cancer Res., 29:969, 1969.

Omenn, G. S.: Pathobiology of ectopic hormone production by neoplasms in man. Pathobiology Annual, 3:177, 1973.

Ossowski, L., et al.: An enzymatic function association with transformation of fibroblasts by oncogenic viruses. II. Mammalian fibroblast cultures transformed by DNA and RNA tumor viruses. J. Exp. Med., 137:112, 1973.

Paul, J.: Metabolic processes in normal and cancer cells. In Ambrose, E. V., and Roe, F. J. C. (eds.): The Biology of Cancer. London, D. van Nostrand, 1966, p. 52.

Peers, F. G., and Linsell, C. A.: Dietary aflatoxins and liver cancer—a population based study in Kenya. Brit. J. Cancer, 27:473, 1973.

Pierce, G. B.: Teratocarcinoma: model for a developmental concept of cancer. In Moscona, A. A., and Monroi, A. (eds.): Current Topics in Developmental Biology. Vol. 2. New York, Academic Press, 1967, p. 223.

Prehn, R. T.: Neoplasia. In Lavia, M. F., and Hill, R. B., Jr. (eds.): Principles of Pathobiology. New York, Oxford University Press, 1971, p. 191.

Rabinowitz, Z., and Sachs, L.: Reversion of properties in cells transformed by polyoma virus. Nature (London), 220:1203, 1968.

Rapp, F.: Question: do herpesviruses cause cancer? Answer: of course they do. J. Nat. Cancer Inst., 50:825, 1973.

Refetoff, S., et al.: Continuing occurrence of thyroid carcinoma after irradiation to the neck in infancy and childhood. New Eng. J. Med., 292:171, 1975.

Ryser, H. P.: Chemical carcinogenesis. New Eng. J. Med., 285:721, 1971.

Sabine, J. R., et al.: Spontaneous tumors in $C3H-A^{vy}$ and $C3H-A^{vy}fB$ mice: High incidence in the United States and low incidence in Australia. J. Nat. Cancer Inst., 50:1237, 1973.

Salaman, M. K., et al.: The combined action of viruses and other carcinogens. In Viruses, Nucleic Acids and Cancer, A Collection of Papers Presented at the 17th Annual Symposium on Fundamental Cancer Research. Baltimore, Williams & Wilkins, 1963, p. 544.

Sandberg, A. A., and Hossfeld, D. K.: Chromosomal abnormalities in human neoplasia. Ann. Rev. Med., *21*:379, 1970.

Sander, J.: Untersuchungen uber die Entstehung cancerogener Nitrosover bindungen im Magen von Versuchstieren und ihre Bedeutung fur den Menschen. Arzneimittel-Forsch., *21*:1572, 1707, 2034, 1971.

Schlom, J., and Spiegelman, S.: Evidence for viral involvement in murine and human mammary adenocarcinoma. Am. J. Clin. Path., *60*:44, 1973.

Segi, M., et al.: Cancer mortality for selected sites in 24 countries. Publication No. 5, Department of Public Health, Japan, 1969, p. 174.

Sivak, A., and Van Duuren, B. L.: Studies with carcinogens and tumor-promoting agents in cell culture. Exp. Cell. Res., *49*:572, 1968.

Slemmer, G.: Host response to pre-malignant mammary tissues. Nat. Cancer. Inst. Monograph, Vol. 35, 1972, p. 57.

Spiegelman, S., et al.: Characterization of the products of RNA-directed DNA polymerases in oncogenic RNA viruses. Nature (London), *227*:563, 1970*a*.

Spiegelman, S., et al.: DNA polymerase activity in oncogenic RNA viruses. Nature (London), *227*:1029, 1970*b*.

Spiegelman, S., et al.: Human cancer and animal viral oncology. Cancer, *34*(Suppl.):1406, 1974.

Sunderman, F. W.: Methyl carcinogenesis in experimental animals. Food Cosmet. Toxicol., *9*:105, 1971.

Svoboda, D., et al.: Invasive tumors induced in rats with actinomycin D. Cancer Res., *30*:2271, 2279, 1970.

Takemoto, K. K., and Stone, L. B.: Transformation of murine cells by two "slow viruses," visna virus and progressive pneumonia virus. J. Virol., *7*:770, 1971.

Temin, H. M.: The protovirus hypothesis: speculations on the significance of RNA-directed DNA synthesis for normal development and for carcinogenesis. J. Nat. Cancer Inst., *46*(2):III–VII, 1971.

Temin, H. M.: The RNA tumor viruses, background and foreground. Proc. Nat. Acad. Sci. U.S.A., *69*:1016, 1972.

Temin, H. M.: Introduction to virus caused cancer. Cancer, *34*(Suppl.):1347, 1974.

Temin, H. M., and Mizutani, S.: RNA-dependent DNA polymerase in virions of Rous sarcoma virus. Nature (London), *226*:1211, 1970.

Temin, H. M., et al.: *In* Growth, Nutrition and Metabolism of Cells in Culture. Vol. 5. New York, Academic Press, 1972, p. 50.

Todaro, G. J., and Huebner, R. J.: The viral oncogene hypothesis: new evidence. Proc. Nat. Acad. Sci. U.S.A., *69*:1009, 1972.

Tokuhata, G. K.: Morbidity and mortality among offspring of breast cancer mothers. Am. J. Epidem., *89*:139, 1969.

United States Congress Joint Committee on Atomic Energy, Subcommittee on Research, Development and Radiation: Radiation exposure of uranium miners. Washington, D.C., Government Printing Office, 1968.

Wallach, D. F. H.: Cellular membranes and tumor behavior. Proc. Nat. Acad. Sci. U.S.A., *61*:868, 1968.

Warren, S.: Radiation carcinogenesis. N.Y. Acad. Sci., *46*:133, 1970.

Weinhouse, S.: Enzyme activities in tumor progression. *In* Edsall, J. T. (ed.): Amino Acids, Proteins and Cancer Biochemistry. New York, Academic Press, 1960, p. 109.

Weinhouse, S.: Metabolism and isozyme alterations in experimental hepatomas. Fed. Proc., *32*:2162, 1973.

Willis, R. A.: The Spread of Tumors in the Human Body. London, Butterworth, 1952.

Zamcheck, N., et al.: Occurrence of gastric cancer among patients with pernicious anemia at the Boston City Hospital. New Eng. J. Med., *252*:1103, 1955.

Zamcheck, N., et al.: Immunologic diagnosis and prognosis of human digestive-tract cancer: carcinoembryonic antigens. New Eng. J. Med., *286*:83, 1972.

Zimmerman, F. K.: Genetic aspects of carcinogenesis. Biochem. Pharmacol., *20*:985, 1971.

zurHausen, H., et al.: Occurrence of Epstein-Barr virus genomes in human lymphoblastoid cell lines. Nature (London), *237*:189, 1972.

CHAPTER 4
Clinical Aspects of Neoplasia

EFFECTS OF TUMOR ON HOST

EFFECTS OF HOST ON TUMOR

PREDISPOSITION TO NEOPLASIA
Geographic and Racial Factors
Age and Sex
Social Customs
Heredity

DIAGNOSIS OF CANCER

MESENCHYMAL AND SKIN TUMORS
Connective Tissue Tumors
Smooth Muscle Tumors
Skin Tumors

Ultimately the importance of neoplasia lies in its effect on people. Since its cause and prevention are unknown, retreat must be made to early diagnosis and treatment. The section which follows presents: (1) the effects of a tumor on the individual host, (2) the host response to the tumor, (3) factors involved in predisposition to neoplasia, (4) certain aspects of the diagnosis of neoplasms and (5) brief descriptions of certain neoplasms common to all tissues (mesenchymal tumors), as well as skin tumors not presented elsewhere in this text.

EFFECTS OF TUMOR ON HOST

Obviously, malignant tumors are far more threatening to the host than are benign ones. Nonetheless, benign tumors are not always entirely innocent. They may cause significant clinical disease by virtue of: (1) location and impingement on adjacent structures; (2) functional activity, such as hormone production; (3) complications such as hemorrhage; and (4) rarely, malignant transformation.

The importance of *location* can be demonstrated by the example of a benign epithelial papilloma growing within the common bile duct and producing obstructive jaundice. Leiomyomata in the uterus may not only induce local symptoms, such as a dragging discomfort in the lower abdomen, but may also cause mechanical difficulties at the time of childbirth. A very small benign tumor in the pituitary gland can compress and destroy the surrounding normal gland and thus give rise to hypopituitarism.

The *production of hormones* is perhaps the most important way in which a benign tumor causes serious clinical disease. Indeed, such functional activity is more characteristic of well differentiated benign tumors than it is of cancers. Only a few examples need be cited since the subject is considered in greater detail in the chapter on endocrine disorders (p. 594). A small adenoma of the pancreatic islets may elaborate sufficient insulin to cause death from hypoglycemia (Fig. 4–1). Hyperaldosteronism (Conn's syndrome), with its attendant hypertension and hypokalemia, is another example of significant clinical disease produced by a benign tumor (adrenal adenoma) that is often no larger than 1 cm. in diameter. A variety of hyperpituitary syndromes, including gigantism and acromegaly, are almost always the consequence of relatively small functioning adenomas of the pituitary gland.

Complications of benign tumors include hemorrhages following ulceration through an overlying epithelial or mucosal surface, infection of ulcerated lesions, pain related to acute hemorrhage within the tumor which stretches the tumor capsule, sudden emergencies provoked by twisting of the stalk of a pedunculated benign neoplasm with consequent infarction, and, finally, intussusception of the small intestine precipitated by a benign mass caught up in propulsive intestinal contractions (p. 483). Clearly, benign tumors are not always innocuous.

Although *malignant transformation* of a benign tumor may occur, it is uncommon. Certain notable exceptions should be cited. Adenomas of the thyroid gland are thought to give

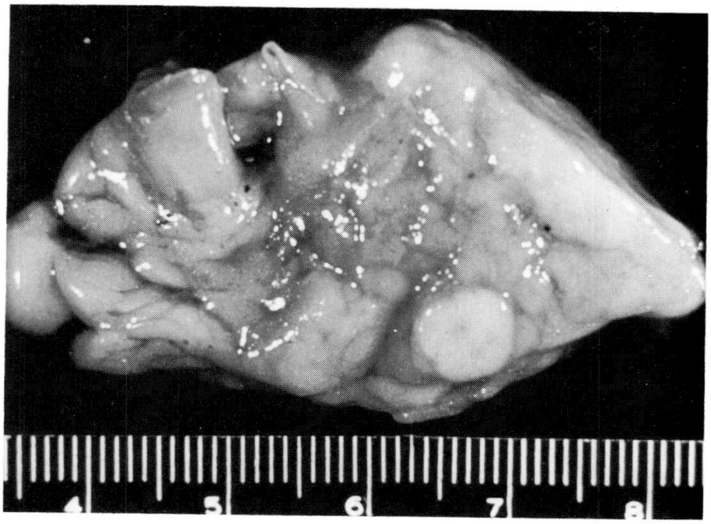

Figure 4–1. A graphic example of the potential significance of a benign tumor. An islet cell adenoma less than 1 cm. in diameter was responsible for fatal hypoglycemia in a young adult.

rise to thyroid cancers in about 10 per cent of cases, and foci of malignant transformation are found in up to 70 to 80 per cent of villous adenomas of the colon (p. 498). In addition to these specific instances, any benign neoplasm may harbor a focus of cancer. When such is discovered, one wonders if the lesion was ever totally benign. Thus, although most benign tumors remain benign, in the individual case this can be established with certainty only by excision and pathologic study of the lesion.

The clinical importance of a cancer is obviously much greater than that of a benign neoplasm. As invasive, destructive lesions, cancers produce a great many local disturbances and frequently develop superimposed complications. They may also produce hormones, but in general do so less often than benign tumors. While most hormonally active cancers arise in endocrine glands, the process of neoplastic transformation may result in ectopic hormone production. Although virtually any cancer may assume hormonal activity, a list of some of the more common hormonally active tumors is provided in Table 4–1.

In addition to the production of hormones, cancers may give rise to a variety of *"paraneoplastic"* syndromes, apparently caused by ill defined circulating products of the neoplasm. Multiple venous thromboses, known as *migratory thrombophlebitis*, sometimes appear in cancer patients, usually those with a primary lesion in the pancreas or lungs. This curious association — *Trousseau's sign* — was first described by this French physician, who tragically diagnosed his own malady as cancer of the pancreas when he developed multiple venous thromboses (Fusco and Rosen, 1966). Peripheral neuropathy and myopathy are sometimes encountered in patients with visceral cancers. No well defined circulating

product or toxin has been established, and the origin of such myoneural changes is still obscure. Cancers of the lung have a propensity for inducing abnormal proliferative changes in the periosteum of the distal phalanges and in the subungual tissues of the nail beds, referred to clinically as "clubbing of the fingertips." Once again no circulating product has been identified but successful resection of the lung cancer is followed by remission of these changes. It should be pointed out, however, that similar changes occur with other chronic lung disorders. Other "paraneoplastic" syndromes will be encountered in the consideration of the cancers of the various organs in the body.

Intriguing as these effects of cancer are, they seldom are direct causes of death. The final cause of death is in some instances clearly evident, as with perforation of the gastrointestinal tract and generalized peritonitis, obstruction of a bronchus leading to overwhelming pulmonary infection, or obstruction of the ureters by an infiltrative cervical carcinoma with consequent renal failure. *Much more often, patients die of progressive weakness, weight loss, anemia and wasting, a picture referred to as cachexia.* The causes of cachexia are still obscure, but many influences may contribute. Patients with advanced cancer often have impaired immune defenses and so are prone to infections. Erosion of the mucosa of the gut or of the endometrium may lead to loss of blood. Infections and hemorrhages may well explain the anemia seen in some patients, but in many terminally ill cancer patients there is no such simple explanation. Similarly, the cause or causes of the weakness and weight loss are obscure. Usually there is some correlation between the size and spread of the cancer and the severity of cachexia.

TABLE 4–1. PRINCIPAL FUNCTIONING TUMORS*

TUMOR	HORMONE PRODUCED	SYNDROME
Pituitary gland adenoma	Growth hormone	Gigantism and acromegaly
	ACTH	Cushing's syndrome
	Prolactin	Forbes-Albright syndrome
Thyroid adenoma	Thyroid hormone	Hyperthyroidism
Parathyroid adenoma or carcinoma	Parathormone	Hyperparathyroidism
Islet cell adenoma or carcinoma	Insulin	Hypoglycemia
	Gastrin	Zollinger-Ellison syndrome
	Glucagon	?Diabetes
	"Diarrheogenic hormone"	"Pancreatic cholera"
Adrenal cortical adenoma or carcinoma	Cortisol	Cushing's syndrome
	Aldosterone	Conn's syndrome
	Estrogen or androgen	Adrenogenital syndrome
Adrenal and extra-adrenal pheochromocytoma; chemo-dectoma; ganglioneuroma; ganglioneuroblastoma; retinoblastoma	Dopamine, norepinephrine and epinephrine	Hypertension, paroxysmal or sustained
Carcinoid tumor; oat-cell carcinoma; islet cell tumor; medullary carcinoma of thyroid	5-hydroxytryptophan, serotonin, kinins	Carcinoid syndrome
Granulosa-theca cell tumor of ovary; primary and meta-static ovarian tumors with "functioning stroma"; Sertoli cell tumor of testis	Estrogen	Estrinism
Sertoli-Leydig cell and lipid cell tumors of ovary; Leydig cell tumor of testis	Androgen	Virilization
Choriocarcinoma and other testicular tumors; carcinoma of lung; hepatoma	Gonadotropins	Gynecomastia
Oat-cell carcinoma of lung; bronchial carcinoid; carcin-oid-like tumor of thymus; islet cell tumor; medullary carcinoma of thyroid	ACTH-like hormone	Cushing's syndrome
Renal cell carcinoma; lung carcinoma; malignant lymphoma	Parathyroid-like hormone	Hyperparathyroidism
Mesothelioma; hepatoma; adrenal cortical carcinoma; other carcinomas	Insulin-like hormone	Hypoglycemia
Renal cell carcinoma; cerebellar hemangioblastoma; uterine leiomyoma; hepatoma	Erythropoietin	Polycythemia (usually erythrocytosis)
Oat-cell carcinoma of lung	Antidiuretic hormone	Schwartz-Bartter syndrome
Spindle cell thymoma	?Erythropoiesis-depressing hormone	Red cell aplasia
Medullary thyroid carcinoma	Calcitonin	Hypocalcemia

*Modified from Ackerman, L. V., and Rosai, J.: The Pathology of Tumors. New York, American Cancer Society, Inc., 1972, p. 45.

Thus, the patient with widespread metastatic disease displays the most extreme forms of wasting. The opposite is important; small localized cancers are usually silent and generally do not cause appreciable weight loss or weakness and so, regrettably, may not be discovered until they are incurable. Rarely, however, cachexia presents in a patient with only a small primary tumor with few, if any, metastases. It is simplistic to attribute cachexia to the inordinate nutritional demands of the cancer. Very few malignant tumors develop more rapidly than or achieve the size of a nine month fetus. And yet very few postpartal mothers find, to their regret, that they weigh less than they did before becoming pregnant. Grief, depression and anxiety, only too natural in the mortally ill patient, may be sufficient explanation for the loss of appetite that is one of the hallmarks of cancer. The suspicion persists, however, that other, still unrecognized mechanisms underlie the cachexia of cancer. Whatever its origin, the tragic wasting induced by advanced cancer commonly heralds the demise of the patient.

EFFECTS OF HOST ON TUMOR

As long ago as 1957 Burnet proposed: "It is by no means inconceivable that small accumulations of tumor cells may develop and because of their possession of new antigenic potentialities provoke an effective immunological reaction with regression of the tumor and no clinical hint of its existence." Since that time, a large body of data has been gathered supporting the concept of "immunological surveillance" as a protective mechanism against cancer (Burnet, 1970). Supporting evidence comes from a number of observations. Spontaneous regression of cancer, disappearance of distant metastases after surgical excision of the primary tumor mass, and the large numbers of tumor cells which can be carried in the peripheral blood following tumor surgery without development of metastases are all consonant with the existence of some defensive mechanism in the host (Piessens, 1970). One specific case reported by Wilson and colleagues (1968) is noteworthy. A patient inadvertently received a kidney transplant bearing neoplastic cells. The patient, who had been maintained on immunosuppressive therapy to prevent immunological rejection of the transplant, developed a tumor that was histologically identical with the cancer that had caused the death of the donor. When the tumor was detected in the transplant recipient, immunosuppressive therapy was stopped. Rapid rejection of the transplanted kidney followed. The rejected kidney with its associated tumor and some lymph node metastases were excised. Despite the fact that some malignant tissue had not been removed, the remaining cancer was spontaneously eliminated by the patient. Further evidence for the role of the immune system as a defensive mechanism in the host comes from the increased incidence of "de novo" tumors in those patients having impaired immune defenses (Kersey et al., 1973; Gatti and Good, 1971). Penn (1974) points out that organ transplant patients receiving immunosuppressive drugs have a 100-fold increased incidence of cancer. Although the increased risk of solid tissue cancers in renal transplant recipients is increased approximately 2.5-fold, the risk of incurring a lymphoma is increased approximately 35-fold. Schwartz (1975) relates this high incidence of lymphomas to some defect of the immune system which leads to failure to terminate lymphoproliferation triggered by any antigenic challenge rather than a breakdown of immunologic surveillance. It has been hypothesized that loss of so-called T-suppressor lymphocytes in the immune apparatus permits the remaining lymphocytes to undergo uncontrolled malignant proliferation (Editorial, 1973). Whatever the interpretation, it is clear that patients having some defect in immunity are at increased risk of developing a cancer, principally in their lymphoid tissues.

There is abundant laboratory evidence of immune responses in man against various forms of cancer. Circulating humoral antibodies and sensitized lymphocytes of the cell-mediated response have been demonstrated in a large number of patients bearing cancers. Indeed, unaffected members of a patient's family may also have antibodies to the antigens of the cancer, a still mysterious but intriguing observation. The cell-mediated response is undoubtedly the more important in the destruction of tumors (just as it is in the rejection of foreign transplants), but humoral antibodies also contribute, sometimes in a surprising fashion. It is clear that some sera of cancer-bearing animals and man contain factors capable of blocking the cell-mediated reaction. At the present time these factors appear to be free tumor antigen, antibodies, or antigen-antibody complexes formed in antigen excess (Baldwin et al., 1974; Hellstrom and Hellstrom, 1974). The Hellstroms (1974) as well as others have documented that while some antibodies act against tumor cells, others participate in blocking sensitized lymphocytes, thus aiding the tumor. To further complicate the problem, antitumor antibodies may coat tumor cells and render them vulnerable to all cells (macrophages, neutrophils, and B-lymphocytes) bearing Fc receptors, and still other factors may "arm" or bestow on macrophages specific tumor cytotoxicity. It is evident that the immune response to tumors is complex and still incompletely understood.

Antibodies and cell-mediated reactions have been demonstrated to a variety of cancers in man, including Burkitt's lymphoma, melanocarcinoma, osteogenic sarcoma and neuroblastoma (Liebowitz and Schwartz, 1973). It is not possible to go into all of the details relevant to each of these neoplasms, but a few points are worthy of note. It has been shown that an antigen derived from one melanocarcinoma stimulates blast transformation of lymphocytes not only from this patient but also from other patients with the same disease. The implication is that all these neoplasms possess identical antigens (Jehn et al., 1970). Similarly, in patients with osteogenic sarcoma, there is a high percentage of reactivity between one patient's serum and the tumors of other patients, again suggesting the presence of identical antigens (Morton et al., 1969). Recalling that in the experimental animal all cancers evoked by a virus have identical antigens, can we postulate a viral etiology of antigenically identical neoplasms in man? Alternatively, the cross reactions might reflect the appearance of identical fetal antigens in similar forms of cancer. Some children with a neuroblastoma have a rapidly progressive downhill course, whereas in others spontaneous regression occurs or the tumor converts to a more benign neoplasm composed of well differentiated ganglion cells—a ganglio-

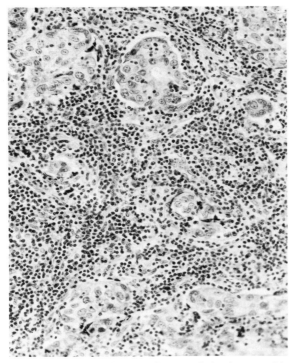

Figure 4–2. Medullary carcinoma of the breast with an intense lymphocytic infiltrate between the nests of tumor cells.

neuroma (Bill, 1969). Could these findings reflect the presence of blocking factors in some, and effective immune responses in the more fortunate patients?

Histologic examination of many human cancers adds additional weight to the evidence that some hosts react against their neoplasms. Lymphocytic infiltrates in and about tumors constitute one of the most striking indications of possible cell-mediated immune responses. Such infiltrates are characteristic of the seminoma of the testis and are also encountered in certain cancers of the breast, colon, lung, melanocarcinoma and others (Fig. 4–2). The correlation between the intensity of the stromal lymphocytic infiltrate and a favorable prognosis in Hodgkin's disease is very striking. One pattern of this disorder, in which there is an abundance of lymphocytes and which is sometimes called "lymphocyte predominance," has on the whole a very good prognosis. With current therapy the great preponderance of patients with this form attain complete arrest of their disease for decades, if not total cure. Conversely, another pattern, in which there are few or no lymphocytes—known as "lymphocyte depletion"—has a poor prognosis (p. 361) (Lukes, 1964). Most of these patients die within five years. The

lymph nodes of drainage in the region of many cancers often display marked reactivity characteristic of that encountered in immune reactions.

All of this immunologic evidence opens two enticing avenues of clinical importance: diagnostic tests for cancer and immunotherapy of cancer. Indeed, some useful diagnostic tests have already been devised. With immunochemical methods it is possible to detect circulating carcinoembryonic antigen (CEA) in many patients with carcinoma of organs derived from endoderm (p. 501) (Gold and Freedman, 1965). Although false positives make testing for CEA of doubtful value as a screening test, it has proved of great value in the postoperative follow-up of patients with neoplasms which produce CEA. When the CEA levels disappear following surgery, the resection has been complete; reappearance of CEA in the circulation indicates recurrence of the tumor.

The hope that immunotherapy can be exploited to control or possibly cure cancer is even more promising. Efforts are now being made to treat a variety of forms of cancer with humoral antibodies and sensitized lymphocytes derived from patients with apparently cured similar neoplasms. Sera and cells derived from close relatives or prepared in animals have also been tried. Recall that close relatives often have elevated titers of antibodies to the tumor. An additional immunologic approach has been the administration to cancer patients of agents such as *Corynebacterium parvum* or BCG (tuberculosis "vaccine"), known to induce cell-mediated reactions. It is theorized that by activating the cell-mediated mechanism in the patient, a more effective immune reaction might conceivably be evoked against the neoplasm. Early results with this form of therapy in patients with melanocarcinoma suggest a significant decrease in the relapse rate following surgical resection of the primary lesion (Gutterman, 1973). Hope runs high that this form of therapy will fulfill its early promise, but to date insufficient data have been gathered for evaluation of the results.

PREDISPOSITION TO NEOPLASIA

It is, fortunately or unfortunately, impossible to predict whether an individual will develop cancer. However, a great many influences have been identified which bear on this possibility. They relate both to the patient's environment and to the patient himself. A discussion of the most important influences follows.

GEOGRAPHIC AND RACIAL FACTORS

Insights into an individual's likelihood of developing a specific form of cancer can be gained from its national prevalence, most accurately expressed in the form of mortality data, recognizing that certain forms are not usually lethal, e.g., cancer of the skin. Analyses of death rates for specific forms of cancer among the nations of the world reveal striking, sometimes startling, differences. For example the age-adjusted death rates in 1975 per 100,000 population for cancer of the breast in the female was estimated to be approximately 22 in the United States, compared to 4 in Japan (American Cancer Society, 1975). Differences in the average number of children per family in these two countries as they reflect cumulative months of pregnancy or, more likely, environmental influences may underlie this striking disparity. This subject is discussed more fully on page 588. The estimated male death rates in 1975 for cancer of the stomach were 9 in the United States, 59 in Chile and 66 in Japan. There is no certain explanation for these puzzling differences. Similarly, primary carcinoma of the liver is the most common cause of cancer deaths in certain regions of Africa, but is a rare disease in Europe and North America. The high death rate of liver cancer in Africa could be related to aflatoxins (p. 513). A long list of such comparisons might be offered, but it suffices to say here that the more we learn about such "geographic pathology," the more certain it becomes that the differences are likely to be environmental rather than hereditary in origin. Table 4–2 indicates that Nisei (second generation Japanese living in the United States) have mortality rates for certain forms of cancer intermediate between natives of Japan and those of the United States. Such data make evident the role of environmental influences on presumed racial or hereditary predisposition. The full significance of environmental impact is best brought out by a remarkable observation made in animals. A highly inbred strain of mice in the United States develops both breast and liver tumors

TABLE 4–3. ESTIMATED NEW CASES OF CANCER IN THE U.S.—1975 (MAJOR SITES)*

SITE	TOTAL	MALE	FEMALE
Colon and rectum	99,000	48,000	51,000
Lung, bronchus and trachea	91,000	72,000	19,000
Breast	88,700	700	88,000
Prostate	56,000	56,000	—
Bladder	28,700	21,000	7700
Corpus uteri	27,000	—	27,000
Stomach	22,900	14,000	8900
Pancreas	21,500	12,000	9500
Leukemia	21,200	12,000	9200
Cervix, invasive	19,000†	—	19,000†
Ovary	17,000	—	17,000
Kidney and other urinary	14,500	9,000	5500
Lymphomas, excluding Hodgkin's	13,900	7500	6400
Liver and biliary passages	11,500	5700	5800
Brain and central nervous system	10,700	5900	4800

*Modified from Cancer statistics, 1975. CA, *25*:10, 1975.
†Carcinoma-in-situ of the uterine cervix not included in totals.
Note: The estimates of new cancer cases are offered as a rough guide and should not be regarded as definitive.

in 100 per cent of animals. The influence here would seem to be genetic. When these animals were transferred to Adelaide, Australia, however, only 17 per cent developed liver tumors. When both food and wood-shavings used for bedding were brought from the United States to these animals in Australia the 100 per cent incidence recurred (Sabine et al., 1973). Clearly environmental factors assume great importance in what at first may appear to be genetic predisposition to cancer and in fact the contribution of heredity to geographic variations has yet to be established.

Even within a given environment certain cancers are more frequent than others, as is indicated in Table 4–3. Such data address the question of what forms of cancer represent the greatest risk to the individual within a specific locale.

AGE AND SEX

Over 80 per cent of all fatal cancers occur in individuals aged 55 or over. There is a small peak in cancer mortality during the first four years of life but the main peak is reached in the sixth and seventh decades, followed by a decline which is probably related to the relatively greater importance of fatal heart disease and strokes among the very aged. Save for bronchogenic carcinoma, which has a well defined environmental association, the neoplasms of advanced years tend to arise in those organs undergoing cyclic or involutional changes. Thus, prostatic cancer is extremely common in men of advanced years and, analogously, breast cancer is a very common

TABLE 4–2. STANDARDIZED MORTALITY RATIOS FOR CANCER IN VARIOUS SITES*

	JAPANESE	NISEI	U.S. WHITE
Stomach	100	38	17
Intestines	100	290	490
Pancreas	100	170	270
Lung, bronchus	100	170	320
Leukemia	100	150	270

*Adapted from Haenszel, W., and Kurihara, M.: Studies of Japanese migrants. I. Mortality from cancer and other diseases among Japanese in the United States. J. Nat. Cancer Inst., *40*: 43, 1968.

malignant neoplasm in American women. Overall, cancer is the second leading cause of death from infancy to age 74. Even among children one to 14 years of age, only accidents cause more deaths.

There are significant sex differences in the predisposition to cancer in general and to specific forms of malignant neoplasia, above and beyond the obvious differences relating to cancers of the genital tracts. The death rate (age-adjusted) for cancer among males in the United States currently hovers about the mark of 150 per 100,000, while for females it is approximately 110 per 100,000. Much of this difference is accounted for by the fact that the death rate from bronchogenic carcinoma among males is four times higher than among females. From Table 4–3 it is evident that males and females have approximately the same annual number of new cases of cancer of the colon and rectum, but for cancers of the lung, bladder, stomach, pancreas and kidney, as well as leukemia, males are more often affected than females. Could some of these differences reflect a greater environmental exposure of males to carcinogenic influences? Whatever the reason, men are at greater risk of dying from cancer than are women.

SOCIAL CUSTOMS

It is sad to realize that even life style and social customs influence an individual's predisposition to cancer. Cigarette smoking and lung cancer is one obvious example. Smoking and alcohol consumption are predisposing agents in cancer of the esophagus. Penile cancer is rare among males circumcised at birth. The incidence of cervical cancer in women rises in proportion to (1) youth at time of first intercourse, (2) frequency of intercourse and (3) the number of consorts. All of these influences may reflect a causative role of Herpes-simplex virus, type 2, and the likelihood of contracting this venereal infection (p. 565). Cancer of the lower lip, attributed to chronic heat injury, is more common among clay pipe smokers. Chewing of betel nuts, a custom in India and other Asian countries, leads to cancer of the oral cavity. It has been said that everything one does for pleasure is fattening, immoral or illegal; to this doleful list we must now add—oncogenic!

HEREDITY

All disease is the consequence of either "nurture" or "nature" or, of course, both. Cancer is no exception. Here we are concerned with the role of "nature" in the predisposition to cancer. In any multifactorial disease such as cancer, it is exceedingly difficult to elucidate the significance of heredity. In the study of inheritance patterns the long generation cycle of man, the limited number of progeny, the lack of pathologic information (proven diagnoses) on many death certificates, and the difficulties in follow-up and in obtaining data on previous generations has made the study of hereditary influences in neoplasia most difficult. Nonetheless, some progress has been made and a few observations can be offered:

(1) *There is probably no hereditary predisposition to cancer in general.*

(2) *Such hereditary influences as have been defined operate independently for specific tumor types.*

(3) *Mendelian inheritance patterns have been identified for a very few forms of cancer and for several pre-cancerous conditions.*

Only a handful of extraordinary families have provided evidence for an inherited predisposition to cancer in general. In these remarkable families there is an increased incidence of adenocarcinoma, primarily of the colon and endometrium; leukemia; lymphoma; and an increased frequency of multiple primary malignant neoplasms as well as an early age of onset of the tumors (Lynch and Krush, 1971). Save for these enigmatic and remarkable instances, families of cancer patients are no more vulnerable to cancer in general than the population at large.

An hereditary predisposition, however, has been noted for certain specific forms of neoplasia. As mentioned earlier, first degree relatives of premenopausal patients with breast cancer have a higher frequency of breast cancer than controls of similar age (Anderson, 1971). Retrospective genetic studies disclose that stomach cancer is two to four times more frequent in first degree relatives of individuals with this malignancy than in controls. This hereditary tendency may in part reflect an association between stomach cancer and blood type A, since individuals with this blood type are about 20 per cent more susceptible to stomach cancer than those with blood groups O, B or AB. A fairly well defined hereditary predisposition to bronchogenic carcinoma has been dissociated from environmental influences. Individuals who have an affected close relative and who smoke have an increased risk of developing lung cancer, greater than that associated with either influence alone. There are many hereditary influences relating to cancer of the large intestine. Two conditions (familial polyposis of the colon and Gardner's syndrome, both autosomal dominant disorders) strongly predispose to cancer of the colon. In the former condition, approximately 40 to 75 per cent of patients develop carcinoma of the colon, and perhaps all would if they lived long enough. In addition, evidence is beginning to accumulate suggesting a predisposition to colonic cancer in specific families free of predisposing non-neoplastic disease. In these families, the cancer often appears at a relatively early age (Anderson, 1970). This condition, now referred to as hereditary adenocarcinomatosis of the colon, does not affect the general population; the predisposition appears to be limited to specific family trees. Other examples might be cited and can be found in the excellent review by Knudson et al. (1974).

Well defined mendelian inheritance patterns have been identified for a few cancers, as well as for certain precancerous disorders (Table 4–4).

It is most important to note that while any of the conditions cited in Table 4–4 may be inherited along mendelian lines, these same neoplasms occur in many patients who provide no history of familial disease (Lynch and Krush, 1971). For example, a large percentage of retinoblastomas appear in the absence of hereditary predisposition. Similarly, only about 3 per cent of all cases of melanocarcinoma have a familial setting; the great preponderance occur sporadically. Mendelian inheritance, therefore, accounts for only a small fraction of the attack rate of neoplasia, even for the specific forms of cancer presented in Table 4–4.

DIAGNOSIS OF CANCER

In a day when man can walk on the moon, it is remarkable that identification of the exact nature of a tumor still depends on subjective morphologic evaluation. Despite the frailty of the method, no better one has yet been devised. The clinician, however shrewd his clinical diagnosis may be, requires more precise identification of the nature of the tumor, which can be provided only by microscopic examination of adequate sections prepared from a representative biopsy of the lesion. As indicated earlier, while the benign or malignant nature of most tumors usually can be confidently assessed histologically, a no man's land of borderline lesions still exists. When 20 microscopic sections from a variety of cervical biopsies were submitted to 25 pathologists, there was very good agreement on some lesions, but those lesions occupying the interstage between atypical dysplasia and carcinoma in situ evoked considerable disagreement. Some pathologists interpreted a particular lesion as benign, while others considered it malignant. From what has been said before, it is obvious that none of the parameters that differentiate benign from malignant neoplasms are always black or white, and for some tumors, all the criteria are gray.

The selection of the biopsy site for a representative sample of a tumor is a critical step in tumor diagnosis. At the margins of frank carcinomas, the borderline epithelial cells may have only somewhat atypical changes not definitely cancerous. The evaluation of a marginal biopsy may therefore fail to assess the complete significance of the lesion. A central biopsy of a cancer, on the other hand, may disclose only tissue that has become necrotic from lack of a blood supply. The removal of an enlarged inguinal node suspected of harboring a metastatic lesion may disclose such severe inflammatory changes as to make interpretation extremely difficult. Considerable responsibility then rests on the surgeon in his selection of an appropriate biopsy site.

There is much to recommend the needle biopsy method for neoplasms since this approach generally obviates the need for anesthesia and for the more complicated aspects of the usual surgical biopsy. In skilled hands, the large needle removes a boring of the appropriate tissue. Since the core of tissue removed is small and the process essentially blind, the validity of the diagnosis rests heavily on the accuracy of the hand and on the brain that guides it.

With both surgical and needle biopsies, a rapid (frozen section) histologic examination can provide within minutes critical information for the appropriate management of the problem. Let us take the example of a breast mass. The biopsy specimen can be rapidly frozen, sectioned, stained, and examined within minutes, while the patient is still under anesthesia. The breast resection, if necessary, can begin immediately. Sometimes the lesion is so borderline it is best to wait for more adequate paraffin sections. The question is often asked whether it is dangerous to manipulate a neoplasm surgically and then wait for several days before definitive surgery or other therapy is instituted. In general, the answer to this question is no. The fear that surgical trauma may liberate emboli which drain through the lymphatic or vascular channels does not appear to be justified. There is no objective evidence from collected data that this course of action produces dissemination of the neoplasm. Although it is true that cancers can be transplanted, as was cited earlier, when usual care is taken, experience has proved the hazard to be very small indeed. Rapidly growing sarcomas in children may be an exception since cases are on record of their having been transplanted. But even in these instances, the necessity for accurate diagnosis, possibly requiring more adequate paraffin sections, far outweighs the risks involved. To amputate a leg on a frozen section diagnosis is a grave responsibility and is better avoided.

Next best to histologic evaluation of a tumor is the *cytologic diagnosis of cancer* previously mentioned (page 77). It is now approximately 40 years since Papanicolaou firmly

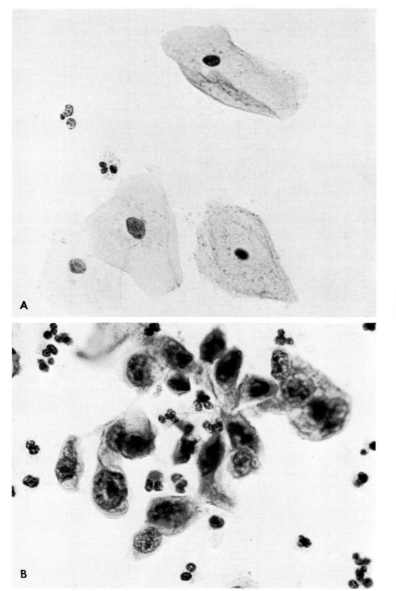

Figure 4–3. Papanicolaou smears of vaginal cytology. *A,* Normal squames. *B,* Class V cancer cells.

established the validity of this method. As was discussed, one of the attributes of cancer cells is their lowered cohesiveness. Cells are shed more readily from tumor surfaces than from normal tissue surfaces. The evaluation of these shed cells for the morphologic features of anaplasia provides a very accurate method for establishing the presence of a tumor (Fig. 4–3). It is standard practice to grade the severity of the cells' atypia as follows.

    Class I. Normal.
    Class II. Probably normal (slight atypia).
    Class III. Doubtful (more severe atypia; probably dysplastic, but possibly anaplastic).
    Class IV. Probably cancer (moderately severe atypia; probably anaplastic).
    Class V. Definitely cancer (clearly anaplastic).

The cytologic technique can be applied to vaginal secretions, sputum, bronchial washings, abdominal fluid (ascites), pleural fluid, abnormal discharges from the nipple of the breast, prostatic secretions and urinary sediment. In competent hands, an 85 to 95 per cent correct positive diagnosis and a 95 to 98 per cent correct negative diagnosis can be achieved (von Haam, 1962). The technique is particularly valuable since it permits the diagnosis of lesions while they are still in situ and therefore not visible on clinical inspection. In the case of vaginal secretions, for example, a small carcinoma high in the endometrial cavity will shed cells long before it becomes an obvious mass. On these grounds, it is now standard medical practice to perform cytologic vaginal smears regularly on all adult female patients. Indeed, where mass screening procedures have been instituted, the results have been most gratifying, with a striking reduction in the morbidity and mortality due to carcinoma of the cervix.

For years there has been a hope that a blood test could be discovered that would disclose the presence of any or all cancers. To date, none has been reported having the specificity and accuracy of the histologic and cytologic methods. The identification of circulating cancer cells in the blood has proved to be of little worth. The false negative error is very large, of the order of 80 per cent, and even when positive the test cannot identify the location of the cancer. Detection of increased levels of circulating hormones may indicate the presence of one of the many tumors which elaborate excessive amounts of hormones (see p. 108). Similarly, certain neoplasms (listed in Table 4–5) produce circulat-

TABLE 4–5. ELEVATED LEVELS OF CIRCULATING PRODUCTS IN DIAGNOSIS OF NEOPLASMS*

Neoplasm	Circulating Product
Enzymes	
Prostatic carcinoma	Acid phosphatase
Cancer of the digestive tract	Regan isoenzyme
Medullary thyroid carcinoma	Histaminase
	Calcitonin
Other Products	
Hepatoma	Alpha fetal globulin
Gastrointestinal carcinoma	Carcinoembryonic antigen
Plasmacytoma	Abnormal globulins
Pancreatic carcinoma	Carcinoembryonic antigen

*Adapted from Robbins, S. L.: Pathologic Basis of Disease. Philadelphia, W. B. Saunders Company, 1974.

ing products which, when detected in the blood, indicate the presence of a tumor. It must be appreciated in evaluating Table 4–5 that not every tumor among the various forms cited elaborates its related product. Carcinoembryonic antigen assay is positive in only 75 per cent of patients with well advanced cancer of the colon and is negative in 50 per cent of patients with small, "early" lesions (Zamcheck et al., 1972). Detectable levels of serum acid phosphatase are usually present only when prostatic cancer has already metastasized to bone. It is believed that the enzyme more freely diffuses into the circulation in the richly vascularized bone marrow. Despite false negative errors, assays for these circulating substances provide valuable diagnostic aids for specific forms of neoplasia. Unfortunately only a small portion of the spectrum of cancers is covered.

MESENCHYMAL AND SKIN TUMORS

Most of the clinically significant forms of benign and malignant neoplasia will be presented in the chapters dealing with specific organs and systems. A few, such as mesenchymal tumors of connective tissue and smooth muscle origin, are so ubiquitous they do not fit into any specific organ presentation and so are considered here. In addition, neoplasms of the skin are presented here since they are not considered elsewhere in this text.

CONNECTIVE TISSUE TUMORS

Tumors arising in connective tissue occur throughout the body. They may take origin from fibrocytes, fibroblasts or the specialized derivatives of mesenchymal tissue, such as fat and muscle. One of the most common of these neoplasms is the *lipoma*. It generally appears in subcutaneous locations as a 3.0 to 5.0 cm., soft, round to oval mass of adult fatty tissue enclosed within a very delicate capsule. The capsule is often so thin that it is easily ruptured during removal. Histologically, these lesions are indistinguishable from normal adipose tissue and the designation "tumor" is only merited by the tumorous accumulation of fat cells enclosed within a delicate capsule. Localized collections of fat not discretely encapsulated may appear in such sites as the spermatic cord, mediastinum and omentum. These lesions probably represent bizarre, aberrant accumulations of fat that are not truly neoplastic. The distinction between these localized overgrowths and true neoplasia is at best arbitrary and academic. On occasion, a benign lipoma may progressively increase in size to encircle such structures as the ureters. Such sluggish engulfment should not be mistaken for invasiveness, since the enclosed structures remain intact. *Liposarcomas* are extremely uncommon lesions. They are most often found in the retroperitoneal region and in the mesentery of the gut. They may achieve massive size and be truly infiltrative lesions which tend to encircle and invade structures and dissect through cleavage planes, making their removal extremely difficult. The liposarcoma may be somewhat more opalescent and gray than the mature lipoma. These qualities are usually imparted by a larger component of fibroblastic and myxomatous elements, mixed with immature and mature fat cells. The histologic diagnosis of a liposarcoma can be extremely difficult since the qualities of anaplasia are far more subtly displayed in these tumors than in many other forms of sarcoma.

The *fibroma* is a common tumor of fibrocytic or fibroblastic origin. It may arise not only in the subcutaneous tissues but anywhere else in the body, from the fibrous sheaths of nerves, vessels, muscles and the fibrous stroma present in all organs. When these fibromas arise within the dermis itself, they are quite distinct from fibromas arising in deeper structures. More about this exception—the dermatofibroma—will be said presently. The common fibroma appears as a rubbery, gray, discrete encapsulated mass. It usually does not exceed 3.0 to 4.0 cm. in diameter. In some locations, these tumors may achieve considerably larger size. On transection, the surface is glistening and gray-white and usually devoid of hemorrhage or necrosis. Histologically, the lesion is composed of mature fibrocytes or fibroblasts having no distinctive orientation. Intercellular collagen may be abundant or scant. As benign lesions, fibromas display no anaplasia and mitoses are

virtually absent. Special stains, such as silver impregnation techniques, will demonstrate reticulin laid down by the fibroblasts, or the phosphotungstic acid–hematoxylin stain may reveal delicate. wavy fibroglial fibrils elaborated by the fibroblast, which is a means of differentiating these spindle cell tumors from those of muscle origin.

Fibromas arising in the dermal connective tissue immediately below the epidermis, are called *dermatofibromas.* In this location, for obscure reasons, the lesions are completely benign cytologically, but are unencapsulated. The margins are poorly demarcated and subtly blend into the surrounding dermis. Often the tumor engulfs hair shafts and other skin adnexa without invading or destroying them The dermatofibroma is easily removed by adequate excision, but it is of interest as an example of a benign yet unencapsulated lesion Dermatofibrosarcomas too tend to remain localized and are generally readily removable.

Fibrosarcomas are the malignant counterpart of the fibroma. These tumors also may occur anywhere in the body but are perhaps most frequent in the soft tissues of the extremities and in the retroperitoneum. They occur as bulky, soft, pearly gray-white infiltrative masses. On transection, the tumor has a characteristic raw fish-flesh appearance. Often there are areas of necrosis or hemorrhage reflecting the rapidity of growth that outstrips the blood supply Histologically. these lesions have variable degrees of anaplasia. Some of the better differentiated fibrosarcomas are made up of quite mature looking fibroblasts and show occasional mitoses and some slight cellular pleomorphism. At the other end of the spectrum, the very anaplastic fibrosarcomas rate among the wildest appearing neoplasms in the body. Massive tumor giant cells, with huge single or multiple nuclei, may be present. Mitoses may be quite frequent and are often very atypical and totally chaotic. Such anarchic lesions are often extremely treacherous, and local recurrence often follows inadequate primary resection. One special pattern of fibrosarcoma, the desmoid, is described on page 646.

SMOOTH MUSCLE TUMORS

The *leiomyoma* is a benign tumor of smooth muscle origin. It may arise anywhere in the body, such as the wall of the intestinal tract or in the walls of arteries, but is particularly common in the uterus and is described in greater detail on page 571. The uterine variety is undoubtedly the most common visceral neo-

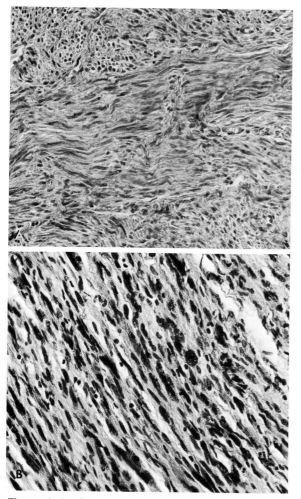

Figure 4–4. A comparison of the well differentiated histology of a leiomyoma (*A*) and a leiomyosarcoma (*B*).

plasm in women. The leiomyomas that arise outside the uterus tend, on the whole, to be small lesions that rarely exceed 2.0 to 3.0 cm. in diameter. They are composed of bands of mature smooth muscle cells closely resembling their normal counterparts.

The leiomyosarcoma may arise in a leiomyoma but more often begins de novo. In common with all cancers the cells display variability in size and shape and the other characteristics already cited in the discussion of anaplasia (Fig. 4–4). These tumors tend to be large, bulky, fleshy masses, often with areas of hemorrhage and necrosis. While infiltrative, their margins on gross inspection may appear deceptively well defined.

SKIN TUMORS

Four specific types of lesions will be considered in this presentation: (1) squamous cell carcinoma, (2) basal cell carcinoma, (3) pigmented nevi and (4) melanocarcinoma.

Skin cancer in general is the most common form of malignant neoplasia. It has been estimated that almost half of all people who reach 65 years of age have had or will have at least one skin cancer. Fortunately, 90 per cent of these lesions are curable by adequate local excision. Among the skin cancers, 30 per cent are squamous cell carcinomas, about 60 per cent are basal cell carcinomas and approximately 2 per cent are melanocarcinomas. The residual 8 per cent includes Kaposi's sarcoma, lymphomas (p. 342), Hodgkin's disease (p. 358) and other forms too rare to merit description here.

Squamous cell carcinomas may arise in any epithelial or mucosal surface made up of stratified squamous epithelium. Thus this form of cancer may occur, for example, in the tongue, lips, esophagus, cervix or vagina. Most, however arise in the skin, usually on the exposed surfaces of the body (90 to 95 per cent). Fair-skinned, blue-eyed, blond individuals who have outdoor occupations are particularly likely to develop this form of cancer. Often these tumors are preceded by so-called actinic (solar) keratosis, a form of dysplasia or anaplasia of the epidermal cells. Actinic radiation therefore is thought to be a very important etiologic agent, but arsenic and coal tars have also been implicated. Protracted chronic inflammation predisposes to squamous cell carcinomas and so this form of cancer is sometimes encountered in the margins of long standing draining sinuses and in old x-ray or burn scars. Sometimes the neoplasm does not appear until decades after the x-ray or thermal injury. You recall that individuals with xeroderma pigmentosum cannot repair DNA and are at particularly high risk of developing skin cancers (p. 101).

Typically, the squamous cell carcinoma begins as a small focus of increased keratinization associated with slight elevation of the lesion. The focus progressively enlarges over the span of months to years to produce a slightly elevated, indurated plateau. When ignored, such lesions may achieve a diameter of 3 to 4 cm., usually accompanied by central ulceration of the cancerous plaque, yielding an ugly necrotic crater rimmed by heaped-up margins of viable tumor. Neglected cases may become deeply invasive, and metastases to regional nodes may appear. However, metastasis to regional nodes occurs in less than 5 per cent of all cases and is rare in lesions less than 1.5 cm. in diameter.

Histologically the squamous cell carcinoma may be confined to an *intraepidermal location, without invasion of the dermis — carcinoma-in-situ (also called Bowen's disease)*—or it may be deeply invasive of the dermis and underlying structures. These cancers also vary from those which are extremely well differentiated (approximately 80 per cent of cases), having keratin pearls (Broder's grade I) (p. 83) to very poorly differentiated tumors with little keratinization, marked anaplasia, tumor giant cell formation and numerous mitoses (Broder's grade IV). The burrowing invasive strands and nests of cells in the well differentiated squamous cell carcinomas tend to replicate the organization of the normal epidermis; basal cells occupy the perimeter of these nests, with progressive maturation of the cells in the centers of the islands. Thus central regions of these tumor nests often exhibit concentric laminated keratinous layers, forming so-called keratin pearls (Fig. 4–5). In contrast, were it not for their location in the skin, it would be difficult to identify the histogenesis of very undifferentiated patterns of squamous cell carcinomas.

The prognosis is more dependent on the size and depth of penetration of the lesion than on the histologic grade, but adequate surgical excision is almost always curative.

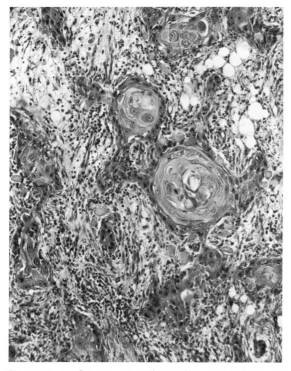

Figure 4–5. Squamous cell carcinoma of the skin. The primary origin of the tumor is not included. Shown are the characteristic invasive cords of cells bearing some resemblance to the squamous cells of the epidermis, which form keratinized epithelial pearls.

Basal cell carcinomas almost never metastasize and so are sometimes called basal cell epitheliomas by dermatologists who do not consider them to be true carcinomas. As with the squamous cell carcinoma, they tend to occur in those with fair skin, usually in areas exposed to the sun. Actinic radiation is an important influence. These cancers arise either in the basal cells of the epidermis or in the pilosebaceous adnexa and occur only on the skin. Mucosal surfaces, such as the lips, tongue and cervix, are never primary sites of these tumors. Grossly they begin as tiny, firm, elevated nodules with an intact overlying surface, and they progressively become small plaques. Even small lesions (less than 1 cm.) soon develop central ulcerations, which are characteristically rimmed by a pearly raised border (rodent ulcers). Some show varying degrees of pigmentation, which make them superficially resemble nevi. Neglected lesions may be locally penetrating, ulcerative and destructive, but in general their progression is slow and indolent, spanning many months to years.

Histologically, basal cell carcinomas usually appear as invasive clusters or strands of compact darkly chromatic spindled cells arising from the deep layers of the epidermis and extending into the superficial dermis. On cross section the strands create numerous nests or islands having a peripheral array of palisaded basal cells strongly resembling their normal forebears, which enclose a uniform collection of spindled forms (Fig. 4–6). Giant cells, striking anaplasia and mitotic figures are conspicuously absent. There are a large number of variations on this basic theme. Some lesions grow as solid masses, invading the dermis or deeper structures. Others are cystic or produce pseudoglandular lacy patterns and still others show maturation of the basal cells to produce keratin-lined microcysts, termed basosquamous carcinoma. Some of these tumors are pigmented, containing melanin granules within many of the epidermal cells. While most basal cell carcinomas are unicentric, on occasion multiple foci of tumor are separated by small zones of normal intervening epidermis. Usually, however, such multicentricity is confined to a relatively localized area (1 to 3 cm) of the skin

Surgical excision. irradiation or adequate cauterization will cure most basal cell carcinomas. Even when the neoplasm extends to the margins of surgical excision only one third of these recur These continue to extend and produce more difficult clinical problems. Ultimately, however, all are amenable to total cure. The presence of keratinization in a basal cell carcinoma does not alter its biologic behavior

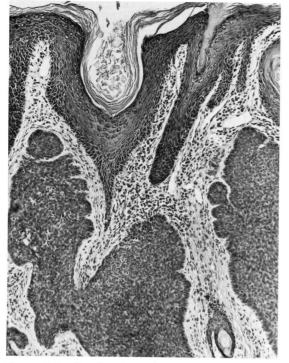

Figure 4–6. Basal cell carcinoma of the skin. The nests of cancer cells are seen in the dermis and are composed of small, tightly packed aggregates having a peripheral layer of neatly palisaded cells.

and so basosquamous patterns do not assume the significance of the somewhat more ominous squamous cell carcinoma which may metastasize.

Nevi and *melanocarcinomas* are considered together because both represent pigmented lesions of the skin which must be differentiated from each other, and also because certain forms of nevi are considered to be important antecedents of melanocarcinoma. All of these pigmented lesions are composed largely of melanocytes (mature melanin-forming cells), melanoblasts (immature melanin-forming cells), and melanophages (macrophages containing phagocytized melanin) (Fitzpatrick and Lerner, 1953). The derivation of the melanocyte was discussed on page 28, and it will suffice here to say that these cells are probably of neuroectodermal origin.

The term *nevus* is often used by dermatologists to apply to any circumscribed new growth of the skin of congenital origin. This definition encompasses melanocytic, vascular and a variety of other developmental anomalies. The pathologist generally uses the term *nevus to specify a developmental anomaly of melanocytes giving rise to a pigmented lesion, more popularly known as a mole.* It should be noted then that nevi are not true neoplasms. It has been estimated that every individual has at least 10 or 20 moles. They generally appear in childhood and enlarge along with the growth of the child; most become stabilized at the time of puberty. As everyone knows, they are extremely variable in appearance, showing every conceivable size, shape, degree of pigmentation and hairiness. A disproportionate number are located in the skin of the head, neck and trunk.

There are three major clinicopathologic types of nevi: (1) junctional, (2) intradermal and (3) compound. They are distinguished by the location of the melanocytes within the epidermis-dermis. In the *junctional nevus* nests of melanocytes are located at the *dermal-epidermal junction* hence the derivation of the term "junctional." The individual melanocytes are usually compact, round or spindled cells bearing a variable amount of finely granular brown to black pigment granules within their cytoplasm. In these benign lesions the nuclei are usually fairly uniform in size and shape. The cytoplasmic pigment granules are actually membrane-bound melanosomes (p. 28). Often the melanocytic nests appear to lie within circular clearings in the epidermis, sharply demarcated from the adjacent epidermal cells. Typically this nevus is flat or slightly elevated, pale brown and non-hairy. The junctional nevus is the most important form, since it is believed to be a precursor to melanocarcinoma.

The *intradermal nevus* is characterized by the location of the melanocytes within the dermis. Here the melanocytes may cluster in nests but are more apt to be scattered diffusely within the dermal connective tissue. The individual cells resemble those described in the junctional nevus but often they are more variable in size and shape and occasional giant cells may be seen. Although some intradermal nevi are very cellular and can be confused histologically with melanocarcinomas, this form of nevus is not thought to be a precursor of melanocarcinoma. It is the most common form of nevi in adults, and often these are hairy, variably pigmented, flat, elevated or papillary and occasionally quite large (4 to 5 cm. in diameter).

The *compound nevus* presents the composite histologic features of the junctional and the intradermal nevus—i.e., the melanocytes are found within both the epidermis and the dermis (Fig. 4–7). Because of their junctional component, these nevi may also give rise to melanocarcinomas. Other forms of nevi have been delineated (Lever, 1967) but are too uncommon to merit inclusion here.

Neither the location of a nevus on the body nor its clinical appearance permits accurate

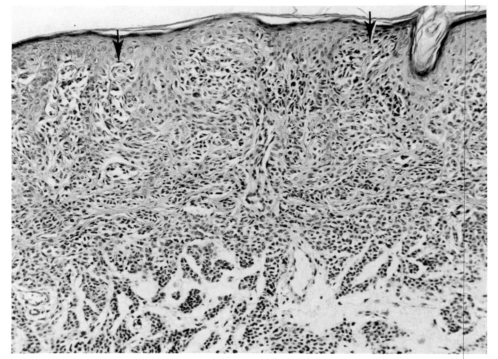

Figure 4–7. A compound nevus. Groups of small regular neval cells are readily evident in the dermis, and small nests of similar cells can be seen within the epidermis (arrows).

differentiation of one type of nevus from another. For unknown reasons, nests of nevus cells within the epidermis at the dermal-epidermal junction (junctional changes) are very common in nevi in children under the age of 10, but these tend to disappear with increasing age. Despite the presence of junctional changes in childhood nevi, they rarely give rise to melanocarcinoma in this age group. Equally mysterious is the fact that in adults junctional nevi either arise or persist more often in the extremities. So it is that nevi in the lower legs, feet, nail beds, palms and soles are very likely to have junctional features. Clinical features which tend to rule out junctional activity include hairiness and polypoid, dome shaped, sessile or pedunculated conformations (Shaffer, 1956). Because nevi are so commonplace, it is comforting to know that the chances that a nevus will become a melanocarcinoma have been estimated to be about 1 in 1,000,000. Most authorities, therefore, do not recommend prophylactic removal of all nevi—virtually an impossible task in the general population. Instead they recommend that lesions in adults so located as to be subject to chronic irritation by belts, straps, collars or underwear, and those on the palms and soles, should be removed.

Some characteristics of malignant transformation include a sudden change in color, diffusion of the pigment beyond the margin of the nevus, rapid growth, ulceration, inflammatory reddening of the margin, satellite foci of pigmentation about the perimeter, bleeding with insignificant trauma and the development of regional adenopathy (Mihm et al., 1973; Davis et al., 1966).

Melanocarcinomas, sometimes called malignant melanomas or more loosely (and incorrectly) melanomas, are important skin cancers which are often highly malignant. The term melanoma is particularly unfortunate, since there is a pigmented lesion of childhood, the juvenile melanoma, which, although it has a certain degree of melanocytic atypicality, is not malignant (McWhorter and Woolner, 1955). Although most melanocarcinomas occur in the skin, rarely they arise in the mucosa of the oral cavity and anus, the retina (intraocular melanocarcinoma) or in other tissues harboring melanocytes. Because melanocarcinomas are relatively uncommon, they are responsible for just under 1 per cent of all cancer deaths. The peak incidence occurs in the sixth decade. Approximately 3 per cent of melanocarcinomas are familial and transmitted by autosomal dominant inheritance. It has been estimated that approximately 50 per cent arise in preexisting nevi, usually of the junctional type and less commonly in compound nevi. As mentioned earlier, despite the frequency of junctional changes in nevi in children under the age of 10, happily melanocarcinomas are uncommon prior to puberty. The most common location for these lesions is the skin of the head and neck, followed by that of the lower extremities. Although most appear as enlarging pigmented skin lesions, some are so undifferentiated as to be unable to produce melanin and are characterized as amelanotic.

Three distinctive clinicopathologic patterns have been delineated (Mihm et al., 1971). The *nodular melanoma* presents as a slightly elevated (more than 2 mm.), firm, deeply pigmented, indurated nodule usually covered at the outset by intact epidermis. In most reported series this pattern carries the worst prognosis and is responsible for death in over half of all patients. The second variant is known as the *superficial spreading melanoma.* It is more common than the nodular variant, tends to produce large, flat, spreading lesions having a variegated appearance, including areas of brown to black pigmentation sometimes interspersed with foci of unpigmented tumor. The margins of these lesions often present small pigmented pseudopods and satellite foci of spread. Less aggressive than the nodular melanoma, this neoplasm kills about one third of its victims. The third variant begins as a lesion known as *Hutchinson's freckle* or *lentigo malignum.* It tends to occur most commonly on sun-exposed areas of elderly whites, particularly on the cheeks. It appears as a flat, slowly growing lesion, often 3 to 4 cm. in diameter, tan-brown, sometimes with foci of deep pigmentation. Of 85 patients with such lesions studied by Wayte and Helwig (1968), 45 developed melanocarcinoma. Thus not all Hutchinson's freckles are cancerous.

The histopathology of the melanocarcinoma is exceedingly variable; it may resemble an undifferentiated carcinoma of either small cell or giant cell type, a lymphoma or a sarcoma. Indeed, the entire range of cytology and anaplasia encountered in all of oncology may be seen in these cases. Certain features, however, are more or less characteristic. The atypical melanocytes are usually pigmented, and some involvement of the junctional zone between dermis and epidermis can almost always be defined. Because the neoplastic melanocytes of the spreading melanoma and those melanocarcinomas arising in a Hutchinson's freckle tend to be confined to the epidermal-dermal location, they are most difficult to differentiate from active junctional nevi. Atypical melanocytes usually have disproportionately large nuclei and nucleoli, and frequently tumor giant cells are evident. In time, penetration of the epidermis almost

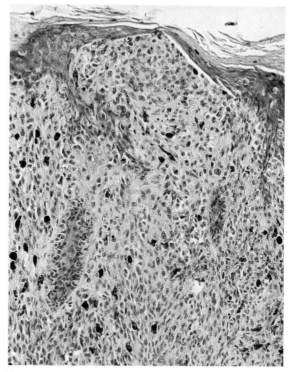

Figure 4–8. Melanocarcinoma. The anaplastic cells have invaded the epidermis and have almost eroded through the surface. The dark cells are filled with melanin pigment.

always occurs, and frequently the neoplastic cells erode through the surface of the skin (Fig. 4–8). Similarly, there is downward spread of the cancerous cells into the dermis. In advanced lesions, there may be deep invasion down to the subcutaneous structures. Most melanocarcinomas are marked by mitoses, an important feature in the differentiation of these malignant neoplasms from nevi. When an atypical mitosis is found in a pigmented lesion, it is almost certainly a melanocarcinoma. Generally a variable amount of lymphocytic infiltrate, found deep to the neoplasm can be taken as an indication of a cell mediated immune reaction to the neoplasm (p. 110), and there is considerable evidence that the heavier the infiltrate the better the prognosis. The histologic differentiation of an actively growing benign nevus from certain melanocarcinomas is most difficult and presents a problem even for the experts.

The clinical behavior of a melanocarcinoma is as variable as its cytology. Some lesions grow rapidly at the local site, yet do not spread to regional nodes or metastasize widely. On the other hand, disseminated metastases to the liver, lungs, brain, heart or bone may develop from a primary skin lesion so small it may require several examinations of the patient to find it. Spontaneous regression of the primary tumor has been recorded even in patients with rapidly advancing metastases. It is difficult, therefore, to express a prognosis for this form of neoplasia. The size of the local lesion, its depth of penetration, regional node involvement and evidence of an immunologic response all modify the prognosis. Until recently, the only form of therapy has been adequate local excision, sometimes with removal of regional nodes. Overall, the five-year survival rate is 40 to 50 per cent with such therapy (Fitzpatrick et al., 1972). At present there is hope that immunotherapy may provide further gains in the control of this form of neoplasia.

EPILOGUE

Many other forms of neoplasia will be considered in the various chapters dealing with specific organs and systems. For each of these tumors it is important to gain a perspective of its biologic nature and significance What is known about possible causative influences? What is the general growth behavior of such neoplasms? What patterns of spread do such tumors tend to follow? What is the cure rate with specific modalities of therapy and what is the five year survival rate? More indolent cancers, such as those of the female breast, may require over five years to kill the patient whereas with highly aggressive neoplasms, such as bronchogenic carcinomas, a five year survival is virtually tantamount to cure. Like people, neoplasms tend to behave in much the same manner as their cohorts, but as with people, individual behavior may sometimes be very aberrant.

REFERENCES

American Cancer Society: Cancer statistics. CA, 25:16–17, Jan./Feb., 1975.

Anderson, D. E.: Genetic varieties of neoplasia. In The University of Texas M. D. Anderson Hospital and Tumor Institute at Houston, 23rd Annual Symposium on Fundamental Cancer Research, 1969. Genetic concepts in neoplasia, p. 85. Baltimore, Williams & Wilkins, 1970.

Anderson, D. E.: Some characteristics of familial breast cancer. Cancer, 28:1500, 1971.

Baldwin, R. W., et al.: Immunity in the tumor-bearing host and its modification by serum factors. Cancer, 34:(Suppl.):1452, 1974.

Bill, A. H.: The implications of immune reactions to neuroblastoma. Surgery, 66:415, 1969.

Burnet, F. M.: Cancer, a biological approach. Brit. Med. J., 1:779, 841, 1957.

Burnet, F. M.: The concept of immunological surveillance. Progr. Exp. Tumor Res., 13:1, 1970.

Davis, N. C., et al.: The macroscopic appearance of malignant melanoma of the skin. Med. J. Aust., 2:883, 1966.

Editorial: Loss of suppressor function as a cause of lymphoid malignancy. Lancet, 2:1174, 1973.

Fitzpatrick, T. B., and Lerner, A. B.: Terminology of pigment cells. Science, 117:640, 1953.

Fitzpatrick, P. J., et al: Malignant melanoma of the head and neck: a clinicopathological study. Can. J. Surg., 15:90, 1972.

Fusco, F. D., and Rosen, S. W.: Gonadotropin-producing anaplastic large-cell carcinomas of the lung. New Eng. J. Med., 275:507, 1966.

Gatti, R. A., and Good, R. A.: Occurrence of malignancy in immunodeficiency diseases. A literature review. Cancer, 28:89, 1971.

Gold, T., and Freedman, S. O.: Demonstration of tumor-specific antigens in human colonic carcinomata by immunological tolerance and absorption techniques. J. Exp. Med., 121:439, 1965.

Gutterman, J. U.: Active immunotherapy with B.C.G. for recurrent malignant melanoma. Lancet, 1:1208, 1973.

Hellstrom, K. E., and Hellstrom, I.: Lymphocyte mediated cytotoxicity and blocking serum activity to tumor antigens. Adv. Immunol., 18:209, 1974.

Jehn, U. W., et al.: Lymphocyte stimulation by soluble antigen from malignant melanoma. New Eng. J. Med., 283:329, 1970.

Kersey, J. H., et al.: Malignancy in individuals with primary immunodeficiency diseases: The immunodeficiency-cancer registry. Proc. Amer. Assoc. Cancer Res., 14:57 (Abstr. 227), 1973.

Knudson, A. G.: Heredity and human cancer. Am. J. Path., 77:77, 1974.

Lever, W. F.: Histopathology of the Skin. 4th ed. Philadelphia, J. B. Lippincott Co., 1967.

Lukes, R. J.: Hodgkin's disease. Prognosis and relationship of histologic features to clinical stage. J.A.M.A., 190:914, 1964.

Lynch, H. T., and Krush, A. J.: Cancer genetics. South. Med. J., 64(Suppl. 1):26, 1971.

McWhorter, H. E., and Woolner, L. B.: Pigmented nevi, juvenile melanomas and malignant melanomas in children. Cancer, 7:564, 1955.

Mihm, M. C., Jr., et al.: The clinical diagnosis, classification and histogenetic concepts of the early stages of cutaneous malignant melanomas. New Eng. J. Med., 284:1078, 1971.

Mihm, M. C., Jr., et al.: Early detection of cutaneous malignant melanoma. A color atlas. New Eng. J. Med., 289:989, 1973.

Morton, D. T., et al.: Immunologic virus studies with human sarcomas. Surgery, 66:152, 1969.

Penn, I.: Chemical immunosuppression and human cancer. Cancer, 34(Suppl.):1474, 1974.

Piessens, W. F.: Evidence for human cancer immunity. Cancer, 26:1212, 1970.

Sabine, J. R., et al.: Spontaneous tumors in C3H-A^{vy} and C3H-A^{vy}fB mice: High incidence in the United States and low incidence in Australia. J. Nat. Cancer Inst., 50:1237, 1973.

Schwartz, R. S.: Another look at immunologic surveillance. New Eng. J. Med., 293:181, 1975.

Shaffer, B.: Identification of malignant potentialities of melanocytic (pigmented) nevus. J.A.M.A., 161:1222, 1956.

von Hamm, E. A.: Comparative study of the accuracy of cancer cell detection by cytologic methods. Acta Cytologica, 6:508, 1962.

Wayte, D. M., and Helwig, E. B.: Melanotic freckles of Hutchinson. Cancer, 21:893, 1968.

Wilson, R. E., et al.: Immunologic rejection of human cancer transplanted with a renal allograft. New Eng. J. Med., 278:479, 1968.

Zamcheck, N., et al.: Immunologic diagnosis and prognosis of human digestive-tract cancer: carcinoembryonic antigens. New Eng. J. Med., 286:83, 1972.

CHAPTER 5
Genetic Diseases

From time immemorial every lover has intuitively known what science now stands on the threshold of proving—his loved one is truly unique. Even seemingly identical, monozygotic female twins probably have biochemical differences as a result of random inactivation of one of the X chromosomes. Within the past decade, remarkable advances, such as improved enzyme assays, precise amino acid sequencing of polypeptides and deep penetrations into the mysteries of the genetic code, have disclosed seemingly endless genotypic and biochemical variations among individuals. Recall that until as recently as 1956, when Tjio and Levan established the correct human chromosome count as 46, it was believed that man possessed 48 chromosomes. Today point mutations can be identified at the level of a single triplet in the sequence of DNA bases. The origin of sickle cell anemia has been traced to the subtlest of mutations, the substitution of one purine base in the DNA sequence for another, resulting in valine rather than glutamic acid being incorporated into the beta hemoglobin chains. More than 100 hemoglobin variants have subsequently been identified, arising in similar point mutations (Vogel, 1969). Over 90 abnormal G-6-PD enzymes have been described arising from mutations among the alleles at the sex-linked locus which governs the synthesis of this enzyme. The genetic code, masked within the chromosomes, is slowly yielding to new sophisticated probes, such as fluorescence staining with quinacrine mustard (and similar agents), giemsa staining after special treatment of the chromosomes, "reverse" banding techniques, autoradiography and cell hybridization. It is now possible to fuse cultured human cells to those derived from animals. These hybrids tend to lose human chromosomes as they replicate. Characterization of the karyotype and enzymes possessed by isolated clones then makes it possible to localize genes coding for specific enzymes. Techniques such as these have led to the identification of each chromosome and to the recognition of translocations that do not alter chromosome morphology, and even have begun to unfold the map of gene loci within the chromosomes (Caspersson et al., 1971; Crossen, 1972; Martin and Hoehn, 1974; Paris Conference, 1972). Such great progress was made in the "horse and buggy" days; imagine what lies ahead in this rocket age of genetic exploration!

Traditionally, the diseases of man have been segregated into three categories: (1) those that are basically genetically determined, (2) those that are almost entirely environmentally determined and (3) those to which both "nature" and "nurture" contribute. Advances in knowledge, however, have tended to blur these distinctions. At one time microbiologic infections were cited as examples of disorders arising wholly from environmental influences. It is now clear, however, that to some extent heredity conditions the immune response and the susceptibility to microbiologic infections (Benacerraf, 1971–1972). Despite these uncertainties, there is a large and ever-growing list of disorders referred to as genetic diseases, whose prevalence is not generally appreciated. It has been estimated that in no fewer than 4 per cent of all live births there is a genetically determined deviation from the norm, and at least 1 per cent of all infants have a major chromosomal abnormality (World Health Organization, 1969). Surveys indicate that as many as one sixth of the pediatric inpatients and 10 per cent of the pediatric outpatients in university hospital populations suffer from disorders of genetic origin (Day and Holmes, 1973). These data only express the tip of the iceberg. Chromosome aberrations have been identified in 25 to 40 per cent of spontaneous abortuses (Carr, 1967). Remember, only those mutations compatible with independent existence constitute the reservoir of genetic disease in the population at large. Many more abortuses must have had gene mutations. The discovery that DNA is not limited to the nucleus, but is present also in the mitochondria, raises the intriguing possibility that some disorders of man may be due to changes in mitochondrial DNA (Borest and Froon, 1969).

It is beyond the scope of this book to review normal human genetics, but excellent brief surveys are available in the current literature (Hirschhorn, 1973; Carter, 1969a). It is necessary, however, to clarify several commonly used terms—hereditary, familial and congenital. *Hereditary* disorders, by definition, are derived from one's parents and are transmitted in the gametes. These arise in mutations, some of which are transmitted through several generations and therefore are *familial*. However, sometimes the mutation occurs during gametogenesis and the parents as well as previous generations are therefore free of the defect. The proband, of course, may be the forebear of affected generations to come. Sometimes the mutations may be lethal or so reduce fertility that further transmission of the defect is prevented. Similarly, genetic diseases with polygenic modes of transmission may disappear as the many mutant genes are diluted by repeated matings with normal individuals. The term *congenital* simply implies "born with." It should be noted that some congenital diseases are not genetic, as for example congenital syphilis. On the other hand, not all genetic diseases are congenital; patients with hereditary Huntington's chorea, for example, begin to manifest their condition only after the third or fourth decade of life.

Genetic disorders fall into three major categories: (1) diseases with polygenic (multifactorial) inheritance; (2) those related to mutant genes of large effect, and (3) those arising in chromosomal aberrations. The first category includes some of the most common disorders of man, such as hypertension and diabetes mellitus. Multifactorial or polygenic inheritance implies that usually both genetic and environmental influences condition the expression of a phenotypic characteristic or disease. The genetic component involves the additive result of multiple genes of small effect; the environmental contribution may be small or large, and in some cases, is required for expression of the phenotypic attribute. The second category, sometimes referred to as mendelian disorders, includes many relatively rare conditions such as the "storage" diseases and inborn errors of metabolism, all resulting from single gene mutations of large effect. Most of these conditions are hereditary and familial. The third category includes disorders which have been shown to be the consequence of numerical or structural abnormalities in the chromosomes.

Each of these three categories will be discussed separately in the material to follow. First, however, we should discuss the causes of mutation and say a few words about some conditions which have variable modes of transmission.

CAUSES OF MUTATION

Up to the present time, lack of precise methods for detecting changes in the genotype has severely limited the study of causes of mutation. Despite all handicaps it is clear that *aging, ionizing radiation, chemical agents and viruses are mutagenic* (Table 5–1). The frequency of so-called "spontaneous" mutations increases with age, as is well documented by the increased frequency of Down's syndrome (p. 159) in the offspring of older mothers. The incidence of this tragic genetic error is approximately 1 in 2000 live births for women under 29 years of age, but rises progressively to 1 in 50 for mothers over 45 years of age (Penrose, 1961). Sperm are produced afresh throughout the life of the post-

TABLE 5–1. CHROMOSOMAL MUTAGENS*

A. Radiation
  1. Human cells in vitro: threshold, 50 r
  2. Human lymphocytes in vivo; threshold, 12 to 35 r
B. Drugs
  1. Affecting human cells
    Alkylating agents: Triethylmelamine, busulfan, nitrogen mustards
    Methotrexate, azathioprine
    Benzene
    Lysergic acid (LSD) (?)
    Streptonigrin
    Bromouracil
    Caffeine
  2. Affecting plant cells
    Caffeine and its analogues
    Phenols, ethyl alcohol and other alcohols
    Menadione, coumarin, etc.
C. Viruses
  1. In vitro effects on mammalian cells
    Herpes simplex
    SV 40 virus
    Adenovirus type 12
    Vaccinia
    Poliomyelitis
    Mumps
    Influenza
    Measles
    Rubella
  2. In vivo effects in humans
    Poliomyelitis
    Measles
    Yellow fever vaccine
    Infectious hepatitis
    Serum hepatitis
    Mumps (?)
    Chickenpox (?)

*Modified from Jensen, M. K.: Chromosome studies in patients treated with azathioprine and amethopterine. Acta Med. Scand., *182*:445, 1967.

pubertal male, but all ova are present from birth. Could this increased likelihood of chromosomal damage reflect the long exposure of ova to environmental factors? Humans, after all, are an ingenious aggregate of some trillions of cells derived by successive mitoses from a fertilized ovum. Small wonder that mitotic errors creep in.

Ionizing radiation has clearly been established as a cause of genetic injury. Evidence is available from all species, including man. The animal studies have been well reviewed by Green (1968). Most of these animal data relate to rates of abortion, size of litters and incidence of congenital anomalies. Chromosomal aberrations can be demonstrated in these animal models (Russell, 1964). In man, direct evidence of radiation injury has come from many sources, among them the survivors of the atomic bombs. Cytogenetic studies have disclosed considerably greater numbers of lymphocytes with altered karyotypes in heavily exposed survivors of Hiroshima and Nagasaki bombings, as well as in infants exposed in utero, than in normal controls (Bloom et al., 1967). Nearly 40 per cent of the infants exposed in utero had chromosomal breaks and

alterations, in contrast with 4 per cent of the controls (Bloom, 1968). Moreover, these data document only the chromosomal alterations; many more gene or point mutations probably occurred, which went undetected. The rate of abortions and stillbirths in those exposed during pregnancy was also significantly higher than in nonexposed controls (Yamazaki et al., 1954).

In addition, as has already been pointed out on page 98, survivors of the atomic blasts have a well-documented increased incidence of leukemia and other forms of cancer, in all probability the result of radiation-induced mutations.

Even the smaller doses of radiant energy employed in radiotherapy may be hazardous. Ankylosing spondylitis, a form of chronic arthritis of the spine, was at one time treated by repeated and heavy doses of radiation. Studies of these patients have disclosed substantial numbers of chromosomal aberrations that have persisted for years after exposure (Buckton et al., 1962). Infants and children who received significant amounts of radiotherapy to the head and neck region developed a higher than chance incidence of thyroid cancer two to three decades later (Duffy and Fitzgerald, 1950; Refetoff et al., 1975). Thus, even therapeutic radiation may be mutagenic. Happily, however, the small amounts of radiation employed in diagnostic radiology have not been implicated to date. Nonetheless, prudence is clearly indicated.

The subject of *chemicals (including drugs) and genetic injury* is a complicated one. A great many agents have been shown to alter the development of the human fetus when the pregnant mother is exposed to sufficiently large quantities. In the great majority of instances, it has been impossible to determine whether damage results from interference with the growth, development and metabolism of the fetus or from genetic mutation (Smithells, 1966). The tragic case of thalidomide is an excellent example. Mothers taking this drug gave birth to infants with striking "seal-limb" deformities, referred to as phocomelia. The few studies performed on chromosomes in the leukocytes of these children have failed to disclose abnormalities. Currently, it is believed that the drug interferes in some way with cell metabolism and hence with cell growth. On the other hand, cytogenetic alterations have been observed both in vitro and in vivo following the use of some chemicals (including drugs), as is indicated in Table 5–1.

A word of caution is in order about the relationship of chemicals and drugs in the production of genetic injury. In most instances the genetic effects of these agents have been studied on cells in tissue culture, and the relevance of the in vitro findings to possible in vivo effects has been seriously challenged. Indeed, it has been shown that even such seemingly innocuous drugs as aspirin may cause chromosomal changes in cell cultures. The question must be raised: Are these in vitro mutations merely a reflection of a non-specific noxious influence and hostile environment on growing cells? If so, in vitro changes may not be applicable to the in vivo action of a drug. Moreover, in vivo alterations do not necessarily imply clinical dysfunction. Our ignorance in these areas is still profound. The issue of lysergic acid diethylamide (LSD) and chromosomal abnormalities is an excellent case in point. This subject is discussed in some detail on page 247. Suffice it to say here that there is no evidence from in vivo studies of lymphocytes that at the blood levels of LSD commonly encountered in habitual users this agent is a true mutagen Similarly, there have been numerous reports in the recent literature of chromosomal breakage resulting from the exposure of human lymphocytes in culture to caffeine (Kuhlmann et al., 1968). However in vivo experiments have documented that even af er the daily administration of relatively large amounts of caffeine, no significant chromosomal damage was seen (Weinstein, 1972). Here again we see that in vitro results cannot be freely extrapolated to in vivo effects.

Viruses have been shown to be mutagenic for a variety of animal cells both in vitro and in vivo (Stich and Yohn, 1970). This fact has already been pointed out in the discussion of oncogenic viruses (p. 93). In addition, many viruses have been shown to induce chromosome aberrations in cultured mammalian and particularly in human cells (see Table 5–1). Chromosomal aberrations have also been identified in the lymphocytes of patients having the following viral infections: viral hepatitis, measles and poliomyelitis, and there are some reports that chickenpox, mumps and infectious mononucleosis may also be implicated (Gripenberg, 1965). It should be noted that all of these studies were based on the older technique of karyotype analysis. It is highly likely that many more associations between viral infection and mutation will be disclosed in the near future. A word of caution, however—whereas congenital malformations are common in infants of mothers who contract rubella in the first trimester of pregnancy, these malformations are attributed to direct viral infection of the developing fetus rather than to induced mutations. No karyotypic alterations have been identified in the malformed children. Such evidence does not,

however, exclude point mutations nor has this problem been submitted to the more rigorous methods of chromosome analysis currently available.

Several rare possible causes of mutation should be mentioned. An increased incidence of mutation has been observed in certain autoimmune states. For example, there is an association between thyroid antibodies and Turner's syndrome (45,XO). Does this imply an immune causation of mutation or the reverse (the mutation causes the autoimmune state)? Still another cause of mutation has been proposed recently—a gene for nondisjunction. Several families have been discovered in which members have more than one kind of aneuploidy. Despite these hypothetic mechanisms, the major causes of mutation are likely to be radiation, chemicals and viruses.

DISORDERS WITH VARIABLE MODES OF TRANSMISSION

Hereditary malformations are forms of genetic disease with an inconstant mode of transmission. Certain common congenital malformations have polygenic modes of transmission whereas others are transmitted by mutant genes of large effect; still others are caused by chromosomal aberrations. Some of the polygenic defects which have a frequency of one or more per 1000 births are listed in Table 5–2. These disorders run in families and present significant risks to blood relatives. First degree relatives of an individual with a hereditary harelip (*proband*) have a 35 to 40 times greater chance of being similarly affected than control populations; the risk for second degree relatives is sevenfold and for third degree relatives threefold. In some malformations of multifactorial inheritance, environmental influences contribute to the expression of the disease. For example, in the infant with a genetic vulnerability to congenital hip dislocation, premature weight bearing or trauma

TABLE 5–2. MALFORMATIONS OCCURRING IN AT LEAST 1 IN 1000 BIRTHS*

DIAGNOSES	INCIDENCE/1000 BIRTHS
Cleft lip (± cleft palate)	1
Congenital heart defects	4–5
Pyloric stenosis	3
Anencephaly	2
Spina bifida cystica	3
Congenital dislocation of the hip	1–3
Talipes equinovarus	1–3

*Modified from Carter, C. O.: Genetics today. Public Health (London), *82*:199, 1968. Courtesy of The Society of Community Medicine.

may unmask the problem. The importance of recognizing these polygenic hereditary traits lies, then, in the possibility of controlling environmental factors contributing to the expression of the disorder. Other hereditary malformations are transmitted by single mutant genes. For the most part, these monogenic errors of morphogenesis take the form of localized lesions affecting a single organ or system, e.g., the fingers, eyes or small intestine. The list of such defects is too long for inclusion here, but has been detailed by Holmes (1974). Mutations so gross that they alter the karyotype almost invariably induce widespread malformations; the best examples are the autosomal trisomies (e.g., Down's syndrome) presented on page 159.

Neoplasia is another disorder which may involve inconstant genetic influence. Here the mutation may be germinal and hereditary or it may be somatic, as has been discussed on page 100. In this earlier discussion it was pointed out that ultimately the induction of cancer probably involves one or more mutations in somatic cells (Knudson, 1973). Susceptibility to environmental oncogenic agents (chemicals, radiation or viruses) is known to be conditioned by the genetic constitution (Rowley, 1974). The development of a cancer, then, may well be a mutational event imposed by some environmental carcinogenic influence on a fertile genetic soil (Ames et al., 1973).

DISORDERS WITH POLYGENIC INHERITANCE

Polygenic (also called multifactorial) inheritance is involved in many of the physiologic characteristics of man, e.g., height, weight, blood pressure and hair color. *It may be defined as a physiologic or pathologic trait governed by the additive effect of many genes of small effect, but conditioned by environmental nongenetic influences.* Even monozygous twins reared separately may achieve different heights because of nutritional or other environmental influences. When assayed in a large population, phenotypic attributes governed by polygenic inheritance fall on a continuous or Gaussian distribution curve. However, diseases related to polygenic inheritance do not conform to Gaussian distributions. Presumably there is some threshold effect so that the disorder becomes manifest only when a certain number of effector genes are involved, as well as conditioning environmental influences. Thus the severity of a disease can vary widely, depending on the number of inherited genes. This variation is referred to as *dosage effect.*

Polygenic disorders run in families, since family members share many of their genes as well as environmental influences. The risk of a disorder's being expressed depends to a large extent on the relationship of the family member to the proband. However, as pointed out, all polygenic disorders involve environmental influences and so risk factors at best are approximations. The concordance rate of a disease in monozygous twins is significantly less than 100 per cent when multifactorial inheritance is involved. However, the chance of concordance in monozygous twins is much higher than that between first degree relatives (parents, siblings or offspring). More about these risk factors will emerge in the later discussion of one of the most important of the polygenic diseases, diabetes mellitus.

It is extremely difficult to establish polygenic inheritance for any disease—much more difficult than for disorders related to mutant genes of large effect or those arising in chromosomal aberrations. Ascribing a disease to polygenic inheritance must be based on familial clusterings and the exclusion of mendelian and chromosomal modes of transmission. *Polygenic diseases are expressed when a sufficient number of mutant genes are inherited, and the severity of the disease varies according to the number of affected genes and the presence of predisposing environmental influences.* Polygenic inheritance is believed to underlie not only diabetes mellitus and hypertension, but also gout, schizophrenia, manic depression, rheumatoid arthritis and certain forms of congenital heart disease, as well as some skeletal abnormalities (Carter, 1968). Hypertension provides an excellent example of polygenic inheritance. There is good evidence that the level of blood pressure of an individual, at least in some part, is under genetic control, apparently governed by multiple genes of small effect. The pressure levels of the population at large fall along a continuous Gaussian curve of distribution. At some arbitrary level of blood pressure, hypertension is said to exist, since pressures above this level are associated with a significant disadvantage to the individual. Similarly, when the maximum blood glucose levels in the general population following a standard glucose load are plotted, they fall on a normal bell-shaped curve of distribution. However, as will become clear, a sufficiently large deviation above the mean strongly suggests the existence of diabetes, or at least the likelihood of developing diabetes, to be discussed next.

DIABETES MELLITUS

Diabetes is a genetically conditioned disorder of insulin kinetics characterized by impaired carbohydrate metabolism with attendant alterations in lipid and protein metabolism. Such a brief characterization vastly oversimplifies this complex and still poorly understood disease. The following five qualifications must be added: (1) The possibility cannot be ruled out that diabetes represents a heterogeneous group of disorders having in common hyperglycemia as a nonspecific manifestation. Certainly two somewhat overlapping but nonetheless distinctive patterns can be recognized — *a growth-onset (ketosis-prone) syndrome, representing about 10 per cent of all patients, and a maturity-onset (ketosis-resistant) pattern (90 per cent).* These two variants may result from different inheritances (a point that will be further explored later). (2) More is involved than merely a lack of insulin: a delayed secretory response, resistance to insulin function in the peripheral tissues and inappropriate glucagon secretion probably all contribute to the disordered metabolism of carbohydrates. (3) While the beta cell dysfunction is certainly in part inherited, environmental influences play a significant role in the expression of the diabetic state. (4) The genetic disease, diabetes mellitus, must be differentiated from secondary diabetes, that is, hyperglycemia resulting from pancreatitis, pancreatic carcinoma, pancreatectomy, Cushing's syndrome, acromegaly, pheochromocytoma or hemochromatosis. It is not certain that these secondary diabetic states have the same clinical implications. (5) Most important, *the diabetic state is associated with a strikingly increased susceptibility to generalized vascular disease, principally atherosclerosis and thickening of the walls of small vessels (microangiopathy).* More will be said about this later.

All diabetics, regardless of their genetic and environmental backgrounds and the age of onset of their disease, have in common an inability to metabolize glucose adequately, a failure that leads to hyperglycemia and in turn to glycosuria. The inability of the cells to metabolize glucose provokes the elaboration of a number of hormones, particularly growth hormone, glucagon, epinephrine, ACTH and cortisol, all of which considerably complicate the metabolic picture. The major source of energy becomes fatty acids, mobilized from triglycerides stored within fat depots. As a consequence, ketone bodies (acetoacetic acid, beta-hydroxybutyric acid and acetone) are produced in excess, sometimes leading to ketosis and ketoacidosis. The mobilization of lipids induces hyperlipidemia, which probably contributes to the development of atherosclerosis. Proteins, from both the diet and tissues, are utilized for gluconeogenesis. Thus, anabolic processes, such as the synthesis of glycogen, triglycerides and proteins, are sacrificed to catabolic activities, including glycogenolysis as well as gluconeogenesis and the mobilization of fats. As a result, the diabetic state, which presumably begins as an insulin defect fans out in ever-widening circles.

Incidence. In 1973 diabetes mellitus was the sixth leading cause of death in the United States. The prevalence of this disease has been increasing rapidly. In the years between 1950 and 1965 the number of known diabetics nearly doubled. Part of this increase may represent better case finding (although perhaps 40 per cent of cases still go undiagnosed), but most of the increased prevalence is real. A generally increased longevity, the improved survival of diabetics, the salvage of diabetic infants who formerly died at birth and other factors all contribute. Since the disease may appear at any age the prevalence in each decade rises progressively through life and is greater than 10 per cent of the total population by the eighth decade (O'Sullivan et al., 1967).

A number of constitutional and environmental factors (*diabetogenic influences*) predispose to diabetes mellitus and significantly affect its incidence. Most important among them is *obesity.* Approximately 80 per cent of maturity-onset diabetics are obese and, conversely, about 60 per cent of markedly overweight individuals have some form of carbohydrate intolerance demonstrable by glucose tolerance tests. Frequently weight loss corrects the carbohydrate metabolic abnormality in the nondiabetic and significantly ameliorates the carbohydrate intolerance in the diabetic. *Increasing age* is also associated with an increased incidence of diabetes. *Pregnancy* is another major diabetogenic influence, its effect being attributed to the appearance of an increased resistance to insulin or some diminished effectiveness of insulin. Overt diabetes so precipitated may revert to a subclinical stage following delivery, but the diabetogenic tendency grows stronger with increasing parity. *All forms of stress, including trauma, infections, hypoxia and hyperthermia,* may unmask diabetes in those harboring the hereditary trait. It is a well recognized clinical phenomenon that the insulin requirements of the diabetic mount significantly during periods of stress, particularly with infections. Stress may produce its effects through the release of catecholamines, which induce glycogenolysis and lipolysis. The glycogenolysis further burdens beta cells and the free fatty acids exert an insulin antagonism. Thus, although the diabetic state is inherited as a genetic trait, the expression of this genotype is conditioned by environmental influences.

Stages of Diabetes. Many years before the disease becomes evident, the existence of the diabetic state often can be detected by biochemical abnormalities indicative of deranged carbohydrate metabolism. For example, an individual apparently free of disease may develop hyperglycemia postprandially, or it may appear with stress. Such an individual is at high risk of developing clinically overt disease, perhaps some years later. Indeed, the family pedigree alone may strongly suggest the presence of the diabetic trait in otherwise healthy individuals. In recognition of these antecedent states, diabetes is classically divided into four stages:

1. *Prediabetes* is a theoretical state applied to an individual who has an identical twin with diabetes, or both of whose parents or several close relatives are affected. Prediabetes may also be suspected in the female with any of these: obesity, a history of miscarriages, large babies at birth or toxemia of pregnancy. Microangiopathy in the eye grounds or subcutaneous microvessels also suggests the existence of prediabetes.

2. *Subclinical diabetes* refers to the stage in which the fasting blood sugar and glucose tolerance test are normal under usual conditions, but pregnancy, emotional disturbances, infections, trauma or the administration of cortisone provokes an abnormal glucose tolerance test.

3. *Latent diabetes* is present when the patient is asymptomatic, may or may not have a normal fasting blood glucose level, but has definite postprandial hyperglycemia and a clearly abnormal glucose tolerance test. Latent diabetes may persist for years and, indeed, the patient may never develop overt disease. However, when diabetogenic influences are imposed on the patient, he is at high risk of developing overt diabetes. Some clinics combine the subclinical and latent stages into a category called *"chemical diabetes."*

4. *Overt or manifest diabetes* is the full-blown clinical syndrome described in the introductory paragraphs. However, many patients, with mild overt diabetes may shift back to latent diabetes with marked weight reduction and, conversely, patients with latent diabetes may relapse to the overt stage during illnesses, only to remit once again into the latent category.

Inheritance. Although it is clearly a genetic disorder, the precise mode of transmission of diabetes mellitus is still uncertain. Three patterns of inheritance are now equally ardently favored: (1) autosomal recessive; (2) polygenic; and (3) heterogenic, implying mutation at one of many possible gene loci.

Autosomal recessive inheritance continues to be a popular hypothesis. A bimodal distribution of abnormal plasma glucose levels would be expected if diabetes were an autosomal recessive condition. Such a distribution has been demonstrated among a tribe of American Indians having a high incidence of diabetes (Rushforth et al., 1971). One would predict from this mode of inheritance that all offspring of two homozygous diabetics must possess the diabetic genotype. However, only about 50 per cent of such offspring have been found to be affected (Kahn et al., 1969). Incomplete penetrance and variation in environmental diabetogenic influences have been invoked as explanations.

Polygenic or multifactorial inheritance is an attractive possibility consonant with many of the findings. This would explain the wide variation in the clinical severity of the disease, as well as the less than 100 per cent incidence of diabetes among offspring of two diabetics. A continuous (unimodal) distribution of blood glucose levels is found in the general population as well as in first degree relatives of diabetics, and this is most compatible with a multifactorial or polygenic trait. Although this theory violates the findings in the tribe of Indians just mentioned (which may be a special case), it is currently in favor.

Heterogeneity, or the proposal that diabetes mellitus represents a group of genetic disorders having as a common denominator deranged insulin metabolism, has recently come to the forefront. Theoretically, insulin function could be deranged at any one of a number of points—in its synthesis, secretion, transport or peripheral action. For example, a mutation in the structural gene might alter the insulin molecule and render it ineffective. Another mutation at a different locus might affect enzymes involved in the release of insulin. Support of the concept of heterogeneity comes from the recent recognition of an increased incidence of diabetes mellitus in a variety of genetic syndromes. For example, an increased prevalence of diabetes mellitus has been found in patients having such hereditary recessive syndromes as Fanconi's anemia (Swift and Sholman, 1972), cystic fibrosis and G-6-PD deficiency, as well as in patients with Turner's syndrome, Klinefelter's syndrome and other chromosomal disorders (Rimoin, 1973). Clearly, these conditions do not all arise from identical mutations, and so it is inferred that one of many genetic aberrations may induce diabetes mellitus.

Although the mode of transmission is still uncertain, sufficient data have been collected to estimate the risk of the development of diabetes when a member of the family is affected (Table 5-3). For unexplained reasons,

TABLE 5–3. RISK OF DEVELOPMENT OF DIABETES WHEN A MEMBER OF THE FAMILY IS DIABETIC*†

MEMBER OF FAMILY AT INCREASED RISK	INCREASED RISK RELATED TO AGE OF PROBAND AT ONSET OF DISEASE		
	0–19 yr. old	20–39 yr. old	>40 yr. old
Parents of proband	2 to 3 times	2 to 3 times	2 to 4 times
Siblings of proband	10 to 14 times	4 to 5 times	2 to 4 times
Child of diabetic father	40 to 41 times	7 to 13 times	2 to 3 times
Child of diabetic mother	18 to 29 times	6 to 9 times	1 to 3 times

*From Simpson, N. E.: Diabetes in the families of diabetics. Canad. Med. Assoc. J., 98:427, 1968.
†Recent work with the HL-A antigens and diabetes by Nerup and associates (Lancet, 2:864, 1974) suggests that there are different risks for different families for "juvenile diabetes" dependent on HL-A types.

offspring are more likely to become diabetic when the father rather than the mother is affected. It must be remembered, however, that because of environmental factors and because the mode of transmission is still uncertain, the risk figures are, at best, inexact.

Pathogenesis. Although the chemical structure of insulin, its biosynthesis and secretory pathways are now understood in elegant detail, and precise immunoassays are available for its quantitation, the nature of the fundamental defect in diabetes mellitus remains a mystery enveloped in controversy. Before turning to this controversy, normal insulin metabolism will be reviewed briefly.

Insulin is a major anabolic hormone. It is necessary for: (1) transmembrane transport of glucose and amino acids, (2) glycogen formation, (3) glucose conversion to triglycerides, (4) nucleic acid synthesis, and (5) protein synthesis. *Its prime metabolic function is to increase the rate of glucose transport into certain cells in the body.* These are the striated muscle cells (including myocardial cells), fibroblasts and fat cells, representing collectively about two thirds of the entire body weight. How insulin effects this transmembrane transport is still uncertain, but it appears to interact with key receptors to activate a carrier system or somehow to render the membrane more permeable to glucose. A lack of insulin, then, impairs intracellular utilization of glucose. It should be noted that insulin does not enhance glucose transport into brain cells, red cells or cells of the intestinal mucosa, liver or renal tubules.

Insulin is synthesized within the beta cells of the pancreas from a long, single chain polypeptide (proinsulin — molecular weight, 9000), the two ends of which are coiled across the middle segment. Linkage of the two ends by disulfide bonds and then excision ("chopping out") of a central segment, known as the C-peptide, by peptidases, yields insulin (molecular weight, 5700) (Steiner et al., 1969). Like all peptides, proinsulin is synthesized on the ri-

bosomes of the rough endoplasmic reticulum, and is then transported through the endoplasmic reticulum to the Golgi apparatus, where it is "packaged" within membrane-bound granules (Lacey, 1970). It is believed, although not definitely established, that some or most of the proinsulin is cleaved in the Golgi apparatus. In any event, the membrane-bound stored insulin (along with some proinsulin and C-peptide) constitutes the granules of the beta cell. The biosynthesis of insulin is principally controlled by the glucose level of the blood which can initiate *both* synthesis and release of insulin into the blood. Proinsulin and C-peptide are secreted into the blood along with insulin. Although proinsulin has a high degree of cross reactivity with insulin in the immunoassay, it has low biologic activity and represents only about 15 per cent of plasma immunoreactive insulin (Goldsmith et al., 1969). There is *no* evidence that the impaired carbohydrate metabolism of diabetes mellitus is related to inability to cleave proinsulin or to the secretion of proinsulin rather than insulin into the blood.

Insulin release occurs as a biphasic process, i.e., it involves two pools of insulin. A rise in the blood glucose levels, for example, calls forth an immediate release of insulin, presumably that stored in the beta granules. If the secretory stimulus persists, a delayed and protracted response follows, which involves active synthesis of insulin. *Among the many substances known to trigger insulin release, glucose is the most important.* Surprisingly, the precise steps involved in glucose-stimulated insulin release are still somewhat uncertain (Taylor, 1972). Two phenomena appear to be involved. The first is an elevation in intracellular calcium ions. How calcium acts is still uncertain, but it is essential to glucose-stimulated insulin release (Sharp et al., 1975). The second phenomenon appears to be some alteration in the cell membrane mediated by an interaction between specific membrane receptors on the beta cell and glucose (Hollenberg and Cuatrecasas, 1975). This in turn activates membrane-bound adenyl cyclase, forming cyclic AMP (cAMP) from ATP within the cell (Charles et al., 1973). It is hypothesized then that cyclic AMP constitutes the "second messenger" or the ultimate intracellular signal which interacts with a microtubular or microfilamentous structure within the beta cell, leading to extrusion of granules (Hardman et al., 1971). Cerasi and Luft (1973) propose that the cAMP pathway has a direct insulin releasing action and intracellular glycolysis acts as an amplifying mechanism. Where calcium would fit into this scheme is not clear. The plethora of theories has yet to yield a unifying concept.

Glucose initiates both synthesis and release of insulin. Other agents, however, including gastrin, secretin, pancreozymin, enteroglucagon, pancreatic glucagon and ACTH, can release insulin through the cAMP pathways. *These other secretory stimuli (including the sulfonylureas) do not initiate insulin synthesis.* The "gut" hormones probably initiate release of insulin following a meal in anticipation of the absorption of glucose. Their effect may also explain why an oral load of glucose results in a higher level of plasma insulin than the same amount of glucose administered intravenously. At least 10 amino acids, but principally arginine, lysine, leucine and phenylalanine, serve as signals for insulin release. These amino acids, particularly arginine, may also act as amplifiers of the glucose signal. The precise steps and signals involved in insulin release are of considerable interest because, as we shall see, one of the major theories of causation of diabetes mellitus involves defective transmission of the insulinogenic signal.

Although the issue of the fundamental defect in diabetes mellitus is still highly controversial, there is general agreement on a few findings.

1. Growth-onset diabetics have an absolute or at least a severe insulin deficiency.

2. Maturity-onset diabetics secrete some insulin but less than normal controls with comparable glycemic stimuli.

3. Maturity-onset diabetics have a delay in the initial rise in plasma insulin levels.

4. Obesity alone, in normals or diabetics, decreases the biologic effectiveness of insulin.

5. Maturity-onset—usually obese—diabetics suffer from some increased resistance to insulin function in the peripheral tissues.

It is widely accepted that both growth-onset (juvenile) and maturity-onset diabetics suffer from inadequate beta cell secretion of insulin, worse in the juveniles than in the maturity-onset diabetics (Kipnis, 1970a; Cerasi and Luft, 1967). Most juvenile diabetics have a substantial reduction in the islet cell mass within the pancreas, sometimes to levels of 10 per cent of controls (Doniach and Morgan, 1973). Beta cell granulation is usually markedly reduced, as is insulin extractable from the pancreas (Wrenshall et al., 1952). Thus, *juvenile diabetics do not respond to oral hypoglycemic agents since they have an absolute deficiency of insulin,* and they are termed "insulin-dependent." However, even growth-onset diabetics secrete *some* insulin during the early stages of their disease, but in ever diminishing amounts as the disease progresses (Rosenbloom, 1970). The evidence therefore suggests that the insulin lack does not stem from a hereditary defect in the ability to synthesize insulin, but rather from progressive deterioration of beta cell function.

A large body of data favors the somewhat more controversial view that *maturity-onset diabetics also generate inadequate amounts of insulin* (Luft, 1968). When the glycemic stimulus is the same in both diabetics and nondiabetics, i.e., when both have identical blood glucose levels, the diabetic secretes significantly (approximately 30 per cent) less insulin than the nondiabetic (Kipnis, 1970b). Maturity-onset disease then is characterized by beta cell dysfunction and inadequate insulin response. However, because this form of the disease continues to be characterized by some insulin secretion, it is termed "non-insulin-dependent." In maturity-onset diabetes the insulin response not only is inadequate but also is delayed. In the normal individual, as the blood glucose level rises, it is quite promptly followed by a parallel increase in insulin levels (Seltzer et al., 1967). Following glucose loading, the peak insulin response occurs in 45 to 60 minutes. In the diabetic, the peak may be delayed as long as 2 hours. This delayed insulin response is taken as further evidence of beta cell dysfunction.

In summary, then, the concept is gaining ground that *both growth-onset diabetes and maturity-onset diabetes are caused by inadequate insulin release because of deficiencies in beta cell function.* The precise nature of the defect, however, is uncertain. At the present time, two differing proposals are most widely accepted: (1) beta cells have some genetic vulnerability to injury and destruction, or (2) there is some impairment in the transmission or reception of the glucose insulinogenic stimulus. Turning to the first proposition, Vracko and Benditt (1974) state: "Diabetes mellitus emerges in the light of new observations as a disorder characterized by a constitutional defect in the make-up of somatic cells manifested by an accelerated rate of cell death and subsequent cell replacement. The evidence suggests that the increased cell turnover is not the primary expression of the cellular defect but rather reflects an increased susceptibility of diabetics' cells to injurious events emanating from the cells' environment." The basis of the genetically transmitted vulnerability to injury is entirely mysterious. However, it is proposed that depending on the severity of the injurious influence, beta cells may suffer a gamut from reversible injury to destruction. The infiltration of islets and surrounding tissue by lymphocytes, sometimes found in both early- and late-onset diabetes, is an apparent reaction to cell death and supports such a proposition (Gepts, 1965; LeCompte and Legg, 1972). If the beta cells are not irreversibly injured, regeneration may occur, resulting in enlargement of preexisting islets and new islet formation. It is of interest in this connection that recent reports document a viral infection prior to the onset of carbohydrate intolerance in some patients (Gamble et al., 1973). Changes in the pancreatic islets following Coxsackie B4 virus infection have been seen which are reminiscent of those encountered in growth-onset diabetes. According to this view, the diabetic state results from an imbalance between the inherited ability of beta cells to sustain injury and adverse environmental influences.

An alternative theory posits failure to release insulin in response to the glucose signal. Cerasi and Luft (1973) point out that diabetics, even most juvenile diabetics, are capable of some insulin response to certain signals, such as arginine and the intestinal hormones. The failure of insulin release appears to be a decrease in "the sensitivity — or affinity — of the beta cell receptor for glucose." So we must leave it that there is general agreement that inadequate insulin release is a basic deficit in diabetes mellitus, but the precise location of the defect is still in doubt.

The possibility of *resistance to insulin in the peripheral tissues, particularly in adipose tissue, has also been invoked as an etiologic influence in diabetes mellitus.* Obesity, as mentioned, is a major diabetogenic influence. Yet there is general agreement that the fasting level of immunoreactive insulin is higher in the serum of obese patients than in that of lean subjects (Bray, 1973). To explain this enigma it is postulated that adipose tissues, more specifically fat cells, do not bind insulin or are somehow resistant to insulin and therefore have impaired uptake of glucose. Recent evidence indicates that the refractoriness of fat cells to insulin *cannot* be attributed to a *total lack* of membrane glucoreceptors (Lockwood et al., 1975). Perhaps enlargement of fat cells leads to fewer receptors per unit area of membrane. It has also been suggested that some

disorder of glucoreceptors affects all tissues throughout the body (Niki et al., 1974; Editorial, 1975), thus offering a possible explanation of the so-called peripheral resistance. Despite these recent observations the fundamental nature of this peripheral resistance is still uncertain. Could it alternatively be due to the production of insulin antagonists? Recently, a single or multiple enzyme defect which leads to abnormally high concentrations of an insulin antagonist derived from growth hormone has been hypothesized (Krahl, 1972). At the present time the hypothesis of peripheral resistance has neither been proved nor disproved.

Recent studies suggest yet another quite provocative theory on the basic nature of diabetes mellitus. The view has been offered that diabetes is not fundamentally a derangement of insulin secretion alone, but rather is a bihormonal disorder also involving oversecretion of glucagon (Unger, 1971; Unger and Orci, 1975). It is proposed that in the diabetic there is excess release of glucagon. Whereas an absolute or relative lack of insulin leads to glucose underutilization, an excess of glucagon induces simultaneously an increased release of glucose — both defects contributing to the hyperglycemia. The bihormonal theory implies that neither the alpha nor the beta cells respond appropriately to the glucose signal (Vinik, 1974). Normally, glucose suppresses release of glucagon from the alpha cells of the pancreas. Conceivably, in the diabetic there is faulty suppression of glucagon release, and it is possible that the hyperglucagonemia is more important, especially in the adult form of the disease, than the insulin defect.

It is impossible within the constraints of space to delve into all the additional pathogenetic hypotheses (some quite seductive) which have been proposed, especially for certain subsets within the phenotypic state called diabetes mellitus. Some of the possibilities include the production of an abnormal insulin, the formation of insulin antagonists which complex with insulin in the circulation and block its function, and an autoimmune reaction against endogenous insulin which simultaneously destroys beta cells (Bottago et al., 1974). Relative to this last proposal, it has recently been noted that juvenile diabetics have a higher incidence of certain HL–A antigens than either control groups or maturity-onset diabetics (Nerup et al., 1974a). It is argued that the linkage of histocompatibility antigens and immune response genes suggests that the juvenile disease may arise as an autoimmune reaction. Indeed, anti-pancreatic cell-mediated immunity has been demonstrated in juvenile diabetics (Nerup et al.,

1974*b*). The failure to find similar HL–A associations with maturity-onset diabetics is taken to mean that the insulin-dependent and non-insulin-dependent forms of the disease have different etiologies and modes of inheritance. Our consideration of the causation of diabetes mellitus must end here, but it is evident that for the present time it is an end without a conclusion.

Morphology. The diabetic at death may have many morphologic changes suggestive of the diagnosis and a few virtually diagnostic findings, or he may have no lesions that might not also be found in age-matched nondiabetics. This variability is poorly understood, but two factors are probably significant: (1) the duration of the disease and (2) the severity of the disease. The duration of diabetes strongly influences the development of anatomic changes. Generally the diabetic with disease of 10 to 15 years' duration develops dermal, renal and retinal microangiopathy, as well as atherosclerosis more severe than that found in age-matched controls. The severity of the metabolic derangement also correlates with the likelihood of morphologic changes, particularly those in the pancreas. In the presentation which follows attention will be focused on those morphologic changes that are most characteristic of diabetes.

Reduplication of Basal Laminae and Microangiopathy. Reduplication of basement membrane is characteristic of diabetes mellitus. When it affects capillaries it produces thickening of their walls, a change referred to as **microangiopathy.** This microvascular alteration is most evident in the capillaries of the skin, skeletal muscle, retina, renal glomeruli and renal medulla. However, reduplication of basal laminae is also seen in such nonvascular structures as renal tubules, Bowman's capsule, peripheral nerves, placenta and possibly other sites (Vracko and Benditt, 1974). The normal basal laminae consist of a relatively uniform layer of extracellular material separating parenchymal or endothelial cells from the surrounding connective tissue stroma. In diabetes this single layer is replaced by concentric layers which often contain cellular debris and droplets of lipids in the small crevices between the multiple layers. Such laminar thickening causes narrowing of the lumina of affected capillaries.

The issue of whether the changes in the basal laminae and the microangiopathy may be found in prediabetes and chemical diabetes is still controversial. **The fundamental question is — are these lesions secondary to the metabolic derangement of the diabetic state (Farid et al., 1973; Spiro, 1973) or instead are they genetic concomitants unrelated to the metabolic derangement (Siperstein et al., 1968)?** The severity of the microangiopathy and nonvascular laminar changes correlates with the duration of the disease rather than its severity. Possibly the genetic vulnerability of the cells to injury leads to cell replication over the span of years and the formation of successive generations of basal laminae. The point should be made that microangiopathy can be found in aged nondiabetic patients, but rarely to the extent seen in all patients with long-standing diabetes, whatever the age at onset of their disease.

Pancreas. The pancreas may show no anatomic changes, particularly in mild maturity-onset disease, or there may be slight atrophy of the islets indistinguishable from that seen in aged nondiabetic individuals. However, in the great majority of patients, one or more characteristic alterations are usually evident: (1) reduction in the size and number of islets, (2) an increase in the size and number of islets, (3) beta cell degranulation, (4) glycogen accumulation within beta cells, (5) amyloid replacement of islets or (6) leukocytic infiltration of the islets. **Reduction in the size and number of islets** may be encountered in two circumstances: (a) in rapidly advancing disease, i.e., in patients who die less than six months after the onset of glucose intolerance and (b) in very long-standing chronic disease. Presumably in the first instance there is rapid and progressive beta cell destruction, while in the latter, progressive cumulative damage ultimately outpaces the capacity for cell renewal and replacement. **An increase in the number and size of islets** is especially characteristic of nondiabetic newborns of diabetic mothers. It is proposed that in this situation the fetal islets undergo hyperplasia in response to the maternal hyperglycemia. Hyperplasia may also be seen, however, in growth-onset and maturity-onset diabetics, presumably as a compensatory response of the beta cells to injury. **Beta cell degranulation** implies depletion of stored insulin. **Glycogen accumulation** appears as small or large, clear cytoplasmic vacuoles within beta cells which show a positive PAS reaction. This change is usually considered to be reversible and a reflection of poor control and long periods of hyperglycemia prior to death. **Amyloid replacement** of islets appears as deposits of pink, amorphous material beginning in and around capillaries and between cells. At advanced stages the islets may be virtually obliterated (Fig. 5–1). Similar lesions may be found in elderly nondiabetics. **Two types of leukocytic infiltration are found in the islets,** principally in growth-onset diabetics. The most common pattern is a heavy lymphocytic infiltrate within and about the islets, a picture referred to as "insulitis." Here an autoimmune immunologic reaction is suspected. Virtually identical inflammatory changes have been found in the islets of cows and rabbits immunized with heterologous insulin. Eosinophilic infiltrates associated with severe regressive and necrotic changes in beta cells may also be found, particularly in diabetic infants who fail to survive the immediate postnatal period.

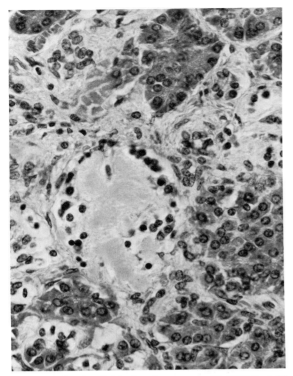

Figure 5–1. Amyloidosis of a pancreatic islet in a 65 year old male with diabetes of 25 years' duration.

Vascular System. Diabetes exacts a heavy toll of the vascular system. Whatever the age at onset, **in the course of 10 to 15 years of the disease, most diabetics have developed significant vascular abnormalities.** Indeed, about 80 per cent of diabetics die of some form of cardiovascular (including renal vascular) disease, compared with 40 to 50 per cent of nondiabetics. Vessels of all sizes are affected, from the aorta down to the smallest arterioles and capillaries (Entmacher et al., 1964).

The aorta and large- and medium-sized arteries suffer from accelerated severe **atherosclerosis.** Since atherosclerosis is a disease common to both diabetics and nondiabetics, it will be discussed in greater detail on page 266.

Myocardial infarction, caused by atherosclerosis of the coronary arteries, is the most common cause of death in diabetics. Significantly, it is almost as common in the diabetic female as it is in the diabetic male. In contrast, myocardial infarction is uncommon in nondiabetic females of reproductive age (p. 295). Gangrene of the lower extremities, as a result of advanced vascular disease, is about 100 times more common in diabetics than in the general population. The larger renal arteries are also subject to severe atherosclerosis. However, the most damaging effect of diabetes on the kidneys is exerted at the level of the glomeruli and the microcirculation. This is the subject of a later discussion.

It is generally believed that the predisposition to vascular disease in diabetes stems from some genetic trait separate from, but in some way related to, the metabolic derangement. In support of this contention, reports cite patients with a strong hereditary background for diabetes, who suffer from accelerated atherosclerosis but who have no demonstrable carbohydrate or lipid abnormalities (Herman and Gorlin, 1965; Ellenberg, 1963). Moreover, as pointed out, the advance of the atherosclerosis correlates better with the duration of the disease than with its severity. Any patient with a 10 year history of diabetes is almost certain to have at least moderate and more often severe atherosclerosis. The development of vascular disease may well be promoted by the hyperlipidemia and hypercholesterolemia so characteristic of diabetes. In addition, diabetics have an increased incidence of hypertension, which is known to accelerate the development of atherosclerosis.

Hyaline arteriolosclerosis, the vascular lesion associated with hypertension (p. 460) is both more prevalent and more severe in diabetics than in nondiabetics. However, it is not specific for diabetes and may be seen in elderly nondiabetics even without hypertension. It takes the form of an amorphous, hyaline thickening of the wall of the arteriole which causes narrowing of the lumen (Fig. 5–2). Not surprisingly, in the diabetic it is related not only to the duration of the disease, but also to the level of the blood pressure. The cause and nature of this vascular change are still uncertain. Al-

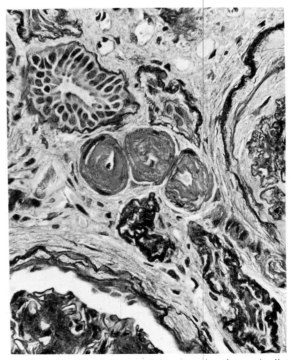

Figure 5–2. Hyaline arteriolosclerosis. A markedly thickened, tortuous afferent arteriole (cut in three planes). The amorphous nature of the thickened vascular wall is evident.

though at one time it was attributed to hypertension, so common among diabetics, a careful study by Bell (1953) noted arteriolosclerosis in 50 per cent of elderly diabetics who did not have hypertension. Recently it has been proposed that the hyaline material comprises deposits of plasma proteins. Presumably these penetrate into the abnormally permeable walls of the arterioles by a process termed insudation (Salinas-Madrigal et al., 1970). This concept relates the arteriolosclerosis to the exudative lesions of the glomerulus described later.

Kidneys. The kidneys are prime targets of diabetes. In fact, renal failure is second only to myocardial infarction as a cause of death from this disease. **Four types of lesions, collectively termed "diabetic nephropathy," are encountered: (1) glomerular lesions; (2) renal vascular lesions, principally arteriolosclerosis; (3) pyelonephritis, including necrotizing papillitis; and (4) glycogen and fatty changes in the tubular epithelium.**

A variety of forms of glomerular involvement may be present: diffuse glomerulosclerosis, nodular glomerulosclerosis (Kimmelstiel-Wilson syndrome), "fibrin caps" and "capsular drops." The last two are sometimes called **exudative lesions.** The sclerotic lesions of the glomeruli destroy renal function and constitute potentially fatal forms of

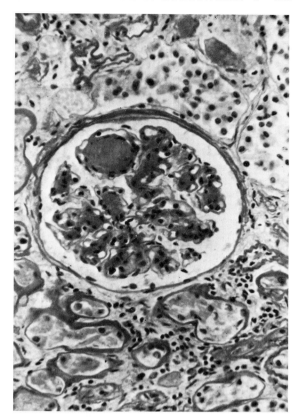

Figure 5–4. Nodular glomerulosclerosis in a patient who had diabetes mellitus for 17 years. The nodule at the upper left of the glomerulus is surrounded by a patent capillary channel. Note the thickening of the basement membranes of the tubules.

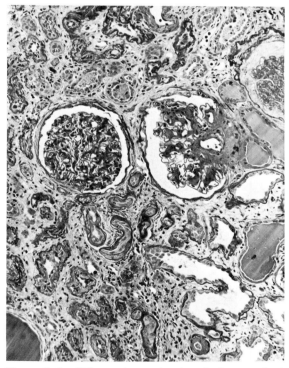

Figure 5–3. Diffuse glomerulosclerosis in a patient who had had diabetes for 16 years. The glomerulus at the right has marked axial thickening, fanning out from the vascular pole. The one on the left, caught in a less advantageous plane, has more delicate, diffuse intercapillary sclerosis.

diabetic nephropathy, but the exudative lesions are largely of diagnostic interest.

Diffuse glomerulosclerosis is found in at least 90 per cent of patients who have had their disease for more than 10 years. It takes the form of thickening of the basement membranes of the glomerular capillaries throughout their entire length, associated with some increased deposition of matrix into the mesangium. The mesangial cells may be overrun by this matrix deposition (Kimmelstiel et al., 1966). The membrane thickenings and matrix deposits are PAS positive. Biochemical analysis of these altered membranes discloses an increase in the hydroxylysine content and in the number of glucosyl-galactose disaccharide units. These changes are related by some authors to the disturbed carbohydrate metabolism (Spiro, 1973). The basement membrane lesions almost always begin in the vascular stalk and sometimes appear to be continuous with the hyaline arteriolosclerosis in the afferent and efferent arterioles (Fig. 5–3). When the diffuse glomerulosclerosis becomes marked, these patients manifest severe proteinuria and the glomerular cells exhibit loss of their foot processes. The nephrotic syndrome (p. 432), characterized by proteinuria, hypoalbuminemia and edema, may ensue. Progression of the glomerulosclerosis can lead to narrowing of the glomerular capillaries and eventual total sclerosis of the glomerular vascular tuft. Since the glomerular involvement is usually diffuse and invariably bilateral, advanced disease often causes renal failure.

Nodular glomerulosclerosis describes a glomerular lesion made distinctive by ball-like deposits of a laminated matrix within the mesangial core of the lobule (Fig. 5—4). These nodules tend to develop in the periphery of the glomerulus, and since they apparently arise within the mesangium, they push the peripheral capillary loops ahead of them. Often these patent loops create halos about the nodule. This lesion also has been referred to as **intercapillary glomerulosclerosis** by Kimmelstiel and Wilson (1936), who first called attention to it. Many object to the designation "intercapillary," because the deposit occurs within the mesangium, which may consist of modified endothelial cells. For this reason the noncommittal designation **Kimmelstiel-Wilson lesion** or **nodular glomerulosclerosis** is preferred. These lesions occur irregularly throughout the kidney and affect random glomeruli, as well as random lobules within a glomerulus. In advanced disease, many nodules are present within a single glomerulus, and most glomeruli become involved. The deposits are PAS positive and contain mucopolysaccharides, lipids and fibrils, as well as collagen fibers, and have the same composition as the matrix deposits of diffuse glomerulosclerosis. Often they contain trapped mesangial cells.

Nodular glomerulosclerosis is encountered in perhaps 10 to 35 per cent of diabetics and is a major cause of morbidity and mortality. Like diffuse glomerulosclerosis, its appearance is related to the duration of the disease. Unlike the diffuse form, **the nodular form of glomerulosclerosis is, for all practical purposes, specific for diabetes.**

In the great preponderance of cases, the nodular lesions are accompanied by diffuse glomerulosclerosis. Advanced arteriolosclerosis generally also is present. Whether the nodular lesion is simply an advanced stage of diffuse glomerulosclerosis or whether the processes are distinct is still a controversial issue (Bloodworth, 1968; Kimmelstiel et al., 1966; Gekkman et al., 1959). In any event, the progression of these two lesions and their constant companion, arteriolosclerosis, usually leads to obliteration of the vascular channels in the glomerulus and to serious, sometimes fatal, impairment of renal function. In the late stages of nodular glomerulosclerosis, adhesions appear between the visceral and parietal layers of Bowman's space, sometimes with considerable proliferation of the glomerular epithelial cells. Interstitial fibrosis and tubular atrophy become marked in advanced cases. Both the diffuse and the nodular forms of glomerulosclerosis induce sufficient ischemia to cause overall fine scarring of the kidneys, marked by a finely granular cortical surface. While diffuse glomerulosclerosis results in a reduction in renal size, nodular glomerulosclerosis may not. **Exudative lesions** take two forms. Glassy, homogeneous, strongly eosinophilic deposits in the parietal layer of Bowman's capsule, called "capsular drops," may hang into the uriniferous space. Similar appearing deposits, termed "fibrin caps," may develop over the outer surface of glomerular capillary loops, between the visceral epithelium of Bowman's capsule and the basement membrane. The nature of both of these lesions is obscure. Recent studies indicate that the "fibrin caps" are somewhat misnamed since they contain all the plasma proteins but only a small amount of fibrin. Although no proof exists, both the capsular drop and the fibrin cap are attributed to excessive leakage of plasma proteins from glomeruli that were severely injured by either diffuse or nodular glomerulosclerosis (Bloodworth, 1963). The fibrin cap is nonspecific and may be encountered in other forms of glomerular disease. The capsular drop, while not pathognomonic, is virtually diagnostic of diabetes.

Renal atherosclerosis and arteriolosclerosis constitute only one part of the systemic involvement of vessels in diabetics. The kidney is one of the most frequently and severely affected organs. However, the changes in the arteries and arterioles are similar to those found throughout the body. **The hyaline arteriolosclerosis affects not only the afferent but also the efferent arteriole.** Such efferent arteriolosclerosis is rarely if ever encountered in nondiabetic persons and is said by some to be virtually diagnostic of diabetes.

Pyelonephritis is an acute or chronic inflammation of the kidneys, which usually begins in the interstitial tissue and then spreads to affect the tubules and—possibly—ultimately the glomeruli. Both the acute and chronic forms of this disease occur in nondiabetics as well as in diabetics, and so they are described more fully on page 441. Suffice it to say here that acute pyelonephritis is essentially a bacterial suppurative inflammation which may cause abscesses. Although chronic pyelonephritis sometimes represents a progression of acute pyelonephritis, other, more complex etiologies may exist. There is some question as to whether these inflammatory disorders are more common in diabetics than in the general population, but in any event, once affected, diabetics tend to have more severe involvements.

One special pattern of acute pyelonephritis, **necrotizing papillitis,** also called **renal medullary necrosis**, is definitely more prevalent in diabetics than in nondiabetics. It is not, however, **limited** to diabetics, but is also seen with obstructions of the urinary tract as well as with analgesic abuse. In a large survey, approximately 60 per cent of the cases of necrotizing papillitis were associated with diabetes. As the term implies, necrotizing papillitis is an acute necrosis of the renal papillae (Fig. 5—5). It is described more fully on page 443. One or more papillae may be involved, bilat-

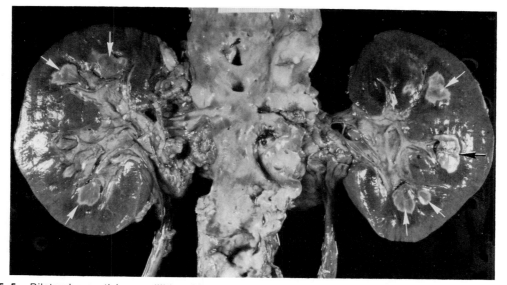

Figure 5-5. Bilateral necrotizing papillitis evidenced by the sharply demarcated areas of pale suppurative necrosis (arrows) in many pyramids of both kidneys.

erally or unilaterally. In the diabetic, bilateral necrosis of all papillae is not uncommon. The infarcted papilla may slough off and be excreted in the urine, permitting a clinical diagnosis by examination of the urinary sediment. When many papillae are involved, medullary necrosis causes acute irreversible renal failure.

Several **tubular lesions** also are encountered in diabetes mellitus. Perhaps the most striking is the deposition of glycogen within the epithelial cells of the distal portions of the proximal convoluted tubules and sometimes in the descending loop of Henle. This lesion is variously termed glycogen infiltration, glycogen nephrosis or Armanni-Ebstein cells (p. 25) (Kimmelstiel, 1966). The glycogen creates clearing of the cytoplasm of the affected cells. Only a distinct cell membrane with a squashed, basally displaced nucleus persists. This condition is believed to be a reflection of severe hyperglycemia and glycosuria for a period of days or weeks prior to death. Experimental evidence indicates that the lesion is reversible. No tubular malfunction has been connected with this tubular change. When glycogen deposits are present, they are virtually diagnostic of diabetes and only need to be differentiated from the far more severe, more diffuse tubular glycogen deposits found in the group of childhood hereditary disorders known as the systemic glycogenoses (p. 151). In addition, tubular basement membrane thickening may be found along with the membrane changes described in the glomeruli. Rarely, a patient who dies in diabetic acidosis may exhibit fatty changes in the proximal convoluted tubules.

Eyes. Visual impairment, sometimes even total blindness, is one of the more feared consequences of long-standing diabetes. This disease is presently responsible for slightly more than 10 per cent of all blindness in the United States. **The ocular involvement may take the form of retinopathy, cataract formation or glaucoma.** Retinopathy, the most common pattern, consists of a constellation of changes which together are considered by many ophthalmologists to be virtually diagnostic of the disease. These include intraretinal or pre-retinal hemorrhages, retinal exudates and edema, as well as venous dilatations and, most important, thickening of the retinal capillaries (microangiopathy), with the development of microaneurysms. The retinal exudates are of both the "soft" (microinfarcts) and "hard" (deposits of plasma proteins and lipids) varieties. The **microaneurysms** are discrete saccular dilatations of retinal-choroidal capillaries which appear through the ophthalmoscope as small red dots. Although their causation is still somewhat uncertain, the view that they represent aneurysmal dilatations at focal points of weakening caused by degeneration of pericytes is favored. Presumably these cells are injured or destroyed when they become trapped in reduplicated layers of basal laminae. It is of interest that about half of the patients with retinal microaneurysms also have nodular glomerulosclerosis. Conversely, **patients who have nodular glomerulosclerosis are almost certain to have retinal microaneurysms.**

Nervous System. The central and peripheral nervous systems are not spared by diabetes. The most frequent pattern of involvement is a **peripheral, symmetrical neuropathy** of the lower extremities, affecting both motor and sensory function, but particularly the latter. Such peripheral neuropathy may be accompanied by visceral neuropathy, producing disturbances in bowel and bladder function, and sometimes sexual impotence. The anatomic changes take the form of myelin degeneration and sometimes damage to the axon itself (see p. 675). The degree to which these changes may be related to the microangiopathy of the vasculature of the nerves is not clear. Neuropathy generally is associated with poorly controlled diabetes, and there is some evidence that those who are under careful control have a lower incidence of this complication.

The **brain,** along with the rest of the body, develops widespread microangiopathy. Such microcirculatory lesions may lead to generalized neuronal degeneration. There is in addition some predisposition to cerebral vascular infarcts and brain hemorrhages, perhaps related to the hypertension seen so often in diabetics. In addition, it must be remembered that hypoglycemia and ketoacidosis may both damage brain cells. Degenerative changes have also been observed in the spinal cord. None of the neurologic disorders, including the peripheral neuropathy, is specific for this disease.

Other Organs. **Hepatic fatty change** (discussed previously on p. 18) **is seen in many long-term diabetics.** In addition, glycogen vacuolation may be found in the nuclei of hepatic cells in about 10 to 20 per cent of cases. **Degenerative changes are encountered in striated muscle,** perhaps related to the microangiopathy or to motor nerve degeneration. It is seen only in long-term diabetics, particularly when the disease has been poorly controlled. In addition to the changes already described in the dermal microcirculation, a variety of lesions may be encountered in the skin. **Skin infections,** manifestations of the vascular insufficiency and predisposition to infection of the diabetic, are perhaps the most common. **Xanthoma diabeticorum** refers to a localized collection in the dermis and subcutis of macrophages filled with lipid (foam cells or xanthoma cells), creating a firm, nontender, usually slightly yellow nodule. They usually appear on the buttocks, on the extensor surfaces of the elbows and knees, and on the back. However, they may occur anywhere on the body. They are not specific for diabetes but are associated with all forms of hyperlipidemia. Another dermatologic change is known as **necrobiosis lipoidica diabeticorum.** This refers to a focal area of necrosis occurring within the dermis and subcutaneous tissues, anywhere on the body. The lesion usually appears as a slightly tender, irregular yellow plaque having a red-violet periphery. Histologically, there are degenerative changes and fragmentation (necrobiosis) of collagen associated with a peripheral nonspecific inflammatory reaction. Foamy histiocytes containing presumably neutral fats, phospholipids and cholesterol are often present in the central lesion. The usual inflammatory infiltrate of lymphocytes, histiocytes and, not infrequently, nonspecific,

foreign body-type giant cells may be found about such a focus. On occasion, a granulomatous reaction develops. Some ascribe this lesion to microangiopathy and loss of blood supply. With progression it may ulcerate through the skin or undergo fibrosis and produce an area of depressed fibrotic induration. Despite its name, this lesion is not limited to the diabetic patient.

It is evident that diabetes is associated with widespread anatomic changes, only a few of which are virtually pathognomonic. **"Insulitis," nodular glomerulosclerosis, glycogen deposits in the renal tubular epithelium, the retinopathy, and arteriolosclerosis in the efferent arterioles of the kidney are virtually diagnostic. Marked atrophy, hyperplasia or amyloid replacement of the islets are strongly suggestive.** Although individually some of these lesions may be found in nondiabetics, when present in combination, the anatomic diagnosis of diabetes can be made with a high level of certainty.

Clinical Correlation. The clinical manifestations of diabetes derive from the two major aspects of this disease (1) the metabolic derangement and (2) the vascular and organ involvements. The growth-onset (ketosis-prone) diabetic is likely to manifest prominent signs and symptoms referable to the metabolic problem early in the course of the disease. Ketoacidosis is an ever-present threat. Sometimes the disease is unsuspected until this medical emergency develops. The classical presentation, however, involves the "three polys"—polyuria, polydipsia, and polyphagia. The hyperglycemia leads to glycosuria, which in turn induces an osmotic diuresis *(polyuria).* This obligatory water loss, combined with the hyperosmolarity resulting from the increased levels of glucose in the blood and interstitial fluids, tends to deplete intracellular water, which is of particular significance in the osmoreceptors of the thirst centers of the brain. Thus arises the intense thirst *(polydipsia)* often seen in these patients. An increased appetite *(polyphagia)* may also be present. The explanation for this is less satisfactory and invokes such tenuous concepts as inability to utilize energy derived from carbohydrates and increased catabolism of fats and proteins. Perhaps it is better to admit that polyphagia is poorly understood. Weight loss and muscle weakness result from the widespread catabolic effects. The combination of polyphagia and weight loss is paradoxical and should always raise the suspicion of diabetes. The increased mobilization of storage fat leads to hyperlipidemia. In summary, then, the "metabolic" consequences of diabetes—particularly marked in the growth-onset form—are manifested *clinically* as polyuria, polydipsia, polyphagia, weight loss and weakness, and *biochemically* as hyperglycemia, glycosuria and hyperlipidemia. Ketoacidosis, with coma, may occur at any time.

In contrast, maturity-onset diabetes is more prominently associated with signs and symptoms secondary to the development of microangiopathy, atherosclerosis, nephropathy, retinopathy and neuropathy, the latter three referred to as the "triopathy of diabetes." *While maturity-onset diabetics also have metabolic derangements, they are usually relatively mild and controllable, and so this form of the disease is not often complicated by ketoacidosis,* unless intercurrent infection or stress imposes new burdens. Atherosclerotic events, such as myocardial infarction, cerebrovascular accidents and gangrene of the leg, are the most threatening and most frequent concomitants of long-standing diabetes. The Joslin Clinic points with pride to "Victory Medal" diabetics without vascular complications after up to 45 years of rigorously controlled diabetes (Chazan et al., 1970). Most diabetologists doubt that metabolic control so directly influences the vascular disease but nonetheless attempt to maintain reasonable metabolic control in the *hope* of ameliorating the vascular problem while at the same time reducing the load on the beta cells of the pancreas.

The glomerular basement membrane changes in diabetes mellitus induce proteinuria sometimes sufficient to cause the nephrotic syndrome (p. 432). In addition, elevated blood pressures are found in up to 80 per cent of diabetics, especially in those who are obese. Increased vascular resistance secondary to the generalized large and small vessel disease may contribute to the hypertension. *The combination of diabetes mellitus, hypertension and edema (resulting from proteinuria) is known as the Kimmelstiel-Wilson (K-W) syndrome.* Although at one time this syndrome was thought to imply the presence of nodular glomerulosclerosis, it is now evident that diffuse glomerulosclerosis is a more likely cause of the striking proteinuria of the K-W syndrome. While the ocular and neurologic complications do not contribute to the mortality of this disease, they bedevil the sufferer with loss or impairment of vision and all manner of sensory and motor nerve deficits.

Diabetics are also plagued by an enhanced susceptibility to infections such as tuberculosis, pneumonia, pyelonephritis and skin infections. Collectively, these cause the deaths of about 5 per cent of diabetic patients. The basis for this susceptibility is still obscure but is certainly not simply related to the increased levels of glucose in the blood. Defensive mechanisms against bacterial invasion, such as phagocytosis, are impaired and so infections tend to be serious. A trivial infection in a toe may be the first event in a long succession of complications (gangrene, bacteremia and pneumonia), ultimately leading to death.

The young diabetic female has her own special set of problems. Prematurity and stillbirths are significantly more common among diabetics than nondiabetics. If the infant is born alive it is usually fat and larger than normal, and has an increased chance of dying. This increased vulnerability is of short duration (1 to 2 weeks) if the infant itself is not diabetic.

The prognosis for the patient with diabetes depends on the age of onset of the disease and its severity. In a recent analysis of over 20,000 diabetics followed for a 26 year period, a significant excess mortality was found in both sexes and at all ages (Kessler, 1971). The excess mortality was greater for females than for males. It was particularly prominent in the age range of 20 to 39 years, when most who died had growth-onset disease. When overt diabetes is manifested prior to 20 years of age, life expectancy is shortened by as much as 20 to 25 years (Knowles et al., 1965; Larsson et al., 1962). However, when the disease becomes manifest after 40 years of age, longevity may only be slightly shortened. The causes of death in order of importance are: myocardial infarction, renal failure, cerebrovascular disease, arteriosclerotic heart disease and infections, followed by a large number of other complications more common in the diabetic than in the nondiabetic, e.g., gangrene of an extremity or mesenteric thrombosis. Fortunately, hypoglycemia and ketoacidosis are rare causes of death today. It is sad to close with the note that the diabetic's life expectancy has not significantly improved over the past three decades and, as mentioned at the outset, this disease continues to be one of the top 10 "killers" in the United States.

GOUT

Gout is a genetic disorder (or rather a group of disorders) of uric acid metabolism leading to hyperuricemia and consequent acute and chronic arthritis. The recurrent but transient attacks of acute arthritis are triggered by the precipitation into the joints of monosodium urate crystals from supersaturated body fluids. Over the span of years, the progressive accumulation of urates and the surrounding intense inflammatory reaction in the joints erodes the articular cartilage, eventually to produce chronic destructive arthritis. Inflammatory foci evoked by focal masses of urates are known as *tophi* — the morphologic hallmarks of gout. Tophi may form in joints and in soft tissues in and about the joints, as well as elsewhere. Whatever its pathophysiology, *the primary biochemical requirement for the development of clinical gout is hyperuricemia.*

It is now clear that gout is a group of phenotypically similar but biochemically and genetically heterogeneous disorders all having in common hyperuricemia. However, only 15 to 25 per cent of hyperuricemic patients develop clinical gout. The great majority of gouty patients (approximately 90 per cent) have as the cause of their hyperuricemia some inborn error of metabolism, and this form of the disease is called *primary* or *idiopathic gout.* In the remainder, the hyperuricemia is secondary to some underlying disease or medication, and this pattern is called *secondary gout.* The articular involvement and morphologic changes are identical in both forms, and so the following presentation deals principally with the idiopathic disease.

Gout is predominantly a disease of males (95 per cent) in their fourth and fifth decades of life. Most affected women are postmenopausal. More than one mode of genetic transmission is involved. It is currently believed that most patients with primary gout acquire their disease through polygenic or multifactorial inheritance. The male preponderance is attributed to the fact that women before menopause normally have lower serum concentrations of urate than men and so are at lower risk. The possibility of autosomal dominant transmission with incomplete penetrance has still not been rigorously excluded. One special subset of gouty patients has an X-linked form of the disease. As will be seen, these patients lack a specific enzyme involved in purine metabolism (Lesch and Nyhan, 1964). Whatever the mode of transmission, the same genetic and metabolic defect(s) are present within the individual family tree (Hauge and Harvold, 1955).

Pathophysiology of Hyperuricemia. There is no universal agreement on the precise normal upper limits of serum urates. Hyperuricemia is best defined as any level of serum urates which induces supersaturation of the serum and other body fluids. Normally saturation occurs at a concentration of 6.4 mg. of sodium urate per 100 ml. serum. However, plasma constituents (possibly mucopolysaccharides) exert urate solubilizing properties so that crystallization of urates does not occur until the urate level in the serum is about 7 mg. per 100 ml. In the United States, the mean serum urate levels for non-gouty populations are approximately 5.0 mg. per 100 ml. for men and 4.5 mg. per 100 ml. for women. In contrast, the mean serum urate level for gouty subjects is approximately 8.5 to 9.0 mg. per 100 ml., ranging to as high as 15 mg. in exceptional instances (Seegmiller et al., 1963).

There is considerable evidence that either increased production or reduced renal excretion of uric acid, or both, may be involved in primary gout. Consideration of these mechanisms requires an understanding of purine and uric acid metabolism (Seegmiller, 1974; Wyngaarden and Kelley, 1972), which can be considered here only summarily. A simplified overview is presented in Figure 5–6. Man, unlike lower animals, lacks uricase, so uric acid constitutes the end product of purine metabolism. Overproduction of uric acid then implies overproduction of purines. The natural nucleotides from which nucleic acids are synthesized, adenylic and guanylic acids, are formed in two major pathways: (1) de novo biosynthesis, and (2) salvage or reutilization pathways. In the *de novo pathway*, phosphoribosyl amidotransferase (PPGTase) catalyzes the formation of 5-phosphoribosyl-1-amine from 5-phosphoribosyl-1-pyrophosphate (PRPP) and glutamine. This is the rate limiting step in the de novo synthesis of purines. The *salvage or reutilization pathways* convert free purine bases from the diet, or from catabolism of nucleic acids, into their respective nucleotides. Such reutilization of free purine bases may occur in two ways, but our interest centers on hypoxanthine-guanine phosphoribosyl transferase (HG-PRTase) and adenine phosphoribosyl transferase. These enzymes, in the presence of PRPP, catalyze the synthesis of guanylic acid from guanine and adenylic acid from adenine. The amidotransferase (PPGTase) involved in the rate limiting step in de novo biosynthesis is subject to inhibition by the products of the salvage pathway, namely the ribonucleotides guanylic acid and adenylic acid. Control points in these metabolic reactions are: the availability of required substrates, the activity of involved enzymes and the concentrations of nucleotide inhibitors. *Recent evidence suggests that overproduction of uric acid in idiopathic gout may arise from three general categories of metabolic abnormalities: (1) defects which increase the level of the critical substrates PRPP or glutamine, or both, (2) a mutant enzyme accounting for increased intrinsic synthetic activity. or (3) decreased inhibition of the de novo pathway.*

Increased levels of PRPP have been identified in some gouty subjects (Wyngaarden, 1974). These increased levels result from two distinctive genetic metabolic defects. In the first, PRPP synthetase mutants overproduce PRPP leading to an increased production of 5-phosphoribosyl-1-amine in the first critical step involved in the de novo pathway (Sperling et al., 1971).

The second defect is a consequence of a deficiency of HG-PRTase. The discovery of the important role of HG-PRTase in primary gout followed the identification of the Lesch-

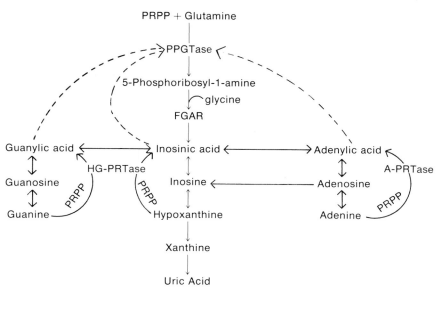

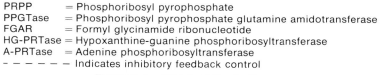

PRPP = Phosphoribosyl pyrophosphate
PPGTase = Phosphoribosyl pyrophosphate glutamine amidotransferase
FGAR = Formyl glycinamide ribonucleotide
HG-PRTase = Hypoxanthine-guanine phosphoribosyltransferase
A-PRTase = Adenine phosphoribosyltransferase
– – – – – Indicates inhibitory feedback control

Figure 5–6. Uric Acid Production

Nyhan syndrome (Seegmiller et al., 1967). This X-linked genetic condition, seen only in males, is characterized by the excretion of excessive amounts of uric acid, severe neurologic disease with mental retardation and sometimes all the clinical manifestations of gout. With an almost total lack of HG-PRTase, the reutilization pathways involving the consumption of PRPP are blocked and the levels of PRPP rise, leading to increased de novo production of uric acid. Less severe deficiencies of this enzyme may occur, and these patients present clinically with severe gouty arthritis beginning in adolescence, associated in some cases with mild neurologic disease (Kelley et al., 1969). Thus, this partial deficiency state identifies an X-linked pattern of gout particularly common in juveniles, characterized by increased levels of PRPP. While increased amounts of glutamine might also induce overproduction of uric acid, to date metabolic defects leading to such have not been identified in gouty patients.

The second category of metabolic disturbances involves some mutation accounting for increased synthetic activity of an enzyme. Indeed, several mutants of the PPGTase (amidotransferase) have been identified which in rare cases result in overproduction of uric acid (Nagy, 1970).

The third category refers to a possible lack of inhibition of the de novo pathway. A deficiency of HG-PRTase with lowered levels of salvage or reutilization of purines to form ribonucleotides not only might lead to elevated levels of PRPP but also might reduce the inhibition of PPGTase, known to be subject to feedback control. Alternatively, mutant amidotransferases might be resistant to inhibition. In either event, the de novo pathway would operate unchecked and lead to increased production of uric acid (Henderson et al., 1968). Therefore, it is evident that *overproduction of uric acid in primary gout is merely a common phenotypic expression of a heterogeneous group of genetic abnormalities*, all of which ultimately evoke overproduction of uric acid. Indeed, other defects as yet unidentified may also contribute.

Primary gout may also arise because of impaired renal excretion of uric acid, either as the sole metabolic derangement or in combination with overproduction of uric acid. The kidney has a remarkably inefficient mechanism for the excretion of urate. It is filtered through the glomerulus, reabsorbed in the proximal tubules and then returned to the urine more distally by a secretory process. Inadequate tubular secretion of uric acid has been observed in some patients with gout, leading to higher serum urate values (Rieselbach and Steele, 1974). Although all of these pathways for the development of hyperuricemia have been identified in gouty patients, it is discouraging to report that they only account for a minority of patients and in most the underlying metabolic defect(s) continue to elude us.

The hyperuricemia of *secondary gout* has many origins. In certain hematopoietic disorders, such as polycythemia, leukemia and myeloid metaplasia, there is excessive cell proliferation. The augmented synthesis of nucleic acids so lowers the level of nucleotides that inhibition of the de novo pathway is reduced. Any cause of renal failure may impair excretion of uric acid, and certain drugs, notably the thiazides, hinder renal excretion as well. In all these situations, the metabolic pool of uric acid is increased and may lead to disease indistinguishable from the idiopathic form.

Morphology. The distinctive morphologic as well as clinical features of gout are: (1) acute arthritis, (2) chronic tophaceous arthritis and (3) tophi in soft tissues.

The **acute arthritis** takes the form of an acute inflammatory synovitis made distinctive by the microcrystals of urates in the joint effusion. In order of frequency, the joints in the following regions are involved, although ultimately any joint in the body may be affected: great toe (90 per cent of patients), instep, ankle, heel, knee and wrist. The sequence of events is as follows. At first microcrystals of urates are precipitated into the synovial fluid and possibly synovial membranes. The crystals are instantly coated with extracellular elements, such as plasma protein. Attracted neutrophils phagocytize the crystals and enclose them within phagocytic vacuoles (Agndelo and Schumacher, 1973). Fusion of the vacuoles with lysosomes brings the coated urates into direct contact with lysosomal enzymes, which digest the protein covering. It is proposed that at this point the crystals form hydrogen bonds with the phagolysosomal membrane, rendering it more permeable (Weissmann, 1974). Lysosomal enzymes leak out, injure the neutrophil and eventually kill it. Thus, the urate crystals are released again only to be phagocytized by other

cells recycling the series of events. The release of lysosomal enzymes and cellular debris constitutes the major stimulus to the acute inflammatory arthritis (Seegmiller et al., 1962; Shirahama and Cohen, 1974). At this stage the synovial membranes are congested, swollen and heavily infiltrated with neutrophils, macrophages, lymphocytes and lesser numbers of plasma cells. When the episode of crystallization abates and the formed crystals are resolubilized, the acute attack remits. Embellishments have been added to this sequence. Kellermeyer (1968) proposes that the negatively charged urate crystals initiate the acute arthritis by activation of Hagemann factor This in turn leads to the release of chemical mediators of the inflammatory response (such as the kinins) and the simultaneous activation of complement. Many questions remain unanswered. Why does crystallization occur principally in the joint spaces and not, for example, in serosal cavities such as the peritoneum or pericardium? What accounts for the involvement of certain joints and not others? In other words, why are there selective sites of formation of tophi? Increased concentrations of urates secondary to slow turnover of fluid in the joint spaces (Simpkin, 1973) and urate binding substances, such as connective tissue mucopolysaccharides, have been proposed to explain the selective sites of involvement, but there are as yet no clear answers to these questions.

Chronic arthritis evolves from the continued pre-

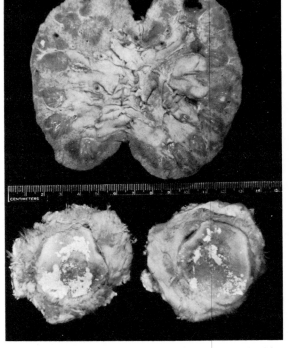

Figure 5–7. Urate depositions in gout. Several white urate deposits are seen within the pyramids of the opened kidney. Below, the white encrustations are seen on the articular surfaces of the patellae.

cipitation of urates in the recurrent attacks of acute arthritis. The urates produce heavy encrustations on the articular surface and some deposits penetrate deeply (Fig. 5—7). Large aggregations of urates are now formed within the subarticular bone or in the soft tissues about the joint. These deposits create the pathognomonic tissue lesion of gout—**the tophus. The tophus is a mass of crystalline or amorphous urates surrounded by an intense inflammatory reaction of histiocytes, lymphocytes and fibroblasts. Large foreign-body type giant cells, which are often wrapped around masses of precipitated salts, are very prominent** (Fig. 5—8). As tophi develop in joints, the articular cartilage and the underlying bone are eroded and progressive destruction of the joint ensues, simulating the changes of advanced osteoarthritis. Indeed, secondary osteoarthritis often supervenes in gouty arthritis.

Tophi are also likely to develop in the periarticular ligaments, tendons, connective tissues, olecranon and patellar bursae and in the ear lobes. Less frequently they appear in the kidneys, skin of the fingertips, palms or soles, nasal cartilages, aorta, myocardium and aortic or mitral valves. Very rarely, tophi develop in the central nervous system, eyes, tongue, larynx, penis and testes (Chung, 1962).

Urate crystals are water soluble, and non-aqueous fixatives, such as absolute alcohol, are necessary to preserve them in histologic sections. When preserved, they are demonstrable with routine or, more effectively, with silver staining techniques (deGalantha, 1935). The crystals are brilliantly anisotropic with polarized light microscopy.

For somewhat obscure reasons, gouty subjects have a predisposition to the development of **generalized vascular disease** of both large and small vessels. Prematurely advanced atherosclerosis is found in 30 to 40 per cent of patients, and often it is quite marked by the time the patients have reached their middle years. A review of the literature has shown that about 45 per cent of gouty deaths result from coronary artery disease. Recently it has been suggested that these patients have some abnormality in lipid metabolism that may be relevant to their predisposition to atherosclerosis (Barlow, 1966). Advanced arteriolosclerosis is also often present, particularly in the kidneys. Hypertension is a frequent concomitant of gout. It is still not clear whether the higher blood pressure is a cause or an effect of the arteriolosclerosis.

The **kidneys** are a prime target in gout. In a review of almost 300 cases, Talbot and Terplan (1960) found some form of renal disease in all but four patients. The renal lesions include pyelonephritis (p. 459), nephrosclerosis (p. 440), tubular aggregations of urates, intertubular deposits in

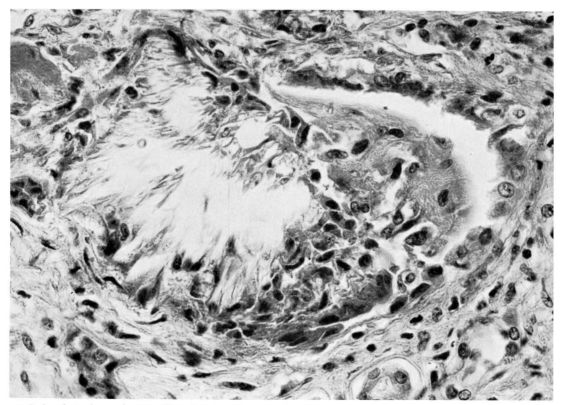

Figure 5—8. A tophus of gout. The deposit of urate crystals is surrounded by an inflammatory reaction of fibroblasts, occasional lymphocytes, and giant cells.

the medulla, uric acid renal stones and, occasionally, well developed tophi. The pyelonephritis may be secondary to the tubular obstruction created by the medullary deposits of urates. A variety of other lesions have also been described, such as acute tubular necrosis, glomerular lesions simulating proliferative glomerulonephritis, and amyloidosis. It should be noted that the renal disease does not necessarily parallel in severity the changes in the joints. Advanced renal changes may be present with minimal or no arthritis, and vice versa.

Clinical Correlation. From the clinical standpoint, gout has many faces. It may disclose its presence by a severe attack of arthritis early in its course, but equally often it smolders as a subclinical disease, nonetheless exacting its toll on the kidneys and blood vessels. Three stages have been delineated. *Stage 1 is designated as hyperuricemic asymptomatic gout.* Silent hyperuricemia is present in 25 to 33 per cent of relatives of patients with the overt disease. *Stage 2 is acute gouty arthritis*, characterized by flare-ups that may last a few days to weeks, but which are followed by complete remissions (intercritical periods) ranging from months to years. *Stage 3 — chronic tophaceous gout —* is the likely sequel to years of recurrent acute arthritis. Persistent disabling joint disease may develop within a few years or only after many decades of acute attacks. Renal symptoms, such as proteinuria, passage of gravel, and azotemia, are encountered in many patients and indeed about 20 per cent of those with chronic gout die of renal failure.

Gout is a very satisfying disease to the physician because the correct diagnosis and appropriate therapy have much to offer the patient.

DISORDERS RELATED TO MUTANT GENES OF LARGE EFFECT

Mutant genes of large effect are responsible for an enormous array of disorders, including inborn errors of metabolism, hemoglobinopathies, hereditary forms of neoplasia and certain endocrinopathies. Approximately 80 to 85 per cent of these conditions are familial, having arisen in a mutation in a past generation which is passed on to new generations according to mendelian laws. The remainder represent new mutants and so there is no family history of the disorder. Some of these disorders are believed to have reached genetic equilibrium, i.e., the loss of genes from the population, due to the failure of affected individuals to have as many children as the population as a whole, is balanced by the addition of new mutations. New mendelian traits are being identified virtually weekly, as can be seen in Table 5–4, drawn from McKusick and Chase (1973). It is evident that an impressive — or to the student of medicine, bewildering — array of mendelian traits was already recognized as of 1973 and the list is doubtless longer now.

An understanding of the characteristic pedigree patterns of these mendelian disorders is absolutely essential to genetic counseling. It is convenient to divide them into autosomal dominant, recessive and X-linked. A list of some of the more common disorders within these categories is offered in Table 5–5. The sections which follow deal separately with each of these categories.

AUTOSOMAL DOMINANT CONDITIONS

Autosomal dominant disorders are transmitted from one generation to the next; both males and females are affected and both males and females can transmit the condition. When an affected person marries an unaffected individual, on the average half the children will have the disease. The parents and siblings may of course be normal if a new mutation is involved. Clearly, the mutant gene is not passed on to subsequent generations if repro-

TABLE 5–4. PROGRESS IN IDENTIFICATION OF MENDELIAN TRAITS AND IN THE NOSOLOGY OF MENDELIAN DISEASE*†

	VERSCHUER (1958)	**McKUSICK's** *Mendelian Inheritance in Man*			
		(1966 ed.)	*(1968 ed.)*	*(1971 ed.)*	*(Jan. 1973)*
Autosomal Dominant	258	269 (+568)	344 (+449)	415 (+528)	498 (+588)
Autosomal Recessive	89	237 (+294)	280 (+349)	365 (+418)	419 (+448)
X-linked	38	68 (+51)	68 (+55)	86 (+64)	92 (+65)
Totals	412	574 (+913) 1487	692 (+853) 1545	866 (+1010) 1876	1009 (+1101) 2110

*From McKusick, V. A., and Chase, G. A.: Human genetics. Ann. Rev. Gen., 7:435, 1973.

†Insofar as is known, the numbers refer to separate loci. The numbers in parentheses refer to loci "in limbo"; i.e., monogenic inheritance of a particular trait has, with some reason, been suggested but proof is not complete.

TABLE 5–5. DISORDERS RELATED TO MUTANT GENES OF LARGE EFFECT

Autosomal Dominant	Autosomal Recessive	Sex-Linked
Marfan's syndrome	Cystic fibrosis	Hemophilia A (classic hemophilia)
Ehlers-Danlos syndrome	Phenylketonuria	Hemophilia B (Christmas disease)
Retinoblastoma	Galactosemia	Glucose-6-phosphate dehydrogenase (G-6-PD) deficiency
Neurofibromatosis	Wilson's disease	
Huntington's chorea	Albinism	Bruton's agammaglobulinemia
Osteogenesis imperfecta ("brittle bones")	Glycogen storage diseases	One form of gout
Milroy's disease (congenital lymphedema)	Mucopolysaccharide storage disease (certain forms)	One form of mucopolysaccharidosis (Hunter's syndrome)
Familial polyposis of the colon		
Hereditary spherocytosis	Lipid storage diseases (Gaucher's, Niemann-Pick, Tay-Sachs)	
Achondroplasia	Sickle cell anemia	
Hereditary hemorrhagic telangiectasia	Thalassemia	

ductive fitness is reduced to zero. Many degrees of reduction in reproductive capability may be seen, however. Some dominant conditions do not invariably manifest themselves in the heterozygote. This phenomenon is usually referred to as incomplete penetrance. Thus it is possible, given a long family history of a disorder, for an affected child to be born of normal parents. Such is the case with retinoblastoma, a highly malignant retinal neoplasm composed of anaplastic, poorly differentiated neuroblasts. This cancer may be genetic or sporadic. Generally, if not always, the genetic form of this neoplasm is present at birth although it may be two or three years before it is discovered (Ladda et al., 1973). When the tumor is multicentric and bilateral, it is almost certain to be hereditary. If the patient survives, nearly half the progeny will be affected, despite the occasional case of incomplete penetrance. This implies dominant inheritance.

MARFAN'S SYNDROME

This autosomal dominant disorder is characterized by defective formation of collagen and elastic fibers as well. The precise nature of the fiber defect still is not clear, but it may involve inadequate or inappropriate cross linking, which reduces elasticity and fiber strength. It is still not certain whether the primary defect involves collagen or elastin (Pinkus et al., 1966), but the similarity of its pathologic physiology to lathyrism (p. 283) in animals suggests a collagen defect as the basic lesion. In lathyrism foods rich in beta aminopropionitriles interfere in some manner with intramolecular cross linkages in collagen (Page and Benditt, 1972). Similarly, in some animals, a copper deficiency induces another

possible model of Marfan's syndrome. Conceivably copper serves as a requisite cofactor for lysine oxidase, which is involved in the cross linkages of collagen and elastin.

Individuals with Marfan's syndrome have manifestations relating to three systems—skeletal, visual and cardiovascular. These patients have a slender, elongated habitus with abnormally long legs and arms, spider-like fingers (arachnodactyly), high arched palate and hyperextensibility of joints. The lens in the eye may suffer dislocation because of weakness of its suspensory ligaments. Most serious, however, are the involvements of the cardiovascular system. Defective formation of collagen and/or elastica in the tunica media of the aorta predisposes to aneurysmal dilatation and dissecting aneurysms (p. 282). The cardiac valves, especially the mitral and aortic, may be excessively distensible and regurgitant (floppy valve syndrome), giving rise to left-sided cardiac failure. Death may occur at any age from aortic rupture. Although some patients with this disorder survive into the seventh and eighth decades, the average age at death is 30 to 40 years.

EHLERS-DANLOS (E-D) SYNDROME

This primary disorder of connective tissue, particularly collagen, is characterized by a wide range of clinical manifestations. Some are variable and appear inconstantly, whereas others, such as joint hypermobility; excessive stretchability, fragility and bruisability of the skin; and a bleeding diathesis, are usually present. Seven variants have been distinguished on the basis of the variable presentations of this syndrome. The first five, in which the exact nature of the biochemical abnormality is obscure, are transmitted as autosomal dominants. Jansen (1955) proposes that in these the organization of collagen fibrils into bundles and of the bundles into a strong network is defective. Alternatively, the possibility of excessive synthesis of elastic fibers in the skin and joint capsules has been raised. Supporting the view that the primary defect is in collagen is the fact that in both the sixth (E-D VI) and seventh (E-D VII) variants, specific enzyme deficits relating to collagen synthesis have been identified. E-D VI is characterized by a deficiency of protocollagen lysyl hydroxylase which leads to inadequate hydroxylation of lysyl residues and defective formation of the intramolecular cross links in collagen (Pinnell et al., 1972). E-D VII involves a defect in procollagen peptidase inducing abnormally long collagen fibers which do not cross link in the normal fashion. These two variants of the Ehlers-Danlos syndrome are inherited as recessives rather than dominants. Whatever the basic nature of the deficit, in all variants the joint hypermobility and excessive stretchability of the skin appear to be the consequence of the altered state of the connective tissue. The bleeding diathesis reasonably is attributed to inadequate support of the microvessels, which renders them vulnerable to rupture.

NEUROFIBROMATOSIS (RECKLINGHAUSEN'S MULTIPLE NEUROFIBROMATOSIS)

Recklinghausen's disease is a rare autosomal dominant condition which can be diagnosed entirely by clinical criteria. Most distinctive is the appearance of *multiple neurofibromas*, usually in the form of pedunculated nodules protruding from the skin. The neurofibromas are discrete, generally unencapsulated, soft nodules composed of a tangled array of all the elements found in peripheral nerves, i.e., Schwann cells, neurites, fibroblasts and possibly perineurial cells. Similar tumors ranging in size from microscopic to monstrous masses may occur in every conceivable site (along nerve trunks, the cauda equina, cranial nerves, in the retroperitoneum, orbit, tongue and gastrointestinal tract, for example). In addition, most patients have pigmented skin lesions known as *cafe au lait spots*. Sometimes these occur overlying a neurofibroma. Solitary cafe au lait spots, often over 1.5 cm. in diameter, are common in normal individuals, but when five or more are present there is a high likelihood of associated neurofibromatosis (Whitehouse, 1966). Infrequently, patients with Recklinghausen's disease have only the cafe au lait spots, an example of variable expressivity of a genetic defect. Besides being a disfiguring condition, neurofibromatosis may be extremely serious, either by virtue of the location of a lesion (e.g., within the cranial vault) or because one or more of the benign neurofibromas becomes transformed into a malignant schwannoma (approximately 1 to 5 per cent of patients). Usually the malignant tumors arise in the large nerve trunks of the neck or extremities. Infrequently, patients with this condition have other associated, presumably genetic disorders, including congenital malformations, pheochromocytomas, medullary carcinomas of the thyroid gland or intracranial neoplasms. It is of interest that nearly half of these patients have no affected relatives and are therefore thought to have new mutations.

AUTOSOMAL RECESSIVE DISORDERS

The great majority of inborn errors of metabolism are transmitted by autosomal recessive inheritance. Such disorders typically occur in offspring of unaffected heterozygous carrier parents, the risk being 1 in 4 (Carter, 1969b). With familial recessive conditions there is an increased frequency of first cousin or other consanguineous marriages among parents of probands. It is now possible in many conditions to identify heterozygous carriers. For example, many of the inborn errors of metabolism are characterized by a total lack or severe deficiency of an enzyme. Heterozygotes often have a partial enzyme defect, but since there is a considerable safety margin relative to the required levels of the enzyme, these carriers are apparently normal clinically. The expression of the identical enzyme deficiency in cultured fibroblasts provides another means of identification of heterozygous carriers. Although fibroblasts normally possess a wide enzymatic spectrum it should be noted that they do not synthesize the enzymes related to phenylketonuria and type I glycogen storage disease and so these conditions cannot be investigated in fibroblast culture (Raivio and Seegmiller, 1972). The culture of cells from amniotic fluid obtained through amniocentesis also provides a method of prenatal diagnosis of many of these biochemical disorders.

About 100 hereditary biochemical abnormalities have been recognized which are transmitted as autosomal recessive traits. Some take the form of missing enzyme syndromes, whereas others are characterized by an alteration in one or more amino acids in a specific protein or enzyme which changes its function or efficacy. Certain of the autosomal recessive conditions are discussed elsewhere: sickle cell disease and related hemoglobinopathies (p. 328) thalassemia (p. 330), and alpha-l-antitrypsin deficiency (p. 388). A few additional disorders are discussed below either because their recognition offers the opportunity for life-saving intervention or because they are among the more common of these genetic diseases.

CYSTIC FIBROSIS

Cystic fibrosis is a systemic disease of infancy or childhood in which there is a fundamental defect in the secretory process of all forms of exocrine glands. Most consistently involved are the eccrine *sweat glands, which elaborate a sweat abnormally high in sodium and chloride. The secretion of mucous glands is also altered, both chemically and physically, resulting in impaired transport of their secretions* (diSant'Agnese and Talamo, 1967). Earlier, attention was focused on the striking morphologic abnormalities in the pancreas evoked by the inspissated mucus within the ducts and so sometimes this condition is still called "fibrocystic disease of the pancreas," or "mucoviscidosis." Like gout, cystic fibrosis is genetically heterogeneous and comprises a group of closely related genetic abnormalities (all transmitted as autosomal recessives) with similar phenotypic expression (Danes and Bearn, 1969). Although the disease is expressed only in the homozygote, biochemical abnormalities have been detected in heterozygotes. Largely a disease of whites, it is also encountered, although rarely, in blacks, principally among those in the United States. It is equally rare among those of Oriental and Mongolian descent. Approximately 1 in 2000 live births in the United States are infants affected with this condition, and so cystic fibrosis is one of the most common, substantially lethal chronic diseases among children in this country.

The plethora of pathogenetic theories makes it obvious that the cause(s) of this disorder is (are) still unknown. Moreover, no single hypothesis offered to date satisfactorily explains all the features of this disorder. The theories attracting greatest attention at the present are: (1) elaboration of a humoral factor which inhibits ciliary motility and also resorption of sodium from exocrine secretions, (2) some basic defect in the movement of ions and water through the exocrine glands and (3) some fundamental abnormality in the process of exocrine secretion.

A *humoral factor* has been demonstrated in the serum which disorganizes ciliary rhythm and function in explants of respiratory epithelium (Spock et al., 1967). This factor, sometimes called anti-ciliary factor, can also be assayed on the cilia of oysters' gills. Presumably it impairs the transport of mucous secretions through exocrine gland ducts and also has been shown to inhibit resorption of sodium from parotid secretions. Recently, however, its significance has been challenged by a study showing that in children with cystic fibrosis clearance of inhaled particles from the ciliated airways in the lungs takes place at rates equal to if not superior to the rates of mucociliary clearance in normal adults (Sanchis, 1973).

Some *dysfunction in ion transport* is offered as the basis for the excessive sodium and chloride content of the sweat, a cardinal feature of this disorder. Mangos and McSherry (1967) have described a factor in the sweat capable of inhibiting sodium reabsorption. In addition, excess calcium concentrations have been identified in exocrine secretions (Gibson et al., 1971). It is suggested that calcium renders mucus more permeable to water, so that water is therefore excessively resorbed, resulting in increased viscosity. At the same time, increased resorption of water from sweat would explain the relative excess of sodium and chloride. However, the theory of deranged ion transport has been challenged by others (Benke et al., 1972).

The third major hypothesis speaks vaguely of some defect in the *process of secretion* and alludes to some fundamental genetic abnormality in secretory cell function. A defect in secretory signals, perhaps involving cyclic AMP, has been suggested, but is without substantial support. The morphologic appearance of the mucous-secreting glands in the respiratory airways and intestines suggests hypersecretion and possibly loss of normal controls. It must be concluded that despite the many theories, the origins of this disorder are far from understood.

The anatomic changes in cystic fibrosis are highly variable and depend on the age of onset and severity of expression of this genetic disorder. Pancreatic abnormalities are present in approximately 80 per cent of patients. These may consist only of accumulations of mucus, leading to dilatation of ducts, or, in more advanced cases, the ducts may become totally plugged causing atrophy of the exocrine glands (Fig. 5–9). The ducts may be converted into cysts separated only by an abundant fibrous stroma, a picture giving rise to the designation "fibrocystic disease of the pancreas." Loss of pancreatic secretion may lead to severe malabsorption, particularly of fats. A resultant lack of vitamin A, a fat-soluble vitamin, may then contribute to squamous metaplasia of the linings of the ducts. Changes similar to those in the pancreas may develop in the salivary glands. Pulmonary lesions are the most serious aspect of this disease. Retention of abnormally viscid mucin within the small airways leads to dilatation of bronchioles and bronchi with secondary infection, so that severe chronic bronchitis (p. 395), bronchiectasis (p. 397) and lung abscesses (p. 398) are frequent sequelae. In over 90 per cent of these patients **Staphylococcus aureus** is the infecting agent, but

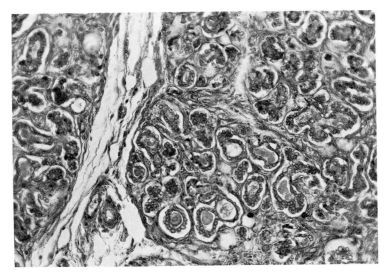

Figure 5–9. Cystic fibrosis of pancreas. The ducts are dilated and plugged with mucin, and the parenchymal glands are totally atrophic and replaced by fibrous tissue. (From Robbins, S. L.: Pathologic Basis of Disease. Philadelphia, W. B. Saunders Company, 1974.)

antibiotic control of this microorganism may lead to superinfection with gram negative bacteria such as *Pseudomonas aeruginosa.* The subtended pulmonary parenchyma may undergo emphysema (p. 386) or atelectasis (p. 377). Obstruction of the small bowel secondary to impacted viscid mucin **(meconium ileus)** is a not uncommon complication in newborns. In approximately 25 per cent of patients inspissation of mucin within the bile ducts impairs the excretion of bile, adding to the malabsorption problems. In time biliary cirrhosis (p. 529) may develop, but only in about 2 per cent of patients. The exocrine glands of the male reproductive tract are affected and in adults this often leads to sterility.

The clinical manifestations of this condition are extremely varied and range from mild to severe, from onset at birth to onset years later, and from syndromes which are predominantly gastrointestinal to those which appear to be cardiopulmonary. As many as 15 per cent of the cases come to clinical attention at birth or soon after because of an attack of meconium ileus. More commonly, manifestations of malabsorption (e.g., large, foul stools, abdominal distention and poor weight gain) appear during the first year of life. The faulty fat absorption may induce deficiency states of the fat-soluble vitamins, resulting in manifestations of avitaminosis A (p. 250), D (p. 251) or K (p. 254). If the child survives these hazards, pulmonary problems such as chronic cough, persistent lung infections, obstructive pulmonary disease and cor pulmonale may make their appearance.

At least three of the four following criteria are required for the diagnosis of cystic fibrosis: (1) increased levels of sodium, and more definitively of chloride, in the sweat; (2) a deficiency of pancreatic enzymes in the duodenal drainage; (3) chronic pulmonary sepsis related to one of the specific microorganisms mentioned, and (4) a family history of the disorder. The prognosis in this condition depends entirely on its severity, age at first diagnosis and effectiveness of management of the many complications. In a recent long-term study, Shwachman and colleagues (1970) found that about one quarter of the patients died before the age of 20 years. Increasingly, patients are surviving into adult life, albeit with pulmonary and gastrointestinal problems. Women with cystic fibrosis are capable of bearing children, but men, as mentioned, are frequently sterile.

PHENYLKETONURIA (PKU)

Homozygotes with this autosomal recessive disorder classically have a total lack of phenylalanine hydroxylase leading to phenylketonuria. Affected babies are normal at birth but within a few weeks develop a rising plasma phenylalanine level, which in some way impairs brain development. Usually by six months of life severe mental retardation becomes all too evident; fewer than 4 per cent of untreated phenylketonuric children have IQ values greater than 50 to 60. About one third of these unfortunate children are never able to walk and two thirds cannot talk. Seizures, other neurologic abnormalities, decreased pigmentation of hair and skin and eczema often accompany the mental retardation in untreated children. Once established, the mental deficit is irreversible, but if PKU is recognized promptly and the patient is placed on a low phenylalanine diet, the hyperphenylalaninemia can be prevented and the retardation of brain development avoided. A number of screening procedures are now available to detect phenylketonuria (Raine, 1974).

The biochemical abnormality in PKU is an inability to convert phenylalanine into tyrosine. In the normal child, less than 50 per cent of the dietary intake of phenylalanine is necessary for protein synthesis. The rest is converted to tyrosine, some of which is involved in the synthesis of melanin. With a block in phenylalanine metabolism, this amino acid is not available for synthesis of melanin and minor shunt pathways come into play, yielding phenylpyruvic acid, phenyllactic acid, phenylacetic acid and o-hydroxyphenylacetic acid, which are excreted in large amounts in the urine in PKU. Some of these abnormal metabolites are excreted in the sweat, and phenylacetic acid in particular imparts a strong musty or "mousy" odor to affected infants.

This inborn error of metabolism is quite common in those of Scandinavian descent and is distinctly uncommon in blacks and in Jews. As with all inborn errors of metabolism, a number of phenotypic variants have been identified. In addition to the classic homozygous disease described above, heterozygotes may have a partial deficiency of phenylalanine hydroxylase and so develop slightly elevated levels of phenylalanine without neurologic impairment. Another so-called "mild" variant has been identified, characterized by elevated plasma phenylalanine levels and phenylketonuria, but no detectable enzyme defect. Mental retardation may or may not develop in this variant. It is hypothesized that these patients have a high tolerance for phenylalanine. This pattern of the disease might reflect a variant in one of the three isoenzymes involved in phenylalanine metabolism. Still other phenotypes have been identified, such as transient phenylketonuria in infants. These children apparently begin life with what appears to be the classic disease, but the metabolic abnormality subsequently disappears. Only the classic homozygous disease has such devastating effect on the central nervous system.

Morphologic changes are limited to the central nervous system, but despite the obvious disastrous functional manifestations, the changes in the brain are inconstant and not striking. Almost always the brain is reduced in weight, and usually there is evidence of focal but widespread demyelination in the white matter, accompanied by focal gliosis (Malamud, 1966). Sometimes these foci are soft and spongy rather than gliotic and indurated (Salguero et al., 1968). There is still no understanding of how phenylalanine excess evokes these changes and, more specifically, deranges myelination. A number of proposals have been made, including inhibition of glucose incorporation into the glycolipids of myelin by phenylalanine metabolites, and general inhibition of glucose metabolism in the brain. Nevertheless, the origin of the central nervous system damage remains obscure.

GALACTOSEMIA

Galactosemia is an autosomal recessive disorder of galactose metabolism. Normally, lactose, the major carbohydrate of mammalian milk, is split into glucose and galactose in the intestinal microvilli by lactase. Galactose is then converted to glucose in three steps, as is detailed in Figure 5–10. *Two variants of galactosemia have been identified. The more common variant is a total lack of galactose-1-phosphate uridyl transferase involved in Reaction 2. The rare variant arises from a deficiency of galactokinase involved in Reaction 1.* Both variants are characterized by similar clinicopathologic changes, but only the transferase deficiency is considered here. As a result of the metabolic block, galactose-1-phosphate accumulates in many locations, including the liver, spleen, lens of the eye, kidney, heart muscle, cerebral cortex and erythrocytes. Alternative metabolic pathways are activated, leading to the production of galactitol, which also accumulates in the tissues (Quan-ma et al., 1968). Heterozygotes may have a mild deficiency but are spared the clinicomorphologic consequences of the homozygote.

The liver, eyes and brain bear the brunt of the damage. The early appearing **hepatomegaly** is largely due to fatty change, but in time widespread scarring may supervene, closely resembling the cirrhosis of alcohol abuse (p. 525). **Opacification of the lens (cataracts)** develops, probably because the lens imbibes water and swells as galactose-1-phosphate or other metabolites of galactose accumulate and increase its tonicity. **Nonspecific alterations appear in the central nervous system,** including loss of nerve cells, gliosis and edema, particularly in the dentate nuclei of the cerebellum and the olivary nuclei of the medulla. Similar changes may occur in the cerebral cortex and white matter (Smetana and Olen, 1962).

(Reaction 1) Galactose + ATP $\xrightleftharpoons{\text{Galactokinase}}$ Galactose-1-phosphate + ADP

(Reaction 2) Galactose-1-phosphate + UDP glucose $\xrightleftharpoons{\text{Galactose-1-phosphate uridyl transferase}}$ UDP galactose + glucose-1-phosphate

(Reaction 3) UDP-galactose $\xrightleftharpoons{\text{UDP-galactose-4-epimerase}}$ UDP-glucose

Figure 5–10. Conversion of galactose to glucose.

There is still no clear understanding of the mechanism of injury to the liver and brain. Toxicity has been imputed to galactose-1-phosphate. Alternatively, galactitol has been indicted as the toxic product. It is also possible that the abnormal galactose metabolism interferes with the formation of galactose-containing cerebral lipids.

Almost from birth these infants fail to thrive. Vomiting and diarrhea appear within a few days of milk ingestion. Jaundice and hepatomegaly usually become evident during the first week of life and may seem to be a continuation of the physiologic jaundice of the newborn. The cataracts develop within a few days of birth, and soon thereafter, within the first 2 to 4 months of life, mental retardation may be detected. Even in untreated infants the mental deficit is usually not as severe as that of phenylketonuria. Involvement of the kidneys may lead to proteinuria and aminoaciduria. As the patients grow older, alternative metabolic pathways for galactose are established and may permit prolonged survival.

Most of the clinical and morphologic changes can be prevented by early removal of galactose from the diet for at least the first two years of life. However, there is evidence in experimental animals that if the mother is mildly galactosemic some mental impairment may occur in utero. Control instituted soon after birth prevents the cataracts and liver damage and permits almost normal mental development. When galactosemia is recognized later, the changes in the lens and liver (if cirrhosis has not occurred) may be reversible, but the mental retardation is irreversible. The diagnosis can be suspected by the demonstration of a reducing sugar other than glucose in the urine, but tests which directly identify the deficiency of the transferase in leukocytes and erythrocytes are more certain. Recently it was observed that transferase can be introduced into cultured fibroblasts derived from patients by infecting these cells with a virus harboring an effective transferase gene (Merrill et al., 1971). To date, there are no reports of the use of this exciting observation in galactosemic patients.

ALBINISM

Albinism need be mentioned only briefly since, happily, it is not a serious clinical disorder. It represents the hereditary inability to synthesize melanin. There are a great many genetic variants of albinism, most of which are transmitted as autosomal recessives, but certain pedigrees suggest dominant transfer and others sex-linked transmission. Preponderant opinion favors the view that the absence of pigmentation results from a deficiency of tyrosine oxidase. This enzyme is involved in the conversion of tyrosine to 3,4-DOPA necessary for the synthesis of melanin. The lack of pigmentation of skin, hair, sclera and iris is only of consequence insofar as it permits light to pour through the unpigmented iris and sclera, thus causing retinal injury. The absence of melanin pigmentation of the skin also makes these patients vulnerable to skin cancer.

WILSON'S DISEASE

This autosomal recessive disorder of copper metabolism is characterized by three principal features: *(1) excessive deposits of copper in liver cells, leading in time to a form of cirrhosis, (2) degenerative changes in the brain, hence the synonym "hepatolenticular disease," and (3) a pathognomonic greenish-brown ring (Kayser-Fleischer ring) at the limbus of the cornea.* The nature of the metabolic error is as yet unestablished. Most of the evidence favors a deficiency in the synthesis of a specific copper-transporting alpha-2-globulin called *ceruloplasmin.* With a deficiency of ceruloplasmin, large amounts of copper are loosely bound to albumin. Ready dissociation of this albumin complex permits copper to be deposited in the tissues of the body, particularly in the liver, brain and cornea. An alternative hypothesis proposes that the mutant gene is responsible for the elaboration of an abnormal protein in the sites of involvement which have an increased affinity for ionic copper. In any event, *a normal or slightly lowered serum copper level, a well defined decrease in serum ceruloplasmin and an increase in albumin-bound copper are characteristic of Wilson's disease.*

Manifestations of liver disease usually become evident after five or six years of life. Early in the course, hepatocellular necrosis is observed, accompanied by the formation of hyaline deposits very similar to those seen in the liver with alcohol abuse (Levi et al., 1967). Electron microscopy discloses an accumulation of copper in the hepatic cell lysosomes, as well as mitochondrial abnormalities (Goldfischer and Sternlieb, 1968). Scarring is a consequence of the hepatocellular necrosis and in time *cirrhosis* develops, which may take the form of either a fine delicate network of fibrous tissue or massive scars resembling postnecrotic cirrhosis (p. 528). Signs of portal hypertension and liver failure may develop, and some children die of their liver disease with few neurologic manifestations.

If the liver disease does not prove fatal, involvement of the brain usually appears sometime during the second decade. The most dramatic findings are cavitations in the lenticular nucleus, in the tip of the frontal lobe and rarely in the dentate nucleus of the cerebellum. This is accompanied by brownish discoloration and often atrophy of the basal nuclei.

Histologically, there is an increase in the size and number of protoplasmic astrocytes, many of which become multinucleated. Degeneration of nerve cells and astrocytes in these areas leads to cavitations. The Kayser-Fleischer ring results from deposits of copper in the cornea and can usually be seen with the naked eye but may require slit-lamp examination. Aminoaciduria and glycosuria as well as other renal tubular abnormalities are virtually always present in patients who have developed neurologic disease.

Happily, despite the fact that the basic metabolic defect is unknown, it is possible to prevent the development of hepatic and brain disease, or in any event significantly improve the condition of patients with established disease by treatment (penicillamine, chelating agents) that reduces the stores of copper in the tissues. The disease can be recognized at an asymptomatic stage by the low serum ceruloplasmin level, which should be sought in children with a family history of this disorder.

GLYCOGEN STORAGE DISORDERS (GLYCOGENOSES)

There are at least 10 "missing enzyme" hereditary syndromes characterized by some metabolic defect either in the synthesis or the degradation of glycogen. All result in the excessive accumulation ("storage") of glycogen or some abnormal form of glycogen in various

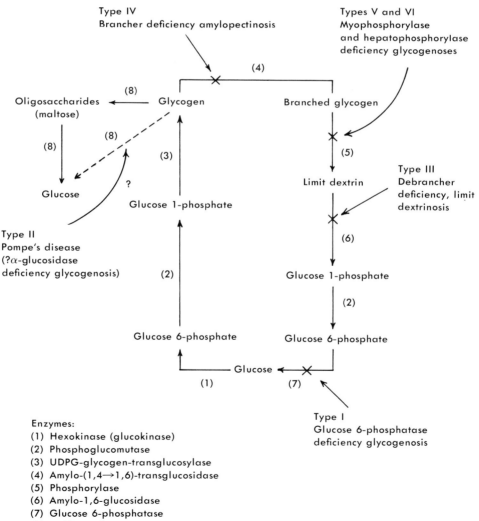

Figure 5–11. The glycogen cycle (schematic) and sites (marked with an x) of genetically determined enzyme "lesions" causing excessive glycogen deposition. (Adapted from Field, R. A.: Glycogen deposition diseases. *In* Stanbury, J. B., Wyngaarden, J. B., and Fredrickson, D. S. [eds.]: The Metabolic Basis of Inherited Disease. New York, The Blakiston Division, McGraw-Hill Book Co., 1966, p. 171.)

tissues and organs of the body.

Glycogen is a very large (molecular weight, 250,000 to 100,000,000), branched-chain polysaccharide of glucose. Its synthesis from and degradation to glucose is summarized in Figure 5–11. *Each of the 10 glycogenoses results from a lack of one of the enzymes involved in this glycogen cycle. The specific tissues and organs affected depend on the particular enzyme involved and its distribution in the body.* Whatever the tissue or cells affected, the glycogen is stored most often within the cytoplasm, sometimes within nuclei, and in one variant within lysosomes. Affected cells become swollen and distended and contain large amounts of PAS positive material. Frequently organomegaly develops as a consequence of the accumulated glycogen. Since all of these inborn errors of metabolism are rare, the 10 forms are summarized in Table 5–6. More details follow on four of the more frequent specific syndromes (McAdams et al., 1974). All, except possibly type IX, are inherited as autosomal recessive disorders.

Type I (glucose-6-phosphatase deficiency, von Gierke's disease) is best remembered as the hepatorenal form of glycogenosis. As a consequence of the block in degradation of gly-

TABLE 5–6. PRINCIPAL FEATURES OF THE GLYCOGENOSES

	TYPE	ENZYME INVOLVED	MORPHOLOGIC CHANGES	CLINICAL MANIFESTATIONS
I	Hepatorenal— von Gierke's disease	Glucose-6-phosphatase	*Hepatomegaly*—intracytoplasmic accumulations of glycogen and small amounts of lipid; intranuclear glycogen. *Renomegaly*—intracytoplasmic accumulations of glycogen in cortical tubular epithelial cells.	Stunted growth, hepato- and renomegaly, hypoglycemia, acidosis, hyperlipidemia.
II	Generalized glycogenosis— Pompe's disease	Lysosomal glucosidase	*Mild hepatomegaly*—ballooning of lysosomes with glycogen creating lacy cytoplasmic pattern. *Cardiomegaly*—glycogen within sarcoplasm and sometimes membrane-bound. *Skeletal muscle*—similar to heart.	Massive cardiomegaly, muscle hypotonia and cardiorespiratory failure.
III	Cori's disease— limit dextrinosis	Debrancher system	Mild to marked *hepatomegaly*—cells similar to type I. Mild to moderate *cardiomegaly*—cells similar to type II. *Skeletal muscle*—similar to type II.	Similar to type I but usually milder.
IV	Brancher glycogenosis	Amylo-1,4→1,6 transglucosidase (brancher enzyme)	Accumulation of abnormal glycogen (*amylopectin*) *in liver cells, cardiac and skeletal muscle and brain*. Intracytoplasmic accumulations of a hyaline, fibrillar, PAS positive material which is diastase resistant. In time, development of *cirrhosis* of liver.	Hepatomegaly, splenomegaly, ascites and liver failure.
V	McArdle's syndrome	Muscle phosphorylase	*Skeletal muscle only*—sarcoplasmic accumulations of glycogen similar to type II.	Muscle weakness, cramping; no rise in blood lactate.
VI		Liver phosphorylase	*Only hepatomegaly*—scattered cytoplasmic vacuoles, occasionally lipid vacuoles; no intranuclear glycogen.	Hepatomegaly, no hypoglycemia or acidosis.
VII		Phosphofructokinase and phosphoglucomutase	*Only skeletal muscle* and erythrocytes studied—sarcoplasmic glycogen similar to that in type II.	Similar to type V.
VIII		No deficiency but apparent inactivity of liver phosphorylase	*Hepatomegaly* as in type I. Accumulation of glycogen in *axon cylinders and synaptic vesicles of brain*.	Hepatomegaly and rapid deterioration of central nervous system function to total decerebration in months or few years.
IX		Deficient activity of phosphorylase kinase	*Hepatomegaly*—similar to type VI.	Two genetic variants, one autosomal recessive, the other sex-linked. Only hepatomegaly in both.
X		cAMP-dependent phosphorylase kinase	*Hepatomegaly*—similar to type VI. *Sarcoplasmic glycogen* similar to type II in skeletal muscle.	Hepatomegaly with vitamin D resistant rickets, Fanconi's syndrome.

cogen, lipids are mobilized, with resultant hyperlipidemia. The hepatomegaly is extreme, resulting from the accumulation not only of glycogen but also of fat in liver cells. The nuclei are often ballooned by glycogen. Kidney enlargement is not frequent, but the tubular epithelium contains considerable glycogen. These infants fail to thrive from birth, have protuberant abdomens and exhibit hypoglycemia when deprived of food for any period of time. The hypoglycemia, although intermittent, may lead to ketosis and convulsions. Some of these patients may develop gout for reasons which are not entirely clear. It has been suggested that a greater than normal fraction of glucose is converted to ribose and then to phosphoribosyl-pyrophosphate, the substrate for production of uric acid. The definitive diagnosis of type I glycogenosis requires proof of markedly reduced glucose-6-phosphatase levels in samples of liver or kidney. In general, these children have growth retardation and many die of infections. However, those who survive childhood frequently show improvement in their metabolic defect and many have normal children.

Type II (glucosidase deficiency, Pompe's disease) is a prototype of a hereditary lysosomal disease. There are other lysosomal disorders which involve the storage of lipids. As a consequence of the lysosomal enzyme deficiency, glycogen accumulates and distends these organelles, in turn inducing ballooning of the liver cells and hepatomegaly. On light microscopy, the membrane-bound, swollen lysosomes impart a lacy appearance to the cytoplasm. Glycogen also accumulates within myocardial cells to produce cardiomegaly. Other striated muscles, including those in the tongue and diaphragm, may be affected, and sometimes abnormal accumulations of glycogen appear in the kidneys and RE cells. Affected children have profound motor weakness and often develop signs of cardiac failure, and so this syndrome is sometimes known as *cardiac glycogenosis* (Fig. 5–12). The definitive diagnosis requires the demonstration of a lack of glucosidase in affected tissues. Heterozygotes can be detected by assay of phytohemagglutinin-stimulated lymphocytes for alpha-glucosidase activity (Hirschhorn et al., 1969).

Type III (debrancher deficiency, limit dextrinosis) closely resembles type I disease but in general is milder. Sometimes the metabolic abnormality clears with age. The lack of debrancher enzyme blocks the degradation of glycogen beyond the branching points, and so the stored glycogen is abnormal in configuration. The hepatic involvement is essentially the same as in type I disease but occasionally a mild periportal fibrosis develops. Sometimes

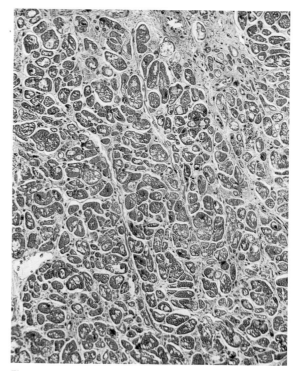

Figure 5–12. Cardiac glycogenosis, manifested as cleared spaces within the myocardial fibers.

the kidneys are also involved. Skeletal muscle and heart are also affected, which differentiate this variant from type I glycogenosis.

Type V (muscle phosphorylase deficiency, McArdle's syndrome) is distinctive for its striking muscle weakness. The enzyme deficiency blocks the release of glucose from glycogen. The motor weakness becomes particularly evident after brief intervals of physical activity. An elevation of blood lactic acid is caused by the inability to metabolize glycogen. Prolonged exercise may result in muscle fiber necrosis, myoglobinuria and acute renal failure (Grunfeld et al., 1972).

LIPID STORAGE DISORDERS

A group of biochemically and genetically distinctive hereditary disorders are characterized by the abnormal accumulation of complex lipids in various cells and tissues in the body. Generically, these are referred to as *lipidoses*. In most, a specific enzyme deficiency or lack has been identified as the basis for the deranged lipid metabolism. Fortunately for both medical students and potential victims, most of these conditions are very rare and are better relegated to special texts (Stanbury, Wyngaarden and Fredrickson, 1972). Only three will be considered briefly here: Gaucher's, Niemann-Pick and Tay-Sachs disease.

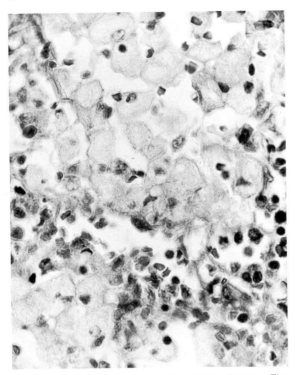

Figure 5–13. The spleen in Gaucher's disease. The large vacuolated cells have a ground glass appearance and contain some faint wavy lines, creating some resemblance to wrinkled tissue paper.

Gaucher's disease exists in three autosomal recessive variants, all of which involve defective metabolism of glucose cerebrosides, more accurately termed glucosyl-ceramides. It is speculated that different mutations affecting the same or closely linked genetic loci are the basis of the variations. Common to all three is deficient activity of a glucocerebrosidase. The absence of glucocerebrosidase leads to an accumulation of ceramides and the formation of so-called *Gaucher cells*. Normally the glycolipids derived from the breakdown of blood cells, particularly erythrocytes, are sequentially degraded. In Gaucher's disease the degradation stops at the level of the glucosyl-ceramides. These macromolecules thus accumulate and circulate in the blood, probably in the form of lipoproteins. They are engulfed by all phagocytic cells in the body, particularly the RE and endothelial cells, as well as macrophages. Alternatively, the partially digested erythrocytes are phagocytized, with subsequent release of the ceramides (Penelli et al., 1969). In any event, *these phagocytes become enlarged, sometimes up to 100 μm. in size, and develop a pathognomonic cytoplasmic appearance, characterized as "wrinkled tissue paper"* (Fig. 5–13). No distinct vacuolation is present. Electron microscopy indicates that the distinctive

cytoplasmic morphology represents secondary lysosomes or residual bodies filled with tubular structures and fibrils (Hibbs et al., 1970). The accumulated ceramides yield a positive PAS stain and the cells are also strongly positive for acid phosphatase.

The most common variant is referred to as *type I adult Gaucher's disease*, distinguished from the other two by *noninvolvement* of the central nervous system. The designation "adult" is somewhat misleading, since the disease may start in childhood and may or may not pursue a benign indolent course. The major clinical features of this form of the disease include massive hepatosplenomegaly, generalized lymphadenopathy and diffuse infiltration of the bone marrow by Gaucher cells, sometimes producing tumorous masses which erode the osseous structure and lead to pathologic fractures.

Type II is best remembered as acute or malignant neuronopathic Gaucher's disease. Although the infant may appear normal at birth, within a few months hepatosplenomegaly, lymphadenopathy and neurologic abnormalities become apparent. The central nervous system damage is progressive, leading to death usually within one to two years. At death, the brain is found to contain ceramide-laden, swollen periadventitial cells, scattered areas of neuronal loss and, in some cases, storage of ceramides in ballooned out swollen neurons. Presumably in the neurons there is a block in the sequential degradation of gangliosides at the level of glucosyl ceramide.

Type III Gaucher's disease represents an intermediate juvenile form, sometimes called "subacute neuronopathic." The course is intermediate between that seen in type I and type II disease, as is the involvement of the brain.

Type I non-neuronopathic Gaucher's disease may occur in any race or ethnic group but is particularly frequent among Ashkenazi Jews. The prevalence of type II among Jews is relatively high, but far less striking than type I. Of the relatively few cases of type III reported in the literature, none has involved Jews. A satisfactory diagnosis of all variants can usually be made by morphologic examination of a bone marrow aspirate or liver biopsy, but definitive diagnosis may require chemical analysis of the stored lipid and determination of the enzyme lack.

Niemann-Pick disease includes a constellation of hereditary syndromes characterized by the accumulation of sphingomyelin in phagocytic cells throughout the body, sometimes including the central nervous system. Sphingomyelin, a constituent of all cells and extracellular lipoproteins, accumulates because the mechanism responsible for its degradation cannot keep pace with its release from obsolescent

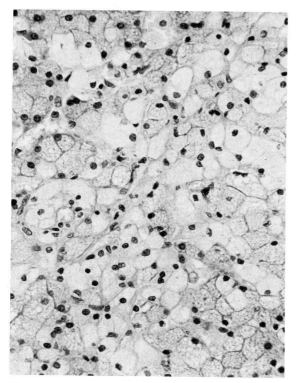

Figure 5–14. Niemann-Pick disease: The foamy vacuolation of the cells in the spleen results from accumulations of sphingomyelin.

cells. The excess is incorporated into all phagocytic cells, usually within secondary lysosomes, which later become transformed to residual bodies. In this manner *the cells become stuffed with droplets or particles of the complex lipid, which impart a fine vacuolation or foaminess to the cytoplasm* (Fig. 5–14). At higher resolution, some of the minute vacuoles can be resolved as myelin figures (Lynn and Terry, 1964). There is also usually a concomitant intracellular accumulation of cholesterol. Histochemical stains are of some help in identifying these lipid-laden cells, which are positive with Sudan black and frequently positive with PAS (Lynn and Terry, 1964). Because of their high content of phagocytic cells, the organs most severely affected are the spleen, liver, bone marrow, lymph nodes, and lungs. The spleen and lymph nodes in particular are virtually replaced by masses of foam cells, which cause considerable enlargement of these structures. In several variants, the central nervous system is also affected, as will be pointed out. At present four distinguishable autosomal recessive patterns of Niemann-Pick disease have been identified, as well as a fifth pattern of indeterminate genetic origin. Collectively they are classified as types A to E (Crocker, 1961).

Type A is the most common and the classical form. It is characterized by onset in infancy, involvement of the viscera and the nervous system, and rapid progression to death nearly always by four years of age. A widespread deficiency of sphingomyelinase is the primary defect. In these children, the ganglion cells throughout the brain are frequently swollen, secondary to deficient catabolism of endogenous sphingomyelin. There may be patchy or widespread myelin degeneration in the white matter. Proliferation of glial cells is variable, but often these cells are also laden with lipid. The entire central nervous system, including the spinal cord and ganglia, are involved in this tragic, inexorable process. Often the ganglion cells in the retina are also affected and degenerate. Since there are no ganglion cells in the fovea of the macula, the vascularization in this area remains visible as a *cherry red spot*, surrounded by the pale, swollen and disintegrating retinal cells.

Type B represents a chronic form without nervous system involvement. These patients develop all the visceral manifestations of type A, with equally early onset. Sphingomyelinase deficiency is present but generally is less severe than in type A. *Type C is closely similar to type A, with involvement of the central nervous system, but the patients have a more prolonged course.* Sometimes the disease begins one to five years following birth. This subacute form of Niemann-Pick disease does not exhibit an apparent lack of sphingomyelinase. *Type D is a special variant restricted to patients of Nova Scotian ancestry* which pursues a clinical course similar to type C. Type E is too ill-defined and uncommon to merit comment.

The diagnosis can often be made on the basis of the hepatosplenomegaly associated with the dramatic evidence of mental deterioration. Bone marrow aspirates and sometimes peripheral white cells will disclose the foamy cytoplasm yielding the histochemical reactions mentioned. More definitive evidence is derived from chemical analysis of affected tissues and enzyme assays in types A and B.

Tay-Sachs disease is one of six forms of *amaurotic (having blindness) idiocy* resulting from the deranged metabolism of gangliosides in nervous tissue (O'Brien et al., 1971). Specific "missing enzymes" have been conclusively identified in only two variants, one of which is Tay-Sachs disease. In this familial inborn error of metabolism a deficiency of hexosaminidase A blocks the degradation of ganglioside G_{M2} [N-acetyl galactosaminyl-(N-acetylneuraminyl)-galactosylglucosyl-N-acyl-sphingosine]. The brain is principally affected since it is most involved in ganglioside metabolism. Storage of G_{M2} occurs within ganglion cells, axis cylinders of nerves and glial cells throughout the central nervous system. Other spingoglycolipids also accumulate. Affected cells appear swollen, possibly foamy and not dissimilar from those in Niemann-Pick disease. Electron microscopy, however, reveals numerous round or oval membranous cytoplasmic bodies which contain acid hydrolases, suggesting that they represent secondary lysosomes or residual bodies (Volk et al., 1968; Adachi et al., 1974). These anatomic changes are found throughout the central nervous system, including the spinal cord, peripheral nerves and autonomic nervous system. The retina is usually involved and discloses the characteristic *cherry red spot* in the fovea of the macula. Occasionally minimal visceral involvement is encountered in Tay-Sachs disease, usually in the form of lipid inclusions in the parenchymal cells of the liver and lipid-laden foam cells in the spleen and lung. Obviously, this variant of G_{M2} gangliosidosis bears many phenotypic similarities to Niemann-Pick disease (type A), but it should be noted that the lipid and enzyme deficiencies are totally dissimilar.

Tay-Sachs disease begins insidiously in infants with weakness, retardation in development and difficulties in feeding. Muscle hypotonia and spasticity is usually evident by the third to fourth month of life as is an exaggerated "startle reaction" (spastic extension of both arms). Visual impairment follows and progresses usually to complete blindness by the end of the first year of life. The unrelenting progression of the neurologic involvement reduces these pathetic infants to tragic caricatures until death provides a release, usually within two to three years.

Two other phenotypic variants of Tay-Sachs disease have been identified in which the same ganglioside (G_{M2}) accumulates. In one there is a deficiency of both hexosaminidase A and B and in the other, more protracted disorder, a partial deficiency of hexosaminidase A and B.

MUCOPOLYSACCHARIDOSES (MPS)

Abnormal storage of acid mucopolysaccharides occurs in a group of hereditary disorders characterized by defective degradation of glycosaminoglycans. A deficiency of a specific protein (corrective factor), probably a "missing enzyme" has been documented in five of these mucopolysaccharidoses (McKusick and Chase, 1973). When cultured fibroblasts from affected individuals are treated with culture medium from normal fibroblasts, the mucopolysaccharide defect is corrected. The therapeutic implications of this observation are currently being tested. Because all of these disorders are extremely rare, they are characterized briefly in Table 5-7.

TABLE 5-7. THE GENETIC MUCOPOLYSACCHARIDOSES*

	DESIGNATION	CLINICAL FEATURES	GENETICS	EXCESSIVE URINARY MPS	SUBSTANCE DEFICIENT
MPS I H	Hurler syndrome	Early clouding of cornea, grave manifestations, death usually before age 10	Homozygous for MPS I H gene	Dermatan sulfate Heparan sulfate	α-L-iduronidase (formerly called Hurler corrective factor)
MPS I S	Scheie syndrome	Stiff joints, cloudy cornea, aortic regurgitation, normal intelligence, ? normal life-span	Homozygous for MPS I S gene	Dermatan sulfate Heparan sulfate	α-L-iduronidase
MPS I H/S	Hurler-Scheie syndrome	Phenotype intermediate between Hurler and Scheie	Genetic compound of MPS I H and I S genes	Dermatan sulfate Heparan sulfate	α-L-iduronidase
MPS II A	Hunter syndrome, severe	No clouding of cornea, milder course than in MPS I H but death usually before age 15 years	Hemizygous for X-linked gene	Dermatan sulfate Heparan sulfate	Sulfo-iduronate sulfatase
MPS II B	Hunter syndrome, mild	Survival to 30's to 50's, fair intelligence	Hemizygous for X-linked allele for mild form	Dermatan sulfate Heparan sulfate	Sulfo-iduronate sulfatase
MPS III A	Sanfilippo syndrome A	Identical phenotype: Mild somatic, severe central nervous system effects	Homozygous for Sanfilippo A gene	Heparan sulfate	Heparan sulfate sulfatase
MPS III B	Sanfilippo syndrome B		Homozygous for Sanfilippo B (at different locus)	Heparan sulfate	N-acetyl-α-D-glucosaminidase
MPS IV	Morquio syndrome (probably more than one allelic form)	Severe bone changes of distinctive type, cloudy cornea, aortic regurgitation	Homozygous for Morquio gene	Keratan sulfate	Unknown

*Modified from McKusick, V. A.: Heritable Disorders of Connective Tissue. 4th ed. St. Louis, C. V. Mosby Co., 1972, p. 525.

All save one of these syndromes are transmitted as autosomal recessives; Hunter's syndrome is X-linked. The most common form, Hurler's syndrome, is more graphically referred to as "gargoylism." The accumulation of mucopolysaccharides occurs in phagocytic cells throughout the body, principally in the spleen, liver, lymph nodes and bone marrow. The involvement of the bones leads to a variety of skeletal deformities, particularly enlargement of the skull, widening and lengthening of the bones of the limbs, distortion of the small bones of the hands and feet, and deformities of the vertebrae. It is the distortion of the facial bones and skull which led to the designation of gargoylism. In all affected tissues, the storage cells are monstrously distended by PAS positive mucopolysaccharides, contained within massively distended lysosomes (Langunoff and Gritzka, 1966). The mucopolysaccharides spill out of the storage cells to appear in the blood and are excreted in excessive amounts in the urine. In transit through the blood, some of the macromolecules are phagocytized by endothelial cells to produce subendothelial plaques. When the coronary arteries and cardiac valves are affected, myocardial infarction or heart failure may supervene and sometimes cause death. This survey of some of the storage diseases emphasizes the far-reaching impact of a single gene mutation.

X-LINKED DISORDERS

Sex-linked, better known as X-linked, disorders are transmitted by heterozygous carrier females virtually only to sons, who of course are hemizygous for the X chromosome. Very rarely a female child is affected if the mother or father transmits a mutant dominant gene or, more commonly, when mother and father both transmit mutant recessive genes. An affected male does not transmit the disorder to sons, but all daughters are carriers. Sons of heterozygous women have, of course, a one in two chance of receiving the mutant gene. As in autosomal recessive conditions, heterozygous carrier women sometimes can be identified. To date, no Y-linked diseases are known. Save for determinants dictating male differentiation, the only characteristic which may be located on the Y-chromosome is the not altogether unpleasant attribute of "hairy ears."

X-linked disorders are much less common than those arising in autosomal mutations. Some of the more important conditions having this mode of transmission are presented elsewhere — glucose-6-phosphate dehydrogenase deficiency (p. 331), hemophilia A (p. 366), hemophilia B (p. 367) and Bruton's agam-maglobulinemia (p. 169). Some variants of inborn errors of metabolism have already been cited as being X-linked — for example, the Lesch-Nyhan syndrome and one pattern of overproduction gout, as well as one form of mucopolysaccharidosis (Hunter's syndrome). Other X-linked disorders, such as Fabry's disease, Duchenne's and Becker's muscular dystrophies and nephrogenic diabetes insipidus, are too uncommon for inclusion here. Without regrets we can proceed then to the next major category of genetic disease.

DISORDERS RELATED TO CHROMOSOMAL ABERRATIONS

Compared to the plethora of conditions related to monogenic mutations, only a relatively few disorders are associated with identifiable aberrations in the karyotype (Heller, 1969). This may well be attributable to the fact that most genetic accidents gross enough to induce an abnormal karyotype are lethal. Chromosomal aberrations may affect either the autosomes or sex chromosomes and involve a change in number or morphology or some internal rearrangement within a chromosome. *Virtually all of the presently recognized diseases associated with an abnormal karyotype involve a change in number or morphology of chromosomes.* Very little is yet known about conditions related to internal rearrangements, perhaps because up to the recent past the technical methods have been so limited.

An abnormal number of chromosomes (aneuploidy) is almost always the result of *nondisjunction* or *anaphase lag.* If either occurs during a meiotic division, an aneuploid gamete results which, when fertilized, develops into an aneuploid fetus. As will be seen, aneuploidy underlies a few clinical conditions. It usually takes the form of an extra autosome or sex chromosome (trisomy). Only one type of monosomy is known in man — Turner's syndrome, 45,XO (loss of an X chromosome). So much genetic information is lost with autosomal monosomy that it is incompatible with life. Postzygotic, mitotic nondisjunction gives rise to *mosaicism* — the presence of more than one karyotypic variety of cell in the same individual. Mitotic nondisjunction or anaphase lag may occur later in life and give rise to an abnormal clone of cells exhibiting all manner of aneuploidy and polyploidy, such as is encountered in some cancers.

A change in chromosome morphology always implies breakage followed by rearrangement. The causes of breakage so far as we know are the same as those giving rise to other genetic mutations. Three autosomal recessive syndromes in which chromosomal

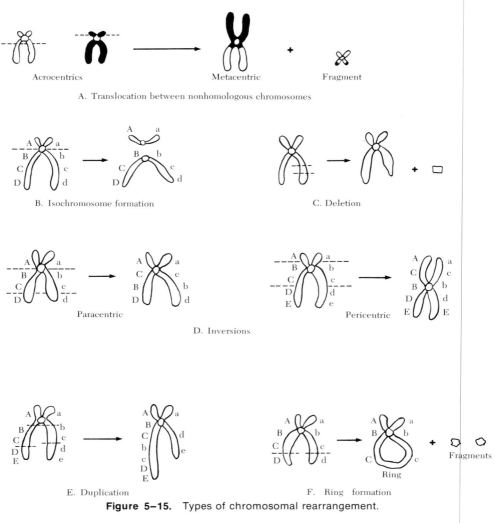

A. Translocation between nonhomologous chromosomes

B. Isochromosome formation

C. Deletion

D. Inversions

Paracentric

Pericentric

E. Duplication

F. Ring formation

Figure 5–15. Types of chromosomal rearrangement.

breakage occurs exceptionally frequently have been identified: Fanconi's anemia, Bloom's syndrome and ataxia telangiectasia. The patterns of chromosomal rearrangement following breakage (diagrammed in Fig. 5–15) are as follows:

Translocation may appear when there are two simultaneous breaks in nonhomologous chromosomes with exchange of the fragments. This is called a balanced translocation. Rarely, a large translocation may involve virtually an entire chromosome, yielding a phenotypically normal individual having only 45 separate chromosomes, one comprising a large translocation chromosome. No genetic information is lost.

Isochromosomes result when the centromere divides horizontally rather than vertically, yielding two new chromosomes.

Deletion involves loss of a portion of a chromosome. A single break may delete a terminal segment. Two interstitial breaks, with reunion of the proximal and distal segments, may result in loss of an intermediate segment. The isolated fragment, which lacks a centromere, almost never survives and thus many genes are lost.

Inversions occur when there are two interstitial breaks in a chromosome and the segment reunites after a complete turnaround, yielding an ACBD genetic sequence (reversal of the BC segment).

A ring chromosome is a variant of a deletion. Following the loss of segments from each of two chromatids they reunite to form a ring.

It is apparent that some of these abnormal morphologies can be readily recognized in a metaphase spread, but an inversion or a subtle deletion might be missed without banding techniques. Against this background we can turn to a consideration of the disorders involving changes in the karyotype.

TABLE 5–8. DISORDERS ASSOCIATED WITH THE AUTOSOMES*

DISORDER	KARYOTYPE EXAMPLES	APPROXIMATE INCIDENCE	MATERNAL AGE	CLINICAL SIGNS IN NEWBORNS
Down's syndrome		1 in 600 births		1. Mental retardation
				2. Flat facial profile
				3. Muscle hypotonia
Trisomy 21 type	47,XX,G+ or 47,XY,G+	Over 95% of cases	Increased	4. Hyperflexibility
				5. Lack of Moro reflex
				6. Abundant neck skin
Translocation type	46,XX,D-t(DqGq)+ 46,XY,G-t(GqGq)+	3–4% of cases	Normal	7. Dysplastic ears
				8. Horizontal palmar crease
				9. Dysplastic pelvis (by x-ray)
Mosaic type	46,XX/47,XX,G+	2–3% of cases	Normal	10. Dysplastic middle phalanx V (by x-ray)
				11. Epicanthic folds
				12. Predisposition to acute leukemia
Edwards' syndrome Trisomy 18E	47,XX,E+ 47,XY,E+	1 in 5000 births	Increased	1. Mental retardation and failure to thrive
				2. Prominent occiput
				3. Micrognathia and low-set ears
				4. Hypertonicity
Translocation type	46,XX,t(DqEq)+		Normal	5. Flexion of fingers (index over third)
				6. Cardiac, renal and intestinal defects
				7. Short sternum and small pelvis
Mosaic type	46,XX/47,XX,E+		Normal	8. Abduction deformity of hip
Patau's syndrome Trisomy 13 D (arhinencephaly)	47,XX,D+ 47,XY,D+	1 in 6000 births Over 80% of cases	Increased	1. Microcephaly and mental retardation
				2. Scalp defect
				3. Microphthalmia
				4. Harelip and cleft palate
				5. Polydactyly
Translocation type	46,XX,D-t(DqDq)+	10% of cases	Normal	6. Rocker-bottom feet
				7. Abnormal ears
Mosaic type	46,XX/47,XX,D+	5% of cases	Normal	8. Apneic spells and myoclonic seizures
				9. Cardiac dextroposition and interventricular septal defect
				10. Extensive visceral defects
"Le cri du chat" (cat-cry) syndrome	46,XX,5p− 46,XY,5p−	Rare	Normal	1. Mental retardation
				2. Microcephaly and round facies
				3. Mewing cry
				4. Epicanthic folds

*From Robbins, S. L.: Pathologic Basis of Disease. Philadelphia, W. B. Saunders Co., 1974.

AUTOSOMAL DISORDERS

Three autosomal trisomies (21, 18 and 13) and one deletion syndrome (*cri du chat*) resulting from partial deletion of the short arm of chromosome 5 were first identified over a decade ago. Within the past few years, an additional trisomy involving chromosome 8 (Caspersson, 1972) and two deletion syndromes involving chromosomes 21 and 22 (Warren, 1973) have been described. Most of these disorders are quite uncommon. All are characterized by clinical features which should permit ready recognition. Some of the features of the four most common entities are presented in Table 5–8. Only trisomy 21 occurs with sufficient frequency to merit further consideration.

DOWN'S SYNDROME (TRISOMY 21)

Down's syndrome is the most common of the chromosomal disorders. It has been known in the past as "mongolism" or "mongolian idiocy." Its incidence is clearly related to maternal age. As was pointed out, it occurs once in 2000 live births in women under 29

years of age, in contrast to 1 in 50 live births for mothers over 45 years of age. The classic features are detailed in Table 5–8. The combination of epicanthic folds and flat facial profile accounted for the older, unfortunate designation "mongolian idiocy." The mental retardation is usually quite extreme, and most children have an IQ between 25 and 50. Ironically these tragically disadvantaged children are usually gentle, shy and amenable to training, and, indeed, more easily managed than their advantaged siblings.

Over 95 per cent of these children have trisomy 21 G, according to the recent classification of chromosomes (Fig. 5–16). With rare exceptions the parents are normal. Approximately 2 per cent of individuals with Down's syndrome are mosaics (trisomy 21/normal) and, depending upon how many cells are affected and what systems are involved, their manifestations vary from those indistinguishable from trisomy 21 to apparent normality (Carr, 1969). The remaining patients have translocations, as detailed in Table 5–8. Forty-six chromosomes are present, but presumably there has been translocation of

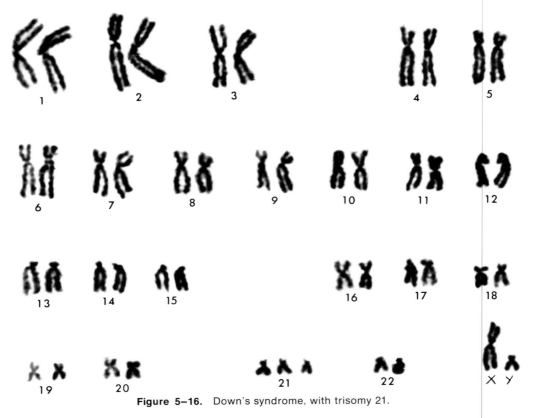

Figure 5–16. Down's syndrome, with trisomy 21.

some segment of chromosome 21 or 22 to another chromosome, usually in group D or group G. *Translocation Down's syndrome is not influenced by maternal age and may be familial.* Clearly, children bearing this mutation may reach adult life and reproduce.

Overall, the prognosis for individuals with Down's syndrome has improved remarkably in the recent past as the result of control of infections. Some children having serious visceral abnormalities die at an early age, others succumb to acute myelogenous leukemia, which is unusually common in Down's syndrome, but the great majority now have an almost normal longevity.

SEX CHROMOSOMAL DISORDERS

A number of abnormal karyotypes involving the sex chromosomes, ranging from 45,XO to 49,XXXXY, are compatible with life (Krmpotic et al., 1970). Indeed, males who are phenotypically normal have been identified with two and even three Y chromosomes. Such extreme karyotypic deviations are not encountered with the autosomes. In large part this latitude relates to two facts: (1) lyonization of X chromosomes and (2) the scant amount of genetic information carried by the Y chromosome. The consideration of lyonization

must begin with the *Barr body or sex chromatin* first described in 1949 (Bertram and Barr, 1949). These investigators called attention to a distinctive clump of chromatin in the nuclei of the neurons of female cats which was not present in males. Soon thereafter it was observed that somatic cells in women bear a chromatin mass in the interphase nuclei about 1 μm. in width which lies adjacent to the nuclear membrane. This chromatin mass now is referred to most often as an X body or Barr body (Fig. 5–17). A "drumstick" nuclear appendage is also found in 5 per cent of the polymorphonuclear cells of the female. Lyon, in 1962, proposed that *the X or Barr body represents one genetically inactivated X chromosome.* This inactivation occurs early in fetal life, about 16 days after conception, and randomly inactivates either X chromosome in the cluster of primitive cells representing the developing zygote. Once inactivated, this chromosome remains genetically neutralized in all of the progeny of these cells. Moreover, it is now established that *all but one X chromosome is inactivated and so a 48,XXXX female has three X or Barr bodies and only one active X chromosome.* This phenomenon explains why the normal female is truly a mosaic with respect to X chromosomal genes and also explains why normal females do not have a double dosage

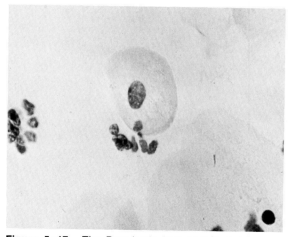

Figure 5–17. The Barr body (sex chromatin) is seen within the nucleus attached to the nuclear membrane at the ten o'clock position.

(as compared with the male) of phenotypic attributes located on the X chromosome. Extra Y chromosomes are readily tolerated because at the present time the only information carried on the Y chromosome appears to relate to male differentiation. It might be noted that whatever the number of X chromosomes the presence of a Y invariably dictates the male phenotype. Recently it has become apparent that male somatic cells carry a Y (sometimes called F) body in interphase nuclei analogous to the X body in the female. The Y body appears as a small, brightly fluorescent spot in interphase nuclei stained with fluorescent dyes and examined with the ultraviolet microscope (Pearson, 1972). It may be absent in about 0.1 per cent of normal males, presumably because the long arm of the Y chromosome is abbreviated (Pearson, 1972). It appears that the genes for male differentiation are located on the short arm of the Y. Indeed, some males have been shown to have two Y bodies (XYY), a karyotype suspected of inducing aggressive antisocial behavior (Editorial, 1974). It is apparent, then, that loss of an X chromosome in the female or the presence of supernumerary X or Y chromosomes, while inducing phenotypic changes, do not have a devastating effect.

The disorders arising in aberrations of sex chromosomes are detailed in Table 5–9. Two of the most common conditions are described briefly.

KLINEFELTER'S SYNDROME

This common form of hypogonadism, also called *testicular dysgenesis*, may be responsible for sterility in the male. Patients usually have a distinctive body habitus with an increase in sole-to-os pubis length, which creates the appearance of an elongated body. Reduced facial and body hair and gynecomastia are also

characteristic. The testes are markedly reduced in size, sometimes to only 2 cm. in greatest length. Along with the testicular atrophy, the serum testosterone levels are usually lower than normal, although the urinary gonadotropin levels are high. The incidence of this condition is estimated to be 1 in 500 live male births. Most patients are 47,XXY and are therefore sex chromatin positive (Fig. 5–18). The extra X chromosome may be of either maternal or paternal origin (Race and Sanger, 1969). Advanced maternal age and history of irradiation of either parent may contribute to the meiotic error resulting in this condition. Some cases of Klinefelter's syndrome have been found to be 48,XXXY or 49,XXXXY; there have also been a variety of mosaic patterns, including 46,XY/47,XXY or 47,XXY/48,XXXY and variations on this theme.

The principal clinical effects of this syndrome are: (1) it often causes sterility and (2) it is sometimes associated with a slight decrease in intelligence. The sterility is due to impaired spermatogenesis, sometimes to the extent of total azospermia. A variety of testicular tubular alterations may be present. Some patients have hyalinization of tubules, so that they appear as ghostlike structures in tissue section. Others show rare, apparently normal testicular tubules mixed with atrophic tubules having virtually no spermatogenic germ cells, the so-called *tubule dysgenesis* pattern. Still others have very embryonic-appearing tubules, as though development had been arrested in early fetal life. In all forms there is prominent Leydig cell hyperplasia. The reduction in intelligence is correlated with the number of extra X chromosomes. Thus, in the most common variant (XXY) the intelligence is nearly normal, but with additional X chromosomes these patients may have significantly subnormal levels of intelligence as well as more severe physical abnormalities, including cryptorchidism, hypospadias, more severe hypoplasia of the testes and skeletal changes.

TURNER'S SYNDROME

This condition is manifested by sexual infantilism, "streak" gonads, abnormally short stature and at least two of the following somatic anomalies: web neck, cubitus valgus (an increase in carrying angle of the arms), shield-like chest with widely spaced nipples, coarctation of the aorta, webbing of the digits or of the axillae, senile facies, high-arched palate, low set ears, and peripheral lymphedema (Krmpotic et al., 1970). Often the existence of this syndrome is unsuspected until puberty, when affected girls fail to develop normal secondary sex characteristics, the genitalia remain infantile, breast development is inade-

TABLE 5-9. DISORDERS ASSOCIATED WITH THE SEX CHROMOSOMES*

Disorder	Karyotype	Chromatin Pattern	Approximate Incidence	Maternal Age	Clinical Signs
Klinefelter's syndrome with mosaicism	47,XXY 46,XY/47,XXY	+ +	1 in 500 male births	Slightly increased	1. Testicular atrophy and azoospermia 2. Increase in sole – os pubis length 3. Gynecomastia 4. Female distribution of hair 5. Mental retardation
Variants of Klinefelter's syndrome	48,XXXY 49,XXXXY 48,XXYY 49,XXXYY	++ +++ + ++	Rare	Increased	1. More severe mental retardation 2. Cryptorchidism 3. Hypospadias 4. Radio-ulnar synostosis
Gonadal dysgenesis (Turner's syndrome) defective second X chromosome	45,X 46,XXp– 46,XXq– 46,XXr 46,XXiq	Negative +(small) +(small) + +(large)	1 in 2000 female births	Normal Normal Normal Normal Normal	1. Short stature 2. Primary amenorrhea 3. Webbing of the neck 4. Cubitus valgus 5. Peripheral lymphedema 6. Broad chest and wide-spaced nipples 7. Low posterior hairline 8. Pigmented nevi 9. Coarctation of the aorta
Mosaicism	46,XX/45,X	Usually +		Normal	
Triple X females Variants	47,XXX 48,XXXX	++ +++	1 in 1000 female births Rare	Increased	1. Mental retardation 2. Menstrual irregularities 3. Many normal and fertile
Double Y males	47,XYY	Negative	Rare	Normal	1. Phenotypically normal 2. Most over 6 feet tall 3. "Increased aggressive behavior"
True hermaphrodites Most cases Some mosaics Rare case of double fertilization	46,XX 46,XX/47,XXY 46,XX/46XY	+ + +	Rare	Normal	1. Testicular and ovarian tissue 2. Varying genital abnormalities

*From Robbins, S. L.: Pathologic Basis of Disease. Philadelphia. W. B. Saunders. Co., 1974.

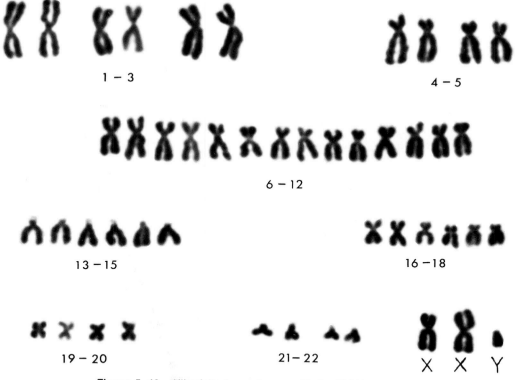

Figure 5–18. Klinefelter's syndrome, with the XXY karyotype.

quate and little pubic hair appears. Most have primary amenorrhea and morphologic examination of the ovaries discloses that they are replaced by white "streaks" of fibrous stroma devoid of follicles. Ovarian estrogen levels are low, and the loss of feedback inhibition leads to elevated pituitary gonadotropins. Intelligence is usually normal but may be slightly reduced.

Approximately 60 per cent of patients have the classic 45,XO karyotype and are therefore chromatin negative. This is the only recognized sex chromosome monosomy. The YO syndrome is presumably incompatible with survival. Other variants of Turner's syndrome have been identified, including 45,XO/46,XX and 45,XO/46,XX/47,XXX (a triclonal mosaicism). Such patients have many chromatin positive cells and manifest changes ranging from the full-blown syndrome to an almost normal phenotype. The fewer the abnormal cells the more normal the patient. Occasionally a patient with gonadal dysgenesis has an apparently normal karyotype and it is assumed that she has suffered some deletion in one of the X chromosomes. In addition to being a cause of sterility in the female, Turner's syndrome is important because of the possibility of underlying anomalous development of the aorta or even the heart.

Although the number of diseases presented in this chapter is not small, it represents only a sample of the many conditions now known to be of genetic origin. It is evident that these disorders range from the relatively innocuous (for example, albinism) to the devastating (such as Tay-Sachs disease), and that they may reach out to affect every organ and system in the body. Without doubt many of the uncertainties expressed today will be clarified in the near future and equally without doubt, the list of genetic diseases is fated to grow much longer.

REFERENCES

Adachi, M., et al.: Ultrastructural studies of 8 cases of fetal Tay-Sachs disease. Lab. Invest., *30*:102, 1974.

Agndelo, C. A., and Schumacher, H. R.: The synovitis of acute gouty arthritis. Hum. Pathol., *4*:265, 1973.

Ames, B. N., et al.: Carcinogens are mutagens: a simple test system for combining liver homogenates for activation and bacteria for detection. Proc. Nat. Acad. Sci. (U.S.A.), *70*:2281, 1973.

Barlow, K. A.: Lipid metabolism in gout. Proc. Roy. Soc. Med., *59*:325, 1966.

Bell, E. T.: Renal vascular disease in diabetes mellitus. Diabetes, *2*:376, 1953.

Benacerraf, B.: The genetic control of specific immune responses. Harvey Lect., *67*:109, 1971–1972.

Benke, P. J., et al.: Transport of labelled compounds in

control and cystic-fibrosis cells in vitro. Lancet, *1*:182, 1972.

Bertram, L. M., and Barr, E. G.: A morphologic distinction between the neurons of the male and female cat and the behavior of the nucleolar satellite during accelerated nuclear protein synthesis. Nature (London), *163*:676, 1949.

Bloodworth, J. M. B., Jr.: Diabetic microangiopathy. Diabetes, *12*:99, 1963.

Bloodworth, J. M. B., Jr.: Diabetes mellitus, extrapancreatic pathology. In Bloodworth, J. M. B., Jr. (ed.): Endocrine Pathology. Baltimore, Williams & Wilkins Co., 1968, p. 330.

Bloom, A. D.: Cytogenetics of the in-utero exposed of Hiroshima and Nagasaki. Lancet, 2:10, 1968.

Bloom, A. D., et al.: Chromosome aberrations in leukocytes of older survivors of the atomic bombings of Hiroshima and Nagasaki. Lancet, *2*:802, 1967.

Borest, T., and Froon, A. M.: Mitochondrial DNA: physical, chemical properties, replication and genetic function. Int. Rev. Cytol., *26*:108, 1969.

Bottago, G. F., et al.: Islet-cell antibodies in diabetes mellitus with autoimmune polyendocrine deficiencies. Lancet, *2*:1279, 1974.

Bray, G. A.: New developments in diabetes. Obesity and insulin resistance. Calif. Med., *119*:22, 1973.

Buckton, K. E., et al.: A study of the chromosome damage persisting after x-ray therapy for ankylosing spondylitis. Lancet, *2*:676, 1962.

Carr, D. H.: Chromosome anomalies as a cause of spontaneous abortion. Am. J. Obstet. Gynec., *97*:283, 1967.

Carr, D. H.: Chromosomal errors and development. Amer. J. Obstet. Gynec., *104*:327, 1969.

Carter, C. O.: Genetics of common disorders. Brit. Med. Bull., *25*:52, 1968.

Carter, C. O.: An ABC of Medical Genetics. Boston, Little, Brown & Co., 1969*a*.

Carter, C. O.: Mutant genes of large effect. Lancet, *1*:1139, 1969*b*.

Caspersson, T.: Four patients with trisomy 8 identified by the fluorescence and giemsa banding techniques. J. Med. Gen., *9*:1, 1972.

Caspersson, T., et al.: The 24 fluorescence patterns of the human metaphase chromosomes: distinguishing characters and variability. Hereditas, *67*:89, 1971.

Cerasi, E., and Luft, R.: "What is inherited—what is added?" Hypothesis for the pathogenesis of diabetes mellitus. Diabetes, *16*:615, 1967.

Cerasi, E., and Luft, R.: Pathogenesis of genetic diabetes mellitus: further development of a hypothesis. Mt. Sinai J. Med., *40*:334, 1973.

Charles, M. A., et al.: Adenosine 3′,5′-monophosphate in pancreatic islets: glucose-induced insulin release. Science, *179*:569, 1973.

Chazan, B. I., et al.: 25 to 45 years of diabetes with and without vascular complications. Diabetologia, *6*:565, 1970.

Chung, E. B.: Histologic changes in gout. Georgetown Med. Bull., *15*:269, 1962.

Crocker, A. C.: The cerebral defect in Tay-Sachs disease and Niemann-Pick disease. J. Neurochem., *7*:69, 1961.

Crossen, P. E.: Giemsa banding patterns of human chromosomes. Clin. Gen., *3*:169, 1972.

Danes, B. S., and Bearn, A. G.: Cystic fibrosis of the pancreas. A study in cell culture. J. Exp. Med., *129*:775, 1969.

Day, N., and Holmes, L. B.: The incidence of genetic disease in a university hospital population. Am. J. Hum. Gen., *25*:237, 1973.

deGalantha, E.: Techniques for preservation and microscopic demonstration of nodules in gout. Am. J. Clin. Path., *5*:165, 1935.

diSant'Agnese, T. A., and Talamo, R. C.: Pathogenesis and physiopathology of cystic fibrosis of the pancreas: fibrocystic disease of the pancreas (mucoviscidosis). New Eng. J. Med., *277*:1287, 1967.

Doniach, I., and Morgan, A. G.: Islets of Langerhans in juvenile diabetes mellitus. Clin. Endocr., *2*:233, 1973.

Duffy, B. J., Jr., and Fitzgerald, P. J.: Thyroid cancer in childhood and adolescence. A report on 28 cases. Cancer, *3*:1018, 1950.

Editorial: What becomes of the XYY male? Lancet, *2*:1297, 1974.

Editorial: Glucoreceptors, insulin release and diabetes. Lancet, *2*:646, 1975.

Ellenberg, M.: Diabetic complications without manifest diabetes. J.A.M.A., *183*:926, 1963.

Entmacher, P. S., et al.: Longevity of diabetic patients in recent years. Diabetes, *13*:373, 1964.

Farid, N. R., et al.: Basement membrane thickness of rectal capillaries in diabetes. Lancet, *1*:837, 1973.

Gamble, D. R., et al.: Coxsackie viruses and diabetes mellitus. Brit. Med. J., *4*:260, 1973.

Gekkman, D. D., et al.: Diabetic nephropathy. A clinical and pathologic study based on renal biopsies. Medicine, *38*:321, 1959.

Gepts, W.: Pathologic anatomy of the pancreas in juvenile diabetes mellitus. Diabetes, *14*:619, 1965.

Gibson, L. E., et al.: Relating mucus, calcium and sweat in a new concept of cystic fibrosis. Pediatrics, *48*:659, 1971.

Goldfischer, S., and Sternlieb, I.: Changes in the distribution of hepatic copper in relation to the progression of Wilson's disease (hepatolenticular degeneration). Am. J. Path., *53*:883, 1968.

Goldsmith, S. J., et al.: Significance of human plasma insulin sephadex fractions. Diabetes, *18*:834, 1969.

Green, E. L.: Genetic effects of radiation on the mammalian population. Am. Rev. Genet., *2*:87, 1968.

Gripenberg, U.: Chromosome studies in some virus infections. Hereditas, *54*:1, 1965.

Grunfeld, J. P., et al.: Acute renal failure in McArdle's disease. Report of two cases. New Eng. J. Med., *286*:1237, 1972.

Hardman, J. C., et al.: Cyclic nucleotides. Ann. Rev. Physiol., *33*:311, 1971.

Hauge, M., and Harvold, B.: Heredity in gout and hyperuricemia. Acta Med. Scand., *152*:247, 1955.

Heller, J. H.: Human chromosome abnormalities as related to physical and mental dysfunction. J. Hered., *60*:239, 1969.

Henderson, J. F., et al.: Variations in purine metabolism of cultured skin fibroblasts from patients with gout. J. Clin. Invest., *47*:1511, 1968.

Herman, M. V., and Gorlin, R.: Premature coronary artery disease and the preclinical diabetic state. Amer. J. Med., *38*:481, 1965.

Hibbs, R. G., et al.: A histochemical and electron microscopic study of Gaucher's cells. Arch. Path., *89*:137, 1970.

Hirschhorn, K.: Human genetics. J.A.M.A., *224*:597, 1973.

Hirschhorn, K., et al.: Pompe's disease: detection of heterozygotes by lymphocyte stimulation. Science, *166*:1632, 1969.

Hollenberg, M. D., and Cuatrecasas, P.: Insulin: interaction with membrane receptors and relationship to cyclic purine nucleotides and cell growth. Fed. Proc., *34*:1556, 1975.

Holmes, L. B.: Inborn errors of morphogenesis: A review of localized hereditary malformations. New Eng. J. Med., *291*:763, 1974.

Jansen, L. H.: The structure of the connective tissue, an explanation of the symptoms of the Ehlers-Danlos syndrome. Dermatologica, *110*:108, 1955.

Kahn, C. B., et al.: Clinical and chemical diabetes in offsping of diabetic couples. New Eng. J. Med., *281*:343, 1969.

Kellermeyer, R. W.: Hagemann factor and acute gouty arthritis. Arch. Rheum., *11*:452, 1968.

Kelley, W. N., et al.: Hypoxanthine-guanine phosphoribosyl transferase deficiency in gout. A review. Ann. Int. Med., *70*:155, 1969.

Kessler, I. I.: Mortality experience of diabetic patients. A 26 year follow up study. Amer. J. Med., *51*:715. 1971.

Kimmelstiel, P.: Diabetic nephropathy. *In* Mostofi, F. K., and Smith, D. E. (eds.): The Kidney. Baltimore, Williams & Wilkins Co., 1966.

Kimmelstiel, P., and Wilson, C.: Intercapillary lesions in the glomeruli of the kidney. Amer. J. Path., *12*:83, 1936.

Kimmelstiel, P., et al.: Glomerular basement membrane in diabetics. Am. J. Clin. Path., *45*:21, 1966.

Kipnis, D. M.: Does diabetes begin with insulin resistance? Adv. Metab. Dis., 6 (Suppl.):171, 1970*a*.

Kipnis, D. M.: Insulin secretion in normal and diabetic individuals. Adv. Int. Med., *16*:103, 1970*b*.

Knowles, H. C., Jr., et al.: The course of juvenile diabetes treated with unmeasured diet. Diabetes, *14*:239, 1965.

Knudson, A. G.: Mutation and human cancer. Adv. Cancer Res., *17*:317, 1973.

Krahl, M. E.: Insulin action at the molecular level. Facts and speculation. Diabetes, *21*:(Suppl. 2):695, 1972.

Krmpotic, E., et al.: Sex chromosome abnormalities. Chicago Med. School Quart., *29*:99, 1970.

Kuhlmann, W., et al.: The mutagenic action of caffeine in higher organisms. Cancer Res., *28*:2375, 1968.

Lacey, P. E.: Beta cell secretion — from the standpoint of a pathologist. Diabetes, *19*:895, 1970.

Ladda, R., et al.: Retinoblastoma: chromosome banding in patients with hereditable tumour. Lancet, 2:506, 1973.

Lagunoff, D., and Gritzka, T. L.: The site of mucopolysaccharide accumulation in Hurler's syndrome. An electron microscopic and histochemical study. Lab. Inves., *15*:1578, 1966.

Larsson, Y., et al.: Longterm prognosis in juvenile diabetes mellitus. Acta Paediat., Suppl. 130, *51*:1, 1962.

LeCompte, P. M., and Legg, M. A.: Insulitis (lymphocytic infiltration of pancreatic islets) in late-onset diabetes. Diabetes, *21*:762, 1972.

Lesch, M., and Nyhan, W. L.: A familial disorder of uric acid metabolism and central nervous system function. Am. J. Med., *36*:561, 1964.

Levi, A. J., et al.: Presymptomatic Wilson's disease. Lancet, 2:575, 1967.

Lockwood, D. H., et al.: Relation of insulin receptors to insulin resistance. Fed. Proc., *34*:1564, 1975.

Luft, R.: Some considerations on the pathogenesis of diabetes mellitus. New Eng. J. Med., *279*:1086, 1968.

Lynn, R., and Terry, R. D.: Lipid histochemistry and electron microscopy in adults: Niemann Pick disease. Am. J. Med., *37*:987, 1964.

Lyon, M. F.: Sex chromatin and gene action in the mammalian X chromosome. Am. J. Hum. Genet., *14*:135, 1962.

Malamud, N.: Neuropathology of phenylketonuria. J. Neuropath. Exp. Neurol., *25*:254, 1966.

Mangos, J. A., and McSherry, N. R.: Sodium transport: inhibitory factor in sweat of patients with cystic fibrosis. Science, *158*:135, 1967.

Martin, G. M., and Hoehn, H.: Genetics in human disease. Hum. Pathol., 5:387, 1974.

McAdams, A. J., et al.: Glycogen storage disease, types I to X. Hum. Pathol., 5:463, 1974.

McKusick, V. A., and Chase, G. A.: Human genetics. Ann. Rev. Genet., *7*:435, 1973.

Merrill, C. R., et al.: Bacterial virus gene expression in human cells. Nature, *233*:398, 1971.

Nagy, M.: Regulation of the biosynthesis of purine nucleotides in *Schizosaccharomyces pombe*. I. Properties of the phosphoribosyl-pyrophosphate glutamine amidotransferase of the wild strain and of a mutant desensitized toward feedback modifiers. Biochim. Biophys. Acta, *198*:471, 1970.

Nerup, J., et al.: HL-A antigens and diabetes mellitus. Lancet, 2:864, 1974*a*.

Nerup, J., et al.: Cell-mediated immunity in diabetes mellitus. Proc. Roy. Soc. Med., *67*:506, 1974*b*.

Niki, A., et al.: Insulin secretion by anomers of D-glucose. Science, *186*:150, 1974.

O'Brien, J. S., et al.: Ganglioside storage diseases. Fed. Proc., *30*:956, 1971.

O'Sullivan, J. B., et al.: The prevalence of diabetes mellitus and related variables: a population study in Sudbury, Mass. J. Chronic Dis., *20*:535, 1967.

Page, R. C., and Benditt, E. P.: Diseases of connective and vascular tissues. IV. The molecular basis for lathyrism. Lab. Invest., *26*:22, 1972.

Paris Conference (1971): Standardization in human cytogenetics. Cytogenetics, *11*:313, 1972.

Pearson, P.: The use of new staining techniques for human chromosome identification. J. Med. Genet., *9*:264, 1972.

Pennelli, N., et al.: The morphogenesis of Gaucher's cells investigated by electron microscopy. Blood, *34*:331, 1969.

Penrose, L. S.: Mongolism. Brit. Med. Bull., *17*:184, 1961.

Pinkus, H., et al.: Histopathology of striae distensae with special reference to striae and wound healing in Marfan's syndrome. J. Invest. Derm., *46*:283, 1966.

Pinnell, S. R., et al.: A new hereditable disorder of connective tissue with hydroxylysine-deficient collagen. New Eng. J. Med., *286*:1013, 1972.

Quan-ma, R., et al.: Galactitol in the tissues of a galactosemic child. Am. J. Dis. Child., *112*:477, 1968.

Race, R. R., and Sanger, R.: Xg and sex chromosome abnormalities. Brit. Med. Bull., *25*:99, 1969.

Raine, D. N.: Inherited metabolic disease. Lancet, 2:996, 1974.

Raivio, K. O., and Seegmiller, J. E.: Genetic diseases of metabolism. Ann. Rev. Biochem., *41*:543, 1972.

Refetoff, S., et al.: Continuing occurrence of thyroid carcinoma after irradiation to the neck in infancy and childhood. New Eng. J. Med., *292*:171, 1975.

Rieselbach, R. E., and Steele, T. H.: Influence of the kidney upon urate homeostasis in health and disease. Am. J. Med., *56*:665, 1974.

Rimoin, D. L.: Genetics of diabetics. Calif. Med., *119*:14, 1973.

Rosenbloom, A. L.: Insulin responses of children with chemical diabetes mellitus. New Eng. J. Med., *282*:1228, 1970.

Rowley, J. D.: Do human tumors show a chromosome pattern specific for each etiologic agent? J. Nat. Cancer Inst., *52*:315, 1974.

Rushforth, N. B., et al.: Diabetes in the Pima Indians. Evidence of bimodality in glucose tolerance distribution. Diabetes, *20*:756, 1971.

Russell, L. B.: Experimental studies on mammalian chromosome aberrations. *In* Pava, C., Frotapessoa, O., and Caldas, L. R. (eds.): Mammalian Cytogenetics and Related Problems in Radiobiology. New York, Pergamon Press, 1964, p. 61.

Salguero, I. F., et al.: Neuropathologic observations in phenylketonuria. Trans. Amer. Neurol. Assoc., *93*:274, 1968.

Salinas-Madrigal, L., et al.: Glomerular and vascular "insudative" lesions of diabetic nephropathy: electron microscopic observations. Am. J. Path., *59*:369, 1970.

Sanchis, J.: Pulmonary mucociliary clearance in cystic fibrosis. New Eng. J. Med., *288*:651, 1973.

Seegmiller, J. E.: Diseases of purine and pyrimidine metabolism. *In* Bondy, P. K., and Rosenberg, L. E. (eds.): Duncan's Diseases of Metabolism. Philadelphia, W. B. Saunders Co., 1974, p. 655.

Seegmiller, J. E., et al.: Inflammatory reactions to sodium urate: its possible relationship to genesis of acute gouty arthritis. J.A.M.A., *180*:469, 1962.

Seegmiller, J. E., et al.: Biochemistry of uric acid and its relation to gout. New Eng. J. Med., *268*:712, 1963.

Seegmiller, J. E., et al.: Enzyme defect associated with a sex-linked human neurological disorder and excessive purine synthesis. Science, *155*:1682, 1967.

Sharp, G. W. G., et al.: Studies on the mechanism of insulin release. Fed. Proc., *34*:1537, 1975.

Shirahama, T., and Cohen, A. S.: Ultrastructural evidence for leakage of lysosomal contents after phagocytosis of monosodium urate crystals: A mechanism of gouty inflammation. Am. J. Path., *76*:501, 1974.

Shwachman, H., et al.: Studies in cystic fibrosis. Report of 130 patients diagnosed under 3 months of age over a 20 year period at the Children's Hospital Medical Center, Boston, Mass. Pediatrics, *46*:335, 1970.

Simpkin, P. A.: Local concentration of urate in the pathogenesis of gout. Lancet, *2*:1295, 1973.

Siperstein, M. D., et al.: Studies of muscle capillary basement membrane in normal subjects, diabetic and prediabetic patients. J. Clin. Invest., *47*:1973, 1968.

Smetana, H. F., and Olen, E.: Hereditary galactose disease. Am. J. Clin. Path., *38*:3, 1962.

Smithells, R. W.: Drugs and human malformations. Adv. Teratol., *1*:251, 1966.

Sperling, O., et al.: Purine base incorporation into erythrocyte nucleotides and erythrocyte phosphoribosyl transferase activity in primary gout. Rev. Eur. Etud. Clin. Biol., *16*:147, 1971.

Spiro, R. G.: Biochemistry of the renal glomerular basement membrane and its alterations in diabetes mellitus. New Eng. J. Med., *288*:1337, 1973.

Spock, A., et al.: Abnormal serum factor in patients with cystic fibrosis of the pancreas. Ped. Res., *1*:173, 1967.

Stanbury, J. B., Wyngaarden, J. B., and Fredrickson, D. S. (eds.): The Metabolic Basis of Inherited Disease, 3rd edition. New York, McGraw-Hill Book Company, 1972.

Steiner, D. P., et al.: Pro-insulin and the biosynthesis of insulin. Recent Progr. Hormone Res., *25*:207, 1969.

Stich, H. F., and Yohn, D. S.: Viruses and chromosomes. Progr. Med. Virol., *12*:78, 1970.

Swift, M., and Sholman, L.: Diabetes mellitus and the gene for Fanconi's anemia. Science, *178*:308, 1972.

Talbot, J. H., and Terplan, K. L.: The kidney in gout. Medicine, *39*:405, 1960.

Taylor, K. W.: The biosynthesis and secretion of insulin. Clin. Endocr. Metab., *1*:601, 1972.

Tjio, J. H., and Levan, A.: The chromosome number of man. Hereditas, *42*:1, 1956.

Unger, R. H.: Glucagon and the insulin: glucagon ratio in diabetes and other catabolic illnesses. Diabetes, *20*:834, 1971.

Unger, R. H., and Orci, L.: The essential role of glucagon in the pathogenesis of diabetes mellitus. Lancet, *1*:15, 1975.

Vinik, A. I.: A unifying hypothesis for hereditary and acquired diabetes. Lancet, *1*:485, 1974.

Vogel, F.: Point mutations and human hemoglobin variants. Humangenetik, *8*:1, 1969.

Volk, B. W., et al.: Some ultrastructural and histochemical aspects of lipidoses. Path. Europ., *3*:200, 1968.

Vracko, R., and Benditt, E. P.: Manifestations of diabetes mellitus — their possible relationships to an underlying cell defect. Am. J. Path., *75*:204, 1974.

Warren, R. J.: Identification by fluorescent microscopy of the abnormal chromosomes associated with the G-deletion syndromes. Am. J. Hum. Genet., *25*:77, 1973.

Weinstein, D.: The effect of caffeine on chromosomes of human lymphocytes. In vivo and in vitro studies. Mutation Res., *16*:391, 1972.

Weissman, G.: Crystals, lysosomes and gout. Adv. Int. Med., *19*:234, 1974.

Whitehouse, D.: Diagnostic value of the cafe-au-lait spot in children. Arch. Dis. Child., *41*:316, 1966.

World Health Organization: Genetic Counseling. WHO Technical Report Series, No. 416, 1969.

Wrenshall, G. A., et al.: Extractable insulin of pancreas. Diabetes, *1*:87, 1952.

Wyngaarden, J. B.: Metabolic defects of primary hyperuricemia and gout. Am. J. Med., *56*:651, 1974.

Wyngaarden, J. B., and Kelley, W. N.: Gout. *In* Stanbury, J. B., Wyngaarden, J. B., and Fredrickson, D. S. (eds.): The Metabolic Basis of Inherited Disease. New York, McGraw-Hill, 1972, p. 889.

Yamazaki, J. N., et al.: Outcome of pregnancy in women exposed to the atomic bomb in Nagasaki. Am. J. Dis. Child., *7*:448, 1954.

CHAPTER 6
Disorders of Immunity

Immunity and immunologic disorders are to contemporary medicine what bacteriology and bacterial diseases were to the medical world of the turn of the century. New diseases, new immunologic insights into the causation of "old diseases," and new vistas of immunotherapy permeate the contemporary medical literature. More than ever it has become apparent that dependent as man is for his survival on the immune system, so vulnerable is he to the wide-ranging disorders in its function. On the one extreme, immunodeficiency states render him an easy prey to infectious diseases. At the other extreme a hyperreactive immune apparatus may seemingly run amok, reacting against "self" to induce life-threatening disease. Put more succinctly, the disorders range from those caused by "too little" to those caused by "too much" immunologic reactivity. To encompass this spectrum, the various immunologic conditions will be considered under the following four headings:

1. Immunodeficiency states.
2. Immunologic mechanisms of tissue injury.
3. Autoimmune diseases.
4. Possible immune disorders.

The important prototypes in each category will be considered in the following sections,

but first a brief recapitulation of the development of the immune system may be of help in understanding the immunodeficiency states (Cooper and Lawton, 1974).

As is now well known, immunologic responsiveness involves two effector mechanisms: humoral antibodies derived from the B-cell system and cell-mediated mechanisms involving T-cells (delayed hypersensitivity). Both depend upon the activity of small lymphocytes ultimately derived from stem cell precursors which in postnatal life reside in the bone marrow. These stem cells differentiate to form at least two distinct lymphocyte populations, one thymus-independent (B-cells) and one thymus-dependent (T-cells). Approximately 60 to 70 per cent of the small lymphocytes in the circulating blood are T-cells and most of the remainder are B-cells. In addition, there are other minor populations such as null cells (not identifiable as belonging to either the B- or T-cell classes), as well as other cells which may represent special classes of lymphocytes. For example, a cell type has been segregated recently which appears to be involved principally in surveillance of hematopoietic precursors. These are called M-cells and it is not certain whether they are macrophages or a subset of lymphocytes.

The thymus, critical to the development of

the T-cell system, is derived from epithelial cells that line the third and fourth pharyngeal pouches in the embryo. Early in embryonic development these epithelial cells begin to specialize and migrate down the neck into the chest to form the definitive thymus. Thymus-dependent T-lymphocytes require either temporary residence in the thymus or exposure to some thymus-derived humoral factor (thymosin). T-cells, as mentioned, constitute the greater part of the circulating pool of small lymphocytes; they are also found in peripheral lymphoid organs, e.g., in the paracortical areas of lymph nodes and periarteriolar lymphocytic sheaths of the spleen. They possess specific surface receptors whose nature has not yet been identified, but according to present evidence the receptors are not immunoglobulins of endogenous origin. In response to antigens to which they are sensitive, T-cells undergo blast transformation (immunoblasts) and rapidly divide to form an expanded population of antigen-sensitive cells.

T-cells subserve many functions. (1) They make a major contribution to immunologic memory because of their long life span. (2) Some are converted into "killer" cells capable of nonphagocytic destruction of target cells—for example, in allogeneic grafts (Henry, 1974). (3) Sensitized lymphocytes release a number of soluble factors such as transfer factor (Editorial, 1973*a*) and lymphokines (e.g., macrophage migration inhibitory factor, a factor mitogenic for other lymphocytes, cytotoxic factor, specific macrophage arming factor and others) (Editorial, 1973*b*). (4) T-cells along with macrophages cooperate with B-lymphocytes in the antibody response to certain antigens designated as thymus-dependent. It is not certain that every sensitized T-lymphocyte can subserve all the above described functions, and special subclasses have been proposed in the belief that there may be a distribution of labor. Possibly T-memory cells belong to a special subclass. T-helper cells would be those involved in cooperation with the B-cell system. T-"killer" cells may perhaps be specialized for the destruction of allogeneic "foreign" cells. In addition, another subset, called T-suppressor cells, may serve to regulate the humoral response of B-cells and also may play a role in regulating T-cell immune responses. We still do not know whether such a division of labor actually exists, but there is much circumstantial evidence for functional heterogeneity among T-cells (Asofsky et al., 1975). It is apparent, then, that failure to develop an effective T-cell system leads to defects in cell-mediated immunity (delayed hypersensitivity) and also to deficiencies in the humoral antibody response,

for which cooperation between B- and T-cells is necessary. The principal role of T-cells is protection against viral, fungal and certain bacterial infections, as well as rejection of "foreign" cells, i.e., graft or possibly tumor rejection.

Recently, a new form of cell-mediated immune reaction now termed "antibody dependent cellular cytotoxicity" (ADCC) has been described. This may be an important mechanism for rejection or destruction of "foreign" target cells (Perlmann et al., 1972). In this reaction, B-cells produce antibodies against graft or tumor cells. These antibodies then coat the target cells. Macrophages, neutrophils, B-cells, "null" lymphocytes and conceivably any other cell form bearing Fc receptors for the specific immunoglobulin attach to the Fc region of the antibody and destroy the target cells. It should be noted then that B-cells as well as other Fc bearing cells participate in cell-mediated destruction of target cells (Von Boxel et al., 1972).

The *B-lymphocytes* constitute a distinct lymphoid system specific for antibody production. Their progenitors are also marrow stem cells. In fowl these cells come under the influence of the bursa of Fabricius, but no comparable organ has yet been identified in man. In addition to those in circulation, B-cells are found within and about the lymphoid follicles of the nodes and spleen, and also diffusely throughout the bone marrow and connective tissues. Upon contact with antigen, they divide and differentiate within three days to become secretory B-lymphocytes and plasma cells synthesizing immunoglobulins (Miller and Phillips, 1975). B-lymphocytes have specific surface receptors, including: membrane-bound immunoglobulin synthesized by B-cells themselves, a receptor for aggregated immunoglobulin (Fc determinant) and a receptor for the third component of complement (C'3). Immunodeficiency states may arise because of defects in the surface receptors of B-cells or because of secretory defects. Thus, one may have the apparent paradox of an adequate number of B-lymphocytes and yet ineffective antibody response.

As is well known, there are five distinct classes of immunoglobulins: IgM, IgG, IgA, IgD and IgE. In the development of the B-cell system the marrow stem cells first give rise to IgM producing cells. Some of these serve as the progenitors of other IgM producing cells, but others give rise to IgG progenitors. The IgG progenitors then yield other IgG secreting cells or give rise to IgA precursors. IgA progenitors then mature to yield more IgA precursor cells. Little is yet known about the involvement of IgD and IgE in this sequence.

This embryologic chronology explains how it is possible for patients to exhibit a selective IgA deficiency despite normal levels of IgM and IgG and why patients deficient in IgM are likely to have concomitant IgG and IgA deficiencies.

IMMUNODEFICIENCY DISEASES

The more we learn about the immune system the more complex it becomes. No less complex is the classification of immunodeficiency states. At one time, in blissful ignorance, these were simply categorized as a lack of B-cells or of T-cells or sometimes of both forms of cells; but alas, many new subtleties have emerged. For example, it is now appreciated that ineffective immune responses may be caused by secretory defects in lymphocytes or as a result of abnormalities in antigen recognition in the face of adequate numbers of lymphocytes. In addition, there are a very few, rare disorders affecting neutrophil function (chronic granulomatous disease) or spleen function, which are sometimes categorized as immunodeficiency states. Since these do not involve immunocompetent cells, they are not considered further here. Despite many complexities, the immunodeficiencies can be broadly subdivided into primary diseases of genetic origin and those secondary to some underlying disorder. At the risk of disconcerting those with orderly minds, the secondary states will be considered first and with great brevity.

SECONDARY IMMUNODEFICIENCIES

These disorders are sometimes encountered in patients with malnutrition, infection, cancer, renal diseases, Hodgkin's disease and sarcoidosis. They may also occur secondary to the use of immunosuppressive drugs, as well as in other conditions (Lessof, 1974). Many of these secondary states can be accounted for by loss of immunoglobulins (as in proteinuric renal diseases), inadequate synthesis of immunoglobulins (as in malnutrition) or loss of lymphocytes (as may occur with systemic infections), but other mechanisms may also be operative. Recently, an immunosuppressive peptide fraction was identified in the serum of cancer patients suffering from T-cell anergy (Glasgow et al., 1974). The basis for the depressed immunity in renal failure not associated with heavy protein loss is totally obscure. While at first glance the depressed immunity might be viewed as a fortunate happenstance in patients about to receive an allogeneic kidney transplant, it also hampers antigenic cross-matching of donor and recipient (p. 177). As a group, the secondary immunodeficiencies are more common than the disorders of genetic origin. They also occur later in life, depending on the underlying disorder. However, they rarely induce as profound a depression of immunoresponsiveness as the primary diseases and so are less often directly responsible for death.

PRIMARY IMMUNODEFICIENCY STATES

The primary immunodeficiencies usually come to attention within the first six to eight months of life because of the vulnerability of the infant to recurrent infections. Although these immune disorders are relatively uncommon, they are often devastating and the infections too often are fatal (Hermans, 1973; Gatti and Seligmann, 1973). Table 6–1 presents a classification of the primary immunodeficiencies. A few of the more common will now be characterized.

X-LINKED (CONGENITAL) AGAMMAGLOBULINEMIA — BRUTON'S DISEASE

This disorder is the counterpart in man of the immune defect produced in birds by neonatal bursectomy. It is one of the more common forms of primary immunodeficiency. As an X-linked disease it is seen almost entirely in males, but sporadic cases have been described in females. It usually does not become apparent until about six months of age, when maternal immunoglobulins are depleted. In most cases recurrent bacterial infections such as acute and chronic pharyngitis, sinusitis, otitis media, bronchitis and pneumonia call attention to the underlying immune defect. Almost always the causative organisms are *Hemophilus influenzae, Streptococcus pyogenes, Staphylococcus aureus* or the pneumococci. The classic form of this disease, first described by Bruton, has the following characteristics: *(1) B-cells are absent or remarkably decreased in the circulation, and the serum levels of all classes of immunoglobulins are depressed. It should be noted that there may not be a total lack of immunoglobulins and therefore sometimes the disease is called X-linked hypogammaglobulinemia. (2) The germinal centers of lymph nodes, Peyer's patches, the appendix and tonsils are underdeveloped or rudimentary. (3) There is a remarkable absence of plasma cells throughout the body. (4) The T-cell system and cell-mediated reactions are entirely normal.*

In addition to the classic presentation, variants have been described. Patients have been observed who have normal or nearly normal numbers of B-cells in the peripheral blood but nonetheless have a total lack or low levels of serum immunoglobulins (Aiuti et al., 1972). The exact meaning of these findings is

TABLE 6-1. CLASSIFICATION OF PRIMARY IMMUNODEFICIENCIES*

DEFICIENCY	CELLULAR DEFECT			INHERITANCE		
	B-Lymphocytes		T-Lymphocytes	X-Linked	Autosomal Recessive	Other[2]
	Absent or Decreased	Easily Detectable or Increased[1]				
X-linked agammaglobulinemia (Bruton's disease)	X	(X)[3]		X		
Thymic hypoplasia (DiGeorge's syndrome)			X			X
Severe combined immuno-deficiency (Swiss-type)	X	X	X	X	X	X
With dysostosis	X	?	X		X	
With adenosine deaminase deficiency	X		X		X	
Immunodeficiency with gener-alized hematopoietic hypo-plasia	X		X		X	
Selective Ig deficiency: IgA	?	X	(X)[3]			X
Others (IgM, IgE)		?				X
X-linked immunodeficiency with increased IgM		X		X		
Immunodeficiency with ataxia telangiectasia		X	X		X	
Immunodeficiency with thrombocytopenia and eczema (Wiskott-Aldrich syndrome)			X	X		
Immunodeficiency with thymoma		X	X			X
Immunodeficiency with normal or hypergammaglobulinemia	X	X	(X)[3]			X
Transient hypogammaglobulinemia of infancy		X				X
Variable immunodeficiencies (largely unclassified and very frequent)	X	X	(X)[3]		(X)[3]	X

*Adapted from Cooper, M. D., et al.: Meeting report of the Second International Workshop in Primary Immunodeficiency Diseases in Man. Clin. Immunol. Immunopathol., 2:416, 1974.

[1]These cells usually show deranged function.

[2]"Other" implies multifactorial or unknown genetic bases or no known genetic basis.

[3](X) indicates less frequent occurrence than X.

still unclear. The lymphocytes may lack specific receptors, and thus be rendered incapable of responding to antigens. Alternatively, non-B-cells incapable of synthesizing immunoglobulins may bear surface markers which lead to their misidentification as B-cells in the circulating blood (Geha et al., 1973). It is evident that the apparent presence of B-lymphocytes in the circulating blood does not rule out the diagnosis of this form of congenital hypogammaglobulinemia.

Autoimmune diseases occur with increased frequency in these patients. Nearly half of these children develop a condition similar to rheumatoid arthritis which clears remarkably with restitutive gammaglobulin therapy. Similarly, lupus erythematosus (p. 184), dermatomyositis (p. 196) and other autoimmune diseases are more common in these patients.

In passing it should be noted that there is an idiopathic late-onset form of primary immunoglobulin deficiency sometimes encountered in adults (Hermans, 1973).

THYMIC HYPOPLASIA (DIGEORGE'S SYNDROME)

This disorder results from a lack of thymic influence on the immune system. *The thymus is usually rudimentary and T-cells are deficient or absent in the circulation. They are similarly depleted in the thymus dependent areas of the lymph nodes and spleen.* Thus, infants with this defect are extremely vulnerable to viral and fungal infections as well as to those bacterial infections requiring T- and B-cell cooperation. The parathyroid glands are also either hypoplastic or totally absent, often leading to tetany from hypocalcemia. The evidence suggests some embryonic defect in the development of the third and fourth pharyngeal pouches, from which both the thymus and parathyroids are derived. The mode of inheritance of this condition is uncertain and, indeed, it may well represent a nonhereditary mutation arising during embryogenesis. Only rarely is more than one child in a family affected. The B-cell system and serum immunoglobulins are entirely unaffected. A few of these infants have additional developmental defects affecting the face, ears and sometimes the heart, adding further evidence of a developmental origin of this disorder. Transplantation of thymic tissue has been remarkably successful in some of these infants, but in others has triggered serious, even fatal, graft-versus-host reactions (Cleveland et al., 1968; Steele et al., 1972).

SEVERE COMBINED IMMUNODEFICIENCY (SWISS-TYPE AGAMMAGLOBULINEMIA)

Severe combined immunodeficiency represents a constellation of syndromes all having in common defects in both humoral and cell-mediated immune responses. At least four variants have been identified, all quite rare. *The most common form, inherited as an autosomal recessive condition, is characterized by a marked decrease in the total circulating lymphocyte population, involving both B- and T-cells.* The thymus is usually hypoplastic and fetal in type or it may be absent. Lymph nodes are difficult to find, markedly reduced in size and lack both germinal centers, which normally contain B-cells, and the paracortical T-cells. The lymphoid tissues of the tonsils, gut and appendix are also markedly hypoplastic (Berry, 1970). A second, X-linked syndrome is essentially the same as that just described except that the lymphopenia is less severe and the prognosis slightly better. A third syndrome, with immunologic deficiencies similar to those encountered in the autosomal recessive disease, is associated with dysostosis (short-limbed dwarfism). A fourth variant, also transmitted as an autosomal recessive disease, involves a deficiency of adenosine deaminase in addition to the combined immunologic defects. Many other, less well characterized variants have now been identified, some with uncertain modes of inheritance. Infants with these severe immunologic handicaps are vulnerable to all forms of infections and most die within the first year of life. One remarkable youngster, however, has survived for years in a germ-free enclosure. Immunologic reconstitution by thymus and bone marrow transplantation has been attempted in many cases and achieved in a few. Regrettably, the risks of fatal graft-versus-host reactions are high in this procedure (De Koning et al., 1969). Some success has also been achieved with bone marrow transplantation alone, suggesting that the underlying basis for this constellation of syndromes is a defect in marrow stem cells. However, the markedly hypoplastic thymus, characteristic of this group of disorders, must also have some bearing on the immunologic deficiency (Yata et al., 1974).

IMMUNODEFICIENCY WITH THROMBOCYTOPENIA AND ECZEMA (WISKOTT-ALDRICH SYNDROME)

This condition is selected for presentation because it demonstrates the complexity of the immunologic findings in some patients with primary immune deficiency syndromes. The Wiskott-Aldrich syndrome, which occurs only in males, is characterized by eczema, thrombocytopenia and recurrent infections. Classically these patients show a poor antibody response to polysaccharide antigens (for example, those derived from pneumococcus types I and II) despite normal responses to other antigens such as tetanus and diphtheria toxoids. In addition, the titers of isohemagluttinins and serum concentrations of IgM are classically low. Serum IgE levels are greatly elevated in some patients. With time, a progressive loss of cell-mediated immunity develops. But despite all of these defects the number of circulating lymphocytes may be normal or near normal. Only when there is well developed loss of T-cell function is lymphopenia found. The pathogenesis of this form of immunodeficiency is still obscure, but much of the evidence is compatible with some defect in antigen handling or recognition. Here, then, is an example of an immunodeficiency in the presence of adequate numbers of immunocompetent cells. Encouraging results have been achieved in the treatment of this syndrome by the administration of transfer factor (Spitler et al., 1972; Griscelli et al., 1973).

Figure 6–1, which schematically indicates the development of the immune system, marks the sites of the genetic defects in the previously described primary immunodeficiencies.

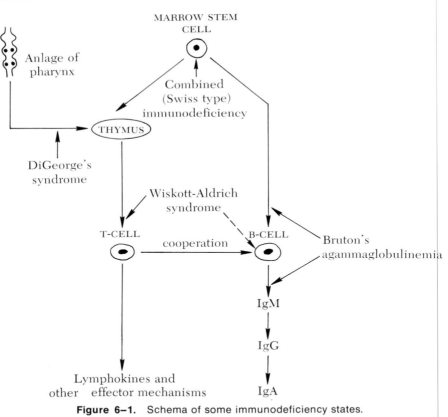

Figure 6–1. Schema of some immunodeficiency states.

IMMUNOLOGIC MECHANISMS OF TISSUE INJURY

Immunologic responses (humoral or cell-mediated) to antigens of either endogenous or exogenous sources can cause tissue damaging reactions. Classically these are called *hypersensitivity reactions* and the resultant tissue lesions *hypersensitivity disease*. The term hypersensitivity, however, is somewhat misleading. It implies abnormal or excessive sensitivity to an antigen. However, hypersensitivity disease may result from perfectly usual or normal immune responses to an antigen, e.g., the rejection of tissue grafts from antigenically dissimilar donors. A better designation for hypersensitivity diseases might be "diseases resulting from immunologically mediated tissue-damaging reactions," but alas, this is too cumbersome a designation.

Disorders resulting from tissue damaging immune reactions have been categorized in a variety of ways, but only two classifications will be reviewed here. The first (Table 6–2) divides the immunologically mediated disorders into three categories on the basis of the source of the offending antigen, i.e., exogenous, homologous or autologous. This classification is of value because it indicates that some disorders—those due to exogenous antigens—are essentially environmental and as such are theoretically preventable. Poison ivy contact dermatitis could be eradicated as a disease by mere avoidance of contact with the plant, as could hay fever resulting from inhalation of plant pollens. On the other hand, many of the most important immune diseases are caused by homologous and autologous antigens intrinsic to man. The disorders triggered by homologous antigens result from the genetic and antigenic dissimilarities between individuals. Transfusion reactions are

TABLE 6–2. IMMUNE DISORDERS CLASSIFIED BY SOURCE OF ANTIGEN

Exogenous	Atopic diseases (e.g., poison ivy contact dermatitis, reactions to plant pollens, sera and drugs)
Homologous	Reactions to isoantigens (e.g., transfusion reactions, erythroblastosis fetalis, transplantation rejection)
Autologous	Autoimmune diseases (e.g., systemic lupus erythematosus, rheumatoid arthritis, Sjögren's syndrome)

TABLE 6–3. MECHANISMS OF IMMUNOLOGICALLY MEDIATED DISORDERS

TYPE	PROTOTYPE DISORDER	IMMUNE MECHANISM
I Anaphylactic type	Anaphylaxis, some forms of bronchial asthma.	Formation of IgE (cytotropic antibody, reagin) → release of vasoactive amines from basophils and mast cells.
II Cytotoxic type	Autoimmune hemolytic anemia, erythroblastosis fetalis, Goodpasture's disease.	Formation of IgG, IgM → binds to antigen on target cell surface → phagocytosis of target cell or lysis of target cell by C′8, 9 fraction of activated complement.
III Immune complex disease	Arthus reaction, serum sickness, systemic lupus erythematosus, certain forms of acute glomeru-lonephritis.	Antigen-antibody complexes → activated complement → attracted neutrophils → release of lysosomal enzymes.
IV Cell-mediated (delayed) hyper-sensitivity	Tuberculosis, contact dermatitis, transplantation rejection.	Sensitized thymus-derived T lymphocytes → release of lymphokines and other effector mechanisms.

examples of immunologic disorders evoked by homologous antigens. Appropriate cross matching of donor and recipient could preclude such reactions. Unfortunately, as will be discussed later (p. 177), we do not yet have enough knowledge to match accurately the donor and recipient for transplantation of organs, nor are we likely to attempt to control erythroblastosis fetalis in the newborn (p. 331) by making blood group compatibility a requisite for marriage. The third category of disorders, those incited by autologous antigens, comprises the important group of autoimmune diseases to be discussed later (p. 182). These diseases appear to arise because of the emergence of immune reactions against "self" antigens.

The second classification (Table 6–3) is based on the immunologic mechanism mediating the disease. This approach is also of great value since it clarifies the manner in which the immune response ultimately causes tissue injury and disease. In type I disease the immune response releases vasoactive amines which act on smooth muscle within organs, thus altering their function. In the type II disorder humoral antibodies participate directly in injuring cells by predisposing them to phagocytosis or to lysis. Type III disorders are best remembered as "immune complex diseases"; here humoral antibodies bind antigens and activate complement. The fractions of complement then attract neutrophils. Ultimately it is the activated complement and the release of neutrophilic lysosomal enzymes which produce the tissue damage. Type IV disorders are examples of tissue injury in which cell-mediated immune responses with sensitized lymphocytes are the ultimate cause of the cellular and tissue injury. Prototypes of each of these immune mechanisms are presented in the succeeding sections.

TYPE I, REAGINIC DISORDER — ANAPHYLAXIS

Anaphylaxis is a potentially fatal immunologic reaction which erupts within minutes of the combination of antigen with a special type of antibody, usually IgE, in individuals or animals having prior sensitization to the antigen. It may occur as a systemic disorder or as a local reaction, but the following remarks will be confined to the systemic pattern. Animal models of this disease can be readily produced, particularly in guinea pigs, by the administration of an antigen as innocuous as egg albumin, followed after a suitable period of two to three weeks by a challenge dose of the same antigen. In man, sensitization usually occurs by a prior inoculation of some agent such as a drug or heterologous serum. One of the more common offenders is penicillin. In some reported cases sensitization occurs very subtly. Patients have been known to become sensitive to horse serum from inhaling horse dander and to antibiotics merely from drinking the milk of antibiotic-treated cows. It should be remembered that the shock dose of antigen may be exceedingly small, as for example the tiny amounts used in ordinary skin testing for various forms of allergy. Anaphylaxis has also been observed in the sensitized individual following a mere insect bite.

For obscure reasons the shock organs, i.e. those reacting to the antigen challenge, vary from one species to another. In man, itching, hives and skin erythema appear within a few minutes, followed shortly thereafter by striking respiratory difficulty resulting presumably from constriction of respiratory bronchioles. Thus the principal shock organ is the lung, more specifically the smooth musculature of the pulmonary blood vessels and the respiratory passages. Laryngeal obstruction may also appear. In addition, the musculature of the entire GI tract may be affected, with resultant vomiting, abdominal cramps and diarrhea (Broder, 1971). The patient may go into shock and even die within the hour. At autopsy the findings may be surprisingly few, consisting principally of pulmonary edema and hemorrhages, sometimes accompanied by hyperdistension of the lungs and right-sided cardiac dilatation (James and Austin, 1964).

The pathogenesis of this immune disorder has been well elucidated. The sensitizing dose of antigen evokes cytotropic antibodies, usually belonging to the IgE class (reagins), which bind to the surface membranes of basophils and mast cells through their Fc regions. Certain classes of IgG can also act as reagins, but their contribution to anaphylaxis in man is not yet resolved. On administration of the challenge dose, *the antigen combines with the cytotropic antibody and triggers degranulation of the mast cells or basophils, with release of contained vasoactive amines, principally histamine and 5-hydroxytryptamine.* Slow reacting substance (SRS-A), capable of inducing contraction of smooth muscle, may also participate in the reaction, but its role is still unclear. The release of vasoactive amines is explosive. It has been speculated that when the reagins bound to mast cells and basophils are cross linked by specific antigen, some membrane signal is transmitted to the intracellular AMP which is involved in the maintenance of the membrane-bound intracellular granules of stored vasoactive agents. Type I immune disease, then, documents the role of antigen-antibody complexes in releasing vasoactive compounds. Complement is not involved.

Anaphylaxis is an important condition to bear in mind since it is capable of causing death within minutes. It has been estimated, for example, that as many as 20 per cent of individuals treated with penicillin develop varying degrees of sensitivity to the drug, each of whom is a potential candidate for an anaphylactic attack. Predisposition to anaphylaxis is found in individuals having other forms of sensitivities, a useful fact to remember when administering medications to patients. The common forms of skin and food allergies, hay fever, and certain forms of asthma are examples of localized anaphylactic (atopic) reactions, also involving IgE. Those sensitive to cherries, for instance, may develop edema of the oral mucosa or skin hives or diarrhea, documenting the vagaries of the shock organ among individuals. Presumably the antigen is absorbed through the gut into the bloodstream and evokes its reaction wherever the reagin is bound to tissue mast cells. When administered in time, antihistaminics and steroids may be effective in controlling the manifestations of atopic diseases.

TYPE II, CYTOTOXIC DISORDER—AUTOIMMUNE HEMOLYTIC ANEMIA

This form of hemolytic anemia, presented in greater detail on page 331, is discussed here only as an example of a cytotoxic immune disorder. In some instances the hemolytic reaction appears spontaneously in otherwise healthy individuals. Occasionally a history of the recent ingestion of drugs such as penicillin, methyl dopa, quinidine, phenacetin or chlorpromazine is obtained. In these cases it is suspected that the drug complexed with red cell antigens to create a "foreign" antigen which initiated the immunologic reaction. In other patients the hemolytic disease occurs following syphilitic, viral or mycoplasmic infection, raising once again the possibility of a haptenic reaction or, alternatively, some cross reaction between microbial antigens and red cell antigens (Feizi et al., 1969). All of these instances are classified as "primary" autoimmune hemolytic anemia to differentiate them from so-called "secondary" autoimmune hemolytic anemia. The latter is encountered in patients having an underlying disorder of the lymphoid system, such as lymphocytic leukemia, lymphoma, sarcoidosis or systemic lupus erythematosus. Whether primary or secondary, *several classes of circulating antibodies appear in autoimmune hemolytic anemia and induce three distinctive immunologic patterns of this disease.* The three classes of antibodies are responsible for three distinctive mechanisms of red cell destruction. The first mechanism is coating of target cells with IgG antibody followed by their opsonic adherence and phagocytosis by cells of the RE system, especially within the spleen. The immune adherence may be mediated by bound C'3. The second mechanism involves another class of IgG or IgM, which activates complement and so releases the direct membrane damaging potential of the C'8,9 fraction of activated complement. Still a third mechanism involving antibody dependent cellular cytotoxicity (p. 168) has been postulated recently. Red cells coated with IgG antibody can be destroyed by nonsensitized reticular cells, lymphocytes or macrophages having Fc receptors for IgG (Perlmann et al., 1972). Whatever immunoglobulin or mechanism is involved, autoimmune hemolytic anemia exemplifies the destructive effect of antibodies on target cells.

TYPE III, IMMUNE COMPLEX DISORDER—ARTHUS REACTION

The Arthus reaction constitutes a focal area of inflammation and necrosis at the site of injection of a soluble antigen into an individual previously sensitized to this antigen. The local inflammatory reaction is mediated by fractions of complement and abetted by ischemia resulting from an acute necrotizing vasculitis in the inflammatory site. *Gross antibody excess and rapid precipitation of the complexes at the site of introduction of the antigen are essential to the pathogenesis of this lesion.* The precise sequence of events is as follows. Initial exposure to an antigen induces the formation of antibodies and a state of sensitization. With the subsequent local injection of antigen, immune complexes which bind and activate complement are precipitated at the site of injection. Anaphylatoxins, released from C′3 and C′5, increase vascular permeability, probably by the release of histamine. Some evidence suggests that an anaphylaxis-like reaction also contributes to the release of histamine, but whether this is mediated by IgE or IgG is not clear. Other fragments of C′3 and the trimolecular complex C′5,6,7 act as chemotactic factors, leading to the aggregation of neutrophils within the abnormally permeable vascular walls. The neutrophils phagocytize the immune complexes and in turn release cytolytic lysosomal enzymes. These simultaneously activate the kinin system, thus further increasing vascular permeability. In this way the small vessels in the area become the focus of a necrotizing vasculitis. The ultimate mediators of injury to the vessel walls and surrounding cells are both the lysosomal enzymes and the C′8,9 activated fraction of complement, which can directly lyse cells. *Plasma proteins seep into the abnormally permeable vessel walls and together with the infiltrated neutrophils create the appearance of fibrinoid necrosis of the vessels* (Fig. 6–2). Platelets become adherent to these injured vessels and often contribute to thrombosis of their lumens. This adds an element of ischemic necrosis to the inflammatory reaction. *Thus, the Arthus reaction is a prototype of tissue injury which is initiated by immune complexes formed in antibody excess and is mediated by complement and neutrophils.*

TYPE III, IMMUNE COMPLEX DISORDER—SERUM SICKNESS

Serum sickness is another form of immune complex disease which differs from the Arthus reaction in that it requires antigen excess. As with the Arthus phenomenon, complement and neutrophils are the critical mediators of the tissue lesions. The consideration of *serum sickness assumes importance because it is a prototype of a group of important immune complex disorders of man which includes systemic lupus erythematosus, some forms of proliferative glomerulonephritis and rheumatoid arthritis.* It may occur as an acute (one shot), self-limited process or in a chronic, more damaging form.

Acute (one shot) serum sickness may follow a single large intravenous injection of a foreign antigen, such as an antitoxin produced in a horse. It has also followed drug administration. Some 8 to 12 days later, urticaria, fever, edema and generalized lymphadenopathy appear. In this acute form of the disease the illness is transient and may or may not be associated with renal involvement and swollen joints, but in any event usually clears spontaneously within a few days. The pathogenesis of this disorder has been well elucidated in rabbits (Dixon et al., 1958 and 1961). When a large dose of foreign protein is administered, antibody begins to appear some five days later. At this time immune complexes are formed in antigen excess, a situation which results in the formation of relatively small soluble complexes, which remain within the circulation. During the next five to seven days continued antibody production leads to the

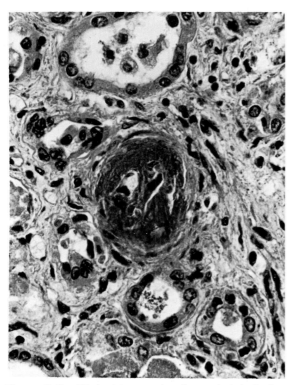

Figure 6–2. Fibrinoid necrosis of an arteriole in the kidney. The structure of the vessel in the midfield is virtually obliterated by an amorphous deposit of plasma proteins. Immunofluorescent stains disclosed fibrin, complement and gamma globulins.

formation of more immune complexes, but the excess of antigen has not yet been cleared. While in the circulation the soluble immune complexes cause clumping of platelets with release of their vasoactive amines, which in turn induce increased vascular permeability. The increased vascular permeability accounts for the urticaria and edema. The generalized lymphadenopathy reflects the systemic immune response. The small soluble complexes penetrate and localize within blood vessel walls throughout the body. Here they bind complement and by the same sequence described in the Arthus reaction induce acute vasculitis. Eventually the build-up of antibody leads to the formation of larger, insoluble immune complexes in the circulation which are cleared by the RE system, thus limiting the entire process. Sometimes a transient renal involvement is seen, as will be described below.

The chronic form of serum sickness results from repeated (or prolonged) exposure to an antigen. Presumably the preformed levels of antibody are not sufficient to clear the newly introduced antigen, and the antigen excess leads to the formation of small soluble complexes in the circulation. The repeated reintroduction of more antigen maintains the antigen excess and the continued presence within the circulation of immune complexes often causes serious damage to the blood vessels, kidneys, joints and heart. *In the blood vessels, acute necrotizing vasculitis similar to that described in the Arthus reaction may develop. The small circulating immune complexes are filtered out of the glomerular capillaries to become trapped between the glomerular basement membrane and the podocytic epithelial cells.* Here they can be visualized readily by immunofluorescent methods or electron microscopy as "lumpy-bumpy" granules which yield positive stains for immunoglobulin, complement (C'3) and sometimes the involved antigen. In this location the immune complexes bind and activate complement; neutrophils are attracted, and their lysosomal enzymes as well as the activated complement injure the glomeruli. This pathogenetic mechanism underlies many important renal diseases and is discussed more fully in Chapter 13. Here it should be noted that the kidney is an innocent bystander since the antigens and the immune complexes are of extrarenal origin. Localization of the immune complexes in the synovia of the joints may induce a form of arthritis closely resembling that seen in rheumatoid arthritis (p. 190). Similarly, the endocardium of the heart, particularly the heart valves, may be injured. Serum sickness is then an example of an immunologic disease affecting many organs in the body which results from the formation of soluble circulating immune complexes.

TYPE IV, CELL-MEDIATED (DELAYED) HYPERSENSITIVITY—TUBERCULOSENSITIVITY

Sensitivity to tuberculin (tuberculoprotein derivative) is a prototype of a T-cell mediated reaction. This form of immune response also characterizes the reactions to certain bacteria, most viruses and fungi, skin contact allergens and the rejection of transplanted tissues. We still do not know why certain antigens, such as tuberculoprotein, evoke a cell-mediated response, whereas others evoke humoral responses. The generalization can be made that large antigens which bear many determinants (multivalent) directly activate B-cells, i.e., are thymus independent. Other antigenic molecules, usually smaller, also evoke humoral antibodies but require an additional signal provided by T-cells and are therefore known as T-dependent antigens. Still other antigens evoke only T-cell responses, for reasons that yet elude us. There are only these few hints. Antigens of low potency which are slowly absorbed tend to evoke T-cell responses. Thus, bacteria which do not produce either powerful exo- or endotoxins, such as the tubercle bacillus, are likely to evoke cell-mediated responses. Similarly, antigens administered along with an adjuvant, such as Freund's, are slowly absorbed and generally cause cell-mediated responses. In the same way the intradermal route of antigen introduction tends to evoke delayed hypersensitivity. In the tuberculin test, for example, the antigen is slowly absorbed from its intradermal site of inoculation.

The classic example of a cell-mediated immune response is a positive Mantoux reaction (tuberculin test) elicited in an individual already sensitized to the tubercle bacillus by a tuberculous infection. Following the intracutaneous injection of tuberculin, a local area of erythema and induration begins to appear at 8 to 12 hours, and reaches a peak (approximately 1 to 2 cm. in diameter) in 2 to 7 days and thereafter slowly subsides. The extremely sensitive individual may develop a larger area of induration and even central necrosis. Histologically the first change is the appearance of mononuclear cells, lymphocytes and macrophages about the blood vessels adjacent to the inoculation (perivascular cuffing). Later some neutrophils may gather but these soon disappear, leaving only the infiltrate of lymphocytes and monocytes (Fig. 6–3). Lymphocytotoxicity may cause the death of tissue cells as well as induce acute vascular necrosis.

The mechanisms by which sensitized lymphocytes are thought to exert their effect on target cells was discussed on page 168. How they destroy or inactivate targets such as viruses, fungi and T-cell allergens (such as

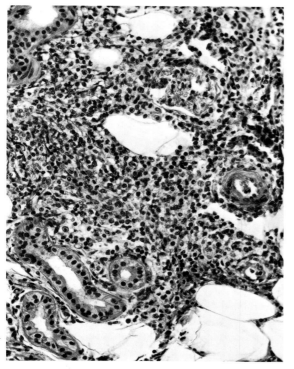

Figure 6–3. A tuberculin reaction in the dermis. There is infiltration of lymphocytes and macrophages about the small vessels and skin adnexa.

those causing contact dermatitis) is still not clear; however, one aspect of the T-cell response has been well documented. In any T-cell immune reaction most of the accumulated lymphocytes at first are not sensitized to the specific antigen. Soon, however, all of the lymphocytes become sensitized and reactive. This recruitment appears to result from elaboration of transfer factor by the minority of the sensitized cells (Lawrence, 1970a). Thus, transfer factor has an amplifying effect, greatly enhancing the magnitude of the T-cell response.

COMBINED TYPES III AND IV DISORDER—TRANSPLANT REJECTION

The immunologic rejection of transplanted tissues involves both humoral and cell-mediated mechanisms. The prospect that worn out or destroyed organs might be replaced is tantalizing and has excited the world. The surgical expertise for the transplantation of skin, kidneys, heart, lungs, liver, spleen, bone marrow and endocrine organs is now well in hand. However, experience has taught that the surgical difficulties, while considerable, are only the tip of the iceberg. It has become increasingly apparent that below the surface lies the vast problem of the im-

mune system with its long memory and implacable reactivity. At the heart of the problem lies our imperfect understanding of the antigenic profile, known as the histocompatibility system, of each individual's cells, and our inability to achieve perfect matches between these tissue antigens in donors and recipients.

All of the nucleated cells of man possess histocompatibility antigens. *Lymphoid cells and epithelial cells of the skin are rich in these antigens; liver, lung and kidney have moderate amounts, whereas the brain, skeletal muscle and probably the heart have only scant amounts.* It should be noted that whereas red cells have none, leukocytes, particularly lymphocytes, are rich in these antigens, and thus these cells provide a ready source of material for tissue typing and cross matching. The antigens, which are glycoprotein in nature, are membrane-bound on the surface of the cells. Each passing year brings to light new complexities within the genetic system, which dictates the amino acid sequences responsible for the antigenic specificity of the glycoproteins. In unraveling the details of this histocompatibility system we have drawn heavily on an analogous system in the mouse. In the mouse, at least 20 chromosomal loci have been identified which regulate the synthesis of histocompatibility antigens. One locus on chromosome 17, termed H-2, governs what appear to be the strongest antigens. These antigens evoke humoral antibodies and so are referred to as H-2 serum determinants. As best we now know, each locus, and particularly the H-2 locus, comprises more than one allele and each allele in turn controls the production of more than one specific antigen. There is, however, considerable overlapping; whereas some antigens appear to be associated with a single allele, others are associated with several alleles. Within the H-2 locus itself two distinct regions dictating serum determinants have been identified. These are separated by immune-response (Ir) genes, other genes which control certain serum proteins as well as genes concerned with the specific antigens apparently involved in accelerated skin graft rejections and the so-called Hh gene involved in the rejection of marrow allografts. More recently it has been established that still other genes (termed lymphocyte determinants or LD) within the same locus govern synthesis of antigenic determinants that evoke only cell-mediated responses. Thus, in addition to the histocompatibility antigens detected by serologic techniques, there now appear to be other histocompatibility antigens which can be detected only by T-cells in mixed lymphocyte cultures.

By analogy with the mouse it is believed that man possesses many genetic loci dictating the production of histocompatibility antigens.

One dominant locus in humans—HL-A—represents the counterpart of the H-2 locus of the mouse inasmuch as it appears to govern the production of the strong histocompatibility antigens. Just as the ABO antigens are the strongest and most important of the red cell antigens, so tissue typing and transplantation is largely dependent on matching of HL-A antigens. In man the HL-A locus is no less complex than its counterpart in the mouse. It encompasses at least two separate subregions, known as LA and Four, governing serologic determinants, a third region governing antigens which evoke cell-mediated responses, sometimes called the LD or MLR (mixed lymphocyte reaction) locus, as well as other genes analogous to those described in the H-2 complex of the mouse. Each of the subregions governing serologic determinants is responsible for the production of a number of antigens, including HL-A1, 2, 3, 9, 10 and 11 in the LA locus and HL-A5, 7, 8, 12 and 13 in the Four subregion. Many more have been identified in the recent past. Many of these antigens, formerly thought to be discrete, have now been shown to be composed of two or more specificities, yielding a bewildering complexity which we need not delve into further here (Morris, 1973a,b). Fortunately the individual can have at most only four of these serotypable antigens; two derived from the mother (one from the LA locus and one from the Four locus) and two similarly derived from the father. The histocompatibility profile of an individual with respect to these HL-A antigens may comprise, for example, HL-A2 and HL-A5 of maternal origin and HL-A9 and HL-A12 of paternal origin. It is entirely possible to inherit the same serologic determinants from mother and father, yielding a histocompatibility profile for the individual of only two or three antigens. Because of the multiplicity of these HL-A antigens the chance of finding a pair of unrelated individuals who have identical antigenic profiles is very small indeed. It is hardly necessary to point out that ABO red cell compatibility must also be considered.

In addition to HL-A antigens which evoke humoral responses, there are also, as mentioned, those evoking cell-mediated reactions. Techniques are not yet available for identifying the individual LD specificities among these antigens, but it is possible to determine the degree of compatibility between the cells of a donor and a recipient by culturing their lymphocytes together. When LD antigenic dissimilarities are present, the lymphocytes undergo blast cell transformation and mitosis. Indeed, there are techniques, so-called one-way cultures, for determining the reactivity of the lymphocytes of the recipient to the antigens borne on the lymphocytes of the donor. Because the genetic loci dictating the HL-A serologic determinants are closely linked on the same chromosome with the loci dictating the LD determinants, it is hoped that HL-A serologically compatible individuals will also possess equal LD compatibility.

The extent of the histocompatibility antigenic differences between donor and recipient—"the antigenic barrier"—conditions the likelihood of a successful transplant. Autografting of skin, for example, evokes no immune reaction and generally is highly successful. Isografts between syngeneic individuals, i.e., identical twins, can be equally successful. As the "antigenic barrier" increases so does the likelihood of rejection. Related individuals, because of their similar genetic backgrounds, are much more likely to be compatible than are unrelated individuals. Indeed, siblings have a 1 in 4 chance of having identical HL-A serologic profiles.

Because of the many problems mentioned concerning precise tissue typing and because appropriate tissues and organs for transplantation are not available in unlimited supply, it is usually necessary in practice to accept less than perfect cross matches and to fall back on immunosuppression to decrease the risk of rejection. Graft rejection can be more or less held at bay by interventions which nonspecifically interfere with the induction or expression of the immune response. For instance, whole body irradiation can, for a period of time, render the recipient immunologically unresponsive, but too often this leads to life-threatening consequences, including profound hematologic disturbances and uncontrolled infections. Cytotoxic and antimetabolite drugs such as azathioprine, methotrexate and nitrogen mustards are employed more commonly. Steroids offer another approach, since they are lympholytic and inhibit the inflammatory reaction. Heterologous antilymphocyte serum, known as antilymphocyte globulin (ALG), also has proved effective in some cases but involves the risk of an immune response to the heterologous protein. Currently two new approaches are being pursued. The first involves an attempt to develop immunologic tolerance in the recipient by the prior administration of repeated small doses of antigen derived from the potential donor. The second, referred to as transplantation enhancement, involves deliberate immunization of the recipient with larger doses of donor antigens in the hope of evoking antibodies which will block the cell-mediated immune response (Elkins et al., 1974). Reference was made earlier to the existence of serum factors which apparently block the immune response to tumor antigens (p. 109).Studies in the mouse suggest that analogous blockade can be induced to prevent transplantation rejection. It is speculated that the antibodies combine with the surface antigens of target cells, which thus are no longer recognized by sensitized lymphocytes. All of these methods have produced significant clinical gains, but the battle has not yet been won. Regrettably, immunosuppression renders the recipient extremely vulnerable to infections. Indeed, infections account for more deaths in transplant recipients than loss of the graft. Immunosuppression has also led, as you recall, to an increased incidence of cancer in the recipients (p. 109). Moreover, immunosuppression can hold the immune response at bay only for as long as the therapy is maintained; the immune system never forgets.

Mechanisms Involved in Rejection. Although both cell-mediated and humoral immune mechanisms are involved in transplant rejection, the former plays the larger role. T-cells sensitized to specific alloantigens are able to kill target cells in vitro, either on contact or by the release of cytotoxic factors. In experimental animals, neonatal thymectomy prolongs the survival of skin transplants, just as grafts in children with genetic thymic deficiency states demonstrate prolonged survival. The question of whether complement is required for this lymphocyte cytotoxicity is as yet unanswered (Berke et al., 1973). Macrophages modified by "macrophage arming factor" produced by sensitized T-cells and "antibody dependent cellular cytotoxicity" (ADCC) involving neutrophils, macrophages, B-cells and indeed any cell bearing Fc receptors may also contribute. Thus a variety of cell-mediated mechanisms participate in the destruction of "foreign" cells.

Humoral antibodies are also capable of destroying transplanted cells. They assume major importance when recipients have been sensitized prior to transplantation. *Presensitization may occur by a prior transplant or by previous transfusions or pregnancy.* In this circumstance the humoral antibodies and complement induce an Arthus-like reaction, resulting in diffuse vascular damage and consequent ischemic necrosis of the transplant. In addition, antibody may complex with and activate complement, and the C'8,9 fraction may then directly attack target cell membranes. Humoral antibodies also participate in the ADCC reaction by coating target cells and thus rendering them vulnerable to direct destruction by white cells. Since this mechanism was only recently identified, its importance in transplant rejection has yet to be established. As mentioned earlier, some humoral antibodies have the paradoxic effect of blocking the rejection reaction, thereby enhancing the survival of transplants.

The contributions of the cellular and humoral mechanisms to the rejection reaction vary with the specific cells or tissue transplanted.

Isolated lymphocytes may be destroyed by humoral antibody alone in cytolytic complement-mediated reactions.

Marrow cells are rejected by cell-mediated mechanisms, but recent evidence suggests that the cells are probably lymphocytes which do not belong to the usual class of T-cells. This separate class of marrow-dependent immunocompetent cells which are either lymphocytes or possibly macrophages has been described by Bennett (1973); this class is responsible for the rejection of allogeneic dispersed hematopoietic cells. Thus, this special class of "M-cells" comes into play when, for example, a patient with leukemia is treated by whole body irradiation and the bone marrow is subsequently reconstituted by an allograft from a genetically dissimilar donor.

Skin has strong histocompatibility antigens. Grafts are rejected almost entirely by T-cell responses. Serum from an animal which has rejected a skin allograft, when transferred to another host, does not usually accelerate the rejection of a skin graft from the same donor. The transfer of lymphocytes, however, strikingly reduces the graft survival.

Vascularized organs such as the kidney, heart and liver are rejected by both cellular and humoral mechanisms. In presensitized individuals, the transplant may be rejected by humoral mechanisms literally within minutes to hours. This phenomenon is termed hyperacute rejection and, as mentioned, involves humoral antibodies, activated complement, vascular injury and ischemic necrosis. Even if presensitization is not present, a large "antigenic barrier" may lead to rapid cell-mediated destruction of transplanted cells and the release of free antigens, which may then secondarily evoke humoral antibodies. As mentioned earlier, visceral organs generally are not rich in histocompatibility antigens. There is a strong suspicion that some of their immunogenicity may reside in leukocytes found within the blood vessels and the interstitial tissues of the organ. Recent work has shown that successful transplantation of the heart can be accomplished in rats across antigenic differences if the hematopoietic cells within the organ can be destroyed (Dittmer and Bennett, 1975). The connective tissue and muscle elements of the heart appear to have low immunogenicity. Confirmation of these results would open new vistas in the transplantation of visceral organs.

The severity of the rejection reaction, length of survival of the graft and the resultant morphologic changes are dependent on the antigenic differences between donor and recipient and on the immunocompetence of the recipient. It must be appreciated that in the present state of the art, tissue typing detects only the HL-A antigens which evoke humoral antibodies. Significant differences in lymphocyte determinants which evoke the more important cell-mediated responses can only be judged approximately by mixed lymphocyte reactions (Thompson et al., 1973). The hope that compatibility as detected by serologic determinants implies equal compatibility with respect to the lymphocyte determinants (because of the close linkage of controlling genes) may be ephemeral. Differing degrees of success in renal transplantation have been reported from Europe and the United States despite apparently comparable levels of histocompatibility as determined by serologic methods (Editorial, 1974). It is speculated that the genetically much more diverse population of the United States may have lesser degrees of linkage between loci controlling serologic and lymphocyte determinants. Another word of caution must be given with respect to tissue typing and matching of donor and recipient. We do not yet know whether all the HL-A antigens are of equal strength and therefore of equal importance. In clinical practice the duration of survival of renal transplants achieved with one dissimilar HL-A serologic determinant is not significantly different from that achieved with two antigenic differences (Opelz et al., 1974). Perhaps these results only mean that the additional mismatched antigen was not sufficiently strong to influence the immune rejection response. Alternatively, *any* dissimilarity in serologic antigens may imply that differences must exist in the more important LD antigens. It is apparent that there is much yet to be learned about tissue typing and matching of donor and recipient.

The immunocompetence of the recipient obviously modifies the intensity of the rejection reaction. For obscure reasons some individuals are innately "poor responders" and so do not mount as effective an immune response as others. These differences are, on the whole, small. Much more important is the level of prophylactic and therapeutic immunosuppression employed. In renal transplantation, for example, any indication of rejection is followed by more intense immunosuppressive therapy. The level of immunosuppression might again be lowered if it appeared that the rejection was checked. The morphologic appearance of grafts therefore reflects the varying levels, over time, of the intensity of the immune response. Even after one or more years of apparently adequate function, changes indicative of acute rejection may be encountered.

Morphology of Rejection Reactions. In the past, two morphologic patterns of rejection were recognized, based on the intensity of the reaction. The term **"first set rejection"** was applied to the initial rejection of a skin allograft; **"second set rejection"** designated the rejection of a second skin allograft from the same donor to the same recipient. It is apparent that "second set rejection" implied a more intense immune response in a recipient previously sensitized to the particular tissue antigens. It is now appreciated that a potential recipient can become sensitized by other pathways, as mentioned on page 179. Thus, this older terminology has been replaced by the terms "hyperacute," "acute," and "chronic" rejection (Russell and Winn, 1970). The morphologic changes in these patterns will be described as they relate to renal transplants. Similar changes would be encountered in any other vascularized visceral organ transplant. Skin grafts, because they contain strong antigens and are not well vascularized, are somewhat special cases and "first set rejection" would more or less resemble the pattern to be described as a less intense acute reaction while "second set rejection" would more closely resemble the more florid hyperacute rejection. But it must be admitted that all categories are at best arbitrary and represent divisions of a continuous spectrum.

Hyperacute rejection may occur within minutes in presensitized individuals. **Basically it is characterized by widespread acute arteritis and arteriolitis, thrombosis of vessels and ischemic necrosis** (Williams et al., 1968; Myburgh et al., 1969). **As indicated earlier, this pattern of rejection is mediated largely by humoral antibodies, which evoke an Arthus-like reaction.** As a consequence of the arterial lesions the graft never becomes vascularized and undergoes ischemic necrosis. The renal allograft becomes mottled, dusky and flaccid and loses its arterial pulsation within minutes of establishing the vascular connections. Virtually all arterioles and arteries exhibit characteristic acute fibrinoid necrosis of their walls, with narrowing or complete occlusion of the lumens by precipitated fibrin and cellular debris. Deposits of IgG, IgM, complement and fibrin can be demonstrated within the vessel walls. The glomeruli are large and swollen and contain deposits of fibrinoid as well as granular debris and fragments of cells within the vascular lumens. Immunoglobulins, C'3 and fibrin can be demonstrated within these glomerular deposits. Acutely involved glomeruli may also be infiltrated with neutrophils if the kidney is left in situ for more than a few minutes. Tubular cells undergo ischemic necrosis and usually the interstitial tissue is edematous and infiltrated with neutrophils and occasional lymphocytes and macrophages. Sometimes, in the less

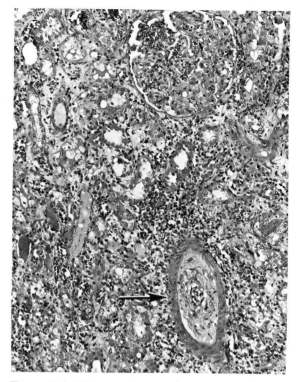

Figure 6–4. Hyperacute transplant rejection of kidney. There is extensive interstitial edema and leukocytic infiltration. The glomerulus at the top is partially necrotic. The blood vessel (arrow) is virtually occluded by marked subintimal edema and fibrosis and the small cleared spaces in the intima contain lipid. There is extensive damage to the tubular epithelial cells.

florid hyperacute reactions, vacuolation of endothelial cells and of intimal muscle cells appears in small to medium-sized arteries. This may produce intimal thickening resembling atherosclerosis (Fig. 6–4). Obviously, the hyperacute rejection results in prompt irreversible destruction of the graft (Rossman et al., 1973).

Acute rejection may occur within days of transplantation in the untreated recipient or may appear suddenly months or even years later when immunosuppression has been employed and is terminated. **The principal mechanism responsible for the rejection is a cell-mediated immune response, but there is evidence that as early as three days after rejection has begun, IgG and IgM antibodies appear in the peritubular capillaries.** As was pointed out the cell-mediated destruction of graft cells releases histocompatibility antigens, which may then evoke a humoral response (Balch and Diethelm, 1972). Although a wide range of morphologic changes may be present, the paramount histologic features in the untreated recipient are a perivascular interstitial infiltration of mononuclear cells (small lymphocytes, macrophages and transformed lymphocytes

or immunoblasts) and a vasculitis involving the peritubular vessels, with resultant ischemic injury and necrosis of tubular cells. The perivascular infiltrate in time becomes widespread and is accompanied by interstitial edema. Plasma cells as well as neutrophils appear later when tubular cells become atrophic or necrotic. The tubules may become converted into narrow cords lined by atrophic epithelium, or they may be virtually totally destroyed. The glomeruli either appear normal or are reduced in size and are often avascular. Frequently the glomerular tufts appear hypercellular or smudged, apparently as a consequence of swelling of endothelial and mesangial cells, which obliterates the normal vascular architecture. The hypercellularity of the glomeruli has been interpreted as recurrence of the glomerulonephritis which was responsible for the destruction of the recipient's own kidneys, but most experts consider it a type of **rejection glomerulopathy.** Occasionally glomerular tufts become partially or completely necrotic as a manifestation of more intense immunologic rejection. Granular deposits of IgG, complement and fibrin are seen by EM in such acutely involved glomeruli. A wide range of vascular changes occurs depending on the intensity of the rejection reaction. In the more florid instances an Arthus-like reaction consisting of an acute arteritis and arteriolitis apparently related to humoral antibodies involves all levels of the arterial system from the major branches to the arterioles. In less severely involved vessels, endothelial swelling, proliferation or necrosis may be evident, accompanied by edema and necrosis of the smooth muscle cells within the media. A polymorphonuclear infiltrate is present within the more acutely affected vessels. As a consequence of these changes the vascular lumens are often narrowed and may even be obliterated. In the more indolent acute reactions the vessel walls undergo fibroproliferative thickening.

Chronic rejection mediated by T-cells may occur months or even years after transplantation. Even in well tolerated grafts, which have functioned for years, lesions indicative of rejection can be found (Hamburger, 1967). The morphologic changes are quite varied. In general they reflect earlier acute vascular lesions which result in vascular narrowing and chronic arterial insufficiency accompanied by the progressive accumulation of sensitized lymphocytes. The glomerulus is the primary site of injury in long-standing functioning renal allografts. Four types of changes are found (Corson, 1972):

1. **Proliferative glomerulopathy,** characterized by hypertrophy and hyperplasia of both endothelial and epithelial cells, accompanied by mesangial thickening. These changes are highly reminiscent of those seen in proliferative glomerulonephritis (p. 436). In time, such glomeruli may undergo obsolescence and atrophy as the capillary lumens are obliterated. The shrunken tuft may then appear as a mass of wavy, closely packed base-

ment membranes which are markedly thickened and smudged.

2. **Membranous lesions,** appearing as diffuse thickening of the glomerular basement membranes with narrowing of the capillary lumens (Busch et al., 1971).

3. **Mixed proliferative and membranous lesions,** partaking of the changes described in the preceding two patterns.

4. **Focal and segmental proliferative changes,** affecting only one or more lobules within occasional glomeruli.

Despite the prolonged survival of kidneys undergoing chronic rejection, the glomeruli (particularly the mesangium) may contain deposits of immunoglobulins, complement and fibrin, although usually these have been cleared by the time the kidney is examined. In chronic rejection the walls of the arteries and arterioles are almost always thickened and fibrotic, and their lumens are thus narrowed. The intima in particular is thickened by edematous fibrous connective tissue and often it contains vacuolated lipid-laden macrophages reminiscent of florid atherosclerosis. Some vessels are reduced to virtual fibrous cords with obliteration of their lumens. As a consequence of these glomerular and vascular changes, there is striking ischemic atrophy of the tubules and an increase in interstitial

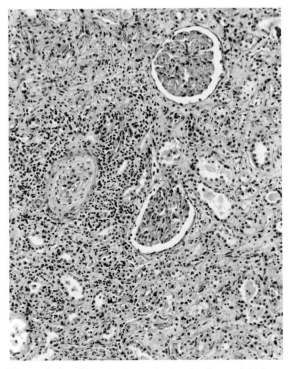

Figure 6–5. Chronic transplant rejection of kidney. There is marked tubular atrophy, increased interstitial fibrosis and mononuclear cell infiltration. The vessel at left center has a markedly thickened wall with virtual obliteration of the lumen. The glomeruli show some ischemic axial thickening.

fibrous tissue. In addition, there is an intense infiltrate of mononuclear cells, predominantly small lymphocytes admixed with large lymphocytes, macrophages and occasional plasma cells. Immunoblasts on the whole are rare. Sometimes there is total atrophy of the tubules, leaving only fields of fibrous tissue heavily infiltrated with leukocytes (Fig. 6–5).

As mentioned earlier, acute changes may be superimposed on chronic changes when, for example, immunosuppression is terminated. Presumably it is the acute rejection which delivers the *coup de grace* to the already damaged kidney. Indeed, chronic rejection may represent the summation of repeated "miniepisodes" of acute rejection.

AUTOIMMUNE DISEASES

An immune reaction against "self" antigens—autoimmunity—is now a well established cause of disease. There is, however, a great deal of controversy over the criteria for establishing a disease as autoimmune in origin. Autoantibodies can be demonstrated in a surprisingly large number of individuals, particularly older individuals, who are apparently entirely free of autoimmune disease. Moreover, even when disease is present, are the autoantibodies causative? Conceivably there is some other cause for the tissue injury, and the immune response is merely secondary to the abnormal release of antigens from injured cells. Autoantibodies can be identified in a significant number of patients with myocardial infarctions, but no one would categorize myocardial infarction as an autoimmune disease. The designation of a condition as an autoimmune disease is then somewhat arbitrary and is based on: (1) evidence of an autoimmune reaction, (2) the judgment that the immunological findings are not merely secondary, and (3) the lack of any other identified cause for the disorder.

Despite uncertainties, a number of conditions have been fairly certainly designated as autoimmune diseases (Table 6–4). They range from *single organ* or *single cell-type disorders,* which involve specific immune reactions directed against one particular organ or cell type, to *multisystem diseases,* characterized by lesions in many organs, associated usually with a multiplicity of autoantibodies or cell-mediated reactions or both. In most of the latter diseases the pathological changes are found principally within the connective tissue and blood vessels of the various organs involved. Thus, these diseases were once called "collagen-vascular diseases" or "connective tissue diseases." As will be seen, the autoimmune reactions in these systemic diseases are not

TABLE 6–4. AUTOIMMUNE DISEASES

SINGLE ORGAN OR CELL TYPE	SYSTEMIC
Probable	*Probable*
Hashimoto's thyroiditis	Systemic lupus erythema-
Autoimmune hemolytic	tosus
anemia	Rheumatoid arthritis
Autoimmune atrophic gas-	Sjögren's syndrome
tritis of pernicious	Reiter's syndrome
anemia	
Autoimmune encephalo-	*Possible*
myelitis	
Autoimmune orchitis	Polymyositis–dermatomyo-
Goodpasture's syndrome*	sitis
Autoimmune thrombo-	Systemic sclerosis
cytopenia	(scleroderma)
Sympathetic ophthalmia	Polyarteritis nodosa
Possible	
Graves disease	
Primary biliary cirrhosis	
Chronic agressive hepatitis	
Ulcerative colitis	
Myasthenia gravis	
Membranous glomerulopathy	

*Target is basement membrane of glomeruli and alveolar walls.

specifically directed against the constituents of connective tissue or blood vessels, but these older designations remain useful since they connote widespread lesions affecting many organs and systems.

The immunologic evidence that the diseases listed in Table 6–4 are indeed the result of autoimmune reactions is more compelling for some than for others. With systemic lupus erythematosus, the presence of a multiplicity of autoantibodies logically explains many of the observed changes. Moreover, the autoantibodies can be identified within the lesions by immunofluorescent and electron microscopic techniques. Few would dispute the assumption that systemic lupus erythematosus is an autoimmune disease. At the other end of the spectrum is polyarteritis nodosa, tenuously held by some authors to be of autoimmune origin. Evidence derives from reasonable facsimiles which can be induced in experimental animals by immunologic methods and by certain similarities between this condition and other, better defined autoimmune diseases. Yet in most affected individuals it has been impossible to document the presence of immunologic reactions directed against the arteries which are the targets in this disease. For this reason some classifications of autoimmune disease would not include polyarteritis nodosa. There must be awareness therefore of the extent of the immunologic evidence for each so-called autoimmune disease.

Only the systemic autoimmune diseases are considered in this chapter. The single-target involvements are more appropriately dis-cussed in the chapters dealing with the specific organ. Before describing individual disorders we should consider the general nature of self-tolerance and theories about its loss.

TOLERANCE AND LOSS OF SELF-TOLERANCE

It is obvious that autoimmunity implies loss of self-tolerance. Regrettably, there is no clear understanding of how self-tolerance is lost, nor indeed is the nature of tolerance well understood. It is clear that *self-tolerance is acquired during embryonic or neonatal life.* Three decades ago Owen (1945) made the epochal observation that nonidentical (dizygotic) twin cattle with shared placental circulations also shared to some extent, and were tolerant of, each other's red cells, i.e., they were red cell chimaeras. He correctly concluded that foreign antigens introduced into a host during embryonic or neonatal life before maturation of the immune apparatus would induce lifelong tolerance to these antigens. Thereafter Burnet (1959) explained this phenomenon by proposing the concept of "forbidden clones," i.e., all clones of immunocompetent cells reactive to antigens to which they were exposed during fetal and neonatal life were "forbidden" and destroyed. According to this theory self-tolerance resulted from destruction during embryologic development of all self-reactive clones. Attractive as this concept may be, it has run into serious difficulties. In the experimental animal it is readily possible to induce immune reactions to autologous tissues by the administration of tissue macerates admixed with Freund's adjuvant (Senyk and Michaeli, 1973; Allison, 1973). The self-reactive clones therefore are indeed present and can be activated. An alternative explanation for the tolerance to "self" antigens suggested that tissue and cellular antigens are sequestered, and so do not come into contact with the immune apparatus. Although this is true of a few tissues—the testes, brain and lens of the eye—there is indisputable evidence that thyroid proteins, for example, are constantly present in low levels in the circulation of all individuals without evoking autoimmune thyroiditis.

Newer concepts suggest that tolerance is a much more complex phenomenon and takes many forms. In addition to the induction of tolerance by inoculation of the newborn, tolerance to most antigens requiring B- and T-cell cooperation can be induced in adults by repeated injections of small amounts of antigen *(low zone tolerance)* or large doses of the antigen *(high zone tolerance).* Low zone tolerance would apply to most tissue antigens which may be present in the circulation from time to time but in very small amounts. High zone tolerance would apply to the plasma proteins, for example. Low zone tolerance is now believed to be a result of unresponsiveness of T-helper cells, which are required for the immune response. Possibly blockade of specific receptors on the T-cells is the basis for their unresponsiveness (Benson and Borel, 1974), but this explanation is still speculative (Weigle, 1973). High zone tolerance may result from the loss of both B- and T-cell responses, but even in this circumstance it is clear that the T-cell tolerance persists much longer than that of the B-cell. Yet other proposals have been invoked as fail-safe mechanisms. T-suppressor cells may block humoral antibody production. By analogy with immune responses to tumors and transplanted tissues, the possibility is raised that serum factors, possibly antibodies, immune complexes or antigens themselves, may block the immune response. These brief remarks merely skim the surface of this vast subject, but it is not profitable to delve more deeply here because at best what obtains today may be disproved tomorrow.

With our imperfect understanding of the nature of self-tolerance it is no surprise that a multiplicity of theories have been invoked to explain its loss and the consequent emergence of autoimmune reactions. Some of the most widely accepted are outlined below.

1. *Alteration of "self" antigens* by exogenous agents. Conceivably drugs, viruses, bacteria, radiant energy or some other mechanism might so alter an autologous antigen that it is no longer recognizable as "self." Alternatively, the *exogenous agent might serve as a new carrier* for a cellular hapten, which evokes antibodies reactive against the hapten.

2. *Microbiologic agents might serve as adjuvants.* A widely held theory proposes that autoimmune diseases are triggered by virus infections. Conceivably the virus serves as an adjuvant and along with self antigens induces a response to the self antigens (Paterson, 1973).

3. *Cross reactions* between exogenous and "self" antigens might result in autoimmune disease. There is evidence that rheumatic heart disease often follows streptococcal infections because an antibody to streptococci also reacts with the sarcolemma of cardiac muscle (McLaughlin et al., 1972).

4. Some form of *immunologic defect* could result in failure to clear antigens or organisms from the body, thus leading to persistent stimulation of the residual immunologic apparatus (Good and Yunis, 1974). Alternatively, persistence of a microbiologic infection might operate through one of the previously mentioned mechanisms.

5. Release of *sequestered self antigens.* There are, as mentioned, a few tissues which truly possess sequestered antigens. For these, injury might release antigens which trigger, for example, autoimmune orchitis or so-called sympathetic ophthalmia.

6. *Emergence of autoreactive clones.* Autoimmune diseases are more frequent in patients suffering from some widespread disorder of the lymphoid system, such as leukemia or lymphoma, or from a chronic viral infection. It is postulated that in such conditions random mutations of proliferating lymphoid cells might lead to a clone of cells reactive against "self." The frequency of autoantibodies in the general population rises progressively with age, and this is possibly related to an increasing predisposition to mutational events in the later years of life.

7. *Loss of T-suppressor cells.* Building on the hypothesis that self-tolerance may in some part be related to the presence of T-suppressor cells which inhibit autoimmune reactions, it is theorized that loss of these cells would abrogate self-tolerance. Indeed, lymphotoxins specifically directed against T-cells have been reported in some autoimmune diseases. These are discussed in more detail on page 186.

8. *Genetic predisposition* to autoimmune disease. There is abundant evidence that immunologic responsiveness is genetically controlled by so-called immune response genes. As is pointed out on page 177, these immune response genes are closely linked on the same chromosome with histocompatibility genes. The following observations relate genetic factors to autoimmune diseases: (a) an increased frequency of autoimmune diseases among individuals having certain HL-A antigens (Grumet et al., 1971), (b) the familial clustering of autoimmune diseases, (c) the increased incidence of autoantibodies in otherwise normal close relatives of affected patients, (d) an increased frequency of autoimmune diseases in women, and (e) the vulnerability of certain strains of animals to autoimmune reactions and the resistance of other strains.

Still other concepts might be cited, but it is already evident that when uncertainties abound, so do theories. Against this general background we turn to the individual systemic autoimmune diseases.

SYSTEMIC LUPUS ERYTHEMATOSUS (SLE)

This is a febrile, inflammatory, multisystem disease of protean manifestations and variable behavior. It is best characterized by the following parameters: (1) *Clinically*, it is an unpredictable remitting, relapsing disease of acute or insidious onset which may involve virtually any organ in the body, but principally affects the skin, kidneys, serosal membranes, joints and heart. (2) *Anatomically,* all sites of involvement have in common vascular lesions with fibrinoid deposits. (3) *Immunologically,* the disease involves a bewildering array of antibodies of presumed autoimmune origin, especially antinuclear antibodies. The clinical presentation of SLE is so variable and bears so many similarities to other autoimmune connective tissue diseases (rheumatoid arthritis, polymyositis-dermatomyositis and others) that it has been necessary to develop diagnostic criteria. Fourteen featues of the disease have been selected, permitting a diagnosis of SLE if four or more are present during any interval of observation (from Cohen et al., 1971).

1. Facial erythema.
2. Discoid lupus rash.
3. Raynaud's phenomenon.
4. Alopecia.
5. Photosensitivity.
6. Oral, nasal or pharyngeal ulceration.
7. Arthritis without deformity.
8. LE cells.
9. Chronic false positive serologic tests for syphilis.
10. Proteinuria (greater than 3.5 gm./day).
11. Cellular casts in the urine.
12. One or both of the following: pleuritis, pericarditis.
13. One or both of the following: psychosis, convulsions.
14. One or more of the following: hemolytic anemia, leukopenia, thrombocytopenia.

At one time SLE was considered to be a fairly rare disease. Better methods of diagnosis and an increased awareness that it may be mild and insidious, however, have made it evident that its prevalence may be as high as 1 case per 10,000 population. There is a strong female preponderance—about 10 to 1. It usually arises in the second and third decades, but may become manifest at any age, even in early childhood (Kornreich and Hanson, 1974).

Etiology and Pathogenesis. A mountain of evidence points toward an autoimmune pathogenesis for SLE, but the cause or causes of the bewildering array of autoimmune reactions in these patients still elude us. First we shall present some of the immunologic findings, followed by the theories which attempt to explain their origins.

A host of autoantibodies have been identified against both nuclear and cytoplasmic components of cells, some of which are neither organ- nor species-specific. *Antinuclear antibodies (ANA)* are directed against soluble and particulate nucleoprotein, both double and single stranded DNA and double and single stranded RNA, as well as a saline extractable nuclear constituent (Sm antigen). The presence of antibody to native, double

stranded DNA is virtually diagnostic of SLE since it is not found in any other "connective tissue disorder." In addition, antibodies have been identified against mitochondria, ribosomes, lysosomes, a soluble cytoplasmic fraction, red cells, white cells, platelets and blood clotting factors (Wiedermann and Miescher, 1965). The ANA are of greatest diagnostic importance. They are reported to be present in 80 to 100 per cent of patients. The various forms of ANA can be differentiated by both serologic and immunofluorescent techniques. When tissue sections, even those from normal individuals, are stained with SLE serum and counterstained with fluorescent anti-immunoglobulin, the following patterns are obtained:

Anti-DNA	Rim or shaggy fluorescence (outlining the periphery of the nucleus).
Anti-nucleoprotein	Homogeneous fluorescence (staining of the entire nucleus).
Anti-Sm	Speckled fluorescence (numerous minute fluorescent points throughout the nucleus).
Anti-RNA	Nucleolar fluorescence.

Cell-mediated immune reactions, as judged by skin testing, have been abnormal in some cases (Goldman et al., 1972), and normal in others (Senyk et al., 1974). In either event, as is discussed below, there is considerable evidence that one of the fundamental immunologic abnormalities in this disease is some defect in T- and B-cell collaboration, leading to abnormal humoral reactions.

Given the presence of all these autoantibodies, we still know little about the mechanism of their emergence. *Three converging lines of investigation hold center stage today: (1) genetic predisposition, (2) a fundamental abnormality in the immune system, particularly involving T-cells, and (3) a latent virus infection.* Other factors may also play some role.

The evidence which supports a genetic predisposition takes many forms. SLE has been encountered in identical twins. SLE and related disorders such as rheumatoid arthritis occur with greater than chance frequency within family groups. Mention was made earlier of the increased incidence of SLE in patients who have genetically determined immunodeficiency states. The incidence of SLE is significantly higher than chance alone would dictate among individuals having certain histocompatibility antigens (McDevitt and

Bodmer, 1972; Grumet et al., 1971). There are many suggestions, then, that some individuals are genetically predisposed to the development of this disease.

Some *fundamental abnormality in the immune system* is a logical and seductive concept. It would appear that these patients are unable to identify antigens as autologous and so react to a host of self antigens. Favored today is the belief that the derangement involves T-lymphocytes. Allison and his co-workers (1971) make the provocative proposal that B-cells are normally capable of recognizing self constituents. However, no immune response occurs in the normal individual because T-cells are tolerant and so do not cooperate with the reactive B-cells. These investigators raise the possibilities that T-cell tolerance is abrogated in SLE or that T-suppressor cells are inactivated or depleted and so do not maintain normal control of B-cell function. Relative to the latter possibility, there are reports in the literature of a reduction in the number of T-lymphocytes in the circulation, and a corresponding increase in the number of "null" cells (having neither B- nor T-cell characteristics) (Scheinberg and Cathcart, 1974). Moreover, lymphotoxins capable of destroying T-cells have been described in up to 80 per cent of patients with SLE (Lies et al., 1973).

There is a good deal of suspicion, unfortunately much of it based on analogy with experimental models, that *viruses provide the trigger mechanism for the emergence of autoimmune reactions* (Phillips, 1974). The search for a viral etiology was particularly stimulated by the clinical and serologic similarities of New Zealand black mouse (NZB) autoimmune disease and human SLE. An RNA leukemia virus can be isolated from these NZB mice. Antigens possessed by this virus have been demonstrated on the cells of some patients with SLE (Schwartz, 1975). There have also been reports of the identification by electron microscopy of "virus-like" particles in the kidneys of humans with SLE (Gyorkey et al., 1972). However it has not been possible to isolate a viral agent even from tissues bearing the "virus-like" structures (Christian and Phillips, 1973). Higher than normal levels of antibodies against various viruses have been reported in SLE, but immunologic "tracks" of a single offending viral agent have not been demonstrated (Rothfield et al., 1973). Possibly a number of viral agents might all be capable of initiating autoimmune reactions. A latent, so-called slow-virus infection might be involved, yielding no detectable immunologic changes. As mentioned earlier, viruses might operate in a number of ways. They could complex as carriers with "self" haptens. By inducing inflammatory reactive changes in lymphoid tissue viral infections might lead to the emergence of autoreactive mutant clones. Ingenious mechanisms have been proposed whereby viruses might inactivate or destroy T-cells and more particularly T-suppressor cells (Messner, 1974; Steinberg, 1974). However, all these theories are still highly speculative.

Other mechanisms have been invoked to explain the development of the autoimmune reactions in SLE. Some patients give a history of ingestion of drugs prior to the onset of their disease. Hydralazine, Procainamide, Dilantin Sodium, reserpine, isoniazid and oral contraceptives are implicated most commonly (Alarcon-Segovia, 1969). It is theorized that these drugs complex with autologous constituents of cells to create "foreign" antigens which evoke antibodies cross reactive with self antigens. Sometimes patients date the onset of their disease to prolonged exposure to sunlight. Could ultraviolet light denature DNA making it antigenic? It has been documented that trace amounts of DNA and indeed anti-DNA immunoglobulins can be found in the sera of many normal individuals. Conceivably, in individuals genetically or immunologically predisposed the chemical alteration induced by ultraviolet light triggers an autoimmune reaction. Other interesting observations might be cited, but at the present time all theories must be viewed as intriguing but still conjectural.

Morphology. The characteristic anatomic features of SLE are: (1) LE cells and LE rosettes, (2) LE (hematoxylin) bodies, (3) acute vasculitis, principally involving small arteries and arterioles, coupled with foci of necrosis and fibrinoid deposition in many tissues and organs, (4) the occasional development of a special form of endocarditis (Libman-Sacks endocarditis), and (5) immune deposits in the kidneys which may assume a distinctive ultrastructural pattern. Most of these anatomic features are microscopic and often are not suspected on gross examination.

LE cells and LE rosettes are the most important microscopic features of systemic lupus erythematosus. They are rarely encountered in tissue sections or in vivo, but are readily elicited by in vitro methods. **Basically the LE cell is any phagocytic leukocyte (neutrophil or macrophage) that has engulfed the denatured nucleus of an injured cell** (Fig. 6–6). Omitting much of the technical detail, the demonstration of LE cells involves the microscopic examination of white cells within clotted blood two hours after withdrawal. Presumably in the act of drawing blood a sufficient number of leukocytes are injured in such a way as to expose their nuclei to the antinuclear antibodies. These denature the nuclei and by binding complement render the denatured nuclei strongly chemotactic

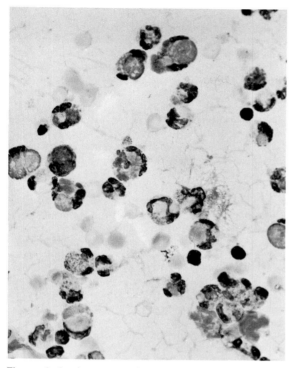

Figure 6–6. Lupus erythematosus (LE) cells: Homogeneous inclusions representing denatured nuclei are seen in many of the polymorphonuclear leukocytes.

for phagocytes. Sometimes the denatured nuclei become surrounded by a cluster of neutrophils, producing an **LE rosette.**

Unlike LE cells, **LE bodies** or **hematoxylin bodies** can be seen within tissue sections. They are round to oval, rose-pink to purple (when stained with hematoxylin and eosin) structures the size of a nucleus, usually found lying free between cells in the margins of areas of tissue necrosis. LE bodies are the in vivo counterpart of in vitro LE cells. It is believed that they too represent injured nuclei which have been extruded and have undergone denaturation by the antinuclear antibodies.

An **acute necrotizing vasculitis** affecting small arteries and arterioles classically is present in affected tissues and organs. These vascular lesions are identical to those encountered in serum sickness, further supporting an immunologic basis for SLE. The arteritis is characterized by necrosis and fibrinoid deposits within the vessel walls. Immunoglobulins, DNA, the third component of complement (C′3) and fibrinogen have been found in the fibrinoid deposits within the arterial and arteriolar lesions. At a later stage, the involved vessels undergo fibrous thickening with luminal narrowing. Frequently a perivascular lymphocytic infiltrate is present, sometimes accompanied by significant edema and an apparent increase in ground substance. Typically foci of fibrinoid deposits in microscopic areas of necrosis are found within the interstitial tissue of affected organs

These foci of necrosis are presumably caused by vascular lesions.

The distribution of organ involvement in several large series was as follows (Dubois, 1966; Harvey et al., 1954):

	Approximate Percentage of Cases
Joints*	85
Kidneys*	60
Heart*	50
Serous membranes*	40
Skin	80
Lymph node enlargement	60
Gastrointestinal tract	30
Central nervous system	30
Liver	25
Spleen	20
Eyes	20
Lungs	15
Peripheral nervous system	10

*Lesions cause major clinical syndromes.

Skin lesions are prominent clinical findings in these patients. Classically the lesion is an erythematous or maculopapular eruption over the malar eminences and/or bridge of the nose, creating a "butterfly" shape. Microscopically the areas of involvement show liquefactive degeneration of the basal layer of the epidermis, edema at the dermoepidermal junction, with swelling and apparent fusion of collagen fibers, and an acute necrotizing vasculitis, with fibrinoid deposits in dermal vessels. In an occasional patient the rash may occur on the neck, chest, back or abdomen and may even be purpuric, bullous or vesicular. Twenty to 30 per cent of patients develop so-called **discoid lupus.** This takes the form of erythematous raised patches with adherent keratotic scaling, which may progress to atrophic scarring. These lesions may be present anywhere on the body. We still do not understand the basis for the variability in the skin lesions.

Serosal membranes, particularly the pericardium and pleura, may exhibit a variety of changes ranging from serous effusions or fibrinous exudation in acute cases to fibrous opacification in chronic cases. During the acute stages of serositis there is microscopic evidence of edema, focal vasculitis with perivascular lymphocytic infiltration, and foci of fibrinoid necrosis, sometimes containing LE bodies. These microscopic changes may be present without grossly visible alterations in the serosal membranes.

The **heart,** when involved, may display quite characteristic small vegetations on the valves, known as **Libman-Sacks endocarditis.** This **nonbacterial verrucose endocarditis** takes the form of single or multiple irregular warty deposits on any valve in the heart. The individual vegetations

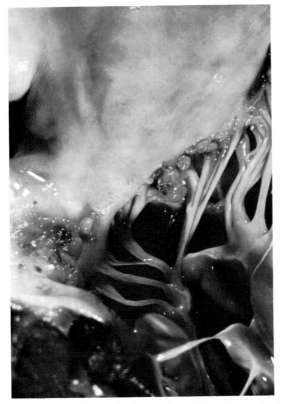

Figure 6–7. Libman-Sacks endocarditis of the mitral valve in lupus erythematosus. The small vegetations attached to the margin of the valve leaflet are easily seen.

range from 1 to 3 mm. in size (Fig. 6–7). **Perhaps the most distinctive feature of this endocarditis is the location of the vegetations on either surface of the leaflets,** i.e., on the surface exposed to the forward flow of the blood or on the underside of the leaflet. Histologic examination of these lesions reveals deposits of fibrinoid associated with a surrounding mononuclear inflammatory reaction. At a later phase, there may be collagenization of the areas of inflammation. Not surprisingly, such fibrinoid contains a variety of plasma proteins, including immunoglobulins (Paronetto and Koffler, 1965). Elsewhere in the heart, the interstitial connective tissue may contain foci of vasculitis, deposits of fibrinoid, mononuclear infiltrates and focal poolings of ground substance in the interstitial tissue of the myocardium.

Kidney involvement is one of the most important anatomic features of SLE, since renal failure is the major cause of death in these patients. The renal damage involves principally the glomeruli and takes a variety of forms: (1) focal glomerulonephritis (focal lupus nephritis) in approximately 40 per cent of patients, (2) diffuse proliferative glomerulonephritis (diffuse lupus nephritis) in approximately 50 per cent of patients, and (3) membranous glomerulopathy (membranous lupus nephritis) in approximately 10 per cent of patients (Mery et al., 1975). Any combination of these patterns may occur in the individual patient, but since focal glomerulonephritis may extend to become diffuse proliferative glomerulonephritis, the two diagnoses are mutually exclusive (Ginzler et al., 1974).

Focal glomerulonephritis implies involvement of only portions of some glomeruli. Typically one or several glomerular tufts within an otherwise normal glomerulus exhibit swelling and proliferation of endothelial and mesangial cells, foci of acute capillary necrosis infiltrated with neutrophils, and sometimes fibrinoid deposits and intracapillary thrombi. Rupture of glomerular capillaries may release red cells into Bowman's space and the renal tubule. Occasionally hematoxylin bodies are found within the renal interstitium. Generally there is no basement membrane thickening in this pattern of renal involvement, nor evidence of crescent formation (see below). Almost always these kidneys are of normal size and color, but occasionally they are dotted by small petechial hemorrhages.

Diffuse proliferative glomerulonephritis is morphologically an extension of focal glomerulonephritis. The anatomic changes are dominated by proliferation of endothelial, mesangial and sometimes epithelial cells. This produces striking hypercellularity of the glomeruli. Sometimes the proliferation of epithelial cells fills Bowman's space to create crescent-shaped masses of cells, not surprisingly referred to as "crescents." In time these changes lead to sclerosis of the glomeruli. Most or all glomeruli are involved in both kidneys, and almost always entire glomeruli are affected. Basement membrane thickening creating "wire loop lesions" may be present, but it is generally not as prominent nor as uniform as in membranous glomerulopathy (p. 434). The pathogenesis of both focal and diffuse proliferative glomerulonephritis involves the deposition of immune complexes within the glomeruli. The immune deposits within the glomeruli in SLE appear first within the mesangium. Later they can be seen on either the endothelial or the epithelial side of the basement membrane or within the mesangium. The subepithelial location is identical to that seen in serum sickness. **The subendothelial location of immune deposits is particularly characteristic of SLE.** This distribution is generally encountered during the acute stages of the disease (Dujovne et al., 1972). The immune deposits contain immunoglobulins, principally IgA and IgM and occasionally IgG, complement and sometimes fibrin. It has been possible to demonstrate DNA as well as anti-DNA within these deposits (Koffler et al., 1967). There is a suspicion that the larger immunoglobulins form large complexes which cannot penetrate the glomerular basement membrane, and thus they assume a subendothelial location. As a consequence of the increased cellularity and basement membrane alterations, the capillary lumens are narrowed or even obliterated, leading to ischemic injury to tubules and interstitial fibrosis. Kidneys so affected may be normal in size and color during the acute stages, but sometimes are enlarged, pale and dotted with punctate cortical hemorrhages. When glomerular sclerosis supervenes, contraction and a diffuse, fine cortical granularity appear. This pattern of glomerulonephritis is very similar to that encountered in serum sickness and poststreptococcal glomerulonephritis. It is essentially an immune complex disease resulting from the deposition of DNA–anti-DNA complexes, and it has as its pathogenesis the sequence of events described in the discussion of serum sickness (p. 175).

Membranous glomerulopathy (membranous glomerulonephritis) is the designation given to glomerular disease in which the principal histologic change consists of widespread thickening of the capillary walls ("wire loop lesions"). Membranous glomerulopathy associated with SLE is very similar if not identical to that encountered in idiopathic membranous glomerulopathy and is described more fully on page 434. Thickening of glomerular capillary walls is the consequence both of the increased deposition of basement membrane-like material and the presence of irregular clumps of immune deposits lying between the glomerular basement membrane and the podocytic epithelial cells. Usually necrosis, thrombi and neutrophils are not prominent in membranous disease and such increased cellularity as is present is mesangial in origin. In advanced cases glomerular sclerosis may supervene.

Joint involvement, although very common clinically, is usually not associated with striking anatomic changes nor with joint deformity. When present it consists of swelling and a nonspecific mononuclear cell infiltration in the synovial membranes, occasionally accompanied by some increase in ground substance and focal areas of fibrinoid necrosis in the subepithelial connective tissue. Grossly the synovial membranes may appear reddened, opaque and somewhat thickened. Erosion of the membranes and destruction of articular cartilage such as occurs with rheumatoid arthritis is exceedingly rare. For this reason, even in advanced cases, permanent disabling joint disease is very uncommon in SLE.

The **spleen** may be of normal size or moderately enlarged. Capsular fibrous thickening is common, as is follicular hyperplasia. Plasma cells are usually numerous in the pulp and can be shown to contain immunoglobulins of the IgG and IgM varieties. One of the most constant alterations, in spleens of both normal and abnormal size, is a marked perivascular fibrosis, producing so-called **onionskin lesions** around the central penicilliary arteries (Fig. 6–8). Immunoglobulins have been localized in these lesions also.

Lymph nodes often are enlarged throughout the body because of nonspecific reactive changes prin-

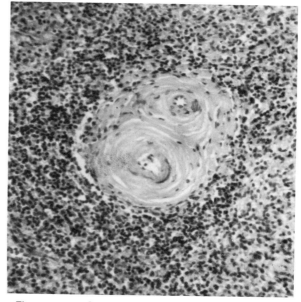

Figure 6–8. Concentric laminated fibrosis about the penicilliary arteries in the spleen, producing so-called "onionskinning."

cipally within the follicular centers. Plasma cells may be seen in the perifollicular collars.

Many **other organs and tissues** may be involved. The changes consist essentially of acute vasculitis of the small vessels, foci of mononuclear infiltrations and fibrinoid deposits. Acute necrotizing vasculitis in the brain and spinal cord may lead either to microinfarcts or microhemorrhages.

Clinical Manifestations. The diagnosis of SLE may be obvious in a young female with a classic butterfly rash over the face, fever, nondeforming pain in one or more of the peripheral joints (feet, ankles, knees, hips, fingers, wrists, elbows, shoulders), pleuritic chest pain and photosensitivity. However, in many patients the presentation of SLE is subtle and puzzling, taking forms such as a febrile illness of unknown origin, abnormal urinary findings, or joint disease masquerading as rheumatoid arthritis or rheumatic fever. Among the diagnostic criteria listed earlier (p. 185) those having the greatest importance are, in descending order: the demonstration of antinuclear antibodies in titers greater than 1:64, LE cells, hemolytic anemia/leukopenia/thrombocytopenia, pleuritis/pericarditis, photosensitivity and Raynaud's phenomenon (p. 278) (Trimble et al., 1974). Antinuclear antibodies (ANA) can be found in 80 to 100 per cent of patients. However, ANA can also be found in 60 to 80 per cent of patients with Sjögren's syndrome, in 80 per cent with scleroderma and in 15 to 25 per cent with adult rheumatoid arthritis, as well as in patients with other autoimmune disorders.

The titer of antibodies does not necessarily correlate with the activity of the disease, but in most patients with acute disease the complement levels are depressed. A variety of findings may point toward renal involvement, including hematuria, red cell casts, proteinuria and, in some cases, the classic nephrotic syndrome (p. 432). Moreover, it has been shown that there is a correlation between the presence of circulating DNA and anti-DNA and glomerular involvement (Schur and Sandson, 1968). Varying levels of azotemia are encountered in those with diffuse proliferative or membranous glomerulopathy, or both. Renal failure accounts for about one quarter of all deaths. Focal glomerulonephritis may produce hematuria but rarely leads to renal failure. The hematologic derangements mentioned may in some cases be the presenting manifestation as well as the dominant clinical problem. In still others, mental aberrations, including psychosis or convulsions, may constitute prominent clinical problems. In addition, patients with SLE often have small retinal exudates (cytoid bodies) and such nonspecific complaints as malaise, anorexia, vomiting and weakness.

The course of SLE is extremely variable and virtually unpredictable. Some unfortunate individuals have an acute onset and follow a progressively downhill course to death within months. More often the disease is characterized by flare-ups and remissions spanning a period of years and even decades. Acute attacks are usually treated by adrenocortical steroids or immunosuppressive drugs, and these drugs often control the acute manifestations. With cessation of therapy the disease eventually reexacerbates. The prognosis appears to have improved significantly in the recent past; approximately 70 to 80 per cent of patients are alive five years after the onset of illness and 60 per cent at 10 years. In some part this apparent improvement derives from the earlier diagnosis and the recognition of milder forms of the disease (Estes and Christian, 1971). Recently it has been shown that the administration of thymic extract (thymosin) appears to transform "null" lymphocytes into functional T-cells (Scheinberg et al., 1975). Still to be determined is whether restoration of T-cell function in these patients will beneficially affect the course of the disease. In addition to renal failure, other important causes of death are diffuse central nervous system involvement, intercurrent infections and uncontrolled acute febrile illness.

RHEUMATOID ARTHRITIS

Rheumatoid arthritis (RA) is a systemic, chronic inflammatory disease which affects principally the joints and sometimes many other organs and tissues throughout the body as well. More specifically *the disease is characterized by a nonsuppurative proliferative synovitis which in time leads to the destruction of articular cartilage and progressive disabling arthritis.* When extra-articular involvement develops—for example, of the skin, heart, blood vessels, muscles and lungs—RA assumes more than a passing resemblance to SLE, scleroderma and polymyositis–dermatomyositis, and, along with these entities, is sometimes referred to as a "connective tissue disease." The course of the disease varies greatly. Sometimes the arthritis is mild and may even clear completely or remain confined to a few joints. In a few cases the disease pursues a rapidly progressive course, marked by relentless, widespread joint destruction. Most often, however, there are repeated remissions and relapses and progressive involvement of additional joints. RA is a very common condition and is variously reported (depending on diagnostic criteria) to affect 0.5 to 3.8 per cent of women and 0.1 to 1.3 per cent of men in the United States (O'Sullivan and Cathcart, 1972). It usually has its onset in young adults but may begin at any age and is 3 to 5 times more common in women than in men. Although still somewhat disputed, the weight of evidence favors some genetic familial predisposition, possibly transmitted by polygenic inheritance (Lawrence, 1970b).

There are many variants of rheumatoid arthritis, all characterized by nonsuppurative inflammatory synovitis and arthritis. These include: juvenile rheumatoid arthritis (Still's disease); ankylosing spondylitis (Marie-Strümpell disease); Felty's syndrome; palindromic rheumatism; Sjögren's syndrome; psoriatic arthritis; arthritis associated with gastrointestinal disease (ulcerative colitis, regional enteritis); arthritis associated with Reiter's syndrome; and arthritis associated with agammaglobulinemia. All of these variants have features distinct from those of the classic form of the disease. Only a few need brief characterization. *Juvenile RA* may begin as early as six weeks of age; often it is accompanied by systemic manifestations such as fever, hepatosplenomegaly, lymphadenopathy, rash and myocarditis. Nonetheless, the prognosis is generally favorable and the disease often subsides spontaneously, with little or no residual joint damage. *Felty's syndrome* comprises the triad of polyarthritis, splenomegaly and leukopenia. In these patients the hematologic problems are often more serious than the joint involvement. *Palindromic rheumatism* is the term used to characterize episodic pain and swelling of joints that last but a few hours to days and then subside, leaving no residual evidence of joint disease. Some of the patients eventually develop mild RA, but in most the disorder clears spontaneously, leaving no traces. When articular involvement suggestive of rheumatoid arthritis is present, these variant syndromes must be kept in mind.

Etiology and Pathogenesis. Although in the final analysis the cause of rheumatoid arthritis is still unknown, an intriguing postulate is widely held. In brief, it proposes that *some antigenic challenge, perhaps a transient synovial infection, results in a local inflammatory synovitis and a consequent humoral immune response. The interaction within the joint of antigen and antibodies activates complement. Retention of antigen within the joint structure at the same time sensitizes T-lymphocytes, and both the humoral and cell-mediated mechanisms lead to the characteristic injury to the joints.* What is the evidence supporting such a contention? Most patients with RA have a serum antibody against IgG belonging to the 19S IgM class, known as *rheumatoid factor (RF)* (Bartfeld and Epstein, 1969). Although RF reacts specifically with IgG, it is not known whether the IgG is unaltered or in some way denatured and thus in a sense is a "foreign" antigen against which B-cells are reactive (Johnson et al., 1975). Recent studies indicate that, in addition to IgM, immunoglobulins of smaller molecular weight—namely, IgG and IgA—may also possess RF activity. It has further been shown that both the antigenic IgG and the RF are synthesized locally by the inflammatory infiltrate of involved synovial membranes (Smiley et al., 1968). Although the serum complement level is normal in patients with RA, the synovial fluid complement level is lowered. Presumably binding of complement by the immune complexes is responsible for lowering of complement levels in the synovial fluid. The complement is then activated through both the classic and the alternative pathways, yielding anaphylactoid and chemotactic fractions. These attract leukocytes, principally neutrophils, into the synovial membrane and joint fluid. The immigrant white cells and the synovial lining cells phagocytize the immune complexes and thus acquire intracytoplasmic granules of IgG and IgM (rheumatoid factor), as well as complement (Britton and Schur, 1971). In the course of such phagocytic activity lysosomal enzymes are released which damage the synovial membranes and evoke a nonsuppurative synovitis (Svaifler, 1974).

There are many suggestions that T-cells also participate in the immune reaction. The inflammatory infiltrate within the involved synovial membranes after the acute phase has peaked is largely composed of macrophages and lymphocytes. Electron microscopic studies indicate that some of the lymphocytes differentiate into plasma cells and are presumably B-cells, whereas others presented ultrastructural details highly suggestive of T-cells (Ziff, 1974). Moreover, lymphokines, particularly macrophage migration inhibitor, have been demonstrated in RA synovial fluid, and there is some evidence that repeated injection of lymphokines into the rabbit knee produces a chronic inflammatory reaction within the synovium.

Granted the large body of data implicating immune reactions, principally humoral, in the inflammatory synovitis, two questions remain. What triggers these immune reactions, and how is the immune reaction translated into the destructive articular lesions? For many years, *microbiologic agents have been proposed as the initiators of the inflammatory synovitis, which then becomes converted into a continuing immune reaction.* Mycoplasmas are associated with arthritis in cattle, goats, chickens and mice, and there have been repeated reports of the isolation of mycoplasmas from RA joint fluid in humans. But there are an even greater number of reports denying such an association (Rodnan, 1973). Attention has turned to viruses, particularly "slow" viruses (Smith and Hamerman, 1969). To date, however, it has not been possible to visualize viral particles in rheumatoid synovium nor to isolate such agents from joint tissues (Ziff, 1971). Nonetheless, because of the similarity between RA and the experimental forms of microbiologic origin, the belief persists that the primary trigger event is an infectious synovitis. The precise mechanism of joint destruction is equally obscure. Lysosomal enzymes and lymphokines have already been alluded to. Collagenases and possibly proteases derived from either immigrant white cells or native proliferating synovial cells are also imputed to participate in the destructive process (Krane, 1974). Certainly the structures within joints, such as cartilage, subchondral bone, synovium, joint capsule, surrounding tendons and ligaments all contain collagen, which is vulnerable to such enzymatic degradation. In addition, a local decrease in pH plus the release of substances such as prostaglandins from inflammatory cells are proposed as contributors to the dissolution of the mineral phase of bone. Despite so many putative destructive mechanisms, hard data are still wanting. Thus, although rheumatoid arthritis is generally viewed as an autoimmune disease, there are still uncertainties about the precise sequence of pathogenetic events.

Morphology. RA is a systemic disease which can cause significant damage to many organs. Its most destructive effects are seen in the joints. Classically it produces symmetric arthritis which affects principally the small joints of the hands and

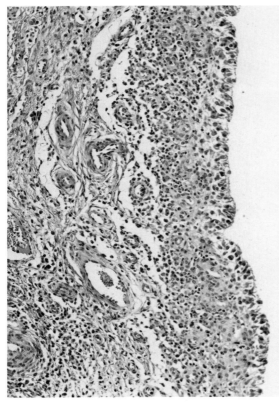

Figure 6–9. Rheumatoid arthritis—the evolving chronic synovitis. Palisaded synoviocytes constitute the surface seen on the right. The subjacent chronic inflammatory mononuclear infiltrate and increased vascularization are evident.

feet, ankles, knees, wrists, elbows, shoulders, temporomandibular joints and sometimes the joints of the vertebral column. Strikingly the hip joints are seldom involved, except in severe, advanced disease. The process begins as a nonspecific inflammatory synovitis characterized by swelling and hypertrophy of the synoviocytes and the sublining connective tissues. More advanced chronic synovitis shows: (1) proliferation of synovial lining cells as well as subjacent cells, often with palisading of synoviocytes; (2) marked hypertrophy of the synovium, with the formation of villi (finger-like projections); (3) lymphocytic and plasma cell infiltration (with perivascular predilection), sometimes with formation of lymphocytic nodules; (4) focal depositions of fibrinoid; and (5) foci of cellular necrosis (Fig. 6–9). The highly vascularized, inflammatory, reduplicated synovium which covers the articular cartilaginous surfaces is known as a **pannus** (mantle). With full-blown inflammatory joint involvement, periarticular soft tissue edema usually develops, which is classically manifested first by fusiform swelling of the proximal interphalangeal joints. Later, swelling of other affected joints may appear. With progression of the disease the ar-

ticular cartilage subjacent to the pannus is eroded and in time virtually destroyed. The subarticular bone may also be attacked and eroded. Eventually the pannus fills the joint space, and subsequent fibrosis and calcification may cause permanent ankylosis. A number of additional changes occur simultaneously.

Early in the disease the synovial fluid is increased in volume, becomes turbid because of the inflammatory infiltrate of neutrophils, and loses some of its mucin content (thus forming a poor mucin clot when mixed with dilute acetic acid). The contained leukocytes exhibit granular inclusions of phagocytized immune complexes, as mentioned previously. Joint motion may cause erosion of the exuberant pannus, leading to bleeding and fibrin clots. The eroded, devascularized cartilage may undergo calcification and fragmentation, adding foreign bodies to the inflammatory process. Osteoarthritis may supervene and compound the articular disability. The periarticular inflammatory response may lead to local myositis, followed by muscle atrophy, and is sometimes accompanied by more remote focal myositis in the form of collections of lymphocytes, plasma cells and occasional epithelioid cells. Collectively, then, the musculoskeletal lesions in progressive disease cause marked motor disability and even permanent crippling disease.

Rheumatoid subcutaneous nodules eventually appear in about one quarter of patients, usually along the extensor surface of the forearm or within the olecranon bursa. They are firm, nontender, oval or rounded masses varying in size to up to 2 cm. in diameter. Less commonly these nodules appear in the Achilles' tendons, on the back of the skull, overlying the ischial tuberosities or along the tibia. They are characterized by a focus of central necrosis surrounded by a palisade of connective tissue cells and macrophages. Sometimes the central focus of necrosis contains deposits of fibrinoid. About the connective tissue palisade there is usually an infiltrate of lymphocytes and occasional plasma cells.

As a systemic disease, a number of other structures may be affected in RA, as indicated below.

Arteries. Acute necrotizing arteritis similar to that in serum sickness (p. 176) in any of the large or small arteries of the body. May lead to thrombosis, with consequent infarction of dependent tissues.

Heart. Fibrinous pericarditis; may progress to fibrous thickening of serosal membranes or fibrous adhesions bridging the pericardial space.

Cardiomyopathy resulting from rheumatoid nodules within myocardium.

Valvular lesions, principally aortic, secondary to rheumatoid granulomas.

Lungs. Serofibrinous pleuritis, with or without effusions.

Multiple pulmonary rheumatoid granulomas.

Progressive interstitial fibrosis.

Pulmonary acute necrotizing arteritis.

Nervous System. Nonspecific peripheral neuropathy associated with mononuclear leukocytic infiltration, chiefly in perineurium.

Rheumatoid nodules in dura mater.

Eye. Uveitis, keratoconjunctivitis, similar to that in Sjögren's syndrome.

Bone. Periosteal rheumatoid nodules.

Lymph Nodes and Spleen. Nonspecific reactive hyperplasia with prominent follicles.

Clinical Course. Although rheumatoid arthritis is basically a symmetrical polyarticular arthritis, the joint involvement is often preceded by constitutional symptoms, such as weakness, malaise, and low grade fever. Occasionally in children there is an "unexplained" high fever. The arthritis first appears insidiously, with aching and stiffness of the joints, particularly in the morning. Although the small joints of the hand (particularly the proximal interphalangeal and metacarpophalangeal joints) usually are affected first, other joints become involved in most cases and sometimes virtually all of the joints of the body, even the hips, are affected. As the disease advances the joints become enlarged, motion is limited and even complete ankylosis may appear. The fingers may become virtually immobilized in a clawlike position, with ulnar deviation (Fig. 6–10). At this stage of the disease, anemia is common. The vasculitis may give rise to Raynaud's phenomenon, chronic leg ulcers and gastrointestinal mucosal erosions, and indeed may cause infarctions in the brain, heart or intestines. It is obvious that with such multisystemic involvement, rheumatoid arthritis must be differentiated from systemic lupus erythematosus, scleroderma, polymyositis–dermatomyositis and rheumatic fever, as well as other forms of arthritis. Critical to this differential diagnosis are: (1) characteristic radiographic findings; (2) sterile, turbid synovial fluid with: decreased viscosity, poor mucin clot formation and inclusion-bearing leukocytes; and (3) rheumatoid factor (85 to 90 per cent of patients). It must be appreciated, however, that rheumatoid factor may also be present with SLE, sarcoidosis, leprosy, syphilis and other connective tissue diseases. Because of the protean nature of RA, diagnostic criteria have been established, as is indicated in Table 6–5.

The clinical course of RA is highly variable. After approximately 10 years, the disease in about half of the patients becomes stabilized or may even regress. Most of the remainder pursue a chronic, remitting, relapsing course (Duthie et al., 1964). After 15 to 20 years, approximately 10 per cent of patients become permanently and severely crippled. RA is the most common cause of systemic amyloidosis. This complication develops in 5 to 10 per cent of these patients, particularly those with protracted severe disease.

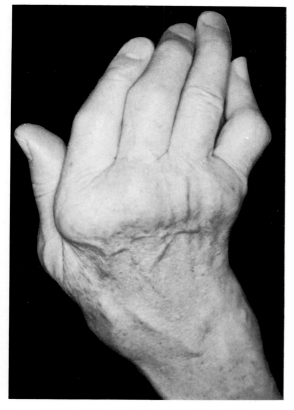

Figure 6–10. Advanced rheumatoid arthritis with marked enlargement of the joints and ulnar deviation of the fingers.

TABLE 6–5. CRITERIA FOR RHEUMATOID ARTHRITIS*

AMERICAN RHEUMATISM ASSOCIATION CRITERIA†	NEW YORK CRITERIA
1. Morning stiffness.	1. History of episode of three painful limb joints.‡
2. Joint tenderness or pain on motion.	2. Swelling, limitation, subluxation or ankylosis of
3. Soft-tissue swelling of one joint.	three limb joints (must include a hand, wrist or
4. Soft-tissue swelling of a second joint (within 3 months).	foot and symmetry of one joint pair, and must exclude distal interphalan-
5. Soft-tissue swelling of symmetrical joints (excludes distal interphalangeal joint).	geal joints, fifth proximal interphalangeal joints, first metatarsophalangeal
6. Subcutaneous nodules.	joints and hips).
7. X-ray changes.	3. X-ray changes (erosions).
8. Serum positive for rheumatoid factors.	4. Serum positive for rheumatoid factors.

*From O'Sullivan, J. B., and Cathcart, E. S.: The prevalence of rheumatoid arthritis. Ann. Int. Med., 76:573, 1972.

†Three or four points = "probable" rheumatoid arthritis; five or more points = "definite" rheumatoid arthritis.

‡Count each joint group (for example, proximal interphalangeal joints) as one joint, scoring each side separately.

SYSTEMIC SCLEROSIS (SCLERODERMA)

Although the designation "scleroderma" is time-honored, this disorder is better called "systemic sclerosis" (SS) since it is characterized by inflammatory and fibrotic changes throughout the interstitium of many organs in the body. *While skin involvement is the usual presenting symptom and eventually appears in approximately 95 per cent of cases, it is the visceral involvement — of the gastrointestinal tract, lungs, kidneys, heart and striated muscles — which produces the major disabilities and threatens life.* The disease may begin at any age, from infancy to the advanced years of life, but most often commences in the third to fifth decades. Women are affected about three times more commonly than men.

SS with its visceral involvement must be differentiated from *localized scleroderma* (also called morphea). The latter entity comprises focal or sometimes generalized sclerotic atrophy confined to the skin. The relationship of this localized disease to SS is unclear; possibly it represents an early form of SS, which in time will spread to internal structures. Such spread has been noted in a few patients.

Etiology and Pathogenesis. There are many hints but no certain proof that systemic sclerosis is of autoimmune origin. Since the morphologic changes always begin in the interstitium of organs it is a prime example of a "connective tissue disease." It also has many clinical and morphologic overlaps with other "connective tissue diseases," such as rheumatoid arthritis, SLE and Sjögren's syndrome, which are fairly well established as immunologic disorders. Indeed, Sjögren's syndrome may appear in patients with SS, adding further fuel to the fire of autoimmunity (Alarcon-Segovia et al., 1974a). A variety of serologic abnormalities are seen in many, but not all, patients. Hypergammaglobulinemia of mild degree is present in about 50 per cent of cases. Antinuclear antibodies have been identified in up to 80 per cent of patients, but generally in lower titers than are present in SLE. Rheumatoid factor is present in approximately 25 per cent of patients. Gamma globulin and complement have been described in the acute vascular lesions which precede the stages of sclerosing fibrosis (Tuffanelli and Winkelmann, 1962).

Attention has also been given to possible cell-mediated reactions. Using the macrophage-migration inhibition test, Hughes and colleagues (1974) have shown that lymphocytes from patients with SS apparently are sensitized to a wide variety of both autologous and homologous antigens. There are additional hints of loss of T-cell tolerance or T-suppressor cell function, and Currie and his associates (1971) have identified lymphocytotoxins in some of these patients which could explain the loss of T-cells. If an immunologic reaction underlies this disorder, what triggers it? As is almost always the case, the theoreticians' friendly virus is called upon. Virus-like particles have been identified in the kidneys of a few patients with systemic sclerosis (Becker, 1968). However, it has not been possible to isolate the agent, and the significance of these particles must be questioned (Haas and Yunis, 1970). Not even the most enthusiastic investigator could claim that a virus-incited immunologic causation for this disease has been established.

The widespread sclerosis of connective tissue in SS raises obvious questions about the possibility of a disorder in connective tissue metabolism. A number of studies have, in the last analysis, failed to disclose any critical abnormalities other than would be anticipated in a disease characterized by excessive collagenization. There is evidence of increased synthesis of collagen and ground substance and an increased proportion of "immature or un-cross-linked collagen" (Winkelmann, 1971). Recent reports point to some defect in cross linking and lead to a suggestion that the collagen is abnormally extractable, but the relevance of these findings is uncertain (Bashey et al., 1975). Once again we must repeat the dreary conclusion — the etiology of this disease is still unknown.

Morphology. Virtually any organ may be affected with SS, but the most prominent changes are found in the skin, musculoskeletal system, gastrointestinal tract, lungs, kidneys and heart (D'Angelo et al., 1969).

The changes in the **skin** almost always begin in the fingers and distal regions of the upper extremities and extend proximally to involve the upper arm, shoulders, neck and face. In advanced cases the entire back and abdomen as well as the lower extremities may be affected. The earliest changes consist only of some dermal edema and possibly some increased ground substance, but as the disease advances, there is considerable increase in dermal collagen, with epidermal atrophy and loss of skin adnexa (Fig. 6–11). The fingers may take on a tapered, claw-like appearance, and the dermal fibrosis may result in limitation of motion in the joints. The sclerotic atrophy of the tips of the fingers often causes resorption of the terminal phalanges of the fingers. Focal and sometimes diffuse subcutaneous calcifications may develop and along with the collagenization induce ulcerations, which may indeed progress to autoamputation of the fingers. The face may take on the appearance of a drawn mask. A variety of superimposed changes may appear, including telangiectases, vitiligo and hyperpigmentation.

The **gastrointestinal tract** is affected in over

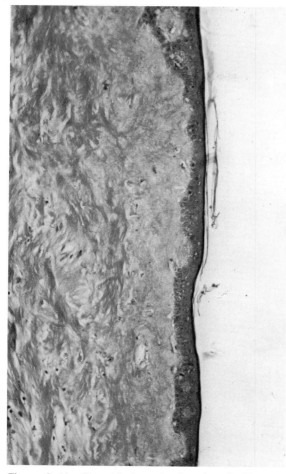

Figure 6–11. The skin in systemic sclerosis. The epidermis is atrophic, adnexal structures have been obliterated, and the dermis has been replaced by dense collagenous, fibrous tissue.

half the patients. The most common manifestation consists of progressive atrophy and fibrosis of the esophageal wall, involving principally the submucosa and muscularis. This may be accompanied by atrophy and ulceration of the overlying mucosa. Almost invariably the small vessels in these areas show progressive thickening of their walls, accompanied by a perivascular infiltrate of lymphocytes. Similar atrophy and fibrosis may occur in the stomach and small bowel. Only rarely is the colon affected.

In the **musculoskeletal system** both joints and muscles are affected. Early in the disease a nonspecific inflammatory synovitis may appear, resembling the early stages of rheumatoid arthritis. With progression the synovium undergoes collagenous sclerosis, followed in some cases by some bony resorption of the subjacent bone. At the same time there is sclerosis in the periarticular connective tissues which limits joint motion. Destruction of joints, such as occurs with rheumatoid arthritis, is quite rare. Focal inflammatory infiltrates followed by fibrosis may appear in the skeletal muscles, and many of these patients develop muscle atrophy.

The **lungs** often develop diffuse interstitial fibrosis of the alveolar septa, accompanied by progressive thickening of the walls of the smaller pulmonary vessels. The fibrosis may lead to the production of microcysts.

The **kidneys** frequently are damaged by a variety of lesions, but it is difficult to interpret the nature of the renal lesions, since most patients with SS and renal involvement have severe hypertension. Localized or diffuse thickening of the glomerular basement membranes, simulating the wire loop changes of SLE, are often seen. Thickening of the walls of the arterioles and small arteries is common, but this is an almost invariable finding in malignant hypertension, whatever the clinical setting. Necrosis and fibrinoid deposits in the small arteries and arterioles have been found in those with more severe renal damage. These vascular changes are often associated with small infarcts. The acute arteriolitis may lead to focal necroses of glomeruli. We can not be certain whether these vascular alterations induce the hypertension or result from it, since patients having pure forms of malignant hypertension (without associated immune disease) have identical vascular lesions.

The **heart** may have focal interstitial fibrosis, principally in the perivascular areas, and occasionally there are perivascular infiltrates of lymphocytes and macrophages. Small intramyocardial arteries and arterioles may show vascular thickening. Because of the changes in the lungs, right sided cardiac hypertrophy (cor pulmonale, p. 309) is often present.

Other sites may be affected, particularly nerve trunks, possibly related to microvascular lesions with ischemic and fibrotic alterations in the perimysium.

Clinical Course. It must be apparent from the described anatomic changes that systemic sclerosis has many of the features of rheumatoid arthritis, SLE and, as will be described, dermatomyositis. It is, however, distinctive in its striking cutaneous changes. Most patients first develop Raynaud's phenomenon, which may be present for many years prior to the appearance of the more definitive changes in the skin. The progressive collagenization of the skin leads to atrophy of the hands, with increasing stiffness and eventually complete immobilization of the joints (Fig. 6–12). The disability becomes more generalized as the trunk and extremities are affected. Muscular weakness and atrophy soon make their appearance, perhaps as a result of limitation of motion imposed by the cutaneous changes, or possibly as a result of intrinsic involvement of the joints and muscles as they suffer progressive interstitial fibrosis. Difficulty in swallowing and gastrointestinal symptoms are inevitable consequences of the changes in the

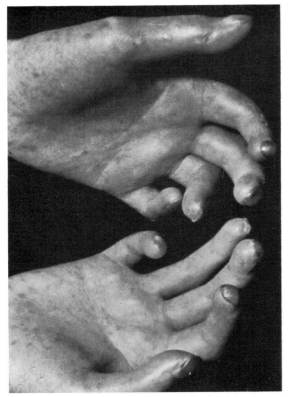

Figure 6–12. Advanced scleroderma. The extensive subcutaneous fibrosis has virtually immobilized the fingers, creating a claw-like flexion deformity.

esophagus and lower gut. Malabsorption may appear as the submucosal atrophy, muscular atrophy and fibrosis extend to the small intestine. Dyspnea and chronic cough reflect the pulmonary changes, and often these patients develop the so-called *stiff lung syndrome*. With advanced pulmonary involvement, secondary pulmonary hypertension may develop, leading in turn to right-sided cardiac dysfunction. Renal functional impairment secondary to both the advance of SS and the concomitant malignant hypertension frequently is marked.

The course of this disease is difficult to predict. In most patients, the disease pursues a steady, slow downhill course over the span of many years, with gradual evolution of the cutaneous lesions and progressive deformity. Many develop crippling limitation of motion of various joints. Involvement of the kidneys, heart or lungs eventually occurs in most cases and accounts for most deaths. In a recent analysis only 35 per cent of the patients survived seven years (Medsger and Masi, 1973). However, in some cases, the disease progresses slowly and, in fact, may become stabilized to permit a normal life span.

POLYMYOSITIS (DERMATOMYOSITIS)

Polymyositis is a chronic inflammatory myopathy of uncertain cause. When a skin rash is also present it is called dermatomyositis. *Clinically* the disease is characterized by muscle weakness and variable degrees of pain, swelling or atrophy of affected muscles, often accompanied by a rash about the eyes, face and extensor surfaces of the limbs. *Anatomically* the dominant features are focal areas of muscle inflammation leading to individual muscle cell atrophy or loss and hypertrophy. The disease may occur at any age from infancy to late life, with bimodal peaks in the age groups of 5 to 15 and 50 to 60 years. *The association of polymyositis–dermatomyositis with visceral cancers is somewhat disputed.* Williams (1959) states that about 15 per cent of cases of polymyositis–dermatomyositis in adults are associated with some form of visceral cancer. Bohan and Peter (1975), on the other hand, state: "Neoplasia may indeed be more frequent in polymyositis–dermatomyositis. However, there are as yet no statistically convincing data to support this notion unequivocally." Overall, females are affected twice as often as males.

The clinical expressions of dermatomyositis are extremely varied. Pearson (1971) has divided these into six syndromes.

1. *Polymyositis in adults:* an insidious onset, usually in females, sometimes accompanied by an atypical skin rash. Patients frequently have an accompanying Raynaud's phenomenon and arthritis, mimicking to a considerable degree SLE, scleroderma or rheumatoid arthritis.

2. *Typical dermatomyositis:* an acute or subacute onset, usually in women, associated with a classic rash on the face, as well as progressive muscular involvement.

3. *Typical dermatomyositis with cancer:* a syndrome resembling type 2, but more common in males.

4. *Childhood dermatomyositis:* an acute or chronic disease, usually with both myositis and rash. Widespread vasculitis affecting the skin leads to ulcerations and sometimes to calcifications; vasculitis within the gastrointestinal tract adds a prominent element of intestinal manifestations.

5. *Acute intermittent myolysis:* an acute, sometimes catastrophic onset characterized by rapidly progressive muscle destruction. May be initiated by a viral infection.

6. *Polymyositis with Sjögren's syndrome* (p. 198).

Etiology and Pathogenesis. The conviction that polymyositis–dermatomyositis is of immunologic origin is growing stronger. Up to the recent past it was largely "guilt by association," because, as will be seen, the clinical and anatomic manifestations of dermatomyositis overlap to a considerable degree those of other "connective tissue diseases," particularly scleroderma, systemic lupus erythematosus, rheumatoid arthritis and Sjögren's syndrome. Since some of these entities have better established immunologic causations, polymyositis–dermatomyositis was assumed without substantial proof also to be an immunologic disease. Moreover, a minority of patients have antinuclear antibodies and some have rheumatoid factor. Within the recent past more substantial documentation of an immunologic mechanism has been offered. Autoantibody to purified human myoglobin has been identified in the sera of some patients with polymyositis (Nishikai and Homma, 1972). Immune complexes and complement have been identified within blood vessels in foci of inflammatory myopathy (Whitaker and Engel, 1972). In addition, and probably of greater significance, is the evidence suggesting cell-mediated immune reactions. T-cells sensitized to muscle antigens have been documented in patients with polymyositis (Saunders et al., 1969). Recently, cell-mediated cytotoxicity to muscle has been reported (Dawkins, 1973). It was shown in vitro that lymphocytes from patients with this disease lysed muscle cells. Ziff and Johnson (1973) state, "To date we can only conclude that lymphocytes from patients with polymyositis are sensitized to release mediators of cellular immunity upon contact with their own or heterologous muscle. Does muscle contain a specific autoantigen? Does it contain an immunogenic infectious agent? Does it contain an antigen that cross reacts with an infectious agent to which the polymyositis patient is sensitized?" Relative to the last query, electron microscopy has disclosed virus-like particles in involved muscle cells in acute dermatomyositis (Ben-Bassat and Machtey, 1972). Moreover, Coxsackie type A virus has been isolated in patients with chronic but nonspecific myositis (Tang et al., 1975). In addition, there is a clinical association between certain viral infections and the onset of the disease. However, no agent has been isolated consistently from well documented cases of polymyositis, and most regard the intracellular particles as damaged organelles (Yunis, 1971).

Although an increased incidence of cancer has been disputed, as pointed out earlier, some patients with polymyositis, particularly those over the age of 50, do have some form of visceral cancer, such as cancer of the lung, stomach, breast, kidney, uterus or ovary, or rarely a lymphoma or thymoma. If the association is more than coincidental, it raises some intriguing etiologic possibilities. Could the tumor antigens evoke an immune reaction which cross reacts with muscle and skin? Alternatively, do both neoplasm and autoimmune disease result from some fundamental derangement in immunologic surveillance, such as loss of T-suppressor cell function? The genesis of polymyositis–dermatomyositis must still be considered uncertain, but increasingly the findings point to an immunologic origin.

Morphology. The major anatomic features of polymyositis–dermatomyositis are the muscle involvement and the skin rash. Classically the disease produces symmetrical myositis first of the limb-girdle muscles and anterior neck flexors, sparing the muscles of the distal extremities. With progression the muscle involvement becomes more global, extending to the distal extremities, pharyngeal muscles, intercostals and the diaphragm. Initially, the involved muscles are only slightly swollen and edematous. In advanced cases, affected muscles become pale gray, atrophic and fibrous. Sometimes focal calcifications appear. Histologically, any or all of the following features may be present: necrosis of muscle cells, phagocytosis of muscle cell fragments, regenerative activity resulting in basophilia of muscle cells with the appearance of

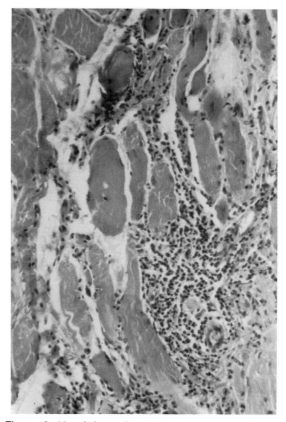

Figure 6–13. A focus in skeletal muscle in polymyositis–dermatomyositis, with loss of some fibers and irregular adjacent atrophy and hypertrophy of others. The inflammatory infiltrate is entirely mononuclear.

large prominent sarcolemmal nuclei and nucleoli, variation in individual fiber size and, usually, a prominent mononuclear inflammatory infiltrate in the sites of involvement (Fig. 6-13).

The skin rash may be quite variable or it may be virtually diagnostic. The classic rash takes the form of a lilac or heliotrope discoloration of the upper eyelids, with periorbital edema, accompanied by a scaling erythematous eruption or dusky red patches over the knuckles, elbows, knees, medial malleoli, forehead, face, neck and upper chest and back. Histologically, dermal edema is seen in the early stages, with mononuclear infiltrates surrounding the dermal vessels. These changes are followed in the later stages by fibrosis and sometimes calcification.

In children, and in some acute involvements in adults, widespread necrotizing vasculitis may be present, involving the lungs, kidneys, heart and other organs. This vasculitis is reminiscent of that encountered in other "connective tissue disorders." These acute lesions may lead to vascular fibrosis. Transitory arthritis may appear during the acute phases of the disease, but the underlying articular changes have not been adequately described. In any event the arthritis is not crippling or deforming.

Clinical Course. Polymyositis–dermatomyositis has, as its principal clinical finding, symmetrical muscular weakness, sometimes insidious, but sometimes acute in onset. Acute cases are often febrile. *The diagnosis cannot be entertained in the absence of muscular involvement.* It usually begins proximally in the shoulders and pelvic girdles and may then extend to the neck and eventually to the arms and legs. This pattern is not invariable. Frequently weakness of the striated muscles of the pharynx leads to difficulty in swallowing. In advanced cases, the muscular atrophy and fibrosis may be totally disabling. The skin rash may or may not be diagnostic. Sometimes the skin and muscle changes become sufficiently advanced and fibrocalcific to induce disabling contractures. Occasionally patients exhibit Raynaud's phenomenon or rheumatoid manifestations. As mentioned, there is considerable overlap of symptoms among SLE, systemic sclerosis and rheumatoid arthritis and, indeed, sometimes these diseases coexist. Moreover, it is hardly necessary to point out that many other muscle disorders (e.g., myasthenia gravis and the muscular dystrophies), may also provide differential diagnoses.

Bohan and Peter (1975) cite five major criteria which may help to define polymyositis–dermatomyositis. These include: (1) *proximal* muscle weakness, (2) characteristic changes on muscle biopsy, (3) elevated muscle enzymes in the serum (creatine phosphokinase, aldolase, transaminases and lactic dehydrogenase), (4) electromyographic abnormalities, and (5) a characteristic skin rash.

The course is characterized by remissions and exacerbations. In about 33 to 50 per cent of cases, the disease slowly progresses over many years to death. Other patients may have long periods of inactivity of the disease and long survival.

SJÖGREN'S SYNDROME

Sjögren's syndrome represents a clinicopathologic syndrome which occurs as an isolated disorder or, more often, develops in patients having another "connective tissue disease." In essence it comprises a triad of findings: (1) keratoconjunctivitis sicca (dry eyes), (2) xerostomia (dry mouth), and (3) an associated connective tissue disorder. Of the 62 patients with Sjögren's syndrome studied by Bloch and colleagues (1965), 32 had rheumatoid arthritis, four had polymyositis–dermatomyositis, three had systemic sclerosis and 23 presented the first two features of the triad unassociated with any other disorder. The designation *"sicca syndrome"* is reserved for those cases in which only the first two features are present. Sjögren's syndrome is of special interest for two reasons. First, it appears to represent a confluence of many of the other immunologic disorders discussed in this chapter. Second, it is of further interest because the intense infiltration of the salivary glands by lymphocytes and macrophages which is characteristic of this condition sometimes gives rise to a lymphoma. This raises the intriguing possibility that persistent immunologic lymphoid hyperactivity may in time initiate neoplasia.

Etiology and Pathogenesis. Sjögren's syndrome is second only to SLE in its multiplicity of serum autoantibodies. Hypergammaglobulinemia is virtually always present (Alarcon-Segovia et al., 1974b). Almost all patients have rheumatoid factor in their sera, even in the absence of demonstrable rheumatoid arthritis. Approximately 70 per cent of patients have antinuclear antibodies, and about 25 per cent have a positive LE cell test. A whole host of additional antibodies have been identified in these patients, including autoantibodies to thyroglobulin, thyroid microsomes, gastric parietal cells, mitochondria, salivary duct cells and other autologous antigens. The basis for all of these humoral immune reactions is still unclear, but there are recent suggestions that the culprit is the T-cell system. The intense lymphoid infiltrates in the salivary glands in this disorder strongly suggest a direct cell-mediated effector mechanism. There is a decrease in the number of T-cells in the circulating blood (Talal, 1974), and it has been suggested that many, if not most, of the lymphocytes within the infiltrates in the tissue lesions are T-cells. From recent studies it ap-

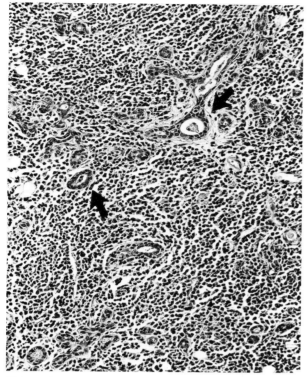

Figure 6–14. Sjögren's syndrome—submandibular gland. The intense lymphocytic and plasma cell infiltration virtually obscures the native architecture. Only a few residual ducts (arrows) can be identified.

pears then that both B- and T-cell systems are involved in the causation of Sjögren's syndrome, but what triggers these immune reactions is not clear. When other explanations are wanting, the twin specters of genetic predisposition and viral infection are raised and may one day be confirmed as causes of this syndrome. At the present time, however, they remain conjectural.

Morphology. The keratoconjunctivitis and xerostomia are the consequence of extensive damage to the lacrimal and salivary glands. Other secretory glands, including those in the nose, pharynx, larynx, trachea, bronchi and vagina, may also be involved. When involved, all exhibit an intense lymphocytic and plasma cell infiltration, with destruction of the native architecture, similar to the changes encountered in Hashimoto's thyroiditis (p. 598) (Fig. 6–14). Sometimes the lymphoid infiltrates create germinal follicles. These changes may be confused with lymphomatous invasion and, as mentioned, in some instances true neoplastic transformation occurs.

The lack of tears in the eyes resulting from the secretory lesions leads to drying of the corneal epithelium, which becomes inflamed, eroded and ulcerated. The oral mucosa may atrophy, with inflammatory fissuring and ulceration. Dryness and crusting of the nose may lead to ulcerations and even perforation of the nasal septum. When the respiratory passages are involved, secondary laryngitis, bronchitis and pneumonitis may appear. Some patients develop esophageal webs similar to those found in the Plummer-Vincent syndrome (p. 466). Atrophic gastritis (p. 473) also may appear. Defects of tubular function are commonly present, probably related to hyperviscosity of the blood, which is secondary to hypergammaglobulinemia. In addition, an interstitial nephritis is found occasionally, but its origin is obscure.

Clinical Course. As was noted at the outset, Sjögren's syndrome is most often seen in conjunction with one of the other "connective tissue diseases." About one third of the cases present only the first two features—the "sicca syndrome." The diagnosis of the sicca syndrome can be made readily by the lack of moisture and by the secondary changes in the eyes and oral cavity. Some patients have mild arthritis, neuropathy and Raynaud's phenomenon. Functional renal tubular defects, when present, include renal tubular acidosis, uricosuria, phosphaturia and generalized aminoaciduria, characteristic of the Fanconi syndrome (Hughes and Whaley, 1972). Serologic findings are merely confirmatory and do not differentiate among the related "connective tissue diseases." Of particular interest is the development of lymphoid cancer, reported in 3 of 58 patients with this disease (Talal and Bunim, 1964). In addition, some patients have had lesions designated as "pseudolymphoma." These comprise marked inflammatory hyperplastic changes within the salivary glands, bordering on the hypercellularity of lymphoid cancer. It would therefore appear that, in this disorder of probable immunologic origin, lymphoid hyperactivity may in time give rise to abnormal pseudolymphomatous proliferations (Talal et al., 1967) and in some cases to true malignant lymphoid tumors.

POLYARTERITIS NODOSA

Polyarteritis nodosa, sometimes called *periarteritis nodosa*, is a disease of medium-sized muscular arteries characterized by necrotizing inflammation of these vessels. The arteritis is peculiarly focal, random and episodic, often producing vascular obstruction and sometimes infarctions in the organ or tissue supplied. This unpredictability results in extremely variable clinical manifestations, reflecting the sites of involvement. In the early descriptions of this disease, aneurysmal dilatation of the necrosed arteries was emphasized, but in the more recently described cases, this is not a prominent feature. This apparent change, as well as others, in the manifestations of the disease, has raised many problems in understanding the nature of polyarteritis nodosa.

Acute necrotizing arteritis (discussed on p. 266) has many origins. It is common as a secondary change in areas of acute inflammation, such as in the wall of an abscess. Acute angiitis or vasculitis is very common in immunologic disorders, including the Arthus reaction and serum sickness, as well as the previously described "connective tissue diseases." Acute vascular necroses also are encountered with hypertension. Wegener's granulomatosis is characterized by acute arteritis and focal granulomatous lesions in the kidneys and upper respiratory tract. It is difficult to differentiate among all these forms of acute arteritis to clearly establish the diagnosis of polyarteritis. The problem is made all the more complex since there are no specific diagnostic features or tests.

Several attempts have been made to classify the acute angiitides. Zeek (1952) divided them only into periarteritis (attributed to hypertension), hypersensitivity angiitis (presumably related to drug sensitization) and allergic granulomatous angiitis. Wigley (1970) proposed the following somewhat more complex classification:

Necrotizing Arteritis
    Acute polyarteritis (older term—hypersensitivity arteritis)
    Chronic polyarteritis (older term—periarteritis nodosa)
Variants of Polyarteritis
    Wegener's granulomatosis
    Allergic granulomatosis
Other Forms of Arteritis
    Temporal arteritis
    Takayasu's disease
Arteritis in Other Diseases
    Rheumatic fever
    Rheumatoid arthritis
    Systemic lupus erythematosus
    Systemic sclerosis

In all of these disorders the morphologic changes within affected arteries are very similar indeed. Thus, the anatomic diagnosis of polyarteritis requires not only appropriate morphologic changes (which are regrettably not pathognomonic) but also exclusion of the other, better defined causes of inflammatory arteritis. Polyarteritis occurs at any age, most often in the elderly, with a *male* preponderance of approximately 3 to 1.

Etiology and Pathogenesis. Determining the etiology of a poorly defined condition is bound to be an unsatisfactory exercise. The possibility must be borne in mind that the disorder now referred to as polyarteritis may represent a number of etiologically separate entities. For many years, hypertension was considered an etiologic factor. However, it is quite clear that elevations of blood pressure do not always antedate the appearance of lesions, and indeed the hypertension may well be attributable to renal vascular involvement and renal ischemia which sometimes appear in the course of the disease. Respiratory infections commonly precede the appearance of the vascular lesions and bacterial and/or viral etiologies have been postulated. Microorganisms might serve as sensitizing mechanisms or instead evoke lesions by direct microbiologic injury.

A variety of observations suggests some form of immunologic causation. Polyarteritis nodosa is sometimes found in association with SLE, scleroderma, dermatomyositis and Sjögren's syndrome. However, Alarcon-Segovia and Brown (1964) question the validity of these associations and whether the arteritis found in these cases truly conforms to polyarteritis. Immunohistochemical studies have revealed a variety of plasma proteins within the lesions in the walls of arteries, including gamma globulin, complement and fibrinogen. However, the presence of these plasma proteins may reflect only nonselective seepage in areas of increased vascular permeability rather than mechanisms of injury. Vascular wall antigens have yielded negative results when tested against the sera of patients with polyarteritis nodosa (Piomelli, 1959). Antinuclear antibodies have been identified in some patients; but one wonders if these were truly cases of polyarteritis or if they were cases of acute arteritis occurring in the course of SLE, for example (Seligmann et al., 1965). An acute arteritis resembling polyarteritis has been described in some patients with hepatitis B (Gocke et al., 1971). The presence of circulating immune complexes containing Australia antigen in these patients also supports an immune causation for the vascular disease.

There are other immunologic hints. Elevated serum gamma globulin levels are found in some cases. The most effective therapy for this disease has been administration of corticosteroids, which are known to suppress immune reactions. Additional important clues are the documented flare-ups of the disorder following a drug reaction, and indeed cases are on record in which repeated administrations of the drug were followed by exacerbations. Here the possibility of some response similar to serum sickness is raised. Experimental observations also offer support. Acute necrotizing arteritis is common in a variety of experimental models of sensitivity reactions to foreign proteins (Rich and Gregory, 1943). Similarities exist between the vascular lesions of polyarteritis and those of viral Aleutian mink disease (Barnett et al., 1968). This animal model also has similarities to SLE, suggesting that the virus serves as a stimulus to an autoimmune reaction. However, the possibility of direct microbiologic injury in these animals has not been excluded. In sum, although there are many immunologic leads, the cause of this disease is still uncertain.

Morphology. The focal necrotizing lesions of polyarteritis nodosa may be found in any artery of medium to small size. In autopsied series, the sites of predilection are: kidneys (80 per cent), heart (70 per cent), liver (65 per cent) and gastrointestinal tract (50 per cent), followed by possible involvement of virtually every other organ in the body. In one large series the lungs were involved in 33 per cent (Rose, 1957), but cases with pulmonary involvement may represent a distinctive variant of the disease, since the lung symptoms often precede the arterial involvement. The inflammatory necroses are randomly distributed in curiously localized, sharply demarcated segments of the artery. Sometimes they involve only a portion of the circumference. In the acute phase of the lesion, the vessel may show subtle thickening and periarterial edema. Later, progressive fibrosis may create discrete **nodulations** at the sites of involvement. Microscopically, the pattern is that of an acute necrotizing inflammation beginning in the intima and inner portion of the media and extending in both directions to involve ultimately the entire thickness of the arterial wall, including the adventitia (Fig. 6–15). During the acute phase of the disease, fibrinoid deposits are prominent in the necrotic vessel walls. At this time, there is an acute inflammatory reaction in which eosinophils may be quite numerous. Thrombosis and rupture are potential sequelae. This acute lesion is later converted into an area of fibroblastic thickening of the involved segment, sometimes with organized obliteration of the lumen and striking periarterial fibrosis. Aneurysmal dilatation of the injured wall may occur but is not common. It should be stressed that individual lesions of varying stages of development—from the earliest inflammatory changes to dense collagenization—may coexist in the same patient at the same time, suggesting that whatever the underlying mechanism may be, it acts asynchronously throughout the body. The principal importance of these arterial lesions is their production of ischemic injury and infarction of tissues and organs. The kidneys bear the brunt of such injury, and in addition to the infarctions, they may also develop foci of glomerular necrosis.

Clinical Course. It is apparent that the clinical signs and symptoms of this disease are as varied as the sites of involvement. Indeed, the diagnosis is often reached by exclusion or because of the erratic multisystem involvement. Polyarteritis nodosa may be of acute onset or may arise insidiously. Most cases pur-

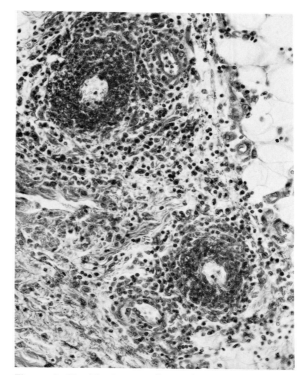

Figure 6–15. The two small vessels disclose an acute necrotizing angiitis virtually destroying the vessel walls. There is an extensive perivascular inflammatory infiltrate.

sue a protracted course, with recurrent flare-ups of activity. During the acute phase, the patient often shows systemic manifestations, such as malaise, fever, weakness and weight loss. Renal involvement is one of the prominent manifestations. Hematuria, albuminuria and sudden costovertebral angle pain may herald focal necroses in the kidneys. Vascular lesions in the gastrointestinal tract produce a wide variety of symptoms, including abdominal pain, diarrhea and melena. Peripheral neuritis or spinal cord involvement is quite frequent. As has been mentioned, a certain number of cases begin with persistent pulmonary infections. These patients, however, often develop granulomatous lesions along with the acute vasculitis (very reminiscent of Wegener's granulomatosis), and it is not certain that they are forms of classic polyarteritis as the term is used here.

The course and outcome of this disease are completely unpredictable. Sometimes it is an acute process which subsides within a few weeks or months, never to recur. More often, the disease persists, with recurrent exacerbations over a course of years, until some vital organ is destroyed.

The diagnosis can only be suspected from the clinical manifestations and must be confirmed by histologic examination. The difficulties inherent in such histologic diagnosis have already been cited. Moreover, the lesions are sharply segmental and unless a nodule can be palpated in a superficial artery, a false negative result may be obtained. Contrariwise, many of the causes of acute arteritis that have already been cited may lead to a false positive diagnosis. Eosinophilia, when present (12 to 50 per cent of cases), is supportive but not diagnostic. Ultimately it is the random, unpredictable distribution of manifestations relating to many systems which is the most distinctive feature of this disease.

POSSIBLE IMMUNE DISORDERS

Immunologic mechanisms are suspected of contributing to a large number of diseases in addition to those already described in this chapter. Some of these entities will be discussed in the chapters dealing with individual organs and systems. One disease—amyloidosis—requires description at this point. New observations provide strong evidence that some derangement in the immune apparatus underlies this disease, and as a systemic disease it cannot be assigned to any single organ or system.

AMYLOIDOSIS

Amyloid is an abnormal amorphous substance, at least in some cases related to the immunoglobulins, which is deposited in many tissues and organs of the body in a variety of clinical settings. Since its first recognition, it has been delineated by its morphologic appearance under the light microscope. With usual tissue stains, amyloid appears as an intercellular pink translucent material. At one time it was thought to be starch-like, hence the designation "amyloid"; however, recent evidence indicates that it is protein in nature. In some patients the proteins have biochemical and immunologic similarities to the light chains of immunoglobulins, but in others the proteins appear not to be of immunoglobulin origin. Despite this biochemical heterogeneity, it has a surprising morphologic uniformity. Amyloid has the additional following properties:

1. With electron microscopy it is seen to have a fibrillar substructure. Amyloid fibrils (the major component) consist of filaments 7.5 nm. in diameter, made up of two or more intertwined subunits (protofibrils) 3.5 nm. in diameter. A second minor component known as the pentagonal unit is about 9 nm. in diameter; these may aggregate in the fashion of stacked doughnuts to create rods.

2. By x-ray diffraction amyloid yields a pattern indicating a beta-pleated sheet conformation.

3. It has an affinity for congo red stain and exhibits metachromasia with crystal violet stain.

4. After congo red staining it yields a green birefringence on polarization microscopy. This property is attributable to the major component—i.e., the amyloid fibrils.

Many proteins may conform to the characteristics just given. It has been shown, for example, that polymerization of insulin and glucagon under appropriate conditions yields fibrils that, when polarized, have the optical properties of amyloid fibrils stained with congo red (Glenner et al., 1973). Thus, biochemically there may well be more than one kind of amyloid (Levin et al., 1973).

The clinical settings in which amyloidosis occurs are, as mentioned, quite variable. Some patients have an underlying disease, in others it appears as an isolated disorder independent of any associated disease, and less commonly it is a component of certain heredofamilial states. It may be widespread throughout the body, or it may occur within a single organ. Numerous attempts have been made to subdivide this wide spectrum into useful clinicoanatomic categories, but regrettably amyloidosis does not divide itself into neat categories. No classification has been universally accepted and so the simplest, composed of four categories, suffices: (1) primary (idiopathic) amyloidosis, (2) secondary amyloidosis, (3) heredofamilial amyloidosis and (4) isolated organ amyloidosis. The first three categories denote systemic distributions. It should be noted that some authors further subdivide primary amyloidosis into two categories, as will be pointed out later. At the risk of doing violence to convention, primary amyloidosis will be described last.

Secondary amyloidosis refers to the development of the disorder in patients having some long-standing underlying disease which causes extensive breakdown of cells and tissues. Major offenders are tuberculosis, rheumatoid arthritis, bronchiectasis, osteomyelitis, syphilis, ulcerative colitis, regional enteritis, and any form of disseminated cancer associated with necrosis of neoplastic or normal tissue.

It is postulated that in these disorders persistent immunologic challenge, resulting from the release of cellular antigens, in some way initiates the formation of amyloid. The amyloid protein in these cases may or may not be homologous with the light chains of immunoglobulins.

Heredofamilial amyloidosis refers to a group of genetic disorders characterized by the deposition of amyloid in various sites throughout the body. The most common of these disorders is familial Mediterranean fever, which has an autosomal recessive mode of transmission. Other, less common syndromes include familial amyloid polyneuropathy, familial amyloid nephropathy, medullary amyloidotic thyroid carcinoma and familial cardiac amyloidosis. In most of these syndromes it has been observed that the amyloid protein is not homologous with immunoglobulin fractions.

Primary (idiopathic) amyloidosis refers to those instances of amyloidosis which are not clearly attributable to some chronic, destructive disease, nor are they hereditary in origin. Some of these patients do have, however, an underlying dyscrasia of B-cells, but most do not. The most common B-cell dyscrasia associated with amyloidosis is called multiple myeloma (a form of plasma cell cancer usually arising within the skeletal system) (p. 355) (Azar, 1966). Abnormally high levels of immunoglobulins, belonging to any one of the five major classes, are present in the plasma of the great majority of patients with this form of B-cell dyscrasia, as well as, sometimes, smaller fragments of the immunoglobulins, composed of either kappa or lambda light chains (Bence-Jones protein). Other B-cell dyscrasias — Waldenström's macroglobulinemia (p. 354), lymphocytic lymphoma (p. 342), and lymphocytic leukemia (p. 349) — are sometimes also associated with abnormal elevations of the gamma globulins and primary amyloidosis. Some experts prefer to segregate these cases with B-cell dyscrasias from the category of primary amyloidosis to create a subset referred to as "amyloidosis associated with malignant B-cell dyscrasia" (Benson et al., 1975). *Most patients with primary amyloidosis do not have an underlying B-cell dyscrasia.* Some of these patients nonetheless have demonstrably elevated levels of immunoglobulins and Bence-Jones proteins, which led to the discovery of an apparently benign plasmacytosis in their bone marrows (Cathcart et al., 1972). This finding has led certain investigators to propose that all cases of primary amyloidosis reflect abnormal plasma cell activity which in some individuals progresses to the stage of producing a plasma cell neoplasm (Osserman, 1965). Not all agree with this point of view and so many workers prefer to call this pattern of amyloidosis "idiopathic." They raise the issue of whether the amyloidosis and the abnormal plasmacytosis both reflect a response to some still unknown challenge (Cohen and Cathcart, 1974). In any event, whether a B-cell dyscrasia is present or not, the proteins in the deposits in primary amyloidosis are usually homologous with the light chains of immunoglobulins.

Isolated organ amyloidosis refers to amyloid deposits in a single organ, most often the heart, tongue, brain, seminal vesicles, or islets of Langerhans in patients with diabetes mellitus. Some of these patients, particularly those with cardiac amyloidosis, are of advanced age. Except for this association, little is known about the interpretation of isolated organ amyloidosis or whether it might in time become systemic in distribution.

NATURE AND ORIGIN OF AMYLOID

The nature and genesis of amyloid has become a subject of great current interest and the literature is replete with confusion and contradiction. A central question is — are all forms of amyloid composed of immunoglobulins? *The weight of evidence favors the view that some amyloid deposits are of immunoglobulin origin, but some are not and in fact vary from one patient to the next in their precise composition.* However, within the individual patient, the amyloid in all organs appears to be of identical composition. Glenner and his co-workers (1972) are largely responsible for an elegant series of studies demonstrating that in at least some patients the amyloid is composed of either kappa or lambda light chains, principally the variable region of these light chains. Amino acid sequencing has documented complete homology between the amino-terminal variable region of the light chains in Bence-Jones protein and the amyloid proteins in these patients. Moreover, it has been possible to cleave the Bence-Jones protein enzymically and then under suitable — nearly physiologic — conditions to obtain a precipitate which has the typical congo red birefringence, electron microscopic fibrillar appearance and x-ray diffraction patterns characteristic of amyloid fibrils (Glenner et al., 1971). Others, however, contend that there are subtle differences in morphology between the in vitro fibril and isolated, purified amyloid fibrils (Shirahama et al., 1973). Despite these doubts there is a wide acceptance of the view that *at least in some patients (largely those with primary amyloidosis and particularly those having an associated B-cell dyscrasia) the amyloid fibrils represent a fragment of light-chain Bence-Jones protein, often lacking some part or all of the constant region of the light chain.* In vivo cleavage of the light chains might be followed by polymerization and deposition, yielding the deposits recognized as amyloid (Glenner and Terry, 1974).

With rare exceptions *the proteins derived from the amyloid deposits in patients having secondary amyloidosis or heredofamilial amyloidosis appear not to be immunoglobulins* (Benditt and Eriksen, 1971). Although amino acid sequencing has failed to demonstrate homology between these non-immunoglobulin amyloid proteins and light chains, it has demonstrated remarkable biochemical uniformity among the amyloid proteins in patients with secondary amyloidosis, with modest variations in one or two amino acids. Recently a third class of amyloid fibril protein, also of non-immunoglobulin origin, has been described (Husby et al., 1974). At the present time it seems wisest to consider amyloid as having one of at least two or possibly three basic compositions, and it is highly likely that future studies will expose even greater variety.

What is the cellular origin of amyloid? It is believed to be produced locally in its sites of deposition at least largely by RE cells or immunocompetent cells. The majority of patients with amyloid disease, whether primary, secondary or heredofamilial in nature, have nonspecific immunoglobulin abnormalities, such as elevated or depressed serum levels of IgG, IgA or IgM. In patients with plasma cell dyscrasias one can obviously point to the immunoglobulin-secreting plasma cells. In those with secondary amyloidosis the prolonged antigenic challenge may activate the immunocompetent cells. However, it is not known whether B-cells alone are deranged or whether cooperating T-cells are involved in the abnormal elaboration of proteins. At the present time there are suggestions that abnormal T-cell high zone tolerance to a specific immunogen may be involved along with B-cells in the genesis of amyloidosis (Hardt and Claesson, 1972).

Morphology. There are no consistently distinctive patterns of organ or tissue distribution of amyloid deposits in any of the categories cited. Nonetheless, a few generalizations can be made. **Secondary amyloidosis tends to yield the most severe systemic involvements.** The kidneys, liver, spleen, lymph nodes, adrenals and thyroid, as well as many other tissues, are classically involved. **Although primary amyloidosis cannot be distinguished from the secondary form by its organ distribution, more often it involves the heart and blood vessels.** In addition, bizarre distributions, such as amyloidosis of the eye, respiratory tract and skin, are encountered more often in patients with primary amyloidosis. However, the same organs affected by secondary amyloidosis, including the kidneys, liver and spleen, may also contain deposits in the primary form of the disease. Therefore, it should be emphasized that the diagnosis of primary amyloidosis requires ruling out the secondary and heredofamilial forms. The localization of amyloid deposits in the **heredofamilial syndromes** is quite varied. In familial Mediterranean fever the amyloidosis may be widespread, involving the kidneys, blood vessels, spleen, respiratory tract and, rarely, the liver. The localization of amyloid in the remaining hereditary syndromes can be inferred from the designations of these entities. **Isolated organ amyloidosis** has already been characterized.

Whatever the clinical setting, the amyloidosis may or may not be apparent on macroscopic examination. Often small amounts are not recognized until the surface of the cut organ is painted with iodine and sulfuric acid. This yields a mahogany brown staining of the amyloid deposits. When amyloid accumulates in larger amounts, frequently the organ is enlarged, and the tissue appears gray, with a waxy, firm consistency. **Histologically, the deposition always begins between cells,** often closely adjacent to basement membranes. As the amyloid progressively accumulates, it encroaches on the cells. In time the depositions surround and destroy the trapped native cells. **Most important for the histologic identification of amyloid is the demonstration with polarization microscopy of birefringence after congo red staining.**

Because of the variability in its distribution, each of the major organ involvements will be described separately.

Amyloidosis of the kidney is the most common and the most serious involvement in the disease. Grossly, the kidney may appear unchanged, it may be abnormally large, pale, gray and firm, or it may be reduced in size. Contracted kidneys generally are found in the advanced stages of the disease. Microscopically, the amyloid deposits are found principally in the glomeruli, but they are also present in the interstitial peritubular tissue, as well as in the walls of the blood vessels. The glomerulus first develops focal deposits within the mesangial matrix, as well as diffuse or nodular thickenings of the basement membranes of the capillary loops. Subsequently, the fibrils appear to stream through and obscure the basement membrane, appearing on the epithelial side as well as the endothelial side (Suzuki et al., 1963). With progression, the deposition encroaches on the capillary lumina and eventually leads to total obliteration of the vascular tuft (Fig. 6–16). The interstitial peritubular deposits frequently are associated with the appearance of amorphous pink casts within the tubular lumina, presumably of proteinaceous nature. Blood vessels of all sizes may develop deposits of amyloid within their walls, often causing marked vascular narrowing. It is this vascular narrowing which presumably leads to the contracture of the kidneys mentioned previously.

Amyloidosis of the spleen often causes moderate or even marked enlargement (200 to 800 gm.). For obscure reasons, one of two patterns may develop. The deposits may be virtually limited to the splenic central arteries and follicles, producing tapioca-like granules on gross examination ("sago spleen"), or the involvement may affect principally the splenic sinuses and eventually extend to the splenic pulp, forming large, sheet-like deposits ("lardaceous spleen"). In both patterns, the spleen exhibits increased consistency and often reveals, on the cut surface, the pale gray, waxy deposits in the distribution described. In both forms of the disease, the early deposit occurs between cells,

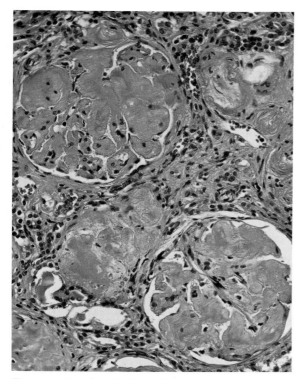

Figure 6–16. Amyloidosis of the kidney. The glomeruli are obliterated by the amorphous amyloid deposit. The vessels (upper right) are also virtually occluded by the deposition within their walls.

usually in close proximity to the littoral cells of the sinuses or within the reticular framework of the splenic cords (Cohen, 1965). With progressive accumulation, the amyloid encroaches on and eventually destroys the contiguous cells.

Amyloidosis of the liver may cause massive enlargement, up to such extraordinary weights as 9000 gm. In such advanced cases, the liver is extremely pale, grayish and waxy on both the external surface and the cut section. Histologically, the deposits appear first in the space of Disse and then progressively enlarge, to encroach on the adjacent hepatic parenchyma and sinusoids. The trapped liver cells are literally squeezed to death and are eventually replaced by sheets of amyloid. The blood vessels, as well as the Kupffer cells, are often involved. It is difficult to believe but normal hepatic function may be preserved even with massive amyloid replacement.

Amyloidosis of the heart may occur either as an isolated organ involvement or as part of a systemic distribution. The isolated form (**senile amyloidosis**) is usually confined to individuals of advanced age. The depositions may not be evident on gross examination, or they may cause minimal to moderate cardiac enlargement. The most characteristic gross findings are gray-pink, dewdrop-like, subendocardial elevations, particularly in the atrial chambers. However, on histologic examination, in addition to these focal subendocardial accumulations, deposits

are frequently found throughout the myocardium, beginning between myocardial fibers and eventually causing their pressure atrophy. Vascular involvement and subepicardial accumulations may also be present. In advanced cases, the myocardial aggregates may cause considerable loss of muscle fibers, with attendant derangements of the cardiac conduction system and cardiac contractility. Cardiac failure is an important cause of death in amyloidosis.

Amyloidosis of the endocrine organs, particularly of the adrenals, thyroid, and pituitary, is common in advanced systemic distributions. In this case also, the amyloid deposition begins in relation to stromal and endothelial cells and progressively encroaches on the parenchymal cells. Surprisingly large amounts of amyloid may be present in any of these endocrine glands without apparent disturbance of function. The adrenal must be almost totally replaced before hypofunction is manifested and, hence, amyloidosis is an uncommon cause of Addison's disease (hypoadrenalism) (p. 610).

Other organs may be involved. Indeed, no organ or tissue of the body is exempt. Deposits may be encountered in the upper and lower respiratory passages, sometimes in nodular masses. The gastrointestinal tract is a relatively favored site, in which amyloid may be found at all levels, sometimes producing tumorous masses that must be distinguished from neoplasms. Depositions in the tongue may produce macroglossia. On the basis of the frequent involvement of the GI tract in systemic cases, gingival, intestinal and rectal biopsies are commonly employed in the diagnosis of suspected cases. The gingival biopsy may be expected to be positive in approximately 60 per cent and the rectal biopsy in 75 per cent of patients having advanced systemic amyloidosis (Blum and Sohar, 1960). It is assumed that in order to obtain frequencies as high as these, congo red staining and polarization microscopy are employed to detect trace amounts, which may be limited to the vascular walls within the tissue examined. The skin, eye and nervous system are also affected. Indeed, amyloid deposits in the peripheral nerves are among the prominent manifestations of one of the hereditary forms of this disease. As was previously mentioned, involvement of the arterial and arteriolar walls may be found in any site in the body.

Clinical Correlation. Amyloidosis may be an unsuspected finding at autopsy in a patient having no apparent related clinical manifestations, or it may be responsible for serious clinical dysfunction and even death. All depends on the particular sites or organs affected and the severity of the involvement. Overall, amyloidosis tends to manifest itself in one of several ways—by renal disease, hepatomegaly, splenomegaly, cardiac abnormalities or alterations in serum or urinary proteins, or both (Cathcart et al., 1972). Renal involvement is usually manifested by proteinuria, protein and cellular casts and, rarely, red cell casts. In some patients the proteinuria is severe enough to induce the nephrotic syndrome (p. 432). Advancement of the renal disease may lead to renal failure, which is the most common related cause of death in these patients. Renal failure in the absence of hypertension should raise a suspicion of amyloidosis. The hepatosplenomegaly rarely causes significant clinical dysfunction, but it may be the presenting finding. Very rarely severe hepatic amyloidosis causes liver failure. Cardiac amyloidosis may represent an isolated organ involvement or be part of a systemic distribution. The most severe forms of cardiac amyloidosis are seen in aged individuals, usually in the eighth and ninth decades of life, as isolated organ involvement. The intramyocardial deposits may manifest themselves as conduction disturbances or as an apparent cardiomyopathy. Sometimes diffuse myocardial amyloidosis masquerades as chronic constrictive pericarditis. Deposits within the coronary arteries may cause narrowing and even consequent myocardial infarction. Abnormalities in the serum gamma globulins, usually a marked elevation in one of the immunoglobulins (creating a so-called M-spike on the electrophoretic analysis) may denote the presence of multiple myeloma or amyloidosis or both.

The diagnosis of amyloidosis may be suspected from the clinical settings and from some of the findings mentioned above. However, more specific tests must often be employed for definitive diagnosis. Severe amyloidosis can be detected by the intravascular injection of known amounts of congo red dye and quantitating the amount of dye taken out of the circulation by the amyloid deposits. However, the test is not very specific and in general is considered to be positive only when 80 per cent or more of the circulating dye is retained within affected tissues. Even at this level, false positive results are sometimes encountered. As mentioned, gingival and rectal biopsies, examined by congo red staining and polarization, are very useful diagnostic procedures. A positive biopsy quite reliably indicates amyloidosis, but a negative biopsy, because of the focal nature of the deposits, does not rule out the diagnosis.

Of recent date there are reports of resolution of amyloid deposits in man following therapeutic control or elimination of the antigenic stimulus in secondary amyloidosis (Lowenstein and Gallo, 1970). If, for example, a chronic inflammatory disease can be resolved or excised, apparent resorption of the deposits follows. At the present time immunosuppressive drugs are being explored as another therapeutic modality.

Widespread amyloidosis must be considered a life-threatening disease. In one study the mean survival after diagnosis was approximately 11 months (Brandt et al., 1968). Obviously in these cases the amyloidosis must have been sufficiently advanced to have permitted diagnosis, and equally obviously milder involvements may produce no clinical symptoms and so may lurk unsuspected for an unknown number of years.

REFERENCES

Aiuti, F., et al.: B-lymphocytes in agammaglobulinemia. Lancet, 2:761, 1972.

Alarcon-Segovia, D.: Drug induced lupus syndromes. Mayo Clin. Proc., 44:664, 1969.

Alarcon-Segovia, D., and Brown, A. L.: Classification and etiologic aspects of necrotizing angiitides: An analytic approach to a confused subject with a critical review of the evidence for hypersensitivity in polyarteritis nodosa. Mayo Clin. Proc., 39:205, 1964.

Alarcon-Segovia, D., et al.: Sjögren's syndrome in progressive systemic sclerosis (scleroderma). Am. J. Med., 57:78, 1974a.

Alarcon-Segovia, D., et al.: Serum hyperviscosity in Sjögren's syndrome. Interactions between IgG and IgG rheumatoid factor. Ann. Int. Med., 80:35, 1974b.

Allison, A. C.: Mechanisms of tolerance in autoimmunity. Ann. Rheum. Dis., 32:283, 1973.

Allison, A. C., et al.: Cooperating and controlling functions of thymic derived lymphocytes in relation to autoimmunity. Lancet, 2:135, 1971.

Asofsky, R., et al.: Panel discussion on T-cell heterogeneity. Fed. Proc., 34:162, 1975.

Azar, H. A.: Amyloidosis and plasma cell disorders. Ann. Rev. Med., 17:49, 1966.

Balch, C. M., and Diethelm, A. G.: The pathophysiology of renal allograft rejections: a collective review. J. Surg. Res., 12:350, 1972.

Barnett, E. V., et al.: Nuclear antigens and antinuclear antibodies in mink sera. Arthritis Rheum., 11:92, 1968.

Bartfeld, H., and Epstein, W. V. (eds.): Rheumatoid factors and their biological significance. Ann. N.Y. Acad. Sci., 168:1, 1969.

Bashey, R. I., et al.: Solubility of collagen from normal and scleroderma fibroblasts in culture. Biochem. Biophys. Res. Commun., 62:303, 1975.

Becker, E. L.: Structural Basis of Renal Disease. New York, Hoeber Medical Division, Harper & Row, 1968, p. 163.

Ben-Bassat, M., and Machtey, I.: Picorna virus-like structures in acute dermatomyositis. Am. J. Clin. Pathol., 58:245, 1972.

Benditt, E. P., and Eriksen, N.: Chemical classes of amyloid substance. Am. J. Path., 65:231, 1971.

Bennett, M.: Prevention of marrow allograft rejection with radioactive strontium: evidence for marrow-dependent effector cells. J. Immunol., 110:510, 1973.

Benson, M. A., and Borel, Y.: The tolerant cell: direct evidence for receptor blockade by tolerogen. J. Immunol., 112:1793, 1974.

Benson, M. D., et al.: Neuropathy, M components and amyloid. Lancet, 1:10, 1975.

Berke, G., et al.: Mechanisms of lymphocyte-mediated cytolysis. Trans. Rev., 17:71, 1973.

Berry, C. L.: Histopathological findings in the combined immunity-deficiency syndrome. J. Clin. Pathol., 23:193, 1970.

Bloch, K. J., et al.: Sjögren's syndrome. A clinical, pathological and serological study of 62 cases. Medicine, 44:187, 1965.

Blum, A., and Sohar, E.: Rectal biopsy for diagnosis of amyloidosis. Am. J. Med. Sci., 240:332, 1960.

Bohan, A., and Peter, J. B.: Polymyositis and dermatomyositis. New Eng. J. Med., 292:343, 405, 1975.

Brandt, K., et al.: A clinical analysis of the course and prognosis of forty-two patients with amyloidosis. Am. J. Med., 44:955, 1968.

Britton, M. C., and Schur, B.: The complement system in rheumatoid synovitis. II. Intracytoplasmic inclusions of immunoglobulins and complement. Arth. Rheum., 14:87, 1971.

Broder, I.: Anaphylaxis. In Movat, H. Z. (ed.): Inflammation, Immunity and Hypersensitivity. New York, Harper & Row, 1971, p. 333.

Burnet, F. M.: Autoimmune disease. I. Modern immunologic concepts. II. Pathology of the immune response. Brit. Med. J., 2:645, 729, 1959.

Busch, G. J., et al.: Human renal allografts: analysis of lesions in long term survivors. Hum. Pathol., 2:253, 1971.

Cathcart, E. S., et al.: Immunoglobulins and amyloidosis. An immunologic study of 62 patients with biopsy proved disease. Am. J. Med., 52:93, 1972.

Christian, C. L., and Phillips, P. E.: Viruses and autoimmunity. Am. J. Med., 54:611, 1973.

Cleveland, W. W., et al.: Foetal thymic transplant in a case of DiGeorge's syndrome. Lancet, 2:1211, 1968.

Cohen, A. S.: The constitution and genesis of amyloid. Int. Rev. Exp. Pathol., 4:159, 1965.

Cohen, A. S., and Cathcart, E. S.: Amyloidosis and immunoglobulins. Adv. Int. Med., 19:41, 1974.

Cohen, A. S., et al.: Diagnostic and Therapeutic Criteria Committee of the American Rheumatism Association: Preliminary criteria for the classification of systemic lupus erythematosus. Bull. Rheum. Dis., 21:643, 1971.

Cooper, M. D., and Lawton, A. R., III: The development of the immune system. Sci. Am., 231:59, 1974.

Cooper, M. D., et al.: Meeting report of the Second International Workshop on Primary Immunodeficiency Diseases in Man. Clin. Immunol. Immunopathol., 2:416, 1974.

Corson, J. M.: The pathologist and the kidney transplant. Pathol. Annu., 7:251, 1972.

Currie, S., et al.: Immunologic aspects of systemic sclerosis: in vitro activity of lymphocytes from patients with the disorder. Brit. J. Dermatol., 84:400, 1971.

D'Angelo, W. A., et al.: Pathologic observations in systemic sclerosis (scleroderma). Am. J. Med., 46:428, 1969.

Dawkins, R. L.: Cell-mediated cytotoxicity to muscle in polymyositis. New Eng. J. Med., 288:434, 1973.

De Koning, J., et al.: Transplantation of bone-marrow cells and fetal thymus in an infant with lymphopenic immunological deficiency. Lancet, 1:1223, 1969.

Dittmer, J., and Bennett, M.: Long-term survival of cardiac allografts in lethally irradiated rats repopulated with host-type hemopoietic cells. Transplantation, 19:295, 1975.

Dixon, F. J., et al.: Pathogenesis of serum sickness. Arch. Pathol., 65:18, 1958.

Dixon, F. J., et al.: Experimental glomerulonephritis: the pathogenesis of a laboratory model resembling the spectrum of human glomerulonephritis. J. Exp. Med., 113:899, 1961.

Dubois, E. L.: Lupus Erythematosus. A Review of the Current Status of Discoid and Systemic Lupus Erythematosus. New York, Blakiston Division, McGraw-Hill Book Co., 1966.

Dujovne, I., et al.: The distribution and character of glomerular deposits in systemic lupus erythematosus. Kidney Internat., 2:33, 1972.

Duthie, J. J., et al.: Course and prognosis in rheumatoid arthritis. Ann. Rheum. Dis., 23:193, 1964.

Editorial: Transfer factor. Lancet, 2:79, 1973a.

Editorial: Lymphokines. Lancet, 1:1490, 1973b.

Editorial: Is HL-A matching worthwhile in kidney transplantation? Lancet, 1:1150, 1974.

Elkins, W. L., et al.: Transplantation tolerance and enhancement. Transplantation, 18:38, 1974.

Estes, D., and Christian, C. L.: The natural history of systemic lupus erythematosus by prospective analysis. Medicine, 50:85, 1971.

Feizi, T., et al.: Cold agglutinin produced in rabbits immunized with Mycoplasma pneumoniae-treated human erythrocytes. Clin. Res., 17:366, 1969.

Gatti, R. A., and Seligmann, M.: The primary immunodeficiency diseases: classification, pathogenesis and treatment. Turk. J. Ped., 15:195, 1973.

Geha, R. S., et al.: Identification and characterization of subpopulations of lymphocytes in human peripheral blood after fractionation on discontinuous gradients of albumin. The cellular defect in X-linked agammaglobulinemia. J. Clin. Invest., 52:1726, 1973.

Ginzler, E. M., et al.: Progression of mesangial and focal to diffuse lupus nephritis. New Eng. J. Med., 291:693, 1974.

Glasgow, A. H., et al.: Association of anergy with an immunosuppressive peptide fraction in the serum of patients with cancer. New Eng. J. Med., 291:1263, 1974.

Glenner, G. G., and Terry, W. D.: Characterization of amyloid. Ann. Rev. Med., 25:131, 1974.

Glenner, G. G., et al.: Creation of "amyloid" fibrils from Bence Jones proteins in vitro. Science, 174:712, 1971.

Glenner, G. G., et al.: The immunoglobulin origin of amyloid. Am. J. Med., 52:141, 1972.

Glenner, G. G., et al.: The structural characteristics of some proteins having the properties of congo red-stained amyloid fibrils. J. Histochem. Cytochem., 21:406, 1973.

Gocke, D. J., et al.: Vasculitis in association with Australia antigen. J. Exp. Med., 134:330, 1971.

Goldman, J. A., et al.: Cellular immunity to nuclear antigens in SLE. J. Clin. Invest., 51:2669, 1972.

Good, R. A., and Yunis, E.: Association of autoimmunity, immunodeficiency and aging in man, rabbits and mice. Fed. Proc., 33:2040, 1974.

Griscelli, C., et al.: Transfer factor therapy in immunodeficiencies. Biomedicine, 18:220, 1973.

Grumet, F. C., et al.: Histocompatibility (HL-A) antigens associated with systemic lupus erythematosus. A possible genetic predisposition to disease. New Eng. J. Med., 285:193, 1971.

Gyorkey, F., et al.: A morphologic study on the occurrence and distribution of structures resembling viral nucleocapsids in collagen diseases. Am. J. Med., 53:148, 1972.

Haas, J. E., and Yunis, E. G.: Tubular inclusions of systemic lupus erythematosus: ultrastructural observations regarding their possible viral nature. Exp. Molec. Pathol., 12:257, 1970.

Hamburger, J. A.: Reappraisal of the concept of organ "rejection." Based on the study of homotransplanted kidneys. Transplantation, 5:870, 1967.

Hardt, F., and Claesson, N. H.: Quantitative studies on the T-cell populations in spleens from amyloidotic and non-amyloidotic mice. Immunology, 22:677, 1972.

Harvey, A. M., et al.: Systemic lupus erythematosus. Review of the literature and clinical analysis of 138 cases. Medicine, 33:291, 1954.

Henry, C. S.: Killer cells. New Eng. J. Med., 291:1357, 1974.

Hermans, P. E.: Immune deficiency diseases. Postgrad. Med., 54:66, 1973.

Hughes, G. R. V., and Whaley, K.: Sjögren's syndrome. Brit. Med. J., 4:533, 1972.

Hughes, P., et al.: Leukocyte-migration inhibition in progressive systemic sclerosis. Brit. J. Dermatol., 91:1, 1974.

Husby, G., et al.: New, third class of amyloid fibril protein. J. Exp. Med., 139:773, 1974.

James, L. P., Jr., and Austin, K. F.: Fatal systemic anaphylaxis in man. New Eng. J. Med., 270:597, 1964.

Johnson, P. M., et al.: Antiglobulin production to altered IgG in rheumatoid arthritis. Lancet, 1:611, 1975.

Koffler, D., et al.: Immunological studies concerning the nephritis of systemic lupus erythematosus. J. Exp. Med., 126:607, 1967.

Kornreich, H. K., and Hanson, V.: The rheumatic diseases of childhood. Curr. Probl. Pediatr., 4:3, 1974.

Krane, S. M.: Joint erosion in rheumatoid arthritis. Arthritis Rheum., 17:306, 1974.

Lawrence, H. S.: Transfer factor and cellular immune deficiency disease. New Eng. J. Med., 283:411, 1970a.

Lawrence, J. S.: Heberden Oration, 1969. Rheumatoid arthritis—nature or nurture? Ann. Rheum. Dis., 29:357, 1970b.

Lessof, M. H.: Immunodeficiency states. Proc. Roy. Soc. Med., 67:530, 1974.

Levin, M., et al.: Immunologic studies of the major non-immunoglobulin protein of amyloid. I. Identification and partial characterization of a related serum component. J. Exp. Med., 138:373, 1973.

Lies, R. B., et al.: Relative T-cell specificity of lymphocytotoxins from patients with SLE. Arthritis Rheum., 16:369, 1973.

Lowenstein, J., and Gallo, G.: Remission of the nephrotic syndrome in renal amyloidosis. New Eng. J. Med., 282:128, 1970.

McDevitt, H. O., and Bodmer, W. F.: Histocompatibility antigens, immune responsiveness and susceptibility to disease. Am. J. Med., 52:1, 1972.

McLaughlin, J. F., et al.: Rheumatic carditis: in vitro response of peripheral blood leukocytes to heart and streptococcal antigens. Arthritis Rheum., 15:600, 1972.

Medsger, T. A., and Masi, A. T.: Survival with scleroderma. II. A life-table analysis of clinical and demographic factors in 358 male U.S. Veteran patients. J. Chron. Dis., 26:647, 1973.

Mery, J. P., et al.: Glomerulonephritis in SLE. New Eng. J. Med., 292:480, 1975.

Messner, R. P.: Clinical aspects of T- and B-lymphocytes in rheumatic disease. Arthritis Rheum., 17:339, 1974.

Miller, R. G., and Phillips, R. A.: Development of B-lymphocytes. Fed. Proc., 34:145, 1975.

Morris, P. J.: Histocompatibility in organ transplantation in man. Pathol. Annu., 3:1, 1973a.

Morris, P. J.: Histocompatibility in organ transplantation. Ann. Roy. Coll. Surg. Eng., 53:324, 1973b.

Myburgh, J. A., et al.: Hyperacute rejection in human kidney allografts—Shwartzman or Arthus reaction. New Eng. J. Med., 281:131, 1969.

Nishikai, M., and Homma, M.: Anti-myoglobin antibody in polymyositis. Lancet, 2:1205, 1972.

Opelz, G., et al.: HL-A and kidney transplants: reexamination. Transplantation, 17:371, 1974.

Osserman, E. F.: Amyloidosis and plasma cell dyscrasia. In Grabar, P., and Miescher, P. A. (eds.): Immunopathology. IVth International Symposium, Montecarlo. New York, Grune and Stratton, Inc., 1965.

O'Sullivan, J. B., and Cathcart, E. S.: The prevalence of rheumatoid arthritis. Ann. Int. Med., 76:573, 1972.

Owen, R. D.: Immunogenetic consequences of vascular anastomoses between bovine twins. Science, 102:400, 1945.

Paronetto, F., and Koffler, D.: Immunofluorescent localization of immunoglobulins. Complement and fibrinogens in human disease. I. Systemic lupus erythematosus. J. Clin. Inves., 44:1657, 1965.

Paterson, T. Y.: Adjuvants, cell-mediated immune responses and autoimmune disease. J. Reticuloendothel. Soc., 14:426, 1973.

Pearson, C. M.: Polymyositis and dermatomyositis. In Santer, M. (ed.): Immunological Diseases. Boston, Little, Brown & Co., 1971, p. 1039.

Perlmann, P., et al.: Lymphocyte-mediated cytotoxicity in vitro. Induction and inhibition by humoral antibody and nature of effector cells. Transp. Rev., 13:91, 1972.

Phillips, P. E.: Viruses and systemic lupus erythematosus. Am. Heart J., 88:120, 1974.

Piomelli, S.: Antigenicity of human vascular endothelium: lack of relationship to the pathogenesis of vasculitis. J. Lab. Clin. Med., 54:241, 1959.

Rich, A. R., and Gregory, J. E.: The experimental demonstration that periarteritis nodosa is a manifestation of hypersensitivity. Bull. Johns Hopkins Hosp., 72:65, 1943.

Rodnan, G. P. (ed.): Primer on rheumatic diseases: rheumatoid arthritis. J.A.M.A., 224:687, 1973.

Rose, G. A.: The natural history of polyarteritis. Brit. Med. J., 2:1148, 1957.

Rossmann, P., et al.: Histology and fine structure of necrotic renal allografts in man. J. Pathol., 110:177, 1973.

Rothfield, N. F., et al.: Clinical and laboratory aspects of raised virus antibody titers in SLE. Ann. Rheum. Dis., 32:238, 1973.

Russell, P. S., and Winn, H. J.: Transplantation. New Eng. J. Med., 282:786, 1970.

Saunders, M., et al.: Lymphocyte-stimulation with muscle homogenate in polymyositis and other muscle-wasting disorders. J. Neurol. Neurosurg. Psychiatry, 32:569, 1969.

Scheinberg, M. A., and Cathcart, E. S.: B-cell and T-cell lymphopenia in systemic lupus erythematosus. Cell. Immunol., 12:309, 1974.

Scheinberg, M. A., et al.: Thymosin-induced reduction of "null cells" in peripheral blood lymphocytes of patients with SLE. Lancet, 1:424, 1975.

Schur, P., and Sandson, J.: Immunological factors and clinical activity in SLE. New Eng. J. Med., 278:533, 1968.

Schwartz, R. S.: Viruses and systemic lupus erythematosus. New Eng. J. Med., 293:132, 1975.

Seligmann, M., et al.: Studies on antinuclear antibodies. Ann. N.Y. Acad. Sci., 124:816, 1965.

Senyk, G., and Michaeli, D.: Induction of cell-mediated immunity and tolerance to homologous collagen in guinea pigs. Demonstration of antigen-reactive cells for a self antigen. J. Immunol., 111:1381, 1973.

Senyk, G., et al.: Cellular immunity in SLE. Arthritis Rheum., 17:553, 1974.

Shirahama, T., et al.: Fibrillar assemblage of variable segments of immunoglobulin-light chains: an electron microscopic study. J. Immunol., 110:21, 1973.

Smiley, J. D., et al.: In vitro synthesis of immunoglobulin by rheumatoid synovial membrane. J. Clin. Invest., 47:624, 1968.

Smith, C., and Hamerman, D.: Significance of persistent differences between normal and rheumatoid synovial membrane cells in culture. Arthritis Rheum., 12:639, 1969.

Spitler, L. E., et al.: The Wiskott-Aldrich syndrome. Results of transfer factor therapy. J. Clin. Invest., 51:3216, 1972.

Steele, R. W., et al.: Familial thymic aplasia. Attempted reconstitution with fetal thymus in a millipore diffusion chamber. New Eng. J. Med., 287:787, 1972.

Steinberg, A. D.: Pathogenesis of autoimmunity in New Zealand mice. V. Loss of thymic suppressor function. Arthritis Rheum., 17:11, 1974.

Suzuki, Y., et al.: The mesangium of renal glomerulus. Electron microscopic studies of pathologic alterations. Am. J. Path., 43:555, 1963.

Svaifler, N. J.: Rheumatoid synovitis, an extravascular immune complex disease. Arthritis Rheum., 17:297, 1974.

Talal, N.: T and B lymphocytes in peripheral blood and tissue lesions in Sjögren's syndrome. J. Clin. Invest., 53:180, 1974.

Talal, N., and Bunim, J. J.: The development of malignant lymphoma in the course of Sjögren's syndrome. Am. J. Med., 36:529, 1964.

Talal, N., et al.: Extrasalivary lymphoid abnormalities in Sjögren's syndrome (reticulum cell sarcoma, "pseudolymphoma," and macroglobulinemia). Am. J. Med., 43:50, 1967.

Tang, T. T., et al.: Chronic myopathy associated with coxsackievirus Type A9; a combined electron microscopical and viral isolation study. New Eng. J. Med., 292:608, 1975.

Thompson, J. S., et al.: Relationship of mixed lymphocyte culture response, HL-A histocompatibility antigens, and renal transplantation. Transp. Proc., 5:1763, 1973.

Trimble, R. B., et al.: Preliminary criteria for the classification of systemic lupus erythematosus (SLE). Evaluation in early diagnosed SLE and rheumatoid arthritis. Arthritis Rheum., *17*:184, 1974.

Tuffanelli, D. L., and Winkelmann, R. K.: Scleroderma and its relationship to the "collagenoses": dermatomyositis, lupus erythematosus, rheumatoid arthritis and Sjögren's syndrome. Am. J. Med. Sci., *243*:133, 1962.

Von Boxel, J., et al.: Antibody-dependent lymphocyte cell-mediated cytotoxicity: no requirement for thymus derived lymphocytes. Science, *175*:194, 1972.

Weigle, W. O.: Different types of immunological unresponsiveness. Adv. Exp. Med. Biol., *29*:357, 1973.

Whitaker, J. N., and Engel, W. K.: Vascular deposits of immunoglobulins and complement in idiopathic inflammatory myopathy. New Eng. J. Med., *286*:333, 1972.

Wiedermann, G., and Miescher, P. A.: Cytoplasmic antibodies in patients with systemic lupus erythematosus. Ann. N.Y. Acad. Sci., *124*:807, 1965.

Wigley, R. D.: The aetiology of polyarteritis nodosa: a review. New Zealand Med. J., *71*:151, 1970.

Williams, G. M., et al.: "Hyperacute" renal-homograft rejection in man. New Eng. J. Med., *279*:611, 1968.

Williams, R. C., Jr.: Dermatomyositis and malignancy: a review of the literature. Ann. Int. Med., *50*:1174, 1959.

Winkelmann, R. K.: Classification and pathogenesis of scleroderma. Mayo Clin. Proc., *46*:83, 1971.

Yata, J., et al.: Lymphocyte subpopulations in immunodeficiency disorders. I. Human thymus-lymphoid tissue antigen. Clin. Immunol. Immunopathol., *2*:519, 1974.

Yunis, E. J.: Inclusion body myositis. Lab. Invest., *25*:240, 1971.

Zeek, P. M.: Periarteritis nodosa. A clinical review. Am. J. Clin. Path., *22*:777, 1952.

Ziff, M.: Viruses and connective tissue diseases. Ann. Int. Med., *75*:951, 1971.

Ziff, M.: Relation of cellular infiltration of rheumatoid synovial membrane to its immune response. Arthritis Rheum., *17*:313, 1974.

Ziff, M., and Johnson, R. L.: Polymyositis and cell-mediated immunity. New Eng. J. Med., *288*:465, 1973.

CHAPTER 7

Fluid and Hemodynamic Derangements

EDEMA

HYPEREMIA OR CONGESTION

HEMORRHAGE

SHOCK

THROMBOSIS
Microcirculatory Thrombosis — Disseminated
    Intravascular Coagulation

EMBOLISM
Fat Embolism

INFARCTION

Survival of cells and tissues is exquisitely dependent on the oxygen contained within a normal blood supply. What may be less apparent is their dependence on a normal fluid balance. Approximately 70 per cent of man's lean body weight is water. This is divided between the intracellular compartment (50 per cent) and the extracellular compartment (interstitial fluid, 15 per cent; plasma water, 5 per cent). Derangements in either blood supply or fluid balance cause some of the most commonly encountered disorders in medical practice: edema, congestion, hemorrhage, shock, and the three interrelated conditions — thrombosis, embolism and infarction. Not only are these disorders common; they are also major causes of mortality. Pulmonary edema is often the terminal event in nearly any form of heart disease. Hemorrhage and shock are virtually daily problems in the emergency room of any large hospital. Thrombosis, embolism and infarction underlie two of the most important disorders in industrialized nations: myocardial infarction and cerebrovascular accidents (strokes). This chapter, then, deals with predominating mechanisms of morbidity and mortality.

EDEMA

The term *edema* refers to the accumulation of abnormal amounts of fluid in the intercellular tissue spaces or body cavities. It may occur as a generalized or a localized disorder. The term *anasarca* is used when the edema is severe and generalized, producing marked swelling of the subcutaneous tissues. Edematous collections in the various serous cavities of the body are given the special designations *hydrothorax, hydropericardium* and *hydroperitoneum* (more commonly called *ascites*). Noninflammatory edema, such as develops in hydrodynamic derangements, is a transudate, low in protein and other colloids, with a specific gravity usually below 1.012. Inflammatory collections of fluid are rich in proteins (see p. 34) and therefore have a higher specific gravity — usually over 1.018. This difference in specific gravity often provides a valuable diagnostic aid.

Edema is the result of an increase in the forces tending to move fluids from the intravascular compartment into the interstitial fluid. The normal interchange of fluid, as proposed by Starling, is regulated by the hydrostatic and osmotic pressures within and without the vascular compartment. At the arteriolar end of the capillary bed, the hydrostatic pressure is about 35 to 40 mm. Hg. At the venular end it falls to 12 to 15 mm. Hg. The colloid osmotic pressure of the plasma is 20 to 25 mm. Hg. The colloid osmotic tension and hydrostatic pressure of the interstitial fluid within the tissue spaces are relatively small and essentially counterbalance each other. Thus, on the basis of these forces, fluid leaves the microcirculation at the arteriolar end of the capillary bed and returns at the venular end. Maintenance of the integrity of the endothelium is critical in this ebb and flow of fluid. Not all of the fluid in the interstitial spaces returns to the venules; some is drained off through the lymphatics, to be returned to the bloodstream only indirectly.

Generalized edema develops whenever there is: (1) an increase in the hydrostatic pressure of the blood, (2) a decrease in osmotic tension of the blood, or (3) an increase in the osmotic tension of the interstitial fluid, a condition almost always related to sodium retention. These derangements are usually encountered in heart failure or renal disease. The pathophysiology involved is presented in the chapters dealing with these organs (p. 289 and p. 428). Starvation may also produce generalized edema, attributed to the low levels of plasma proteins. However, the severity of the edema correlates poorly with the colloid osmotic pressure of the plasma; loss of fat, atrophy of muscles and the development of loose tissue spaces may contribute. Severe generalized liver disease, such as cirrhosis of the liver, is sometimes accompanied by generalized edema, attributed here to inadequate synthesis of serum proteins. Protein-losing enteropathies and malabsorption syndromes also occasionally cause sufficient hypoproteinemia to induce generalized edema.

Localized edema most often is the result of (1) a local increase in the hydrostatic pressure of the blood, (2) an increase in capillary permeability, or (3) a local obstruction to lymphatic drainage. The two most common causes of localized edema are inflammation, with its increased endothelial permeability, and impaired venous outflow. As discussed in Chapter 2, sites of inflammation are characterized by "tumor" (swelling), which is caused by the escape of intravascular fluid. Very soon plasma proteins leak out and convert the edema fluid to an inflammatory exudate, thus increasing the interstitial osmotic pressure. Impaired venous outflow is most frequently encountered in the lower extremities, secondary to the development of obstructive thromboses (p. 223) or varicosities (p. 278). This leads to an increase in the local hydrostatic pressure. Any blockage or destruction of a group of lymph nodes or lymphatics by neoplastic or inflammatory processes or by surgical procedures causes significant edema in the drainage area involved. Carcinoma of the breast, for example, is frequently treated by removal of the entire breast, the pectoral muscles and the lymph nodes in the axilla. Consequently, postoperative edema in the arm often follows such surgery and sometimes is a very troublesome clinical problem. Perhaps the most graphic example of localized edema due to lymphatic obstruction is produced by the parasitic infection called *filariasis*. In this case the worms gain entrance to the subcutaneous tissues, usually in the feet, drain to the regional nodes in the inguinal region, and there induce massive fibrosis in the lymph nodes and lymphatic channels. The resultant edema of the lower extremities and external genitalia is so extreme it is called *elephantiasis*. Lymphatic channels may be congenitally absent or malformed in a variety of familial disorders. These are discussed further on page 279. One such condition is Milroy's disease, involving lymphatic abnormalities, usually in one or both of the lower extremities, with consequent severe edema of the affected part.

Morphology. The morphologic changes of edema are much more evident grossly than microscopically. Although any organ or tissue in the body may be involved, edema is encountered most often in three sites: the subcutaneous tissues, usually in the lower extremities; the lungs; and the brain.

Subcutaneous edema of the lower parts of the body is a prominent manifestation of cardiac failure, particularly failure of the right ventricle. Although right ventricular failure obviously affects the entire systemic venous return to the heart, edema is most prominent in the lower extremities because they are subject to the highest hydrostatic pressures. If the patient is confined to bed, sacral edema may become evident. **Since the distribution of the edema is influenced by gravity, it is termed "dependent." Edema produced by renal dysfunction** tends to be more severe and usually results from loss of plasma proteins, which lowers the colloid osmotic pressure in the blood. The most extreme instances of hypoproteinemia are found in the **nephrotic syndrome**, caused by a group of renal diseases which involve abnormal permeability of the glomeruli to plasma proteins, with consequent heavy proteinuria (p. 432). All subcutaneous tissues may be affected, particularly in the lower extremities and the loose tissue about the eyes **(periorbital edema)**. Such generalized edema merits the designation **anasarca**. Finger pressure over edematous subcutaneous tissue will squeeze out the fluid and produce pitted depressions, hence the common clinical term **pitting edema.** Incision of edematous subcutaneous tissues will disclose an increased oozing of interstitial fluid, but it is usually slight and difficult to appreciate.

Microscopically, it may be extremely difficult to detect the increase of interstitial fluid in the subcutaneous connective tissue. Occasionally, a fine granular precipitate (a residuum of the trace amounts of protein in the edema fluid) is seen between the separated connective tissue fibers and cells. The cells of edematous tissues (i.e., the epithelial cells, fat cells and muscle cells) may also become enlarged because of increased amounts of fluid, but these changes cannot be detected by simple microscopic examination and require more precise quantitative methods. Dilatation of lymphatics may be present.

The **lungs,** composed of a loose, honeycombed

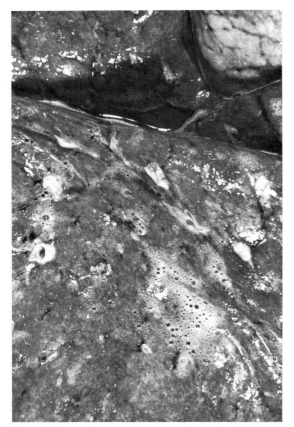

Figure 7–1. Pulmonary edema. A close-up view of the transected surface of a very wet lung, from which frothy edema fluid exudes.

tissue, are particularly susceptible to edema. **Pulmonary edema** is a prominent manifestation of left ventricular failure (Fig. 7–1). These changes are described more fully in the consideration of congestive heart failure on page 289.

Edema of the **brain** is encountered in a variety of clinical circumstances, such as brain trauma, meningitis, encephalitis, hypertensive crises and any form of obstruction to the venous outflow of the brain. This condition is described on page 642.

Solid organs, such as the liver and kidneys, may be involved when edema is systemic in distribution. Such involvement is evidenced only by a slight increase in size and weight, and possibly by some pallor. The capsule may be tense. The changes are rarely sufficiently well marked to be clearly identified by inspection, and the scales provide the most reliable indication. Microscopically, there is only some increase in cell size and in the intercellular spaces, but it is rarely detectable by light microscopy. At the level of the electron microscope, there may be dilatation of the cisternae of the ER and some increase in cell sap between the organelles.

Clinical Correlation. Edema may give rise to only minor clinical problems, or it may be lethal. Edema of the subcutaneous tissues in cardiac or renal failure is important chiefly because it indicates underlying disease, but sometimes it impairs healing of wounds or infections. Since edema of the lungs (pulmonary edema) impairs normal ventilatory function, it may be lethal. The fluid first collects within the alveolar walls around the capillaries, producing an "alveolocapillary block" in oxygen diffusion. The impact on ventilatory function may seem out of proportion to the relatively small amounts of fluid required to produce such a block. In the later stages, when the fluid collects within the alveolar spaces, it creates a favorable soil for bacterial infection, termed *hypostatic pneumonia.* Edema of the brain can be a serious clinical problem and, indeed, may cause death if it is sufficiently marked. The increased mass of brain substance may cause herniation of the cerebellar tonsils into the foramen magnum or may cause shearing stresses on the blood supply to the brain stem. Both conditions secondarily impinge upon medullary centers to cause death.

HYPEREMIA OR CONGESTION

These synonyms refer to a local increased volume of blood caused by dilatation of the small vessels. *Active hyperemia* results from an augmented arterial inflow, such as occurs in the muscles during exercise, at sites of inflammation and in the pleasing neurovascular dilatation termed blushing. *Passive congestion* results from diminished venous outflow such as follows cardiac failure or obstructive venous disease. Thus, in cardiac failure the appearance of edema is almost always accompanied by passive congestion, giving rise to the more appropriate designation *congestion and edema. Chronic passive congestion of the lungs is one of the most reliable postmortem indicators of left ventricular cardiac failure.* When congestion is encountered in the lower extremities, the legs are abnormally cool and either pale, owing to the predominance of edema, or dusky blue-gray, owing to the venous congestion accompanying the edema.

HEMORRHAGE

Hemorrhage obviously implies rupture of a blood vessel. Rupture of a large artery or vein is almost always caused by some form of injury, such as trauma, atherosclerosis or inflammatory or neoplastic erosion of the vessel wall. Rupture of a large artery in the brain is a frequent cause of death in hypertensive patients (Fig. 7–2). An increased tendency to

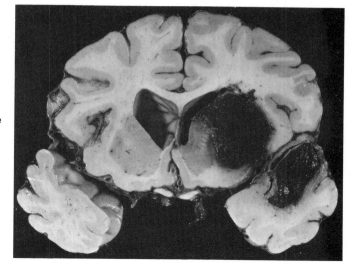

Figure 7–2. A fatal intracerebral hemorrhage in a 65 year old hypertensive male.

hemorrhage is encountered in a wide variety of clinical disorders, known collectively as the *hemorrhagic diatheses*. These are discussed in Chapter 11.

Hemorrhages may be external and exsanguinating. When the blood is trapped within the tissues of the body, the accumulation is referred to as a *hematoma*. Rupture of the aorta, for example, in a dissecting or atherosclerotic aneurysm, may cause a massive retroperitoneal hematoma with sufficient loss of blood to cause death. When the blood accumulates in one of the body cavities it is referred to as *hemothorax, hemopericardium, hemoperitoneum* or *hemarthrosis*. Minute hemorrhages into the skin, mucous membranes or serosal surfaces are known as *petechiae*. Slightly larger hemorrhages are designated *purpura*. When a large (over 1 to 2 cm. in diameter) subcutaneous hematoma appears, it may be called an *ecchymosis*. The common bruise is a good example of an ecchymosis. The released hemoglobin is converted into bilirubin and eventually into hemosiderin. Sometimes when the tissue at the site of the hemorrhage is hypoxic, some of the released hemoglobin is converted to an iron-free, rhombic crystalline brown pigment, *hematoidin*, which is virtually identical chemically with bilirubin. Hematoidin therefore generally is encountered when occlusion of a vessel leads simultaneously to hemorrhage and ischemia, described later as an infarct (p. 227). Patients sustaining a large hemorrhage, such as massive gastrointestinal bleeding, a pulmonary hemorrhage or infarct (p. 228) or a hematoma, sometimes become jaundiced because of the breakdown of red cells and subsequent release of bilirubin.

The significance of hemorrhage depends on the volume of blood loss, the rate of loss and the site of hemorrhage. Sudden losses of up to 20 per cent of the blood volume and slow losses of even larger amounts may have little clinical significance. Larger or more acute losses may induce hemorrhagic (hypovolemic) shock (p. 214). The site of the hemorrhage is, of course, important. A hemorrhage which would be trivial in the subcutaneous tissues may cause death when located in the brain stem. Repeated external hemorrhages (i.e., those in which the blood is shed—as from the skin, gastrointestinal tract or female genital tract) represent losses not only of blood volume but also of valuable iron. Usually the small but repeated volume losses are rapidly corrected by movement of water from the interstitial spaces into the vascular compartment, but the chronic loss of iron may lead to an iron deficiency anemia. In contrast, when the red cells are retained, as occurs with hemorrhages into the body cavities, joints or tissues, the iron can be recaptured for synthesis of hemoglobin.

SHOCK

Shock is best viewed as a constellation of syndromes precipitated by any massive insult to the body, such as profuse hemorrhage, severe trauma or burns, extensive myocardial infarction, cardiac tamponade, massive pulmonary embolism or uncontrolled bacterial sepsis. All of these medical emergencies lead to life-threatening derangements in the homeostasis of all cells in the body. In some instances, as for example profuse hemorrhage, the patient presents an ashen gray pallor, cool clammy skin, weak thready pulse, tachycardia, rapid respiration, obtunded sensorium, oliguria and hypotension. In other circumstances, for example, uncontrolled bacterial sepsis, the patient may have a flushed, warm, dry skin. Occasionally, there is no obtundation and the patient remains alert, oriented and, indeed, anxious. Clearly there is no constant clinical syndrome which characterizes all patients in shock. To find a common denominator one must delve down to the level of cellular metabolic changes. At this level *shock has been defined as a syndrome characterized by "inadequate blood flow to vital organs or the inability of the tissues of these organs to utilize oxygen and other nutrients"* (MacLean, 1972). These derangements lead to a metabolic lactic acidosis, a feature characterizing all forms of shock. The origins of these functional derangements will become evident in the consideration of the pathophysiology of shock.

Classification and Pathophysiology. Many classifications of shock are based on the inciting clinical event, e.g., traumatic shock, surgical shock, septic shock and burn shock. Basically, however, all forms of shock can be divided according to four pathophysiologic mechanisms: (1) hypovolemic shock, (2) cardiogenic shock, (3) septic shock, and (4) neurogenic shock. It is important to emphasize here that each patient is a pathophysiologic tangle unto himself and several mechanisms may contribute to the shock state in the individual patient. Although the fundamental defect may be loss of blood volume (hypovolemic shock), pain may introduce neurogenic mechanisms and bacterial infections may add the element of septic shock.

Hypovolemic shock follows the acute loss of a critical fraction of the plasma volume. The most obvious cause of hypovolemic shock is massive hemorrhage *(hemorrhagic shock)*. The extent of hemorrhage necessary to induce shock varies with the rate of loss, the cardiopulmonary status of the patient prior to shock, the hemoglobin level of the blood and the degree of trauma associated with the hemorrhage. A relatively slow loss of even 40 per cent of the blood volume is better tolerated than an acute loss of 20 per cent. Selective loss of plasma may also cause hypovolemic shock. Plasma volume may be acutely reduced by an outpouring of exudate into an extensive burn or into a large wound, giving rise to the clinical patterns *burn shock, traumatic shock and wound shock.* Blood volume depletion which occurs during surgery, either from hemorrhage, drying of tissues or fluid exudation is referred to as *surgical shock* or sometimes *postoperative shock.*

The fall in blood volume in hypovolemic shock is associated with a diminished venous return to the heart, low central venous pressure, low cardiac output and hypotension. At one time it was postulated that myocardial contractility deteriorated in hypovolemic shock and some vague "myocardial depressant factor" was invoked, but recent studies do not confirm such a mechanism (Forrester et al., 1969). With the loss of blood volume, a train of compensatory mechanisms comes into play. Fluid is mobilized from the extravascular compartment at rates of up to 1 liter per hour (Carey et al., 1971). Vasomotor centers in the medulla are signalled. Depressed vagal activity and augmented sympathetic activity simultaneously increase the force and rate of cardiac contraction and constrict arterioles and veins, increasing the peripheral resistance. If the initial reflex vasoconstriction is prolonged, it is followed in time by fatigue and atony of the resistance vessels (arterioles). When this happens, the peripheral microcirculation dilates. This is augmented by the metabolic acidosis and various vasodilator substances, such as histamine and the kinins. However, sphincteric control of the venous outflow, which is less sensitive to metabolic acidosis, often persists and creates, in effect, a massive stagnant pooling in the capillary and venular beds (Rhoads and Dudrick, 1966). Transudation of plasma results, with further depletion of blood volume.

The lowered blood volume simultaneously leads to the release of increased amounts of the antidiuretic and adrenocorticotropic hormones, as well as aldosterone and catecholamines. The vasomotor activity and the catecholamines reduce the blood flow to the skin, kidneys, muscles and splanchnic viscera, thus shunting blood to the heart and brain. The renal cortex is particularly deprived since reduction in blood flow is accompanied by redistribution in favor of the medulla. Thus, glomerular filtration and urine output are depressed, the latter sometimes to remarkably low levels.

The impaired perfusion of the peripheral tissues has a number of deleterious effects on the cells. Oxygen depletion forces the cell to revert to glycolytic pathways, thus forming large amounts of pyruvic acid. The pyruvate is then converted to lactic acid, and this produces the lactic acidosis referred to earlier (Moss and Saletta, 1974). As with any hypoxic injury the cellular derangements fan out in ever-widening circles. Increased permeability, leakage of sodium into and potassium out of the cell, depletion of ATP and impairment of mitochondrial function, as well as other biomolecular dysfunctions, all follow (Baue et al., 1974). The acidosis throws an increased burden on the lungs; the cellular hypoxia impairs uptake and metabolism of glucose, inducing hyperglycemia; the slowed blood flow and hemoconcentration (when plasma fluid is lost) increase the viscosity of the blood and further impair perfusion; and red cell aggregation and alterations in the clotting factors may lead to hypercoagulability, perhaps with a bleeding diathesis. Other changes might be detailed but it is sufficient to paraphrase Haldane: hypoxia not only stops the machine but also wrecks the machinery.

Cardiogenic, sometimes called central, shock is best considered as "pump failure." Most often it is caused by myocardial infarction and indeed accounts for many of the deaths during the acute phase of this medical emergency. Cardiogenic shock occurs in about 12 per cent of patients who have a myocardial infarct and carries an 80 per cent mortality rate, despite present-day interventions. This form of shock may also result from cardiac tamponade (p. 311), acute arrythmias, surgical or spontaneous damage to the cardiac valves, massive pulmonary embolism, fulminating myocarditis or any other form of severe myocardial injury.

Patients in cardiogenic shock generally are hypotensive as a result of low cardiac output and stroke volume. Most, but not all, have an elevated central venous pressure. Compensatory mechanisms similar to those described in hypovolemic shock are activated. Similarly, sympathetic vasoconstriction with poor perfusion of the peripheral tissues, low urine output, reversion from aerobic to anaerobic metabolism, elevated blood lactate levels and fall in blood pH are all present (Haddy, 1970).

Not all patients with cardiogenic shock have an increased central venous pressure and low cardiac output. Some may have a normal or even high cardiac output, normal or low central venous pressure and a normal or low peripheral resistance (Weil and Shubin, 1968). Much depends on the size of the infarct, duration of the shock and durability of the reflex compensatory mechanisms. With a small infarct, cardiac output may remain normal. *It is apparent, then, that cardiogenic shock may involve more than pump failure,* but whatever the precise pathway the result is impaired cellular perfusion and cellular function (as described in hypovolemic shock).

Septic shock, also known as *gram-negative bacteremic shock or endotoxic shock,* almost always is caused by an uncontrolled blood-borne infection, usually by gram-negative organisms. The common causative organisms are, in order of frequency: *Escherichia coli, Klebsiella* and *Proteus* organisms. The source of these bacteremias is usually an infection in the urinary tract (50 to 60 per cent) or in the gastrointestinal tract (25 to 35 per cent), although postabortion and postpartum infections (5 per cent), burn infections and indeed any infection may also serve as a source for the bacteremia (Hassen, 1973). Occasionally, septic shock follows gram-positive bacteremia—for example, from a staphylococcal infection—and it may then be referred to as *exotoxic shock.*

Understanding of the pathophysiology of septic shock is still incomplete, perhaps because the hemodynamic changes are so inconstant. Some patients develop what is called *hyperdynamic* or *warm shock* while others develop a *hypodynamic state.* The hyperdynamic pattern is generally characterized by hypotension, tachycardia, low to high cardiac output and high to low central venous pressure. As with shock from any cause, there is a lactic acidosis. These patients often have an elevated plasma volume and reduced peripheral resistance, leading to widespread vasodilatation. Thus the skin is warm, dry and flushed, with a ruddy cyanotic hue. No satisfactory understanding of this constellation of findings has been achieved. When administered to animals, endotoxin, a lipopolysaccharide, activates the complement system and vasoactive substances such as anaphylatoxins, histamine, and the kinins, which cause widespread vasodilatation (Weil and Shubin, 1967). It has been suggested that the hypotension and circulatory insufficiency are secondary to the trapping of large volumes of blood in the splanchnic and liver beds, leading to a so-called *stagnant anoxia.* Other explanations of endotoxic shock have been offered; possibly the endotoxin activates the clotting system, leading to disseminated intravascular coagulation (DIC). Indeed, Hardaway and colleagues (1967) contend that DIC is a major factor in the evolution of most forms of shock, particularly septic shock. Whether DIC initiates the shock state or merely perpetuates it is still uncertain. Recently attention has turned toward the possibility that the endotoxin directly damages cells and peripheral organs. Ultrastructural changes in hepatic mitochondria, depression of mitochondrial respiration, impaired membrane transport and a direct deleterious effect upon the heart, kidneys and other organs have been identified in septic shock (White et al., 1973; Baue et al., 1973). According to this view septic shock implies defective oxygen consumption by cells and, conceivably, injury to vasomotor centers secondary to direct bacterial action. Thus, even though organ perfusion may be adequate, the cells may not be able to utilize the oxygen delivered to them. Whatever the precise pathway it is clear that these patients suffer from widespread cellular injury and lactic acidosis similar to that encountered in other forms of shock.

Some patients with septic shock develop a *hypodynamic state,* which strongly suggests hypovolemic shock. They have hypotension, low cardiac output, low central venous pressure, increased peripheral resistance, low urine output and cold, clammy or even cyanotic extremities. Conceivably, in these instances sequestration of blood in the atonic vessels of the splanchnic and liver beds, with loss of effective circulating blood volume, is the dominant mechanism.

Neurogenic shock, although uncommon, is sometimes encountered in patients receiving general anesthetics, spinal anesthesia or epidural blocks. It is postulated that the neural control mechanisms which maintain vascular tone are interrupted. As a result, peripheral resistance is reduced, leading in turn to peripheral pooling and loss of effective circulating blood volume. Shock may also follow severe pain, such as occurs in biliary colic or ureteral colic while passing a calculus. An experimental model of neurogenic shock can be produced in animals. When an extremity is crushed and tourniquets are applied to prevent fluid loss, circulatory collapse may develop. However, if the nerves to the extremity are sectioned before the injury shock does not follow. The mechanisms here are poorly understood and are vaguely attributed to vasodilatation of the peripheral microcirculation. Neurogenic shock is a true circulatory collapse and should not be confused with fainting, which has sometimes also been called neurogenic shock. Perhaps fainting can be considered a mild and very transient form of neurogenic shock, but there is no loss of effective circulating blood volume, except perhaps transiently to the brain, and no alteration in the pumping mechanism. Indeed, the trigger is often the mere sight of blood.

At this point it is necessary to clarify an inappropriate term—*irreversible shock.* It has been applied to the progressive hemodynamic deterioration that sometimes follows the acute phase of shock and leads to death despite all efforts to reverse the process by treatment (Lillehei et al., 1964). The concept derives from experiments on dogs. It has been shown that if a dog is bled to shock levels and the blood is not replaced for approximately 4 hours, about 95 per cent of the animals will develop shock which cannot be reversed despite return of all of the shed blood. Earlier replacement of the blood usually brings about complete recovery of the animal. Some patients, after a period of time in shock, develop a similar refractory state of circulatory failure and many die despite heroic therapeutic efforts. Often death results from the inability to control the basic disease responsible for the onset of the shock. The patient who has a massive myocardial infarct followed by cardiogenic shock has a grave prognosis because the loss of myocardial function is irreversible. In others the persistence of uncontrollable sepsis leads to the progressive circulatory deterioration. But even in the absence of such well-defined causes a downward spiral sometimes supervenes. Fine and associates (1959) propose that when any form of shock has been present for some time, gram-negative endotoxins are released from the injured gut into the circulation. Since the damaged liver cannot clear these endotoxins, an element of endotoxic shock is added to the underlying derangement. Others maintain that DIC is responsible for the later deterioration, and still others postulate the release of lysosomal enzymes from hypoxic tissues (Janoff et al., 1962). Perhaps the simplest explanation is that cellular hypoxia and widespread cellular damage convert the microcirculation into a sponge with an unlimited capacity to sequester and leak the already diminished blood volume. Despite these speculations, *no patient is in irreversible shock until he dies,* and indeed, some patients for whom hope had waned eventually walked out of the hospital.

Morphology of Shock. Abnormal changes may be found in virtually any tissue or organ of the patient in shock, but the most prominent lesions are encountered in the lungs, kidneys, adrenals, heart, liver and gastrointestinal tract (McGovern, 1971).

The **lungs** manifest a variety of pathologic changes, including congestion, interstitial edema, intra-alveolar edema and, rarely, hyaline membrane formation. These changes are collectively referred to as "shock lung." The lungs are usually heavy, red and boggy. Secondary infection may create foci of bronchopneumonic consolidation. The edema may accumulate only within the alveolar wall. It is proposed that the collagen within the alveolar septa develops an increased affinity for sodium, followed by an increased affinity for water (Moss et al., 1973), but increased capillary permeability undoubtedly contributes to the development of edema (Teplitz, 1968). This is sometimes accompanied by lifting of the alveolar lining cells from the underlying basement membrane. Occasionally scattered microthrombi are found in proximity to these septal changes. Whatever the mechanism, the interstitial edema reduces the pliability of the septal walls and so gives rise to the "stiff lung syndrome," as well as to an alveolocapillary block. When intra-alveolar fluid accumulates it not only worsens the respiratory deficit but also provides a fertile soil for bacterial infection. The cause of the development of hyaline membranes along the alveolar septa is a controversial subject. They may result from leakage of fibrinogen from abnormally permeable septal capillaries, but many patients are administered relatively pure concentrations of oxygen, and the hyaline membranes may be a consequence of oxygen toxicity (Soloway et al., 1969).

The **kidneys** are especially vulnerable to the injurious effects of shock and indeed acute renal failure is one of the most important late causes of death from severe shock. Morphologic changes begin within about 24 hours and become more marked over the next 7 to 10 days in the more severe cases. The renal lesion has been known by a host of terms, of which the most widely used is **acute tubular necrosis (ATN)**. Older designations include shock kidneys, hypoxic nephrosis, lower nephron nephrosis and hemoglobinuric nephrosis. ATN embraces two distinctive patterns: (1) ischemic injury, the common form encountered in shock, and (2) a nephrotoxic pattern, usually caused by toxic agents which damage tubular epithelial cells. Both forms are discussed in greater detail on page 446. Our principal interest here is the hypotensive or ischemic pattern, also designated **tubulorrhexis** by Oliver and his associates (1951). The kidneys may be relatively normal in gross appearance, or the cortex may appear pale and swollen, in contrast to red, dusky pyramids. Histologically a variety of tubular changes may be present, ranging from swelling of the epithelial cells to fatty change, frank necrosis and even complete disruption of the tubule with fragmentation of its basement membrane (hence the designation "tubulorrhexis"). These tubular alterations are distributed randomly throughout the kidney but principally affect the terminal portions of the proximal convoluted tubules and the distal convoluted tubules. They have been attributed to vasoconstriction and shunting of blood from cortex to medulla and to ischemia. Similar damage may be found in the loops of Henle

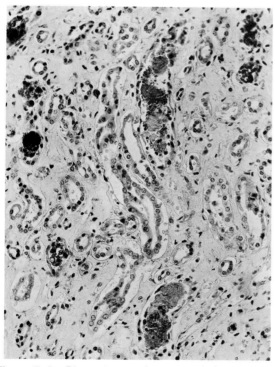

Figure 7–3. Pigment casts in acute tubular necrosis occupy many of the collecting tubules. The tubular epithelial cells are in disarray as a result of cellular necrosis followed by regeneration.

and sometimes in the collecting tubules. Casts within tubules are prominent features of ATN. These take the form of hyaline, proteinaceous or pigment casts most often deposited in the distal convoluted and collecting tubules (Fig. 7–3). The pigment is most often hemoglobin but may be myoglobin if there has been a crushing injury.

The ultrastructural changes in the damaged tubular epithelial cells consist of mitochondrial swelling and other degenerative changes in these organelles, microvacuolation of the ground substance of the cytoplasm, and swelling and distortion of the endoplasmic reticulum. **Focal tubular basement membrane rupture and destruction are prominent changes seen with the electron microscope.** Interstitial edema, mild to pronounced, is usually one of the most striking features of the lesion during the acute phase. Interstitial aggregates of mononuclear inflammatory cells, including lymphocytes, plasma cells and histiocytes, often appear about the tubulorrhectic foci. To this point, the changes described relate to the acute phase of the renal lesions. After about seven to 10 days, the interstitial edema begins to subside and the mononuclear infiltrates slowly disappear. The most striking change is the regeneration of tubular cells, which can lead to complete restoration of the preexisting architecture during the following weeks.

The glomeruli are unaffected in most cases of shock. However, in endotoxic shock, thromboses within glomerular capillaries are sometimes encountered, presumably as a manifestation of DIC (Dalgaard, 1960). Infrequently patients in shock develop bilateral cortical necrosis, in which there is necrosis of almost the entire cortex. This fatal complication usually implies the development of DIC (p. 363).

The **adrenals** play a prominent role in the response of the body to any form of stress. During adaptation to shock, the lipids stored in the cortical cells are mobilized, and the usual vacuolated cells filled with stored lipids are transformed to a nonvacuolated, actively metabolic state. Although the lipids appear to be depleted, this is not a regressive alteration; rather, it is a reflection of synthesis of steroids in response to an increased demand. These changes constitute, in essence, the reaction of the adrenals to all forms of stress. Scattered necrosis of isolated cortical cells may create apparent lumina or "pseudotubules."

The **intestines** may develop striking changes, sometimes designated as **ischemic enterocolitis** or **acute hemorrhagic enteropathy**. There may be involvement of any part of the gut from jejunum to rectum, but the sites of predilection are the splenic flexure and descending colon. Even in an affected segment of intestine the lesions may be focal, appearing initially on the summits of the mucosal ridges. The macroscopic changes take the form of edema and thickening of the intestinal wall, accompanied by hemorrhagic congestion or even su-

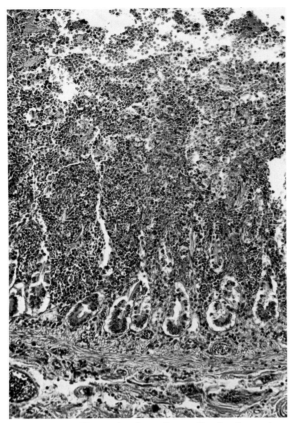

Figure 7–4. Hemorrhagic enteropathy in the colon. The superficial mucosa is entirely obscured by the extensive hemorrhage; only the bases of the colonic glands are visible. The submucosa is unaffected.

perficial ulceration and shedding of the mucosa. The microscopic changes may be relatively minor (focal dilatation of submucosal capillaries and venules, accompanied by submucosal edema) or more extensive (hemorrhagic extravasation of red cells and in some cases massive hemorrhage and necrosis of the mucosal lining cells) (Fig. 7–4). In some cases thrombi are found within the massively distended vessels. It should be noted that the muscularis and serosa are usually unaffected, differentiating this lesion from infarction (Ming, 1965). These intestinal changes have been attributed to underperfusion of the intestines. Presumably the lowered effective circulating blood volume induces splanchnic vasoconstriction, followed in time by loss of vasomotor tone possibly resulting from the tissue hypoxia or release of vasoactive amines. Extreme vasodilatation and hemorrhagic necrosis ensue. In passing, it might be noted that similar changes may be encountered in states of low cardiac output (severe cardiac failure or arrhythmias). In these cases antecedent treatment with large doses of digitalis or norepinephrine may in some way potentiate the development of the intestinal lesions.

Many **other organs** develop pathologic changes during shock. Fatty change appears in the myocardial fibers and may even be accompanied by focal necrotizing lesions. The liver cells may develop fatty change beginning in the center of the lobules and sometimes extending throughout the entire lobule. The brain, because of its extreme vulnerability to oxygen deficit, may suffer widespread neuronal injury, referred to as **anoxic** or **hypoxic encephalopathy** (p. 647). It is this neuronal damage which accounts for the obtundation or even coma sometimes encountered in shock patients. When DIC supervenes, many other organs may be affected, including the pituitary, pancreas and skin.

Clinical Course. The course of the patient in shock is beset with hazards and pitfalls at every step. The initial phase, lasting about 36 hours, is usually dominated by the inciting medical, surgical or obstetric event. During this phase the circulatory failure and peripheral hypoxia threaten death from cerebral ischemia or cardiac failure. If these hazards are avoided, metabolic acidosis, shifts in electrolyte levels and pulmonary edema rear their ugly heads. Indeed, the lungs may become a critical target organ. The metabolic acidosis leads to compensatory hyperventilation and in some patients to a subsequent respiratory alkalosis. However, often the respiratory compensatory effort is largely unsuccessful, in part because of a decreased tidal volume, the increased work of air exchange and increased arteriovenous pulmonary shunting. The excessive effort to achieve a given level of alveolar ventilation is attributed to the "stiff lung syndrome" (Proctor et al., 1970).

A second phase, dominated by renal dysfunction, may appear anytime from the second to the sixth day. *Reduction of the renal blood flow* to as low as 10 per cent or less of the cardiac output (normal, 25 per cent) occurs in all forms of shock (Strauch et al., 1967). Urine output falls dramatically, often to only a few milliliters per day. The oliguria, a classic clinical feature of shock, may last only a few days or may persist for as long as 3 weeks; indeed, the severity of the oliguria is a good parameter of the severity of the shock state and of the effectiveness of therapy. The clinical picture now is dominated by the signs and symptoms of uremia, fluid overload, hyperkalemia and acidosis. Fortunately, ATN is reversible and with appropriate therapy most patients can be maintained during the period of renal shutdown and fully recover from this phase.

The third or diuretic phase is ushered in by a steady increase in urine volume, reaching possibly 3 liters per day over the course of a few days. This urinary flood heralds the regeneration of the tubular epithelium, but because it is still incomplete, tubular function is imperfect and serious electrolyte imbalances may occur. There also appears to be an increased vulnerability to infections during this phase, and about 25 per cent of deaths from ATN occur during the diuretic phase.

If these hazards are successfully overcome the patient may be expected to improve progressively. Indeed, with modern methods of care, patients who do not die of the precipitating catastrophe have an excellent chance of recovering from shock. Implicit in this prognosis is the ability to control the primary cause of the shock. Thus, patients with hypovolemic and traumatic shock have a better prognosis than those with cardiogenic or septic shock, in whom the fatality rate may be as high as 70 to 80 per cent.

THROMBOSIS

The formation, in blood vessels or the heart, of a blood clot is known as thrombosis, and the mass itself is termed a thrombus. Blood clotting, which may be life-saving when it plugs a severed vessel, may be life-threatening when it occurs within the intact vascular system and occludes a vessel supplying a vital structure. In addition, some part or all of the thrombus may break loose to create an *embolus* that flows downstream to lodge at a distant site. Thrombosis and embolism are then closely interrelated, as is indicated by the commonly used

term *thromboembolism.* The potential consequence of both thrombosis and embolism is ischemic necrosis of cells and tissue, known as *infarction.* First we shall consider the subject of thrombosis and in later sections embolism and infarction.

Pathogenesis. Thrombosis is basically intravascular clotting. As is well known, the maintenance of the fluidity of the blood is one of the most delicately balanced of the homeostatic mechanisms. Involved are forces predisposing to clotting and preventive influences. A standard diagram of the clotting sequence and some of the protective influences is offered in Figure 7–5.

There is considerable controversy over the precise steps involved in the formation of a thrombus and the events which initiate this sequence. There is general agreement, however, that *three influences are important: (1) local injury to arteries, veins or the heart, (2) stasis or turbulence of blood flow, and (3) alterations (hypercoagulability) of the blood itself.* Any one of this triad may play a dominant role in the individual instance, but probably at least two are required to induce a thrombus.

Vascular injury plays a dominant role in the formation of thrombi in arteries and in the heart. This is amply documented by the fact that thrombi on the arterial side of the circulation almost invariably are located at sites of inflammatory injury of vessels or atherosclerotic damage to arterial walls, and within cardiac

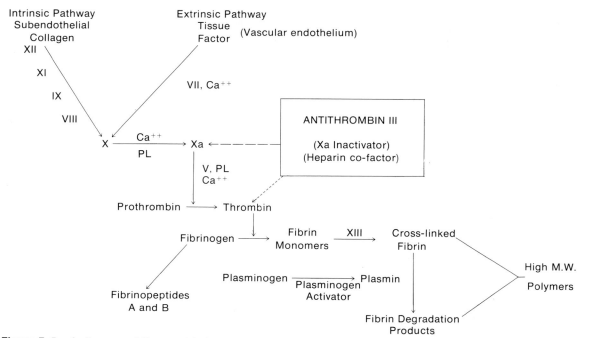

Figure 7–5. A diagram of the coagulation and fibrinolytic system emphasizing the role of inhibitors to activated clotting factors. Ca^{++}, calcium; PL, phospholipid; and Xa, activated factor X. From Handin, R. I.: Thromboembolic complications of pregnancy and oral contraceptives. Progr. Cardiovasc. Dis. *16*:395, 1974.

chambers contiguous to myocardial infarcts or other forms of endocardial injury. Moreover, the formation of a clot in the severed end of any vessel is clear documentation of the role of vascular injury in initiating thrombosis. Although the precise sequence of events is still somewhat controversial, most of the evidence suggests that *following endothelial cell injury, platelets adhere to subendothelial collagen or to recently described noncollagenous microfibrils to create a platelet nidus* (Stemerman et al., 1971). Other pathways which might lead to adherence of platelets have been elegantly detailed by Jorgensen (1971). They include release of adenosine diphosphate (a potent initiator of platelet aggregation) from damaged endothelial cells, exposure of basement membrane by damage to endothelial cells and widening of interendothelial cell junctions. Adenosine diphosphate (ADP) is also released from damaged red cells, as well as from the adherent platelets, and this augments the buildup of the platelet nidus. The initial aggregation of platelets is reversible and dissociation might occur were it not for intercurrent events. Small amounts of thrombin are formed which induce a so-called "release reaction" in platelets, which leads to their irreversible aggregation. Two pathways may be involved in the generation of thrombin: (1) activation of Hageman factor (XII) by exposed collagen, which triggers the intrinsic pathway, or (2) release of tissue factor (thromboplastin) from injured endothelium, involving the extrinsic pathway (Zeldis et al., 1972). Other possible inducers of the "release reaction" are ADP, catecholamines, serotonin and polymerizing fibrin (Jorgensen, 1971). The "release reaction" involves rupture of platelet membranes, with release of intraplatelet granules, lysosomal enzymes, more ADP and intraplatelet fibrinogen. The released lysosomal enzymes are of particular interest since they may contribute to further endothelial injury. Thus, a number of factors come into play which potentiate the buildup of a platelet mass. Thereafter, with the formation of thrombin, fibrin is laid down to complete the development of the intravascular clot. *The evolution of a thrombus thus begins with the adherence of platelets at sites of vascular injury, followed by the buildup first of a reversible aggregation of platelets, then the formation of an irreversible platelet mass, in turn leading to the standard clotting sequence, possibly through both the intrinsic and extrinsic pathways.*

Homeostatic mechanisms protect against such intravascular clotting. Activated clotting factors are cleared in the liver. The naturally occurring antithrombin III not only inhibits the action of thrombin but also inhibits activated factor X. Inactivation of factor X is of great importance since even small amounts generate massive amounts of fibrin in an autocatalytic reaction. Fibrin, once precipitated, absorbs large amounts of thrombin, which retards the continued polymerization of fibrinogen. Perhaps the most important of the protective mechanisms is the fibrinolytic system. Activated plasmin (fibrinolysin) not only digests fibrin but also yields fibrin split products, which have anticoagulant effects (Deykin, 1970). It is indeed fortunate that there are such protective mechanisms against thrombosis when one considers the innumerable trivial injuries encountered daily.

Stasis and turbulence constitute the second feature of the triad. Although vessel injury may trigger platelet aggregation, it is unlikely that a larger mass could build up without alteration in the normal blood flow. It has been observed repeatedly in the experimental animal that although a small thrombus may begin in an injured vessel, it is swept off and fails to evolve unless there is concomitant alteration in flow. Both turbulence and stasis bring the formed elements of the blood, such as platelets, into contact with the endothelial surface. *Stasis probably plays a dominant role in veins because of their low velocity flow.* Hume and associates (1970) have elegantly documented the origin of venous thrombi in the sinuses behind valve cusps. Presumably small aggregates of platelets accumulate here and initiate blood clotting. A similar phenomenon probably occurs in the auricular appendages of the heart when there is atrial fibrillation or massive dilatation of the atria as, for example, with mitral stenosis. In contrast, in the usual high velocity flow of the heart and arteries, turbulence and the development of vortices assume major importance. The shear stress on the intimal surface created by friction has been shown to deform or even destroy the endothelial lining (Fry, 1969). Conceivably, ADP is released from mechanically damaged platelets and red cells. Thus, thrombi are prone to develop where the intima is most damaged, e.g., in arteries with atherosclerotic roughening of their intimal surfaces and in abnormal dilatations of arteries and the heart wall, known as *aneurysms.*

Stasis alone, however, probably will not trigger the formation of a coagulum. Wessler (1968) pointed out that, in the experimental animal, careful sequestration of a length of a vein between ligatures did not result in thrombosis. In his experimental model, he found it necessary to activate the clotting mechanism simultaneously. When he induced hypercoagulability within the isolated segment by the injection of aged serum (which he postulates contains some thrombus inducing factor), thrombosis followed.

Hypercoagulability, the third component of

the triad, although strongly suspected, has proved to be an elusive phenomenon to confirm in man. It can be demonstrated easily in the test tube and can be established fairly clearly in the laboratory animal. It has been defined as "a state in which activated clotting factors normally absent from circulating blood are either released from tissue directly into the circulation or are formed intravascularly" (Wessler, 1971). Support for its existence derives from the relative rarity of thromboses among patients with congenital marked deficiencies of specific clotting factors, the prophylactic efficacy of anticoagulant drugs and documented elevations of clotting factors in the plasma of patients subject to thromboses. For example, it has been shown that patients during the first postpartum month or those taking antiovulatory drugs having a high estrogen content (both situations associated with a thrombotic tendency) have increases in factors VII and X. Likewise, a number of changes have been identified in the blood of postoperative patients who are also known to have an increased risk of venous thrombosis. These include an increased number of platelets, increased platelet adhesiveness, increased concentrations of fibrinogen and factor VII and a shortened clotting time of whole blood or plasma (Ygge, 1970). There are, however, a number of objections to inferring hypercoagulability from these alterations in the blood. Thromboses have been observed in patients with low levels of factors I, V, VII, VIII and XII. In fact, John Hageman, the proband of Hageman factor deficiency, died from a pulmonary embolus (Ratnoff et al., 1968). During pregnancy, particularly in the third trimester, elevations of the same coagulation factors found in the immediate postpartum period occur, yet the incidence of thromboses within the leg veins is five to six times higher during the first postpartum month than during the antepartum period. Adjusting for the difference in time intervals the risk of developing venous thrombosis increases approximately 50 times during the first month after delivery. Wessler (1971) suggests that perhaps· the explanation of these discordant observations lies in the fact that the mere *levels* of the clotting factors are not important, but rather the determining element is the level of *activated* factors. In support of this view, he has shown that trace amounts of activated factor X are much more potent in inducing hypercoagulability than relatively massive amounts of unactivated factor X. However, there are not many studies on levels of activated clotting factors in patients who subsequently develop a thrombosis. In summary, then, the phenomenon of hypercoagulability may indeed be valid and not yet confirmed in man because appropriate parameters have not been measured.

Morphology of Thrombi. Thrombi may develop anywhere in the cardiovascular system: in the chambers of the heart, arteries, veins or capillaries. All are essentially intravascular clots, the composition, size and shape of which are dictated by their site of origin. Those arising in the arterial side of the circulation (including the heart) differ somewhat from those arising in the venous side. Arterial or cardiac thrombi usually begin at a site where there is turbulence of flow either because of some lesion or where a vessel bifurcates or branches. Classically the arterial thrombus is a dry, friable tangled gray mass which on transection usually discloses darker gray lines of aggregated platelets interspersed between paler layers of coagulated fibrin. These lamellations are known as the **lines of Zahn.** Because they are largely composed of platelets and fibrin, **arterial thrombi are known as white or conglutination thrombi.** When arterial thrombi arise in the capacious chambers of the heart or in the aorta they are usually applied to one wall of the underlying structure and thus are termed **mural thrombi.** Mural thrombi also develop in abnormal dilatations of arteries (aneurysms). In arteries smaller than the aorta the thrombus usually builds up rapidly until it completely obstructs the lumen, producing a so-called **occlusive thrombus.** Any artery may be affected, but the most common and most important sites of involvement in order of frequency are: coronary, cerebral, femoral, iliac, popliteal and mesenteric arteries. **Unless otherwise designated the use of the term "thrombus" implies the occlusive type.**

Venous thrombosis, also known as **phlebothrombosis,** is almost invariably occlusive. In fact, the thrombus often creates a long cast of the lumen of the vein. In the slower moving blood of the veins, the coagulation simulates that in a test tube. Thus, these thrombi have a much richer admixture of erythrocytes and are therefore known as **red, coagulative** or **stasis thrombi.** On transection laminations are not well developed, but tangled strands of fibrin can usually be seen. **Phlebothrombosis most commonly affects the veins of the lower extremities (90 per cent) in approximately the following order of frequency: deep calf, femoral, popliteal and iliac veins.** Less commonly venous thrombi may develop in the periprostatic plexus, or the ovarian and periuterine veins (Hume et al., 1970). Rarely, they occur in the portal vein or its radicles or in the dural sinuses.

Coagulation thrombi can be readily confused with postmortem clots at autopsy. The postmortem clot forms a cast of the vessel, but it is rubbery and gelatinous. The dependent portions of the clot where the red cells have settled by gravity tend to resemble dark red "currant jelly." The supernatant, free of red cells, has a yellow "chicken fat" appearance. Characteristically the postmortem clot is not attached to the underlying wall. In contrast, coagulation thrombi are more firm, almost always have a point of attachment, and on transection disclose tangled strands of pale gray fibrin.

Arterial and venous thrombi vary enormously in size. They range from small, irregular, roughly spherical masses to enormously elongated, snake-like structures which are formed when a long tail builds up behind the occluding head. In the arterial circulation the tail builds up retrograde to the direction of flow. On the venous side the tail extends in the direction of the blood flow, i.e., toward the heart. Often such propagations extend to the next major vascular branch.

A small or large area of attachment to the underlying vessel or heart wall is characteristic of all thromboses. Frequently the attachment is most firm at the point of origin, and the propagating tail may or may not be attached. It is this loosely attached tail which, in veins, is most likely to fragment to create an embolus. On the arterial side of the circulation, embolization usually implies detachment of the entire or almost the entire thrombus.

In special circumstances thrombi may be deposited on the heart valves. Blood-borne infections may attack heart valves (**bacterial** or **infective endocarditis**), creating ideal sites for the development of thrombotic masses. These masses, laden with microorganisms, are referred to as vegetations. Less commonly, noninfective, **verrucous endocarditis** may appear in patients who have systemic lupus erythematosus (p. 187). Wasted, gravely debilitated patients who have disseminated cancer or another chronic fatal disease may develop aseptic thrombotic vegetations on their heart valves termed **marantic vegetations.** In this condition hypercoagulability of the blood is invoked as the causative mechanism.

If a patient survives the immediate effects of vascular obstruction what happens to the thrombus over the course of days and weeks? One of the following sequences evolves: (1) the thrombus may propagate and eventually cause obstruction of some critical vessel, (2) it may embolize, (3) it may be removed by fibrinolytic activity, or (4) it may undergo organization and become recanalized — that is, incorporated within the vessel wall. The first two eventualities need no further comment here. There is evidence that fibrinolytic removal may occur. By angiography, pulmonary thromboemboli have been observed to shrink rapidly and even be totally lysed soon after their development (Sabiston, 1968). Such a happy outcome usually occurs within the first day or two, presumably because as the thrombus ages and the fibrin undergoes continued polymerization, it is more resistant to proteolysis. This sequence implies that the patient survives the immediate insult and retains a fairly adequate level of blood flow in the environs of the thrombotic mass. Blood flow past the thrombus may well be maintained since fresh thrombi contract slightly, providing a narrow slit-like channel through which blood may flow. If fibrinolysis does not occur within the first few days it is unlikely to take place later.

When a thrombus persists in situ for a few days it incites an inflammatory reaction in the underlying vessel or cardiac wall. The catalytic enzymes released from platelets may contribute to the injury and consequent inflammatory reaction. Fibroblasts and capillary buds invade the thrombus, producing a more firm anchorage. The ingrowth eventually works its way along the entire length of the mass. In the course of time, perhaps over a period of weeks to months, the thrombus undergoes **organization** and is transformed to firm connective tissue. Not infrequently, the newly formed capillary channels interconnect to create thoroughfares from one end of the thrombus to the other, through which blood may flow, reestablishing to some extent the continuity of the lumen of the original vessel. This process is known as **recanalization** of the thrombus (Fig. 7–6). In time the exposed surfaces of the thrombus become covered by endothelium, and to a large extent, therefore, the mass becomes incorporated into the vessel wall as a permanent

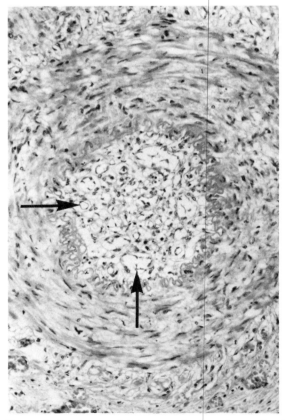

Figure 7–6. A completely organized and canalized thromboembolus within an artery. The newly formed connective tissue is perforated by numerous vascular channels, several of which are marked by arrows.

residuum. Nonetheless, blood flow is reestablished by the recanalization process. Occasionally, instead of becoming organized, the center of a thrombus undergoes lytic digestion to produce so-called **puriform** (resembling pus) **softening.** This sequence is particularly likely in large thrombi within aneurysmal dilatations or within the mural thrombi of the heart. It hardly needs to be pointed out that if a bacteremia occurs, such puriform softening is an ideal culture medium, which may convert the thrombus into a septic mass of pus.

Clinical Correlation.   The clinical implications of thromboses are: (1) *they cause obstruction of arteries and veins,* and (2) *they provide possible sources of emboli.* Venous thrombi pose somewhat different threats from those arising in the arterial side of the circulation. Pulmonary embolization is their most feared consequence. While this disorder is discussed in more detail on pages 226 and 380, it suffices to say here that it is often fatal. Venous thrombosis may, of course, cause occlusive disease and thus block venous drainage. Clinically significant venous obstruction due to occlusive thrombosis is encountered most often in the deep veins of the legs or the portal vein. Portal vein thrombosis is considered on page 533.

Occlusive thrombosis of leg veins may affect the major outflow vessels or superficial varicosities. The latter may be painful and disabling and cause slight edema of the foot and lower leg, but only rarely do they embolize. However, the edema and impaired venous drainage predispose the skin to infections from slight trauma and to the development of varicose ulcers. When major outflow vessels (such as the popliteal, femoral or iliac veins) are affected, edema of the leg and distention of the more distal veins often develop. In addition, pain and tenderness on compression of the calf muscles *(Homan's sign)* may be present because most of these thrombi arise in the muscular veins of the lower leg. However, clinical studies indicate that Homan's sign is not a reliable indicator of deep vein thrombosis, since many patients without thrombi present this finding and others with thrombi do not. Indeed, recent studies using special techniques such as the administration of labeled fibrinogen for the demonstration of thrombi disclose that only one third to one sixth of patients present signs and symptoms of their thromboses. At one time it was postulated that patients who had local pain and tenderness had *thrombophlebitis,* whereas those with silent lesions had *phlebothrombosis.* Thrombophlebitis was conceived of as some mysterious primary inflammatory disease of the veins secondarily causing thrombosis. It was held that thrombophlebitis was a less grave disorder since the primary inflammation was

likely to induce firm attachment of the thrombus, lessening the risk of embolization. It is apparent now, however, that since thrombi themselves initiate an inflammatory reaction in the underlying vein wall the distinction between phlebothrombosis and thrombophlebitis is artificial.

As mentioned earlier, the most serious aspect of venous thrombosis is its potential for giving rise to emboli. *Pulmonary embolization is a major contributing cause of death in 10 to 20 per cent of all hospital deaths.* Thrombosis of the deep veins of the calf muscles or the major outflow veins of the leg (popliteal, femoral and iliac) is referred to as *deep venous thrombophlebitis,* and is the source of 95 per cent of pulmonary emboli. The patients at greatest risk of suffering such vascular complications are described in the following paragraphs.

Clinical correlates associated with venous thrombosis are: advanced age, prolonged bed rest, immobilization, cardiac failure, severe trauma or burns, postoperative and postpartum states, disseminated cancer and, in fact, all serious illnesses. Although controversy persists, as will soon be made clear, most of the evidence suggests that the use of oral contraceptive pills also increases the risk of venous thrombosis. Advanced age, bed rest and immobilization all contribute to the hazard, probably because there is increased stasis of blood in the veins of the lower leg with reduced physical activity. The muscles of the leg facilitate venous return by their milking action. Indeed, relatively young individuals have been known to develop venous thrombi after long plane flights or with prolonged standing. Cardiac failure is an obvious cause of sluggish venous circulation. All forms of trauma, particularly fractures of the hip and burns, increase the likelihood of phlebothrombosis. Trauma usually implies reduced activity, injury to vessels and possibly hypercoagulability of the blood. Hip fractures almost always occur in the elderly and often require prolonged bed rest and immobilization. In a series of 125 injured and burned patients, Sevitt (1962) encountered the following: 65 per cent of all patients had venous thrombi; of those with thrombi 74 per cent had involvement of the veins of the calf, 70 per cent had pelvic or thigh vein thrombi and 37 per cent had popliteal vein involvement. The increased vulnerability of postoperative patients to thrombosis is clearly documented in a recent report from England indicating that as many as 61 per cent of elderly postoperative patients had phlebothrombosis (Flanc et al., 1968). Surgery inevitably traumatizes vessels; most patients are elderly and some may have cardiac failure.

Thrombosis is so common during the first

postpartum month that it has received the specific designation *"milk-leg"* or *phlegmasia alba dolens* (painful white leg). It must be admitted that the explanation of this increased vulnerability still eludes us, as was discussed on page 221. Could the trauma of labor contribute? All is speculative, but the hazard is unmistakable.

Few subjects have aroused more impassioned controversy in the literature than the relationship of oral contraceptive pills to thrombosis. This controversy is treated in greater depth on page 240. Here it is sufficient to say that opinions encompass those contending that there is no enhanced risk of thrombosis with the use of "the pill" and the view that the incidence of thrombosis is increased. The weight of evidence favors the latter opinion. A recent large-scale prospective study initiated by The Royal College of General Practitioners in England indicates, in an interim report, a five- to six-fold increased incidence in the users of oral contraceptives (Royal College of General Practitioners, 1974; Editorial, 1974). There is also an impressive array of retrospective reports which indicate an increased risk of thrombosis associated with the use of contraceptive pills. Drill (1972), among others, however, points out that retrospective studies do not provide critical evidence since they can only suggest a possible association but not prove a causal relationship. Moreover, a well designed recent prospective study in Puerto Rico found no increased risk associated with the use of oral contraceptives (Fuertes-de la Haba et al., 1971). So the controversy persists.

Patients with cancer are likely to develop venous thrombi. Trousseau first called attention to this relationship, hence it is sometimes known as *Trousseau's sign.* At first, the increased frequency of venous thrombosis was thought to be restricted to pancreatic and other deeply situated abdominal cancers. It now appears to be characteristic of all forms of cancer and has been attributed to the release of tissue factors from necrotic tumors, affecting blood coagulability. At one time this entity was dignified by the name *"migratory thrombophlebitis,"* but it is doubtful whether it represents more than a thrombotic diathesis.

When thrombi arise in the cardiac chambers, aorta or aneurysmal dilatations, they are almost always of the mural type. Thus, they do not constitute occlusive disease, but they do often yield fragments which embolize. The principal sites of lodgment of such emboli are: (1) brain, (2) kidneys, (3) legs, and (4) spleen. Although it must be admitted that any tissue or organ may be affected, the brain and kidneys constitute prime targets because of the large volume of blood flow to these organs. The iliac, femoral and more distal arteries are vulnerable because they represent the terminus of the aortic flow. Embolization of course carries the risk of infarction, as is discussed in a later section (p. 227).

Thrombosis of atherosclerotic coronary, cerebral or renal arteries or of the major arteries of the leg accounts for some of the gravest consequences of atherosclerosis. One need only recall that coronary thrombosis plays an important role in the pathogenesis of myocardial infarction, the most common cause of death in industrialized nations.

Thrombi in the arterial side of the circulation are particularly likely to develop in patients with myocardial infarction, rheumatic heart disease, florid atherosclerosis and aneurysmal dilatations of the aorta or other major arteries (Fig. 7–7). Myocardial infarction usually is associated with damage to the adjacent endocardium, providing a site for the origin of a thrombus. Stasis and turbulence within the affected cardiac chamber are usually present because of dyskinetic contraction of the myocardium or the development of cardiac irregularities. Advanced age, bed rest and impaired circulation add further hazards.

Florid atherosclerosis, particularly common in diabetes mellitus, and aneurysmal dilatations are prime contributors to the develop-

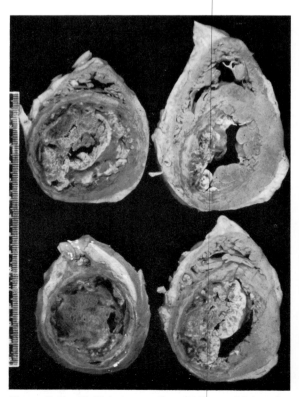

Figure 7–7. Multiple transections of the ventricles of a heart with a recent myocardial infarction. The left ventricle is virtually filled with thrombus, particularly toward the apex of the heart.

ment of thromboses within the arterial circulation. In aneurysms the thrombus often fills the abnormal dilatation up to the original level of the vessel wall. Not infrequently prominent laminations can be seen on cross section of such thrombi, and surprisingly the freshest thrombus may be deeply situated adjacent to the aneurysmal wall. Presumably as the thrombus forms it contracts, providing a small slit-like dead space which can refill with blood and thrombose.

Although many "high risk" clinical disorders have been cited, it should be made clear that thrombosis may occur in any clinical setting. Indeed, thrombosis and consequent embolism sometimes occur in otherwise healthy, active young individuals with no apparent provocation. This is an unpredictable, puzzling disorder of quixotic nature.

MICROCIRCULATORY THROMBOSIS—DISSEMINATED INTRAVASCULAR COAGULATION (DIC)

In many disease states minute thrombi develop in widely dispersed sites within arterioles, capillaries and venules, hence the designation DIC. The thrombi are largely platelet aggregates, perhaps admixed with some fibrin. They are rarely visible grossly and are detected only on microscopic examination. Mustard and Packham (1970) have shown that platelets can be rendered more adhesive and more vulnerable to aggregation by endotoxins, immune complexes, viruses, catecholamines, serotonin, trypsin and thrombin. Once platelets are activated they release platelet factor 3, a surface phospholipid which triggers or accelerates the coagulation mechanism. Microcirculatory thrombosis, therefore, is encountered in any situation in which enhanced platelet adhesiveness comes into play. It is best considered, then, as a complication of many disorders and a mechanism involved in many diseases rather than an entity unto itself. The clinical settings in which DIC is encountered range from obstetric complications to immune reactions, infections, extensive burns, trauma and a host of other entities. This subject is considered in more detail on page 363. Because random capillary beds may be affected, DIC can induce serious clinical dysfunction as well as tissue damage, but rarely infarction.

EMBOLISM

Embolism refers to occlusion of some part of the cardiovascular system by the impaction of a foreign mass (embolus) *transported to the site through the bloodstream.* The great majority of emboli represent some part or the whole of a dislodged thrombus, hence the commonly used term *thromboembolism.* Much less commonly, embolization is produced by droplets of fat, undissolved air or gas bubbles, tumor fragments, bits of bone marrow or any other foreign substance that gains entry to the bloodstream (such as a bullet). Collectively, these unusual forms of embolism account for less than 1 per cent of all instances, and so, unless otherwise indicated, embolism is considered to be thrombotic in origin.

Embolism may occur within either the venous or the arterial system. *In approximately 95 per cent of instances, venous emboli arise from thrombi* within the veins of the leg in the locations previously mentioned (p. 221). They drain through progressively larger channels, usually pass through the right heart and become lodged in the pulmonary circulation (Fig. 7–8). Regrettably, not one but many emboli may become dislodged, often at recurrent intervals. Thus, the patient who has one pulmonary embolus has a high risk of having more. Indeed, at times the pulmonary circula-

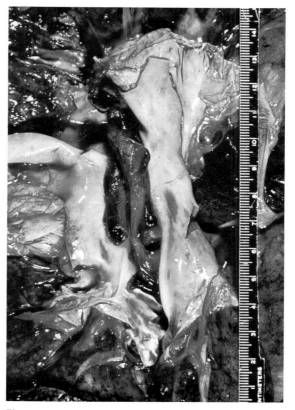

Figure 7–8. The opened major pulmonary arteries in the root of the lung. A large, coiled embolus having the diameter of one of the large veins in the leg was the cause of the sudden death of this patient.

tion is peppered by a shower of small fragments. Rarely, a large, snakelike mass may become coiled upon itself and lodge in one of the valvular orifices of the right side of the heart. Alternatively, it may impinge on the bifurcation of the main pulmonary artery and sit astride the two major subdivisions, thus creating a *saddle embolus*. The size of the vessel occluded obviously depends on the size of the mass. Very infrequently, when congenital malformations of the heart produce right-to-left shunts, venous emboli may enter the left heart chambers and thus gain access to the arterial system. This phenomenon is known as *paradoxical embolism*.

Pulmonary embolism is the most serious form of thromboembolic disease. It is an extremely common clinical problem. Fresh pulmonary emboli have been identified in approximately one fourth to one third of unselected autopsies on patients dying in general hospitals (Freiman, 1965; Freiman et al., 1965; Davis and Sasahara, 1968; Morrell and Dunnill, 1968). It was thought to be the major or contributing cause of 10 to 20 per cent of hospital deaths and the most common cause of sudden unexpected death (Smith et al., 1965; Kucera, 1968; Roberts, 1963). However, not all pulmonary emboli are fatal. Much depends on the size of the occluded vessel and on the status of the patient's cardiovascular system. Large emboli are often fatal because they produce massive strain on the right side of the heart (*acute cor pulmonale*), or sudden severe hypoxemia as the blood flow to the pulmonary capillary system is blocked. Death may be literally instantaneous, with insufficient time for ischemic damage to the pulmonary tissues to develop. Fortunately, however, many pulmonary emboli, even though large, permit some flow about their margins and then contract sufficiently to enhance the flow, ultimately becoming resolved (Soloff and Rodman, 1967). This sequence usually is encountered in the young patient who is capable of withstanding the initial assault (Sabiston, 1968), but there are no accurate data on its frequency. It is therefore important to recognize that *the consequence of embolism is not always infarction nor even lasting occlusion of a vessel* (Fred et al., 1966). Smaller emboli may pass into one of the second or third order branches of the pulmonary arterial system to cause either *pulmonary hemorrhage* or *pulmonary infarction*. In younger patients with good cardiac function, the bronchial circulation may be sufficient to maintain the vitality of the lung tissue, even though the pulmonary arterial supply is cut off. Intra-alveolar hemorrhage is then the result. In the patient with marginal or inadequate cardiac function, the bronchial circulation does not suffice to keep the tissues alive, and infarction occurs. It should be noted, therefore, that *pulmonary embolism is not synonymous with pulmonary infarction*. The clinical implications of this often catastrophic pulmonary complication are discussed in greater detail in Chapter 12.

Arterial emboli most commonly arise from intracardiac mural thrombi. Less often they take origin from mural thrombi in an aortic aneurysm or from those overlying atherosclerotic plaques in the aorta or some other large artery. Infrequently, arterial emboli arise from fragmentation of a vegetation on a heart valve (discussed in more detail on page 229). Occlusive thrombi in arteries of medium to small size rarely embolize, since they are usually firmly lodged at their sites of origin. In contrast to venous emboli, arterial masses usually follow a shorter pathway, since they travel through vessels of progressively diminishing caliber. The site of lodgment depends to a considerable extent on the point of origin of the thromboembolus and the volume of blood flow through an organ or tissue. The consequences of such embolism are somewhat dependent on the richness of the vascular supply of the affected tissue, its vulnerability to ischemia and the caliber of the vessel occluded. These considerations are dealt with on page 229.

FAT EMBOLISM

Occlusion of some part of the microcirculation by minute fat globules can be demonstrated morphologically in 90 to 100 per cent of patients who die following a fracture, whether or not the fracture is the cause of death (Sevitt, 1966). It is especially common with fractures of the shafts of the long bones, which have fatty marrows. There is good evidence that the fat gains access to the circulation by rupture of the marrow vascular sinusoids and indeed sometimes the fat globules are accompanied by bits of bone marrow bearing hematopoietic cells (*marrow emboli*). Despite the frequency of fat embolism with fractures, only rarely are there signs or symptoms attributable to the microembolism.

When fat embolism produces clinical symptoms it presents in one of two patterns: a pulmonary syndrome or a central nervous system syndrome. The size of the fat globules determines which of the two syndromes will appear. When the individual globules are relatively large they are trapped in the lungs. Dyspnea (difficulty in breathing), tachypnea (increased respiratory rate), tachycardia, cyanosis and, in extreme cases, death may follow. If the emboli are smaller, they pass through the lung circulation and are distributed throughout the arterial circulation, where they tend to produce untoward effects only in the brain. The brain disturbance is manifested by anxiety, restlessness and confusion, perhaps progressing to coma and even death. Both syndromes may be accompanied by a petechial skin rash (Editorial, 1972).

Fat embolism sometimes can be demonstrated as a histologic finding in the absence of trauma. It has been described in association with pancreatitis, osteomyelitis, diabetes, prolonged treatment with steroids and burns. In these circumstances it is usually an incidental autopsy finding and has not caused clinical manifestations. It is postulated that the stress incurred by the underlying disease alters the blood in some way, leading to coalescence of fat chylomicrons (Tedeschi et al., 1968; Tedeschi et al., 1971). Presumably it is the quantity and size of the fat emboli which determine their clinical significance, and it appears that fracture of bones introduces more and larger fat emboli.

Whatever the setting, the demonstration of fat emboli in tissues requires special techniques using frozen sections and fat stains, because the emboli are dissolved out of vessels by the usual solvents employed in paraffin embedding of tissues. Sometimes the microemboli can be identified in the gross specimen by gentle pressure on fresh tissue slices under saline. This releases minute droplets of fat that float to the surface.

The phenomenon of embolization is of theoretic significance since it demonstrates the capacity of showers of microemboli to induce widespread microcirculatory derangements and sometimes death. However, for reemphasis, the mere histologic demonstration of fat globules in tissues has no clinical significance since even quite severe embolism may be without effect.

INFARCTION

An infarct is a localized area of ischemic necrosis within a tissue or organ produced by occlusion of either its arterial supply or its venous drainage. Nearly all infarcts result from thrombotic or embolic occlusion, but rarely infarction may be caused by other mechanisms, such as ballooning of an atheroma secondary to hemorrhage within a plaque. Other rare causes include twisting of an organ, such as the ovary or a loop of bowel, compression of the blood supply of a loop of bowel in a hernial sac or trapping of a viscus under a peritoneal adhesion. In these last mentioned situations the veins alone or both the veins and arteries may be blocked, but often the final occlusive episode is thrombotic closure of the already narrowed vessel. However, vascular occlusion does not always product infarction, as will become clear later.

Nearly 99 per cent of infarcts are caused by thromboembolic events and almost all are the result of arterial occlusions. Emboli arising in the heart or major arteries must impact in arteries. Similarly, venous thromboemboli lodge in the pulmonary arterial system and so cause arterial infarcts. Although venous thrombosis may cause infarction of some tissue or organ, more often it merely induces venous obstruction. Usually bypass channels develop, providing some outflow from the area, which in turn permits some improvement in the arterial inflow. Infarcts are more likely in organs having a single venous outflow channel, such as the testis and ovary.

Infarcts are crudely divided into two types — white (anemic) and red (hemorrhagic). This differentiation is quite arbitrary and is based merely upon the amount of hemorrhage which occurs in the area of infarction at the moment of vascular occlusion. This in turn depends on the solidity of the tissue involved and on the type of vascular compromise (venous or arterial). Most infarcts in solid organs result from arterial occlusion and are white or pale. The solidity of the tissue limits the amount of hemorrhage into the area of ischemic necrosis. **The heart, spleen and kidneys exemplify solid, compact organs that develop white or pale infarcts. In contrast, the lung usually suffers hemorrhagic or red infarction** (Fig. 7–9). This loose, spongy organ permits blood to collect in the infarct from the anastomotic capillary circulation in the margins of the necrotic area. Hemorrhagic infarction is also encountered in those organs in which the venous outflow is limited to the obstructed vessel and in which bypass channels cannot develop. The ovary and the testis are the best examples of such. The entire ovarian blood supply and outflow passes through the mesovarium, and the testicular venous drainage traverses the spermatic cord. A twist in either of these organs may occlude only the thin-walled venous outflow tract. Similarly, hemorrhagic venous infarction may be encountered in loops of the intestine or in the brain (from bilateral occlusion of the jugular veins). Another uncommon mechanism for hemorrhagic infarction of the brain deserves passing mention. An arterial embolus may impact in a large artery such as the middle cerebral and induce a large area of nonhemorrhagic infarction. Subsequently, the embolus may shatter and the small fragments may move onward into smaller vessels, permitting "reflow" and hemorrhage into the primary area of ischemia.

All infarcts, red and white, tend to be wedge-shaped, with the occluded vessel at the apex and the periphery of the organ forming the base. Sometimes the margins are quite irregular, reflecting the pattern of vascular supply from adjacent vessels. When the base is a serosal surface, there is often a covering fibrinous exudate. At the outset, all infarcts are poorly defined and slightly hemorrhagic. In solid organs in which the lesions have relatively little hemorrhage, the contained red cells are laked and the released hemoglobin either diffuses out or is transformed to hemosiderin. **Thus, in the course of approximately 48 hours, infarcts in solid organs become progressively more pale and more sharply delimited** (Fig. 7–10). In spongy organs, such as the lungs, too many red cells are present to permit the lesion ever to become pale. The infarct is at first spongy and cyanotic (red-blue). Over the course of a few days, it becomes more firm and brown, reflecting the development of hemosiderin pigment. The margins of both types of infarcts, in the course of a few days, become progressively better defined. The delimitation is produced by the fibroblastic wall demarcating the destroyed tissue from the surrounding vital substance. Fibrosis progressively extends inward and converts the lesion to a scar that is usually much smaller than the fresh infarct because of the contraction of the fibrous tissue (Sheehan and Davis, 1958 and 1959). The time required for such organization depends on the size of the lesion.

The dominant histologic characteristic of infarction is ischemic coagulative necrosis of affected cells (page 23). It should be noted, however, that if the patient dies immediately after

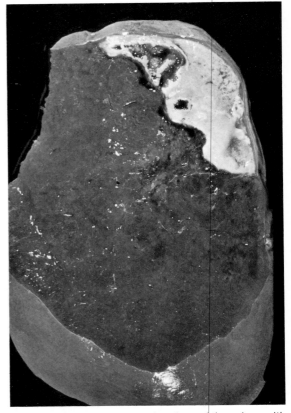

Figure 7–10. The transected surface of the spleen with a one-week-old pale, sharply demarcated infarct. One portion has undergone cystic softening.

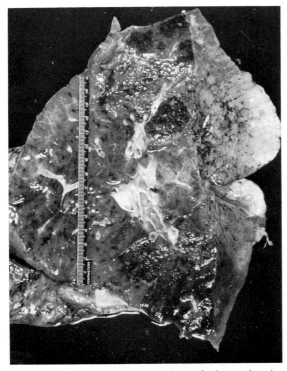

Figure 7–9. The transected surface of a lung, showing several dark hemorrhagic infarcts most evident at the apex and lower right. The infarction is recent and poorly demarcated from the adjacent, preserved lung substance.

having sustained the infarction, insufficient time may have elapsed to permit the enzymic alterations in cells that follow cell death. Thus, for example, in sudden death after myocardial infarction both light and electron microscopy may disclose no demonstrable cytologic or histologic changes in the heart. The dynamic sequence and time required for the appearance of changes following cell death have been described in Chapter 1, to which reference should be made for an understanding of this important consideration. In hemorrhagic or red infarcts, the suffusion of red cells often seems to obliterate the native underlying architecture. In this connection, the pulmonary hemorrhage is distinguished from an infarct by preservation of the native structure. Only the alveolar spaces are filled with red cells; the alveolar walls, blood vessels and stroma are preserved.

Most infarcts are ultimately replaced by scar tissue, which often contains hemosiderin and occasionally hematoidin pigment as residua of the broken down red cells. In the present usage of the term infarct, regeneration is not possible even though the parenchymal cells affected have such capability, because all structures, including fibroblastic stroma and framework, are destroyed. Thus, an infarct implies a more destructive lesion than ischemic necrosis of only parenchymal cells, in which stroma and framework are preserved. The time required for repair of an infarct depends on many factors, particularly on the size of the lesion, the adequacy of the still preserved blood supply supporting the fibroproliferative response, and the availability of the nutrients required for the proliferation of fibroblasts and blood vessels.

When an infarct is produced by an infected embolus (**septic embolus**), as may occur with a fragment of a bacterial vegetation from a heart valve, or when organisms of bacteremic origin seed the area of devitalized tissue, the infarct virtually is converted to an abscess.

Factors Conditioning the Development of an Infarct.
Occlusion of an artery or vein may have little or no effect on the involved tissue, or it may cause death of the tissue, and indeed of the individual. *The major determinants include: (1) the nature of the vascular supply, (2) the rate of development of the occlusion, (3) the vulnerability of the tissue to hypoxia, and (4) the oxygen carrying capacity of the blood.*

Nature of Vascular Supply. The availability of an *alternative or newly acquired source of blood supply* is perhaps the most important factor in determining whether occlusion of a vessel will cause damage.

As was indicated previously, blockage of a small radicle of the pulmonary arterial tree may be without effect in a young person having a normal bronchial circulation. The same applies to the liver, with its double blood supply of hepatic artery and portal vein. In the young, healthy individual, occlusion of one point in the circle of Willis may be without effect if the patient's vessels are not narrowed by preexistent disease. Infarction or gangrene of the hand or forearm is almost never encountered, because of the double arterial supply through the radial and ulnar arteries, with their numerous interconnections. Such could occur only if both major arteries were simultaneously occluded.

Newly acquired *collateral circulation* may be equally effective in preventing infarction. The coronary arterial supply to the myocardium is an excellent case in point. Small anastomoses normally exist between the three major coronary trunks—i.e., the left anterior descending, the left circumflex and the right coronary arteries. If one of these trunks is slowly narrowed, as by an atheroma, these anastomoses may enlarge sufficiently to prevent infarction, even though the major coronary artery is eventually occluded. Such collateral circulation is of great importance in understanding the pathogenesis of myocardial infarction; this topic is discussed in greater detail on page 293.

Rate of Development of Occlusion. Slowly developing occlusions are less likely to cause infarction since they provide an opportunity for alternative pathways of flow and anastomotic bypass channels to develop. The rate of development is of particular importance in instances in which the occlusion is preceded by atherosclerotic narrowing of the vessel, as in the heart. One may find, therefore, a totally occluded coronary artery without an infarct in the dependent myocardium. Presumably the stenosis developed very slowly before the final thrombotic episode. Obviously embolic occlusions occur acutely and thus tend to have more serious consequences.

Vulnerability of Tissue to Hypoxia. The susceptibility of the tissue to hypoxia conditions the likelihood of infarction. Ganglion cells of the nervous system undergo irreversible damage when deprived of their blood supply for 3 to 4 minutes. When microcirculatory occlusion is produced in the heart and there is no blood supply at the level of the individual muscle fiber, not even from collateral channels, myocardial cells die within approximately 5 minutes. In contrast, the fibroblasts within the myocardium are unaffected and are quite resistant to hypoxia. The epithelial cells of the proximal renal tubules are much more vulnerable to hypoxia than are the other segments of the nephron.

The functional activity of a tissue influences its vulnerability to ischemia. If a large artery of the lower leg is occluded, infarction (in this setting termed *gangrene*), can sometimes be prevented by cooling the leg to lower the metabolic needs of the tissue. In contrast, there is no rest for the heart, and the best that can be accomplished is to strive for basal levels that bring supply and demand into closer balance.

Oxygen Carrying Capacity of Blood. The *oxygen level of the blood* will obviously be of significance in determining the effect of vascular occlusion or narrowing. The anemic or cyanotic patient tolerates arterial insufficiency less well than does the normal patient. Occlusion of a small vessel might lead to an infarction in those so handicapped, whereas it would be without effect at normal levels of oxygen transport. In this way, cardiac decompensation with its circulatory stasis and possibly reduced levels of oxygen saturation of the blood contribute to, and indeed may be critical in, determining whether the patient with a pulmonary arterial occlusion will develop only a pulmonary hemorrhage or an infarction.

Clinical Correlation.
Infarction of tissues underlies some of the most frequent as well as most serious clinical disorders. The two most common forms of infarction are myocardial and pulmonary. The primary cause of death today in the United States and in other industrialized nations is coronary heart disease, and the great preponderance of these deaths re-

sult from myocardial infarction. Less awesome, but still gravely significant, is pulmonary infarction. Many large surveys cite it as responsible for death in one in every seven hospitalized patients. Infarction of the brain (encephalomalacia) (p. 651) is another very common "infarct killer." Infarction of the small or large intestine happily is not a common disease, but when it does occur, it is frequently fatal. Less grave, but nonetheless productive of clinical signs and symptoms and possibly of serious disease, are renal and splenic infarcts.

Infarctions tend to have a special gravity because they are most common in patients least able to withstand them. Thus, infarcts tend to occur in aged individuals with advanced atherosclerosis or cardiac decompensation. The postoperative and postdelivery periods are also times of increased vulnerability. The anemic or cyanotic patient is often fragile and poorly prepared for further insult. Thus, the triad of thrombosis, embolism and infarction resembles the proverbial vultures always hovering over the heads of those least able to withstand the attack.

REFERENCES

Baue, A. E., et al.: Impairment of cell membrane transport during shock and after treatment. Ann. Surg., *178*:412, 1973.

Baue, A. E., et al.: Cellular alterations with shock and ischemia. Angiology, *25*:31, 1974.

Carey, L. C., et al.: Hemorrhagic shock. Curr. Probl. Surg., *3*:48, January, 1971.

Dalgaard, O. Z.: An electron microscopic study on glomeruli in renal biopsies taken from human shock kidney. Lab. Invest., *9*:364, 1960.

Davis, W. C., and Sasahara, A. A.: Management of pulmonary embolism in the postoperative patient. Surg. Clin. N. Amer., *48*:869, 1968.

Deykin, D.: Local and systemic factors in the pathogenesis of thrombosis. Calif. Med., *112*:31, 1970.

Drill, V. A.: Oral contraceptives and thromboembolic disease. J.A.M.A., *219*:583, 1972.

Editorial: Fat embolism. Lancet, *1*:672, 1972.

Editorial: Oral contraceptives and health. Lancet, *1*:1147, 1974.

Fine, J., et al.: The bacterial factor in traumatic shock. New Eng. J. Med., *260*:214, 1959.

Flanc, C., et al.: The detection of venous thrombosis of the legs using I-125 labelled fibrinogen. Brit. J. Surg., *55*:742, 1968.

Forrester, J. A., et al.: Dissociation between myocardial contractility and pump performance in hemorrhagic shock. Circulation, *40* (Suppl. 3):81, 1969.

Fred, H. L., et al.: Rapid resolution of pulmonary thromboemboli in man. J.A.M.A., *196*:1137, 1966.

Freiman, D. G.: Pathologic observations on experimental and human thromboembolism. *In* Sasahara, A. A., and Stein, M. (Eds.): Pulmonary Embolic Disease. New York, Grune & Stratton, 1965.

Freiman, D. G., et al.: Frequency of pulmonary embolism in man. New Eng. J. Med., *272*:1278, 1965.

Fry, D. L.: Certain chemorheologic considerations regarding the blood vascular interface with particular reference to coronary artery disease. Circulation, *39/40* (Suppl IV):38, 1969.

Fuertes-de la Haba, A., et al.: Thrombophlebitis among oral and nonoral contraceptive users. Obstet. Gynec., *38*:259, 1971.

Haddy, F. J.: Pathophysiology and therapy of the shock of myocardial infarction. Ann. Int. Med., *73*:809, 1970.

Handin, R. I.: Thromboembolic complications of pregnancy and oral contraceptives. Progr. Cardiovasc. Dis., *16*:395, 1974.

Hardaway, R. M., et al.: Intensive study and treatment of shock in man. J.A.M.A., *199*:779, 1967.

Hassen, A.: Gram negative bacteremic shock. Med. Clin. N. Amer., *57*:1403, 1973.

Hume, M., et al.: Venous Thrombosis and Pulmonary Embolism. Cambridge, Mass., Harvard University Press, 1970, p. 25.

Janoff, A., et al.: Pathogenesis of experimental shock. IV. Studies on lysosomes in normal and tolerant animals subjected to lethal trauma and endotoxemia. J. Exp. Med., *116*:451, 1962.

Jorgensen, L.: Mechanisms of thrombosis. Pathobiology Annual, *1*:139, 1971.

Kucera, M.: Some problems of venous thromboembolism in patients with heart disease. Rev. Czech. Med., *14*:1, 1968.

Lillehei, R. C., et al.: The nature of irreversible shock: Experimental and clinical observations. Ann. Surg., *160*:682, 1964.

McGovern, V. J.: Shock. Pathol. Annu., *6*:279, 1971.

MacLean, L. D.: Shock: causes and management of circulatory collapse. *In* Sabiston, D. C., Jr. (ed.): Textbook of Surgery. Philadelphia, W. B. Saunders Co., 1972, p. 67.

Ming, S. C.: Hemorrhagic necrosis of the gastrointestinal tract and its relation to cardiovascular status. Circulation, *32*:332, 1965.

Morrell, M. T., and Dunnill, M. S.: The postmortem incidence of pulmonary embolism in a hospital population. Brit. J. Surg., *55*:347, 1968.

Moss, G. S., and Saletta, J. D.: Traumatic shock in man. New Eng. J. Med., *290*:724, 1974.

Moss, G. S., et al.: Effect of hemorrhagic shock on pulmonary interstitial sodium distribution in the primate lung. Ann. Surg., *177*:211, 1973.

Mustard, J. F., and Packham, M. A.: Thromboembolism — a manifestation of the response of blood to injury. Circulation, *62*:1, 1970.

Oliver, J., et al.: The pathogenesis of acute renal failure associated with traumatic and toxic injury. Renal ischemia, nephrotoxic damage and ischemuric episode. J. Clin. Invest., *30*:1307, 1951.

Proctor, H. J., et al.: An analysis of pulmonary function following non-thoracic trauma with recommendations for therapy. Ann. Surg., *172*:180, 1970.

Ratnoff, O. D., et al.: The demise of John Hageman. New Eng. J. Med., *279*:760, 1968.

Rhoads, J. E., and Dudrick, S. J.: Hypovolemic shock. Postgrad. Med., *39*:3, 1966.

Roberts, G. H.: Venous thrombosis in hospital patients: a post mortem study. Scot. Med. J., *8*:11, 1963.

Royal College of General Practitioners: Oral contraceptives and health: an interim report from the Oral Contraception Study of the Royal College of General Practitioners. London, Pittman Medical, 1974, p. 98.

Sabiston, D. C.: Pulmonary embolism. Surg. Gynec. Obstet., *126*:1075, 1968.

Sevitt, S.: Venous thrombosis and pulmonary embolism. Am. J. Med., *33*:703, 1962.

Sevitt, S.: The boundaries between physiology, pathology, and irreversibility after injury. Lancet, *2*:1203, 1966.

Sheehan, H. L., and Davis, J. C.: Complete permanent renal ischemia. J. Path. Bact., *76*:569, 1958.

Sheehan, H. L., and Davis, J. C.: Patchy permanent renal ischemia. J. Path. Bact., *77*:33, 1959.

Smith, G. T., et al.: Post mortem quantitative studies of pulmonary embolism. *In* Sasahara, A. A., and Stein, M. (Eds.): Pulmonary Embolic Disease. New York, Grune & Stratton, 1965.

Soloff, L. A., and Rodman, T.: Acute pulmonary embolism. Am. Heart J., *74*:710, 1967.

Soloway, H. B., et al.: Adult hyaline membrane disease. Relationship of oxygen therapy. Ann. Surg., *168*:937, 1969.

Stemerman, M. B., et al.: The subendothelial microfibril and platelet adhesion. Lab. Invest., *24*:179, 1971.

Strauch, M., et al.: Effects of septic shock on renal function in humans. Ann. Surg., *165*:518, 1967.

Tedeschi, C. G., et al.: Fat macroglobulinemia and fat embolism. Surg. Gynec. Obstet., *126*:83, 1968.

Tedeschi, L. G., et al.: Fat particles in plasma. The macroglobule: its relevance to the concept of fat embolism. Hum. Pathol., *2*:165, 1971.

Teplitz, C.: The ultrastructural basis for pulmonary pathophysiology following trauma. J. Trauma, *8*:700, 1968.

Weil, M. H., and Shubin, H. S.: Diagnosis and Treatment of Shock. Baltimore, Williams & Wilkins Co., 1967.

Weil, M. H., and Shubin, H. S.: Shock following acute myocardial infarction. Current understanding of the hemodynamic mechanism. Progr. Cardiovasc. Dis., *11*:1, 1968.

Wessler, S.: Experimental thrombosis. Clin. Obstet. Gynec., *11*:197, 1968.

Wessler, S.: The role of hypercoagulability in venous and arterial thrombosis. Cardiovasc. Clin., *3*:1, 1971.

White, R. R., et al.: Hepatic ultrastructure in endotoxemia, hemorrhage and hypoxia: emphasis on mitochondrial changes. Surgery, *73*:525, 1973.

Ygge, J.: Changes in blood coagulation in fibrinolysis during the post operative period. Am. J. Surg., *119*:225, 1970.

Zeldis, S. M., et al.: Tissue factor (thromboplastin): localization to plasma membranes by peroxidase-conjugated antibodies. Science, *175*:766, 1972.

CHAPTER 8
Environmental Pathology

In this day of awakened interest in ecology, the deteriorating environment and its impact on health are of ever greater concern. The world-wide problems of overpopulation, air pollution, shortages of food and potable water and dwindling sources of energy threaten the survival of the human race. The array of diseases in which environmental influences play a role is almost limitless and primarily includes all those of microbiologic, nutritional and toxicologic origin, as well as those resulting from physical injury. A select few, which involve obvious environmental impact, are presented here under these headings: physical injuries, chemical injuries and nutritional disorders.

PHYSICAL INJURIES

Physical energy in its many forms (mechanical violence, changes in atmospheric pressure, changes in temperature and electromagnetic energy) is responsible for a staggering number of injuries and deaths. Mechanical violence such as occurs in automobile accidents is, of course, the most common form of physical injury. The resultant traumatic lesions, e.g., hematomas, contusions, lacerations and fractures, are too varied to describe here, but account for an enormous morbidity and mortality, particularly in affluent nations. Among the other forms of injury produced by physical energy, only thermal burns and overexposure to radiation are of sufficient frequency and gravity to merit further consideration.

THERMAL BURNS

Although theoretically burns are totally preventable, year in and year out they continue to be important causes of morbidity and mortality. They are particularly lamentable because very often children and young adults are involved. Their clinical significance depends on two factors: the proportion of the body surface involved and the depth of the burn. The *extent* of a burn is generally expressed as a percentage of the total body surface as judged by the use of topographic tables. With regard to their *depth*, burns are divided into "partial-thickness" or "full-thickness" lesions. Partial-thickness burns may be further subdivided into first degree and second degree categories.

The *local and immediate effects* of burns stem not only from destruction of cells and tissue, but also from resultant microcirculatory changes (Shea et al., 1973). With *first degree burns,* such as occur with a sunburn, only superficial layers of the epidermis are devitalized. With *second degree burns* the epidermis is destroyed, but some of the skin appendages remain viable. With all partial-thickness burns a characteristic inflammatory response ensues in the dermis, marked by congestion and increased permeability in the microcirculation, accompanied by varying intensities of leukocytic exudation. Full-thickness burns, also referred to as *third degree burns,* are characterized by destruction of at least the epidermis and dermis, including all of the dermal appendages from which reepithelialization can occur. Deeper structures may, of course, also be affected. Restoration of the epidermis in full-thickness burns usually requires skin grafting. Microcirculatory changes in the base of a full-thickness burn are more intense. The inflammatory response is located in the most superficial layer of the viable tissue, be it subcutaneous fat and fibrous, or muscle.

Fluid losses resulting from the burn may well have greater significance than the loss of cells and tissue. Increased vascular permeability may be due to direct damage to vessels. However, the release of the vasoactive chemical mediators of the inflammatory response (such as histamine and the kinins), which lead to increased permeability and exudation, is often more important. With first degree burns, the inflammatory exudation may be limited to trivial blisters, but deeper burns may weep copiously for days. There is, in addition, considerable evaporation of water from large denuded wounds. The loss of fluids, plasma proteins and electrolytes may be trivial or life-threatening, depending on the extent and depth of the burn. Together, evaporation of water and inflammatory exudation may account for a 40 to 50 per cent reduction in the plasma volume within 3 to 6 hours in patients who have burns covering 40 per cent of their body surface. This depletion of plasma volume reflects not only loss of water and plasma proteins, but also hemolysis of red cells as they pass through the damaged tissue. As much as 50 per cent of the total red cell mass may be destroyed.

Although the healing of the burn site and the fluid losses are serious problems, usually the *secondary systemic ramifications* of burns are even more threatening to life than are the immediate effects. Almost inevitably wounds are contaminated by microorganisms (Moncrief, 1973). Staphylococci are the usual initial contaminants and within 48 hours may reach a level of 10^8 organisms per gram of tissue in the superficial necrotic tissue and inflammatory exudate. Toward the end of the first week these gram-positive organisms are usually replaced by gram-negative bacilli, most often *Pseudomonas aeruginosa.* The gram-negative bacteria tend to invade blood vessel walls and produce a bacteremia. The combination of bacteremia and endotoxemia accounted for 74 per cent of fatalities in a recent study of severely burned patients (Teplitz, 1969). Not only is the burn wound colonized by organisms, but the normal skin also is widely contaminated and so septic phlebitis at venipuncture sites and around intravenous catheters and tracheostomies is very frequent.

Shock is another grave sequel to severe burns. It is usually a consequence of the hypovolemia or sepsis or both (p. 213).

Pulmonary edema (p. 289) develops in approximately 30 per cent of severely burned patients (Morris and Spitzer, 1971). These pulmonary changes may be attributable to shock, to the inhalation of smoke and noxious gases by patients trapped in burning buildings or to cardiac insufficiency induced by hypovolemia.

Acute gastroduodenal stress ulcers may develop in as many as half the patients dying of burn wounds. These are referred to as *Curling's ulcers* (p. 469). They are commonly multiple, small, superficial and scattered throughout the body or fundus of the stomach and sometimes the duodenum. Perforation of one of these lesions may be the cause of death.

Many other late complications may develop, such as renal failure (secondary to shock-induced acute tubular necrosis), laryngeal edema from inhaled smoke and other noxious gases, as well as infections in the many viscera affected in shock. It is evident that even when burned patients survive the immediate effects of the injury they run a gamut of potentially lethal complications.

RADIATION INJURIES

Radiant energy is a double-edged sword. It provides an invaluable means of clinical diagnosis and sometimes a curative mode of therapy, but at the same time it is a potent mutagen and destroyer of cells and of life.

We will not go into great detail about the physics of radiation; it is sufficient to say here that radiation may occur in two forms: (1) electromagnetic waves (x-rays and gamma rays), and (2) energetic charged particles (alpha, beta [also known as electrons], protons, neutrons, pi-mesons and heavy ions, as well as other high energy particles). Details on these forms of radiant energy are available in the excellent monograph by Rubin and Casarett (1968).

The qualitative effects upon cells of the different forms of radiant energy are similar, but there is great variation in their patterns of energy deposition within exposed tissues. The neutral particles (neutrons, x- and gamma rays) lose energy in infrequent random collisions, generally leading to a nearly exponential reduction of energy deposition in progressively deeper levels of tissue, but nevertheless with substantial penetration to significant depths. Charged particles (electrons, alpha particles, protons and pi-mesons) mostly lose energy by innumerable multiple collisions with electrons in the target material. These collisions "leach" energy from the incident particles until they come to rest. The pattern of energy deposition is quite constant along the course of penetration of the particles. However, charged particles have a sharply limited depth of penetration. Near the end of their range, when the charged particles have a low velocity, the rate of energy deposition per unit path length *(linear energy transfer, LET)* rises, leading to a region of increased local dose, referred to as the Bragg peak of ionization. The precise depth of penetration of these charged particles depends on their energy. Beta particles from radioisotopes generally have penetrations in tissue measured in millimeters. Alpha particles from radioisotopes have even shorter ranges, having their greatest effect on the epidermis. However, charged particles accelerated to high energies (by a cyclotron, for example) can readily penetrate more than 20 cm. of tissue.

The *energy deposition of radiation* at a given point in tissue is known as the radiation *dose.* The unit of dose is the *rad (r),* defined as the deposition of 100 ergs of energy per gram of irradiated material. The output of radiation sources, especially x-ray machines and therapy units, is often defined in terms of *exposure,* the unit of which is the *roentgen (R).* The roentgen is defined as the exposure which, under certain defined conditions, would liberate 1 electrostatic unit of positive ions from 1 cc. of air. Air, exposed to 1 R of radiation, receives a dose of 0.87 rad.

The activity of radioactive isotopes is quantitated in terms of their instantaneous rate of disintegration, measured in *curies (Ci),* and their half-life. One curie of radioactive isotope suffers 3.7×10^{10} disintegrations per second. One half of the atoms will have disintegrated during one "half-life" of the isotope. Knowledge of the activity and half-life of the isotope is not adequate to determine the exposure at a given distance from the source, since this depends on the nature and energy of the emitted radiation(s). This is expressed by the "specific gamma ray constant," defined as the exposure rate (in R/hr) at one meter from a 1 Ci source, and is a constant which typifies a given isotope.

Regardless of the primary source of the radiant energy, it exerts its biologic effect by the ionization of cellular atoms and molecules with which it collides. However, the fundamental mechanism by which radiation energy causes this ionization is still unknown. Two proposals have been made: (1) the *direct* or *target theory,* and (2) the *indirect action theory.* The target theory proposes direct hits on sensitive vital molecules within the cell, e.g., the linkages and bonds within the DNA molecule (Hutchinson, 1966). The indirect theory proposes instead that radiant energy causes ionization of the cellular water, leading to the formation of free "hot" radicals (such as hydroxy and peroxide radicals) that secondarily interact with vital molecules. The mode of interaction may well depend on the LET of the radiation.

Another radiobiologic enigma is the *latency of radiation.* It is clear that the transfer of energy to a target atom or molecule occurs within microfractions of a second, yet its biologic effect, functional or morphologic, may not become evident for decades. Radiation-related cancers were discovered in some survivors of the atomic bombs of Hiroshima and Nagasaki more than 20 years after the bombings (Jablon et al., 1971). Does this imply sequential intracellular interactions eventually extending to some crucial molecule or function, or instead is the first physicochemical dislocation so minor that it exerts a detectable effect only through potentiating ever more severe mutations in successive generations of cells?

EFFECTS OF RADIATION ON CELLS

Four considerations are of major importance in determining the extent of injury induced by radiation: (1) the dosage, (2) the rate of dose delivery, (3) the LET of the radiation, and (4) the vulnerability of the cells to radiation injury. Other things being equal, damage is proportional to the dose. However, the *rate of delivery of radiant energy* significantly modifies its effect, especially when it is delivered in divided doses or fractions, as is the practice in radiotherapy. It is well documented, for example, that cells are able to repair some DNA damage. If sufficient time elapses after the initial radiation-induced injury, the cell may have almost completely recovered by the time it receives a second exposure and there would be no cumulative effect (Russell et al., 1958). Divided dosages, then, have cumulative effect only to the extent that recovery in the interval is incomplete. Radiotherapy of tumors takes advantage of the fact that in general normal cells appear to be capable of more rapid recovery and not to suffer the same cumulative radiation effects as do tumor cells. Thus, they are less severely injured by repeated exposures to radiation.

The *radiobiological effectiveness (RBE)* of radiation is a dose-modifying factor which depends on LET. Generally, as LET increases, a lesser dose of radiation is required to achieve a given biological end-point, i.e., the RBE increases. Moreover, the ability to recover from radiation damage depends on the LET, being greater for lower LET radiations. Also, the relative insensitivity of hypoxic cells to low LET radiations is less important at high LET levels.

The *radiosensitivity of cells and tissues* is determined by the inherent response of the cells to a pulse of radiation, by the kinetics of cellular repair between radiation exposures and by the proliferative state of the cells. Even cells of the same kind and condition express a wide range of severity of injury in response to a given exposure to radiation. Radiation energy is absorbed in an apparently random way rather than in a uniform fashion. Ionizations within one cell might be lethal, whereas in another cell there might be no critical damage. Although there are many potential intracellular targets, DNA is thought to be the most vulnerable target of radiation. For this reason the induction of *post-irradiation cell necrosis is most closely correlated with the reproductive activity of cells.* Although cells are at all times vulnerable to radiation their sensitivity can vary markedly with their phase in the mitotic cycle. For many cells the G_2 phase, when RNA and protein synthesis occur, is most sensitive (Casarett, 1972). Unless the dose of radiation has been massive, cells already in mitosis at the time of irradiation complete their division but may be unable to undergo subsequent mitosis. Thus, rapidly dividing, undifferentiated cancers are generally more responsive to radiotherapy than slowly growing, well differentiated cancers. The same principle applies to the various normal cells of the body which have been divided into three categories of radiosensitivity.

Most vulnerable to radiation injury are the rapidly dividing cells of the body, i.e., precursor hematopoietic cells, cells in the crypts of the intestinal mucosa, spermatogonia, granulosal cells of the developing and mature ovarian follicles, basal cells of the epidermis, germinal cells of the gastric and holocrine glands, short-lived lymphocytes and dividing cells in stratified squamous epithelia.

Moderately radiosensitive are connective tissue cells, glia, endothelium and growing cartilage and bone.

Relatively resistant to radiation are the parenchymal cells of most of the glands and ducts of the body, muscle cells, nerve cells, mature cartilage and bone cells and renal tubular epithelium.

Despite this hierarchy, all cells can be injured or destroyed with sufficient exposure to radiation energy.

The morphologic changes induced within cells by irradiation are not distinctive or qualitatively different from those encountered with injury caused by other agents. Both the cytoplasm and the nucleus are affected. The initial response takes the form of cellular swelling; cytoplasmic vacuolization; mitochondrial enlargement; and distortion, disruption, swelling and fragmentation of the endoplasmic reticulum. However, lysosomes appear to be relatively resistant and sometimes are increased in number (Ghidoni, 1967). The nuclei swell, become vacuolated and in severely affected cells undergo pyknosis or karyorrhexis. Both nuclear membrane and plasma membrane disruption occur in heavily irradiated cells. All manner of chromosomal damage may be seen in cells undergoing division, including deletions, breaks, translocations, interadherence and fragmentation of chromosomes. Mitotic figures become disorderly or even chaotic. Unquestionably, other more subtle mutations at the level of individual genes must also be present. **It is this damage to the genetic apparatus of the cell which underlies the lethality, oncogenicity and mutagenicity of radiation energy.** It might be noted in passing that the cytoplasmic, nuclear and mitotic changes seen in irradiated cells make them closely resemble cancer cells, a problem that plagues the pathologist when evaluating post-irradiation tissues for the possible persistence of tumor cells.

Much of the effect of radiation on both normal and tumorous tissue is mediated by radiation injury of the vasculature and connective tissue cells. During the immediate post-irradiation period blood vessels may show only dilatation, accounting for the erythema of the skin seen so often following radiotherapy. Later (or with more intense exposure) endothelial cells undergo swelling, vacuolation and even destruction. With time, heavily damaged vessels may rupture, thrombose or undergo progressive fibrosis and narrowing of their lumina. The contiguous connective tissue also becomes increasingly sclerotic. In this way the dependent parenchymal cells are deprived of their nutrition and thus undergo atrophy or die. These stromal changes and the associated parenchymal atrophy are very much like those encountered in aging.

EFFECTS OF RADIATION ON ORGAN SYSTEMS

The radiopathology of certain organs and systems is worthy of separate description either because of their frequent involvement or because of their particular vulnerability.

The skin is usually involved in radiation injury because it is in the pathway of most forms of radiotherapy. Post-irradiation erythema, beginning in 2 to 3 days and reaching a peak in two to three weeks, is commonly encountered in patients receiving cancer radiotherapy. Later, blotchy hyperpigmentation or depigmentation, hyperkeratosis, epilation, skin atrophy, dermal and subcutaneous fibrosis and telangiectases may appear. When the skin is severely affected, post-irradiation ulcerations may develop as long as five years later. Development of squamous cell cancers, in one instance 56 years after exposure, is another, more serious result (Cade, 1957).

The **hematopoietic and lymphoid systems,** because they contain rapidly dividing cells, are extremely susceptible to radiation injury. Nonlethal total body irradiation may induce striking lymphopenia within hours, followed in the course of the next day or two by shrinkage of the lymph nodes and spleen. Granulocytopenia and thrombocytopenia do not appear until the end of the first week, and anemia appears about two to three weeks later. All of these changes are reversible if the patient survives.

The **germ cells** in both sexes are extremely radiosensitive, and sterility may be a residual effect of radiation injury. However, identical dosages of radiation are more likely to produce sterility in the female than in the male. The progressive vulnerability of cells in the male in descending order is: spermatogonia, spermatocytes, spermatids and spermatozoa. In the female the follicular granulosal cells and germ cells are most vulnerable. It should be noted in passing that cancer of the endometrium and the endometrium itself are more sensitive to radiation than the smooth muscle of the uterine wall. This fact permits the use of intracavitary radon needles for the therapy of endometrial carcinoma.

The **lungs** may be damaged by radiation to the chest. As is the case with all blood vessels, the rich vascularization of the alveolar septa is vulnerable to radiation injury. Endothelial damage may lead at first to increased permeability with severe congestion, edema and pulmonary hemorrhages. Later progressive fibrosis and sclerosis of the pulmonary septa develop (Fig. 8–1).

The **mucosal epithelium of the entire gastrointestinal tract** is exquisitely radiosensitive and is sometimes severely damaged in the course of radiation treatment of intra-abdominal malignant tumors. The early changes range from swelling and vacuolization of intestinal mucosal cells, accompanied by mild hyperemia of the submucosal vasculature, to total necrosis and ulceration of the mucosa. Later, mucosal atrophy and fibrosis, and even interstitial fibrosis throughout the muscularis, may result. The fibrosis may be so severe as to cause strictures at any level of the bowel, particularly in the esophagus and rectum. With the high rate of turnover of intestinal epithelium, it is not unanticipated that abnormal mitoses and all manner of chromosomal damage may be encountered.

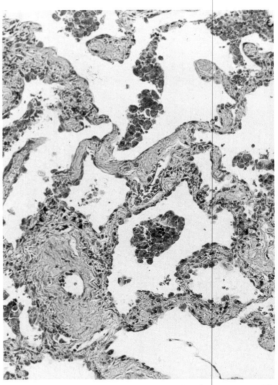

Figure 8–1. Radiation pneumonitis, late stage. The alveolar walls are fibrosed and the small vessel (lower left) shows marked collagenous fibrosis and thickening of its wall. Desquamated macrophages are seen within the alveolar spaces.

Total body radiation, such as occurred when the atomic bombs were dropped on Japan, has devastating effects. As little as 100 rads of radiation to the entire body will induce nausea, vomiting and changes in the circulating blood. To place this dosage in some perspective, it must be appreciated that 5000 to 6000 rads are commonly employed in carefully delimited fields and in divided doses in the therapy of cancers. The lethal range of total body radiation begins at 500 rads and death is almost certain at 1000 rads. Nausea, vomiting, diarrhea, loss of appetite, fever and thirst appear very soon after such dosages. One of three fatal syndromes may then develop; these have been called: (1) the bone marrow syndrome, (2) the intestinal syndrome, and (3) the central nervous system syndrome (Rubin and Casarett, 1968). The *bone marrow syndrome,* as can be anticipated, is dominated by a striking reduction in the number of circulating lymphocytes, platelets, neutrophils and eventually red cells. In most of these cases a bleeding diathesis or infection causes death. The *intestinal syndrome* is characterized by the gastrointestinal manifestations already described, but diarrhea with loss of fluids and electrolytes is primarily responsible for death.

The *central nervous system syndrome* generally does not appear until the dosage of total body radiation reaches the level of 2000 to 5000 rads. In these cases convulsions and death occur within hours to days, even before manifestations of bone marrow or intestinal involvement appear. If the total body irradiation is not immediately fatal, irreversible aplastic anemia, cataract formation in the lens of the eye, developmental and mental defects in children and an increased incidence of cancer may appear later (Steer, 1971). A recent study of survivors of the atomic bombings indicates that nearly 30 years later, in addition to an increased frequency of malignant neoplasms (discussed below), stunted growth and development in exposed children, microencephaly in children of exposed mothers, diabetes mellitus and accelerated aging, as well as other changes, continue to appear (Belsky, 1973; Anderson et al., 1974).

In closing this discussion of the potentials of radiation, even when used therapeutically, its oncogenicity must be emphasized. An increased incidence of thyroid cancer appeared in young adults exposed to radiation in and about the head and neck during childhood (p. 601). An increased incidence of liver carcinoma has followed the now abandoned use of Thorotrast (a radioactive dye used to outline the biliary tract). Osteogenic sarcoma has occurred in radium-dial painters (p. 625). A ten- to fifty-fold increased incidence of leukemia, particularly the acute myelogenous form, has been reported in the long-term survivors of the atomic bombs. A less striking increase in the incidence of solid tissue neoplasms has also been reported (Brill et al., 1962; Jablon et al., 1971). Therapeutic radiation, like all treatment modalities, underscores the validity of the admonition—"be sure that the treatment is not worse than the disease."

CHEMICAL INJURIES

Virtually all of the known chemical agents (including therapeutic drugs) have at one time or another been known to cause injury or death in man. Many mechanisms are involved in chemically induced cellular and tissue damage. In some instances the agent is highly toxic—a poison—and will cause injury to every individual exposed to a sufficient quantity. In other instances the injury is mediated by an immune (allergic) reaction to the agent. Some agents, mostly therapeutic drugs, have well defined undesirable side effects which are accepted as the price to be paid for the greater therapeutic gains to be achieved. The most dramatic examples of the injurious potential of chemical agents are the more than 6000 suicides which occur annually in the United States and are attributable to chemical agents, including drugs. Table 8–1 presents the doleful list of agents indicted in such deaths. Perhaps even more frightening are the more than 100,000 instances which occur annually in the United States of the ingestion of toxic substances by children under five years of age. Unhappily about 4000 of these accidents result in death; some idea of the range of the hazards can be obtained from Table 8–2, which lists the amazing array of agents that find their way into unsuspecting mouths.

THERAPEUTIC AGENTS

Most would not deny that drugs are usually beneficial. They alleviate symptoms and help

TABLE 8–1.   SUICIDES FROM POISONING*

CHEMICAL AGENT	NUMBER OF DEATHS	TOTAL NUMBER OF DEATHS
I. Suicide from poisoning by solid or liquid substances		3659
Barbituric acid and derivatives	1810	
Salicylates and congeners	72	
Psychotherapeutic agents	179	
Other and unspecified drugs	915	
Corrosive aromatics	11	
Strychnine	22	
Lye and potash (caustic alkali)	53	
Arsenic and its compounds	39	
Fluorides	18	
Other and unspecified solid and liquid substances	540	
II. Suicide from poisoning by gas for domestic use	61	61
III. Suicide from poisoning by other gases		2398
Motor vehicle exhaust gas	2041	
Other carbon monoxide	336	
Other and unspecified gases and vapors	21	
Total		6118

*Derived from Vital Statistics of the United States, 1969. Bethesda, Md., U.S. Department of Health, Education and Welfare, 1974.

TABLE 8-2. CATEGORIES OF SUBSTANCES MOST FREQUENTLY INGESTED BY CHILDREN UNDER 5 YEARS OF AGE REPORTED BY POISON CONTROL CENTERS (1971–1973)*†

TYPE OF SUBSTANCE	1973 No.	1973 %	1972 No.	1972 %	1971 No.	1971 %
1. Aspirin	6576	6.5	8146	7.8	8529	10.1
Baby	4275	4.2	5305	5.1	5773	6.8
Adult	1098	1.1	1322	1.3	1165	1.4
Unspecified	1203	1.2	1519	1.4	1591	1.9
2. Soaps, Detergents, Cleaners	5513	5.4	5940	5.7	4359	5.2
3. Plants (excluding mushrooms and toadstools)	5394	5.3	4759	4.5	4059	4.8
4. Vitamins, Minerals	5146	5.1	5320	5.1	4053	4.8
5. Antihistamines, Cold Medicines	4770	4.7	4355	4.1	3246	3.8
6. Perfume, Cologne, Toilet Water	3062	3.0	3108	3.0	2281	2.7
7. Household Disinfectants, Deodorizers	3059	3.0	3301	3.1	2670	3.2
8. Miscellaneous Internal Medicines	3040	3.0	3186	3.0	2607	3.1
9. Psychopharmacologic Agents	3010	3.0	2998	2.9	2486	3.0
10. Household Bleach	2636	2.6	2794	2.7	2142	2.5
11. Chemicals	2286	2.3	2382	2.3	1593	1.9
12. Miscellaneous Analgesics	2218	2.2	2220	2.1	1856	2.2
13. Insecticides (excluding mothballs)	2136	2.1	2306	2.2	1886	2.2
14. Hormones	2050	2.0	1970	1.9	1692	2.0
15. Liquid Polish or Wax	1996	2.0	1872	1.8	1342	1.6
16. Liniments	1982	2.0	2133	2.0	1415	1.7
17. Glues, Adhesives	1827	1.8	1866	1.8	1475	1.7
18. Cosmetic Lotions, Creams	1801	1.8	1783	1.7	1300	1.5
19. Miscellaneous Products	1800	1.8	1941	1.9	1398	1.7
20. Medicine Combinations	1741	1.7	1865	1.8	1654	2.0
21. Acids, Alkalies	1662	1.6	1815	1.7	1406	1.7
22. Miscellaneous External Medicines	1596	1.6	1587	1.5	1203	1.4
23. Fingernail Preparations	1517	1.5	1191	1.1	806	1.0
24. Rodenticides	1483	1.5	1508	1.4	1274	1.5
25. Antiseptic Medication	1417	1.4	1346	1.3	1142	1.4

*From the National Clearinghouse for Poison Control Centers Bulletin. Bethesda, Md., U.S. Department of Health, Education and Welfare, Food and Drug Administration. Tabulations of 1973 Reports. May–June, 1974.

†Source: Individual case reports submitted to the National Clearinghouse for Poison Control Centers, 1973: 117,589 reports from 517 Centers in 45 States‡; 1972; 105,018 reports from 548 Centers in 47 States‡; 1971; 84,370 reports from 505 Centers in 47 States.‡
‡Includes District of Columbia, Canal Zone, Virgin Islands, and military bases abroad.

cure disease. Unfortunately their injury-producing potential sometimes is forgotten. Any of the mechanisms mentioned above may be involved in drug-induced injury. A sufficient quantity of aspirin (a sort of noncaloric candy as used by millions) can kill. Halothane, a widely used anesthetic, may cause fatal massive hepatic necrosis. Most often the liver damage follows multiple exposures to the agent and an allergic reaction is postulated, but sometimes death occurs with the first exposure and is attributed to an idiosyncratic reaction (p. 518). Immune reactions to drugs are much more commonplace than is generally appreciated, particularly in patients having some history of hypersensitivity. In a study of 740 patients with atopic (allergic) respiratory disease (such as hay fever), 17 per cent of the patients had untoward reactions to drugs (Miller, 1967). Penicillin was the worst offender and accounted for more than half of these reactions. As mentioned earlier, sometimes the tissue damage comprises a well known and accepted side effect of the drug. For example, alkylating agents (such as nitrogen mustards, cyclophosphamide, and so forth) and antimetabolites (such as azathio-

prine, methotrexate, and others) which are used in antitumor therapy cause damage to the hematopoietic system. A few of the drugs most commonly implicated in untoward reactions (excluding unpredictable allergic reactions) will be discussed briefly; other less common offenders are cited in Table 8-3.

SALICYLATES

Aspirin (acetylsalicylic acid) and oil of wintergreen (methylsalicylate) are highly toxic drugs despite the casual attitude toward their use. Aspirin continues to be the single harmful substance most frequently ingested by children. Happily the use of safety packaging and increased public awareness have brought about a remarkable decline (75 per cent) in the number of poisonings attributable to this agent over the past decade. As little as 2 to 4 grams of aspirin (1 gram = 15 grains or three adult aspirin) or 5 ml. of oil of wintergreen may be fatal in infants. Fifteen grams of aspirin in one dose may kill an adult. Acute poisonings are rapidly followed by stimulation of the respiratory centers. The hyperventilation first induces a respiratory alkalosis, but this may be replaced later by a metabolic

FIGURE 8–3. REACTIONS TO SOME COMMON DRUGS

Antibacterial Agents	
Sulfonamides	Bile stasis, focal liver necrosis.
Tetracycline	Fatty change in liver, focal necrosis of renal and pancreatic epithelium.
Chloramphenicol	Aplastic anemia, granulocytopenia, thrombocytopenia.
Neomycin	Malabsorption syndromes.
Antitubercular Agents	
Para-aminosalicylic acid (PAS)	Focal to massive liver necrosis.
Isoniazid	Fatty change, focal necroses of liver.
Steroids	
Methyltestosterone	Centrilobular bile stasis, jaundice.
Oral contraceptives	Centrilobular bile stasis, jaundice, cerebrovascular disease, venous thrombosis, myocardial infarction, ? liver adenoma.
Miscellaneous	
Chlorpromazine	Bile stasis, focal liver necrosis.
Phenylbutazone	Focal to massive liver necrosis, aplastic anemia.
Hydralazine	Systemic lupus erythematosus-like syndrome.
Phenacetin	Hemolytic anemia, methemoglobinemia, chronic interstitial nephritis with necrotizing papillitis.

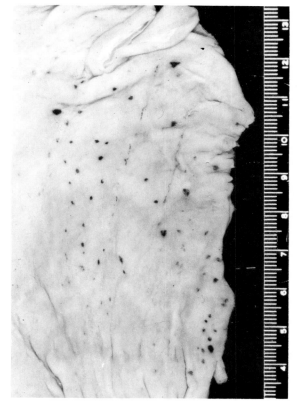

Figure 8–2. A close-up of numerous small acute mucosal erosions caused by chronic ingestion of aspirin.

acidosis. The respiratory alkalosis is associated with hypokalemia which may, in fatal cases, be the cause of death. If the victim survives, a hemorrhagic ulcerative gastroenteritis may develop as a consequence of the irritative effects of ingested salicylates (Fig. 8–2). Inhibition of platelet aggregation, another action of salicylates, sometimes induces a hemorrhagic diathesis which takes the form of petechial or ecchymotic hemorrhages in the skin, serosal surfaces and meninges. Chronic interstitial nephritis is occasionally encountered in those who, over the course of years, have taken large amounts of proprietary preparations containing both aspirin and phenacetin (p. 444). Which of these two analgesics is responsible is still in dispute, but some investigators have indicted aspirin as the culprit.

BARBITURATES

Barbiturates continue to lead the list of therapeutic agents causing death from overdosage. Most of these deaths are suicides, but in a recent analysis a surprisingly large number (approximately one third) were considered accidental (Drug Abuse Warning Network, 1973). Some of these accidental deaths may be attributable to the wide range of individual susceptibilities to barbiturates and to the synergistic depressant effects of alcohol and barbiturates on the central nervous system. Underlying liver disease which impairs the metabolism of barbiturates may also contribute to these accidental deaths. In addition, it is reputed that individuals on barbiturates may be sufficiently sedated to forget how much they have taken and so continue to take additional medication at frequent intervals until fatal levels are reached. This phenomenon is termed "barbiturate automatism" and it is probably a factor in many deaths from barbiturate overdosage. Because of all these variables it is difficult to establish threshold fatal dosages of the barbiturates. Even in the absence of predisposing influences, as little as 2 to 3 gm. of a short acting barbiturate or 5 gm. of a long acting agent taken in one dose may cause death. There are, however, rare reports of recovery following larger dosages.

The morphologic changes in fatal cases depend on the rapidity of death and may be surprisingly few. Barbiturates depress central nervous system function, affecting first the cerebral cortex, then progressively lower levels of the CNS, depending on the dosage. With the ingestion of sufficiently large amounts, death is produced by paralysis of the medullary control of respiration. In patients who survive longer, severe skin reactions similar to exfoliative dermatitis and acute inflammatory lesions of arteries similar to polyarteritis nodosa (p. 199) may appear. The skin lesions often take the form of large bullae, sometimes referred to as barbiturate "blisters." Other inconstant changes include hypoxic injury to the renal tubular epithelium, bronchopneumonia and hypoxic damage to ganglion cells in the brain. All of these last cited alterations reflect respiratory depression and appear only in patients who survive for some time following the poisoning.

ORAL CONTRACEPTIVES

Few subjects in medicine are more "in the eye of the storm" than the risks involved in oral contraception. The accumulated data to this time yield contradictory conclusions, possibly resulting from differences in population samples and from changes which have been introduced into the composition of many "pills," in particular lowered estrogen levels relative to the amount of progesterone. It must also be remembered that we do not yet know the results either of the long-term use of these agents or of possible delayed effects decades after cessation of their use. Drugs, especially hormones, sometimes have very late sequelae—witness the appearance of adenocarcinoma of the vagina in adolescent offspring of mothers who had taken stilbestrol while pregnant (p. 563). Even at the present time the benefits must be weighed against the known risks. To quote a recent editorial, "Oral contraceptive medication carries a small but definite risk to health. The incidence of venous thrombosis, pulmonary embolism and stroke is increased about five fold to six fold in users and a wide variety of metabolic effects have cast further doubt on the long term safety of oral contraceptive drugs" (Editorial, 1974). Despite this view, the controversy with respect to venous thrombosis and pulmonary embolism, which is also discussed on page 224, continues to swirl. Notwithstanding reports to the contrary, the weight of evidence indicates a statistically valid correlation between oral contraceptive drugs and increased venous thrombosis and pulmonary embolism. Moreover, an increased risk of cerebral ischemia or thrombosis following the use of oral contraceptive agents appears to be reasonably well established at the present time. In a collaborative study from 12 university hospitals in the United States, the relative risk of cerebral ischemia or thrombosis was estimated to be about nine times greater for women who use this mode of contraception than for those who do not (Collaborative Group for the Study of Stroke in Young Women, 1973). Recently, a three to five times increased risk of myocardial infarction has been cited in long term users of the "pill." An increased incidence of liver adenomas has also been identified in these individuals (Baum et al., 1973); and Janerich and colleagues (1974) state: "Recently evidence has been offered of an etiologic relation between oral contraceptives and birth defects, specifically limb anomalies." A number of other physiologic and metabolic changes have been described such as slight deterioration of glucose tolerance, an increased incidence of hypertension, a rise in serum triglycerides and cholesterol concentrations and an increased incidence of jaundice, as well as other findings, but none can be considered well established and they require additional confirmation. On the positive side no evidence has been found of an association between the use of oral contraceptives and carcinoma of either the breast or uterus, and indeed a slight protective effect is suspected (Vessey et al., 1972). Although many physicians and properly informed women would not agree, one report concludes that "the estimated risk at the present time of using the "Pill" is one that a properly informed woman would be happy to take" (Royal College of General Practitioners, 1974). If this method of contraception is chosen, obviously it is necessary to weigh the apparent risks against the hazards involved in other methods of contraception and the risks of unwanted pregnancies with each form of contraception.

NONTHERAPEUTIC AGENTS

ETHYL ALCOHOL

The chronic consumption of excessive amounts of ethanol is a major public health problem which, it is believed, affects the quality and length of life of over eight million Americans. Thus, in addition to the social and economic implications of alcoholism, it is a serious medical problem. Alcoholism can be separated into three clinical syndromes: (1) drunkenness, (2) acute alcoholic intoxication, and (3) chronic alcoholism. Drunkenness contributes to more than 50 per cent of fatal automobile accidents. Acute alcoholic intoxication is responsible for a significant number of deaths. Chronic alcoholism has wide-ranging effects and is almost invariably associated with protein malnutrition, vitamin deficiencies, impaired immunologic responsiveness, enhanced susceptibility to infections and direct toxicity on cells. There is a growing body of evidence suggesting that alcohol directly injures liver cells, in time inducing alcoholic cirrhosis (discussed more fully on p. 525). Chronic alcoholism also has serious effects on other organs, as will be pointed out below.

A few words are in order on the metabolism of alcohol, but for more detail, reference should be made to the recent review of this subject by Hawkins and Kalant (1972). Alcohol is rapidly absorbed in the empty stomach; food slows the rate of absorption. Only 5 per cent of the absorbed alcohol is excreted through the skin, lungs and kidneys; the remainder is transported through the blood to the liver, where ultimately it is metabolized to CO_2 and water. There are three principal enzyme systems capable of oxidizing ethanol: (1) alcohol dehydrogenase (ADH), (2) microsomal ethanol oxidizing system (MEOS), and (3) catalase. Of these three pathways it is the ADH system which is responsible for the metabolism of almost all absorbed ethanol. ADH is found principally in the soluble fraction of liver cells. It is an NAD-dependent zinc-containing enzyme which catalyzes the initial oxidation of ethanol to acetaldehyde. The reoxidation of hepatic NADH is the rate limiting factor in the kinetics of ethanol oxidation; thus, a significant decrease in hepatic NAD-NADH ratios retards the oxidation of ethanol. The contribution of the MEOS and catalase systems to the metabolism of alcohol in man has not been definitely established. The rate of ethanol metabolism is markedly increased in both animals and man following chronic ethanol consumption (Israel et al., 1975). This adaptive phenomenon is poorly understood, but in some way reflects the increased capacity of the liver to reoxidize NADH. The increased metabolism of ethanol in chronic alcoholics generates larger amounts of acetaldehyde. This compound may be toxic and account for some of the injurious effects of chronic ethanol consumption (Cederbaum and Rubin, 1975). In any event such increased rates of ethanol metabolism as have been reported in habitual users of alcohol are not sufficient to explain the considerable degree of tolerance demonstrated by chronic alcoholics in the performance of perceptual and motor tasks. Mendelson (1970) proposes instead some vaguely defined central nervous system adaptation to elevated blood levels of ethanol which acts at a functional or behavioral level.

The physiologic and pharmacologic effects of alcohol are directly related to the blood levels, although tolerance introduces some modifications. The precise statutory blood levels of alcohol indicative of drunkenness vary from one state to another, but in general 100 to 150 mg. per 100 ml. is considered intoxicating. Approximately 500 mg. per 100 ml. is usually fatal. Save for the insane freak who gulps down a whole bottle of whiskey at one time, it is almost impossible to achieve a fatal blood level because blessed stupor usually intervenes. To place these figures in some perspective, note that if an individual of average size, not engaged in heavy physical activity, consumes four or five one ounce drinks on an empty stomach, he usually develops a blood alcohol level of 100 mg. per 100 ml. or more.

Despite the striking—sometimes ludicrous, sometimes pathetic—effects of alcohol on behavior there are remarkably few morphologic changes directly attributable to this agent. As mentioned earlier, there is substantial evidence that alcohol is a direct hepatotoxin. Acute and chronic pancreatitis is common among chronic alcoholics, but it is not certain that this is related to direct toxicity. Some evidence suggests that instead it is more closely correlated with the malnutrition and low protein intake so common in these individuals (Mezey et al., 1970). Recently it has been proposed that ethanol alone may induce a macrocytic anemia, not related to concomitant deficiencies of the B vitamins (Wu et al., 1974). In addition there are numerous reports of myocardial changes attributed to ethanol toxicity alone, including alcoholic cardiomyopathy (p. 305) (Hognestad and Teisberg, 1973). However, the question persists as to whether other nutritional disturbances, such as protein or thiamine deficiencies, contribute to or perhaps cause the cardiac lesion. In fact, recently a controlled study in animals did not support the concept that alcohol is directly toxic to the heart (Hall and Rowlands, 1970), and the issue remains unresolved. The same doubts persist about the impact of ethanol on the nervous system. Clearly it acts as a depressant or inhibitor of neuronal function, affecting first the cerebral cortex and then progressively the lower centers. The stimulation commonly ascribed to alcohol was once thought to be related only to inhibition of cortical controls, but there is some evidence that alcohol may also stimulate the release of catecholamines and thus have direct stimulant actions (Murphree, 1973). However, when sufficiently high blood levels are reached, vital centers in the medulla are depressed, and respiratory arrest may follow. Despite all of these functional effects the evidence that ethanol produces specific morphologic changes in the brain or peripheral nerves is scanty indeed. It is well known that chronic alcoholics may develop Wernicke's syndrome (p. 255), Korsakoff's dementia, cerebellar degeneration and peripheral neuropathy, but most investigators ascribe these disorders to concomitant nutritional deficiencies, principally of the complex of B vitamins (Victor and Adams, 1953). However, a recent study raises the possibility that peripheral neuropathy and striated muscle dysfunction may be attributed to alcohol alone (Mayer, 1973). It is evident that the difficulties in ascribing lesions in man directly to alcohol stems from the almost invariable association of chronic alcoholism with chronic malnutrition.

METHYL ALCOHOL

Methyl alcohol may be ingested (either accidentally or with suicidal intent) or inhaled as toxic fumes in industrial exposure. When swallowed it causes patchy edema and hemorrhages in the stomach. Inhalation causes similar edema and hemorrhages in the lung tissues, chiefly in the subpleural regions. The major effects of methanol, however, are manifested in the eye. After absorption methanol is oxidized to formaldehyde and formic acid, and both substances cause degeneration of the receptor cells of the retina. Rarely, degeneration of the optic disc and nerve follows. It has been suggested that the eye, with its high water content, is the major site of damage because absorbed methyl alcohol is distributed in the various organs in proportion to their water content. Swelling of the brain and brain stem may also occur, accompanied by swelling and various regressive changes in cortical ganglion cells. Many patients manifest severe acidosis, the basis for which is still uncertain. Severe intoxication may also be associated with pancreatic changes, such as interstitial edema and acinar cell degranulation and swelling. As a consequence of these anatomic changes patients with methyl alcohol poisoning present with visual impairment ranging from mild blurring to total blindness, abdominal pain, headache, nausea and central nervous system symptoms—from dizziness and convulsions to coma. If the victim recovers, the central nervous system manifestations may regress, but about 10 to 20 per cent of patients have some residual visual impairment.

CARBON MONOXIDE

Inhalation of carbon monoxide continues to be a favorite mode of suicide, albeit less popular than the ingestion of barbiturates. Accidental deaths from the inhalation of automobile exhaust or the fumes from almost any incompletely combusted carbon fuel are also all too frequent. Relatively low levels of this gas may be fatal. For example, the inhalation of a 1 per cent concentration by a physically active individual with a high respiratory rate may prove fatal within 10 to 20 minutes (ordinary illuminating gas contains approximately 16 per cent carbon monoxide and automobile exhaust contains about 7 per cent). Thus, a car engine left running in a small closed garage may produce fatal levels of carbon monoxide within as little as 5 minutes. Carbon monoxide has a 200 to 300 times greater affinity for hemoglobin than oxygen and forms a stable carboxyhemoglobin, which is removed from the blood slowly by the pressure and mass action of inspired oxygen. Thus, absorption of this gas is cumulative (over weeks to months) and toxic effects depend on the level, frequency and duration of exposure.

Acute fatal intoxication is marked by a cherry red hyperemia of all tissues, sometimes accompanied by petechial hemorrhages in serosal surfaces and the white matter of the cerebral hemispheres. If the patient survives a day or two, the findings of anoxic encephalopathy (p. 647) appear. Most characteristic is symmetrical degeneration of the basal ganglia, especially the lenticular nuclei. Occasionally hypoxic injury to the myocardium, liver or tubular cells of the kidneys is found, but in most cases death occurs too rapidly to permit the full development of these changes.

Chronic carbon monoxide poisoning may occur from prolonged or repeated inhalation of low levels of the gas. The carboxyhemoglobin accumulates, as mentioned, and when approximately 30 per cent of the hemoglobin is saturated with carbon monoxide, symptoms begin to appear. Levels of 60 to 70 per cent generally are fatal. The central nervous system changes in chronic poisoning resemble those described in the acute form. In addition, chronically exposed patients are more likely to manifest renal, hepatic or cardiac failure due to hypoxic injury to parenchymal cells even weeks after the last exposure.

The clinical manifestations of carbon monoxide poisoning are most invidious and often the victim is unaware of his plight. First drowsiness, somnolence and mental confusion set in, so that even in accidental intoxication the victim may be so confused he is unable to help himself. As the blood levels of carboxyhemoglobin rise the victim lapses into coma and eventually the central nervous system damage causes death. In nonfatal poisonings central nervous system residuals such as impairment of memory, vision, hearing and speech may persist.

LEAD

Lead poisoning *(plumbism)* stands out as a classic example of an environmental disease. It occurs in an acute or chronic form. Acute poisoning generally follows the ingestion of some soluble lead salt with suicidal intent or accidental heavy respiratory industrial exposure. This form of the disease is happily uncommon today because there are so many "better" ways to commit suicide and because the hazards of industrial exposure are well recognized and largely controlled. Chronic plumbism, however, continues to be a menace, particularly to children. Lead is stored in the body and the progressive accumulation of small amounts may lead to toxic levels. It is no exaggeration to say that in this modern world it is almost impossible to escape exposure to lead. The exhaust of automobiles using gasoline with lead additives is the greatest source of contamination in the environment. It has been estimated that in North America more than 200,000 tons of lead annually are spewed into the air from this source (Goyer, 1971). The average adult in the United States has a blood level of lead of about 25 μg. per 100 ml.; toxic levels are 80 μg. per 100 ml. Children are at particular risk because in addition to air pollution they may ingest dangerous amounts of lead from lead-based paints, city dirt and dust, lead-laden ceramic glazes and even from chewing newspapers and magazines bearing red and orange print which is particularly rich in lead (Lin-Fu, 1973). A recent survey revealed that approximately 26 per cent of children had blood levels of at least 40 μg. of lead per 100 ml. (Gilsinn, 1972). The "silent epidemic," as chronic lead poisoning in children has been called, is not confined to the slums. Up to 40 per cent of those with significantly elevated blood lead levels come from the suburbs or even from rural areas. Adults are not immune from chronic plumbism. Not only did 3 per cent of the general population in six large cities in the United States have levels of 40 μg. per 100 ml. or over, but also nearly one quarter of gas station workers and two thirds of garage mechanics were similarly burdened.

The principal anatomic and clinical effects of lead poisoning are on the hematopoietic, gastrointestinal and nervous systems, as well as on the kidneys. The red cells become coated with lead salts, which damage their cell membranes and lead to increased fragility and hemolysis. Furthermore, lead has been shown to interfere with hemoglobin synthesis at an early step involving the enzyme delta aminolevulinic acid dehydratase. *Extensive basophilic stippling of the red cells is seen, the significance of which is unclear.* Although severe abdominal colic is characteristic of plumbism, the only morphologic finding in the gastrointestinal tract is the *"lead line"*—a line of discoloration at the dental margins of the gingivae, presumably resulting from the local formation and precipitation of lead sulfide. In the brain, widespread degeneration of the cortical and ganglionic neurons is accompanied by diffuse edema of the gray and white matter (Fig. 8–3). The peripheral nerve lesions take the form of myelin degeneration of the axis cylinders of those motor nerves supplying the most actively used muscles of the body. The extensor muscles of the wrist and fingers ordinarily are the first and most severely affected, followed by paralysis of the peroneal muscles. Clinically, this results in finger, wrist and foot drop. Renal changes are not as prominent as the CNS and hematopoietic effects just described, but proximal tubular dysfunction (the

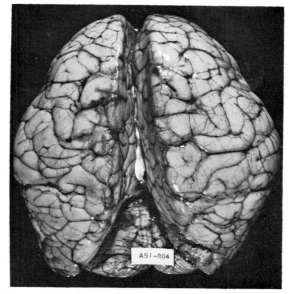

Figure 8–3. Cerebral edema in lead poisoning. The gyri are flattened and widened and the sulci are narrowed and relatively inapparent. (From Robbins, S. L.: Pathologic Basis of Disease. Philadelphia, W. B. Saunders Company, 1974.)

Fanconi syndrome) may appear, presumably because lead interferes with the function of certain enzymes. A characteristic finding in chronic plumbism is the development of acid-fast intranuclear inclusions thought to be lead-protein complexes in the epithelial cells of the proximal tubules.

The diagnosis of plumbism is supported by the demonstration of red cell stippling, the lead line in the mouth and increased x-ray density of the epiphyseal ends of the bones in children, which is caused by the deposition of lead in these sites (Fig. 8–4). Usually the diagnosis can be firmly established by the identification of lead in the urine.

MERCURY

Mercury compounds are protein precipitants and cause tissue injury principally by inactivating enzymes involved in cellular respiration, particularly the cytochrome oxidases. They also complex with sulfhydryl and phosphoryl groups and by this mechanism damage cellular membranes. A syndrome of acute poisoning is sometimes distinguished from that of chronic poisoning. The acute form of poisoning usually presents with dysarthria, ataxia and constricted visual fields. In contrast chronic poisoning begins more insidiously, with the development of tremors, mental changes (lack of attention, loss of memory, decline of intellect, emotional instability), dermatitis, gingivitis, gastroenteritis and heavy proteinuria, sometimes inducing the nephro-

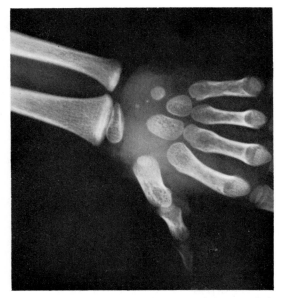

Figure 8–4. Lead deposits in the epiphyses of the wrist have caused a marked increase in their radiodensity so that they are as radiopaque as the cortical bone. (From Robbins, S. L.: Pathologic Basis of Disease. Philadelphia, W. B. Saunders Company, 1974.)

tic syndrome (p. 432). In the past, toxicity resulting from the intake of inorganic compounds was thought to differ from that caused by organic compounds. Case reports now attest to the fact that whether the metal is organic or inorganic the major determinants of the clinical and morphologic changes in mercury poisoning are the rate of accumulation and the ultimate level of mercury within the tissues (Kark et al., 1971). Unlike lead, mercury is not stored in the body and most is excreted fairly rapidly in the urine and feces. Thus, the concentration in the tissues depends on the *intensity* as well as the *duration* of exposure to compounds of mercury, be they inorganic or organic.

Acute poisoning is seen with accidental ingestion of soluble inorganic or organic salts; the latter are widely used in fungicides. Rarely, acute poisoning results from the inhalation of concentrated vapors of volatilized metallic mercury. Chronic poisoning is the consequence of the slow incremental accumulation of mercury compounds, sometimes from the long-term ingestion of contaminated meat or fish, or from the inhalation of industrial dusts or vapors. Only a few years ago there was an outbreak of mercury poisoning in Japan, causing worldwide concern about the danger of eating canned fish processed there. Subsequently it was shown that industrial mercury wastes had been diverted into the coastal waters, heavily contaminating the fish on which the nearby population sub-

sisted. Control of the industrial contamination promptly corrected the problem, but only after a tragic morbidity and mortality had been inflicted. Similarly, the consumption of meat from animals maintained on grains and fodder heavily contaminated with mercury-bearing fungicides has produced cases of mercury poisoning.

The pathologic changes induced by mercury poisoning are found principally in the oral cavity, colon, kidneys and brain. Small amounts of absorbed mercury are excreted through the saliva and this stimulates excessive salivation with deposition of mercury or mercury salts along the gingival margin, resulting in a discoloration closely resembling the "lead line." Gingivitis and destruction of the alveolar bone about the teeth may cause loosening of the teeth. When mercury is ingested, focal to massive confluent necrosis of the gastric epithelium may appear. Similar lesions may occur in the colon as the mercury is excreted. As it is excreted through the urine, mercury produces striking changes in the kidneys ranging from cellular swelling to necrosis of the proximal convoluted tubular cells. If the victim survives long enough, the damaged tubular epithelial cells may undergo calcification. The cytoplasm of injured cells is often filled with eosinophilic droplets attributed to the resorption of protein from the glomerular filtrate. As mentioned, the proteinuria may be sufficiently marked to induce the nephrotic syndrome. This is correlated with glomerular basement membrane damage seen under the electron microscope as basement membrane thickening. In fatal poisonings with organic compounds a variety of changes appear in the central nervous system, including atrophy of the calcarine fissure, enlargement of the occipital horns of the lateral ventricles, atrophy of the cerebellar folia and occasionally scattered foci of atrophy throughout the cerebral cortex (Takeuchi et al., 1962). No morphologic studies are available on the effects of inorganic mercury poisoning on the brain, but the symptoms of these patients make it highly likely that the changes are similar to those encountered with organic compounds. In closing, it should be pointed out that metallic mercury is not absorbable and so swallowing the mercury from a broken thermometer or dental amalgam filling will not cause mercury poisoning.

ARSENIC

Arsenic in its various forms—salts, oxides and arsene gas—is a very potent poison. Arsenic binds rapidly with sulfhydryl groups, and this accounts for the fact that in cases of poisoning it can be detected in hair, nails and the surface squames of the skin. The lethal action of arsenic probably relates to its combining with sulfhydryl groups in intracellular respiratory enzymes. Depending on the levels absorbed, three patterns of toxicity are encountered: (1) fulminating, (2) acute, and (3) chronic.

Fulminating arsenic poisoning implies death within hours following the absorption of massive doses. It is almost always encountered in suicides or homicides caused by the ingestion of a relatively soluble oxide of arsenic. The mode of death appears to be profound depression of the central nervous system with paralysis of vasomotor control, which leads to a fatal reduction in the effective circulating blood volume.

Acute arsenic poisoning implies survival for at least 24 hours and up to one week. This syndrome is usually encountered in those accidentally exposed during the course of their work to heavy concentrations of arsene gas or to dusts containing soluble arsenic compounds. The major anatomic changes are found in the vascular system, skin, brain and gastrointestinal tract. Acute necrosis of the microvasculature leads to petechial hemorrhages in the skin and serous membranes, often accompanied by visceral hyperemia. When the poison is absorbed through the gastrointestinal tract the changes range from congestion and edema of the mucosa of the stomach to hemorrhagic necrosis and ulceration of large areas of the stomach lining. When gastric ulcerations are present, implying high levels of toxicity, similar lesions may occur in lower levels of the intestinal tract. The most serious lesions appear in the brain over a period of 2 to 3 days. They take the form of meningeal petechial hemorrhages, diffuse cerebral edema and focal areas of infarction where injured vessels have thrombosed. Fatty change may appear in the parenchymal cells of the kidneys and liver, sometimes accompanied by fatty change of the myocardium.

The clinical manifestations of acute poisoning largely depend on the amount of arsenic absorbed and on the duration of survival. With large dosages the symptoms are quite similar to those of fulminating poisoning, save that the patient survives longer. Smaller dosages and longer survival permit the appearance of marked vomiting, then severe persistent watery diarrhea, followed in time by obtundation and vascular collapse. The petechial hemorrhages in the skin in such a syndrome should provide a clue to the appropriate diagnosis.

Chronic arsenic poisoning results from daily exposure to small amounts of this element, such as may occur in industry or from the repeated ingestion of small amounts of arsenical compounds commonly used as pesticides and fungicides. With this slow progressive intoxication the principal changes are found in the gastrointestinal tract, skin and peripheral nerves. Congestion, edema and small superficial ulcerations may develop in the stomach or small intestine. A variety of dermatologic changes may appear, including loss of hair, a maculopapular rash and focal or confluent areas of hyperpigmentation and hyperkeratosis of the palms and soles (*arsenical dermatitis*). Demyelination of peripheral nerves often leads to symmetric numbness, paresthesias and sometimes muscle weakness. The clinical diagnosis of chronic arsenic poisoning rests largely on the demonstration of increased levels of arsenic in hair, nails or tissues. The diagnosis can sometimes be suspected by the distinctive skin changes accompanied by the neurologic manifestations.

"STREET DRUGS"

No consideration of environmental pathology would be complete without some reference to marijuana (cannabis), heroin and lysergic acid diethylamide (LSD). The literature on these agents is vast, contradictory and often evangelical. It is perhaps wisest to admit at the outset that although the literature is replete with dire warnings, most are based on shaky evidence. A few of the better established findings follow.

Marijuana generally is classified as a hallucinogen, but in animal experiments it seems, ambiguously, to partake of the properties of a stimulant, sedative, tranquilizer and narcotic. In mice, for example, it potentiates both barbiturates (prolonging sleeping time) and amphetamines (increasing excitement) (Pillard, 1970). The potency of marijuana resides in its content of cannabinoids, particularly tetrahydrocannibol (THC) found in the cannabis resin. There are striking differences (up to 70 times) in the content of THC in marijuana plants derived from different parts of the world.

A wide variety of untoward reactions has been attributed to marijuana and THC. Prolongation of the action of barbiturates has been ascribed to inhibition of liver microsomes, and indeed the habitual marijuana smoker is likely to metabolize a considerable range of drugs more slowly (Paton and Pertwee, 1972). There is evidence that marijuana reduces sympathetic vasomotor tone, resulting in peripheral vasodilatation (particularly noticeable in the conjunctivae), postural hypotension and tachycardia. Smoke derived from marijuana contains a tar which is carcinogenic when painted on mouse skin (Magus and Harris, 1971). Fetal resorption, stunting and congenital anomalies have been produced in the offspring of rats, mice, rabbits and hamsters by injecting cannabis resin extracts early in pregnancy (Geber and Schramm, 1969). However, no comparable findings in humans, such as an increased rate of birth defects or chromosomal abnormalities in offspring, have been described in habitual users of marijuana. Mild liver dysfunction and parenchymal disorganization were identified in eight of 12 regular marijuana smokers who had not taken intravenous drugs or used alcohol to excess (Kew et al., 1969). The most serious ramifications of the use of marijuana, however, relate to its possible effects on the central nervous system and behavior. Changes in memory, perception, concentration, mood and a variety of other psychologic parameters have been described, but are exceedingly difficult to quantify. Other, more serious functional disturbances have also been attributed to marijuana, including acute psychosis, severe loss of motivation and attacks of anxiety. More objectively, electroencephalographic alterations in the form of hypersynchronous discharges, sometimes termed epileptiform, have been reported. Paton (1973) suggests, "the action of the drug is to impair transmitter output particularly at inhibitory synapses, so that it reduces selective processing . . . and allows release phenomena and synchronous—possibly reverberatory—discharges." At the time of this writing more rigorously controlled data are appearing in the daily press of similar findings in subhuman primates. Despite all these functional alterations no morphologic changes have been described in the central nervous systems of chronic users. In addition to the legal issues, the medical evidence is probably sufficient to justify prudence in the use of this agent.

Narcotic analgesics (included among the psychotherapeutic agents in Table 8–1) occupy second place among the causes of death from therapeutic agents. Among the narcotic analgesics are morphine, heroin, methadone and codeine, but most of the deaths can be laid at the doorstep of heroin. In contrast to barbiturate deaths, most of which are intentional, 80 to 90 per cent of the fatalities caused by narcotic analgesics result from accidental overdosage in drug addicts. Drug abuse, principally of heroin, has become the leading cause of death in New York City in the age range of 15 to 35 years. In 1939, in New York City, drugs were responsible for approximately 50 deaths per year; by 1969 the number had skyrocketed to 1016 (Baden, 1971).

Although the evidence that heroin may be lethal is incontrovertible, it is very difficult to isolate its morphologic effects from those of other narcotic agents. Drug addicts do not

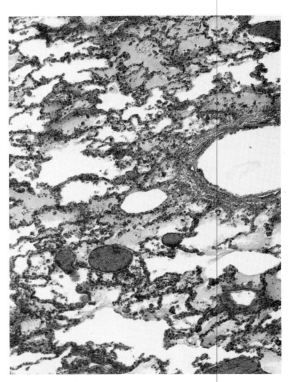

Figure 8–5. Patchy pulmonary edema and atelectasis of the alveoli of the lung in a heroin addict.

usually restrict their appetites to a single agent, and so it is often impossible to ascribe consequent morbidity or mortality to a specific drug. Street drugs are frequently "cut" or contaminated with all manner of white powders, including talc, quinine and starch. Many of the untoward reactions suggest hypersensitivity responses, possibly to the drug but equally likely to the contaminants. Bacterial and viral contamination is often introduced in the course of "mainlining" these hard drugs. So the pathology attributed to heroin abuse among addicts must be viewed with considerable caution.

Nonetheless, heroin is generally thought to be responsible for a distinctive pattern of pulmonary changes called "narcotic lung" (Siegel, 1972). In fatalities the lungs are often heavy and wet. Microscopically there is patchy pulmonary congestion and edema, made distinctive by focal atelectasis, emphysema, hemorrhages and accumulations of mononuclear cells within the alveoli and alveolar walls (Fig. 8–5). There is a possibility that these pulmonary changes represent an anaphylaxis-like reaction, since sometimes death occurs within minutes and the victim is found with the needle still in place (Werner, 1969). The occasional finding of diffuse necrotizing angiitis, virtually indistinguishable from polyarteritis nodosa, supports the concept that hypersensi-

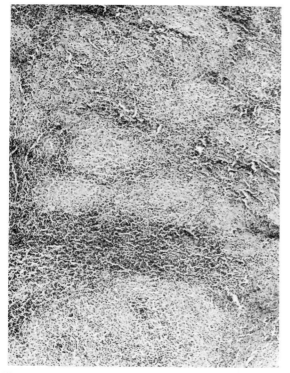

Figure 8–6. The pale foci are numerous granulomata within the spleen of a heroin addict.

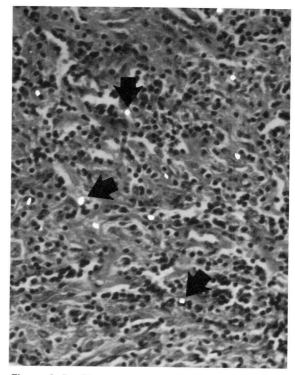

Figure 8–7. The spleen in a heroin addict viewed under partially polarized light. The numerous white flecks scattered throughout represent doubly refractile fragments of talc (arrows).

tivity may be involved in producing the pulmonary damage. In those who die 12 to 24 hours after the onset of respiratory difficulties, florid bacterial bronchopneumonia may be seen. Foreign body granulomata are sometimes found in the lungs, liver, spleen, lymph nodes and bone marrow of drug addicts (Fig. 8–6). Most likely, these represent reactions to contaminants such as talc, cornstarch and cotton fibers. Foreign body giant cells may be present within the granulomata, sometimes enclosing doubly refractile, crystalline fragments of talc (Hopkins and Taylor, 1970) (Fig. 8–7). For obscure reasons, the gallbladder is often distended and filled with thick mucoid bile. Even more striking is the frequent finding of marked (up to ten-fold) enlargement of the portahepatic and peripancreatic lymph nodes. The lymphadenopathy has been attributed to an immunologic reaction against some degradation product of heroin produced in the liver (Edland, 1972). No hepatic parenchymal changes have been identified which are attributable to heroin alone. Such hepatic dysfunction as may be present has been ascribed to the high incidence of viral hepatitis and the frequent history of alcoholism among heroin users (Stimmel, 1972). Some addicts have developed focal and segmental glomerulosclerosis involving the deposition of IgM and the third com-

ponent of complement within the sclerotic foci, associated with the nephrotic syndrome. This finding raises once again the likelihood of an immune response against heroin, a metabolite or conceivably one of the contaminants, rather than direct toxicity (Sreepada Rao et al., 1974).

Perhaps the greatest threat associated with heroin abuse comes with the use, or more properly the misuse, of "the needle." Viral hepatitis (p. 247) has assumed near epidemic proportions among habitual users of hard drugs. Tetanus, infective endocarditis, skin infections, lung abscesses, tuberculosis and septic thrombophlebitis are other unpleasant concomitants of this form of addiction. In the face of all these problems it is of interest that no morphologic changes in the central nervous system have been directly related to this "mind-manipulating" drug. Although cerebral edema, meningeal congestion and petechiae, and occasionally neuronal injury, may be seen, these are more reasonably attributed to the hypoxia caused by the marked pulmonary edema, compounded possibly by respiratory depression.

Lysergic acid diethylamide (LSD) appears to have become less "fashionable" than it once was. Although psychologists and sociologists can wax fervent about its behavioral and psychologic consequences, very few morphologic abnormalities can be ascribed to it with certainty. Most of the controversy has centered on the possible genetic damage induced by this agent. The literature is replete with claims that LSD induces chromosomal damage and equally replete with counterclaims. Supporting the view that LSD induces chromosomal damage are the in vitro studies of Cohen and associates (1967) and Corey and associates (1970), as well as the in vivo studies of Cohen and colleagues (1968) and Nielsen and associates (1969). The in vitro studies are highly suspect since it has been shown that the introduction of a number of seemingly innocent substances, such as antibiotics, aspirin, benzene, caffeine or even water—unless twice distilled—into tissue cultures of leukocytes will induce chromosomal aberrations. An equally impressive array of in vitro and in vivo studies could be marshaled to show that LSD has no significant effects on chromosomes (Dorrance et al., 1970; Tjio et al., 1969). In some part this controversy arises from the difficulties in establishing rigorously controlled in vivo studies, including data on subjects before beginning use of LSD, followed by observations collected after intensive use of the drug. Moreover, many of the studies have been performed on individuals who obtained their LSD "on the street," and such drugs often are highly contaminated and impure. A scholarly review of this problem has recently appeared, which presents additional evidence that no significant chromosomal aberrations were observed in a controlled study using pure LSD (Fernandez et al., 1973). Thus, on balance, the evidence fails to incriminate this all too potent hallucingoen as a mutagen.

NUTRITIONAL DISORDERS

It is bitterly ironic that malnutrition—indeed starvation—is still rampant in impoverished countries at a time when obesity is near epidemic in privileged societies. Protein-calorie malnutrition is the world's dominant nutritional disorder, afflicting approximately half its population (Brown, 1971). It is the consequence of a dietary lack in the total quantity or quality of food. Such gross malnutrition is often accompanied by deficiencies in one or more of the vitamins (avitaminoses may, of course, develop despite an adequate protein and calorie intake). The problem has its roots in stark socioeconomic realities. With the population increase outpacing the availability of the food supply, it would appear that the problem can only get worse.

Nutritional inadequacies may occur as primary or secondary deficiency states. A *primary deficiency* implies an inadequate dietary intake, tragically common in many countries. Even in affluent societies, including the United States and Europe, poverty, ignorance, faddism and psychologic factors may contribute to a primary deficiency state. *Secondary deficiencies* may develop in the midst of plenty, as a consequence of any of five conditions:

1. *The malabsorption syndrome* (p. 488) is seen in a large group of diseases that have in common interference with intestinal absorption, and in parasitic infections, in which the intruder deprives the host of essential nutrients.

2. *Interference with storage* is encountered in severe liver disease, since many of the vitamins are stored in the liver. Reserves, which can be called upon during periods of negative balance, may be inadequate.

3. *Increased losses* are uncommon and are encountered only in extreme examples of chronic excessive sweating, diarrhea or diuresis. Lactation is another pathway by which vitamins may be lost to a nursing mother.

4. *Increased requirements* for protein and vitamins are encountered during periods of rapid growth, especially during childhood and pregnancy, infections and times of prolonged, increased physical activity.

5. *Inhibition of utilization* is caused by substances that block either the absorption or the metabolic activity of vitamins. The best example is avidin in uncooked egg white, which, by combining with biotin (one of the B vitamin fractions), blocks its absorption.

Any of the circumstances just cited may lead to a secondary deficiency in localities where there is no lack of food. Thus, avitaminoses are encountered sporadically in the wealthy as well as endemically in the impoverished.

PROTEIN-CALORIE MALNUTRITION

Protein-calorie malnutrition takes one of three forms: (1) marasmus, (2) kwashiorkor, or (3) nutritional growth failure. *Marasmus is a state of malnutrition resulting from a deficiency of calories. Kwashiorkor results from a dietary deficiency of protein despite an adequate caloric intake.* The term kwashiorkor is derived from the Ghanian language and means "the sickness which the old one gets when the next baby is born," i.e., when the elder child is deprived of breast feeding and weaned largely on a diet of carbohydrates. *Nutritional growth failure may be defined simply as retardation of normal growth and development due to inadequacies in the diet.* All three forms of protein-calorie malnutrition are widely prevalent in nearly all developing countries in Asia, Africa and the Americas and also in some of the economically less favored countries in Europe. These deficiency states have their greatest impact on children. Some idea of the prevalence of these conditions can be gained from the estimate that the *majority* of children in central Africa in the second and third years of life suffer from marasmus or kwashiorkor. The nutritional inadequacies wreak a heavy toll in lives. World surveys disclose an unmistakable correlation between infant mortality rates and inadequate nutrition. Contrast the infant mortality rates of 16 to 30 per 1000 live births of most industrialized nations with rates that vary from 60 to 150 per 1000 live births in poorer nations, where protein-calorie malnutrition is a constant concomitant of life (Patwardhan, 1964). The significance of these infant mortality rates is underscored by the fact that 50 per cent of *all* deaths in these less favored areas of the world occur in children under 5 years of age. The terminal event is usually an infection, although surprisingly not some exotic tropical infection. The five principal immediate causes of preschool mortality in these countries are, in order of importance: (1) gastroenteritis, (2) influenza, (3) measles, (4) whooping cough and (5) bronchitis.

Marasmus is an extreme state of emaciation which usually presents within the first year of life. The defect in this condition is more in weight than in height. The all too obvious physical features of children with this condition comprise loss of subcutaneous fat, thin musculature, and heads much too large for the wasted bodies. It should be noted that, in contrast to kwashiorkor, **marasmus is not characterized by edema.**

Kwashiorkor is characterized by generalized edema, short stature, hair changes (in pigmentation, tensile strength, loosening of the roots and sometimes alternating bands of depigmentation and pigmentation, creating the so-called "flag sign"), pallor and intestinal disturbances, usually diarrhea. In contrast to marasmus, there may be a deceptive plumpness imparted by the generalized edema. Other manifestations which may or may not be present include skin lesions (areas of depigmentation or hyperpigmentation, which create a so-called "crazy pavement" appearance), hepatomegaly, anemia and manifestations of vitamin deficiencies.

The organ changes in these two syndromes involve principally the liver, gastrointestinal mucosa and hematopoietic system. Kwashiorkor, but not marasmus, is characterized by fatty change in the liver, probably due to decreased synthesis of lipoproteins. There is no evidence that these children ever develop cirrhosis, and with an adequate diet the fat in the liver completely disappears. The mucosa of the small bowel in kwashiorkor is usually atrophic, and in severe cases it may show complete loss of microvilli and villi. There is an accompanying loss of small intestinal enzymes, most often manifested as disaccharidase deficiency. Thus, these infants respond poorly to a diet of milk because of the enzyme deficiency. Despite the mucosal atrophy, no other absorptive defects are consistently present. An adequate diet and control of intercurrent infections permit recovery of the normal gastrointestinal mucosa. Anemia of the normochromic normocytic type is almost always present with both marasmus and kwashiorkor. The anemia is often made worse by concomitant intestinal parasites, such as hookworms, that deprive the host of iron and folic acid. Thus, in some of these infants, when protein therapy is administered a folic acid or iron deficiency, or both, is unmasked. The bone marrow usually shows erythroid hypoplasia and a disturbed erythroid-myeloid ratio. Complete remission of all the above changes in marasmus and kwashiorkor can be achieved with an adequate diet and control of infections.

The effect of protein malnutrition on mental development and performance is still a controversial issue. Most of the evidence indicates that if the child is six months or older, protein-calorie malnutrition does not produce any irreversible damage to the brain. Maternal malnutrition during pregnancy, however, may be more important. Furthermore, it is suspected that other economic and social deprivations which almost always accompany protein-calorie malnutrition play at least as important a role as the diet.

VITAMIN DEFICIENCIES

When protein-calorie nutrition is relatively adequate other, more specific nutritional deficiencies may become apparent. Man requires approximately 50 to 60 essential nutrients, including minerals, certain fatty acids, specific amino acids and vitamins, for optimal health. Understandably, deficiencies of vitamins are prevalent in impoverished areas of the world and contribute significantly to the mortality of patients with kwashiorkor or marasmus. For example, in one study reported from Jordan, patients with protein-calorie malnutrition without manifestations of vitamin A deficiency had a mortality of only 15 per cent; but when a deficiency of vitamin A was also present 56 per cent of the patients died (McLaren et al., 1965). Avitaminoses in such settings represent primary deficiencies based on the quantity and quality of the food; however, it should be remembered that avitaminoses may develop as secondary deficiency states for any of the reasons cited in the introductory part of this section. Thus, individuals who appear deceptively well nourished may nonetheless be suffering from a deficiency of one or more vitamins.

In the sections which follow the fat soluble

vitamins—A, D, E and K—are discussed first, followed by a consideration of the water soluble vitamins—C and the major constituents of the B complex.

VITAMIN A

(Deficiency States: Night Blindness, Xerophthalmia, Keratomalacia, Epithelial Keratinizing Metaplasia, Disturbances in Bone Growth)

In animals vitamin A deficiency has widespread metabolic effects, involving virtually all systems, including maintenance of normal growth of the skeletal system. However, in man the more or less established roles of vitamin A involve the visual process and possibly the maintenance of membranes. In the following discussion the nomenclature adopted by the International Union of Pure and Applied Chemistry will be used. Retinol signifies pure vitamin A alcohol, retinyl ester refers to vitamin A ester and retinal means vitamin A aldehyde.

Retinol is available to man in the normal diet in two forms: as the vitamin itself or in the form of provitamin precursors, the carotenes. Both are present in vegetables containing yellow pigments as well as in liver and animal fats such as butter fat or cod liver oil. Beta carotene, the most important of the carotenoids, is partly cleaved in the intestinal mucosa into two molecules of retinal. A deficiency of dietary fat impairs the absorption of the carotenoids just as a deficiency of dietary proteins affects the absorption of preformed vitamin A (retinol). Details of the metabolism of vitamin A are available in the excellent review by Roels (1970), but it suffices for our purposes here to say that after absorption, large amounts are normally stored in the liver, and severe liver disease may impair its storage. Whereas avitaminosis A sometimes occurs as a primary deficiency state after long periods of deprivation, it may also represent a secondary deficiency state as a consequence of disorders affecting fat absorption, such as biliary tract diseases, pancreatic disease, sprue or severe intestinal disease.

The role of vitamin A in the visual process is fairly well understood. The human retina contains two distinct photoreceptor systems: the rods, sensitive to light of low intensity, and the cones, responsive to high intensity light and colors. Retinal is the prosthetic group of the photosensitive pigment in both rods and cones. The major difference between this photosensitive pigment in the rods (rhodopsin) and in the cones (iodopsin) resides in the nature of the protein bound to it. The visual process involves isomerization in the dark of all-trans retinal to the 11-cis form, which in combination with opsin forms rhodopsin. With the absorption of light, the 11-cis isomer is converted back to the all-trans form. Energy for this reaction is supplied by the light quanta. In the course of this energy exchange potential differences arise which are transmitted via the optic nerve to the brain and result in visual perception. During this cyclic transformation some of the retinal may be reduced to retinol and be lost to the reaction. Accordingly, small amounts of vitamin A must constantly be fed into the visual process. With inadequate blood levels of vitamin A, the small amounts of retinal involved in rod vision are rapidly depleted and vision in low intensity light is lost (night blindness).

In addition to its role in the visual process, some believe that vitamin A is required for the maintenance of the integrity of cell membranes as well as of the membranes of ultrastructures (Lucy et al., 1963). A role in the conversion of cholesterol to cortisone and possibly a role in the synthesis of mucopolysaccharides have also been suspected but not clearly established. The significance of these possible actions in the prevention of disease is still obscure.

The disease states associated with a deficiency of vitamin A include night blindness (nyctalopia), epithelial metaplasia, xerophthalmia and keratomalacia. The role of vitamin A in the prevention of night blindness has already been discussed. It should, however, be pointed out that diseases of the retina may also produce impaired vision that is sometimes mistakenly interpreted as a manifestation of avitaminosis A.

In some as yet poorly understood fashion, this vitamin appears to be necessary for the preservation of certain specialized epithelial surfaces, such as the mucous membranes of the eyes, the mucosa of the respiratory, gastrointestinal and genitourinary tracts, and the lining epithelia of gland ducts and ducts of the skin appendages. When a significant lack of vitamin A occurs, keratinization of the mucosa of the conjunctiva results. This keratinization causes replacement of the normal moist mucosal surfaces with a dry, granular, roughened epithelium (**xerophthalmia**), on which keratin debris may accumulate to produce whitish plaques known as **Bitot's spots**. When the keratinization occurs on the corneal mucosa, it causes impairment of vision. Such surfaces are prone to irritation and inflammation and often develop ulcerations, which may extend into the cornea to thus induce softening and opacity of the cornea, referred to as **keratomalacia**. Secondary infections may lead to involvement of the iris and lens. The mucosa of the oral cavity and vagina may also become keratinized. Columnar epithelium may become transformed to stratified squamous epithelium, as for example in the respiratory passages. The inappropriate epithelium impairs normal defenses. Mucus secretion and ciliary action are lost in the bronchi and bronchioles and secondary pulmonary infections are therefore common. When the lining of the collecting system of the kidney becomes keratinized, the desquamated keratin debris may provide a nidus for the formation of urinary tract stones. Formerly hyperkeratinization of the skin was attributed to vitamin A deficiency. Now, however, it is considered more likely that it is related to a deficiency of an essential fatty acid. Although disturbed bone growth is a prominent manifestation of experimentally induced vitamin A deficiency in animals, no similar skeletal abnormalities have been identified in man.

Isolated reports can be found of hypervitaminosis A of both acute (Braun, 1962) and chronic (Jeghers and Marraro, 1956) forms. These reactions are extremely uncommon, but they should be kept in mind when massive doses of this agent are administered.

VITAMIN D

(Deficiency States: Rickets and Osteomalacia)

Children are especially vulnerable to vitamin D deficiency because of the demands of their rapidly growing bones. The deficiency state is termed *rickets* and is characterized by abnormalities of both endochondral and membranous bone formation. In adults, on

the other hand, cartilaginous bone growth has ceased and therefore a deficiency of vitamin D results primarily in deranged membranous bone formation *(osteomalacia)*.

Several closely related fat soluble compounds have antirachitic effect, the most important being vitamin D_3 (cholecalciferol). This compound can be derived from certain fish oils and animal livers but surprisingly it is not abundant in other natural dietary sources. Man, however, also has endogenous sources of cholecalciferol since it is formed in the skin by the ultraviolet irradiation of the physiological precursor 7-dehydrocholesterol. In the hope that no child will read this book it can be divulged that one theory proposes that 7-dehydrocholesterol is secreted by sebaceous glands onto the skin surface and is converted there by ultraviolet irradiation to cholecalciferol, which is then reabsorbed. If such a process were involved it would argue strongly against bathing too frequently! Fortunately there is considerable evidence that the antirachitic range of ultraviolet light readily penetrates the superficial layers of the skin and can transform 7-dehydrocholesterol in the deeper layers. However, save for those living out-

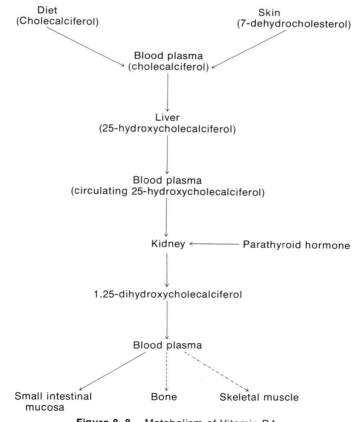

Figure 8-8. Metabolism of Vitamin D.*

*Modified from Wasserman, R. H., and Taylor, A. N.: Metabolic roles of fat soluble vitamins D, E and K. Ann. Rev. Biochem., *41*:179, 1972.

doors in tropical climes, some dietary supply of vitamin D is necessary.

It is now amply documented that cholecalciferol, whatever its origin, is not the active antirachitic metabolite. It undergoes a complex sequence of transformations, as outlined in Figure 8–8. More details are available in the reviews by Stamp (1973), Codicek (1974) and DeLuca (1975). Whether absorbed in the diet or derived from the skin, cholecalciferol is transported in the blood to the liver, where it is converted to 25-hydroxycholecalciferol (25-OH-D_3). This is then transported on a protein carrier to the kidney, where under certain circumstances it is further hydroxylated to 1,25-dihydroxycholecalciferol [1,25-$(\text{OH})_2\text{-D}_3$], presently believed to be the active antirachitic agent. The principal end-organ effect of 1,25-$(\text{OH})_2\text{-D}_3$ is to enhance calcium and inorganic phosphate (Pi) absorption in the small intestine. The increased calcium absorption requires the synthesis of a calcium-binding protein (CaBP) involved in the transport of calcium across the mucosa. The weight of evidence suggests that 1,25-$(\text{OH})_2\text{-D}_3$ is required for the transcription of the messenger RNA of CaBP.

Calcium homeostasis is, of course, also influenced by the release of parathormone (PTH) from the parathyroid glands. The interaction between PTH and 1,25-$(\text{OH})_2\text{-D}_3$ is complicated, but much has been learned about it within the past few years. First, as we shall see, in many cases PTH is necessary for the synthesis of 1,25-$(\text{OH})_2\text{-D}_3$ by the kidneys. It should be emphasized that the kidneys do not always convert 25-OH-D_3 into 1,25-$(\text{OH})_2$-D_3. Indeed, when serum calcium and Pi levels are normal, 25-OH-D_3 is instead converted by the kidneys to a relatively inactive metabolite, 24,25-$(\text{OH})_2\text{-D}_3$. What, then, stimulates the synthesis of the active antirachitic metabolite? The evidence is that this metabolic pathway is triggered by either of two situations: (1) decreased serum calcium levels *plus increased PTH*, or (2) decreased serum Pi levels. Not only does a lowered serum calcium level induce the formation of 1,25-$(\text{OH})_2\text{-D}_3$, which exerts its effect on the small intestine, but in addition two other effects occur: (a) together 1,25-$(\text{OH})_2\text{-D}_3$ and PTH cause increased mobilization of calcium and Pi from the bone, and (b) in the kidneys, PTH causes greatly increased calcium reabsorption with concomitant loss of Pi. The net effect of these changes on the intestine, bone and kidneys is an increased serum level of calcium and a relatively stable serum Pi level (DeLuca, 1975). Thus the active form of vitamin D, by helping to maintain normal serum calcium levels, is necessary for normal bone mineralization. Normal calcium levels are also necessary for mus-

cle contraction. Whether vitamin D has a *direct* role in the mineralization of osteoid in the absence of PTH is uncertain, as is indicated by the broken arrow in Figure 8–8.

The most common cause of rickets in childhood is a dietary deficiency of vitamin D. Osteomalacia in the adult, however, may develop despite a diet adequate in vitamin D. *Malabsorption states* may induce faulty absorption of all fats, including vitamin D. Osteomalacia therefore may develop with steatorrhea from any cause, including the postgastrectomy state, hepatobiliary disease, pancreatic dysfunction and intrinsic intestinal disease. Indeed, osteomalacia has been reported in about 1 per cent of males and 4 per cent of females following gastrectomy. *Chronic renal insufficiency* may also lead to skeletal abnormalities, collectively referred to as renal osteodystrophy (p. 428), which essentially resembles osteomalacia. With our increased understanding of the normal metabolism of vitamin D, the nature of the relationship between chronic renal disease and bone abnormalities becomes clearer. Presumably the kidneys are no longer able to synthesize adequate amounts of the active metabolite 1,25-$(\text{OH})_2\text{-D}_3$. The new understanding of vitamin D metabolism further explains why patients with marked renal damage develop secondary hyperparathyroidism (p. 616). When 1,25-$(\text{OH})_2\text{-D}_3$ cannot be synthesized, the full load of maintaining the blood calcium levels falls on the parathyroid glands which at first hyperfunction and then undergo hyperplasia.

The basic change with both rickets and osteomalacia is an excess of poorly mineralized osteoid tissue. For somewhat mysterious reasons, it seems that the increase in osteoid matrix is absolute as well as relative and, indeed, these patients may have thickened, albeit poorly mineralized, bones.

Rickets involves a greater range of histologic changes than does osteomalacia because of the involvement of endochondral ossification. These changes are:

1. Failure of deposition of calcium into the cartilage—i.e., failure of provisional calcification.

2. Failure of the cartilage cells to mature and disintegrate or be destroyed, with resultant overgrowth of cartilage.

3. Persistence of distorted, irregular masses of cartilage, many of which project into the marrow cavity.

4. Deposition of osteoid matrix on cartilaginous remnants, with formation of a disorderly, totally disrupted osteochondral junction (Fig. 8–9).

5. Abnormal overgrowth of capillaries and fibroblasts into the disorganized zone.

6. Bending, compression and microfractures of soft, weakly supported osteoid and cartilaginous tissue, with resultant skeletal deformities.

The gross skeletal deformities depend to a large

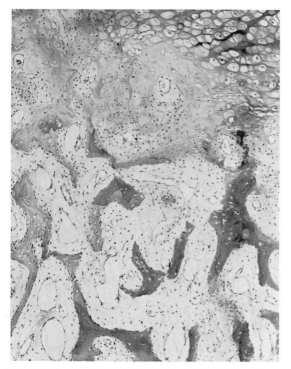

Figure 8–9. A detail of a rachitic costochondral junction. The palisade of cartilage is lost. Some of the trabeculae are old, well formed bone, but the paler ones consist of unmineralized osteoid tissue. (From Robbins, S. L.: Pathologic Basis of Disease. Philadelphia, W. B. Saunders Company, 1974.)

extent on the stress to which individual bones are subjected, which, in turn, is related to the age of the child. During infancy, the nonambulatory child places greatest stress upon the head and chest. Often, the abnormally soft cranium can be buckled under pressure, recoiling back into position with release of pressure. This clinical sign is known as **craniotabes.** An excess of osteoid tissue produces **frontal bossing** and a squared appearance to the head. Chest deformities include the **rachitic rosary,** caused by overgrowth of osteoid tissue at the costochondral junctions; **the pigeon-breast deformity,** resulting from collapse of the ribs with relative protrusion of the sternum; and **Harrison's groove,** produced by the inward pull on the ribs at the margin of the diaphragm. When the child with full-blown rickets begins to ambulate, additional deformities occur in the spine, pelvis and long bones. Lumbar lordosis and bowing of the legs are common.

The changes of osteomalacia are similar to those of rickets, but they tend to be confined to defects in membranous bone formation. The inadequate mineralization leads to an excess of osteoid matrix; thus, although the bony structure is more coarse, it is nonetheless abnormally weak. Deformities of weight-bearing bones are common. Although pathologic fractures occur, they are often

incomplete because of the decreased brittleness of the bones.

In addition to obvious deformities, the clinical features of vitamin D deficiency include bone pain and muscle weakness. X-rays may simply show abnormally radiolucent bone and thus be indistinguishable from x-rays of osteoporosis, or they may demonstrate a mosaic pattern (*pseudofractures* or *Looser's zones*) that is also seen with other bone diseases, principally osteitis deformans (p. 623). Characteristically, serum alkaline phosphatase is elevated because of the osteoblastic activity, while serum calcium and phosphorus may be either normal or low. *These blood values serve to distinguish vitamin D deficiency from osteoporosis, but they may further confuse it with osteitis deformans, which also causes an elevated serum alkaline phosphatase. Ultimately, the conclusive diagnostic criterion is the response of the patient to vitamin D supplementation or more accurately to 1,25-(OH)$_2$-D$_3$ or its synthetic analogue.*

VITAMIN E

Although vitamin E has been shown to be an essential fat soluble nutrient for many species of animals, there is only one bit of evidence that it is essential to man. Only recently a disease in premature infants has been attributed to a deficiency of vitamin E. It was reported that some infants of low birth weight placed on artificial formulas developed edema, decreased erythrocyte survival time, anemia and reticulocytosis. This syndrome was reversed when their diets were supplemented with vitamin E (Ritchie et al., 1968). With this exception, the situation with respect to vitamin E is well expressed in the following statement: "Vitamin E is one of those embarrassing vitamins that has been identified, isolated and synthesized by physiologists and biochemists and then handed to the medical profession with the suggestion that a use should be found for it, without any satisfactory evidence to show that human beings are ever deficient of it or even that it is a necessary nutrient for man" (Davidson and Passmore, 1970). Nonetheless, recommended daily allowances (10 to 15 I.U. for children, 20 to 30 I.U. for adults) have been set.

Of the eight naturally occurring forms of vitamin E (four tocopherols and four tocotrienols), alpha tocopherol possesses the greatest biological activity and in animals appears to be the active metabolite. A bewildering array of functional and anatomic alterations has been identified in vitamin E deficient rats, rabbits, chickens, sheep and dogs, including testicular damage with sterility; abnormalities of gestation; degenerative changes in nervous tissue, liver and skeletal muscles; hemolytic anemias; impaired collagen and enzyme synthesis; derangements in membranes, endoplasmic reticulum and mitochondria; as well as many other diverse changes (Scott, 1970). The manner in which a deficiency of vitamin E induces such various alterations is still poorly understood. The amount of vitamin E in the diet required to prevent signs of some of these deficiency states depends on the quantity of polyunsaturated fatty acids in the diet. It is well established that the tocopherols are powerful antioxidants. Curiously, in some cases in animals synthetic antioxidants, coenzyme Q, selenium and some sulfur amino acids are capable of reversing the manifestations of an E deficiency. For example, animals maintained on a vitamin E deficient diet develop a yellow to brown pigment *(ceroid)* in adipose tissue. The pigment is thought to be produced by polymerization of polyunsaturated fatty acid peroxides with lipoproteins. The development of the pigmentation can be prevented by restoration of vitamin E to the diet or by the administration of antioxidants. On the other hand, the muscular dystrophy which appears in rabbits, guinea pigs and other animals on a vitamin E deficient diet is not reversed by antioxidants but is responsive only to vitamin E. Similarly, this vitamin has been shown to be involved in the maintenance of cell membranes in animals, but synthetic antioxidants cannot substitute for the vitamin itself in this biologic action.

Because of the many wide-ranging effects of vitamin E deficiency in animals, attempts have repeatedly been made to implicate an avitaminosis E in related diseases in man. Thus, vitamin E has been advised for the treatment of muscular dystrophies, sterility in the male, habitual abortion, cardiomyopathies and many other conditions ranging from acne to cancer, but without any evidence that it has had beneficial effect (Tappel, 1973). Despite the suspicion that in man this vitamin must have an as yet undiscovered primary function, to date the only disease state clearly associated with its deficiency is the hemolytic anemia in formula-fed infants of low birth weight.

VITAMIN K

(Deficiency State: Hypoprothrombinemia)

Vitamin K is needed by the liver in order to synthesize not only prothrombin (factor II) but also factors VII, IX and X. Nonetheless, vitamin K deficiency is commonly known as "*hypoprothrombinemia.*" All of these factors are necessary to maintain normal blood clotting, and a deficiency of any one leads to a hemorrhagic diathesis and prolongation of the one stage prothrombin test of Quick. Thus, the Quick prothrombin test does not indicate whether one or all four factors are deficient.

Vitamin K exists in three forms: K_1 (phylloquinone), K_2 (menaquinone) and K_3 (menadione). The first two occur naturally in green plants and animal tissues and are formed by intestinal microorganisms. K_3 is a synthetic product. All are fat soluble, and their uptake from the small intestine therefore depends on normal fat absorption. Thus, even when adequate amounts of the vitamin are present in the gut, absorption is dependent on bile salts, bile acids and pancreatic enzymes, as well as a normal intestinal mucosal surface.

The mode of action of vitamin K is not well understood, although most evidence suggests that it is involved, at the postribosomal level, in the synthesis of the specific clotting factors mentioned above (Suttie, 1969). Conceivably, vitamin K attaches to a polypeptide chain or to some unrecognized prosthetic group. Alternatively, it may modify the amino acid residues to form calcium binding sites (Suttie, 1973; Johnson et al., 1971). An abnormal prothrombin and an abnormal factor IX have been detected in blood from vitamin K deficient or anticoagulant-treated individuals. These might represent precursor proteins lacking the prosthetic group or calcium binding sites.

The clinical importance of vitamin K depends on the severity of the deficiency. Only profound hypoprothrombinemia induces a significant bleeding diathesis. Moderate reductions in the prothrombin level may be entirely unimportant. Indeed, dicumarol, an antagonist of vitamin K, is safely used clinically as an anticoagulant. With severe hypoprothrombinemia, however, the patient is vulnerable to massive hemorrhage with any trauma, no matter how trivial. Common sites for these hemorrhages are operative wounds, particularly those incurred during the surgical relief of obstructive jaundice, with its associated malabsorption of vitamin K. Petechial bleeding may also occur into the skin, mucous membranes (particularly in the intestinal tract) and serosal surfaces, and in any other organ or cavity of the body. When these affect vital structures, such as the brain, they may cause death.

VITAMIN B COMPLEX

The B vitamins (or B complex) are a group of water soluble substances often found together in such foods as yeast, grains, rice, vegetables, fish and meats. This group plays a vital role in energy releasing mechanisms and in hematopoiesis. The energy releasing reactions provide the sources of the high energy bonds of ATP, and so deficiencies of B vitamins tend to induce changes in tissues having high levels of metabolic activity and rapid turnover. Thus, stomatitis, gastritis, and blood and bone marrow disorders are common features of vitamin B deficiencies. Degenerative disorders of the brain and nerves are also characteristic of these deficiency states because nervous tissue is totally dependent on glucose for its energy requirements. Since the B vitamins are water soluble, their absorption is unaffected by malabsorption states which do not involve derangements in the intestinal mucosa. In contrast, the fat soluble vitamins are affected by all malabsorption states.

With these very brief remarks on a vastly complex subject, we may turn to a consideration of the major members of the B complex.

Thiamine (Vitamin B₁) (Deficiency State: Beriberi). Thiamine deficiency gives rise to a condition known as *beriberi.* As a water soluble vitamin, thiamine is readily absorbed from dietary sources. However, only small amounts are stored, so a constant supply is necessary. Beriberi is common in the economically deprived areas of the world, particularly where grains and rice are the dietary staples and where these foods are largely depleted of their thiamine content by methods of processing or preparation, such as polishing of rice. In the United States and Europe thiamine deficiency is uncommon, because of the widely prevalent practice of fortifying foods with vitamin supplements. However, occasional instances of a deficiency state are encountered: in the alcoholic, during pregnancy (when there is increased utilization of the vitamin), and when there is decreased intake as a result of loss of appetite, vomiting or intrinsic intestinal disease.

Beriberi may present as one of three syndromes: a wet form *characterized by cardiovascular failure and peripheral edema, a* dry form *characterized by peripheral neuritis, with paralysis and atrophy of muscles, and a* cerebral form, *also known as Wernicke's syndrome.* In all these presentations the first manifestations of thiamine deficiency are loss of appetite and vomiting, which create an obvious vicious circle.

The fundamental defect in wet beriberi is cardiac failure. The heart is often flabby, dilated and somewhat pale. The dilatation may affect both sides, but it is often more prominent on the right, perhaps because the myocardium on this side is less well developed. A variety of subtle microscopic changes have been described in animals but are rarely seen in man. These include myocardial cell swelling, hydropic vacuolation and, rarely, single cell necroses. Perhaps the most consistent are increased interstitial edema and ground substance, which spread the myocardial fibers apart. In cases of long duration the interstitial edema is replaced by a loose connective tissue. Peripheral edema is encountered secondary to cardiac failure (p. 292). Because the thiamine deficiency induces dilatation of peripheral capillaries and arterioles, these patients have a *shortened circulation time* despite the cardiac failure, giving rise to the term *high-output failure.* As is evident, the morphologic changes are not highly distinctive. The diagnosis can be suspected by the presence of high output failure, by exclusion of other causes of the cardiac failure and by a history of inadequate thiamine intake. It is confirmed by a beneficial response to the administration of thiamine.

Dry beriberi presents essentially as an ascending, bilateral, symmetrical polyneuritis. It may progress to the point of toe and foot drop, as well as wrist drop. A variety of muscular symptoms appear, including tenderness, increased irritability and eventually atrophy. The changes in the peripheral nerves are not distinctive and consist of degeneration of the myelin sheaths, which can, of course, lead to fragmentation of the axis cylinders and loss of nerve conduction. The peripheral neuropathy may extend centrally to involve the spinal cord. Such cases may also have brain involvement, but this is more characteristic of the cerebral pattern, known as Wernicke's disease.

Wernicke's disease takes the form of focal symmetrical degenerations and hemorrhages in the paramedian and paraventricular nuclei of the thalamus and hypothalamus, the mamillary bodies, and about the nuclei of origin of the cranial nerves supplying the extraocular muscles. The myelinated structures suffer to a greater extent than the nerve cells, and undergo swelling and demyelination, accompanied by regressive alterations in the glial cells about these fibers. The ganglion cells in these areas undergo a variety of degenerative changes and may die. Commonly, petechial hemorrhages occur in and about the areas of destruction. In thiamine deficient brain tissue, biochemical studies disclose loss of vital enzyme functions involved in energy metabolism and myelin maintenance (Dreyfus, 1973). Since these patients are also frequently deficient in other members of the B complex, it is not possible to attribute the brain lesions definitely to thiamine. Nonetheless, a striking therapeutic response usually follows the administration of vitamin B₁. No toxicity has been recognized from overdosage.

Riboflavin (Vitamin B₂) (Deficiency State: Ariboflavinosis). Riboflavin in its phosphorylated form is an essential component of cellular respiratory enzymes and so is involved in the oxidative metabolism of all cells. Evidence suggests that it is stored in relatively large amounts, and so deficiency states appear only after long periods (months) of inadequate dietary intake.

The clinical signs of ariboflavinosis are poorly defined and frequently are accompanied by manifestations of deficiencies of the other members of the B complex. When full-blown, *ariboflavinosis is manifested by lesions involving the lips, tongue, skin and perhaps the eyes.* The lip lesions can be characterized as *angular stomatitis.* Pallor or redness appears at the angles of the lips and is followed by desquamation and painful fissuring. Essentially similar changes occur along the vermilion borders of the lips as well, a condition referred to as *cheilosis.* It must be emphasized that these changes are not specific and also may be found in aged individuals with poor dentition, who show chronic drooling and maceration of the lips and angles of the mouth. *The tongue lesion (glossitis) results from atrophy of the mucosa, with loss of filiform papillae.* Often the fungiform papillae are enlarged, producing a pebbled appearance. Such atrophy of the tongue mucosa, along with a superficial submucosal inflammation, induces a bright red or magenta color. *A greasy, scaling dermatitis* may appear over the nasolabial folds and may extend in a butterfly distribution over the cheeks and face, particularly about the ears. Skin lesions also develop on the scrotum and vulva. In this context, it should be noted that nicotinamide deficiency (pellagra) also induces skin lesions, and deficiencies of both riboflavin and nicotinamide often occur concomitantly. *The development of changes in the eyes related to riboflavin deficiency is still somewhat controversial,* but in some more or less carefully controlled studies in human volunteers, a diet lacking only this vitamin induced proliferation of the limbic plexus of vessels, which extended into the superficial layers of the cornea, producing corneal vascularization. A keratitis may follow and induce corneal opacities.

No toxicity has been recognized from the daily administration of large doses of riboflavin.

Nicotinic Acid (Nicotinamide, Niacin, Pellagra-preventive Factor) (Deficiency State: Pellagra). Nicotinamide plays an essential role in electron transport involved in cellular respiration. The clinical syndrome produced by a deficiency of nicotinic acid or its amide is designated *pellagra* (the name is derived from *pelle,* "skin," and *agra,* "rough"). From time immemorial, *pellagra has been remembered by the three D's—dermatitis, diarrhea and dementia.* The dermatitis is usually bilaterally symmetrical and is found on the areas of the body that are exposed to light, trauma and heat. It may also occur in protected areas, such as the elbows and knees, and in the body folds in the perineal region, under the breasts and under a fat abdominal panniculus (sites of irritation). The changes comprise at first redness, thickening and roughening of the skin, which may be followed by extensive scaling and desquama-

tion, producing fissures and chronic inflammation. Depigmentation or increased pigmentation may develop, resulting in a mottled rash of pigmented scaling areas alternating with depigmented, shiny, atrophic areas. Similar lesions may occur in the mucous membranes of the mouth and vagina. *The tongue often becomes red, swollen and beefy, reminiscent of the black tongue found in pellagrous animals. The diarrhea is presumed to be caused by atrophy of the columnar epithelium of the gastrointestinal tract mucosa, followed by submucosal inflammation. The atrophy may be followed by ulceration. The dementia is based upon regressive changes in the ganglion cells of the brain, accompanied by degeneration of the tracts of the spinal cord.* In advanced cases, the spinal cord lesions come to resemble the alterations in the posterior spinal columns found in pernicious anemia. The resemblance of the cord lesions to those of the vitamin B_{12} deficiency of pernicious anemia has raised the suspicion that pellagra is not a simple nicotinic acid deficiency but may involve other members of the B complex.

No serious overdosage effect has been identified, but when nicotinic acid is administered to patients it produces a rapid vasodilator effect which is somewhat disturbing, but not harmful. The sensations of heat, flushing and itching pass within an hour.

Pyridoxine (Vitamin B$_6$). Despite the evidence from experimental animals, it has been exceedingly difficult to delineate a clear-cut clinical syndrome of pyridoxine deficiency. This vitamin is abundantly present in most foods, and so primary deficiencies are uncommon save in those having gross malnutrition. Secondary deficiencies may arise from the administration of antagonists, with intrinsic intestinal disease, or with excessive alcohol intake. Drugs believed to act as pyridoxine antagonists include 1-dopa (used in Parkinsonism), antihypertensives, oral contraceptives and isoniazid (used in the treatment of tuberculosis).

The evidence for a pyridoxine deficiency syndrome in man is fragmentary. Infants who had been kept on a commercial milk formula developed convulsions, and it was subsequently discovered that sterilization of the formula had destroyed the natural pyridoxine content. The addition of this vitamin to the preparation solved the problem. In 1953, Vilter and his colleagues induced a pyridoxine deficiency in volunteers by the administration of an antagonist. These volunteers developed irritability and a seborrhea-like dermatitis. Others manifested *glossitis, cheilosis and polyneuritis, reminiscent of the changes induced by riboflavin deficiency.* These manifestations cleared on the administration of pyridoxine alone. It has also been shown that certain forms of hypochromic anemia unresponsive to iron and to all the usual hematopoietic agents can promptly be alleviated by the administration of pyridoxine. It must be kept in mind, however, that a pure pyridoxine deficiency is exceedingly uncommon; more often it is only one part of the larger problem of inadequate intake of many members of the B complex.

Other B Vitamins. *Folic acid* and *cobalamin (B₁₂)* are required for normal maturation of red cells. In their absence, megaloblastic anemias develop. Absorption of vitamin B_{12} is necessary for the prevention of pernicious anemia. A deficiency of folic acid produces a macrocytic megaloblastic anemia closely resembling pernicious anemia. These are considered in more detail in Chapter 11.

VITAMIN C
(Deficiency State: Scurvy)

A deficiency of vitamin C gives rise to *scurvy.* Since it is water soluble, vitamin C (l-ascorbic acid) is readily and rapidly absorbed from the intestines. Absorption is thus little affected by malabsorption states not involving the intestinal mucosa. Ascorbic acid is widely distributed in fruits and vegetables and is stored in considerable amounts in the various organs in direct proportion to their metabolic activity. It is found in decreasing order of concentration in the pituitary, adrenal cortex, corpus luteum and thymus, and in smaller amounts in almost all of the viscera. Early studies suggested that body stores are sufficient to protect against scurvy for a deprivation period as long as five to six months, but a recent report lowers this time lag to approximately three months (Hodges, 1971).

Many physiologic functions have been ascribed to vitamin C, a six-carbon compound closely related to glucose. Its physiologic activity is thought to be related to its function as a reducing agent. It is believed to be necessary for the normal metabolism of phenylalanine, tyrosine and dihydroxyphenylalanine. A drop in alkaline phosphatase activity of the plasma, bone and other tissues has been noted in deficient animals. The high levels of stored ascorbic acid in the adrenal cortex suggest that this vitamin is involved in some way in the formation of corticosteroids. Vitamin C is essential for the formation of collagen, ground substance, osteoid, dentin and intercellular cement substance. These functions are of principal importance with respect to the manifestations of scurvy. Whereas its exact role in the synthesis of most of these products is still somewhat uncertain, much is known about its function in the synthesis of collagen: (1) In the absence of vitamin C, fibroblasts (and osteoblasts and odontoblasts as well) revert to more undifferentiated cell types, which appear to have lost their capacity for fibrogen-

esis. (2) Vitamin C is necessary for the formation of fibrils of procollagen, as is discussed in more detail on page 61. (3) Some evidence suggests that ascorbic acid is involved in the maintenance of collagen, retarding its resorption. In any event, a delay in wound healing and a poorly formed collagenous scar with low tensile strength are characteristic of scurvy (Edwards and Dunphy, 1958).

Recently Pauling (1970) proposed that high doses of vitamin C (up to 1 gm. per day) prevent the common cold. The literature now is replete with reports affirming and disproving this claim. The collected data leave much to be desired. The dosage of vitamin C varies from one report to another. In addition, the common cold is not a well defined entity but rather a constellation of respiratory illnesses with ill-defined manifestations. Is a "sniffle" a cold, or must there be a significant rise in temperature? Small wonder that the reported results on the effectiveness of vitamin C in preventing the common cold vary. On balance, recent reports suggest that dosages of 1 gm. per day reduce the total days of disability in the experimental group, compared with controls receiving placebos (Anderson et al., 1972; Coulehan et al., 1974). There is also the suggestion that the number of episodes of respiratory illness are reduced (Charleston and Clegg, 1972) and, strangely, that vitamin C has greater effectiveness in females than in males (Wilson and Loh, 1973). However, before this regimen is embraced too fervently, note should be taken of concerns that large doses of vitamin C may be hazardous (Goldsmith, 1971; Beaton and Whalen, 1971; Rhead and Schrauzer, 1971). Large doses of ascorbic acid may increase urinary excretion of oxalates and thus favor the formation of kidney and bladder stones. Moreover, chronic ingestion of large amounts of vitamin C may increase the requirement for this nutrient and paradoxically induce scurvy when normal intake is resumed.

To return to more solid ground, scurvy shows a bimodal peak incidence — in children between the ages of 6 months and 2 years, who are subsisting on unsupplemented processed formulas, and in the very aged, who are on inadequate or bizarre diets. For obscure reasons, the deficiency tends to become manifest in the spring and fall. *As a result of defective connective tissue formation, scorbutic individuals demonstrate alterations in the integrity of capillary walls, in bone formation and in wound healing.*

The cohesion of the endothelial cells in the capillary walls is diminished, very likely by the loss of supportive connective tissue, since the existence of intercellular cement substance has been chal-

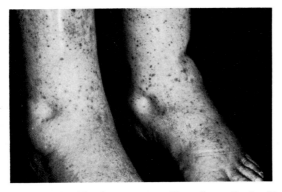

Figure 8–10. The lower extremities of a patient with marked malnutrition, nutritional edema and petechial hemorrhages related to low levels of vitamin C. (From Robbins, S. L.: Pathologic Basis of Disease. Philadelphia, W. B. Saunders Company, 1974.)

lenged. The result is that even the minor trauma of daily life causes rupture of these vessels, with consequent hemorrhage. **This bleeding diathesis is one of the most striking anatomic and clinical manifestations of scurvy** (Fig. 8–10). Rupture of the capillary walls is, of course, most likely when venous pressures are increased. An example of this is the sudden rash of skin petechiae which develops distal to the cuff as the blood pressure is taken. Indeed, it forms the basis for the diagnostic tourniquet test. Histologically, scorbutic vessels appear normal, since the alterations are submicroscopic. When hemorrhage occurs, favored sites are the subperiosteum and subcutaneous tissues (producing petechiae or ecchymoses) and the joints of the lower extremities. Extensive subperiosteal hematomas are common, as are nosebleeds. Hemorrhages into the conjunctivae, eyeballs, brain and kidneys are also encountered. Bleeding into the gastrointestinal tract may produce melena. In addition, the gingivae characteristically become edematous, spongy and hemorrhagic, presumably on the basis of vascular fragility. Secondary bacterial infections (gingivitis) often follow.

Defective bone formation and maintenance result from the deficient elaboration of osteoid matrix. Mineralization remains normal. The palisade of cartilage cells is formed as usual and is provisionally calcified, but the osteoblasts are incapable of forming bone matrix. Resorption of the cartilage is then retarded and as a consequence, long, irregular spicules of overgrown cartilage project into the marrow shaft. The resultant disorganization of the epiphyseal line of growth is similar to that seen with rickets. The persistent cartilage ultimately becomes patchily or completely calcified, without the intermediate formation of osteoid matrix. Since calcified cartilage is an inadequate structural substitute for normal bone, this poorly formed material is subject to compression and distortion by the stresses of weight bearing and muscle tension. Pathologic fractures may occur,

complicated by the bleeding diathesis. Resorption of alveolar bone causes the teeth to loosen, fall out or become malaligned.

The failure of collagen formation is most directly evident in the poor wound repair of scorbutic patients. Although fibroblastic proliferation occurs, the granulation tissue is relatively devoid of collagen. The reparative process results, then, in a loose cellular connective tissue of diminished tensile strength. Contributing to this poor wound healing is the bleeding tendency of the newly formed capillaries. Similarly, walling off of infections is inadequate with scurvy, so that abscesses are not surrounded by the normal collagenous barrier, and the infection therefore is not sharply delimited.

Clinically, scurvy first becomes manifest by the insidious appearance of vague signs and symptoms, such as anorexia, weight loss, listlessness and, in infants, retarded development. Typically there is an anemia, which may be megaloblastic and respond to folic acid, or normocytic and of controversial origin. Affected infants tend to lie quietly with their legs flexed onto the abdomen, presumably to relieve tension on the muscles, tendons and fasciae. The first definitive findings usually result from the bleeding diathesis and include most strikingly the appearance of petechiae or ecchymoses in the skin. Intra-articular or subperiosteal hemorrhages may cause painful swelling of a joint or extremity. The diagnosis is confirmed by bone x-rays, low plasma levels of vitamin C, urinary excretion measurements following administration of vitamin C (saturation test) and increased capillary fragility (positive tourniquet test). Bleeding time and coagulation time are usually normal.

OBESITY

Obesity, although less tragic than the malnutrition of a deficiency state, is nonetheless another form of nutritional disorder. Obesity has been defined as "adiposity in excess of that consistent with good health" (Albrink, 1974). The problem with this definition is the difficulty in determining the relationship between excessive body fat and poor health. For this reason the pejorative term "obese" might better be restricted to those with noticeably excessive body fat. Actuaries estimate that perhaps 20 per cent of the population of the United States is overweight in terms of height and weight relationships, and about one fifth of these individuals are in the range of 20 to 25 per cent too heavy for their height. It is not merely an adult problem. Excessive weight has been called the most prevalent nutritional disturbance in the United Kingdom, involving about 3 per cent of British schoolchildren (Editorial, 1970). In a study in New York, approximately 10 per cent of schoolboys were considered overweight, and curiously children in the lower socioeconomic classes were affected more often than those of more wealthy parents. This distribution also applies to adults (Goldblatt et al., 1972).

As stated, a basic question is the extent to which excessive fat stores impair health. A recent critical evaluation of this issue contends that obesity has been erroneously blamed for contributing to many forms of disease, and points out that weight reduction only rarely has been shown to be a useful treatment for disease (Mann, 1974). The only disorders in which excessive fat stores clearly play some causal role are: diabetes mellitus, hypertension, cerebrovascular disease and respiratory insufficiency.

Diabetes is definitely more likely to be found in the obese, other factors being equal. Individuals who are significantly overweight require more insulin to utilize the same amounts of glucose than do lean individuals. Hyperinsulinemia is a characteristic of those with excessive body fat stores. It appears that in obese individuals peripheral tissues such as fat and muscle have impaired utilization of glucose and as a consequence obesity frequently precedes maturity-onset diabetes (West and Kalbfleisch, 1971).

High blood pressure is also more common among the obese. The mechanism by which adiposity contributes to high blood pressure is still poorly understood, but probably involves an increase in circulating blood volume and an increase in cardiac stroke volume. Obesity also places a hemodynamic load on the heart by increasing the amount of tissue to be perfused.

The incidence of *cerebrovascular disease* is increased in the obese. However, it has not been possible to segregate the effects of the frequently concomitant hypertension from the influence of adiposity alone. In a prospective study, men overweight at the age of 20 and gaining 30 or more pounds thereafter had two times the incidence of cerebrovascular disease of thin men who did not gain such weight (Heyden et al., 1971).

Respiratory symptoms often develop in very obese individuals. Because of the increased body fat stores, a greater effort is required to achieve a given negative intrathoracic pressure with inspiration. Thus, the obese individual generally has a reduced tidal volume and in extreme cases there may be carbon dioxide retention and somnolence (the *Pickwickian syndrome*).

Surprisingly, no direct correlation between obesity and accelerated atherosclerosis has been demonstrated (Heyden et al., 1971; Keys et al., 1972). When the independent variables of hypertension, diabetes and hyperlipidemia are excluded, there is no convincing actuarial data that obesity has any impact on the development of atherosclerosis or myocardial infarction. Nonetheless, the frequency of angina pectoris and sudden death from coronary heart disease do correlate with obesity. Here again the correlation may well be with the hyperlipidemia and diabetes, which are known to predispose to coronary artery atherosclerosis (Damon et al., 1969).

In closing this brief sortie into environmental disease, it is plainly evident that only the surface has been scratched. Indeed, save for disorders of genetic origin alone, every other condition discussed in this text must be considered to be of environmental origin, at least in part.

REFERENCES

Albrink, M. J.: Overnutrition and the fat cell. *In* Bondy, P. K., and Rosenberg, L. E.: Duncan's Diseases of Metabolism, 7th edition. W. B. Saunders Co., Philadelphia, 1974, p. 426.

Anderson, R. E., et al.: Aging in Hiroshima and Nagasaki atomic bomb survivors: speculations based upon the age specific mortality of persons with malignant neoplasms. Am. J. Pathol., *75*:1, 1974.

Anderson, T. W., et al.: Vitamin C and the common cold: a double blind study. Can. Med. Assoc. J., *107*:503, 1972.

Baden, M. M.: Narcotic abuse: a medical examiner's view. *In* Wecht, C. H. (ed.): Legal Medicine Annual. New York, Appleton-Century-Crofts, 1971.

Baum, J. K., et al.: Possible association between hepatomas and oral contraceptives. Lancet, 2:926, 1973.

Beaton, G. H., and Whalen, S.: Vitamin C in the common cold. Can. Med. Assoc. J., *105*:355, 1971.

Belsky, J. L.: The health of atomic bomb survivors: a decade of examinations in a fixed population. Yale J. Biol. Med., *46*:284, 1973.

Braun, I. G.: Vitamin A. Excess, deficiency, requirements, metabolism and misuse. Pediatr. Clin. North Amer., *9*:935, 1962.

Brill, A. B., et al.: Leukemia in man following exposure to ionizing radiation. A summary of the findings in Hiroshima and Nagasaki and a comparison with other human experience. Ann. Int. Med., *56*:590, 1962.

Brown, C. B.: The incidence of protein-calorie malnutrition of early childhood. Guys Hosp. Rep., *120*:129, 1971.

Cade, S.: Radiation induced cancer in man. Brit. J. Radiol., *30*:393, 1957.

Casarett, G. W.: Radiation injury. Surg. Ann., *4*:103, 1972.

Cederbaum, A. I., and Rubin, E.: Molecular injury to mitochondria produced by ethanol and acetaldehyde. Fed. Proc., *34*:2045, 1975.

Charleston, S. S., and Clegg, K. M.: Ascorbic acid and the common cold. Lancet, *1*:1401, 1972.

Codicek, E.: The story of vitamin D from vitamin to hormone. Lancet, *1*:325, 1974.

Cohen, M. M., et al.: Chromosomal damage to human leukocytes induced by LSD. Science, *155*:1417, 1967.

Cohen, M. M., et al.: The effect of LSD on the chromosomes of children exposed in utero. Pediatr. Res., *2*:486, 1968.

Collaborative Group for the Study of Stroke in Young Women: Oral contraception and increased risk of cerebral ischemia or thrombosis. New Eng. J. Med., *288*:871, 1973.

Corey, M. J., et al.: Chromosome studies on patients in vivo and cells in vitro treated with lysergic acid diethylamide. New Eng. J. Med., *282*:939, 1970.

Coulehan, J. L., et al.: Vitamin C prophylaxis in a boarding school. New Eng. J. Med., *290*:6, 1974.

Damon, A., et al.: Predicting coronary heart disease from body measurements of Framingham males. J. Chronic Dis., *21*:781, 1969.

Davidson, S., and Passmore, R.: Human Nutrition and Dietetics. Baltimore, Williams & Wilkins Co., 1970.

DeLuca, H. F.: The kidney as an endocrine organ involved in the function of vitamin D. Am. J. Med., *58*:39, 1975.

Dorrance, D., et al.: In vivo effects of illicit hallucinogens on human lymphocyte chromosomes. J.A.M.A., *212*:1488, 1970.

Dreyfus, P. M.: Thoughts on the pathophysiology of Wernicke's disease. Ann. N.Y. Acad. Sci., *215*:367, 1973.

Drug Abuse Warning Network (DAWN I): Analysis. Interim Report. BNDD contract # 72–47. Washington, D.C., Drug Enforcement Administration, U.S. Department of Justice, November, 1973, p. 73.

Editorial: The overweight child. Brit. Med. J., *1*:64, 1970.

Editorial: Oral contraceptives and health. Lancet, *1*:1147, 1974.

Edland, J. F.: Liver disease in heroin addicts. Hum. Pathol., *2*:75, 1972.

Edwards, L. C., and Dunphy, J. E.: Wound healing. New Eng. J. Med., *259*:224, 275, 1958.

Fernandez, J., et al.: LSD, an in vivo retrospective chromosome study. Ann. Hum. Genetics, London, *37*:81, 1973.

Geber, W. F., and Schramm, L. C.: Effect of marijuana extract on fetal hamsters and rabbits. Toxicol. Appl. Pharmacol., *14*:276, 1969.

Ghidoni, J. J.: Light and electron microscopic study of primate liver 36–48 hours after high doses of 32 million electronvolt protons. Lab. Invest., *16*:268, 1967.

Gilsinn, J.: Estimates of the nature and extent of lead paint poisoning in the United States (NBS TN–746). Washington, D.C., Department of Commerce, National Bureau of Standards, December, 1972.

Goldblatt, P. B., et al.: Social factors in obesity. J.A.M.A., *192*:1039, 1972.

Goldsmith, G. A.: Common cold: prevention and treatment with ascorbic acid not effective. J.A.M.A., *216*:337, 1971.

Goyer, R. A.: Lead toxicity. A problem in environmental pathology. Am. J. Path., *64*:167, 1971.

Hall, J. L., and Rowlands, D. T., Jr.: Cardiotoxicity of alcohol. An electron microscopic study in the rat. Am. J. Pathol., *60*:153, 1970.

Hawkins, R. D., and Kalent, H.: The metabolism of ethanol and its metabolic effects. Pharmacol. Rev., *24*:67, 1972.

Heyden, S., et al.: Weight and weight history in relation to cerebrovascular and ischemic heart disease. Arch. Int. Med., *128*:956, 1971.

Hodges, R. E.: Clinical manifestations of ascorbic acid deficiency in man. Am. J. Clin. Nutr., *24*:432, 1971.

Hognestad, J., and Teisberg, P.: Heart pathology in chronic alcoholism. Acta Pathol. Microbiol. Scand., *81*:315, 1973.

Hopkins, G. B., and Taylor, D. E.: Pulmonary talc granulomatosis. Amer. Rev. Resp. Dis., *101*:101, 1970.

Hutchinson, F.: The molecular basis for radiation effects on cells. Cancer Res., *26*:2045, 1966.

Israel, Y., et al.: Liver hypermetabolic state after chronic ethanol consumption. Fed. Proc., *34*:2052, 1975.

Isselbacher, K. J., and Carter, E. A.: Ethanol oxidation by liver microsomes: evidence against a separate and distinct enzyme system. Biochem. Biophys. Res. Comm., *39*:530, 1970.

Janerich, D. T., et al.: Oral contraceptives and congenital limb-reduction defects. New Eng. J. Med., *291*:697, 1974.

Jablon, S., et al.: Cancer in Japanese exposed as children to atomic bombs. Lancet, *1*:927, 1971.

Jeghers, H., and Marraro, H.: Hypervitaminosis A, its broadening spectrum. Amer. J. Clin. Nutr., *4*:603, 1956.

Johnson, H. V., et al.: Vitamin K and the biosynthesis of the glycoprotein prothrombin. Biochem. Biophys. Res. Comm., *43*:1040, 1971.

Kark, R. A. P., et al.: Mercury poisoning and its treatment with n-acetyl-d, l-penicillamine. New Eng. J. Med., *285*:10, 1971.

Kew, M. C., et al.: Possible hepatoxicity of cannabis. Lancet, *1*:578, 1969.

Keys, A., et al.: Coronary heart disease: overweight and obesity as risk factors. Ann. Int. Med., *77*:15, 1972.

Lin-Fu, J. S.: Vulnerability of children to lead exposure and toxicity. New Eng. J. Med., *289*:1229, 1289, 1973.

Lucy, J. A., et al.: Studies on the mode of action of excess vitamin A. Mitochondrial swelling. Biochem. J., *89*:419, 1963.

Magus, R. D., and Harris, L. S.: Carcinogenic potential of marihuana smoke condensate. Fed. Proc., *30*:279, 1971.

Mann, G. V.: The influence of obesity on health. New Eng. J. Med., *291*:178, 226, 1974.

Mayer, R. F.: Recent studies in man and animal of peripheral nerve and muscle dysfunction associated with chronic alcoholism. Ann. N.Y. Acad. Sci., *215*:370, 1973.

McLaren, D. S., et al.: Xerophthalmia in Jordan. Am. J. Clin. Nutr., *17*:117, 1965.

Mendelson, J. H.: Biologic concomitants of alcoholism. New Eng. J. Med., *283*:24, 71, 1970.

Mezey, E. J., et al.: Pancreatic function and intestinal absorption in chronic alcoholism. Gastroenterology, *59*:657, 1970.

Miller, F. F.: History of drug sensitivity in atopic persons. J. Allerg., *40*:46, 1967.

Moncrief, J. A.: Burns. New Eng. J. Med., *288*:444, 1973.

Morris, A. H., and Spitzer, K. W.: Pulmonary pathophysiologic changes following thermal injury. U.S. Army Institute of Surgical Research Annual Research Progress Report. Fort Sam, Houston, Texas, Brooke Army Medical Center, 1971, Section 52, p. 1.

Murphree, H. B.: Electroencephalographic and other evidence for mixed depressant and stimulant actions of alcoholic beverages. Ann. N.Y. Acad. Sci., *215*:325, 1973.

Nielsen, J., et al.: Chromosome abnormalities in patients treated with chlorpromazine, perphenazine and lysergide. Brit. Med. J., *2*:634, 1969.

Omdahl, J. L., et al.: Regulation of metabolism of 25-hydroxycholecalciferol by kidney tissue in vitro by dietary calcium. Nature: New Biology, *237*:63, 1972.

Paton, W. D. M.: Cannabis and its problems. Proc. Roy. Soc. Med., *66*:718, 1973.

Paton, W. D. M., and Pertwee, R. G.: Effect of cannabis and certain of its constituents on pentobarbitone sleeping time and phenazone metabolism. Brit. J. Pharm., *44*:250, 1972.

Patwardhan, V. N.: *In* Proceedings of the Sixth International Congress on Nutrition. Edinburgh, Livingstone, 1964.

Pauling, L.: Vitamin C and the Common Cold. San Francisco, W. H. Freeman and Co., 1970.

Pillard, R. C.: Marijuana. New Eng. J. Med., *283*:294, 1970.

Rasmussen, H., et al.: Hormonal control of the renal conversion of 25-hydroxycholecalciferol to 1,25-dihydroxycholecalciferol. J. Clin. Invest., *51*:2502, 1972.

Rhead, W. J., and Schrauzer, G. N.: Risks of long term ascorbic acid overdosage. Nutr. Rev., *29*:262, 1971.

Ritchie, J. H., et al.: Edema and hemolytic anemia in premature infants. A vitamin E deficiency syndrome. New Eng. J. Med., *279*:1185, 1968.

Roels, O. A.: Vitamin A physiology. J.A.M.A., *214*:1097, 1970.

Royal College of General Practitioners: Oral contraceptives and health. An interim report from the Oral Contraception Study of the Royal College of General Practitioners. London, Pitmann Medical, 1974.

Rubin, P., and Casarett, G. W.: Clinical Radiation and Pathology. Philadelphia, W. B. Saunders Co., 1968.

Russell, W. L., et al.: Radiation dose rate and mutation frequency. Science, *128*:1546, 1958.

Scott, M. L.: *In* DeLuca, H. F., and Suttie, J. W.: The Fat Soluble Vitamins. Madison, Wisc., University of Wisconsin Press, 1970, p. 355.

Shea, S. M., et al.: Microvascular ultrastructure in thermal injury: a reconsideration of the role of mediators. Microvasc. Res., *5*:87, 1973.

Siegel, H.: Human pulmonary pathology associated with narcotic and other addictive drugs. Hum. Pathol., *2*:55, 1972.

Sreepada Rao, T. K., et al.: Natural history of heroin associated nephropathy. New Eng. J. Med., *290*:19, 1974.

Stamp, T. C. B.: Vitamin D metabolism. Recent advances. Arch. Dis. Child., *48*:2, 1973.

Steer, A.: Symposium: the delayed consequences of exposure to ionizing radiation. Pathology studies at the Atomic Bomb Casualty Commission, Hiroshima and Nagasaki, 1945–1970—"other tumors." Hum. Pathol., *2*:541, 1971.

Stimmel, B.: Hepatic dysfunction in heroin addicts: the role of alcohol. J.A.M.A., *222*:811, 1972.

Suttie, J. W.: Control of clotting factor biosynthetics by vitamin K. Fed. Proc., *28*:1696, 1969.

Suttie, J. W.: Mechanism of action of vitamin K. Demonstration of a liver precursor. Science, *179*:192, 1973.

Takeuchi, P., et al.: A pathological study of Minamata disease in Japan. Acta Neuropath. (Berlin), *2*:40, 1962.

Tappel, A. L.: Vitamin E. Nutr. Today, *8*:4, 1973.

Teplitz, C.: Pathology of burns. *In* Artz, C. P., and Moncrief, J. A. (eds.): Treatment of Burns, 2nd ed. Philadelphia, W. B. Saunders Co., 1969.

Tjio, J. H., et al.: LSD and chromosomes: a controlled experiment. J.A.M.A., *210*:849, 1969.

Vessey, M. P., et al.: Oral contraceptives and breast neoplasia: a retrospective study. Br. Med. J., *3*:719, 1972.

Victor, M., and Adams, R. D.: The effect of alcohol on the nervous system. Assoc. Res. Nerv. Ment. Dis. Proc., *32*:526, 1953.

Vilter, R. W., et al.: The effect of vitamin B_6 deficiency induced by desoxypyridoxine in human beings. J. Lab. Clin. Med., *42*:335, 1953.

Werner, A.: Near fatal hyperacute reaction to intravenously administered heroin. J.A.M.A., *207*:2277, 1969.

West, K. M., and Kalbfleisch, J. M.: Influence of nutritional factors on prevalence of diabetes. Diabetes, *20*:99, 1971.

Wilson, C. W. M., and Loh, H. S.: Common cold and vitamin C. Lancet, *1*:638, 1973.

Wu, A., et al.: Alcoholism and anemia. Lancet, *1*:829, 1974.

PART

TWO

In the remaining chapters of this book, diseases of specific organ systems will be considered. We do not intend to discuss at length rare and exotic afflictions. Rather, our emphasis is on those disorders which actually affect large numbers of people. The chart below listing major causes of death in the United States in 1973 is offered so that you may keep your sense of balance in the event that we occasionally lose ours. Some idea of the interesting changes in the relative importance of various diseases can be gained by comparing these data with those for 1937. The data for 1967 are also given, since these were the figures used in the first edition of this book. We thought it of interest that even in the few intervening years, there have been appreciable changes in the leading causes of death. Coronary heart disease has continued to grow in importance. The addition of cirrhosis of the liver and of chronic obstructive pulmonary disease to the "top ten" are sobering indications of the influence of alcohol and cigarettes on our collective health.

CAUSES OF DEATH IN THE UNITED STATES (EXCLUDING NEONATAL CAUSES)

1973*	PER CENT	1967†	PER CENT	1937†	PER CENT
Coronary heart disease	34.5	Coronary heart disease	30.9	Cancer	10.0
Cancer	17.9	Cancer	16.8	Cerebrovascular accidents	
Cerebrovascular accidents		Cerebrovascular accidents		(CVA)	7.7
(CVA)	10.9	(CVA)	10.9	Pneumonia	7.6
Accidents	5.8	Accidents	6.1	Accidents	7.2
Pneumonia	2.8	Hypertension	3.3	Nephritis	7.1
Diabetes	1.8	Pneumonia	3.0	Coronary heart disease	4.8
Cirrhosis of the liver	1.7	Endocarditis and myocarditis	2.8	Tuberculosis	4.4
Generalized arteriosclerosis	1.7	Early infancy	2.6	Influenza	2.6
Early infancy	1.6	Generalized arteriosclerosis	2.0	Diabetes	2.1
Chronic obstructive pul-		Diabetes	1.9	Generalized arteriosclerosis	
monary disease	1.5	Other	19.7	and hypertension	1.6
Other	19.8			Other	44.9
Total deaths	1,977,000	Total deaths	1,851,323	Total deaths	1,450,427

*Adapted from Annual Summary for 1973, HRA 74–1120, 22, 13, June 27, 1974.

†Vital Statistics of the United States, 1937, 1967. Washington, D.C., Department of Health, Education and Welfare, Public Health Service, 1937, 1969.

CHAPTER 9

The Vascular System

It is customary to consider vascular disease according to whether arteries, veins or lymphatic channels are affected. Here, however, most of the entities will be treated according to clinical manifestations. As will be seen, this departure from traditional treatment is more apparent than real. In general, most vascular diseases cause occlusion of the channel. Obviously, because of differences in function, the clinical consequences of arterial occlusion tend to be quite different from those following blockage of veins or lymphatic channels. Thus, arterial diseases fall naturally under the heading *ischemia,* and venous and lymphatic diseases under the heading *localized congestion and edema.*

Aneurysms (abnormal dilatation of arteries) will be discussed separately. In contrast to most vascular diseases, these lesions do not produce occlusion of the artery, but are significant principally because of their liability to rupture.

The tumors, which as a group are relatively infrequent, are also considered separately.

ISCHEMIA

When diseases of the arteries impair flow — by thrombosis, inflammatory changes or spasm — the tissues served by the affected vessel become ischemic. Regrettably, the vascular disease itself is usually totally silent. A case in point is the man who leaves his doctor's office after a complete examination with a clean bill of health and develops an occlusion of a silently but severely narrowed coronary artery, and dies of myocardial infarction. Symptoms of arterial disease, then, are generally referable to ischemia, and include functional disturbances, pain resulting from infarctions and trophic changes with ulceration of the overlying skin. By far the most important of the arterial diseases is *arteriosclerosis.* Unfortunately, this term, which literally means "hardening of the arteries," can refer to three entirely different entities — *atherosclerosis,* which is overwhelmingly the most important, and which is characterized by the formation of intimal fatty deposits; *Mönckeberg's calcific sclerosis,* which is characterized by calcification of the tunica media of muscular arteries; and *arteriolosclerosis,* or arteriolar thickening seen with diabetes and hypertension (p. 459). *Common usage has largely rendered arteriosclerosis and atherosclerosis synonymous.*

Second in importance to atherosclerosis as a cause of arterial disease and ischemia are the arteritides. Occasionally these are caused by simple bacterial invasion, either from a neighboring infection or from a septicemia. The resultant lesion is a nonspecific inflammatory process. When a focus in the aorta — usually an ulcerated atheroma or a mural thrombus — is seeded hematogenously, the process is specifically designated *bacterial endaortitis.* Such a lesion may cause rupture or weakening of the aortic wall, with the formation of a *mycotic aneurysm.*

TABLE 9–1. SYSTEMIC NECROTIZING ANGIITIDES

Necrotizing Angiitis	Vessels Involved	Organ or Tissues Affected
Hypersensitivity angiitis (serum sickness, Arthus lesion)	Arterioles, capillaries, venules	All organs and tissues (skin, muscles, heart, kidneys, lungs)
Rheumatic arteritis	Medium and large arteries	Aorta and branches, pulmonary vessels, cerebral, coronary vessels
Rheumatoid arteritis	Arterioles, medium and large arteries	Mostly extremities, hands and fingers (Raynaud's phenomenon), coronary, cerebral, mesenteric arteries, widespread
Systemic lupus erythematosus	Arterioles, capillaries	Kidneys, skin, heart, muscles, nerves; may be widespread
	Splenic arterioles	Spleen
Systemic sclerosis (often not present)	Arterioles	Kidneys. skin. lungs. may be widespread
Polyarteritis nodosa	Medium arteries and arterioles	Gastrointestinal tract, mesentery, liver, gallbladder, kidney, pancreas, lung, muscles, other sites
Malignant hypertensive arteriolosclerosis	Arterioles	Kidney, retina, pancreas, adrenals, gallbladder; may be widespread
Wegener's granulomatosis	Arterioles, veins	Lungs, kidneys, upper respiratory tract; occasionally systemic
Giant cell arteritis	Medium arteries	Usually temporal, ophthalmic and cranial arteries; may be widespread
Takayasu's arteritis	Large and medium arteries	Aortic arch, pulmonary artery, origins of aortic branches

More often, the arteritis belongs to a group of systemic disorders characterized by multifocal arterial lesions. This group is collectively known as the *nonsuppurative necrotizing arteritides* or *angiitides*. Most are suspected of having an immunologic basis, and some, such as hypersensitivity angiitis or the angiitis associated with SLE, are of known immunologic pathogenesis. In some cases immunohistochemical studies have supported such a pathogenesis by demonstrating gamma globulin and complement in the vascular lesions. Often other serum proteins are present as well, but these most probably permeate an already injured vessel wall. Sometimes only fibrinogen is present in the vessel wall, compatible with either a nonimmunologic or a delayed hypersensitivity basis for the lesion (Paronetto, 1969). Most of these necrotizing angiitides are discussed in Chapter 6. Here, only two necrotizing arteritides are discussed—giant cell arteritis and Takayasu's arteritis. However, because of the confusion often engendered by the large number of very similar angiitides of probable or possible immune origin, a table of salient and distinguishing characteristics has been prepared (Table 9–1).

There remain two miscellaneous entities which cause arterial occlusion and ischemia.

One is the non-necrotizing vasculitis, *thromboangiitis obliterans*, and the other is a rather mysterious disorder called *Raynaud's disease*.

ATHEROSCLEROSIS

Atherosclerosis is the most prevalent disorder of mankind. Although it is global in distribution, it has become virtually epidemic in the affluent nations, affecting all ages above infancy and both sexes to some degree. Fortunately, in a good many affected individuals it does not cause serious disease. The magnitude of the problem is impressively documented by the following data. In 1973 there were about 1,977,000 deaths in the United States; about 1,037,460 (52 per cent) were due to cardiovascular disease, most of which was caused by atherosclerosis. In contrast, in 1937 there were 1,450,427 total deaths, and only 204,570 (14 per cent) were caused by cardiovascular disease. Since the severity of atherosclerosis progresses with advancing years, some of this awesome increase may result from longer life expectancy and control of the other streams of mortality, such as infectious disease. But the entire increase cannot be so simply explained. Whatever the reasons, ath-

TABLE 9–1. CONTINUED

PRINCIPAL MORPHOLOGIC FEATURES	IMMUNOGLOBULINS AND COMPLEMENT IN LESIONS	WHITE CELL REACTION	IMMUNOLOGIC PATHOGENESIS
Acute necrotizing vasculitis with fibrinoid necrosis of entire wall; white cell reaction; often thrombosis of lumen	Frequent	Neutrophils	Yes; immune complex disease
Similar to hypersensitivity angiitis	—	Neutrophils	Probable; immune complex disease
Similar to hypersensitivity angiitis	—	Neutrophils and monocytes	Probable; immune complex disease
Similar to hypersensitivity angiitis "Onion-skinning"	Frequent	Neutrophils	Probable; immune complex disease
Similar to hypersensitivity angiitis; or "onion-skinning"	Occasional	Neutrophils and eosinophils	Possible
Similar to hypersensitivity angiitis	Frequent	Neutrophils and eosinophils	Possible
Acute necrosis with fibrinoid reaction; often associated with intimal and medial cell proliferation and thickening of walls ("onion-skinning")	Often	Scant neutrophils	Possible
Similar to hypersensitivity angiitis; associated with granulomas in tissues	Occasional	Neutrophils, occasionally eosinophils, histiocytes	Possible
Disruption of elastic lamina, with most intense reaction in the intima and media; later permeates wall; giant cells engulf elastic fiber fragments, occasionally thrombosis of lumen	Infrequent	Neutrophils rare; lymphocytes, histiocytes and occasionally plasma cells	Possible
Mononuclear cuffing of vasa vasorum; later infiltration of adventitia and media; finally sclerosis of entire wall and thrombosis, sometimes with granulomas	—	Lymphocytes and plasma cells; later neutrophils	Possible

erosclerosis is obviously the major challenge in clinical medicine among the affluent populations of the world.

Atherosclerosis affects the tunica intima and secondarily the tunica media of the aorta and arteries of large and medium size. *Basically the disorder comprises the development of focal fibrofatty elevated plaques or thickenings, called atheromas, within the intima and inner portion of the media. As the disorder advances, the atheromas undergo a variety of complications—calcification, internal hemorrhages, ulceration, and sometimes superimposed thrombosis.* The enormous significance of these arterial lesions resides primarily in their potential to produce arterial narrowing (stenosis) and occlusion. *Thus, atherosclerosis, often with superimposed thrombosis, is the usual cause of coronary heart disease (CHD) (the most important form of which is myocardial infarction); cerebrovascular accidents (CVA) (infarcts or hemorrhages in the brain); and gangrene of the lower extremities (arteriosclerosis obliterans).* These organ injuries give atherosclerosis its terrible importance.

Epidemiology. Because the etiology of atherosclerosis is still unknown, much attention has been paid to its epidemiology in the hope of discovering clues to its causation. Many influences condition the incidence of this dis-

order, but two are preeminent: *(1) clinically significant atherosclerosis is most common in affluent areas of the world, and (2) in these areas, it becomes more prevalent with aging.* The geographic differences are striking. High prevalence and severity are found in the United States, Great Britain, Australia, New Zealand and the Scandinavian countries, for example, with relatively low prevalence and severity in many countries in Central and South America, as well as in the economically deprived populations of India and Africa (Tejada et al., 1968). These differences are believed to be environmental rather than genetic in origin.

Within vulnerable geographic areas, a number of influences have been identified as contributing to the development and severity of atherosclerosis. These have been elucidated by long-term prospective studies, principally the Framingham Heart Study, carried out in Framingham, Massachusetts. It should be understood that the identification of atherosclerosis in these studies depends largely on the development of its two most serious clinical complications—coronary heart disease (CHD), including myocardial infarction (MI), and cerebrovascular accidents (CVA). As will be seen, most of the influences which have been identified as contributing to atherosclerosis are more likely to be present with increasing age. Nevertheless, the presence of all of them together would explain only a part of the marked increase in the incidence of clinical atherosclerosis which occurs with age. Clearly, the fact of aging itself somehow predisposes to the progression of this disease. Age, then, can be considered the most important single risk factor within vulnerable geographic areas. Interestingly, despite the fact that clinically overt atherosclerosis is a disease of aging, there is much evidence that it has its subclinical beginnings in the pediatric age group (Blumenthal and Jesse, 1973). This likelihood will be further explored in the discussion of its etiology and pathogenesis. Suffice it to say here that minimal fatty deposits in the aorta—termed *fatty streaks*—seem to be present in all infants over the age of 1 year in all parts of the world; whereas these may remain static or even regress in low-prevalence populations, they may be the precursors of atherosclerosis in others.

Granted that residence in certain affluent areas of the world and increasing age define the population at risk, it remains true that not all members of this population develop clinically significant atherosclerosis. Within the same town, some individuals of 80 years of age have less extensive atherosclerosis than others 30 years of age. What, then, are the other predisposing epidemiologic factors (risk factors) correlated with atherosclerosis? *The most important are: (1) elevated serum lipoproteins, (2) increasing blood pressure, (3) cigarette smoking, and (4) elevated blood sugar levels.* The strength of the association between each of these factors and atherosclerosis varies somewhat with sex and age. For example, among men hyperlipoproteinemia is more important than hypertension, whereas the reverse is true among women. In addition, hyperlipoproteinemia exerts its greatest influence in the younger age groups, whereas hypertension becomes more significant with advancing age. The presence of two or more of these risk factors is potentiating—that is, the total increase in risk is greater than the sum of the risks contributed by each factor. The presence of all four major risk factors increases the probability of developing coronary heart disease thirteenfold over the control population (Kannel, 1974).

In some individuals, the presence of risk factors (and an increased vulnerability to atherosclerosis) stems indirectly from another disease process. For example, people with the nephrotic syndrome (p. 432) or hypothyroidism (p. 605) develop elevated serum lipoprotein levels and accelerated atherosclerosis. Diabetics, with their tendency toward elevated

blood sugar levels, are notoriously prone to develop atherosclerosis. Perhaps most dramatic are the individuals with familial hyperlipoproteinemia, in whom severe atherosclerosis typically develops in early life, even in childhood. These interesting genetic disorders will be discussed further in the section dealing with etiology and pathogenesis. Even among otherwise healthy individuals in whom there is no clear-cut genetic disorder, *there would seem to be some more subtle genetic predisposition to the major risk factors, hence to atherosclerosis* (Goldstein, 1973). Thus, there are families in which early death from an MI is frequent, and other families whose members typically live to extreme old age with only minimal evidence of atherosclerosis. Indeed, the risk of death from an MI to first-degree male relatives of men who have died before age 55 from an MI is five times that of the control population (Blumenthal and Jesse, 1973).

Serum lipoprotein levels and blood pressure—the two strongest of the risk factors other than age—are in general lower among premenopausal women than among men. Accordingly, women seem to be protected against atherosclerosis during their reproductive years. The coronary arteries show this sex differential more than the aorta or the arteries supplying the brain. Unless there is a definite underlying predisposition, an MI (the most lethal form of CHD) is rare in premenopausal women. After the age of about 50 years, lipoprotein and blood pressure levels in women increase rapidly and ultimately overtake those of men. While the incidence of MI in women concomitantly increases after this age, it still does not reach that of men until extreme old age. The incidence of CVA in women becomes equal to that in men at an earlier age than that of MI (Kannel, 1974).

In addition to the four major risk factors mentioned, there are a number of other influences which have been less clearly established as predisposing toward the development of atherosclerosis. These include a stressful and competitive life style (Type A personality structure), lack of regular physical exercise, soft drinking water, high serum uric acid levels, and a relatively high intake of saturated fats. Obesity is probably not an important influence, except insofar as it may in extreme cases predispose to hypertension or diabetes (Mann, 1974).

It is important to remember that epidemiologic studies reveal influences that are correlated with atherosclerosis, but they can only offer clues to the etiology, and they tell nothing of the pathogenesis. About all that can be said for certain in this regard is that *none of the risk factors mentioned has been identified as either necessary or sufficient for the development of ath-*

erosclerosis. The precise initiating event and the reasons for progression remain subjects · of lively speculation and controversy. Before discussing this aspect of atherosclerosis, the morphology of the lesions will be described since an understanding of morphology is necessary for consideration of the pathogenesis.

Morphology. As mentioned, **the fundamental lesion of atherosclerosis is the atheroma.** Its chronologic evolution will be described to provide an overview of the lesion from origin to advanced stage. **All atheromas begin as intimal lesions which in their progression eventually extend to affect the adjacent media.** It should be recalled that the intima is a narrow zone having on its luminal surface a covering of endothelium. Subjacent to this is a layer of ground substance containing elastic and collagen fibers intermixed with elongated cells, now recognized as "multipotential mesenchymal cells." These cells are capable of synthesizing collagen and elastic fibers as well as smooth muscle filaments. They are either identical or closely related to smooth muscle cells and are often termed **myointimal cells** (Getz et al., 1969). These cells play an important role in the development of the atheroma. The deeper boundary of the tunica intima is demarcated by a feltwork of elastic fibers known as the internal elastic membrane. At birth, the tunica intima is extremely narrow, but with age it progressively accumulates more ground substance, more fibers and more myointimal cells.

The nature of the earliest change in the atheromatous lesion is still an issue of controversy. Many believe that the initial event is some form of injury to the vessel wall resulting in increased permeability of the endothelium and reactive proliferation of the myointimal cells. A number of causes for such injury have been postulated. These include hemodynamic forces, immunologic events and platelet dysfunction with adherence of platelets and fibrin to the endothelial surface (Poston and Davies, 1974; Carvalho, 1974). Whether vascular injury is the initial event and, if so, what the nature of the injury is, are matters of dispute to be considered later. Changes in the activity of enzymes within the arterial wall have also been described. These occur with advancing age, and it is difficult to say whether they precede or result from atherosclerotic changes (Zemplenyi, 1974). **Controversy and biochemistry aside, most would agree that the earliest *visible* alterations in atherosclerotic vessels include proliferation of myointimal cells and the appearance of small vacuoles, presumably lipids, within micropinocytotic vesicles apparently traversing the endothelial cells.** Subsequently, small vesicles appear within the myointimal cells. Others have described at this stage poorly defined alterations in the endothelial basement membrane and subjacent ground substance. **With progression, focal clusters of myointimal cells become ballooned out by cytoplasmic accumulations of lipids to create "foam cells" (so**

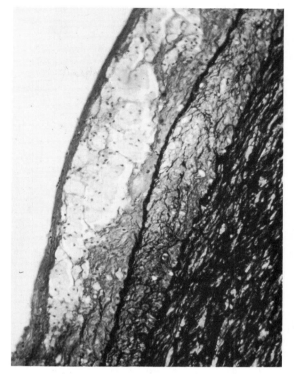

Figure 9–1. Atherosclerosis of the aorta. An early developmental atheroma showing a nest of intimal lipophages.

called because of the apparent foaminess of their cytoplasm) (Fig. 9–1). **Such focal aggregations produce minimally elevated, yellow, "fatty streaks" on the endothelial surface of the affected artery.** Later we shall consider how the lipid accumulates in these cells. Does it filter in from the plasma lipids or is it endogenously synthesized? With progression of the disease, the focal aggregation of foam cells accumulates on its luminal surface a cap of fibrocollagenous tissue, now in all likelihood creating a bulge into the lumen of the vessel. This fibrous cap may extend virtually to enclose the aggregation of foam cells. With time, the foam cells become necrotic, and the center of the atheroma is converted to an accumulation of fatty, pultaceous debris. The rich content of cholesterol is evident in the form of needle-like cholesterol crystals within this debris. A number of pathways may now be followed. Progressive fibrosis may convert the fatty atheroma to a fibrous scar. Calcification frequently ensues. This is seen as irregular amorphous deposits of basophilic precipitate in the center and margins of the fatty atheroma. At the outer margin of the lesion, neovascular formations develop by the ingrowth of the vasa vasorum from the more deeply situated preexisting blood supply of the arterial wall. Hemorrhages may occur within the atheroma, in time releasing hemosiderin pigment. The atheroma may ulcerate through the endothelial surface, releasing its soft, grumous fatty debris. With such ulceration, overlying thrombosis is common. When thrombosis occurs in the aorta, it is of the mural type, but when thrombosis is initiated in smaller vessels, such as the coronary arteries, it often completely occludes the vessel. **All these later stages, that is, the development of fibrosis, calcification, hemorrhage and ulceration, are associated with encroachment of the atheroma on the vascular lumen; hence they are collectively referred to as "raised lesions." These changes are also designated "complicated lesions"** (Fig. 9–2). As they become raised, they at the same time encroach on the underlying tunica media and cause atrophy of the muscle and elastic fibers, thereby weakening the arterial wall. Large lesions may damage the tunica media very deeply and, not infrequently, adventitial scarring appears, with aggregations of lymphocytes about the vasa vasorum. It is clear, then, from the evolution of atheromas that they have three important consequences: **(1) They encroach on the vascular lumen, (2) they provide**

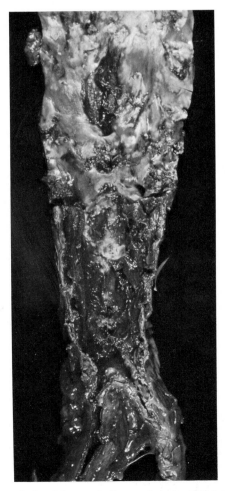

Figure 9–2. Advanced atherosclerosis of the abdominal aorta (iliac bifurcation is at bottom). Many of the ulcerated plaques are covered by mural thrombus.

sites for the initiation of thrombosis and embolism, and (3) they damage the media and weaken the arterial wall.

Turning to the macroscopic features of atherosclerosis, the sites of most severe involvement are the aorta, the coronary and cerebral arteries and major branches of the aorta, such as the innominate, common carotid, renal and iliac arteries. The pulmonary arteries are affected only when the blood pressure is elevated within the pulmonary circuit (pulmonary hypertension). As mentioned, the earliest observable lesions are the fatty streaks. These appear as barely visible, round, oval, crescentic or maplike yellow discolorations on the endothelial surface. They may be slightly elevated. Visualization is greatly enhanced by Sudan IV staining of the entire vessel. Fatty streaks are first seen in infancy and early childhood, during which period they are largely restricted to the aortic ring and arch. Subsequently, they appear in the descending thoracic and abdominal aorta, and by the age of 10 years they cover about 10 per cent of the surface of the aorta. These lesions probably remain reversible until the third decade. Indeed, many of the fatty streaks probably do regress, since, as we shall see, the distribution of typical full-blown atheromatous lesions is somewhat different from that of the fatty streaks. In particular, the fatty streaks in the aortic arch tend to regress. However, in vulnerable populations some of the fatty streaks apparently remain as the precursors of atheromas. Fatty streaks appear in the coronary arteries in the second decade. Persistence is characteristic of the lesions in the coronary arteries. Beginning in the third decade, those lesions destined to progress develop necrotic centers and a surrounding fibrous cap. This is most likely the point of irreversibility. Further complications ensue over the fourth decade, including calcification, hemorrhage, ulceration and thrombosis. **Thus, by the age of 40 years, most individuals in vulnerable populations have very badly damaged major arteries.** That this damage occurs entirely silently in the bloom of youth makes it the more ominous.

The distribution of the full-blown atheromatous lesions is, as mentioned, somewhat different from that of the fatty streaks. **In the aorta, the regions affected in order of decreasing severity are the abdominal aorta, the descending portion of the thoracic arch and the transverse portion.** For unknown reasons, the root of the aorta just above the aortic valve is generally spared. Although these lesions are fairly randomly distributed in the aorta, they appear to be most numerous in areas of maximal stress — branch points and points of fixation (e.g., the posterior wall of the aorta, where it is fixed to the prevertebral tissue) (Fig. 9–3). **In the coronary arteries, the proximal 6 to 8 cm. are the most severely affected regions.** It is important to note at this point that although the atheromatous involvement of the aorta and the

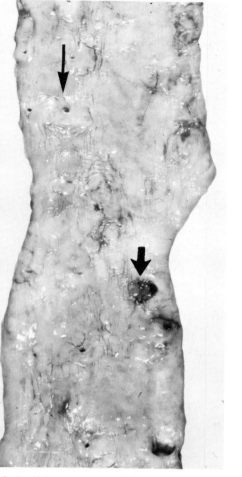

Figure 9–3. Atherosclerosis of the aorta. Virtually the entire intimal surface is involved. Note the well developed atheroma enclosing the mouth of one of the intercostal arteries (small arrow) and the small mural thrombus (large arrow).

smaller arteries tends to develop at about the same rate and to the same degree, this is by no means invariable. **Not infrequently, the aorta is severely involved while the coronary and cerebral atherosclerosis is minimal, and vice versa.** As these early atheromatous streaks evolve and accumulate more lipid, they become soft, yellow, elevated plaques which are clearly seen to bulge into the vascular lumen. The complications already mentioned create areas of gritty white calcification, firm gray-white induration or ulcerated excavations, often covered by thrombi. In the aorta, these complications do not significantly encroach upon the vascular diameter, but in smaller arteries, such as the coronary and cerebral vessels, they obviously impinge upon the lumen. The fibrosis and calcification render the affected vessels inelastic, irregular and tortuous. Smaller arteries may be converted into rigid "pipe stems." The weakening of the media often gives rise to aneurysmal dilata-

tion of the affected vessel. This is particularly common in the abdominal aorta and iliac arteries and results in **atherosclerotic aneurysms** (p. 280). When the disease becomes advanced, with many complicated lesions, it is sometimes designated **endarteritis obliterans**, a poor term, since this is not basically an inflammatory disorder.

Before closing the discussion of gross morphology, a few words are in order about the difficulties in quantitating the severity of atherosclerosis. It is obviously a matter of great importance to determine whether current attempts at control of the disease have had any effect. It has been exceedingly difficult to devise accurate methods of quantitation. It is usual to grade the severity of disease in a large vessel such as the aorta on the basis of the proportion of the intimal surface involved by atheromas, taking into account the relative number of fatty streaks and raised lesions. Obviously the latter are given greater weight. In smaller arteries, although the same approach may be used, it is also important to assess the level of thickening of the arterial wall, as well as the severity of the luminal narrowing. For further details on this problem, reference should be made to the extensive writings of Strong and McGill (Strong and McGill, 1963; McGill, 1968).

Etiology and Pathogenesis. It hardly needs to be stated that the cause of atherosclerosis is unknown. It is, in fact, such a ubiquitous process that some believe it is not a distinct disorder but an inescapable consequence of aging. However, its variable severity in populations and among individuals makes it eminently clear that there are factors other than aging which at least contribute to the development of atherosclerosis. Some of the pathogenetic concepts will be considered here briefly, but it should be remembered that this subject fills volumes and no attempt can be made here to be exhaustive. Most would accept the statement that an abnormal accumulation of lipoproteins, particularly of cholesterol, in the arterial wall is an essential component of atherosclerosis. Whether it is the initiating event is considerably more doubtful. Nor is the source of this accumulation of lipoproteins clear. The favored concept is that the lipoproteins filter in from the blood (filtration theory), but it has also been suggested or that they are endogenously synthesized or that they are released from platelets trapped within the developing lesion. As we shall see, all three pathways might be operative, in conjunction with a diminished capacity of the arterial wall to metabolize and clear the lipoproteins. *Serum lipoprotein levels are probably of major importance in tipping the balance toward accumulation.* Supporting this view is the fact that the most reliable way to produce a reasonable model of this disease in laboratory animals is by a variety of interventions which have in common elevations of serum lipoprotein levels (Wissler and Vesselinovitch, 1968). Moreover, as pointed out, familial hyperlipoproteinemia in humans is uniformly associated with accelerated atherosclerosis. It is appropriate to consider this group of genetic disorders here, since the lipoprotein disturbances encountered in them may be simulated in "normal" individuals—that is, in those who do not have a clear-cut genetic disorder. In these individuals, the hyperlipoproteinemia may be related simply to dietary excess or imbalance. If diet can cause hyperlipoproteinemia, this would present the alluring possibility that regardless of the initiating event in atherosclerosis, the disease may be controllable through dietary manipulations. Before we can discuss the various types of familial hyperlipoproteinemia, a few details about the blood lipids should be recalled.

Lipids are not present in the free state in plasma. They are conjugated with each other and with carrier proteins. All abnormalities in plasma lipids can be related to abnormalities in the type and quantity of lipoproteins. The lipoproteins contain cholesterol, phospholipids and fatty acids (some as esters). They can be separated into classes by ultracentrifugation or by electrophoresis. Four fractions are identifiable in the ultracentrifugate. In order of increasing density, these are chylomicrons, very low density lipoprotein (VLDL), low density lipoprotein (LDL) and high density lipoprotein (HDL). All studies indicate that the high density lipoproteins are not important in the genesis of atherosclerosis. The least dense, the chylomicrons, have the highest Svedberg flotation (Sf) values.

On paper electrophoresis, the chylomicrons do not migrate. In plasma from a normal fasting adult, a densely stained band migrates with the beta globulins. These comprise the beta (low density) lipoproteins. Farther along the strip is found a band migrating with the alpha globulins, comprising the alpha lipoproteins. These are the high density lipoproteins previously cited as not being germane to our discussion. In some individuals, a band less rapidly moving than the beta fraction may be visible, which is known as the pre-beta lipoproteins. These are identical to the very low density lipoproteins already mentioned. Some of these interrelationships are given in Table 9–2, but for more details, the authoritative review by Fredrickson and his colleagues (1967) should be consulted.

Table 9–2 emphasizes that all fractions contain cholesterol and glycerides and that the molecular size and density of the three classes vary widely. Some time ago, Gofman and his associates (1949) proposed that specific clinical syndromes occur in association with an increase in each of these three fractions.

Fredrickson described five types of hyperlipoproteinemia, but subsequently his Type II was subdivided, creating six types of hyperlipoproteinemia, as shown in Table 9–3 (Beaumont et al., 1970; Fredrickson et al., 1967). Whereas these were originally described as genetic disorders in which there may be some environmental influences, Types I, IIB and IV are now thought to be related most often to dietary excess or imbalance. The last two types of hyperlipoproteinemia are of principal interest to us—because they are largely environmental, because they are prevalent and because they are strongly correlated with atherosclerosis. Although Type IIA (familial hypercholesterolemia) is, in contrast, almost completely genetically determined, it too is fairly common. In London, 17 per cent of men and 8 per cent of women were found to have some type of hyperlipoproteinemia, most frequently Types IV, IIA and IIB (Lewis et al., 1974). Type IV hyperlipoproteinemia, also known as pre-beta hyperlipoproteinemia, is clearly associated with obesity and a high dietary intake of calories, principally carbohydrates and fats. Even more striking than the elevations of cholesterol in this pattern are the increases in triglycerides. In this group are found those with diabetes mellitus, abnormal glucose tolerance curves and gout. The plasma lipoprotein levels in Type IV are gratifyingly reduced when there is general restriction of caloric intake, particularly of carbohy-

TABLE 9–2. MAJOR PLASMA LIPOPROTEINS

	CHYLOMICRONS	PRE-BETA LIPOPROTEINS (VLDL)	BETA LIPOPROTEINS (LDL)
Density	0.94	0.98	1.03
Sf class	10,000	20–400	0–20
Greatest molecular diameter	5,000	700	350
Per cent composition			
Protein	2	10	21
Phospholipid	7	22	22
Cholesterol (including esters)	10	20	50
Glycerides	80	55	10

TABLE 9–3. HYPERLIPOPROTEINEMIA*

Type	Familiar Name	Prevalence	Lipoprotein Abnormality	Cholesterol Level	Triglyceride Level	Cause	Coronary Disease Risk
Normal			None; beta > alpha > pre-beta; chylomicra absent	<220 mg. per 100 ml.	150 mg. per 100 ml.	Moderation in all things	
I	Exogenous or dietary hypertriglyceridemia	Rare	Chylomicra present	+ or normal	+++	Dietary fat not cleared from plasma	+
IIA	Hypercholesterolemia (familial)	Moderately common	Beta lipoprotein raised	++	Normal	? Hereditary metabolic defect	+++
IIB	Overindulgence hyperlipidemia	Common	Beta and pre-beta raised	+ to ++	+ to ++	Long-term dietary excess; ? + hereditary element occasionally	+++
III	Familial hyperlipidemia	Rare	Broad beta present	++	++	Hereditary metabolic defect	+++
IV	Endogenous hypertriglyceridemia	Common	Pre-beta raised	+	++	Excessive intake of carbohydrates	++
V	Mixed (types I and IV) endogenous-exogenous hypertriglyceridemia	Fairly common	Chylomicra present and pre-beta raised	+	+++	? Metabolic defect	+

*From World Health Organization: Classification of hyperlipidaemias and hyperproteinaemias. Bull. W. H. O., 43:891, 1970.

drates. Type IIB hyperlipoproteinemia is well-named "overindulgence hyperlipoproteinemia." Here, both cholesterol and triglycerides are elevated, but dietary control of both fats and carbohydrates in most cases will bring about substantial improvement in the serum lipoprotein levels. It should be emphasized at this point that in almost all patients an elevation of one class of lipoproteins is associated with some abnormality in the others. The various forms of hyperlipoproteinemia, therefore, are not pure states but overlap considerably.

At this point we might reiterate three conclusions concerning the etiology and pathogenesis of atherosclerosis which are more or less secure. First, the accumulation of lipoproteins within the arterial wall is the dominant process in the progression of atherosclerosis. Second, these lipoproteins are identical to those in the blood. Third—and least secure—serum lipoprotein levels may in most cases be related to diet. Still, the basic question remains unanswered: What *initiates* the accumulation of lipoproteins within the arterial wall? You will recall that it was mentioned in the description of the morphology that many consider some form of vascular injury to be the initial event. This view is supported by the fact that myointimal cell proliferation with intimal thickening occurs very early in the genesis of fatty streaks (Ross and Glomset, 1973). An attractive and cohesive theory postulates that such proliferation is a reaction to long-standing hemodynamic forces—including suction, shearing or turbulence—to which certain portions of the larger arteries are subjected. Thickening of the intima would then tend to render it and the subjacent tunica media relatively hypoxic since this portion of the arterial wall depends on imbibition for its oxygen supply. It has been suggested that the role of cigarette smoking lies in its tendency to increase the relative hypoxia of the arterial wall through the displacement of oxygen in the blood by carbon monoxide (Astrup and Kjeldsen, 1974). Such hypoxia would in turn lead to diminished activities of the enzymes responsible for metabolizing or mobilizing lipoproteins. At the same time, an increase in endothelial permeability due to trauma would enhance the penetration of lipoproteins from the blood into the arterial wall. The accumulation of lipoproteins would then represent a disturbance of balance between, on the one hand, the lipoproteins entering from the blood plus those endogenously synthesized within the vessel wall and, on the other hand, the capacity of the intimal cells to clear those lipoproteins. What can be said in support of this theory? Perhaps most importantly, it offers an explanation for the well-documented effect of blood pressure on the risk of developing atherosclerosis. Clearly, the higher the blood pressure, the greater the hemodynamic forces acting on the arterial wall. At the other extreme, a very low blood pressure, such as that in the normal pulmonary circuit, seems to confer protection. Conceivably, within the systemic circuit, any blood pressure above shock levels is "hypertensive" with respect to the development of atherosclerosis. Such a view is in accord with the observed fact that the risk of atherosclerosis increases roughly linearly with blood pressure and does not suddenly rise at a critical "hypertensive" level (Kannel, 1974).

Many forms of vascular injury other than that due to hemodynamic forces have also been suggested as the initial event in the genesis of atherosclerosis. Perhaps different ones may be operative in different cases. In experimental animals, radiation injury to the endothelium was found to enhance the effect of a high cholesterol diet in the induction of atherosclerotic lesions (Lee et al., 1974). Similarly, immunization potentiated the effect of a high-cholesterol diet in experimental animals (Levy, 1967). Accordingly, it has been suggested that in humans the deposition of immune complexes in the endothelium may be of importance in the initiation of atherosclerosis. These immune complexes would provoke endothelial proliferation, as well as an increased permeability. In support of this theory is an unexpectedly high prevalence of circulating antibodies against milk in patients who have experienced an MI (Davies et al., 1974). However, known examples of immune-complex disease, such as serum sickness and SLE, show a predilection for small and medium-sized arteries, not for large arteries. If atherosclerosis were related to the presence of circulating immune complexes, it would certainly constitute a mysterious exception to this predilection. Alternatively, it has been suggested that elevated levels of serum lipoproteins might alone have an irritative effect on the arterial walls, possibly through a metabolite (Altschule, 1974). Abnormal platelet adherence has also been considered to be the injurious process, *(thrombogenic hypothesis)* (Duguid, 1948). According to this hypothesis, a layer of platelets and fibrin becomes attached to the endothelium. Possibly by releasing vasoactive amines, such as histamine and 5-hydroxytryptamine, the platelets then render the endothelium more permeable to lipoproteins. Be that as it may, in the course of organization the platelets would become covered by new endothelium and thus be incorporated into the arterial wall. Here they would add their own contained lipids to the development of the atheroma. Again, cigarette smoking might contribute, this time by augmenting a thrombotic diathesis. An entirely different type of vascular "injury" is suggested by the recent evidence that atherosclerotic plaques may be monoclonal in origin—that is, they each arise from only one myointimal cell (Benditt and Benditt, 1973). This finding would indicate that the guilty cell had undergone a mutation, possibly caused by a chemical mutagen or by a virus. Such a mutagen or virus would obviously be virtually ubiquitous, at least in populations with a high prevalence of atherosclerosis.

We should conclude this discussion of the etiology and pathogenesis by admitting that a neat theory does not a truth make. Sadly, despite the wealth of epidemiologic data and the existence of theories which more or less comfortably fit the facts, the cause of atherosclerosis remains unknown. In this state of ignorance, it is perfectly reasonable to attempt to halt the disease during its progression rather than at its inception. The emphasis on serum lipoproteins and the study of other risk factors and their manipulation constitute attempts to approach the problem in this manner.

Clinical Correlation. Atherosclerosis is an insidious disorder. Throughout much of its long evolution, *the arterial changes develop silently and cannot be detected by ordinary clinical examination. It makes its presence known by (1) causing ischemia of some vital organ, such as the heart or brain, (2) predisposing to thrombosis of an important artery, (3) becoming the site of origin for an embolus, or (4) weakening an arterial wall, usually the aorta, resulting in an aneurysm.* The importance of these clinical effects is amply documented by some of the data cited earlier in this discussion and by the introductory material to Chapter 10. Accordingly, there is intense worldwide interest in methods to reduce this toll. The therapeutic attack is two-pronged. One focuses on the prevention of atheromas and the other on prevention of the thrombotic complications.

Few controversies have so sharply divided the medical community as that relating to the control of atherosclerosis by modification of the diet and blood lipid levels. Implicit in this controversy is the view that, in the United States and other economically developed countries, there is a nearly universal "environmental hyperlipoproteinemia," induced, at least in part, by dietary habits. Although there are some genetic hyperlipoproteinemias, these clearly do not account for the great preponderance of patients. The modifications of the diet that have been proposed are so numerous as to be beyond our scope. In general they take the form of lowering the total caloric intake, lowering fat intake, substituting polyunsaturated dietary fat for saturated fat and restricting carbohydrate intake. A low cholesterol intake is one of the principal goals of these diet modifications. However, there are those who claim that lowering of the cholesterol intake is of little benefit, since endogenous synthesis in the liver will increase, holding the plasma levels almost constant. On the other hand, most evidence indicates quite unequivocally that cholesterol in the human diet exerts a significant effect on plasma levels (Connor et al., 1961). The use of polyunsaturated fats has also been a matter of controversy, since it was shown in a National Diet–Heart Study Group report (1968) that a given amount of cholesterol in a diet containing only saturated fats exerts a much greater effect on plasma cholesterol levels than does the same amount of cholesterol added to a diet low in saturated fats and high in polyunsaturated fats.

Even if dietary intervention does lower serum lipoprotein levels, will this in turn lead to the arrest or even the regression of atherosclerosis? This is one of the more pressing questions concerning the disorder. A number of studies are under way to determine an answer. Although the results are controversial and by no means conclusive, there is some evidence from long-term prospective studies that dietary manipulation can lower the mortality from CHD (Miettinen et al., 1972; Bierenbaum et al., 1973). More conclusively, it has been shown in laboratory animals that fatty streaks do regress with dietary manipulation (Eggen et al., 1974; Tucker et al., 1971). Perhaps the human studies have been relatively disappointing because they were carried out on adults, long past the fatty streak stage. In this sense, atherosclerosis might properly be considered a pediatric problem, and the thrust of our preventive efforts best directed toward this age group.

MÖNCKEBERG'S MEDIAL CALCIFIC SCLEROSIS (MEDIAL CALCINOSIS)

This is a lesion of very little clinical significance, which is characterized by focal calcifications and even bone formation within the tunica media of medium-sized muscular arteries. The lumen of the vessel is not narrowed. This lesion is confined to the elderly, being rare under the age of 50. Both sexes are affected.

Although the genesis of medial calcinosis is still obscure, experimental work indicates that the calcification may in some way be related to prolonged vasotonic influences.

The vessels most severely affected are the femoral, tibial, radial and ulnar arteries, those supplying the genital tract, and the coronary arteries. Grossly, the calcification often takes the form of discrete transverse rings, which create a nodularity on palpation. Sometimes the vessel is converted for some length into a rigid, calcified tube. Histologically, the calcium deposits appear either as focal basophilic granular precipitates or as encircling solid masses which destroy the underlying architecture of the tunica media. Often bone and even marrow formation is present within the calcified deposits. Typically, there is no inflammatory reaction, and the tunica intima and tunica adventitia are unaffected.

Since these medial lesions do not encroach on the vessel lumen, there is no interference with normal blood flow. They are of interest largely for the dramatic picture they present on x-ray and on palpation of superficial vessels. Medial calcinosis is, however, frequently associated with the other forms of arteriosclerosis and is thought to predispose to atherosclerosis.

GIANT CELL ARTERITIS (TEMPORAL ARTERITIS, CRANIAL ARTERITIS)

Giant cell arteritis is a patchy granulomatous inflammation which affects large and medium-sized arteries anywhere in the body (Editorial, 1967; Wilske and Healey, 1967). At one time, it was thought to be largely limited to the cranial arteries, especially the temporal arteries, but it is now clear that any major vessel may be involved, and the entity might therefore best be referred to as giant cell arteritis. The disease is one of old age, and is infrequently found in persons under the age of 55 years.

Etiology and Pathogenesis. Although an immunologic pathogenesis has never been proved, giant cell arteritis is usually considered, along with the other necrotizing arteritides, to have an immune basis. This thesis is supported by abnormalities in serum proteins, sometimes including elevated gamma globulins, and by the remarkable response of these patients to corticosteroid treatment. An infectious etiology has been proposed, perhaps triggering an immune process. However, it should be emphasized that the etiology and pathogenesis are not known, and there remain puzzling differences between this disorder and arteritides of known immune origin.

Morphology. Vessels which may be affected include the aorta and all its branches, including the coronaries, and the temporal and other cranial arteries. The affected vessels develop nodular enlargements which may be palpable in certain locations, such as the temple. Sometimes the overlying skin is red and edematous.

It has long been thought that the initial histologic change is degeneration and fragmentation of the internal elastic membrane. However, recently it has been suggested that the initial patho-

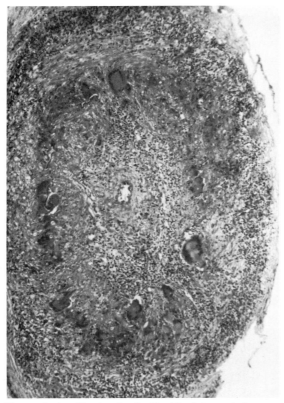

Figure 9–4. Giant cell arteritis. The intense inflammatory reaction with numerous giant cells has virtually obliterated the architecture of the arterial wall and caused marked stenosis of the lumen.

logic change is degeneration of the smooth muscle cells of the media, with **secondary** destruction of elastic fibers and inflammation (Reinecke and Kuwabara, 1969). In either case, the internal elastic membrane is damaged and the elastic fiber fragments excite a foreign body reaction, along with a mononuclear infiltration (Fig. 9–4). Unlike polyarteritis nodosa, giant cell arteritis does not involve large numbers of neutrophils or eosinophils. Typical granulomatous formations develop. The intima undergoes fibrous thickening at the expense of the lumen. Eventually, the reaction permeates the media and may extend out to the adventitia. Thrombus formation regularly follows the intimal damage, and organization of the thrombus contributes to the obliteration of the lumen. With healing, the inflammatory infiltrate and giant cells disappear, and the tunica media is replaced by fibrous tissue. The lumen is occupied by recanalized, organized thrombus.

Clinical Course. The clinical manifestations of giant cell arteritis are extremely variable and depend on the site of arterial involvement. Often the disease is heralded by a flu-like syndrome, with weakness, malaise, low-grade fever and weight loss. More specific symptoms tend to be referable either to the eyes or to the muscles. When cranial vessels are principally involved, especially the ophthalmic artery, visual disturbances, including sudden blindness, may develop. Temporal artery involvement typically produces severe throbbing pain and tenderness over the vessel. In contrast, a more generalized somatic involvement often causes diffuse muscle pain on motion. This pattern, once thought to be a distinct disease entity, is known as *polymyalgia rheumatica* or *polymyalgia arteritica.* It is not an uncommon disorder, having a prevalence similar to that of gout. *Takayasu's arteritis,* to be described later, may also, in some cases, represent a pattern of giant cell arteritis, but this is controversial.

Diagnosis may be made by biopsy, but since the process is patchy a negative biopsy does not rule out giant cell arteritis. A valuable diagnostic point is the extremely high erythrocyte sedimentation rate (ESR), averaging over 100 mm. per hour, which is typical of this disease.

Although ischemia may produce disastrous effects, such as sudden blindness, myocardial ischemia or neurologic derangements, giant cell arteritis is, in general, a relatively benign disease, which usually follows a chronic course, leading eventually to remission. When serious complications do occur, it is imperative to establish the diagnosis within hours, since prompt corticosteroid therapy typically produces a dramatic reversal of the process. In a small proportion of cases, the disease is fatal.

TAKAYASU'S ARTERITIS (PULSELESS DISEASE)

Encroachment on the origins of the great vessels of the aortic arch, known as the *aortic arch syndrome,* occurs in a variety of disorders, including atherosclerosis, syphilitic aortitis, dissecting aneurysm, SLE and giant cell arteritis. Clinically there is weakening of the radial pulse, with ischemia of the upper part of the body, often accompanied by hypertension in the lower extremities. In many cases this syndrome results from an idiopathic arteritis which principally affects young women between the ages of 15 and 45 years, known as *Takayasu's arteritis* or "pulseless disease." Although classically Takayasu's arteritis involves the aortic arch, in 32 per cent of cases it also affects the remainder of the aorta and its branches, and in 12 per cent it is limited to the descending thoracic and abdominal aorta (Nakao et al., 1967; Roberts and Wibin, 1966; Judge, 1962).

Etiology and Pathogenesis. Although the etiology of Takayasu's arteritis is unknown, the rather variable histologic findings have raised the suspicion that there may be multiple etiologies. The presence of a positive tuberculin test and often overt tuberculosis in a large proportion of these cases suggests the possibility of a tuberculous etiology (Nasu, 1963). However, neither tubercle bacilli nor any other microorganisms have been found in the arterial lesions. In one study, five in seven patients were found to have circulating anti-artery antibodies, but whether these antibodies represent cause or effect is unclear.

Morphology. The gross changes are usually limited to a marked irregular mural thickening of the aortic arch and the proximal segments of the great vessels, resulting in severe stenosis. In approximately 50 per cent of cases, the pulmonary artery is also involved. Histologically the early changes consist of an adventitial mononuclear infiltrate surrounding the vasa vasorum. These alterations are similar to those of syphilitic aortitis. However, unlike the case with the luetic lesion, a diffuse polymorphonuclear infiltration and later a mononuclear infiltration soon appear in the media. Less frequently there are granulomatous changes resembling tuberculosis, with Langhans' giant cells and sometimes central caseating necrosis. Sometimes the medial reaction contains foreign body giant cells, and in these cases the lesion may be histologically very similar to giant cell arteritis. **In general, however, giant cell arteritis begins at the junction of intima and media, whereas Takayasu's arteritis begins at the junction of adventitia and media.** In the course of time, the intima becomes markedly sclerotic and thickened, as do the media and adventitia. The fibrosing reaction thickens the wall three- or fourfold and narrows the vascular lumen. The mouths of the exiting branches are sometimes reduced to slits. Final occlusion of the vessel is usually caused by a thrombus, which then undergoes organization. By this time, the inflammatory changes have largely disappeared and are replaced by fibrous scarring of the vessel wall.

Clinical Course. About two thirds of patients with Takayasu's arteritis develop nonspecific symptoms, including malaise, low-grade fever, weight loss and nausea, usually a few weeks before the onset of localizing symptoms. There may also be a variety of cardiopulmonary symptoms, including palpitations and dyspnea. With the narrowing of the mouths of the aortic branches or the development of vessel occlusion, ischemia of the upper body—particularly of the brain—follows and leads to dizziness, syncope, visual disturbances and paresthesias. As with giant cell arteritis, there are serum protein abnormalities, usually elevation of the alpha-2 and gamma globulins, as well as a very high erythrocyte sedimentation rate (ESR), which correlates well with activity of the disease. In contrast to the case with giant cell arteritis,

however, response to corticosteroids is not so uniform nor so dramatic. The clinical course is variable. Of 84 patients followed from six months to 40 years, the conditions of 60 remained unchanged, 12 improved, six worsened and six died from their disease.

THROMBOANGIITIS OBLITERANS (BUERGER'S DISEASE)

This is a remitting, relapsing inflammatory arterial disorder characterized by recurrent thrombosis of medium-sized vessels, principally the tibial and radial arteries. Although it is primarily an arterial disease, adjacent veins and nerves are also involved. The lesion occurs almost always in cigarette smokers, usually young men between the ages of 25 and 50 years. Only extremely rarely has it been reported in nonsmokers or in women (Williams, 1969).

Etiology and Pathogenesis. Some have maintained that thromboangiitis obliterans is not a separate disease entity, but merely represents thrombosis with a secondary inflammatory reaction in vessels already narrowed by atheromatous lesions. However, many aspects of the disorder—including its predilection for young men, its regular association with smoking, the frequent involvement of arms as well as legs, the absence of generalized atherosclerosis in most cases, and the histology—contrast sharply with the usual features of atheromatous peripheral vascular disease. Hence, thromboangiitis obliterans is most probably a distinct entity.

The etiology and pathogenesis are unknown. Buerger postulated an infectious agent, but this has not been substantiated. Despite the correlation between thromboangiitis obliterans and cigarette smoking, it is not clear whether tobacco is somehow causative or merely aggravating, as it is with peripheral vascular insufficiency from any cause. Other questions remain. If the disease is primarily a thrombotic one, as most workers believe, why is the inflammatory response inappropriately intense? Some have suggested two basic derangements—one a hypercoagulable state with episodic thromboses, and the other a focal allergic response to either the thrombus or its breakdown products.

Morphology. Almost invariably, thromboangiitis begins in arteries and secondarily extends to affect contiguous veins and nerves. The affected segment of vessel is firm and indurated. At the site of the lesion, there is a thrombus showing varying stages of organization and recanalization. With the light microscope, the thrombus itself is seen to contain small microabscesses. The adjacent vessel wall shows a nonspecific inflammatory infiltrate, with remarkable preservation of the underlying architecture. With progression, the inflammatory response extends to the tunica adventitia and, in due course, fibrosis with periarterial scarring envelops the adjacent vessels and nerves. **This fibrous encasement of all three structures — artery, vein and nerve — is an important distinguishing characteristic of thromboangiitis obliterans.**

Clinical Course. Often full-blown thromboangiitis obliterans is preceded by recurrent episodes of patchy thrombophlebitis of superficial veins. Eventually, with involvement of the tibial or, less frequently, the radial artery the characteristic manifestations of ischemia ensue. Typically, there is pain in the affected limb, even at rest. When first seen by a physician, many of these patients have chronic ulcerations of their toes or feet, and often the disease progresses to gangrene of the lower leg, necessitating amputation (Eadie et al., 1968). As the underlying thrombus becomes recanalized, total occlusion gives way to partial resumption of blood flow, and the findings abate somewhat, only to recur when a new lesion develops. Cessation of cigarette smoking often brings dramatic relief from further attacks.

RAYNAUD'S DISEASE

Raynaud's disease (as opposed to Raynaud's phenomenon) refers to paroxysmal pallor or cyanosis of acral parts (usually the digits of the hands, sometimes those of the feet, and infrequently the tip of the nose or the ears) caused by intense spasm of local small arteries and arterioles. It is an idiopathic disease, principally of otherwise healthy young women. In contrast, *Raynaud's phenomenon* refers to arterial insufficiency of the acral parts secondary to another disorder — for example, SLE or systemic sclerosis. Although the etiology of Raynaud's disease is unknown, it would appear to be based on an exaggeration of normal central and local vasomotor responses to cold or to emotion. Anatomically, the involved vessels are normal until late in the course, when prolonged vasospasm may cause secondary intimal thickening.

In the classic case, the paroxysms are first noticed in cold weather, and may initially be infrequent. The fingers of both hands become virtually white as the arteries constrict, then cyanotic as the blood stagnates in the capillaries distal to the constriction, later hyperemic as normal blood flow resumes when the hands are again warmed. These changes are most pronounced toward the tips of the fingers. The course of Raynaud's disease is variable. Often it remains static for years, and constitutes no more than a nuisance for the patient, who must avoid situations likely to precipitate an attack. In some cases, the dis-

order subsides spontaneously. Occasionally patients develop a progressive disease, having some degree of cyanosis at all times. Eventually trophic changes and ulcerations appear in the skin, and even areas of gangrene at the fingertips.

LOCALIZED CONGESTION AND EDEMA

Diseases of the veins and lymphatic channels are usually characterized by congestion or edema, or both, distal to the lesion. The exact syndrome varies, of course, depending on the site of the lesion and the size and importance of the vessel involved.

Thrombophlebitis, one of the most common of venous diseases, was discussed on page 219. The *Budd-Chiari syndrome*, caused by obstruction of the hepatic vein, is described on page 533.

VARICOSE VEINS

Varicose veins are abnormally dilated tortuous veins, caused by increased intraluminal pressure and, to a lesser extent, by loss of support of the vessel wall. *Although any vein in the body may be affected, the superficial veins of the leg are by far the most frequently involved.* This predilection is due to the high venous pressure in the legs when they are dependent, coupled with the relatively poor tissue support for the superficial, as opposed to the deep, veins. Even in otherwise normal individuals, these factors produce a tendency toward the development of varices with advancing age and its attendant loss of tissue tone, atrophy of muscles and degenerative changes within the vessel walls. Indeed, this disorder is seen in approximately 50 per cent of individuals over the age of 50 years. There exists a familial tendency toward the development of varicose veins relatively early in life. Because of the venous stasis in the lower legs caused by pregnancy, females develop varicose veins more often than do males.

In addition to the normal burdens on the veins of the legs, any condition that compresses or obstructs veins, causing local increases in intraluminal pressure, clearly increases the risk of varix formation distal to the obstruction. Hence, intravascular thrombosis, tumors which impinge on veins and the wearing of tightly encircling garments or surgical dressings all promote the development of varicosities, in the legs or elsewhere.

Attention should be called to two special sites of varix formation. Hemorrhoids result from varicose dilatation of the hemorrhoidal plexus of veins at the anorectal junction. The causative mechanism is presumed to be prolonged pelvic congestion resulting, for example, from repeated pregnancies or chronic constipation and straining at stools. An important cause of hemorrhoids is portal hypertension due usually to cirrhosis of the liver (page 523).

The second and more important special site of varicosities is the esophagus, and this form is encountered virtually only in patients with cirrhosis of the liver and its attendant portal hypertension. Rupture of an esophageal varix may be more serious than the primary liver disease itself (page 468).

Morphology. The affected veins are dilated, tortuous and elongated. Characteristically, the dilatation is irregular, with nodular or fusiform distentions and even aneurysmal pouchings. Accompanying this asymmetric dilatation, there is marked variation in the thickness of the vessel wall. Thinning is seen at the points of maximal dilatation, while compensatory hypertrophy of the media and fibrosis of the wall may produce thickening in a neighboring segment. Valvular deformities (thickening, rolling and shortening of the cusps) are common, as is intraluminal thrombosis. Microscopically, the changes are quite minimal and consist of variations in the thickness of the wall of the vein. Smooth muscle hypertrophy and subintimal fibrosis are apparent in the areas of compensatory hypertrophy. Frequently there is degeneration of the elastic tissue in the major veins and spotty calcifications within the media (**phlebosclerosis**).

Clinical Course. Sometimes distention of the veins in the legs is painful, although most often early varicose veins are asymptomatic. As the valves become incompetent, a vicious circle is established, with the resultant venous stasis further increasing intraluminal pressure. Marked venous congestion with edema may occur. Such edema impairs circulation, rendering the affected tissues extremely vulnerable to injury. In these severe cases, trophic changes, stasis dermatitis, cellulitis and chronic ulceration are common. Although varicose veins frequently thrombose, embolization to the lungs is uncommon from the superficial leg veins. Hemorrhoids, as is well known, not only are uncomfortable, but also may be a source of bleeding. Sometimes they thrombose and in this distended state are prone to painful ulceration.

OBSTRUCTION OF SUPERIOR VENA CAVA (SUPERIOR VENA CAVAL SYNDROME)

This dramatic entity is usually caused by neoplasms which compress or invade the superior vena cava. Most commonly, a primary bronchogenic carcinoma or a mediastinal lymphoma is the underlying lesion. Occasionally, other disorders, such as an aortic aneurysm, may impinge on the superior vena cava. Regardless of the cause, the consequent obstruction produces a distinctive clinical complex, referred to as the *superior vena caval syndrome.* It is manifested by dusky cyanosis and marked dilatation of the veins of the head, neck and arms. Commonly, the pulmonary vessels are also compressed, and consequently respiratory distress may develop.

OBSTRUCTION OF INFERIOR VENA CAVA (INFERIOR VENA CAVAL SYNDROME)

This is analogous to the superior vena caval syndrome and may be caused by many of the same processes. Neoplasms may either compress or penetrate the walls of the inferior vena cava. In addition, one of the most common causes of inferior vena caval obstruction is propagation of a clot upward from the femoral or iliac veins. Certain tumors, particularly the hepatocarcinoma and the renal cell carcinoma, show a striking tendency to grow within the lumina of the veins, extending ultimately into the inferior vena cava.

As would be anticipated, obstruction to the inferior vena cava induces marked edema of the legs, distention of the superficial collateral veins of the lower abdomen, and, when the renal veins are involved, massive proteinuria.

LYMPHEDEMA

Any occlusion of lymphatic vessels is followed by the abnormal accumulation of interstitial fluid distal to the obstruction, referred to as *lymphedema.* This process is entirely analogous to the formation of edema as a result of venous obstruction. Although there are a few primary lymphatic disorders which produce lymphedema, most often the lymphatic blockage is secondary.

The most common causes of secondary lymphedema are: (1) spread of malignant tumors, with obstruction of either the lymphatic channels or nodes of drainage, (2) radical surgical procedures with removal of regional groups of lymph nodes, as, for example, the removal of axillary nodes in radical mastectomy, (3) postradiation fibrosis, (4) filariasis, and (5) postinflammatory scarring of lymphatic channels.

Primary lymphedema may occur as an isolated congenital defect (*simple congenital lymphedema*), or it may be familial, in which case it is known as *Milroy's disease* or *heredofamilial congenital lymphedema.* Both entities are presumed to be caused by faulty development of lymphatic channels, possibly with poor structural strength, permitting abnormal dilatation and incompetence of the lymphatic valves. Classically, these disorders involve the lower extremities, although they may affect other areas, sometimes in a rather sharply limited, bizarre distribution. Both simple congenital lymphedema and Milroy's disease are present from birth. In contrast, a third form of primary lymphedema, known as *lymphedema praecox*, appears between the ages of 10 and 25 years, usually in females. The etiology is unknown. This disorder begins in one or both feet, and the edema slowly accumulates throughout life, so that the involved extremity may increase to many times its normal size, and the process may extend upward to affect the trunk. Although the size of the limb may produce some disability, more serious complications are unusual.

Morphology. With lymphedema from any cause, the morphologic changes within the lymphatics consist of dilatation distal to the point of obstruction, accompanied by increases of interstitial fluid. Persistence of edema leads to interstitial fibrosis, most evident subcutaneously. The thickened skin assumes the texture of orange peel, a finding termed "peau d'orange." Enlargement of the affected part, brawny induration, cellulitis and chronic skin ulcers are common sequelae to lymphedema, as they are to varicose veins.

Clinical Course. With secondary lymphedema, the clinical picture is usually that of the underlying disorder. Although lymphedema itself is disfiguring and disabling, it is rarely life-threatening. However, persistent ulcers with secondary infection may present serious clinical problems.

ANEURYSMS

Abnormal dilatations of arteries are called aneurysms. They develop wherever there is marked weakening of an arterial wall. Any artery may be affected by a wide variety of disorders, including congenital defects, local infections (mycotic aneurysms), trauma (traumatic aneurysms or arteriovenous aneurysms) or systemic diseases that weaken arterial walls. The most important aneurysms occur in the aorta, and for these atherosclerosis, syphilis and medionecrosis are the principal causes. Congenital defects of the intracranial arteries, termed *berry aneurysms*, are also fairly frequent. They represent an important cause of cerebrovascular accidents (CVA) and, as such, are discussed on page 650.

ATHEROSCLEROTIC ANEURYSM

As the incidence of tertiary cardiovascular syphilis has declined, atherosclerosis has become the most common cause of aortic aneurysms. They are most frequent in males (5:1 ratio) after the fifth decade of life. Although any site in the aorta may be affected, including the thoracic aorta, the great preponderance of these lesions occurs in the abdominal aorta, usually below the renal arteries. *Until proved otherwise, an abdominal aneurysm is assumed to be atherosclerotic in origin.* Occasionally, several separate dilatations occur, and not infrequently aortic lesions are accompanied by additional aneurysms in the iliac arteries.

Atherosclerotic aneurysms take the form of saccular (balloon-like), cylindroid or fusiform swellings, sometimes up to 15 cm. in greatest diameter and of variable length (up to 25 cm.) (Fig. 9–5). As would be expected, there is severe complicated atherosclerosis at these sites, which destroys the underlying tunica media and thus produces the weakening of the aortic wall. Mural thrombus frequently is found within the aneurysmal sac. In the saccular forms, the thrombus may completely fill the outpouching up to the level of the surrounding aortic wall. The elongated fusiform or cylindroid patterns more often have layers of mural thrombus that only partially fill the dilatation.

The clinical consequences of these aneurysms depend principally on their location and size. Occlusion of the iliac, renal, or mesenteric arteries may result either from pressure of the aneurysmal sac or from propagation of the thrombus. The thrombus may embolize. As enlarging pulsatile masses, these aneurysms not only simulate tumors, but also progressively erode adjacent structures, such as the vertebral bodies. They have been known to erode the wall of the gut or, when they occur in the thorax, the wall of the trachea or esophagus. Rupture is the most feared consequence and is related to the size of the dilatation. In general, when they are less than 6 cm. in diameter, these aneurysms rarely rupture, whereas 80 per cent of patients with larger lesions die of rupture within a year of their diagnosis. Fortunately, since most such aneurysms occur below the level of the renal arteries, some can be resected and replaced with prosthetic arterial channels, with excellent results.

SYPHILITIC (LUETIC) AORTITIS AND ANEURYSM

As will be pointed out in the general discussion of syphilis in Chapter 16, the tertiary stage of the disease shows a predilection for the cardiovascular and nervous systems. Fortunately, with better control and treatment of syphilis in its early stages, these involvements are becoming rare. Before discussing the cardiovascular lesion, which is termed *syphilitic aortitis*, reference should be made to Chapter 16 for the basic tissue reactions incited by *Trepo-*

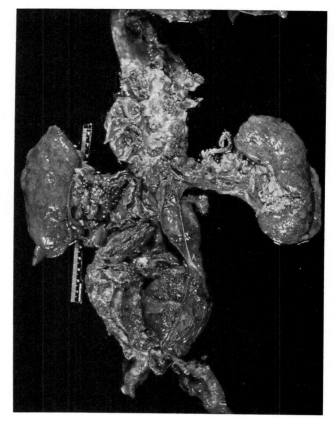

Figure 9–5. Atherosclerotic aneurysm of the abdominal aorta situated below the renal arteries and above the iliac bifurcation. The atherosclerosis throughout the aorta is far advanced. Some mural thrombus layers the back wall of the aneurysm.

nema pallidum (i.e., *obliterative endarteritis, perivascular cuffing* and *gumma formation*).

Although obliterative endarteritis in teritary syphilis may involve small vessels in any part of the body, it is clinically most devastating when it affects the vasa vasorum of the aorta. Such involvement gives rise to thoracic aortitis, which in turn leads to the aneurysmal dilatation of the aorta and the aortic valve ring characteristic of full-blown cardiovascular syphilis. Since this sequel to *T. pallidum* infection does not manifest itself until 15 to 20 years after contraction of the infection, it is seen most frequently in the age range of 40 to 55 years. Males are involved three times as often as females.

Morphology. Syphilitic aortitis is almost always confined to the thoracic aorta, usually to the ascending and transverse portions, and rarely extends below the diaphragm. The earliest changes are obliterative endarteritis with perivascular cuffing of the vasa vasorum by plasma cells. The narrowing of these nutrient arteries leads to ischemic destruction of the elastic tissue and smooth muscle of the media and intima. Inflammatory vascularization and fibrous scarring follow. Grossly, these medial and intimal scars appear as subendothelial, pearly gray, elevated plaques, 1 to 3 cm. in diameter, which bulge into the aortic lumen. With contraction of the irregular scars, longitudinal wrinkling or "tree-barking" of the intervening intimal surface ensues. More importantly, the scarring may envelop and narrow the ostia of vessels arising from the aorta, including those of the coronary arteries. Luetic aortitis thus constitutes one of the causes of coronary artery insufficiency and myocardial infarction, albeit rarely.

With destruction of the tunica media, the aorta loses its elastic support, and tends to become dilated, producing a syphilitic aneurysm. It should be pointed out that, for unknown reasons, secondary atherosclerotic involvement of these damaged areas is almost invariable and may contribute to the weakening of the aortic wall. Because the luetic aortitis usually extends to the very origin of the aorta, the atherosclerosis usually begins right at the base of the aortic valves (Fig. 9–6). In sharp contrast, atherosclerosis, when uncomplicated by lues, almost never involves the root of the aorta. **Even when complicated by atherosclerosis, the location of these aneurysms in the thorax tends to distinguish them from typical atherosclerotic aneurysms, which rarely affect the aortic arch but usually develop in the abdominal aorta.** Syphilitic aneurysms are sometimes enormous, achieving a diameter of 15 to 20 cm. They may be saccular, fusiform or cylindroid. The dilatation commonly extends proximally to include the aortic

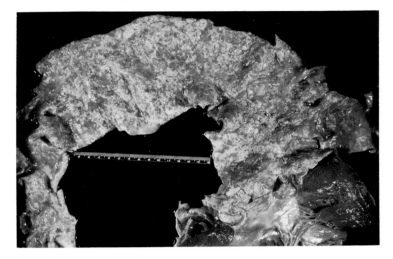

Figure 9–6. Syphilitic aortitis, with superimposed florid atherosclerosis. The heart is seen in the lower right. The lesions begin at the aortic valve and are most marked in the thoracic region, where there is some aneurysmal widening of the aorta.

valve ring. As a consequence, the valvular commissures are widened and the valve leaflets are stretched, so that their free margins tend to roll and become thickened. Incompetence of the valve results. The increased work of the left ventricle leads to marked, sometimes extraordinary, hypertrophy and dilatation of this chamber, with resultant heart weights of up to 1000 gm. Such hearts are known as **"cor bovinum."** The coronary ostia, which normally are hidden from view in the sinuses of Valsalva, become exposed as the leaflets roll back on themselves. The combination of intimal damage resulting both from the luetic and from the atherosclerotic involvement, and abnormal dilatation with its attendant turbulence, often leads to mural thrombosis within the aneurysm. Rupture of the aneurysm may occur, but this is rare.

Clinical Course. Syphilitic aortitis with aneurysmal dilatation may give rise to (1) respiratory difficulties as a result of encroachment on the lungs and airways, (2) difficulty in swallowing, owing to compression of the esophagus, (3) persistent brassy cough, from pressure on the recurrent laryngeal nerve, (4) pain, caused by erosion of bone (ribs and vertebral bodies), and (5) cardiac disease. As the aneurysm leads to dilatation of the aortic valve, there is typically a loud diastolic murmur and widening of the pulse pressure to produce a bounding pulse (Corrigan's pulse). Most patients with syphilitic aneurysms die of congestive heart failure secondary to involvement of the aortic valve. Other causes of death include rupture of the aneurysm, with fatal hemorrhage, and erosion of vital contiguous structures, such as the bronchi or esophagus, by the expanding pulsatile mass.

IDIOPATHIC CYSTIC MEDIAL NECROSIS (MEDIONECROSIS) — DISSECTING ANEURYSM

This disorder is characterized by focal but widespread destruction of the elastic and muscular tissue of the media of the aortic wall. Infrequently, other large arteries, including the coronaries, are involved. By weakening the aortic wall, the focal lesions predispose to aneurysmal dilatation, but more often they lead to hemorrhage within the media, with longitudinal dissection of the blood along laminar planes. This is known as a *dissecting aneurysm.* In one study, the average age at which medionecrosis was discovered was 47 years, but the range was wide, from 27 years to 70 years. Males outnumbered females 9 to 1 (Layman and Wang, 1968).

Etiology and Pathogenesis. The cause or causes of medionecrosis are unknown. For years it was ascribed to disease of the vasa vasorum, either atherosclerotic or hypertensive, which led to hypoxia of the tunica media. However, such a sequence has not been confirmed, and the frequent finding of normal appearing vasa vasorum would argue against it. It is true, however, that most patients with a dissecting aneurysm have hypertension. Whether the hypertension actually plays a causative role in the development of the underlying medionecrosis, or whether it merely predisposes toward dissection by subjecting an already diseased aorta to greater stress, is not clear. The frequent finding of medionecrosis proximal to a congenital coarctation of the aorta, where severe local hypertension exists, has been offered as support of some causative relationship.

Current evidence, however, suggests that medionecrosis results from a metabolic defect in the synthesis of the connective tissue fibers (collagen and elastin) in the tunica media. In addition to occurring as a seemingly isolated lesion in middle-aged males and with coarctation of the aorta, medionecrosis is a common feature of Marfan's syndrome and develops with more than chance frequency in "normal" pregnancies and in extreme old age. The association with Marfan's syndrome has led to the thesis that medionecrosis represents a congenital defect in connective tissue metabolism. Indeed, it has been suggested that medionecrosis is simply a forme fruste or milder expression of Marfan's syndrome. On the other hand, experimental data point out that medionecrosis can be an acquired metabolic abnormality. Although it is known that turkeys may develop medionecrosis spontaneously, these fowl show an increased frequency of the lesion when treated with estrogens. A similar finding of increased incidence during human pregnancy has been attributed to a "loosening" effect of estrogens on connective tissue. Feeding experimental animals food rich in beta aminopropionitrile also produces lesions similar to medionecrosis *(lathyrism)*. These lathyrogenic agents block the cross linkages in collagen and elastin fibers and thus impair their tensile strength (Bornstein, 1970). Although this sort of toxic exposure is unlikely in man, conceivably some metabolic error in the formation of these fibers leads to the same defect in the clinical disease. Experimental copper deficiency also leads to medionecrosis, and it has been postulated that a derangement in copper metabolism, hence a deficiency of copper dependent enzymes in the aortic media, may underlie the human disease. In summary, the multitude and diversity of etiologic theories would seem to indicate that idiopathic cystic medial necrosis is indeed idiopathic. Quite possibly, several pathways may lead to impairment of normal connective tissue metabolism and the development of this lesion.

Not only is the cause of medionecrosis controversial, but the initiation of the complicating dissecting aneurysm is also unclear. It is most widely believed that the hemorrhage originates in rupture of the vasa vasorum, which lose their external tissue support as the tunica media about them degenerates. However, others believe that, as the weakened aortic wall undergoes abnormal dilatation, there may be tearing of the tunica intima, which permits blood to enter the tunica media from the lumen and dissect along the laminar planes.

Morphology. The microscopic lesion is characterized by poorly delineated focal defects within the tunica media, filled with metachromatic acid mucopolysaccharides. Most striking is the destruction of elastic fibers within these defects. The lesions are most pronounced in the outer half of the tunica media, and they totally destroy the normal laminar pattern. Although the lesions are called "cystic," the defects are not demarcated by well defined margins and, moreover, they are usually widely scattered, with completely normal intervening areas of aortic wall. Typically, there is

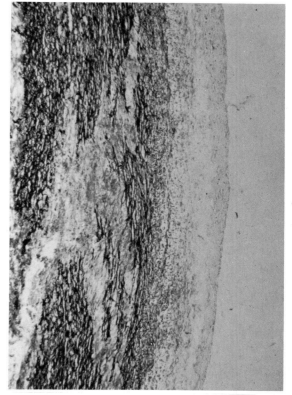

Figure 9–7. Cystic medionecrosis of the aorta. The intima is to the right. An elastic tissue stain accentuates the elastica of the media. The irregular cleftlike area devoid of elastica represents the focus of medionecrosis. Note the absence of inflammatory reaction.

no inflammatory response to the destructive process. Indeed, it can be said in general that these lesions are subtle and rather easily overlooked, unless elastic tissue stains are employed (Fig. 9–7).

In the absence of dissection, the aorta may appear grossly normal, or there may be simple aneurysmal dilatation of the weakened wall. When the dilatation extends proximally to the aortic valve ring, aortic regurgitation with secondary ventricular hypertrophy ensues. In this respect, medionecrosis is similar to syphilitic aortitis, which was discussed previously.

When dissections occur, they usually begin in the ascending portion and extend toward the heart as well as distally along the length of the aorta. Sometimes the proximal dissection extends into and about the coronary arteries. Although the length of the dissection is quite variable, not infrequently the entire aorta is traversed, with progression into the iliac and femoral arteries (Fig. 9–8). The renal arteries may similarly be involved, sometimes with total compression of their lumina. The intramural hemorrhage may occur over the entire circumference or only over a part of it. Characteristically, the plane of dissection cleaves the outer one-third

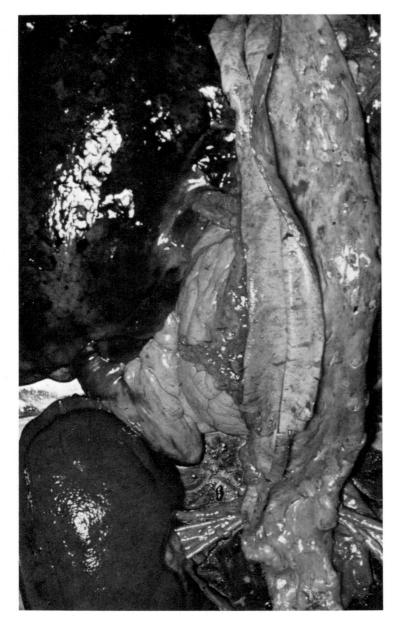

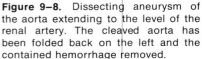

Figure 9-8. Dissecting aneurysm of the aorta extending to the level of the renal artery. The cleaved aorta has been folded back on the left and the contained hemorrhage removed.

of the tunica media from the inner two-thirds. The amount of contained hemorrhage is variable, but may be quite massive. Usually, but not invariably, the hemorrhage ruptures through the inner layers of the tunica media and the tunica intima to enter the lumen of the aorta. In 90 per cent of cases, the resulting intimal tear is found in the ascending aorta, 5 to 10 cm. from the aortic valve. There may also be a distal intimal tear, but this is less frequent. Quite rarely, the proximal and distal tears provide ingress and egress to the blood flow and a functional channel is formed, which may even become endothelialized to form a **double barreled aorta.** Most patients are not so fortunate, and eventually—in almost all cases—external

hemorrhage occurs into the periadventitial tissues or serosal cavities, usually the pericardium.

Clinical Course. Cystic medial necrosis may be asymptomatic until dissection occurs. With dissection, there is characteristically a sudden onset of excruciating pain, usually beginning in the anterior chest and, in classic cases, radiating to the back and moving downward as the dissection progresses. The intensity of this pain often leads to the misdiagnosis of acute myocardial infarction or of perforated peptic ulcer. The pain is often episodic and recurrent as bouts of advancing dissection occur. As the origins of the aortic branches become involved in the process, a multitude of seemingly bizarre findings evolve. Compression of the small vertebral branches may cause striking sensory and motor changes in the lower half of the body. Involvement of the renal arteries may cause hematuria, flank pain and oliguria, and sometimes dissection into the walls of the renal artery compresses its lumen and renal infarction results. Rarely, a myocardial infarction results from dissection into and about a coronary artery.

Unequal compression of major arteries leading to the limbs may produce sudden changes or inequalities in blood pressures. Radiography may disclose a widened ascending aorta and sometimes a double aortic shadow. Retrograde aortography confirms the diagnosis by revealing the aortic wall to be abnormally thick.

Despite this classical pattern of an asymptomatic patient who suddenly develops calamitous indications of dissection, there exist a number of individuals with medionecrosis who come to medical attention because of more or less subtle manifestations of congestive heart failure resulting from aneurysmal dilatation of the aortic valve ring. Surprisingly, at surgery a number of such patients were found to have intimal tears with or without concomitant dissection, yet they had never experienced pain (Layman and Wang, 1968).

Without vigorous intervention, a dissecting aneurysm is almost invariably fatal. Death is most often caused by rupture into the pericardial, pleural or peritoneal sac. According to a review by Hirst and his colleagues (1958), 3 per cent of these patients die immediately, 21 per cent die within 24 hours, 60 per cent die within two weeks and 90 per cent die within three months. With intensive antihypertensive therapy or prosthetic replacement of a dissected segment, the prognosis is much brighter. A three-year survival of 60 per cent has been reported with antihypertensive therapy (Palmer and Wheat, 1967; Wheat et al., 1969). If the dissection begins distal to the subclavian artery, the prognosis is much better than if it begins in the ascending aorta. It has been estimated that about 5 per cent of patients with dissecting aneurysm have the good fortune to develop a second complete channel and survive in this way (Shennan, 1934).

ARTERIOVENOUS FISTULA (ANEURYSM)

Abnormal communications between arteries and accompanying veins may arise as developmental defects, from rupture of an arterial aneurysm into the adjacent vein, from penetrating injuries that pierce the walls of both artery and vein and permit an artificial communication, and from inflammatory necrosis of adjacent vessels. The connection between the vessels may be formed by the canalization of a thrombus, or it may be constructed of an aneurysmal sac. When a fistula takes the form of a tangled mass of intercommunicating vessels, it is designated a *cirsoid aneurysm*. The clinical significance of all these fistulae lies not only in their vulnerability to hemorrhage, but also in the added burden they may place on the heart by short-circuiting blood from the arterial to the venous system. This last mentioned consequence may also occur with those arteriovenous communications that are present in the lungs.

TUMORS

Tumors of vessels (blood or lymphatic) span a wide range of patterns, from those that reproduce vascular channels to those that are solid masses of endothelial cells, sometimes admixed with fibroblasts. Those containing channels may have large sinusoids and be called cavernous hemangiomas (or lymphangiomas), or the channels may be smaller and the tumors termed capillary hemangiomas (or lymphangiomas). Presentation of two special tumors, the glomangioma and Kaposi's sarcoma, as well as the non-neoplastic lesion, telangiectasis, concludes the chapter.

ANGIOMA

The *hemangiomas* and *lymphangiomas* most probably arise as hamartomatous growths which are present from birth and enlarge along with bodily development, often becoming static when the individual reaches maturity. Small (1 to 2 cm.) *cavernous hemangiomas* are most frequent in the liver. The *cavernous lymphangiomas (cystic hygromas)* are encountered most often in the subcutaneous tissues of the axilla and neck and although they are benign, they insinuate between the deeper structures and are exceedingly difficult to excise. Only the *capillary hemangioma* and the *sclerosing hemangioma* are seen with sufficient frequency to warrant description. As will be seen, these two lesions may simply represent stages of the same process.

A **capillary hemangioma** is an unencapsulated tangle of closely packed capillaries separated by a scant connective tissue stroma. It is in continuity with normal vascular channels through solitary afferent and efferent vessels, and thus it is filled with fluid blood. However, thrombosis and fibrous organization within some of the component capillaries is common. The lining endothelial cells appear normal. Although any organ or tissue may be involved, capillary hemangiomas usually occur in the skin, subcutaneous tissues or mucous membranes of the oral cavity and lips. On gross inspection, they appear as bright red to blue lesions, ranging from a few millimeters to several centimeters in diameter, and may be level with the surface of the surrounding tissue, slightly elevated or—occasionally—even pedunculated. Uncommonly, capillary hemangiomas take the form of large, flat, maplike discolorations covering large areas of the face or upper parts of the body, known as **"port wine stains."**

Clinically, all of these lesions are of significance only in their tendency to traumatic ulceration or bleeding, and in their possible confusion with more important neoplasms.

The *sclerosing hemangioma* is believed by many to represent a capillary hemangioma which, by progressive proliferation of endothelial cells and connective tissue stroma, has become transformed over a period of years into a solidly cellular tumor. Such an origin explains their infrequency before adulthood. Others, however, deny a vascular origin for these tumors and refer to them as *dermatofibromas* or *histiocytomas.*

In any event, because of their rich endowment with fibroblasts and histiocytes, sclerosing hemangiomas are usually pale gray to yellow-tan, rather than red-blue. They have the same size and distribution as the capillary hemangiomas. The lesions are unencapsulated and appear as whorling bundles of spindle cells. Careful search will usually disclose central cores of almost obliterated vascular channels. The identification of these vascular remnants is necessary for the diagnosis. Also characteristic of the sclerosing hemangioma is the presence of scattered or nested macrophages with a foamy granular cytoplasm (lipophages). Presumably these cells derive their appearance from imbibing the lipid breakdown products of blood.

GLOMANGIOMA

This is a small, benign tumor which arises from the cells of a *glomus body,* a specialized structure which regulates arteriolar flow according to variations in temperature.

Glomus bodies may be located anywhere in the skin, but they are most commonly found in the distal fingers and toes, especially under the nails. They are supplied with an afferent artery, arteriovenous anastomoses and efferent veins. Surrounding the anastomoses are apparently specialized pericyte cells, which are plump and round to polygonal, resembling epithelial cells. The nuclei are round, quite regular and deeply chromatic. The tumors are small, of the order of 5 mm. in diameter. When in the skin, they are slightly elevated, rounded, red-blue, firm nodules. Under the nail, they appear as minute foci of fresh hemorrhage. Histologically, these lesions are composed of branching vascular channels in a connective tissue stroma, surrounded by masses of neoplastic glomus cells. These neoplastic cells resemble in all respects normal glomus cells.

Glomangiomas are distinctive by virtue of their red-blue color and their exquisite painfulness.

KAPOSI'S SARCOMA (MULTIPLE IDIOPATHIC HEMORRHAGIC SARCOMATOSIS)

This rather mysterious multicentric tumor is considered here because of its probable vascular origin.

The skin is the characteristic site of involvement, although in about 10 per cent of cases visceral lesions are also present. Early cases have been described which show multiple disseminated skin lesions resembling either benign capillary hemangiomas or vascularized chronic inflammatory foci. Over the course of time, repeated biopsies have disclosed a progressive sarcomatous transformation. When full-blown, the lesions appear grossly as multiple, purplish to brown, subcutaneous plaques or nodules, often with a verrucose surface. Histologically, the following four components are seen: (1) Endothelial cell proliferation, either as cellular sheets or as new vessel formations, (2) extravascular hemorrhage with hemosiderin deposition, (3) anaplastic fibroblastic proliferation, and (4) a granulation-like inflammatory reaction.

The clinical course is extremely indolent, and the patient often dies of unrelated causes, although occasionally lesions are aggressive and assume the characteristics of other sarcomas.

TELANGIECTASIS

This term refers to focal red-blue lesions created by the abnormal dilatation of *preexisting* small vessels. *As such, telangiectases are not true neoplasms.* In many of these lesions, a small, central, dilated vessel can be seen surrounded by radiating fine channels. This is understandably called a *spider telangiectasis.*

Most commonly, telangiectases are seen in pregnant women and in patients with chronic liver disease. In both instances, it is thought that they are in some way evoked by hyperestrinism.

Multiple, small, aneurysmal telangiectases distributed over the skin and mucous membranes may be transmitted as an autosomal dominant trait. This extremely uncommon disorder is known as *hereditary hemorrhagic telangiectasia (Rendu-Osler-Weber disease).* It is present from birth.

This hereditary disorder is characterized by discrete or coalescent, small, red-blue lesions, usually less than 5 mm. in diameter, directly beneath the skin and mucosal surfaces of the oral cavity, lips and alimentary, respiratory and urinary tracts. Lesions may also be found in the liver, brain and spleen. Microscopically, these vascular anomalies consist of dilated capillary or venular channels, usually filled with fluid blood, and lined by a single layer of endothelial cells.

Typically, the disease is characterized by recurrent hemorrhages from rupture of the many superficial lesions. Although these hemorrhages are usually readily controlled, they have occasionally proved fatal when they arise in deeply situated lesions in vital organs.

REFERENCES

Albrink, M. J., and Man, E. B.: Serum triglycerides. Arch. Int. Med., *103*:4, 1959.

Altschule, M. D.: The etiology of atherosclerosis. Med. Clin. North Amer., *58*:397, 1974.

Astrup, P., and Kjeldsen, K.: Carbon monoxide, smoking and atherosclerosis. Med. Clin. North Amer., *58*:323, 1974.

Beaumont, J. L., et al.: World Health Organization: Classification of hyperlipidemias and hyperproteinemias. Bull. WHO, *43*:891, 1970.

Benditt, E. P., and Benditt, J. M.: Evidence for a monoclonal origin of human atherosclerotic plaques. Proc. Nat. Acad. Sci., *70*:1753, 1973.

Bierenbaum, M. L., et al.: Ten-year experience of modified-fat diets on younger men with coronary heart disease. Lancet, *1*:1404, 1973.

Blumenthal, S., and Jesse, M. J.: Prevention of atherosclerosis: a pediatric problem. Hospital Practice, April, 1973.

Bornstein, P.: The cross linking of collagen and elastin and its inhibition in osteolathyrism. Am. J. Med., *49*:429, 1970.

Carvalho, A. C. A., et al.: Platelet function in hyperlipoproteinemia. New Engl. J. Med., *290*:434, 1974.

Connor, W. E., et al.: The serum lipids in men receiving high cholesterol and cholesterol free diets. J. Clin. Invest., *40*:894, 1961.

Davies, D. F., et al.: Food antibodies and myocardial infarction. Lancet, *1*:1012, 1974.

Dayton, S., and Pearce, M. L.: Prevention of coronary heart disease and other complications of atherosclerosis modified by diet. Am. J. Med., *46*:751, 1969.

Duguid, J. B.: Thrombosis as a factor in atherosclerosis. J. Path. Bact., *60*:57, 1948.

Eadie, D. G. A., et al.: Buerger's disease. A clinical and pathologic re-examination. Brit. J. Surg., *55*:452, 1968.

Editorial: Cranial arteritis and polymyalgia rheumatica. Lancet, *2*:926, 1967.

Eggen, D. A., et al.: Regression of diet-induced fatty streaks in rhesus monkeys. Lab. Invest., *31*:294, 1974.

Fredrickson, D. S., et al.: Fat transport in lipoproteins. An integrated approach to mechanisms and disorders. New Eng. J. Med., *276*:34, 94, 148, 215, 273, 1967.

Furman, R. H., et al.: Gonadal hormones, blood lipids and ischemic heart disease. In Miras, C. H., Howard, A. N., and Paoletti, R. S. (eds.): Progress in Biochemical Pharmacology. Recent Advances in Atherosclerosis. New York, S. Karger, 1968.

Getz, G. S., et al.: A dynamic pathology of atherosclerosis. Am. J. Med., *46*:657, 1969.

Gofman, J. W., et al.: Ultracentrifugal studies on lipoproteins of human serum. J. Biol. Chem., *179*:973, 1949.

Goldstein, J. L.: Genetic aspects of hyperlipidemia in coronary heart disease. Hospital Practice, October, 1973.

Guidry, M., et al.: Lipid pattern in experimental canine atherosclerosis. Circ. Res., *14*:61, 1964.

Hirst, A. E., et al.: Dissecting aneurysms of the aorta. A review of 505 cases. Medicine, *37*:217, 1958.

Judge, R. D., et al.: Takayasu's arteritis and the aortic arch syndrome. Am. J. Med., *32*:379, 1962.

Kannel, W. B.: The role of cholesterol in coronary atherogenesis. Med. Clin. North Amer., *58*:363, 1974.

Kingsbury, K. J.: Polyunsaturated fatty acids and myocardial infarction. Lancet, *2*:1325, 1969.

Layman, T. E., and Wang, Y.: Idiopathic cystic medionecrosis and aneurysmal dilatation of the ascending aorta. Med. Clin. North Amer., *52*:1145, 1968.

Lee, K. T., et al.: Genesis of atherosclerosis in swine fed high fat-cholesterol diets. Med. Clin. North Amer., *58*:281, 1974.

Levy, L.: A form of immunological atherosclerosis. In DiLuzio, N. R., and Paoletti, R. (eds.): The Reticuloendothelial System and Atherosclerosis. Proceedings of an International Symposium on Atherosclerosis and the Reticuloendothelial System, held in Como, Italy, Sept. 8–10, 1966. New York, Plenum Press, 1967, p. 426. (Series: Advances in Experimental Medicine and Biology, Vol. I).

Lewis, B., et al.: Frequency of risk factors for ischemic heart disease in a healthy British population. Lancet, *1*:141, 1974.

Mann, G. V.: The influence of obesity on health. New Eng. J. Med., *291*:226, 1974.

McGill, H. C. (ed.): The geographic pathology of atherosclerosis. Lab. Invest., *18*:465, 1968.

Miettinen, M., et al.: Effect of cholesterol-lowering diet on mortality from coronary heart-disease and other causes. A twelve-year clinical trial in men and women. Lancet, *2*:835, 1972.

Nakao, K., et al.: Takayasu's arteritis. Clinical report of 84 cases and immunological studies of seven cases. Circulation, *35*:1141, 1967.

Nasu, T.: Pathology of pulseless disease. Angiology, *14*:225, 1963.

National Diet–Heart Study Research Group: The National Diet–Heart Study Final Report. Circulation, *37*, Suppl. 1, 1968.

Palmer, R. F., and Wheat, M. W., Jr.: Treatment of dissecting aneurysms of the aorta. Ann. Thorac. Surg., *4*:38, 1967.

Paronetto, F.: Systemic nonsuppurative necrotizing angiitis. In Miescher, P. A., and Muller-Eberhard, H. J. (eds.): Textbook of Immunopathology. New York, Grune & Stratton, 1969, p. 722.

Poston, R. N., and Davies, D. F.: Immunity and inflammation in the pathogenesis of atherosclerosis. Atherosclerosis, *19*:353, 1974.

Reinecke, R. D., and Kuwabara, T.: Temporal arteritis. Arch. Ophthal., *82*:446, 1969.

Roberts, W. C., and Wibin, E. A.: Idiopathic panaortitis, supra-aortic arteritis, granulomatous myocarditis and pericarditis. Am. J. Med., *41*:453, 1966.

Ross, R., and Glomset, J. A.: Atherosclerosis and the arterial smooth muscle cell. Science, *180*:1332, 1973.

Shennan, T.: Medical Research Council, Special Report Series #193. London, His Majesty's Stationery Office, 1934, p. 138.

Strong, J. P., and McGill, H. C.: Natural history of aortic atherosclerosis. Relationship to race, sex and coronary lesions in New Orleans. J. Exp. Molec. Path., *2* (Suppl. 1):15, 1963.

Tejada, C., et al.: Distribution of coronary and aortic atherosclerosis by geographic location, race and sex. Lab. Invest., *18*:509, 1968.

Tucker, C. F., et al.: Regression of early cholesterol-induced aortic lesions in rhesus monkeys. Am. J. Path., *65*:493, 1971.

Wheat, M. W., Jr., et al.: Acute dissecting aneurysms of the aorta. Treatment and results in 64 patients. J. Thorac. Cardiovasc. Surg., *58*:344, 1969.

Williams, G.: Recent views on Buerger's disease. J. Clin. Path., *22*:573, 1969.

Wilske, K. R., and Healey, L. A.: Polymyalgia rheumatica. A manifestation of systemic giant cell arteritis. Ann. Int. Med., *66*:77, 1967.

Wissler, R. W., and Vesselinovitch, D.: Experimental models of human atherosclerosis. Ann. N.Y. Acad. Sci., *149*:907, 1968.

Zemplenyi, T.: Vascular enzymes and the relevance of their study to problems of atherogenesis. Med. Clin. North Amer., *58*:293, 1974.

CHAPTER 10

The Heart

Heart disease is today the leading cause of morbidity and mortality in the affluent nations. Approximately 38 per cent of all deaths in the United States in 1973 were attributable to heart disease, and of these over 90 per cent were caused by coronary heart disease (CHD) (myocardial injury due to insufficient oxygen delivery by the coronary arteries). The full significance of these data is made evident by the United States Vital Statistics report of the causes of mortality in 1973. Among a total of 1,977,000 deaths from all causes, heart disease accounted for 754,460. The five major forms of heart disease and their relative contributions to death from heart disease are:

Coronary heart
disease   682,910 (90.5 per cent)
Rheumatic heart
disease   13,580 (1.8 per cent)
Hypertensive heart
disease   13,200 (1.7 per cent)
Endocarditis and
myocarditis   4870 (0.6 per cent)
Other   39,900 (5.3 per cent)

These commanding data clearly show that the story of heart disease in the United States is very largely the story of CHD, which in turn is almost always the consequence of coronary atherosclerosis. *CHD alone accounts for about 35 per cent of the total mortality in the United States.* Moreover, in recent years it has shown an increasing predilection for affecting relatively young individuals, in the fifth and sixth decades of life. There is, however, a bright note in the consideration of heart disease in general. In recent years there has been a gratifying decline in the death rates from heart disease other than CHD. This, then, leaves CHD, by default, of increasingly overwhelming relative importance (the big enchilada).

Death from heart disease is usually a direct result either of disturbances in cardiac rhythm or of progressive weakening of the pump. Frequently one leads to the other. All the major diseases of the heart to be discussed in this chapter may be associated with various arrhythmias, such as atrial fibrillation or extrasystoles. Disturbances in cardiac rhythm occur when the normal conduction pathways are interrupted by necrosis, inflammation or fibrosis, or when some local metabolic derangement produces a focus of electrical irritability. As such, arrhythmias, although dramatic, are of little help in identifying the specific pathologic lesion. Similarly, all the major cardiac diseases, when sufficiently severe, may interfere with the capacity of the heart to function as a pump. Through either pathway the clinical syndrome known as congestive heart failure (CHF) may ensue and dominate the clinical picture. Because this ultimate consequence of all major forms of heart disease is a rather complex syndrome with protean effects, we will describe CHF in some detail before discussing each disease separately.

CONGESTIVE HEART FAILURE (CHF)

Congestive heart failure refers to a clinical syndrome resulting from diminished cardiac stroke volume, with inability of the cardiac output to keep pace with the venous return. This eventually results in blood damming back into the venous system, with concomitant diminished filling of the arterial tree. The fundamental derangement may be impaired myocardial contractility, as with intrinsic myocardial disease, or an increased work load placed upon the heart as with, say, valvular incompetence (Dodge and Baxley, 1968). Not infrequently, both factors are operative. In any case, an imbalance results between the work demanded of the heart and its ability to perform that work. Initially, compensatory mechanisms may enable cardiac output and cardiac filling to be maintained, even after venous congestion has become manifest. Usually the first of these compensatory processes is the development of myocardial hypertrophy. Although the contractile activity per unit weight of the hypertrophied muscle is still below normal, the increased mass permits an overall increase in work capacity (Pool and Braunwald, 1968). If this proves insufficient to maintain cardiac function, further compensatory mechanisms are called into play. These include the development of an increased end-diastolic volume with consequent increased stroke volume, according to Starling's Law, and an increased total blood volume through renal retention of salt and water. In addition, cardiac ouptut is enhanced by increased levels of circulating catecholamines. Eventually, however, the compensatory mechanisms cease to be effective and, indeed, come to constitute an added burden on an already overtaxed organ. Myocardial hypertrophy becomes detrimental because of the increased oxygen requirements of the enlarged muscle mass (Bing et al., 1968). The heart becomes dilated beyond the point at which adequate myocar-

dial tension can be generated. Starling's Law then no longer applies and the stroke volume decreases rather than increases. The additional blood volume produces marked congestion, further stressing the heart. Ultimately, cardiac output must fall.

The principal morphologic changes, as well as the signs and symptoms that characterize CHF, are produced by the secondary effects of the failing circulation upon the various organs supplied by the heart. Grossly, the heart shows only hypertrophy and dilatation, along with the changes of the underlying disease.

Usually the two sides of the heart do not begin to fail simultaneously. Although the heart is a single organ, to some extent it acts as two distinct anatomic and functional entities. Under various pathologic stresses, one side — or, rarely, even one chamber — may fail before the other, so that from the clinical standpoint left-sided and right-sided failure may occur separately. However, since the vascular system is a closed circuit, failure of one side cannot exist for long without eventually producing excessive strain upon the other, terminating in total heart failure. Nevertheless, the clearest understanding of the pathologic physiology is derived from considering failure of each side separately.

LEFT-SIDED HEART FAILURE

As will be discussed, left-sided heart failure is most often caused by (1) coronary heart disease, (2) aortic and mitral valvular diseases (rheumatic heart disease, calcific aortic stenosis, congenital heart disease, infective endocarditis and syphilitic heart disease), and (3) hypertension. Except with obstruction at the mitral valve, the left ventricle is usually dilated, sometimes quite massively. With mitral stenosis, the dilatation is confined to the left atrium. The distant effects of left-sided failure are manifested most prominently in the lungs, although function of the kidneys and brain may also be markedly impaired.

Lungs. With the progressive damming of blood within the pulmonary circulation, pressure in the pulmonary veins mounts and is ultimately transmitted to the capillaries. Normally, hydrostatic pressure in the pulmonary capillaries ranges between 6 and 9 mm. Hg. With increases to 25 or 30 mm. Hg, congestion followed by frank edema occurs. The lung is particularly vulnerable to the development of edema because its loose honeycomb structure exerts no significant tissue pressure against the escape of fluids.

At first the transudate is limited to perivascular "cuffing." Later, there is thickening of the alveolar walls as fluid accumulates within them. Finally, the transudate overflows into the alveoli **(pulmonary edema)** (Fig. 10—1). Not infrequently, transudate

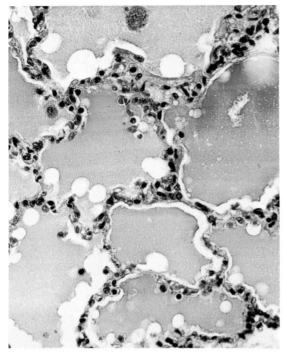

Figure 10–1. The lung in congestive heart failure. The alveolar spaces are filled with a proteinaceous transudate.

accumulates within the pleural space, producing a gross pleural effusion.

The edema appears as an intra-alveolar granular precipitate, with accompanying widening of the alveolar septa. The congestion causes dilatation of the alveolar capillaries. In the more advanced cases, the capillaries may become tortuous, with small aneurysmal outpouchings, and rhexis may produce small hemorrhages into the alveolar spaces. In these cases, the lining epithelial cells become hypertrophied and cuboidal. Such severe changes are most often seen in association with mitral stenosis. As a result of alveolar hemorrhages, hemosiderin laden macrophages, termed "heart failure cells," appear in the alveolar spaces. The chronic persistence of septal edema often induces fibrosis within the alveolar walls. This fibrosis, together with the accumulation of hemosiderin, is designated "brown induration of the lungs." The weight of the lung is increased up to 700 or 800 gm. (normal, 350 to 400 gm.). The most severely affected areas, principally the lower lobes, are soggy and subcrepitant. Sectioning of such lungs permits the free escape of a frothy hemorrhagic fluid. All these changes predispose to secondary bacterial invasion, with resultant bronchopneumonia, which in this setting is often referred to as **hypostatic pneumonia.**

These anatomic changes produce striking clinical manifestations. Dyspnea on exertion is usually the earliest complaint of patients in left-sided heart failure. Later, shortness of breath is present even at rest. The pathogenesis of this dyspnea might simply be ascribed to inadequate oxygenation of the blood flowing through the functionally impaired lungs. However, numerous studies indicate that the probable explanation is much more complex and in all likelihood involves hypoxemia of the respiratory center and carotid sinus, but more importantly encroachment on the vital capacity of the lungs produced by the congestive vascular distention Cyanosis may be present because of the impaired oxygenation of the blood, but it is usually minimal in left-sided failure. A characteristic and therefore highly important symptom of left-sided failure is *paroxysmal nocturnal dyspnea*, the sudden onset of respiratory distress which wakens the patient from sleep. The pathogenesis of this phenomenon is not completely understood, but several factors may be operative. With recumbency, there is decreased venous pressure in the dependent portions of the body, hence gradual resorption of tissue edema. The movement of fluid from the interstitium back into the vascular space produces an augmented blood volume, which in turn is reflected in an increase in pulmonary congestion. Moreover, there is less functional pulmonary reserve in the recumbent position than in the erect posture, because the resting position of the diaphragm is higher, encroaching on the vital capacity of the lungs. It is also possible that during sleep the irritability of the central nervous system is depressed and may permit the accumulation of edema fluid without evoking such normal defense mechanisms as coughing. As failure becomes more advanced, the patient becomes unable to sleep at all in the recumbent position—i.e., he becomes *orthopneic*—and must prop himself up with pillows. Cough is a common accompaniment of left-sided failure and, in severe cases, may raise frothy, blood-tinged sputum.

Kidneys. The hemodynamic derangements occurring with left-sided heart failure may markedly affect the kidneys. Decreased blood flow to the renal arteries, along with venous congestion, leads to sludging within the kidney, with consequent hypoxia and a reduction in arteriolar pulse pressure and glomerular filtration rate. Plasma renin and angiotensin levels are elevated. As the glomerular filtration rate falls, renal retention of salt and water occurs. Increased tubular reabsorption contributes to the sodium retention. Teleologically, this may be looked upon as the response of the kidneys to what they interpret as hypovolemia. Salt and water retention is further enhanced by the augmented secretion of adrenal mineralocorticoids, particularly aldosterone. The elaboration of these steroids may represent a nonspecific stress response, as well as a compensatory response to the diminished perfusion of the kidneys. The consequent increase in total blood volume eventually adds considerably to the load upon the heart and contributes to the generalized edema. With severe disturbances in renal blood flow, impaired excretion of nitrogenous products may cause azotemia, known as *prerenal azotemia* (p. 428).

Brain. Cerebral hypoxia may give rise to many symptoms, such as irritability, loss of attention span and restlessness, which may even progress to stupor and coma. These symptoms, however, are encountered only in far advanced congestive heart failure.

RIGHT-SIDED HEART FAILURE

Right-sided heart failure occurs in relatively pure form in only a few diseases. Usually it is combined with left-sided failure because any increase in pressure in the pulmonary circulation incident to left-sided failure must inevitably produce an increased burden on the right side of the heart. The causes of right-sided failure, then, must include all those which create left heart failure, particularly lesions such as mitral stenosis, which produce great increases in the pulmonary pressure.

Fairly *pure* right-sided failure most often occurs with *cor pulmonale*, i.e., right ventricular strain produced by intrinsic disease of the lungs or pulmonary vasculature. In these cases, the right ventricle is burdened by increased resistance within the pulmonary circuit. Dilatation of the heart is confined to the right ventricle and atrium. Other and less common causes of right-sided heart failure include myocardial infarction of the right ventricle and diffuse myocarditis, which appears to affect the right ventricle more often than the left for reasons to be presented later. Rarely, right-sided failure is caused by tricuspid or pulmonic valvular lesions. Clinically, constrictive pericarditis simulates right-sided failure by the damming of blood back into the systemic venous system, although the right ventricle itself may be normal.

The major morphologic and clinical effects of right-sided failure differ from those of left-sided failure in that pulmonary congestion is minimal whereas engorgement of the systemic and portal systems is more pronounced. It should be remembered, however, that in both instances the twin problems of systemic venous congestion and impaired cardiac output remain qualitatively the same. The major organs affected by right-sided heart failure are the liver, spleen, kidneys, subcutaneous tissues, brain and entire portal area of venous drainage.

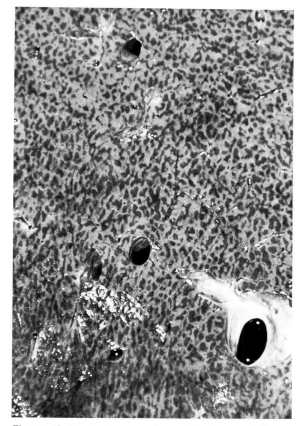

Figure 10–2. A close-up view of the transected surface of the liver with marked chronic passive congestion—the so-called nutmeg pattern.

Liver. The liver is usually slightly increased in size and weight and on sectioning displays a prominent "nutmeg" pattern (Fig. 10–2). This descriptive term refers to congestive red accentuation of the center of the liver lobules surrounded by the paler, sometimes fatty, peripheral regions of the liver lobule. There may be some widening of the space of Disse microscopically, as well as enlargement and congestion of the central veins and central portions of the vascular sinusoids. The liver cells in the central region may become somewhat atrophic as a result of the pressure of the distended vascular sinusoids. Together, these changes are called **chronic passive congestion** of the liver. If the congestive failure is severe and rapidly developing, the passive congestion may lead to rupture of the sinusoids, with actual necrosis of the liver cells, producing **central hemorrhagic necrosis.** If the patient does not die of the usually severe cardiac failure, in time the central areas become fibrotic, creating so-called **cardiac sclerosis,** also known as **cardiac cirrhosis.**

Spleen. Splenic congestion produces a large, heavy organ, which is tense and cyanotic. On section, blood freely exudes and the tissue collapses, so that the capsule becomes wrinkled. Microscopically, there may be marked sinusoidal dilatation, accompanied by areas of recent hemorrhage and possibly deposits of hemosiderin pigment. With long-standing congestion, the enlarged spleen may achieve weights of 500 to 600 gm. (normal, ~150 gm.), and the long-standing edema may produce fibrous thickening of the sinusoidal walls. The areas of previous hemorrhage are now transformed to hemosiderin deposits, to create the firm, meaty organ characteristic of **congestive splenomegaly.**

Kidneys. Congestion and hypoxia of the kidneys are more marked with right-sided heart failure than with left, leading to greater fluid retention and more pronounced prerenal azotemia.

Subcutaneous Tissues. Some degree of peripheral edema of dependent portions of the body occurs regularly. Indeed, ankle edema may be considered a hallmark of CHF. In severe or long-standing cases, edema may be quite massive and generalized, a condition termed *anasarca.* Of probable significance in the perpetuation of edema is the diminished clearing of plasma aldosterone by the congested liver. This contributes to the elevated levels of this hormone (Genest et al., 1968).

Brain. Symptoms essentially identical with those described in left-sided failure may occur, representing venous congestion and hypoxia of the central nervous system.

Portal System of Drainage. Splenic congestion has already been described. In addition, abnormal accumulations of transudate in the peritoneal cavity may give rise to ascites. Congestion of the gut may cause intestinal disturbances.

In summary, right-sided heart failure presents essentially as a venous congestive syndrome, with hepatic and splenic enlargement, peripheral edema and ascites. In contrast to left-sided failure, respiratory symptoms may be absent or quite insignificant. *It is to be emphasized at this point that although the consideration of heart failure has been divided into two functional units, in the usual case of frank chronic cardiac decompensation, these early stages have already passed, and the patient presents with the picture of full-blown CHF, encompassing the clinical syndromes of both right and left heart failure.*

In the remainder of this chapter, the major diseases of the heart will be considered individually, beginning with the most important—CHD. The other heart diseases are divided into four categories, according to their typical clinical presentation. As was previously mentioned, virtually all the important diseases of the heart may lead to CHF. A few diseases, however, characteristically *first* manifest themselves by the development of CHF without prominent accompanying signs or symptoms. These will be discussed under the heading, *"Congestive Heart Failure as a First Manifestation of Cardiac Disease."* Another set of disorders arises from derangements outside the heart, such as hypertension, but secondary CHF ultimately becomes dominant. This group will be presented under the heading, *"Congestive Heart Failure from Extracardiac Disease."* The last two categories are reserved for those lesions which characteristically make themselves known by rather dramatic signs or symptoms before the onset of CHF. One category comprises those diseases presenting with pain (*"Chest Pain as a First Manifestation of Cardiac Disease"*), and the remaining one includes the many entities which are first discovered by the presence of a heart murmur (*"Heart Murmurs as a First Manifestation of Cardiac Disease"*). As with all arbitrary classifications, these four headings do not represent a perfect fit, nor do all instances of a particular disease conform to the prototype. The structure is designed simply to provide a useful tool for remembering the various entities and their clinical correlates.

CORONARY HEART DISEASE (CHD)

The term CHD is the generic designation for three forms of cardiac disease which result from insufficient coronary blood flow: (1) arteriosclerotic heart disease, (2) myocardial infarction, and (3) angina pectoris. In the vast majority of cases, such insufficient blood flow results from atherosclerotic narrowing of the coronary arteries, with or without occlusions. The three patterns represent a continuum, but they are differentiated by the speed of development of the coronary insufficiency, the ultimate severity of the narrowing, including the possibility of superimposed thrombosis, the size of the vessel or vessels most severely affected and the existence and adequacy of intercoronary anastomoses.

The staggering importance of CHD as a cause of death in affluent societies was emphasized at the beginning of this chapter. Nevertheless, despite the ennui almost universally engendered by statistics, a few more are offered here to document the scale of the growing threat from CHD. Until the 1920's CHD was virtually unknown, and its study was certainly not a part of the standard medical curriculum (Editorial, 1974a). By 1937, it had become the sixth leading cause of death in the United States, being responsible for a modest 4.8 per cent of all mortalities. In 1973, as we have seen, CHD was causing a phenomenal 35 per cent of all deaths, reflecting an absolute increase in incidence across all age groups. By contrast, cancer, the second most important cause of death and itself a major scourge, was in that year responsible for only about half as many deaths.

Arteriosclerotic heart disease (ASHD) evolves from slow, progressing narrowing of the coronary arteries occurring over the span of years. The dependent myocardium is slowly deprived of an adequate vascular supply and so undergoes atrophy, with individual fiber necrosis leading to diffuse small areas of scattered fibrosis. Large areas of acute ischemic necrosis are *not* found except insofar as the patient with ASHD may (as he often does) develop an intercurrent myocardial infarct.

Myocardial infarction (MI) is the catastrophic form of CHD and, as its name implies, results from sudden inadequacy of the coronary flow. Until recently, this was thought nearly always to be precipitated by a thrombotic occlusion of a main coronary trunk, superimposed on underlying severe atherosclerosis. However, as we shall see, this and many other cherished beliefs concerning MI have been called into question. Suffice it to say here that the best evidence now indicates that the thrombosis may be the result rather than the cause of infarction (Robbins, 1974; Spain and Breadess, 1970; Erhardt et al., 1973).

Angina pectoris (AP) falls between the two previously described patterns of CHD. It is actually a symptom complex consisting of severe paroxysmal chest pain resulting from transient ischemia that falls precariously short of ischemic necrosis.

Obviously, there is much overlapping among these three patterns, and the patient with ASHD is in danger of attacks of angina or the development of a myocardial infarct. By the same token, attacks of angina carry the ominous threat that the ischemia will at some time be more than transient and thus result in an infarct.

The three patterns of CHD are most likely to be caused by atherosclerosis of the coronary arteries. Infrequently, however, other conditions may cause coronary arterial insufficiency. These include aortic valve disease, cardiac arrhythmias (which seriously impair coronary filling), luetic aortitis (which narrows the orifices of the coronary arteries), profound anemia, shock, thyrotoxicosis, dissecting aneurysms of the coronary arteries and—even more rarely—systemic arterial diseases, such as polyarteritis nodosa involving the coronary arteries. Surprisingly, recent arteriographic studies indicate that about 10 per cent of patients with MI or AP have apparently normal coronary arteries and no obvious cause for their disease (Kahn and Haywood, 1974; Editorial, 1974*b*).

The genesis and prevalence of atherosclerosis are considered on page 266. Here we limit the consideration to how this generalized arterial disease affects the coronary arteries. The coronary arteries are one of the prime points of attack of atherosclerosis. The atheromatous involvement usually affects all three major trunks of the coronary system, frequently but not necessarily in equal measure. It is uncommon to find single coronary artery disease. It is even more rare to find a single atheroma as an occlusive lesion in an otherwise minimally affected artery. The atheromatous lesions are most severe in the first 6 cm. of all three trunks, but they continue to be present to a lesser degree in the more distal extensions. In all forms of CHD, atherosclerotic lesions are often complicated—i.e., fibrotic, calcified, or ulcerated—and they sometimes have superimposed thromboses.

Intercoronary anastomoses, usually less than 40 μm. in diameter, exist in virtually all hearts. With severe coronary atherosclerosis or with chronic hypoxia from any cause these tiny channels enlarge to provide augmented blood flow to the deprived areas of the myocardium. Regrettably, their flow capacity is limited. Moreover, whether they are capable of sufficiently rapid enlargement to compensate for a sudden occlusion is questionable (Bloor, 1974).

It has been pointed out in the discussion of the enigma of atherosclerosis that a number of factors potentiate or accelerate its development. Since CHD is usually the result of atherosclerosis, the risk factors are the same. The most important of these are: elevated blood pressure, elevated serum lipoproteins, cigarette smoking and elevated serum glucose (Kannel, 1974). Reference should be made to page 267 for a discussion of the risk factors. In addition, individuals exhibiting what has become known as the Type A behavior pattern—characterized by competitiveness, perfectionism and feelings of struggle against the limitations of time and the insensitivity of the environment (traits which surely characterize readers of this text)—are about twice as vulnerable to CHD as are their more relaxed peers (Jenkins et al., 1974). Physical activity may confer some protection (Paffenbarger and Hale, 1975). *Against this background we can now turn to more complete descriptions of the three forms of CHD.*

ARTERIOSCLEROTIC HEART DISEASE (ASHD)

Since atherosclerosis with its slow, patchy narrowing of the coronary arteries is an almost invariable accompaniment of advancing years, ASHD is by far the most common clinical as well as anatomic type of cardiac disease. However, it is less lethal than MI, and so accounts for fewer than half of all deaths from CHD. Some clinicians have used the term *senile heart disease (presbycardia)* to imply that the reduction in heart size with clinical manifestations of cardiac decompensation that is encountered so frequently in the very old is merely part of the aging process. However, at autopsy these individuals are almost invariably found to have some atherosclerosis of the coronary arteries with accompanying myocardial and valvular fibrosis, and it is unlikely that cardiac decompensation occurs solely as a result of "senile" changes.

A word of caution is in order. Because of its frequency, there is a tendency to diagnose ASHD in all instances of congestive heart failure in older individuals. This tendency should be resisted, since other causes of CHF may be found in the later decades of life. It should also be pointed out that the mere anatomic presence of minor degrees of coronary atherosclerosis does not warrant the diagnosis of ASHD. In the affluent countries even individuals 20 years old have minimal atherosclerotic lesions; heart disease does not exist until the arterial narrowing damages the myocardium or valves or both. Only when narrowing becomes extreme, usually occluding more than 70 per cent of the lumen of a major vessel, are the myocardium or valves affected.

Morphology. The pathognomonic anatomic criteria of this entity are atherosclerotic involvement of the coronary arteries and diffuse myocardial fibrosis. Left-sided valvular changes are frequent but not invariable. The heart is usually smaller than normal, but it may be of usual size. The coronary atherosclerosis is usually diffuse, producing narrowing of all three major trunks of the coronary arteries. Total occlusion is uncommon in the absence of myocardial infarction, but may be present. When total occlusion without infarction does occur it is presumed that collateral circulation has become sufficiently well developed to supply the ischemic areas. Calcification may convert the arteries into rigid pipestem structures. With severe ASHD, there is grossly apparent fibrotic streaking of the transected myocardium. Sometimes the regions of preserved thinned myocardium appear unusually brown **(brown atrophy)**. When there is involvement of the mitral valve, it takes the form of calcification of the mitral annulus. In advanced cases, calcific nodular masses encircle the mitral leaflets at their base. Calcification affects the aortic valve in a somewhat different pattern. Here, rounded nodular calcific masses accumulate within the sinuses of Valsalva and between the cusps of the aortic valve, obliterating the commissures and rendering the valve stenotic. This form of aortic stenosis, also called **Mönckeberg's aortic stenosis**, may resemble the healed calcified stage of rheumatic valvulitis or congenital aortic stenosis, and the distinction cannot always be made with certainty.

The microscopic features of ASHD are minimal, consisting only of patchy scarring of the myocardium. Although individual muscle fibers may be separated by fibrotic tissue, usually the scarring occurs principally around vessels and in the preexisting fibrous septa (Fig. 10–3). The myofibers may be smaller than normal and contain lipofuscin pigment, creating the grossly visible brown atrophy of the heart. The valvular changes comprise collagenous fibrous thickening enclosing the basophilic deposits of calcium.

Clinical Course. Arteriosclerotic heart disease tends to progress slowly over the course of many years, manifesting itself only during periods of stress, such as with intercurrent infections. Usually it remains largely asymptomatic, and frequently it is discovered only as an incidental finding at autopsy. Eventually, however, if the patient does not succumb from other causes, sustained CHF develops. When scarring involves the cardiac conduction system, various arrhythmias may occur. Concomitant angina pectoris is common. Often, death results from a supervening MI or from a cardiac arrhythmia.

Congestive heart failure caused by ASHD is most often initially left-sided, due to the rela-

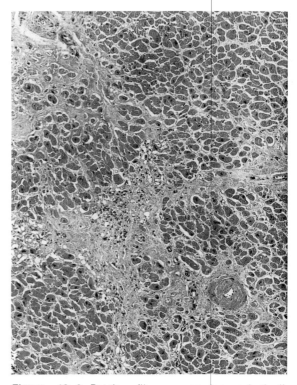

Figure 10–3. Patchy fibrous scarring principally about blood vessels of the myocardium in arteriosclerotic heart disease.

tively greater demands on the left ventricle. Moreover, the thinner right ventricle appears to be less vulnerable to coronary arterial narrowing. Perhaps the transmural thebesian system is sufficient to sustain at least partially the thinner muscle mass. Right-sided CHF, however, ultimately follows chronic left-sided failure. Decompensation may develop insidiously or more or less acutely following a precipitating episode, such as pneumonia. At one time, the prognosis after the onset of right-sided decompensation was poor, with survival time of only one to two years. However, with effective therapy, including sodium restriction and the administration of diuretics and digitalis glycosides, patients may survive comfortably for many years. The outlook is relatively better, of course, if there is a precipitating factor which can be modified.

MYOCARDIAL INFARCTION (MI)

Ischemic necrosis of the myocardium, or myocardial infarction, is the most dramatic and lethal clinical pattern of CHD. It causes over half of all deaths from CHD and therefore represents the single most frequent cause of death in the United States and other affluent countries. In about 90 per cent of cases there is severe and widespread atherosclerotic involvement of the coronary arteries, and this is presumably the basic lesion. Complete occlusion of one of these compromised vessels by a thrombosis may be the precipitating event in some cases, but cannot be documented in many. Nevertheless, there is almost certainly some sudden event which unfavorably alters the balance between the metabolic demands of the myocardium and the capacity of the coronary arteries to satisfy those demands. Possibly as a consequence of such imbalance, electrical instability of the heart may in many cases play an early role in the development of an MI.

Unlike ASHD, MI shows a definite male preponderance, about 3:1 overall. This vulnerability of males is most striking in the younger age groups, with a male-female ratio of about 6:1 between the ages of 33 and 55 years. Women during reproductive life are remarkably resistant. Thereafter, the ratio steadily diminishes and approaches 1:1 in extreme old age. The peak incidence in males is reached in the sixth decade, after which it plateaus. The peak in females is not reached until the eighth decade.

Etiology and Pathogenesis. The search for the causation of any disease can be an arduous process. It is particularly discouraging when a long-accepted theory (or dogma) is found wanting, and the search must begin virtually anew. To some extent this is the situation with MI. For many years the conventional wisdom was that an MI is a sudden definitive event caused by total occlusion of a major coronary artery, usually by a thrombus superimposed on a complicated atheromatous plaque. Over the years, however, repeated analyses have failed to demonstrate occlusive coronary thrombosis in a significant percentage (20 to 50 per cent) of patients dying from an MI (Robbins, 1974). Recently, it has been shown that the frequency of thrombosis increases with the duration of survival. Thus, in one series, thrombosis was found in only 16 per cent of those who died less than one hour after the onset of an MI. In contrast, among those who survived for more than 24 hours, thrombosis was found in 54 per cent (Spain and Bradess, 1970). These figures would suggest that the formation of a thrombus can be *secondary* to the MI and not causative. Such a concept is supported by the finding in six of seven patients that ^{125}I-labeled fibrinogen given *after* the clinical onset of MI was subsequently found within coronary thrombi. The radioactive fibrinogen was evenly dispersed throughout the thrombi and not limited to the periphery. This distribution argues against the possibility that it was simply incorporated into preexisting thrombi (Erhardt, 1973). Even though thrombosis may not be the initiating event in most cases of MI, it remains true that the coronary arteries of MI victims are the site of severe chronic atherosclerosis in about 90 to 95 per cent of cases. What, then, triggers the acute episode? And what of the 5 to 10 per cent who do not show unusually severe coronary atherosclerosis?

In order to find the answers to these and other questions, much attention is now being given to patients who die very suddenly, before reaching a hospital—presumably from an MI. As we shall see, this is a highly important group of patients, not only because of what we can learn from them, but also because of their sheer numbers. It has only recently been appreciated that *sudden cardiac death (SCD)* occurs in about 25 per cent of patients with CHD and accounts for well over half the mortality (Turner and Ball, 1973; Rapaport, 1974). Autopsy studies on these patients do confirm the presence of severe and longstanding multivessel coronary atherosclerosis in the vast majority (Baroldi, 1969). However, in one recent study, *acute* lesions of the coronary arteries were found in only 58 per cent. These most often took the form of a ruptured atheromatous plaque, sometimes with superimposed thrombosis. Thrombosis alone was found less often (Liberthson et al., 1974). This leaves 42 per cent with only old atheromatous lesions, hence with no apparent acute event as a cause for SCD. We shall return to our consideration of the coronary arteries later.

What of the heart muscle itself in SCD? It is to be expected that histologic evidence of infarction would be lacking, since changes visible with the light microscope require at least four hours' survival to develop. However, sophisticated histochemical and biochemical studies do show evidence of early myocardial ischemia in about 80 per cent of patients with SCD (Lie et al., 1971; Zugibe et al., 1966). Moreover, there are a number of patients with SCD who are successfully resuscitated by rescue teams—reversed SCD, if you will. After resuscitation it might be expected that these patients would go on to show the electrocardiographic (ECG) changes of a fresh MI. Curiously, a study of 80 such resuscitated patients revealed ECG changes consistent with an acute MI or with ischemia without actual infarction in only 65 (81 per cent) of these patients. *No new ECG changes were seen in 15 (19 per cent)* (Liberthson et al., 1974). These figures are consistent with the 80 per cent incidence of ischemia or infarction found by histochemical and biochemical studies, cited above. To summarize, it would appear that an acute lesion in the coronary arteries is present in about 58 per cent of these patients, and acute ischemia or infarction of the heart muscle occurs in about 80 per cent. In a minority of cases, then, it would seem that SCD occurs not only without apparent cause, but also without apparent damage other than death! In this regard, it is of interest that about 20 per cent of patients with SCD were found by histologic studies to have an older MI—between one day and several weeks old. Perhaps in these cases the SCD was a complication of the earlier "silent" MI. Since SCD does not always imply an acute occlusive event in a coronary artery with a consequent MI, what *is* its immediate cause? *The only constant finding in SCD is cardiac arrhythmia;* when there was time for ECG monitoring arrhythmias were found in all such patients (Liberthson et al., 1974).

What of the more typical MI's, those which do not involve SCD? Can we assume that these are caused by essentially the same factors that cause SCD, but with a happier outcome? The answer is probably yes. Certainly transient arrhythmias are an almost invariable finding in these cases, too; they simply happen not to be immediately lethal. As mentioned earlier, the coronary arteries are severely atheromatous in about 90 to 95 per cent of patients with an MI (leaving 5 to 10 per cent with normal or near normal coronary arteries). The frequency of thrombosis rises with the duration of survival. Although ECG and serum enzyme determinations (to be described) indicate the presence of infarction by

definition, infarction is not the clear-cut event it was once thought to be. The majority of MI patients experience prodromal symptoms—fatigue, increasing angina or overt CHF—for a period of days to weeks before the acute episode. Nor is the extent of tissue necrosis suddenly and irrevocably determined at the time of the clinical onset. Rather, it becomes defined over the following several days (Braunwald, 1974; Editorial, 1974c; Maroko, 1974). The evidence for this is derived from serial determinations of enzymes released into the serum from the damaged myocardium *(CPK disappearance curve)*, and from serial measurements of the ECG S–T segment elevation at various points on the precordium *(S–T segment mapping)*. Both of these parameters indicate the size and pattern of tissue necrosis. Most studies indicate that the initial damage is patchy and consists of an irregular area of irreversibly injured tissue containing islands of more or less viable tissue. Over the next several days the local balance of oxygen supply and demand probably determines whether these islands succumb and whether the margins of the infarct are extended. Consistent with this patchy evolution was the finding that 12 of 14 patients with a transmural anterior MI underwent an apparent extension of their infarction an average of six days after the initial event (Reid et al., 1974). Moreover, as we shall see later, there is evidence that intervening to alter the balance between oxygen supply and demand can actually limit the extension of an MI.

What are we to make of all the findings and surmises we have presented up to this point? This question can be considered in two parts. First, what causes the initial clinical episode we recognize as an MI? And second, what is the correlation between it and actual ischemic necrosis of the myocardium? Perhaps the most reasonable conclusion is that *there are many causes of an MI.* These certainly include the orthodox one—that is, total occlusion of a coronary artery by a thrombus. Occlusion may also be produced by rupture of an atheromatous plaque or by hemorrhage into it. The possibility of small platelet aggregates involving multiple smaller coronary vessels is now receiving considerable attention (Wu and Hoak, 1974). But what of the cases in which there is no demonstrable occlusion? Conceivably these may involve localized spasm of a coronary artery or the formation of a thrombus followed by very rapid recanalization (MacAlpin, 1974; Khan and Haywood, 1974). It is also to be emphasized that in patients with severely atheromatous coronary arteries, any sudden increase in myocardial demands, such as that produced by physical or emotional stress, may lead to an MI. Any of these pathways leads not only to ischemia of the myocardium, but also to a local accumulation of lactic acid, with a drop in pH. Even without actual necrosis of the myocardium, these metabolic derangements could produce functional disturbances, such as an arrhythmia or even complete cessation of contraction. Such functional disturbances would then augment the ischemia by diminishing coronary artery filling. It is of interest that reduced coronary flow would then predispose to thrombosis. Such a sequence of events might explain the observation, cited earlier, that the frequency of thrombosis is apparently correlated with the duration of survival after an MI. Obviously, many questions concerning the development of an MI remain unanswered. About all that can be said with any degree of certainty is that whereas a coronary thrombosis may be sufficient to produce an MI, it apparently is not always necessary; in short, the causation of an MI is a good deal more complicated than we once believed.

Morphology. When an MI is associated with acute occlusion of a main coronary artery, the occlusion is usually found within the first 6 cm. of the vessel. The arteries involved and the resultant areas of infarction are as follows:

Right coronary artery	(40 per cent)	Posterior wall of left ventricle; posterior part of interventricular septum
Left anterior descending coronary artery	(40 per cent)	Anterior wall of left ventricle; anterior part of interventricular septum
Left circumflex coronary artery	(20 per cent)	Lateral wall of left ventricle

The right ventricle and the atria are also affected in about 5 per cent of left ventricular infarcts. Presumably, the vulnerability of the left ventricle reflects the greater demands of its thicker wall and heavier work load.

Most myocardial infarcts extend throughout the thickness of the myocardium to involve the contiguous epicardium and endocardium. Small infarcts, however, may be confined to the central muscle mass. Those localized to the subendocardial zone are termed **Zahn's infarcts.** All usually have an irregular perimeter, dictated by the pattern of the interdigitating vascular supply.

Both the gross and microscopic changes are entirely analogous to those of ischemic or coagulative necrosis occurring anywhere in the body. The first

indication of damage to be apparent by gross examination is a slight pallor appearing from 18 to 24 hours after the occlusion. Between the second and fourth days, the necrotic focus becomes more sharply defined, with a hyperemic border, and the central portion becomes yellow-brown and soft as a result of beginning fatty change. By the tenth day, fatty change is well developed and the infarct is quite yellow and maximally soft, often containing areas of hemorrhage. At about the tenth day, an ingrowth of vascularized, fibrotic scar tissue becomes apparent at the margin of the infarct (Fig. 10–4). Replacement of necrotic muscle continues toward the center of the lesion and is usually complete by the seventh week.

A fibrinous or serofibrinous pericarditis develops in about 11 per cent of patients between the second and fourth day (Niarchos and McKendrick, 1973). This may be localized to the region overlying the necrotic area, or it may be generalized, in which case it is speculated to be of autoimmune origin. With healing of the infarct, the pericarditis usually resolves, but occasionally it organizes to produce permanent fibrous adhesions. Involvement of the ventricular endocardium often results in

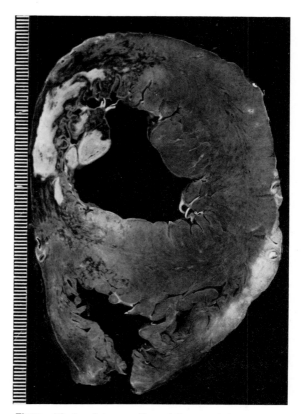

Figure 10–4. A transection of the ventricles to expose the 10- to 14-day-old myocardial infarct seen on the left. The pale, sharply demarcated fatty areas are surrounded by a darker rim of vascularized, fibrous, early repair.

mural thrombosis, as well as in dense fibrous thickening.

Because so many deaths from MI occur shortly after the onset, the search for very early histologic changes has assumed great importance. Traditionally, it has been held that diagnostic changes cannot be appreciated with the light microscope for at least four hours. At about this time, coagulation of the myocardial fibers gradually becomes apparent, usually accompanied by some interstitial edema, fresh hemorrhage and scant marginal neutrophilic exudation. However, it has recently been suggested that other, more subtle histologic changes may be seen much earlier, perhaps within an hour after the onset of ischemia (Bouchardy and Majno, 1974). These changes consist of a **stretching and waviness of the myocardial fibers at the border of the ischemic area.** It is thought that the ischemic area ceases to function within a minute of its oxygen deprivation. With each systole, then, there is a forceful tug on this inert area, which stretches and buckles the fibers nearest the periphery. Those fibers at the center of the ischemic area are less affected since here the pull comes equally from all directions. The wavy fibers show elongation of their nuclei, and soon thereafter there is increased eosinophilia of their cytoplasm. Between the area of waviness and the normal tissue, **contraction bands** may become prominent. These are bands of deep eosinophilia spanning the width of a myocardial fiber. They are thought to represent fusion of several adjacent sarcomeres as a result of spasm of the myocardial fiber. It is not known whether these very early histologic changes are irreversible. With the appearance of coagulative necrosis, however, the injury is clearly irreversible. Over the subsequent days, the nuclei of the myocardial cells become pyknotic and the cytoplasm shrinks, loses its striations and becomes filled with finely dispersed fat droplets. The growing neutrophilic infiltrate becomes admixed with mononuclear leukocytes, and the cellular debris is removed by phagocytosis (Fig. 10–5). Previous hemorrhage may be reflected by deposits of hemosiderin pigment. Fibrous replacement is fairly complete by six weeks, although the scar tissue is still highly vascular and will require months to become collagenous.

Cell death, of course, occurs long before the classical changes of coagulative necrosis become apparent. Even before cell death occurs there are profound metabolic and functional derangements. These very early events may be discernible by electron microscopy and histochemical studies, but these methods of investigation are possible only on properly preserved or very fresh tissue. They have, however, given us much information about the very early course of an MI. The precise duration of ischemia required to produce irreversible damage is unknown. Experimental studies in dogs indicate that the changes produced by ligature of

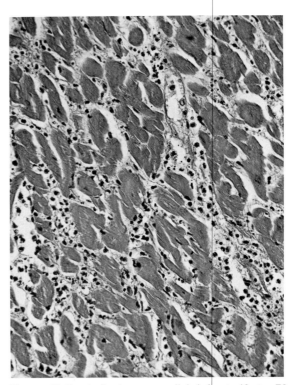

Figure 10–5. A fresh myocardial infarct 48 to 72 hours old. All the fibers have undergone coagulative necrosis, nuclei have disappeared and there is an interstitial inflammatory reaction with edema and neutrophil infiltration.

a coronary artery for 20 minutes are reversible. After 40 minutes of ligature, however, about half the cells in the affected area are irreversibly injured (Kloner et al., 1974.) Interestingly, the ischemic area ceases to contract within only a minute of ligature, indicating the rapid development of a severe, albeit reversible, metabolic disturbance. These time intervals are somewhat different in other experimental animals, so extrapolation to humans should be made with caution. Nonetheless, in humans, as in experimental animals, electron microscopic and histochemical changes are appreciable within minutes to an hour. The earliest and most obvious electron microscopic changes involve the mitochondria. These become swollen, the cristae are distorted and even fragmented and dense granules appear within the matrix. In addition, there is slight swelling of the entire cell, a depletion of glycogen and relaxation of the myofibrils, with the appearance of prominent I bands. Vacuoles may form within the cytoplasm, sometimes appearing as blebs under the sarcolemmal membrane. Clumping of chromatin at the periphery of the nuclei becomes evident. At about the same time, histochemical studies show a marked loss of intracellular enzyme activity. The most sensitive indices are the reductions in glutaminase I and in beta-hydroxybutyrate dehydrogenase (Morales

TABLE 10–1. SEQUENCE OF CHANGES IN MYOCARDIAL INFARCTION

TIME	ELECTRON MICROSCOPE	HISTOCHEMISTRY	LIGHT MICROSCOPE	GROSS CHANGES
0–2 hours	Mitochondrial swelling and granules; distortion of cristae	↓ Glutaminase I and β-hydroxybutyrate dehydrogenase; ↓ K and ↑ Na⁺ and Ca⁺⁺	?Waviness of fibers at border	
4–12 hours	Relaxation of myofibrils (prominent I-bands); aggregation and margination of nuclear chromatin		Beginning coagulation; edema; hemorrhage; marginal neutrophils	
18–24 hours			Continuing coagulation (pyknosis of nuclei; shrunken eosinophilic cytoplasm)	Pallor
24–48 hours			Total coagulative necrosis with loss of nuclei and striations; heavy interstitial infiltrate of neutrophils and mononuclear leukocytes	Pallor, sometimes hyperemia
2–4 days			Beginning fatty change	Hyperemic border; central yellow-brown softening; pericarditis (11 per cent)
10 days			Well developed fatty changes	Maximally yellow and soft; beginning scarring at margins
7th week				Scarring complete

and Fine, 1966). Other dehydrogenases are subsequently depleted, including malate, lactate and succinate. The increased permeability of the membranes leads to a rapid efflux of potassium, as well as an influx of sodium and calcium. The calcium accumulates principally in the mitochondria, where it appears within the dense granules mentioned earlier. The enzymes which leak out of the damaged myocardial cells escape into the serum, providing important diagnostic tests, as we shall see later.

Table 10–1 summarizes the morphologic changes of an MI as determined by gross examination, by light microscopy and, in the very early stages, by electron microscopy and histochemistry.

Clinical Course. The onset of an MI is usually sudden and devastating, with intense, crushing substernal or precordial pain, often radiating to the left shoulder, arm or jaw. The pain is frequently accompanied by diaphoresis, some degree of breathlessness and marked anxiety. There may be nausea and vomiting. As mentioned, this calamitous event is usually preceded by a period of days to weeks of prodromal symptoms. The most common of these symptoms is undue fatigue ("low-output syndrome"), but there may also be a change in the pattern of preexisting angina pectoris, or there may be the onset of dyspnea.

Occasionally, the clinical manifestations of an acute MI are trivial and passed off by the patient as "indigestion." The onset may also be entirely asymptomatic. In these cases, it may be discovered only much later by a routine ECG. It is difficult to ascertain how often an asymptomatic MI occurs, but the autopsy data on patients with SCD would indicate that they are more frequent than formerly appreciated.

After the onset of an MI, one of several pathways may be followed. About 20 to 25 per cent of patients die before reaching the hospital (Turner and Ball, 1973). Among the remaining patients, the course of an MI may be uneventful, with gradual subsidence of symptoms and progressive healing, or it may be dominated by one or both of two types of sequelae: electrical derangements or pump failure. Disturbances in rate, rhythm or conduction occur so commonly that they are virtually an inherent part of the process. Such arrhythmias have been reported in up to 90 per cent of carefully monitored patients (Lown et al., 1969). They are most common at the very outset, and are almost always responsible for the early deaths. The most frequent arrhythmias are ventricular and atrial extrasystoles, sinus tachycardia and sinus bradycardia. The most lethal are complete heart block, ventricular fibrillation and sinus tachycardia

(Jewitt et al., 1969). Because these disturbances are often reversible, reflecting sudden metabolic changes or only transient inflammatory involvement of portions of the conduction system, the deaths they cause are largely preventable and thus are particularly to be lamented (Stannard and Sloman, 1969).

With or without arrhythmias, the clinical picture may be dominated by the onset of pump failure, manifested as CHF. *Some* degree of left ventricular failure is an almost invariable accompaniment of an MI. Even when there are no clinical manifestations, careful studies demonstrate pulmonary vascular congestion and transudation into the interstitial space (Hales and Kazemi, 1974). In over 60 per cent of patients, CHF is clinically apparent, but this may be very transient (Lown et al., 1969). In some patients, however, overt *pulmonary edema* develops and this considerably worsens the prognosis.

Acute failure of the left ventricle implies not only pulmonary congestion, but a diminished cardiac output as well. Commonly there is some drop in blood pressure. This, too, is often of little consequence. However, when over 40 per cent of the left ventricle is infarcted, a profound drop in cardiac output results, constituting *cardiogenic shock* (Page et al., 1971). This occurs in about 12 per cent of patients. The onset of cardiogenic shock is of particularly grave import since 80 per cent of patients who develop it do not survive. When pulmonary edema and cardiogenic shock occur concomitantly, as occasionally they do, they constitute even more difficult therapeutic problems and the outlook for the patient is bleak indeed.

Among the more typical patients who are followed from the inception of pain, the diagnosis is confirmed by the following findings: (1) elevation of serum levels of myocardial enzymes, including creatine phosphokinase (CPK) within 4 to 8 hours, glutamic oxaloacetic transaminase (SGOT) within 12 to 24 hours and lactic dehydrogenase (LDH) within 24 to 72 hours; (2) nonspecific inflammatory responses, such as leukocytosis, elevated C-reactive protein levels and an increased erythrocyte sedimentation rate (ESR), all within 24 hours; and (3) specific serial electrocardiographic changes, characterized first by elevation of the S–T segment, within 24 hours, followed by the development of abnormal Q-waves and inversion of the T-waves.

The later complications of myocardial infarction include: (1) Rupture of the infarcted portion of the heart, which occurs most often in the week following infarction, when the ischemic focus is maximally soft. When the rupture communicates with the pericardial sac, tamponade and death follow at once. Rarely, rupture of the interventricular septum produces a left-to-right shunt and severe strain on the right heart. (2) Rupture of a papillary muscle, leading to severe mitral regurgitation with a loud murmur. (3) The development of a ventricular aneurysm at the point of scarring. (4) Various thromboembolic phenomena, which may arise from mural thrombi within the heart or from thrombosis in the deep veins of the legs, which develops during prolonged bed rest.

As mentioned, about 20 to 25 per cent of patients with an MI die before reaching the hospital (SCD). Of those who reach the hospital alive, about 15 per cent succumb during the first month, giving a total one-month mortality of 30 to 40 per cent (Lie et al., 1975; Thygesen et al., 1974). The risk of death is greatest at the onset, and declines rapidly with each minute. The current use of electronic monitoring and intensive coronary care has measurably improved the survival rates of those who reach a hospital. An important challenge for the future is to control the electrical failures that contribute so heavily to deaths within the first hour or two. Moreover, the possibility that intervening to alter the balance between oxygen supply and demand can actually limit the size of an MI offers another challenge. This is of great practical importance, since the smaller the infarct, the better the prognosis (Braunwald, 1974). In experimental animals good results have been obtained by a variety of measures. These include the administration of agents to block beta-adrenergic receptors in the heart in order to prevent stimulation by endogenous catecholamines; the administration of vasodilators in order to lower the outflow impedence against which the heart works; and the administration of oxygen itself (Braunwald, 1974; Maroko, 1974). Recently similar interventions in humans have yielded promising results (Mueller et al., 1974; Shell and Sobel, 1974).

The prognosis is better for patients experiencing their first MI than it is for those who have had one or more prior episodes (Lie et al., 1975). Males and females have an equal chance for survival (Badger et al., 1968).

Among those who survive for a month, the mortality remains about 5 per cent per year for the next 5 years, then gradually diminishes toward control rates. The major cause of these late fatalities is sudden death, possibly from a new MI with a lethal arrhythmia. Next most important is CHF resulting from the residual effects of the MI. Figure 10–6 summarizes the clinical course of patients with an MI.

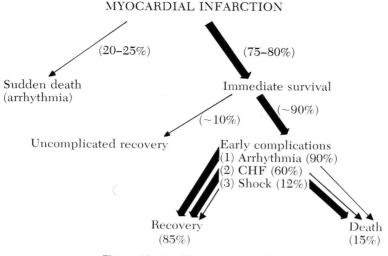

Figure 10–6. Clinical course of MI.

ANGINA PECTORIS (AP)

Angina pectoris is a clinical syndrome characterized by paroxysmal chest pain, which can be precipitated by effort and alleviated by rest. Occasionally, as will be cited later, other specific factors trigger attacks of angina. By definition there are no acute irreversible changes. The pain is usually substernal or precordial, often radiating to the left shoulder and arm or to the jaw. The electrocardiogram may either remain normal or be transiently abnormal. These attacks are thought to be caused by a sudden imbalance between myocardial demands and the capacity of the coronary arteries to fulfill those demands. Thus, angina pectoris constitutes one of the three patterns of CHD.

The underlying condition usually responsible for such a limited coronary reserve is atherosclerosis of the coronary arteries. However, other conditions predispose to angina pectoris, particularly those which in some way diminish diastolic filling of the coronary arteries. In about 10 per cent of patients with AP, arteriographic studies fail to show any abnormality of the coronary arteries (Editorial, 1974b). The daily circumstances which precipitate a paroxysm of pain are usually those which acutely increase the demands of the myocardium, transiently outstripping its vascular reserve. Exertion is the most important of these circumstances. The story of the elderly man who suddenly experiences chest pain while running to catch a train is an old

one. Emotion, pain, cold weather, cigarette smoking, heavy meals and hypoglycemia have all been recognized as precipitating factors.

On occasion, patients have developed attacks of AP while at rest or in situations not clearly associated with increased myocardial demands. Two mechanisms are postulated as causes for the paroxysm of pain in these cases: (1) spasm of the coronary arteries, and (2) occlusion of small branches, rapidly compensated by collateral anastomotic flow, and resulting in only temporary ischemia. At the outset, it should be made clear that the two mechanisms are not mutually exclusive, and both may in fact be operative, either within the same individual or in different individuals. Segmental spasms of the coronary arteries have indeed been seen during angiographic x-ray studies. At times these spasms have evoked characteristic anginal pain, but surprisingly at other times they have gone unnoticed by the patient. It is reasonable to speculate that the severity of the spasm, the underlying adequacy of the coronary flow, and the prior existence of enlarged collateral anastomotic channels may determine whether the vasospasm induces anginal pain or not. The second postulated mechanism—i.e., multiple occlusions of small branches—arises as a result of studies by Blumgart and his colleagues (1941). In a series of postmortem examinations on patients with angina pectoris, multiple small arterial occlusions were almost invariably found. It was, of course, not possible to relate the occlusions directly to the attacks of pain, and indeed small vessel occlusions are a frequent finding in advanced coronary artery atherosclerosis. Both views await substantiation. There is an important distinction between the two explanations. Vasospasm theoretically is reversible. Small vessel occlusions, on the other hand, are likely to be irreversible, and imply that with each anginal attack the coronary flow to the heart is progressively limited. The syndrome of angina pectoris in these cases is important not only for the discomfort it creates, but also because it identifies patients who have an increased risk of subsequent myocardial infarction or sudden death.

CONGESTIVE HEART FAILURE AS A FIRST MANIFESTATION OF CARDIAC DISEASE

Congestive heart failure is characteristically the first indication of the following three disorders of the heart: (1) *arteriosclerotic (or atherosclerotic) heart disease (ASHD)*, (2) a large group of myocardial diseases known collectively as the *cardiomyopathies*, and (3) *endocardial fibroelastosis*. The onset of CHF may be fulminant or, more often, insidious. Although ASHD frequently produces a soft systolic murmur in the aortic area before the onset of CHF, this is a common finding with advancing age, and does not necessarily connote significant disease. Late in the course of all three entities, when CHF is well advanced, dilatation of the heart widens the mitral and sometimes the tricuspid valves, producing murmurs of regurgitation. *Nevertheless, loud heart murmurs are characteristically absent in the early stages of these three entities.* ASHD has already been discussed (p. 293). The other disorders will be presented in this section.

CARDIOMYOPATHIES

This term refers to any dysfunction of the myocardium not attributable to CHD, valvular disease, hypertension, or pulmonary heart disease. Such an umbrella term covers a multitude of diverse entities which have in common the myocardium as the sole or at least the major target of injury. Whereas the reported incidence of the cardiomyopathies is low relative to other heart disease, there is a widespread belief that large numbers of cases escape diagnosis. Such underdiagnosis probably results in large part from the common tendency to ascribe all heart disease in older patients to CHD. In addition, the cardiomyopathies are often either subclinical or secondary to and overshadowed by disease elsewhere in the body.

It should not be surprising (even if alarming) that attempts to arrive at a classification of these diverse entities have yielded mixed, often conflicting results. Perhaps the most meaningful and widely accepted classification divides the primary myocardial disorders into those which are inflammatory and those which are not. Accordingly, *myocarditis* (inflammatory cardiomyopathy), characterized principally by a prominent inflammatory reaction, is regarded separately from the other cardiomyopathies *(degenerative cardiomyopathies)*, which are characterized by myofiber degeneration and fibrosis, with surprisingly little inflammatory reaction. In addition to the histologic distinction, this classification offers the further advantage of being clinically applicable. Thus, myocarditis is usually an acute process of either infectious or immune etiology. In contrast, the degenerative cardiomyopathies (often referred to simply as cardiomyopathies) tend to pursue an insidious chronic course and are most often idiopathic. There is a very great deal of overlapping, however, and in any given case the categorization may be uncertain. Moreover, there is much speculation that the degenerative cardiomyopathies in many cases simply represent the residua of subclinical cases of myocarditis.

A second system of classification of the cardiomyopathies is based on pathophysiology. According to this system, the abnormalities are of three types: (1) *congestive*, (2) *hypertrophic*, or (3) *obliterative* (Robbins, 1974.) The congestive pattern is probably the most common, and is characterized by simple biventricular dilatation of the heart. The hypertrophic pattern is less clear-cut. It includes those cases involving an increase in the thickness of the free wall of the left ventricle, as well as a largely familial form characterized by asymmetric hypertrophy of the ventricular septum. This latter condition results in obstruction of the outflow tract, presumably by the hypertrophied muscle mass. More will be said about this condition later. Least common of the three pathophysiologic patterns is the obliterative form. This is characterized by encroachment on the ventricular cavity by scarring, with a consequent reduction in filling capacity. The prototype of this pattern is *endomyocardial fibrosis*, a disease peculiar to certain parts of Africa, where it affects principally children and young adults. Although the cause is unknown, it is thought by some to be related to nutritional deficiencies.

We shall now discuss myocarditis separately from the other cardiomyopathies, and refer in both discussions to the pathophysiologic pattern where appropriate.

MYOCARDITIS

The incidence of myocarditis in clinical and postmortem studies depends considerably on the diagnostic criteria used. Wenger (1968) has reported it to be present in from 4 per cent to 10 per cent of routine necropsies. The general experience would favor the lower end of this range in incidence. It is most often a relatively unimportant accompaniment of a systemic disease and in this case is known as *secondary myocarditis.* In other instances, when the heart is solely or predominantly involved, the disease is referred to as *primary myocarditis.* Of the primary myocarditides, some have known causes, whereas others are idiopathic.

Secondary myocarditis has been described in connection with a wide variety of systemic diseases and almost every known bacterial, viral, rickettsial, fungal and parasitic infection. Usually it is a transient and minor part of the systemic process, and often it is altogether asymptomatic and detected only by serial ECG's. When symptoms do occur, they may take the form of "postinfectious asthenia"—that is, fatigue and malaise during convalescence from an infectious disease. With more severe myocardial involvement, there may be symptoms referable to the heart. By far the most important of the causative systemic diseases is *rheumatic fever,* which will be discussed later in this chapter. Less frequently, other *"connective tissue disorders,"* such as SLE, systemic sclerosis and polymyositis–dermatomyositis, are associated with myocarditis. Secondary myocarditis may also be caused by *bacterial diseases,* such as typhoid fever, diphtheria and scarlet fever, and by *viral infections,* especially with the Coxsackie and ECHO viruses, as well as the viruses causing influenza, polio, mumps, measles and mononucleosis. *Parasitic infections* may also affect the myocardium. Important among these are Chagas' disease, toxoplasmosis and trichinosis. Some of the agents cause damage to the myocardium through direct invasion, others through the elaboration of a toxin, and still others through hypersensitivity mechanisms. In many cases, particularly those involving some of the viruses, the pathogenetic mechanism is unknown (Wenger, 1968; Friedberg, 1966).

Primary myocarditis may be caused by many agents, including some of the same ones associated with secondary myocarditis. Principal among them are the Coxsackie viruses, *Toxoplasma gondii* and *Trypanosoma cruzi* (the protozoan causing Chagas' disease). Primary myocarditis may also be caused by some of the ECHO and influenza viruses.

With improvement in virologic techniques the Coxsackie viruses, Group B, Types 1 to 5, have only recently been recognized as the single most important cause of primary myocarditis. They are also a frequent cause of pericarditis, and probably of valvulitis as well. Antigens of these highly cardiotropic viruses have been demonstrated within the myocardial fibers of 17 of 55 autopsy subjects (Burch et al., 1967). This study was selective only in that it was weighted toward the younger age groups; there was no selection for patients who had died of heart disease. All 17 patients with Coxsackie antigen showed chronic focal interstitial myocarditis, although most had no history of symptoms referable to the heart. In a similar autopsy study limited to infants and children, 29 of 50 were imputed to have evidence of interstitial myocarditis; in 12 of these, Coxsackie B antigens were found (Burch and Giles, 1972). When Coxsackie myocarditis is symptomatic, it appears most frequently in children and young adults, and affects males twice as often as females. Often there is a history of an upper respiratory infection, followed by a latent period of several days. Among adults, the disease is usually associated with pericarditis and appears to be a relatively benign, self-limited process. However, mysterious sudden death in young adults may occasionally be caused by Coxsackie myocarditis. Coxsackie B myocarditis acquired in intrauterine or neonatal life is more likely to be a rapidly fatal disease than the disease acquired in adulthood (Blattner, 1968; Lerner, 1968). However, it has been suggested that in some cases Coxsackie viruses acquired in utero may remain dormant (in a manner analogous to the herpes viruses), and produce overt disease only when activated by "conditioning" factors, such as intercurrent infection (Burch et al., 1967).

Toxoplasma gondii usually causes systemic infections both in those without known predisposition and in debilitated patients or in those taking drugs which alter normal flora or suppress immune mechanisms. Increasingly it is being recognized as a cause of primary myocarditis or pericarditis. Probably the majority of these cardiac involvements follow a subclinical systemic infection. Pseudocysts containing these organisms may be found in myocardial fibers during postmortem examinations of patients who were not known to have heart disease. In other cases, toxoplasma myocarditis may become symptomatic after a long period of latency; and in still others—unlike most cases of myocarditis—a chronic, protracted course may be followed. As with Coxsackie B viruses, toxoplasma organisms may be acquired in utero (Theologides and Kennedy, 1969).

Chagas' disease, of which myocardial involvement is the most important aspect in about 80 per cent of patients, affects up to half of the population in endemic areas of South America. About 10 per cent of these patients die during the acute phase. Their hearts show the protozoans contained within pseudocysts. A heavy infiltrate of polymorphonuclear leukocytes, as well as focal myocardial fiber necrosis, principally about the parasites, is seen (Fig. 10–7). In other cases, the disease appears to subside, followed by a latent period of 10 to 20 years before the chronic phase of the myocarditis becomes manifest. A still larger group of patients develops the chronic phase of the disease without a history of an antecedent acute infection. In these more protracted instances, the inflammatory reaction is diffuse, in the form of widespread interstitial mononuclear infiltrations, often accompanied by interstitial and focal fibrosis (Prata, 1968). In one endemic area, Chagas' disease has been reported as causing about 25 per cent of all deaths in persons between the ages of 25 and 44 years (Fejfar, 1968).

Idiopathic myocarditis refers to those sporadic cases of myocarditis which occur without discernible cause in previously healthy individuals. A rapidly fatal form of idiopathic myocarditis is known as *Fiedler's myocarditis* or more recently as *giant cell myocarditis.* This type affects males more frequently than females, with a peak incidence in the third decade. Commonly, there is a concurrent or previous respiratory infection. Myocardial failure is intractable and death usually ensues within weeks (Friedberg, 1966). Whether or not

Fiedler's myocarditis is indeed a specific entity, however, is not clear. Possibly it simply represents more severe involvement by any of a number of unknown etiologic agents. It is thought that as routine diagnostic procedures for virus infections become more widespread, much of what has heretofore been called idiopathic myocarditis will emerge as viral myocarditis.

Morphology. Most of the myocarditides produce essentially similar anatomic changes, which will be described here as characteristic of the group as a whole. Minor variations in the morphologic picture depend on the etiologic agent. Sometimes the heart appears grossly normal; however, more often it is both hypertrophied and dilated, with an increase in weight up to about 700 gm. (normal, 350 to 400 gm.). Although all chambers of the heart may be affected, the right side is generally more dilated and flabby. The myocardium often discloses areas of pallor or yellowish mottling. The thickening of the ventricular wall may be masked by the cardiac dilatation.

Histologically, there is always some inflammatory infiltrate, usually associated with some edema. The nature of the infiltrate is highly variable. In the more acute processes, such as those caused by direct bacterial invasion or the fulminant forms of Chagas' disease, it may be composed chiefly of polymorphonuclear leukocytes. In other cases, principally those of viral origin, there may be a predominantly mononuclear inflammatory response (Fig. 10–8). Occasionally there are large numbers of eosinophils and granulomatous formations with giant cells, particularly in certain patterns of

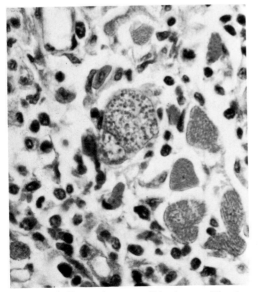

Figure 10–7. Chagas' myocarditis. A parasitized myocardial fiber is evident in mid-field.

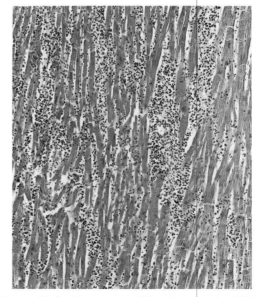

Figure 10–8. Viral myocarditis. A heavy interstitial infiltration of lymphocytes separates many of the myocardial fibers.

Fiedler's (giant cell) myocarditis. When involvement is more chronic, such as with long-standing Chagas' disease and with toxoplasmic myocarditis, a fibrous reaction may be seen. Although the myofibers themselves often appear normal, in many of the myocarditides degenerative changes of varying intensity are often seen, including cellular swelling, fatty change and sometimes actual necrosis. The extent of the myofiber injury correlates better with the severity of the attack than with the specific etiology. Similarly, the intensity of the inflammatory infiltrate versus the amount of fibrous scarring is a function of the chronicity of the disease.

Clinical Course. The clinical picture of myocarditis is extremely variable. In many cases, it is asymptomatic or overshadowed by a systemic disorder. Transient ECG abnormalities may be the only indication of its presence. Acute *symptomatic* myocarditis often manifests itself as malaise, dyspnea and low-grade fever, with tachycardia more marked than the fever alone would warrant. A gallop rhythm is usually present, and there may be a murmur of mitral insufficiency as a result of widening of the mitral valve as the heart dilates. Conduction defects are common, most often taking the form of varying degrees of atrioventricular block. Other arrhythmias may also occur. With advanced disease, CHF involving both ventricles ensues. This is most often manifested clinically as failure of the right side of the heart, since the symptoms of full-blown left-sided heart failure are dependent to some extent on a relatively healthy right ventricle. In most cases, myocarditis is transient, and the symptoms subside after one to two months. A five-year follow-up study of a number of these patients, however, showed that 25 per cent had persistent symptoms, usually precordial pain and fatigue, 20 per cent had cardiomegaly as seen by chest x-ray and 19 per cent had abnormal electrocardiograms at rest (Bengtsson, 1968). It is increasingly speculated that many of the cases to be discussed as idiopathic degenerative cardiomyopathy may represent previous unrecognized or subclinical forms of myocarditis.

DEGENERATIVE CARDIOMYOPATHY

These cardiomyopathies, as opposed to myocarditis, are principally degenerative lesions of the myocardium which lead to the insidious development of progressively intractable CHF. Like the myocarditides, they may be considered as secondary or primary. Almost all primary cardiomyopathies are idiopathic.

Secondary cardiomyopathy is the term applied to a large number of essentially noninflammatory systemic disorders which involve the myocardium and lead to myocardial failure.

Most of these systemic disorders have been discussed elsewhere in this book. Their range may be suggested by the following outline:

1. Metabolic and nutritional disorders: Protein-calorie deficiency states; beriberi heart disease; anemia; endocrine disorders, such as thyrotoxicosis, myxedema and acromegaly; hypo- and hyperkalemia.

2. Infiltrative processes: Amyloidosis; hemochromatosis; the glycogen storage disorders; the mucopolysaccharidoses (Hurler's syndrome).

3. Neuromuscular diseases: Friedreich's disease; progressive muscular dystrophy; myotonia dystrophica.

4. Toxic involvements: Emetine; chloroform; carbon tetrachloride; arsenic; phosphorus; bacterial toxins.

Primary cardiomyopathy may be sporadic or it may occur in one of three specific clinical settings: (1) in association with alcoholism *(alcoholic cardiomyopathy)*, (2) during the puerperium or in late pregnancy *(peripartal cardiomyopathy)*, or (3) as a familial disorder *(familial cardiomyopathy)*. These will be discussed separately in some detail.

Alcoholic cardiomyopathy occurs independently of either thiamine deficiency, which causes beriberi heart disease, or generalized malnutrition. These patients often are well nourished and rarely have concomitant serious liver disease. It has been suggested that either the alcohol itself or some other constituent of alcoholic beverages has a direct toxic effect on the myocardium. In addition, skeletal muscle may be affected. A higher incidence of alcoholic cardiomyopathy has been noted in patients with sickle cell trait. It has been postulated that the acidosis resulting from high alcohol intake leads to sickling of erythrocytes within the small vessels of the myocardium. The diffuse ischemia in turn leads to myocardial degeneration. Such sickling has been found at autopsy of patients who have died with alcoholic cardiomyopathy. The predisposition of individuals with sickle cell trait, then, would explain the reported high incidence of this form of cardiomyopathy in blacks (Fleischer and Rubler, 1968). It has also been suggested that alcoholism acts as a "conditioning" factor in activating latent viruses, which in turn affect the myocardium (Burch and Giles, 1972; Ward and Ward, 1974). To further complicate the issue, the very existence of alcoholic cardiomyopathy has been called into question. Some workers maintain that the concurrence of alcoholism and cardiomyopathy may be no more than coincidence.

Peripartal cardiomyopathy refers to the onset of myocardial failure in previously healthy women during the puerperium or, less frequently, in late pregnancy. It is most common in the first two months after childbirth, although it may have its onset as much as six months later. The incidence is higher in blacks and in persons inhabiting tropical areas. As with alcoholism, it has been suggested that the role of pregnancy is merely to activate a latent cardiotropic virus.

Familial cardiomyopathy refers to the appearance of myocardial disease within several members of a kinship. Most often the pathophysiologic pattern is hypertrophic, although this is not invariably so, even within the same family. Included among the familial cardiomyopathies is the entity known as *idiopathic hypertrophic subaortic stenosis (IHSS)*, also called hypertrophic obstructive cardiomyopathy. Probably most cases of this disorder represent an autosomal dominant trait with a high degree of penetrance (Clark et al., 1973). Since the morphology and clinical course of IHSS differ somewhat from the other cardiomyopathies, a few words will be said about it here. With the light microscope, the myofibers are seen to be hypertrophied and markedly unaligned (Roberts and Ferrans, 1975). Histochemical studies show them to contain increased amounts of norepinephrine as well as lysosomal and mitochondrial enzymes. This entity is unique among the causes of myocardial insufficiency in that it is aggravated by drugs which increase myocardial contractility, since these increase the obstruction to the outflow tract. Presumably this obstruction is caused by the hypertrophied muscle mass, although this mechanism has recently been questioned (Rossen et al., 1974). Syncope and angina pectoris resulting from increased oxygen demands of the hypertrophied muscle are characteristic early symptoms. Congestive heart failure may ensue later, but it is less regularly associated with this entity than with the other cardiomyopathies. Although the prognosis with IHSS is, in general, better than that with the other cardiomyopathies, sudden death is a relatively common phenomenon and the most frequent form of death (Hardarson et al., 1973).

When primary cardiomyopathy arises sporadically—that is, not in association with alcoholism, the peripartal state or a familial tendency—it usually involves adults over the age of 35 years. Possibly some of these cases are unappreciated instances of alcoholic cardiomyopathy. Others may represent varying degrees of protein-calorie deficiency. It has been established that such nutritional deficiency states may affect the heart relatively early, causing myofiber atrophy (Ramalingaswami, 1968). In most instances, however, such a search for hidden causes is unrewarding. It is suspected that episodes of myocarditis, often subclinical, may in many cases be the basis for the development of idiopathic degenerative cardiomyopathy years later. Conceivably, residual myocardial fibrosis in these patients later augments the effect of atherosclerotic heart disease or of alcohol on myocardial function. Alternatively, a virus or viruses might incite the formation of antibodies against the myocardium (Editorial, 1974d). Whether or not *all* idiopathic cardiomyopathies can be attributed to earlier myocarditis is speculative, however. Attempts to demonstrate cardiac autoantibodies in these cases have yielded mixed results, perhaps reflecting the mixed etiologies of this entity. Even when such antibodies are present, it remains unclear whether they are of pathogenetic significance or are merely a nonspecific reflection of underlying myocardial damage (Kaplan and Frengley, 1969).

Morphology. Most of the cardiomyopathies produce similar morphologic changes. The outstanding exception is IHSS, which has been described. Grossly, the alterations of the cardiomyopathies are much like those of the myocarditides. The heart is usually dilated, soft and flabby. Commonly, all chambers are affected. Although concomitant hypertrophy is usual, with heart weights over 400 gm., some forms of cardiomyopathy, such as that resulting from protein-calorie deficiencies, may lead to predominant atrophy, with consequent reduced heart weights. The cardiomyopathies, then, may be **congestive** or **hypertrophic.** The myocardium is pale and there may be diffuse or focal areas of fibrosis. Patchy endothelial fibrosis and mural thrombi, especially in the auricular appendages, are common. With the light microscope the changes are rather undramatic and may be quite subtle. Typically, the myocardial fibers develop considerable variations in size, with hypertrophic fibers lying adjacent to atrophic or degenerating fibers. The nuclei, too, lose their uniformity and some become pyknotic, whereas others are large and bizarre in shape (Edington and Hutt, 1968). The cytoplasm shows varying degrees of degenerative changes, running the gamut from cloudy swelling through vacuolation and fatty change to hyalinization with loss of striation. There may be areas of necrosis. Although scattered mononuclear leukocytes may be seen, they are not present in large numbers and are a minor part of the picture (Egan et al., 1968). With the electron microscope, mitochondrial swelling with fragmentation of the cristae is evident. There is also swelling of the sarcoplasmic reticulum and myofibrillar disruption. Histochemical studies have demonstrated reduced amounts of many of the myocardial oxidative enzymes.

Clinical Course. Because the degenerative cardiomyopathies constitute such a large and diverse group of disorders, any description of the clinical course is of necessity a generalized one, to which there will be exceptions. It can be said, however, that most cardiomyopathies are characterized by the relatively early development of CHF. The clinical setting, of course, varies from amyloidosis to acute poisoning to alcoholism to apparently complete normalcy. Heart failure may be predominantly right-sided or, particularly with alcoholic cardiomyopathy, it may initially be left-sided. Commonly, there is failure of both ventricles, and the presenting event may be either systemic venous congestion or pulmonary congestion. As was pointed out in the discussion of the myocarditides, biventricular failure tends to manifest itself principally as right ventricular failure. Transient arrhythmias, such as extrasystoles or atrial fibrillation, are common, but sustained arrhythmias are unusual. The prognosis is variable, depending to a large extent on the presence and nature of underlying disorders. Although there is no cure for most of the cardiomyopathies, some of them, such as peripartal cardiomyopathy, subside spontaneously in a significant proportion of cases. Others, such as alcoholic cardiomyopathy, are reversible early in their course, when the inciting influence is removed. In most cases, however, there is temporary improvement with therapy, but heart failure tends to recur and ultimately becomes refractory. The course may be fulminant, lasting only a few months, or it may extend over a period of years. Death is most often caused by refractory CHF, but it may be a result of serious arrhythmias, of complete heart block or of thromboembolic phenomena, resulting from the frequent presence of mural thrombi within the heart.

ENDOCARDIAL FIBROELASTOSIS

This disease is characterized by marked fibrous and elastic thickening of the endocardium, extending superficially into the immediately subjacent myocardium. It is the most important cause of death from CHF in infants between the ages of one and two years (Friedberg, 1966). Although many cases are associated with congenital malformations of the heart—principally aortic stenosis, coarctation of the aorta, atresia of the pulmonary and aortic valves, anomalous origin of the left coronary artery and ventricular hypoplasia—it occurs *most* frequently in hearts that are otherwise normal (Moller et al., 1964). The etiology and pathogenesis are unknown. It has been persuasively argued that the primary derangement involves increased intracardiac pressure resulting in hypertrophy and dilatation of the heart, followed by endocardial fibrotic and elastic proliferation, much as the walls of muscular arteries become thickened

with systemic hypertension (Black-Schaffer, 1957). Supporting this thesis is the observation that the lesion tends to occur with those congenital anomalies which cause elevations of intracardiac pressure, and it affects principally chambers subjected to the greatest increases in pressure (Bryan and Oppenheimer, 1969). Moreover, the lesion has been described in the left atrium of adults with rheumatic mitral stenosis and in the right ventricle of those with pulmonic stenosis resulting from the carcinoid syndrome (see page 504) (Clark et al., 1968). Conceivably, the apparently primary form of this disease (i.e., occurring in the absence of other malformations) results from transient increases in intracardiac pressure, possibly during intrauterine life. Other theories invoke intrauterine hypoxia or a genetic metabolic defect as the cause of the lesion. Some consider endocardial fibroelastosis as overlapping to a large extent with the myocarditides. These authorities emphasize the finding of concomitant myocardial changes in the majority of cases while, conversely, alterations suggestive of endocardial fibroelastosis may be seen in many cases of myocarditis. Hastreiter and Miller (1964) suggest intrauterine or neonatal Coxsackie B infection as the cause, and indeed this agent has been identified in the heart muscle in 13 of 28 of these patients at autopsy.

Morphology. Endocardial fibroelastosis appears as a diffuse or patchy, pearly-white thickening of the mural endocardium, predominantly of the left ventricle (Fig. 10–9). However, the left atrium, right ventricle and right atrium, in this order of frequency, may also be involved. The endocardial lining may thus attain a depth up to 10 times normal. Mural thrombi sometimes overlie these fibrous areas. In many cases, the endocardial fibrosis extends into the mitral and aortic valves, which thus become thickened and stenotic. Almost invariably, the heart is enlarged and dilated. Histologically, there is a marked increase of collagenous and elastic fibers on the endocardial surface which may extend into the myocardium. The fibers generally run parallel to the surface. Occasionally, scattered lymphocytes and focal necroses in the underlying myocardium may be seen. Still and Boult (1956) have contended that by electron microscopy a thin layer of fibrin may be seen overlying the involved areas in the early stages, supporting the inflammatory theories of causation.

Clinical Course. The significance of this lesion depends upon the extent of involvement. When focal, it may have no functional importance and permit normal longevity. When severe, however, it produces intractable CHF. This may be especially fulminant in infants and may lead to death within hours of the first noticeable manifestations. Unless there are concomitant congenital anomalies or markedly

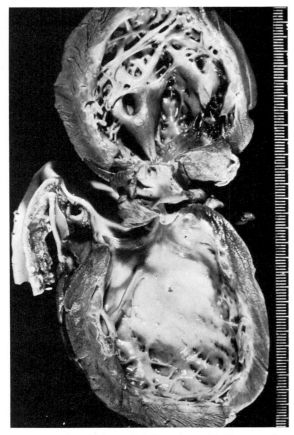

Figure 10–9. Endocardial fibroelastosis. The anterior wall of the left ventricle has been lifted to expose the white, opaque, fibrous subendocardial layer, which can be seen covering the entire surface of the chamber. The fibrosis extends superficially into the adjacent myocardium.

fibrotic valves, a heart murmur is not usually present until the heart has begun to dilate. About 50 per cent of these patients do not respond to treatment, and death follows.

CONGESTIVE HEART FAILURE FROM EXTRACARDIAC DISEASE

Two major forms of cardiac involvement, *hypertensive heart disease* and *cor pulmonale*, are not diseases primary to the heart, but rather refer to effects on the heart of disease that is primary elsewhere in the body. Moreover, the similarity between these two entities does not end there. In both instances, failure of an otherwise healthy heart results from hypertension. With hypertensive heart disease, the elevation in blood pressure is systemic and the left ventricle eventually can no longer carry the extra burden of expelling blood against an abnormally great pressure head. The case of

cor pulmonale is analogous. Here, as mentioned earlier, the hypertension is in the pulmonary circuit and it is the right ventricle which carries the increased work load and eventually fails. In both instances, the primary disorder is often discovered before heart failure ensues. Systemic hypertension may be found on a routine physical examination. Cor pulmonale usually is preceded by years of symptomatic chronic pulmonary disease, manifested by cough and shortness of breath, although occasionally the lung disorder is first brought to light by the seemingly mysterious onset of CHF. The valves are unaffected in both these diseases and, by definition, the CHF cannot be accounted for by significant ASHD. It should be pointed out that, as in the case of ASHD, there is an imbalance between the blood supply to the heart and the amount required for the work it must perform. In the case of ASHD, it is the blood supply which dwindles, whereas with both hypertensive heart disease and cor pulmonale the needs of the heart increase.

Much less frequently, CHF from extracardiac disease is caused by *luetic (syphilitic) aortitis*. This was discussed in Chapter 9.

HYPERTENSIVE HEART DISEASE

This term refers to the secondary effects on the heart of prolonged, sustained systemic hypertension. Remarks here are limited to a brief description of the anatomic effects on the heart, since hypertension in general will be discussed on page 456.

Hypertensive heart disease is characterized anatomically principally by thickening of the left ventricle, with an accompanying increase in the weight of the heart. The left ventricular wall may reach a thickness of more than 2.5 cm., and the weight of the heart may be increased to 500 to 700 gm. Thickening occurs inwardly at the expense of the left ventricular chamber and is therefore referred to as **concentric hypertrophy**. With the onset of CHF, however, the heart begins to dilate and for the first time cardiac enlargement is discernible by chest x-ray or clinical examination. As dilatation progresses, the left ventricular wall becomes progressively stretched and thinned, which may obscure the preexistent thickening.

Although the diameter of the individual myofibrils is increased, the muscle fibers do not usually appear abnormally large on light microscopic examination. At the level of the electron microscope, it has been shown that the hypertrophy of increased work load results in many changes, including increased numbers and enlargement of mitochondria and increased synthesis of myofibrils (Pelosi and Agliati, 1968). There are no specific light microscopic characteristics of hypertensive heart disease.

It should be emphasized that the anatomic diagnosis of hypertensive heart disease can be made only in the absence of structural abnormalities, which may themselves lead to increased cardiac work load with consequent myocardial hypertrophy. Even then, there must also be a history of hypertension or the presence of typical hypertensive vascular changes to establish the diagnosis, since the cardiomyopathies, too, may produce cardiac enlargement without apparent cause.

COR PULMONALE

Cor pulmonale is defined as right ventricular hypertrophy, with or without CHF, caused by pulmonary hypertension from primary disease within the lung substance or within its vessels. It is an important cause of death from these disorders.

Nearly any long-standing lung disease may lead to cor pulmonale, including chronic obstructive pulmonary disease (chronic bronchitis and primary emphysema), the pneumoconioses, idiopathic interstitial fibrosis and bronchiectasis. These entities produce pulmonary hypertension, in part simply through destruction of portions of the pulmonary vascular bed, which results in increased flow through the remaining vessels, and in part through the vasoconstrictive effects of hypoxemia and respiratory acidosis.

Abnormalities of the pulmonary vasculature constitute a second and more direct cause of pulmonary hypertension. Paramount in this category are multiple or large pulmonary emboli. Intrinsic pulmonary vascular disease is a less frequent cause of pulmonary hypertension. Most often such intrinsic disease is caused by an idiopathic disorder known as *primary pulmonary vascular sclerosis* (p. 381). Rarely it rep-

resents pulmonary involvement by one of the necrotizing angiitides, such as polyarteritis nodosa or Wegener's granulomatosis.

Uncommonly, cor pulmonale is caused by *skeletal or neuromuscular derangements* which interfere with normal ventilation, e.g., severe kyphoscoliosis, poliomyelitis, the muscular dystrophies and the Pickwickian syndrome. Presumably these act through pulmonary vasoconstriction induced by the hypoxemia and acidosis that they produce.

It is apparent that the common denominator in all the previously mentioned disorders is pulmonary hypertension. In general, cor pulmonale is asymptomatic until right-sided congestive heart failure ensues. Until then, the picture is usually dominated by the primary disorder.

The morphologic changes associated with cor pulmonale are entirely analogous to those of hypertensive heart disease, with the right ventricle rather than the left ventricle being primarily affected. The right ventricle may thicken up to 1.5 cm., and thus it may achieve virtually the same dimensions as the left ventricle (Fig. 10–10).

It should be noted in passing that right ventricular hypertrophy often develops secondary to left-sided CHF. Cardiac congenital malformations may produce left-to-right shunts and consequent hypertrophy of the right ventricle. Such changes are not included within the present definition of cor pulmonale.

PAIN

Most heart diseases do not produce pain. However, severe and often catastrophic pain is a prominent although not invariable feature of myocardial infarction (MI). Angina pectoris (AP), the first cousin of MI, is by definition

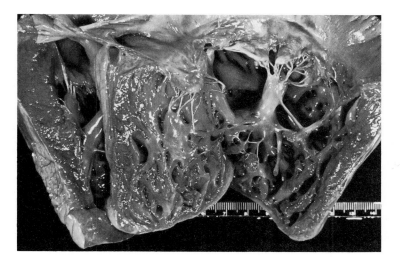

Figure 10–10. Cor pulmonale. The right ventricle and tricuspid valve have been opened to expose the thickened wall and trabeculae carneae. Compare with the thickness of the wall of the left ventricle, seen on the extreme left.

chest pain secondary to transient myocardial ischemia without infarction. This diagnosis, then, rests uniquely on the presence of pain. Thus, among the various disorders of the heart, these two entities stand well apart from the others by virtue of the importance and the intensity of the pain they evoke. To a far lesser degree, the various forms of pericarditis also evoke pain—but seldom of such magnitude as to be confused with MI or AP. However, since MI and AP were discussed earlier, only pericarditis will be presented under this heading.

It is important to remember that chest pain is often produced by extracardiac diseases, such as pulmonary embolism, dissecting aneurysm, esophagitis, and various pulmonary lesions. On occasion, it may be difficult to distinguish the pain evoked by these disorders from that produced by cardiac disease.

PERICARDITIS

Inflammation of the pericardium occurs in a multitude of clinical settings. Thus, it is seen in any age group and in either sex, although males are affected somewhat more often than are females. Like myocarditis, pericarditis may be either *secondary* or *primary.* Secondary pericarditis refers to a relatively insignificant aspect of a more generalized derangement. When pericarditis dominates the clinical picture, it is termed primary. Most primary pericarditis is *idiopathic.* Because of the considerable overlap between the etiologies of secondary and primary pericarditis, a discussion based on this classification is less meaningful than in the case of the myocarditides. A second arrangement divides pericarditis into *acute, subacute* and *chronic* forms. Here again, however, the overlap in causation of these forms is great. Moreover, in many cases the subacute and chronic phases simply evolve from the much more common acute form. An anatomic system of classification is also widely used. This system is based on the character of the inflammatory exudate. Thus, pericarditis may be: *(1) serous, (2) serofibrinous, (3) fibrinous, (4) suppurative, or (5) hemorrhagic.* There is, as we shall see, a good deal of correlation between these anatomic patterns and the causation of pericarditis. In some cases, however, the type of inflammatory exudate is more a function of the severity of injury than of the etiology.

Etiology and Pathogenesis. The principal etiologies are shown in Table 10–2, along with the frequencies of some of the more important causes of the *acute* form.

When pericardial involvement is a relatively minor aspect of a larger disorder, such as with SLE, it is described in the section dealing with

TABLE 10–2. CAUSES OF PERICARDITIS*

	PER CENT
1. Infectious pericarditis:	
Bacterial	16
Tuberculous	7
Viral	?
Mycotic and protozoan	?
2. Metabolic pericarditis:	
Uremic	17
Cholesterol	
Myxedematous (noninflammatory)	
3. Neoplastic pericarditis	8
4. Acute myocardial infarction	11
5. Traumatic pericarditis	3
6. Hypersensitivity pericarditis (either exogenous or endogenous antigens):	
Rheumatic fever	11
Other autoimmune diseases (SLE, rheumatoid arthritis, scleroderma, polyarteritis)	3
Serum sickness, drug reactions	
The postcardiotomy, postmyocardial infarction and posttraumatic syndromes	
7. Idiopathic pericarditis	23

*From Sodeman and Smith (1958).

the basic disease. The comments here are chiefly concerned with those forms listed in Table 10–2 that constitute the primary clinical problem.

Bacteria may reach the pericardium either by direct spread from contiguous structures, such as the esophagus or pleura, or by hematogenous or lymphatic seeding. In recent years, bacterial pericarditis has markedly declined in incidence, although staphylococcal and tuberculous causations remain important. Among children, especially, staphylococcal pericarditis is relatively frequent and is almost always associated with either pneumonia or osteomyelitis (Evans, 1961). Obviously, whether septic pericardial involvement dominates the clinical picture or is a small part of it is variable.

As bacterial pericarditis has declined in importance, fungi, protozoa and, most especially, viruses have taken on new importance as causes of pericardial disease. Very often there is an associated myocarditis (Evans, 1961). *Coccidioides immitis, Histoplasma capsulatum,* and *Candida albicans,* among the fungi, and *Toxoplasma gondii,* among the protozoa, may produce apparently primary pericardial involvement and should be suspected in cases of idiopathic pericarditis. Even more than the fungi and protozoa, the viruses are gaining increasing importance as causes of primary pericarditis. Indeed, some workers believe that viruses cause most, if not all, cases of acute idiopathic pericarditis (Burch and Giles, 1972). Among known cases of viral pericarditis, those caused by the Coxsackie B viruses, influenza A and B viruses, some of the ECHO viruses and the Epstein-Barr virus (in association with mononucleosis) are particularly important. The pathogenesis of viral pericarditis is not clear. Frequently it follows an acute upper respiratory infection, but whether or not the causative viruses then spread to the pericardium is not known. There is some support for the view that many viruses do not directly invade pericardial tissue, but rather in some way incite a hypersensitivity phenomenon, which in turn involves the pericardium.

Among the metabolic pericarditides, that resulting from uremia occurs most frequently and is described on page 429. A rare form of metabolic pericarditis, of unknown etiology, is termed "cholesterol pericarditis" because of the presence of cholesterol crystals in the intrapericardial fluid. Myxedema, too, causes an accumulation of fluid in the pericardial cavity, termed an *effusion*, but this is noninflammatory, hence it does not represent a true pericarditis.

Primary tumors of the pericardium are extremely rare. Neoplastic pericarditis, then, almost always stems from direct or metastatic spread of tumors arising outside the pericardial sac. Most often, direct spread is from mediastinal lymphomas or from bronchogenic or esophageal carcinomas. Although metastases from any organ in the body may involve the pericardium, such spread is in general an infrequent occurrence.

The pericarditis accompanying acute myocardial infarction is described on page 297.

Traumatic pericarditis is a relatively common sequela to nonpenetrating chest trauma, and reflects either mild contusions to the epicardial surface of the heart or the presence of blood in the pericardial sac, which acts as a chemical irritant just as it does in the pleural or peritoneal cavities. Infrequently, penetrating chest wounds introduce bacteria directly into the pericardial cavity, producing a suppurative pericarditis.

The pericardium, like the other serosal membranes, is peculiarly vulnerable to hypersensitivity states. The major immune diseases are discussed in Chapter 6. Rheumatic fever, a particularly important cause of pericarditis in children, is discussed elsewhere in this chapter. Suffice it here to describe briefly the postcardiotomy, postmyocardial infarction (post-MI) and posttraumatic syndromes, all of which are presumed to be based on an immune mechanism. All are characterized by pericarditis, usually with a significant collection of fluid in the pericardial sac, and are often accompanied by pleuritis and, less frequently, by pneumonitis. Postcardiotomy pericarditis usually develops two to five weeks following any heart surgery involving wide excision of the pericardium. In one series, this sequela occurred in 30 of 100 patients who had undergone open heart surgery (Engle and Ito, 1961). A small number of patients develop a similar syndrome two to five weeks following MI or trauma to the pericardium. Clinically, these three entities are virtually identical, manifesting themselves as fever and chest pain, which subside either spontaneously or with corticosteroid therapy. All have a marked tendency to recur periodically, sometimes for months or even years. *It must be remembered that in all three cases, the initial inciting event—namely, cardiotomy, MI or pericardial trauma—is itself often associated with an immediate, transient pericarditis, which should not be confused with the later-developing immune syndrome.* In most cases, these patients have high serum titers of autoantibodies to heart tissue. It has been suggested that antigens released from damaged myocardial tissue evoke the formation of antibodies, and that the inflammation is mediated by soluble antigen-antibody complexes (Versey and Gabriel, 1974).

The largest single category of pericarditis is idiopathic. However, with improved diagnostic measures, particularly for the isolation of viruses, fewer cases are now being assigned to the idiopathic group. Undoubtedly many cases of idiopathic pericarditis are in reality viral, possibly the Coxsackie viruses being most important. It should be remembered that viral and immune etiologies are not mutually exclusive, since it is suspected that viral pericarditis does not always represent direct invasion by the organisms.

Morphology. The various etiologies are expressed in a variety of morphologic patterns. The term "acute pericarditis" usually refers to a **serous, fibrinous** or **serofibrinous** inflammation. It is characterized by a small intrapericardial exudative effusion, usually not greater than 200 ml., containing gray-yellow strands or clumps of fibrin. Frequently a fine granular precipitate of fibrin is deposited on the serosal surfaces. This may cause adherence of the two layers of the pericardium, described as "bread and butter" pericarditis because the shaggy pericardial surfaces, when separated, resemble lavishly buttered slices of bread (see Fig. 2–7, p. 46). Such a condition is encountered in rheumatic fever, MI and sometimes in the immune and viral forms of pericarditis. Microscopically, the subserosal inflammation is nonspecific and consists of both polymorphonuclear and mononuclear leukocytes. A **suppurative** effusion almost always denotes the presence of bacteria or fungi. With neoplastic involvement, the exudate is usually **hemorrhagic**. Tuberculosis evokes a **caseous** exudate.

Occasionally large amounts of pericardial effusion may accumulate. When the volume is massive, sometimes over a liter, or when the accumulation is rapid, diastolic filling may be impaired, a condition known as **cardiac tamponade**. Such large effusions are particularly likely with the more subacute to chronic processes, such as tuberculous, neoplastic or immune pericarditis (Schwartz et al., 1963).

The late sequelae of these acute involvements are somewhat dependent on the severity of the reaction and on the specific etiology. In general, the serous and fibrinous patterns resolve completely. Infrequently, organization of fibrinous exudate yields delicate, bridging fibrous strands or shiny opaque thickenings of the pericardial surfaces, but neither change is of much clinical consequence. The suppurative bacterial and caseous tuberculous reactions are more grave. While these, too, may resolve, more often they lead to fibrous obliteration of the pericardial cavity, with adherence of the parietal pericardium to surrounding structures. This pattern of scarring is termed **adhesive mediastinopericarditis** and produces severe cardiac strain, since the heart with each systolic contraction works not only against the parietal pericardium but also against the attached surrounding structures. Diffuse organization within the pericardial sac may create the entity known as **chronic constrictive pericarditis**. This is characterized by encasement of the heart within a dense fibrous scar which, while not attached to surrounding structures, cannot expand adequately during diastole and thus interferes with cardiac function. The fibrosis may constrict the venae cavae as they enter the heart to produce the clinical syndrome known as **Pick's disease**, which is characterized by hepatosplenomegaly and ascites. This pattern of scarring is probably most common with tuberculous pericarditis (Wood, 1961), although it is also known to occur relatively rapidly a few months following some cases of acute idiopathic pericarditis (Robertson and Arnold, 1962). In about 50 per cent of cases, the fibrous enclosure becomes calcified. When this calcification is diffuse, it produces the appearance of a plaster mold encasing the heart, known as **concretio cordis** (Holmes and Fowler, 1968).

Clinical Course. Much of the clinical picture has already been described in discussing the various etiologies as well as the pattern of scarring. With acute fibrinous pericarditis, the principal symptom is the acute onset of chest pain, although the pain may be minimal or absent in up to 50 per cent of cases. Usually there is associated malaise and fever. The pain may be very similar to that of angina pectoris or MI, but tends to be distinguishable in having a pleuritic component as a result of a commonly associated pleuritis. The pain is often intensified by body movements and relieved by sitting or leaning forward. The presence of a pericardial friction rub is pathognomonic, but it may be very evanescent. In most cases, the process subsides spontaneously within a few weeks, but it tends to recur.

Principal among the complications of pericarditis are the accumulations of large effusions with resultant tamponade, embarassment of the venous return to the heart, and the development of chronic adhesive or constrictive pericarditis.

HYDROPERICARDIUM AND HEMOPERICARDIUM

Hydropericardium refers to the noninflammatory accumulation of a transudate within the pericardial cavity. As such, it is analogous to the passive accumulation of fluid in the pleural cavity *(hydrothorax)* and in the peritoneum *(ascites)*, with considerable overlap of etiologies. The most important cause of hydropericardium is increased venous pressure from congestive heart failure. Indeed, fluid in the pericardium from this cause is more common than from all the inflammatory etiologies. Other states associated with hydropericardium include severe hypoproteinemia from any cause and hypervolemia.

The term *hemopericadium* denotes the presence of pure blood in the pericardial sac, rather than the admixture of blood and inflammatory exudate that is seen with hemorrhagic pericarditis. The most frequent causes of hemopericardium, excluding trauma, are myocardial infarction with rupture (60 per cent), aortic aneurysms with dissection or rupture into the pericardium (33 per cent), eroding malignant tumors (4 per cent) and blood dyscrasias (3 per cent) (Barbour et al., 1961).

HEART MURMURS

Any process interfering with the normal streamlined flow of blood through the heart and great vessels may produce audible turbulence, called a heart murmur. This is encountered in incompetence or stenosis of any of the heart valves, or when normal flow patterns are disrupted, such as occurs in some forms of congenital heart disease. A large variety of cardiac lesions may produce heart murmurs. Here we are concerned with those diseases in which a murmur is usually the first clinical manifestation of cardiac involvement. The most important of these are (1) rheumatic heart disease, (2) infective endocarditis, and (3) congenital heart disease. Far less frequently murmurs are caused by (4) nonbacterial thrombotic endocarditis, (5) Libman-Sacks endocarditis, (6) the carcinoid syndrome, and (7) myxoma of the heart. It should be made clear that many of these diseases are systemic in nature as, for example, rheumatic fever and systemic lupus erythematosus (of which Libman-Sacks endocarditis is only a part). However, in these as well as in the other disorders listed above, the first clue to cardiac involvement is typically the discovery of a heart murmur.

RHEUMATIC FEVER

Rheumatic fever is a systemic, nonsuppurative, inflammatory disease, often recurrent, which is most likely related to prior infection with group A beta hemolytic streptococci. Although the pathogenesis is not completely clear, the disease probably represents an immune reaction in some way induced by the streptococcus. The joints, heart, skin, serosa, blood vessels and lungs are predominantly affected, in variable combinations. Although the joints are the single most frequent site of involvement and initially of most distress to the patient, *the importance of rheumatic fever derives entirely from its capacity to cause severe damage to the heart.* Its effects on other parts of the body are nearly always benign and transient.

Although rheumatic fever may occur at any age, 90 per cent of patients have their first attack between the ages of 5 and 15 years. It is infrequent under the age of 4 years (Glancy et al., 1969). Males and females are affected equally. The incidence is higher among the poor, a fact which seems to be most strongly correlated with overcrowded living conditions. There are no inherent racial differences in susceptibility (Gordis et al., 1969).

Over the past several decades in the United States, the incidence, morbidity and death rate from rheumatic fever and its sequela, *rheumatic heart disease*, have rapidly and steadily declined. A study of a large number of college freshmen over the years 1956 through 1965 showed that the number of those with a history of rheumatic fever, or with heart disease attributable to rheumatic fever, declined from a prevalence rate of 17 per 1000 students to 11 per 1000. It is of interest that about a third gave no history of antecedent rheumatic fever. This is understandable if it is realized that rheumatic fever, as well as the preceding streptococcal infection, frequently is asymptomatic (Perry et al., 1968; Stollerman and Pearce, 1968). Even more dramatic than the decline in incidence of this disease is the fall in death rate. By 1960, the death rate from rheumatic fever between the ages of 5 and 25 years had fallen nearly 90 per cent from the 1920 level. The decline in the incidence and mortality of rheumatic fever can largely be attributed to antibiotic treatment and prophylaxis of streptococcal infections. Improved socioeconomic conditions and changes in the inherent virulence of the streptococcus may also contribute. Despite these heartening trends, rheumatic fever with its sequela is still an important cause of death in school-age children.

Etiology and Pathogenesis. Rheumatic fever develops from one to four weeks following the inciting streptococcal infection, which is usually a pharyngitis. Unlike acute glomerulonephritis (see p. 436), this disease may result from infection with any strain of the group A beta hemolytic streptococci. Although nearly 50 per cent of patients with rheumatic fever give no history of an antecedent acute infection and, furthermore, have negative throat cultures at the time they seek medical attention, *serologic* evidence of recent streptococcal infection is present in well over 95 per cent of these patients. Elevated titers of antistreptolysin O (ASO) are present in about 85 per cent of patients with rheumatic fever, and most of the remainder have high titers of antistreptokinase (ASK), antideoxyribonuclease B (anti-DNase B), anti-NADase or antihyaluronidase. The streptococcus is further implicated by large-scale studies showing that rheumatic fever can be prevented by antibiotic treatment as late as 7 days after the onset of a streptococcal infection (Quie and Ayoub, 1968). Moreover, rheumatic fever does not recur when streptococcal infections are prevented by prophylactic antibiotics.

That the streptococci play some role in the development of rheumatic fever, then, seems clear. The nature of their role, however, is controversial (Robbins, 1974). Some believe that they act merely to unmask or activate latent viruses which are the actual causes of rheumatic fever (Burch and Giles, 1972). In support of this view is the fact that components of the group A streptococcus have been shown to have strong immunosuppressant effects, which could release dormant viruses (Malakian and Schwab, 1968). Certainly there is abundant clinical opportunity for such synergistic action, since streptococci are frequent secondary invaders in cases of viral pharyngitis. Alternatively, it has been suggested that many cases of chronic valvular disease once thought to stem from rheumatic fever may in fact have been caused by viruses alone. There is much evidence, both from experimental and from human studies, that viruses can produce valvulitis (Ward and Ward, 1974; Burch et al., 1967). Nevertheless, it seems clear that, for the reasons mentioned earlier, in most cases of rheumatic heart disease the streptococci do play an essential role.

If we assume that the streptococci act alone, and not in concert with viruses, what is the pathogenetic mechanism by which they produce rheumatic fever?

It was long ago demonstrated conclusively that the lesions of rheumatic fever are sterile, hence they do not result from direct bacterial invasion. The latent period between streptococcal infection and the onset of rheumatic fever, as well as other characteristics of the disease, suggest an immunologic reaction (Dudding et al., 1968). Antibodies against heart tissue, which will localize principally in and just beneath the sarcolemma, have been found in the sera of from 25 to 63 per cent of patients with acute rheumatic fever, in 12 to 21 per cent of those with inactive rheumatic heart disease and in none to only 4 per cent of healthy controls (Kaplan and Frengley, 1969). Moreover, other studies have shown that the sera in more than 50 per cent of patients with rheumatic fever or inactive rheumatic heart disease, as well as in 24 per cent of those with proved uncomplicated streptococcal infection, contain antibodies to the streptococcus that are cross reactive with myocardial and skeletal muscle tissue, as well as with the smooth muscle of the endocardium and vessel walls. Several antibodies may be involved, and those affecting the heart valves are probably different from those affecting the myocardium. One antibody which is cross reactive to streptococcal group A polysaccharide and to the glycoprotein of the heart valves has been isolated (Joorabchi, 1969). Another streptococcal antigen, the M protein, is thought to combine with a heart determinant to form a carrier-hapten antigen which elicits antibodies. Some of these antibodies against heart tissue can be detected at the time of diagnosis. However, other antibodies appear later during the course of the disease, and presumably these represent a nonspecific response to tissue injury. Whether or not the earlier developing antibodies are of pathogenetic significance is unclear. Conceivably, the streptococcus initially damages the heart by some other mechanism, and antibodies which develop as a response to tissue injury then perpetuate that damage. It is of interest that, although similar antibodies are known to occur in postcardiotomy patients, they develop more commonly in those whose surgery was for rheumatic heart disease. This would indicate that the presence of autoantibodies in patients with rheumatic fever cannot entirely be ascribed to tissue trauma.

Only 3 per cent of patients with untreated streptococcal infection develop rheumatic fever. The reason for this selectivity is unknown. It has recently been shown that whereas the lymphocytes of normal individuals are stimulated by streptolysin S toward mitotic activity and blast formation (*transformation*), lymphocytes of patients with rheumatic fever tend to remain relatively quiescent (Gery et al., 1968). Possibly those patients who are vulnerable to rheumatic fever suffer from some prior immunologic derangement. It also appears that rheumatic fever develops only in individuals who have had prior sensitizing exposures to streptococcal infections. This would explain the rarity of the disease in infants and very young children.

Among patients who have already had an initial attack of rheumatic fever, the risk of a recurrence following a new streptococcal infection is very high—a 50 to 65 per cent chance. Whether these patients were inherently just as vulnerable even before their first attack, or whether an initial episode of rheumatic fever increases vulnerability, is unknown. The latter explanation is favored by the decline in the risk of recurrence with the passage of time after the initial attack.

Morphology. The basic and pathognomonic morphologic lesion of rheumatic fever is the Aschoff body. When it is fully evolved, it comprises a focus of fibrinoid material surrounded by a characteristic cellular infiltrate. In active rheumatic fever, the Aschoff body is classically found in the heart. Similar lesions, however, may be seen in the synovia of the joints, in and about joint capsules, tendons and fascia and, less often, in other connective tissues of the body. The Aschoff body represents a localized area of tissue necrosis containing fibrinoid material. Most believe the primary necrosis involves connective tissue, but some still contend that it represents injured muscle fibers. The development of the Aschoff body proceeds through three phases: the early **exudative phase**, the intermediate **proliferative phase** and the late **healed phase. Only the proliferative phase is diagnostic.** During the exudative phase, the central focus of necrosis is surrounded by leukocytes, chiefly neutrophils, with scattered lymphocytes, plasma cells and histiocytes. The proliferative phase is characterized by a central focus of swollen, frayed, necrotic collagen in which fibrinoid is deposited, enclosed within a rim of inflammatory cells. The cellular zone contains large differentiated mesenchymal cells known as **Anitschkow myocytes** and occasional multinucleate **Aschoff giant cells,** as well as mononuclear leukocytes and fibroblasts (Fig. 10–11). The Anitschkow myocytes are known as "caterpillar cells" because the nuclear chromatin is aggregated into the center of the nucleus in the form of a slender, wavy ribbon with innumerable fine, leglike projections. An abundant basophilic cytoplasm with cytoplasmic processes encloses the nucleus. The origin of these cells is controversial. Most consider them to be altered fibroblasts, rather than modified myocytes (Wagner and Siew, 1970). The Aschoff giant cells are considerably larger and have one or two nuclei or a folded multilobular nucleus with prominent nucleoli. The healed phase of the Aschoff body results from progressive hyalinization and fibrosis of the lesion, and is discernible only as a focus of nonspecific scarring. The significance of the Aschoff body is not known. Immunofluorescent studies show that the antibodies against heart tissue, when present, are unrelated in location to the Aschoff bodies (Kaplan, 1969). Moreover, diagnostic Aschoff bodies are frequently encountered in hearts in the apparent absence of signs of activity of the disease. Either these lesions persist long

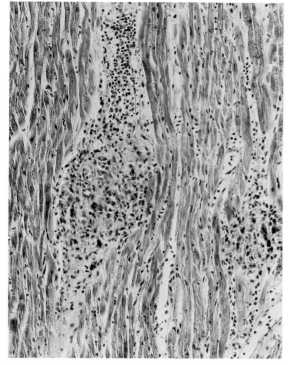

Figure 10–11. Microscopic detail of two Aschoff bodies in the myocardium in acute rheumatic heart disease. The variability in the size of the cells within the foci reflects the mixed composition of fibroblasts, myocytes, giant cells and occasionally mononuclear leukocytes.

after clinical signs of activity have abated, or latent activity may be present without producing clinically apparent evidence.

Heart. Rheumatic heart disease develops with the initial attack of rheumatic fever in about 50 per cent of cases. Usually the cardiac involvement affects all three layers—the pericardium, myocardium and endocardium—simultaneously. However, the layers may be involved singly or in any combination.

During the acute stage, the **pericarditis** takes the form of a diffuse, nonspecific, fibrinous or serofibrinous inflammation. This is described on page 311.

Myocardial involvement is responsible for most deaths during the **acute** phase of rheumatic fever, and it is largely in the myocardium that the classic Aschoff bodies are found. Gross alterations in the myocardium are minimal and are confined usually to a flabby softening and dilatation of the heart. The Aschoff bodies are found principally in the interfascicular fibrous septa, in the perivascular connective tissue and in the subendothelial region. A histologic diagnosis may be difficult unless Aschoff bodies in the pathognomonic proliferative phase are found.

Most deaths from rheumatic fever occur long after the acute disease has subsided and result from endocardial involvement, principally of the heart valves. Although any of the four valves may be affected, the mitral valve alone is affected in nearly 50 per cent of cases, and the mitral and aortic valves together in an approximately equal number of cases. Occasionally a trivalvular pattern occurs, when the tricuspid valve is affected along with the mitral and aortic valves. It was once thought that isolated aortic valve involvement was fairly common, but it is now believed that such aortic disease is probably only rarely rheumatic in origin (Morrow et al., 1968). During the early, acute phase of rheumatic fever, the leaflets of the affected valve or valves become red, swollen and thickened. Later, a row of tiny, 1 to 2 mm., wartlike, rubbery to friable vegetations, called **verrucae,** form along the lines of closure of the valve leaflets on the surface exposed to the forward flow of blood. These vegetations probably result from erosion of the inflamed endocardial surface where the leaflets impinge upon each other. Similar verrucae may occur along the chordae tendineae of the atrioventricular valves. Histologic examination of these lesions may reveal only precipitated fibrinoid material and nonspecific inflammatory cells. However, often the underlying valve has a palisade of altered fibroblasts intermixed with mononuclear white cells, resembling to some extent the Aschoff body. As organization of the endocardial inflammation takes place, the valvular leaflets become thickened, fibrotic, shortened and blunted. Fibrous bridging across the valvular commissures may produce a rigid "fish-mouth" or "buttonhole" stenotic deformity. The chordae tendineae also become thickened, fused and shortened (Fig. 10–12). With the passage of time, focal calcifications may develop in the affected valves. Sometimes nodular calcific masses virtually fill the sinuses of Valsalva behind the aortic valve, a pattern characteristic of aortic stenosis from other causes as well. When the mitral stenosis is tight, the left atrium progressively dilates and often a thrombus forms within the auricular appendage. The mural endocardium may develop plaque-like thickenings, usually of the atria, called **MacCallum's plaques.** Microscopically, these show pooling of ground substance, sometimes accompanied by Aschoff bodies. In time they tend to undergo fibrosis, leaving only a maplike area of endocardial thickening and wrinkling.

Joints. About 75 per cent of patients with rheumatic fever have rheumatic arthritis. During the early clinical phases of joint involvement, the synovial membranes are thickened, red and granular, and frequently they are ulcerated. Histologically, increased amounts of ground substance, foci of fibrinoid deposition and lesions resembling Aschoff bodies have been described in the synovial membranes and occasionally in the joint capsules, tendons, fasciae and muscle sheaths. These changes are largely reversible, and rheumatic arthritis is classically transient.

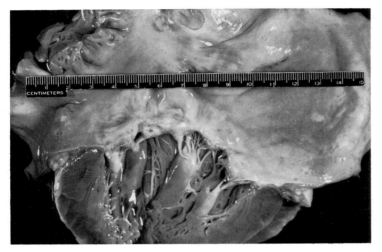

Figure 10-12. Chronic (healed) mitral valvulitis in rheumatic heart disease. The opened valve is markedly thickened, the leaflets have fused and the chordae tendineae are cordlike and shortened. The left atrium is greatly dilated and shows fibrous thickening of the endocardium as a result of chronic distention.

Skin. A minority of patients with rheumatic fever have skin lesions, classically either **subcutaneous nodules** or a rash known as **erythema marginatum.** The subcutaneous nodules are most often found overlying the extensor tendons of the extremities, at the wrists, elbows, ankles and knees. Several or only one of these sites may be involved. The nodules vary in size from 1 to 4 cm. in diameter and are sharply circumscribed, freely moveable, painless masses, often associated with inflammatory hyperemia of the overlying skin. Histologically, they represent large areas of fibrinoid and necrosis resembling confluent Aschoff bodies. Erythema marginatum refers to large, macular, maplike lesions which occur chiefly on the trunk and tend to be migratory.

Blood Vessels. Any of the blood vessels may show foci of acute exudative necrosis accompanied by a polymorphonuclear exudate. These lesions closely resemble the changes of hypersensitivity angiitis and polyarteritis nodosa, but they are distinctive in their tendency to remain localized to the intima. Rheumatic vasculitis is usually an inconspicuous component of rheumatic fever.

Lungs. The lungs occasionally show a nonspecific interstitial pneumonitis similar to that of viral pneumonia. The alveolar septa are thickened by edema and infiltrations of mononuclear leukocytes. Often the alveoli themselves contain a proteinaceous precipitate and fibrin, which may be layered on the alveolar walls to produce hyaline membranes.

Clinical Course. The onset of rheumatic fever may be sudden and stormy, with fever, tachycardia and painful, swollen joints; or it may be insidious and subtle, manifested only by malaise and low-grade fever. When the disease is preceded by a clinically overt streptococcal infection, this has characteristically subsided before the onset of rheumatic fever. *None of the clinical or laboratory features of rheumatic fever is specific for this disease.* The diagnosis must therefore be based on the presence of a constellation of findings. On this basis, the clinical manifestations of rheumatic fever are divided into "major criteria" and the still less specific "minor criteria" (Jones, 1944). It is generally accepted that a diagnosis can be based on the presence of at least two of the major criteria, or on one major and two minor criteria. *Major criteria include polyarthritis, carditis, subcutaneous nodules, erythema marginatum and the presence of the spasmodic involuntary muscle movements termed chorea.* The minor criteria include various indications of a prior streptococcal infection, such as elevated antibody titers to the streptococcal antigens; nonspecific reflections of an inflammatory process, such as leukocytosis, fever and an elevated erythrocyte sedimentation rate; and indirect suggestions of arthritis or carditis, such as arthralgias or a prolonged PR interval on the electrocardiogram. Because patients with a first attack of rheumatic fever are vulnerable to recurrences, a history of rheumatic fever should be weighed heavily when entertaining the diagnosis.

The younger the patient, the more likely it is that there is involvement of the heart. The presence of carditis is indicated by the development of a heart murmur, as a result of either valvular disease or acute myocarditis with dilatation of the heart. Other manifestations of myocarditis, such as arrhythmias and conduction disturbances, may also be present. The combination of auricular thrombosis and atrial fibrillation predisposes to embolization of fragments of the clot.

The prognosis for survival of the acute attack of rheumatic fever is good. Death occurs in only 1 per cent of cases, usually from fulminant myocarditis. The long-term prognosis depends on the presence and severity of the initial carditis. When there is no carditis during the initial attack, almost all patients remain free of rheumatic heart disease, even over long periods of follow-up. Most deaths occur many years after the initial episode, in the so-called healed phase of rheumatic fever, and are attributable to valvular deformities, principally mitral stenosis. During this long phase of compensated heart disease, the heart murmur may be the only indication of cardiac involvement. It was at one time thought that the valves were progressively damaged by the steady continuation of a smoldering rheumatic process. However, it is more likely that progressive valvular disease can be attributed to subclinical exacerbations, as well as to evolving fibrotic reactions and a steadily diminishing tolerance to the hemodynamic derangements. Women show a greater tendency toward progressive valvular scarring than do men and, probably for this reason, they are more vulnerable to long-standing mitral stenosis (Stollerman and Pearce, 1968).

The long-term outlook for patients with cardiac involvement once was poor. However, with antibiotic prophylaxis and successful valvular surgery or prosthetic replacement of damaged valves, the prognosis now is considerably brighter. Without surgery, the 10-year survival rate among patients with mild stenosis of the mitral valve is about 84 per cent. If the initial mitral damage is severe, 10-year survival rate is low. Death from rheumatic heart disease usually results from intractable congestive heart failure. Other frequent causes of death include cerebral embolization, recurrent acute attacks and pneumonia superimposed on long-standing pulmonary congestion. About 4 per cent of a group of patients with rheumatic heart disease developed infective endocarditis over a 10-year period, and this, too, may be a cause of death (Quinn, 1968).

INFECTIVE (VEGETATIVE) ENDOCARDITIS

This form of endocarditis is caused by colonization of the heart, usually the valves, by any of a variety of organisms—including bacteria, fungi, rickettsiae and perhaps viruses. It is one of the most serious of all infections. Usually the organism becomes established at a site already damaged by previous heart disease, but in a minority of cases completely normal heart valves are attacked. Most important among the predisposing lesions are rheumatic heart disease, which underlies about 65 per cent of cases of infective endocarditis, and congenital malformations (principally septal defects and bicuspid aortic valves), which account for about 25 per cent of cases (Hayward, 1973; Quinn, 1968). Occasionally the underlying process is atherosclerotic valvular disease or luetic aortitis. In recent years, the introduction of new and more potent antibiotics, the widespread use of immunosuppres-

sant drugs and, perhaps most importantly, the advent of cardiac surgery have all altered the profile of this form of endocarditis. The nature of the causative organisms has changed dramatically, as will be shown later. In addition, as rheumatic heart disease declines in prevalence and as early corrective surgery for congenital heart malformations becomes widespread, these conditions are becoming correspondingly less important as causes of infective endocarditis. At the same time, atherosclerotic valvular disease is rapidly becoming more important as a predisposing factor. It is not surprising, then, that infective endocarditis, which was once a disease of young people, is now most common in patients over the age of 40 years. Despite these changes, however, the overall incidence of infective endocarditis remains about the same, accounting for approximately 1 per cent of cases of cardiac disease. Surprisingly, after an initial sharp drop in mortality with the introduction of antibiotics, the prognosis, too, has remained unaltered over the past 25 years (Hayward, 1973).

Etiology and Pathogenesis. The following list, drawn from a study of 100 cases of *bacterial* endocarditis between the years 1956 and 1965, shows the frequencies of causative bacteria (Weinstein and Lerner, 1966). Organisms other than bacteria, although becoming increasingly important as causes of infective endocarditis, still account for a relatively small proportion of cases.

	Per Cent
A. Streptococci	
1. *S. viridans*	27
2. Microaerophilic	13
3. *S. faecalis* (enterococci)	8
4. Anaerobic	3
5. Beta hemolytic	3
6. Nonhemolytic	2
B. Staphylococci	
1. *S. aureus*	20
2. *S. albus*	3
C. Negative cultures	14
D. Miscellaneous (one case per organism)	7

Although *S. viridans* is clearly the most common etiologic agent, its frequency has declined markedly in the antibiotic era. Formerly it was responsible for well over 80 per cent of all cases. The pneumococcus, gonococcus and meningococcus have virtually disappeared as important causes of bacterial endocarditis, because they are relatively easily eliminated at their primary site of infection by appropriate antibiotic therapy. As these organisms have declined in importance, other gram-positive cocci, principally the antibiotic resistant staphylococci, the microaerophilic streptococci and the enterococci, have replaced them. The fungi, too, find their lot improved and a wide variety of them, including *Candida albicans*, *Aspergillus fumigatus*, *Histoplasma capsulatum* and *Cryptococcus neoformans*, are being isolated as causes of endocarditis. While gram-negative septicemia is being seen more frequently, the incidence of gram-negative endocarditis fortunately remains relatively small, a fact presumably reflecting the normally high level of circulating antibodies against most gram-negative organisms. Under appropriate conditions, however, virtually any organism may cause endocarditis. In a significant proportion of cases, repeated blood cultures fail to yield a causative organism. In some instances, the causative agent is a strict anaerobe and is difficult to isolate bacteriologically. It has also been suggested that infection with protoplasts or possibly viruses provides another source of endocarditis difficult to diagnose, although this theory has not yet been substantiated. Possibly some cases of marantic endocarditis, to be discussed later, are misdiagnosed as infective endocarditis (Hayward, 1973).

Two factors are of major importance in the development and nature of infective endocarditis: (1) the vulnerability of the patient, and (2) the portal of entrance of the organism into the bloodstream. At one time, bacterial endocarditis was rather rigidly classified as either acute or subacute, according to the virulence of the causative organism. The more common subacute bacterial endocarditis (SBE) was thought to be largely restricted to patients with preexistent valvular lesions, who were thus rendered more vulnerable to relatively avirulent organisms. Acute bacterial endocarditis, by contrast, was caused by virulent organisms, and most often it affected those with normal hearts. Although this view is largely correct, it tends to oversimplify the factor of individual susceptibility. Whereas individuals with normal hearts are highly resistant to endocarditis produced by avirulent organisms, they are not totally immune to the subacute form, especially when the inoculum is large and continuous, as from a contaminated intravenous catheter. On the other hand, those with prior valvular disease are clearly not thereby protected from virulent organisms.

The important modes of entry of the causative organisms are through: (1) dental manipulation, (2) urinary tract instrumentation, (3) respiratory and skin infections, (4) peripartal sepsis, (5) burns, (6) heart surgery, and (7) intravenous catheters. The last two are of increasing importance. Certain clinical situations are fraught with danger. In recent years, as many as 10 to 15 per cent of endocarditis cases have followed cardiotomy. These involve the direct implantation of antibiotic-resistant bacteria or fungi on the exposed surfaces of the heart or on valve prostheses. Frequently, these organisms are coagulase-negative strains of the staphylococci, but often other, extremely bizarre organisms are involved. Pelvic surgery and urologic procedures regrettably provide portals of entry for the gram-negative rods and the enterococci. Drug addicts and patients with polyethylene intravenous catheters that remain in place for long periods of time are prime candidates for the development of infective endocarditis because of the direct introduction of large inocula into the blood with consequent seeding of the heart valves. In general, it can be said that the subacute form of infective endocarditis most often results from spread of the body's normal flora following trauma—for example, after dental procedures. In contrast, acute infective endocarditis usually originates from an active infection elsewhere in the body, such as pneumonia.

Morphology. The anatomic changes of infective endocarditis are usually readily evident. The basic lesion consists of friable, rather bulky masses of the causative organisms, enmeshed in clotted blood, hanging from the leaflets of the affected valves (Fig. 10–13). **These vegetations may be as large as several centimeters in diameter, may occur singly or in a haphazard fashion and usually are located at the free margins of the valve leaflets. In contrast, the vegetations of rheumatic heart disease are considerably smaller and are found in an ordered array at the lines of valve closure, rather than at the free margins.** When infective endocarditis complicates previous heart disease, the vegetations form in the low-pressure pockets created by the preexistent anatomic deformity. Thus, in cases of aortic insufficiency they tend to form on the ventricular edge of the valve leaflets, and in ventricular septal defect they are seen along the right ventricular surface of the defect (Weinstein and Schlesinger, 1974).

In general, the most frequent sites of involvement are the left-sided valves. The aortic valve is involved in 42 per cent of these cases, the mitral valve in 31 per cent, and both in 27 per cent (Buchbinder and Roberts, 1972). In a small number of cases, the valves of the right side of the heart are involved.

Histologically, there is little to be seen save for the irregular, amorphous, tangled mass of fibrin strands, platelets and blood cell debris that, along with the masses of bacteria, constitute the vegetation. The underlying leaflet shows the anticipated vascularization and nonspecific inflammatory response. The bacteria may be extremely difficult to identify and often are deeply buried within the

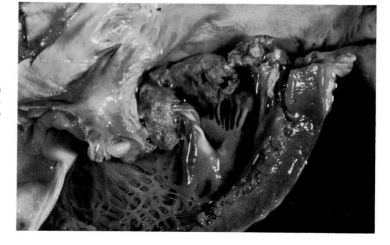

Figure 10–13. Bacterial (vegetative) endocarditis of the mitral valve (streptococcal). The thickened chordae tendineae suggest a preexistent rheumatic disease. The vegetations engulf the mitral leaflets.

vegetation, a situation that explains the difficulty in controlling these infections by antibiotic therapy once they are well developed.

A number of sequelae may ensue. Sometimes the vegetations cause perforation of the underlying valve leaflet or erosion of the chordae tendineae. Suppurative pericarditis may result from direct penetration of the heart wall. In a happy minority of cases, there is spontaneous healing, with progressive organization, fibrosis and calcification of the vegetations. More often, the disease follows a relentless course, with widespread involvement of other tissues. Dissemination of the organisms and fragments of the vegetations through the blood produces small hemorrhages, abscesses or infarction in any tissue or organ of the body.

Renal complications occur so frequently in this disease as virtually to constitute an integral part of the disorder. In 33 to 50 per cent of patients with bacterial endocarditis, the kidneys develop one of many patterns of involvement. Infarctions occur secondary to embolization. More often, glomerular lesions appear, ranging from focal glomerulonephritis (formerly called focal embolic glomerulonephritis) to diffuse proliferative glomerulonephritis. Both forms of glomerulopathy are now considered to represent immune-complex diseases engendered by the immune response of the host to the cardiac infection. Direct embolization of bacteria to the glomeruli has largely been ruled out as a pathogenetic mechanism. The renal lesions are discussed on pages 436 and 437.

Clinical Course. The two dominant clinical features of infective endocarditis are: (1) prolonged fever, and (2) changing cardiac murmurs. In the acute form of the disease the fever may be high and accompanied by chills and leukocytosis. More often the disease is subacute. The changing character of the murmurs, which reflects the buildup and fragmentation of the vegetations, is extremely important, since many patients with this disease have preexistent murmurs. Because the changes in the murmurs may be subtle, the presence of intermittent fever for longer than a week with no apparent cause in a patient with preexistent valvular disease may be reason enough to begin empiric therapy for infective endocarditis. Other manifestations of this disease occur relatively late. They include such vague constitutional symptoms as anorexia, weight loss and weakness. Anemia is common. From the focus of infection on the heart valves, the blood is continuously seeded with the causative organisms, producing metastatic dissemination to distant tissues and organs. Such seeding may give rise to truly protean manifestations of disease, often referable to other organs and thus easily misinterpreted. This embolization frequently leads to abscesses or infarctions, particularly in the spleen, kidneys, brain and joints. Thus, splenomegaly with left upper quadrant pain, hematuria, joint pains and almost any neurologic deficit may be caused by this disease (Ziment, 1969). In addition, mycotic aneurysms may occur in any vessel. Seeding of the nail beds and of the skin produces small petechial hemorrhages, known as "splinter hemorrhages," or microabscesses. Proteinuria and particularly hematuria reflect the development of renal lesions. It has been suggested that not only the renal disease but also other small-vessel manifestations of infective endocarditis may represent immune-complex endarteritis rather than true embolic phenomena (Hayward, 1973). Positive blood cultures establish the diagnosis and can be obtained, in most cases, with repeated attempts. Sometimes, despite repeated negative blood cultures, the diagnosis must be based on the clinical syndrome, and empiric treatment must be instituted promptly.

Before the antibiotic era infective endocarditis was almost invariably fatal. For the past 25 years the overall mortality has remained about 30 per cent. However, if those cases secondary to cardiac surgery—as well as the more fulminant cases and those for which no organism is isolated—are excluded, the mortality is continuing to fall and is now about 14 per cent (Hayward, 1973). The most common cause of death is intractable congestive heart failure due to valvular damage. Cerebral embolism and diffuse glomerulonephritis are less frequent causes of death.

CONGENITAL HEART DISEASE

The exact incidence of congenital heart disease is unknown, but probably it is present in fewer than 1 per cent of live births (Friedberg, 1966). Among children under the age of four years, when rheumatic fever is rare, congenital malformations are the most common form of heart disease. Even among school-age children, the incidence of rheumatic heart disease has declined to the extent that congenital heart disease now is of approximately equal importance. The cause of cardiac anomalies is, in most cases, not clear, but in general they are thought to arise from an interplay of both genetic and environmental factors. Dominant genetic transmission is thought to be involved in atrial septal defects. Other lesions possibly depend on recessively inherited predispositions. Certain environmental hazards are well established, such as contraction by the mother of *rubella* (German measles) during the first trimester of pregnancy, or her ingestion of certain drugs. Influenza, syphilis, tuberculosis and toxoplasmosis in the mother are also suspected of contributing to anomalous development of the fetal heart.

There are a large number of congenital anomalies of the heart. Amost all of them have in common interference with the normal streamlined flow of blood through the chambers of the heart and the great vessels. The resultant turbulence creates heart murmurs that are usually fairly dramatic. In many cases, blood is short-circuited through defects in the heart or great vessels. This diverts blood either toward the systemic circuit or toward the pulmonary circuit. *When blood is shunted from right to left (i.e., toward the systemic vasculature), without passing through the pulmonary tree, the blood is only partially oxygenated and cyanosis is prominent, usually from birth. In contrast, when the blood is short-circuited from left to right, a larger than normal volume of blood reaches the lungs, and there is initially no cyanosis.* However, the resultant pulmonary hypertension, which is eventually transmitted to the right side of the heart, may cause reversal of the shunt. At this point, late in the course, a cyanotic condition termed *cyanose tardive* develops.

The following list, compiled from Friedberg (1966) and from Wood and his colleagues (1954), indicates the most important congenital anomalies, their relative frequencies, and whether they are associated with early cyanosis. The frequencies given are necessarily approximate. Individuals with the more serious lesions die relatively early, hence the reported incidences vary markedly from study to study, according to the age range of the patients.

	Per Cent
A. Congenital anomalies without cyanosis (although there may be cyanose tardive)	
1. Ventricular septal defects (Roger's disease)	20–30
2. Atrial septal defects (variant: Lutembacher's disease)	10
3. Patent ductus arteriosus	13
4. Coarctation of the aorta	10
5. Isolated pulmonic stenosis	10
6. Isolated aortic stenosis	?
7. Anomalies of the coronary arteries	?
B. Congenital anomalies with cyanosis	
1. Transposition of the great vessels	10
2. Tetralogy of Fallot (variant: Eisenmenger's complex)	10

VENTRICULAR SEPTAL DEFECTS

This defect occurs near the atrioventricular septum. It may be minute or as large as several centimeters in diameter. The condition results from a failure of complete fusion of the interventricular septum with the membrane which grows downward from the partition separating the bulbus arteriosus into an aorta and pulmonary artery. A loud systolic murmur, sometimes referred to as a *machinery murmur*, results. Depending upon the size of the defect, life expectancy may be normal or materially reduced. Patients with large, uncorrected defects die in infancy. Those with moderate defects may survive until middle age. In most cases, surgical correction is possible. Since the flow of blood is initially from left to right, right ventricular enlargement develops. Areas of endocardial thickening, called *jet lesions*, may develop in the right ventricle at the point where the jet stream impinges upon the lining of the right ventricular chamber. Eventually pulmonary hypertension with pulmonary vascular sclerosis develops and may become sufficiently severe to cause reversal of blood flow through the defect. Right-sided heart failure is the most common cause of death, followed by vegetative endocarditis on the margins of the defect or on the right ventricular jet lesions.

A variation of this lesion, complete failure of interventricular septal development, creates a common ventricle that is termed *cor triloculare biatriatum.*

ATRIAL SEPTAL DEFECTS

Normally, the atrial septum is created from two adjacent membranes, each with small defects which do not overlie each other. Within the first three months of life, these two membranes usually fuse. Occasionally both membranes are incomplete, but the septum is functionally intact because of the flaplike effect of the membranes when the pressure in the left atrium is higher than the pressure in the right. When these defects are abnormally large, they may overlap each other, creating a hole in the septum. These atrial septal defects occur in females more frequently than in males. They tend to be relatively benign; survival into middle age is usual. Death may occur from right-sided heart failure, *paradoxic embolism* (a condition in which emboli pass through the defect from the right to the left side of the heart into the systemic circulation) or vegetative endocarditis. Surgical correction is commonly successful.

When the septum fails to develop altogether, a common atrium results, a condition known as *cor triloculare biventriculare.*

Occasionally, mitral stenosis of congenital or acquired origin accompanies an atrial septal defect, creating the entity known as *Lutembacher's disease.* The associated mitral stenosis in these cases leads to increased left atrial pressure, resulting in a more marked overload of the right side of the heart than with simple interatrial defects. The attendant pulmonary congestion and vascular sclerosis are also more severe. However, reversal of flow through the defect occurs relatively later, and thus the development of cyanosis is delayed. This lesion too is amenable to surgical correction.

PATENT DUCTUS ARTERIOSUS

Anatomic closure of the ductus arteriosus, which joins the pulmonary artery to the aorta just distal to the origin of the innominate, carotid and subclavian arteries, usually occurs by the third month of life, but sometimes it is delayed for up to a year. When it remains patent, there is shunting of blood from the aorta to the pulmonary artery. This anomaly occurs most often in females. Although it may exist as a solitary lesion, more often it is associated with other congenital malformations. As will be seen later, the patency of the ductus may be life-saving with these multiple anomalies. The morphology of the ductus is quite variable. It may be a distinct vessel, with a length of 1 to 2 cm. and a diameter of 1 to 10 mm., which bridges a gap between the aorta and the pulmonary arterial trunk. In other cases, however, the ductus is merely represented by a fenestration between the apposed pulmonary and aortic trunks.

The most striking clinical feature of a persistent ductus arteriosus is a loud, continuous systolic and diastolic murmur, which has been variously described as machinery-like, humming, sawing, and "train-in-tunnel." The prognosis is relatively good, with average survival to middle age. Death usually results from right-sided heart failure or from vegetative endocarditis. This malformation is readily corrected by surgery.

COARCTATION OF THE AORTA

This anomaly, which shows a striking male preponderance, is of two forms. The *infantile form* is characterized by severe narrowing of the aorta proximal to the ductus arteriosus, which remains patent. The persistence of the ductus arteriosus, then, permits blood to reach the systemic vasculature from the pulmonary artery, while at the same time some of the excessive pulmonary pressure is relieved. Nevertheless, infants with coarctation of the aorta usually die soon after birth, unless surgical repair is accomplished.

Adult coarctation involves a portion of the aorta distal to the ductus arteriosus. Narrowing is less severe and involves a much shorter segment, often appearing as a prominent inner ring or an almost complete membrane. The ductus arteriosus is characteristically closed. In nearly 50 per cent of cases, there is a coexistent bicuspid aortic valve. This adult coarctation anomaly may remain asymptomatic. When symptoms occur, they are usually referable to the severe hypertension in the arterial system proximal to the constriction, with concomitant hypotension distal to the narrowing. Dilated and tortuous collateral vessels develop to the lower half of the body. Prominent among these collaterals are the intercostal arteries which, as they enlarge, cause notching of the ribs. The markedly elevated pressure in the aorta proximal to the coarctation often leads to aortic medionecrosis and dissecting aneurysm (p. 282). Unless coarctation is surgically corrected, death usually occurs before middle age and is attributable most often to rupture of a dissecting aneurysm in the proximal aorta, bacterial invasion of the aorta at the point of narrowing (endarteritis), cerebral hemorrhage from local hypertension or left-sided congestive heart failure.

ISOLATED PULMONIC STENOSIS, ISOLATED AORTIC STENOSIS

These are being recognized with increasing frequency. Often, these stenotic valves are bicuspid. The course of both lesions is extremely variable, depending upon the degree of stenosis.

Symptoms of pulmonic stenosis are dyspnea on exertion and fatigability. Fifty per cent of

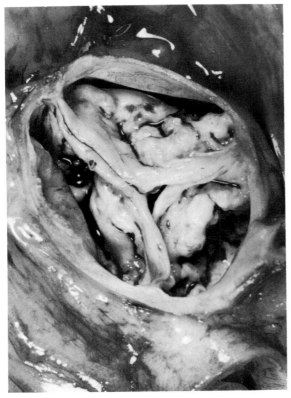

Figure 10–14. Calcific aortic stenosis. A view looking down on the markedly deformed unopened valve with thickened cusps and calcific masses within the sinuses of Valsalva.

these patients die in childhood, usually from right-sided heart failure.

The incidence of congenital aortic stenosis is not known, in part because this anomaly has often been mistakenly attributed to rheumatic heart disease. Recently, it has been suggested that isolated aortic stenosis is probably only rarely caused by rheumatic fever. *Aortic stenosis is probably more often (1) congenital, (2) atherosclerotic, or (3) viral* (Ward and Ward, 1974). *These three forms often cannot be distinguished, so the contribution of each is uncertain* (Fig. 10–14). The congenitally anomalous aortic valve becomes increasingly stenotic with time, as a result of severe calcification. Symptoms such as dyspnea, fatigue and angina pectoris usually develop by early adulthood. Eventually, left-sided CHF develops, and from this point the lesion is rapidly fatal. Occasionally, aortic stenosis first manifests itself in sudden death.

ANOMALIES OF THE CORONARY ARTERIES

A variety of possible anomalies of the coronary arteries may occur, including multiple ostia and unusual sites of origin from the aorta. These are usually without functional significance. However, quite rarely, one or both coronary arteries take their origin from the pulmonary artery rather than from the aorta, and unoxygenated blood is thus delivered to the myocardium. This results in progressive ischemic changes, with eventual heart failure. It will be remembered that this form of congenital anomaly is sometimes associated with endocardial fibroelastosis.

TRANSPOSITION OF THE GREAT VESSELS

This is an extremely grave anomaly, affecting males more often than females. It is characterized by reversed positions of the aorta and pulmonary artery. The cyanosis is usually apparent from birth, along with poor feeding and breathlessness. Most of these infants rapidly develop CHF and die. Longer survival is permitted if there are coexistent anomalies, such as septal defects or a patent ductus arteriosus, which allow communication between the pulmonary and the systemic circuits. Surgical correction is difficult and has a high mortality rate.

A variation of this anomaly, termed *"corrected transposition of the great vessels,"* involves transposition of the ventricles as well as of the aorta and pulmonary artery, so that the aorta emerges from a right-sided ventricle which receives blood from the left atrium, and the pulmonary artery emerges from a left-sided ventricle, which receives blood from the right atrium. Thus, since the aorta receives oxygenated blood and the pulmonary artery unoxygenated blood, the circulation is essentially normal and the anomaly is merely a curiosity.

TETRALOGY OF FALLOT

This is the most common form of cyanotic congenital heart disease that permits survival to adult life. Its components are: (1) a ventricular septal defect, (2) a dextroposed aorta which overrides the septal defect and receives blood from both the right and left ventricles, (3) pulmonic stenosis, and (4) consequent right ventricular hypertrophy. It probably results from anomalous development of the septum, which also affects the relative size and positions of the aorta and pulmonary artery. The course and prognosis of the tetralogy of Fallot vary with the degree of pulmonic stenosis. When this is severe, survival is possible only with a concomitant patent ductus arteriosus, which allows blood to enter the pulmonary vascular bed. Most often, the lesion is manifest from infancy, with cyanosis, dyspnea, clubbing of the fingers and poor feeding and development. Often, cyanosis and dyspnea occur in paroxysms, which arise for no apparent reason, frequently followed by syncope. Unless the condition is amenable to surgical correction or alleviation, the prognosis is generally poor, although it is somewhat better than in transposition of the great vessels. Most patients die in childhood or early adulthood; survival to middle age rarely occurs. Death commonly results from intercurrent respiratory infections, and sometimes from vegetative endocarditis.

The *Eisenmenger complex* is a variant of the tetralogy of Fallot, differing in that pulmonic stenosis is not present. Despite dextroposition of the aorta, some of these patients actually show dilatation of the pulmonary artery. Confusingly, the term Eisenmenger complex is also applied to right-to-left shunting through septal defects when there is pulmonary hypertension of unknown cause.

NONBACTERIAL THROMBOTIC ENDOCARDITIS (MARANTIC ENDOCARDITIS)

This disorder is characterized by the deposition of small masses of fibrin and other blood elements upon the valve leaflets, usually but not necessarily on the left side of the heart. **These vegetations are small, about 1 to 5 mm. in diameter, and resemble those of rheumatic fever, even in their tendency to become aligned along the line of closure of the leaflet.**

The significance and interpretation of these lesions are controversial. In most instances, they are found in patients who have died from a long, debilitating illness, such as cancer or congestive heart failure, hence the adjective "marantic" (wasting). In these instances, the valvular changes are thought to be agonal. Less frequently this form of endocarditis occurs in elderly individuals who are not suffering from a terminal disease or in young people subjected to stress, such as concentration camp inmates. These individuals may follow a clinical course not unlike that of subacute infective endocarditis (Hayward, 1973). It has been proposed that the disorder may be related to an increased tendency toward clotting (hypercoagulable state) (MacDonald and Robbins, 1957).

NONBACTERIAL VERRUCOSE ENDOCARDITIS (LIBMAN-SACKS DISEASE)

Nonbacterial verrucose endocarditis refers to the valvular lesions associated with systemic lupus erythematosus (SLE), and reference should be made to the discussion of this disorder on page 184.

CARCINOID SYNDROME

The carcinoid syndrome is characterized by transient paroxysms of hypotension, cyanosis, bronchoconstriction and diarrhea in patients with argentaffin tumors. Often there are associated lesions of the valves of the right side of the heart, producing murmurs. This interesting syndrome is discussed on page 504.

MYXOMA OF THE HEART

This benign tumor is the most common neoplasm of the heart and the only one to occur sufficiently frequently to warrant description in this chapter. However, it remains one of the least common causes of heart murmur. Myxomas most often develop between the ages of 30 and 60 years, and affect women twice as often as men. It should be stressed that some do not consider the cardiac myxoma a true neoplasm, but rather an organized mural clot.

At any rate, they appear as globular or polypoid masses, arising from the endocardial surface and projecting into the cardiac chambers, most often in the left atrium. Some are sessile, but many are attached by a slender stalk, permitting them to move freely in the blood, sometimes to act as ball-valve obstructions to the heart valves. They are usually covered by a thin glistening endothelial layer and have a semitranslucent, yellow-gray, gelatinous transected surface. Microscopically, they are composed of an abundant acellular ground substance in which are found widely separated spindle or stellate cells resembling fibroblasts or myxoma cells. Scattered within the ground substance are occasional smooth muscle cells, pigmented macrophages, and extracellular hemosiderin. Vessels of varying size are also present, some well developed, others having large cavernous lumina.

The vascular components and the variety of cell types led to the concept that these lesions are actually organizing thrombi. However, a recent electron microscopic study suggests instead that myxomas are true neoplasms arising in multipotential mesenchymal cells capable of differentiating along all the cell lines mentioned (Ferrans and Roberts, 1973).

REFERENCES

Badger, G. F., et al.: Myocardial infarctions in the practices of a group of private physicians. III. J. Chronic Dis., *21*:467, 1968.

Barbour, B. H., et al.: Nontraumatic hemopericardium. An analysis of 105 cases. Am. J. Cardiol., *7*:102, 1961.

Baroldi, G.: Lack of correlation between coronary thrombosis and myocardial infarction or sudden "coronary" heart death. Ann. N.Y. Acad. Sci., *156*:504, 1969.

Bengtsson, E.: Myocarditis and cardiomyopathy. Clinical aspects. Cardiologia, *52*:97, 1968.

Bing, R. J., et al.: What is cardiac failure? Am. J. Cardiol., *22*:2, 1968.

Black, S., et al.: Role of surgery in the treatment of primary infective endocarditis. Am. J. Med., *56*:357, 1974.

Black-Schaffer, B.: Infantile endocardial fibroelastosis. Arch. Path., *63*:281, 1957.

Blattner, R. J.: Myopericarditis associated with Coxsackie virus infection. J. Pediat., *73*:932, 1968.

Bloor, C. M.: Functional significance of the coronary collateral circulation. Am. J. Path., *76*:561, 1974.

Blumgart, H. L., et al.: Angina pectoris, coronary failure and acute myocardial infarction; the role of coronary occlusions and collateral circulation. J.A.M.A., *116*:91, 1941.

Bouchardy, B., and Majno, G.: Histopathology of early myocardial infarcts. Am. J. Path., *74*:301, 1974.

Braunwald, E.: Reduction of myocardial-infarct size. New Eng. J. Med., *291*:525, 1974.

Bryan, C. S., and Oppenheimer, E. H.: Ventricular endocardial fibroelastosis. Basis for its presence or absence in cases of pulmonic and aortic atresia. Arch. Path., *87*:82, 1969.

Buchbinder, N. A., and Roberts, W. C.: Left-sided valvular active infective endocarditis. A study of forty-five necropsy patients. Am. J. Med., *53*:20, 1972.

Burch, G. E., and Giles, T. D.: The role of viruses in the production of heart disease. Am. J. Cardiol., *29*:231, 1972.

Burch, G. E., et al.: Coxsackie B viral myocarditis and valvulitis identified in routine autopsy specimens by immunofluorescent techniques. Am. Heart J., *74*:13, 1967.

Cherubin, C. E., and Neu, H. C.: Infective endocarditis at the Presbyterian Hospital in New York City from 1938–1967. Am. J. Med., *51*:83, 1971.

Clark, C. E., et al.: Familial prevalence and genetic transmission of idiopathic hypertrophic subaortic stenosis. New Eng. J. Med., *289*:709, 1973.

Clark, J. G., et al.: Endocardial fibrosis. Detection by cardiac pacing. Circulation, *38*:1136, 1968.

Dodge, H. T., and Baxley, W. A.: Hemodynamic aspects of heart failure. Amer. J. Cardiol., *22*:24, 1968.

Dudding, B. A., and Ayoub, E. M.: Persistence of streptococcal group A antibody in patients with rheumatic valvular disease. J. Exp. Med., *128*:1081, 1968.

Edington, G. M., and Hutt, M. S. R.: Idiopathic cardiomegaly. Cardiologia (Basel), *52*:33, 1968.

Editorial: Myocardial infarction then and now. Lancet, *1*:395, 1974*a*.

Editorial: Myocardial ischemia without coronary arterial disease. Lancet, *2*:702, 1974*b*.

Editorial: Beta-blockade and size of acute myocardial infarction. Lancet, *2*:813, 1974*c*.

Editorial: Viruses and heart-disease. Lancet, *2*:991, 1974*d*.

Egan, J. D., et al.: Metabolic acidosis in primary myocardial disease. Amer. J. Cardiol., *22*:516, 1968.

Engle, M. A., and Ito, T.: The postpericardiotomy syndrome. Amer. J. Cardiol., *7*:73, 1961.

Erhardt, L. R., et al.: Incorporation of ^{125}I-labeled fibrinogen into coronary arterial thrombi in acute myocardial infarction in man. Lancet, *1*:387, 1973.

Evans, E.: Symposium on pericarditis. Introduction. Amer. J. Cardiol., *7*:1, 1961.

Fabricium-Bjerre, N.: Cardiac arrest following acute myocardial infarction. Acta. Med. Scand., *195*:261, 1974.

Fejfar, Z.: Cardiomyopathies—an international problem. Cardiologia (Basel), *52*:9, 1968.

Ferrans, V. J., and Roberts, W. C.: Structural features of cardiac myxomas. Histology, histochemistry and electron microscopy. Hum. Pathol., *4*:111, 1973.

Fleischer, R. A., and Rubler, S.: Primary cardiomyopathy in nonanemic patients. Association with sickle cell trait. Amer. J. Cardiol., *22*:532, 1968.

Friedberg, C. K.: Diseases of the Heart, 3rd. ed. Philadelphia, W. B. Saunders Co., 1966.

Fuster, V., et al.: Angiographic patterns early in the onset of the coronary syndromes. Am. J. Cardiol., *33*:138, 1974.

Genest, J., et al.: Endocrine factors in congestive heart failure. Amer. J. Cardiol., *22*:35, 1968.

Gery, I., et al.: Transformation of lymphocytes from patients with rheumatic fever by streptolysin. J. Clin. Exp. Immun., *3*:717, 1968.

Glancy, D. L., et al.: Fatal acute rheumatic fever in childhood despite corticosteroid therapy. Amer. Heart J., *77*:534, 1969.

Goodwin, J. F.: Obstructive cardiomyopathy. Cardiologia, *52*:69, 1968.

Gordis, L., et al.: Studies in the epidemiology and preventability of rheumatic fever. II. Socio-economic factors and the incidence of acute attacks. J. Chronic Dis., *21*:655, 1969.

Hales, C. A., and Kazemi, H.: Small-airways function in myocardial infarction. New Eng. J. Med., *290*:761, 1974.

Hardarson, T., et al.: Prognosis and mortality of hypertrophic obstructive cardiomyopathy. Lancet, *2*:1462, 1973.

Hastreiter, A. R., and Miller, R. A.: Management of primary endomyocardial disease. The myocarditis-endocardial fibroelastosis syndrome. Med. Clin. North Amer., *11*:401, 1964.

Hayward, G. W.: Infective endocarditis: a changing disease. Brit. Med. J., *2*:706, 764, 1973.

Holmes, J. C., and Fowler, N. O.: Diagnosis of pericarditis. Postgrad. Med., *44*:92, 1968.

Jenkins, C. D., et al.: Prediction of clinical coronary heart disease by a test for the coronary-prone behavior pattern. New Eng. J. Med., *290*:1271, 1974.

Jewitt, D. E., et al.: Incidence and management of supraventricular arrhythmias after acute myocardial infarction. Amer. Heart J., *77*:290, 1969.

Jones, T. D.: Diagnosis of rheumatic fever. J.A.M.A., *126*:481, 1944.

Joorabchi, B.: Pathogenesis of rheumatic fever. Clin. Pediat., *8*:405, 1969.

Kannel, W. B.: The role of cholesterol in coronary atherogenesis. Med. Clin. North Amer., *58*:363, 1974.

Kaplan, M. N.: Symposium on immunity and the heart. Introduction. Amer. J. Cardiol., *24*:457, 1969.

Kaplan, M. H., and Frengley, J. D.: Autoimmunity to the heart in cardiac disease. Current concepts of the relation of autoimmunity to rheumatic fever, postcardiotomy and postinfarction syndrome and cardiomyopathies. Amer. J. Cardiol., *24*:429, 1969.

Khan, A. H., and Haywood, L. J.: Myocardial infarction in nine patients with radiologically patent coronary arteries. New Eng. J. Med., *291*:427, 1974.

Kloner, R. A., et al.: Effect of a transient period of ischemia on myocardial cells. Am. J. Path., *74*:399, 1974.

Lerner, A. M.: Virus myopericarditis. Ann. Int. Med., *69*:1068, 1968.

Liberthson, R. R., et al.: Pathophysiologic observations in prehospital ventricular fibrillation and sudden cardiac death. Circulation, *49*:790, 1974.

Lie, J. T., et al.: Morphologic evidence of myocardial ischemia in sudden, unexpected death from coronary heart disease. Circulation, *44* (Suppl. II):II–45, 1971.

Lie, K. I., et al.: Immediate prognosis in recurrent myocardial infarction. Lancet, *1*:647, 1975.

Liebow, I. M., and Badger, G. F.: Myocardial infarction in the practices of a group of private physicians. A comparison of patients with and without diabetes. I. The first sixty days. J. Chronic Dis., *16*:1013, 1963.

Lown, B., et al.: Coronary and precoronary care. Amer. J. Med., *46*:705, 1969.

MacAlpin, R. N.: Fugitive coronary occlusion. New Eng. J. Med., *291*:470, 1974.

MacDonald, R. A., and Robbins, S. L.: The significance of nonbacterial thrombotic endocarditis: an autopsy and clinical study of 78 cases. Ann. Int. Med., *46*:255, 1957.

Malakian, A., and Schwab, J. H.: Immunosuppressant from group A streptococci. Science, *159*:880, 1968.

Maroko, P. R.: Assessing myocardial damage in acute infarcts. New Eng. J. Med., *290*:158, 1974.

Mather, H. G., et al.: Acute myocardial infarction: home and hospital treatment. Brit. Med. J., *3*:334, 1971.

Moller, J. G., et al.: Endocardial fibroelastosis. A clinical and anatomic study of 47 patients with emphasis on its relationship to mitral insufficiency. Circulation, *30*:759, 1964.

Morales, A. R., and Fine, G.: Early human myocardial infarction. Arch. Path., *82*:9, 1966.

Morrow, A. G., et al.: Obstruction to left ventricular outflow: Current concepts of management and operative treatment. Ann. Int. Med., *69*:1255, 1968.

Mueller, H. S., et al.: Propranolol in the treatment of acute myocardial infarction. Effect on myocardial oxygenation and hemodynamics. Circulation, *49*:1078, 1974.

Neal, R. W., et al.: Pathophysiological classification of cor pulmonale, with general remarks on therapy. Mod. Concepts Cardiovasc. Dis., *37*:107, 1968.

Niarchos, A. P., and McKendrick, C. S.: Prognosis of pericarditis after acute myocardial infarction. Brit. Heart J., *35*:49, 1973.

Paffenbarger, R. S., Jr., and Hale, W. E.: Work activity and coronary heart mortality. New Eng. J. Med., *292*:545, 1975.

Page, D. L., et al.: Myocardial changes associated with cardiogenic shock. New Eng. J. Med., *285*:133, 1971.

Pelosi, G., and Agliati, G.: The heart muscle in functional overload and hypoxia. A biochemical and ultrastructural study. Lab. Invest., *18*:86, 1968.

Perry, L. W., et al.: Rheumatic fever and rheumatic heart disease among U.S. college freshmen, 1956–65. Public Health Reports, *83*:919, 1968.

Pool, P. E., and Braunwald, E.: Fundamental mechanisms in congestive heart failure. Amer. J. Cardiol., *22*:7, 1968.

Prata, A.: Chagas' heart disease. Cardiologia (Basel), *52*:79, 1968.

Quie, P. G., and Ayoub, E. M.: Rheumatic fever. Postgrad. Med., *44*:73, 1968.

Quinn, E. L.: Bacterial endocarditis. Postgrad. Med., *44*:82, 1968.

Ramalingaswami, V.: Nutrition and the heart. Cardiologia (Basel), *52*:57, 1968.

Rapaport, E.: Prehospital ventricular defibrillation. New Eng. J. Med., *291*:358, 1974.

Reid, P. R., et al.: Myocardial infarct extension detected by precordial ST-segment mapping. New Eng. J. Med., *290*:123, 1974.

Robbins, S. L.: Cardiac pathology—a look at the last five years. Hum. Pathol., *5*:9, 1974.

Roberts, W. C., and Ferrans, V. J.: Pathologic anatomy of the cardiomyopathies. Hum. Pathol., *6*:287, 1975.

Robertson, R., and Arnold, C. R.: Constrictive pericarditis with particular reference to etiology. Circulation, *26*:525, 1962.

Rossen, R. M., et al.: Ventricular systolic septal thickening and excursion in idiopathic hypertrophic subaortic stenosis. New Eng. J. Med., *291*:1317, 1974.

Schwartz, M. J., et al.: Pericardial biopsy. Arch. Int. Med., *112*:917, 1963.

Shell, W. E., and Sobel, B. E.: Protection of jeopardized ischemic myocardium by reduction of ventricular afterload. New Eng. J. Med., *291*:481, 1974.

Sodeman, W. A., and Smith, R. H.: Re-evaluation of the diagnostic criteria for acute pericarditis. Amer. J. Med. Sci., *235*:672, 1958.

Sonnenblick, E. H., et al.: The ultrastructural basis of Starling's law of the heart. The role of the sarcomere in determining ventricular size and stroke volume. Am. Heart J., *68*:336, 1964.

Sonnenblick, E. H., et al.: The ultrastructure of the heart in systole and diastole. Circ. Res., *21*:423, 1967.

Spain, D. M., and Bradess, V. A.: Sudden death from coronary heart disease: survival time, frequency of thrombi and cigarette smoking. Dis. Chest, *58*:107, 1970.

Stannard, M., and Sloman, G.: Ventricular fibrillation in acute myocardial infarction: Prognosis following successful resuscitation. Amer. Heart J., *77*:573, 1969.

Still, W. J. S., and Boult, E. H.: Pathogenesis of endocardial fibroelastosis. Lancet, *2*:117, 1956.

Stollerman, G. H., and Pearce, I. A.: Changing epidemiology of rheumatic fever and acute glomerulonephritis. Adv. Int. Med., *14*:201, 1968.

Theologides, A., and Kennedy, B. J.: Toxoplasmic myocarditis and pericarditis. Amer. J. Med., *47*:169, 1969.

Thygesen, K., et al.: Prognosis after first myocardial infarction. Acta Med. Scand., *195*:253, 1974.

Turner, R., and Ball, K.: Prevention of coronary heart disease. Lancet, *2*:1137, 1973.

Versey, J. M. B., and Gabriel, R.: Soluble-complex formation after myocardial infarction. Lancet, *2*:493, 1974.

Vital Statistics of the United States, 1967. Washington, D.C., United States Department of Health, Education, and Welfare, Public Health Service, 1967.

Wagner, B. M., and Siew, S.: Studies in rheumatic fever. Significance of the human Anitschkow cell. Hum. Pathol., *1*:45, 1970.

Ward, C., and Ward, A. M.: Acquired valvular heart disease in patients who keep pet birds. Lancet, *2*:734, 1974.

Weinstein, L., and Lerner, P. I.: Infective endocarditis in the antibiotic era. New Eng. J. Med., *274*:199, 1966.

Weinstein, L., and Schlesinger, J. J.: Pathoanatomic, pathophysiologic and clinical correlations in endocarditis. New Eng. J. Med., *291*:832, 1974.

Wenger, N. K.: Infectious myocarditis. Postgrad. Med., *44*:105, 1968.

Wood, P., et al.: Ventricular septal defect with a note on acyanotic Fallot's tetralogy. Brit. Heart J., *16*:387, 1954.

Wood, P.: Chronic constrictive pericarditis. Am. J. Cardiol., *7*:48, 1961.

Wu, K. K., and Hoak, J. C.: A new method for the quantitative detection of platelet aggregates in patients with arterial insufficiency. Lancet, *2*:924, 1974.

Ziment, I.: Nervous system complications in bacterial endocarditis. Amer. J. Med., *47*:593, 1969.

Zugibe, F. T., et al.: Determination of myocardial alterations at autopsy in the absence of gross and microscopic changes. Arch. Path., *8*:409, 1966.

CHAPTER 11

The Hematopoietic and Lymphoid Systems

Disorders of the hematopoietic and lymphoid systems encompass a wide range of diseases. They may affect primarily the red cells, the white cells or the hemostatic mechanisms. *Red cell disorders* are usually reflected in *anemia. White cell disorders*, in contrast, most often involve overgrowth, usually malignant. Sometimes these white cell diseases are divided into *myeloproliferative* and *lymphoproliferative* disorders, depending on whether the basic derangement is in the bone marrow or in the lymphoid tissue. However, it is becoming increasingly apparent that this distinction is not always easily made. Therefore, in this chapter we shall consider the white cell disorders together in a single section. Hemostatic derangements result in *hemorrhagic diatheses.* Finally, a group of *miscellaneous disorders*, most of which prominently involve the spleen, are discussed at the end of the chapter.

RED CELL DISORDERS

As mentioned, disorders of the red cells usually result in some form of anemia, although there are exceptions to this rule, such as polycythemia vera. *Anemia* may be considered as a reduction below normal levels of hemoglobin-red cell mass, with consequent impaired delivery of oxygen to the tissues. (Although hemodilution may cause a decrease in hemoglobin-red cell *concentration*, these special cases are not usually associated with impaired oxygenation.) Fundamentally, all anemias are caused by one of the following mechanisms:

A. *Increased losses of red cells*
  1. Hemorrhage
  2. Increased rate of red cell destruction (hemolytic anemias)

B. *Decreased production of red cells*
   1. Nutritional deficiencies
   2. Bone marrow suppression

Those anemias caused by increased losses of red cells are in general associated with a hypercellular and functionally hyperactive bone marrow, which is nevertheless unable to keep pace with the abnormal losses. On the other hand, when the basic derangement is decreased production of red cells, the bone marrow may present a variable picture. Although by definition it is *functionally* hypoactive, it may be hypocellular, normocellular or, as with vitamin B_{12} deficiency, even hypercellular.

HEMORRHAGE—BLOOD LOSS ANEMIA

With acute blood loss, the immediate threat to the patient is hypovolemia with shock, rather than anemia (see p. 213). If the patient survives, hemodilution begins at once and reaches its full effect within 2 to 3 days, unmasking the extent of the red cell loss. Eventually, the red cells are completely replaced, provided that iron stores are sufficient. Although this involves some increased marrow function, it is rarely of a degree to convert areas of inactive fatty marrow into functional marrow. Internal hemorrhages, such as intraperitoneal bleeding, permit total recapture of the iron. On the other hand, with external bleeding, the iron is lost. In these cases, unless there are adequate iron stores, replacement of the red cells is incomplete and iron deficiency anemia results (see p. 334).

Iron deficiency also results from chronic insidious blood loss. In these cases, iron stores are the limiting factor, since both hemodilution and marrow expansion are well able to keep pace with the slow loss of blood.

INCREASED RATE OF RED CELL DESTRUCTION—THE HEMOLYTIC ANEMIAS

Shortened survival of red cells may be due either to inherent defects in the erythrocyte (*intracorpuscular* hemolytic anemia), which are usually inherited, or to external influences (*extracorpuscular* hemolytic anemia), which are usually acquired. The following important disorders will be discussed in this section:

A. Intracorpuscular defects
   1. Hereditary spherocytosis
   2. Sickle cell anemia
   3. Thalassemia
   4. Glucose-6-phosphate dehydrogenase (G-6-PD) deficiency
B. Extracorpuscular abnormalities
   1. Autoimmune hemolytic disease
   2. Toxic, bacterial and physical destruction of red cells
   3. Erythroblastosis fetalis
   4. Malaria

Before proceeding to discuss the various disorders individually, we will here describe certain features common to all hemolytic anemias. All hemolytic anemias are characterized by (1) increased rate of red blood cell destruction, and (2) retention by the body of the products of red cell destruction, including iron. Since the iron is conserved and recycled readily, there is little to limit efforts of the marrow to keep pace with the hemolysis. Consequently, these anemias are almost invariably associated with marked hypercellularity and expansion of the active marrow (*erythron*) into the fatty areas. Sometimes there is also extramedullary hematopoiesis in the liver and spleen. While the shape of the erythrocytes in many of these disorders is bizarre, by and large the mean corpuscular volume (MCV) and mean corpuscular hemoglobin concentration (MCHC) are normal. One of the most striking features of the hemolytic anemias is the hyperactivity of the RE system, which must phagocytize the defective or damaged red cells. Since the *spleen* plays a major role in this process, it is often enlarged, sometimes quite massively.

When the destruction of red cells is intravascular and massive, *hemoglobinemia* with *hemoglobinuria* may result. In these cases, *acute tubular necrosis (ATN)* occasionally follows (see p. 446). Conversion of the heme pigment to bilirubin may lead to *jaundice*, as well as to *cholelithiasis* (see p. 508).

Because the pathways for the excretion of excess iron are limited, there is a tendency in hemolytic anemias for abnormal amounts of iron to accumulate. The iron is deposited in many organs and tissues in the form of *hemosiderin*, which is generally believed to represent insoluble aggregates of ferritin. Since the hemolytic anemias are the most important cause of widespread hemosiderin deposition (*hemosiderosis*), this iron storage disorder will be discussed in some detail here. The hemosiderin first accumulates within the RE cells, where it appears as golden-brown cytoplasmic granules. With the electron microscope, the granules are seen to be membrane-bound within phagosomes. The iron content of hemosiderin is demonstrable by the Prussian blue reaction, in which colorless potassium ferrocyanide applied to the tissue is converted by the iron to blue-black ferriferrocyanide. *Local* hemosiderosis occurs in a number of situations, such as hematomas and hemorrhagic infarcts, which involve the breakdown of extravasated blood. In fact, it is hemosiderin that accounts for the yellowish discoloration which develops several days after a bruise of the skin. *Systemic hemosiderosis*, however, most often results from hemolytic anemia. The tendency toward hemosiderosis is compounded when red cell transfusions are given, adding to the already increased iron stores. Other causes of systemic hemosiderosis are more difficult to define. It appears that the regulation of iron absorption from the gastrointestinal tract is imperfect. Extreme excesses of dietary iron have been shown to lead to an increase in the *absolute* amounts of iron absorbed, even though there is a drop in the percentage absorbed. Excess iron absorption from the GI tract also occurs with underlying liver disease and with alcoholism. Impaired utilization of iron may also lead to hemosiderosis. Evidently this occurs with thalassemia and sideroblastic anemia, both of which involve a defect in hemoglobin synthesis. Whatever the cause, the sites of deposition of hemosiderin in systemic hemosiderosis include the RE cells throughout the body, the spleen, liver, renal tubular lining cells, pancreas and, indeed, in some cases virtually every organ of the body. Only when the RE cells are overloaded does iron enter parenchymal cells in significant amounts. When the accumulations are sufficiently advanced, they impart a brown color to the affected organs. *It is of interest that despite the large accumulation of hemosiderin pigment, hemosiderosis is not known to produce any damage or dysfunction of the involved cells.* This apparent banality of hemosiderosis is in contrast to *hemochromatosis* (p. 530), a disease which also involves the abnormal accumulation of iron but which may lead to severe morbidity and even death. The relationship between these two disorders, if any, is controversial. Some view systemic hemosiderosis as an important step toward the development of hemochromatosis. However, a contrary opinion holds that hemosiderosis does not progress to hemochromatosis unless some concomitant derangement, such as cirrhosis of the liver, is present.

HEREDITARY SPHEROCYTOSIS

The erythrocytes in this hereditary disorder are spherical rather than biconcave, hence they have an increased osmotic fragility. The disorder is transmitted as a dominant trait and affects all races, although most cases occur in whites, particularly those of northern European ancestry.

Etiology and Pathogenesis. The precise pathogenesis of the defect is not entirely clear. Most likely, these erythrocytes have an abnormally permeable cell envelope, which permits the influx of excess sodium. Continued accumulation of sodium within the cell then induces progressive spheroidal dilatation of the erythrocyte with eventual rupture (Jacob and Jandl, 1964). This explanation, however, does not account for the observed fact that splenectomy in these patients abolishes the hemolytic process. In some way, the spleen must play an important role, either directly, by destroying

the red cells, or indirectly, by rendering them vulnerable to destruction (Emerson, 1954). Conceivably sequestration within the spleen with increased anaerobic glycolysis deprives the sodium pump of energy, and so the spherocytes reach the point of hemolysis in this organ (Jacob and Jandl, 1964).

Morphology. On smears the red cells lack the central zone of pallor because of their spheroidal shape. Since the anemia with hereditary spherocytosis is often quite severe, expansion of the erythron is marked and may even cause resorption of the inner layers of cortical bone, with new appositional growth on the outer layers. An irregular, nubbly subperiosteal outer layer may thus be formed, most pronounced on the vault of the skull, where the perpendicular rays of radiodensity on x-ray resemble a "crew haircut."

Splenomegaly is more extreme in this than in any other form of hemolytic anemia. Weights are usually between 500 and 1000 gm., but may be more. The enlargement of the spleen results from striking congestion of the cords of Billroth, leaving the splenic sinuses virtually empty. Phagocytized red cells are frequently seen within hypertrophied sinusoidal lining cells or reticular cord cells. These phagocytic cells may assume multinucleated giant forms. In long-standing cases, hemosiderosis is prominent within the spleen.

The general features of hemolytic anemias described earlier are present with this disorder. In particular, cholelithiasis occurs in from 50 to 85 per cent of these patients.

Clinical Course. Usually hereditary spherocytosis, despite its congenital nature, does not manifest itself until adult life. In some cases, however, it becomes apparent soon after birth. The severity of the disorder is thus highly variable. Asymptomatic cases occur, as well as those characterized by a profound anemia. In general, the anemia is moderate, with red cell counts between 3,000,000 and 3,500,000 per mm.[3] In severe cases, "hemolytic crises" may develop, consisting of a wave of massive hemolysis accompanied by fever, abdominal pain, vomiting and hypotension. Occasionally, these episodes are associated with a mysterious cessation of bone marrow function with consequent thrombocytopenia and leukopenia. *Hereditary spherocytosis is cured by splenectomy.* In the absence of this measure, most cases take a long chronic course; however, a hemolytic crisis may be fatal.

SICKLE CELL ANEMIA (AND OTHER HEMOGLOBINOPATHIES)

The hemoglobinopathies are a group of hereditary disorders characterized by the presence of an abnormal hemoglobin. The prototype and most important of these disorders is sickle cell anemia (*hemoglobin S disease*), which is caused by a genetic defect that is virtually limited to blacks. The morphologic and clinical aspects of this form of anemia will be described briefly here. First, it should be remembered that hemoglobin S results from the hereditary substitution of valine for glutamic acid in the beta polypeptide chains of hemoglobin A. Hemoglobin A, as you will recall, contains two alpha chains and two beta chains ($\alpha_2\beta_2$). It has recently been proposed that an intramolecular hydrophobic bond forms between the two substituted valines in the beta chains, creating an alteration in stereoconfiguration which permits rigid molecular stacking within the red cell. This stacking (*tactoid* formation) distorts the thin membranous envelope of the red cell, particularly at low oxygen tensions (Gabuzda, 1971). Various proportions of Hb-S and normal Hb-A are possible, depending on whether the individual is homozygous or heterozygous. The tendency toward sickling is dependent upon both the amount of Hb-S present in the erythrocyte and the level of oxygen tension. Thus, cells with 100 per cent Hb-S will sickle at normal oxygen tensions, but as the level of Hb-S falls and Hb-A rises, there must be progressively lower oxygen tensions to induce sickling. *In the homozygous individual, 80 to 100 per cent of the hemoglobin is in the Hb-S form, sickling occurs at ordinary oxygen tensions and these patients are said to have sickle cell disease. On the other hand, heterozygous individuals have only 25 to 40 per cent Hb-S, sickling only occurs with unusually low oxygen tensions and the entity is known as sickle cell trait.* The trait is fortunately much more common than the disease. Approximately 8 to 11 per cent of American blacks, and possibly as many as 45 per cent of African blacks, have the trait. However, only 1 in 350 black Americans is homozygous for hemoglobin S and thus has the full-blown disease.

When red cells sickle, they encounter mechanical difficulties in moving through small vessels. The consequent stasis and jamming of these abnormal red cells lead to thromboses and tissue anoxia. Moreover, their increased mechanical fragility results in hemolysis.

Morphology. The anatomic alterations stem from the following three aspects of the disease: (1) hemolysis with resultant anemia, (2) increased release of hemoglobin with bilirubin formation, and (3) capillary stasis with thrombosis. When tissue sections are fixed in formalin so that anaerobiosis develops before complete fixation, sickled red cells are evident as bizarre elongated, spindled or boat-shaped structures. Both the severe anemia and the vascular stasis lead to hypoxic fatty changes in the heart, liver and renal tubules. Fatty marrow is activated. The hypercellularity of the marrow occurs principally at the level of the

normoblasts. Extramedullary hematopoiesis may appear in the spleen and liver. X-rays of the skull often show the "crew-cut" appearance described earlier.

In children there is moderate splenomegaly — up to 500 gm. — caused by congestion of the red pulp with masses of red cells sickled and jammed together. Eventually this splenic erythrostasis leads to enough hypoxic tissue damage, sometimes with frank infarction, to create a shrunken fibrotic spleen. This process is termed **autosplenectomy**, and is seen in all long-standing adult cases. Ultimately, only a small nubbin of fibrous tissue remains of the spleen.

Vascular congestion, thrombosis and infarction may affect any organ (Fig. 11--1). Approximately 50 per cent of adult patients develop leg ulcers because of hypoxia of the subcutaneous tissues. Cor pulmonale may result from thromboses in the pulmonary vessels. As with the other hemolytic anemias, hemosiderosis and gallstones are common.

Clinical Course. Sickle cell disease usually becomes apparent in the second or third year of life, as fetal hemoglobin (Hb-F) is gradually replaced by Hb-S. The anemia is severe, with red cell counts of the order of 2,500,000 per mm.[3] From the time of onset, the process runs an unremitting course, punctuated by sudden episodes of exacerbation of the anemia accompanied by pain. These "sickle cell crises"

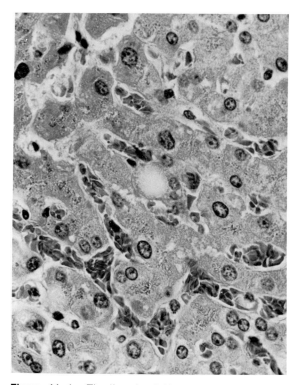

Figure 11-1. The liver in sickle cell anemia. The hepatic sinusoids are stuffed with the misshapen red cells, many of which assume sickle forms. Similar changes occur in other organs, including the spleen.

are thought to be related to poorly understood paroxysms of hemolysis associated with transient depression of the bone marrow. The pain is usually localized to the abdomen (sometimes simulating an acute abdomen), to some portion of the skeletal system or to the central nervous system. Headaches, stiff neck, convulsions, hemiplegia or coma may occur.

The remainder of the clinical findings depend largely on the areas most severely affected by thromboses and hypoxia. Leg ulcers have been mentioned. Cardiac abnormalities resulting from myocardial hypoxia have been reported in up to 90 per cent of adult patients. Although some degree of hepatomegaly is characteristic, *splenomegaly is not found in adults because of autosplenectomy.*

With the full-blown sickle cell *disease*, at least some sickled erythrocytes can be seen on ordinary peripheral blood smear. Ultimately the diagnosis depends on the electrophoretic demonstration of Hb-S. The prognosis is grave, and most patients die before the age of 30 years, usually from thrombosis of a major vessel within some vital structure or from central nervous system damage. Sickle cell *trait*, in contrast, generally remains entirely asymptomatic unless unusual circumstances, such as a plane flight in an unpressurized craft, lead to abnormally low oxygen tensions. Recently attempts have been made to treat sickle cell disease with such agents as glucose-urea solutions or sodium cyanate, which theoretically block the intramolecular bonding between the abnormal beta chains. However, the effect of this form of therapy on the long-term outlook for patients with sickle cell anemia is still uncertain (Editorial, 1974a).

THALASSEMIA

This is a heterogeneous group of disorders characterized by an inherited defect in the *rate* of synthesis of the globin chains in hemoglobin A ($\alpha_2\beta_2$). Diminished alpha chain synthesis is termed *alpha thalassemia;* similarly, *beta thalassemia* results from a decrease in beta globin synthesis (Ingram and Stretton, 1959). The latter is more common, and it is to this pattern that the unqualified term *thalassemia* refers. The result of a beta chain deficit is not only a relative excess of alpha chains within the erythrocytes but also a compensatory increase in Hb-F ($\alpha_2\gamma_2$ or fetal hemoglobin) and Hb-A$_2$ ($\alpha_2\delta_2$). In contrast, a deficit in alpha chains cannot be similarly compensated. Moreover, since alpha thalassemia would affect Hb-F, the fetus would be jeopardized. Perhaps this is the reason for its relative infrequency, at least in the homozygous form.

Beta thalassemia occurs in either a homozygous form (*thalassemia major* or *Cooley's anemia*) or a heterozygous form (*thalassemia minor*). With either, however, the degree of beta chain deficit and the clinical severity are highly variable. The disease was first noted in high frequency among Mediterranean peoples, hence its name (*thalassos*, "sea"). Subsequently, it has also been described in areas of central Africa and southern Asia, as well as among American blacks.

Etiology and Pathogenesis. The fundamental defect with beta thalassemia is not precisely known. Possibly it involves derangements in the regulatory genes controlling the synthesis of beta globin. It has also been persuasively argued that the defect occurs in the structural beta chain gene, such that a defective RNA is produced, which may actually occupy and block the ribosomes (Ingram, 1963). Whatever the fundamental derangement, in both the heterozygote and the homozygote there is a variable degree of beta chain deficit, more severe in the latter than in the former. Hemolysis seems to result not directly from the deficit in beta globin and the consequent reduction in Hb-A, but rather from the relative excess in unstable alpha globin (Weatherall et al., 1969; Vigi et al., 1969). Indeed, the inclusion bodies seen in these red cells are probably aggregates of alpha globin which become associated with the cell membrane. It is thought that they cause hemolysis by altering membrane permeability, possibly by mechanical damage, or perhaps by combining with membrane sulfhydryl (SH) groups (Weatherall et al., 1969).

Morphology. Thalassemia major is characterized by a severe microcytic hypochromic anemia, with red cell counts as low as 1,000,000 per mm.[3] **It should be noted that the reduced mean corpuscular volume (MCV) and mean corpuscular hemoglobin concentration (MCHC) contrast with those of the other hemolytic anemias.** This is accompanied by a decreased capacity for iron utilization with systemic hemosiderosis. Blood smears show a variety of abnormal red cell forms, including markedly immature cells, poikilocytosis and anisocytosis, stippled cells and target cells.

The anatomic changes are those of all hemolytic anemias, but especially prominent are hyperactivity of the bone marrow and splenomegaly. The erythron is expanded to the fetal level, and thus all the fatty marrow may be reactivated. In the red cell series, there is a striking shift toward primitive forms, including erythroblasts and stem cells. A "crew-cut" appearance is seen on skull x-ray as the expanded marrow stimulates neoosteogenesis. In thalassemia, the splenomegaly results from marked extramedullary hematopoiesis, which may also produce hepatomegaly.

Clinical Course. Thalassemia major manifests itself as soon as Hb-F is normally replaced by Hb-A. These children fail to develop normally and are retarded almost from birth. They are sustained only by repeated blood transfusions, and infrequently survive to adulthood. However, milder patterns occasionally are seen. With thalassemia minor there is usually only a mild microcytic hypochromic anemia, which may be discovered only on routine examination. Occasionally the anemia of thalassemia minor is severe and splenomegaly may be present. In general, however, these patients have a normal life expectancy. Of interest is the fact that in both thalassemia major and minor there is a reduced, not increased, osmotic fragility.

GLUCOSE-6-PHOSPHATE DEHYDROGENASE (G-6-PD) DEFICIENCY

A miscellaneous group of congenital hemolytic anemias is based on enzyme deficiencies within the erythrocytes. The prototype and most important of these anemias is caused by an hereditary deficit in G-6-PD, the genetic background for which was mentioned on page 123. This disorder remains asymptomatic unless certain drugs or foods are ingested; only then is a hemolytic anemia precipitated. The list of offending agents continues to grow longer and includes primaquine, quinine, quinidine, some of the sulfonamides, nitrofurantoin, probenecid, vitamin K derivatives, aspirin, phenacetin and fava beans. The induced hemolysis is acute and of variable severity. *However, in all cases it is self-limited, even when the offending agent is continued, since only the older erythrocytes are affected.* As the bone marrow replaces the hemolyzed cells with new red cells, hemolysis becomes insignificant.

AUTOIMMUNE HEMOLYTIC ANEMIA

The nature and pathogenesis of autoimmune hemolytic anemia were discussed on page 174. There it was pointed out that in some patients the disorder arises apparently spontaneously (*idiopathic autoimmune hemolytic anemia*); in the remainder, it is associated with one of a variety of other diseases. These latter conditions include other "autoimmune" diseases such as SLE; the lymphoproliferative disorders; certain interstitial infections, such as that caused by *Mycoplasma pneumoniae*; and the ingestion of some drugs such as alpha methyl DOPA. In a recent review, Dacie (1970) proposed that autoantibodies against a patient's own red cells may arise by one of the following mechanisms:

1. Modification of red cell antigens by, for example, viruses or drugs, so that they become "foreign" to the patient.
2. Formation of antibodies against exogenous antigens, which cross react with the red cells.

3. Enhanced antibody-forming capacity, possibly on a genetic basis.
4. Spontaneous appearance of forbidden clones.

Of particular interest with regard to the last of these mechanisms is the fact that most patients with idiopathic autoimmune hemolytic anemia have some degree of immunoglobulin deficiency, principally diminished IgA levels. Similar deficiencies are also found in those patients whose hemolytic anemia is associated with other autoimmune diseases or with the lymphoproliferative disorders (Blajchman et al., 1969). It has been suggested that in these cases the immune deficit, even when subtle, permits the emergence of a forbidden clone. Thus, the individual patient may have an autoimmune hemolytic anemia, another autoimmune disorder or a lymphoproliferative disorder, singly or in any combination. This hypothesis is carried one step further by Zuelzer and his colleagues, who found a high incidence of cytomegalovirus in children with immune deficiencies and autoimmune hemolytic anemia. They postulated that because of the immune deficit, these children are susceptible to latent viral infections, which in turn induce formation of antibodies that cross react with red cells (Zuelzer et al., 1970).

The anatomic changes are those of all hemolytic disorders, which have been discussed earlier. Clinically, autoimmune hemolytic anemia is similar to the other hemolytic anemias, although it is quite variable in its severity. It yields a positive Coombs test (a technique for detecting antibody coating of red cells). When the anemia is secondary to a disease such as primary atypical pneumonia, it is self-limited; that which is associated with the ingestion of alpha methyl DOPA subsides when the drug is discontinued. In other instances, particularly when the disorder is idiopathic, the hemolysis may be life-threatening and respond only to large doses of corticosteroids. Splenectomy may be helpful in selected cases.

TOXIC, BACTERIAL AND PHYSICAL DESTRUCTION OF RED CELLS

Hemolytic anemia may result from a variety of nonimmune extracorpuscular causes, including the direct toxic effects of phenylhydrazine, heavy metals, hemolysins of bacterial origin and such physical agents as thermal injury and ionizing radiation. *In this category is the hemolytic anemia of lead poisoning* (plumbism), discussed on page 242.

ERYTHROBLASTOSIS FETALIS (HEMOLYTIC DISEASE OF THE NEWBORN)

This disorder results from hemolysis of red cells in the fetus or newborn by maternal antibodies developed against "foreign" antigens in the fetal red cells. Most cases are caused by an ABO blood group incompatibility between mother and child. On the other hand, while Rh incompatibility is a less frequent cause, it tends to produce the more serious expressions of the disease. The exact incidence of erythroblastosis fetalis is difficult to determine, probably because of the wide range of severity and the possible confusion of the milder cases with physiologic jaundice. The incidence of ABO hemolytic disease has been variously given as 1 in 180 births (Halbrecht, 1951) to 1 in 30 births (Rosenfield and Ohno, 1955). Almost always, this form of the disease involves an infant with blood group A or B and a group O mother, as will be discussed later. Probably 1 in 5 such infants develops some degree of hemolytic disease (Mollison, 1967). Disease caused by Rh incompatibility is probably less than half as common but, as was mentioned, is usually more severe.

Etiology and Pathogenesis. The underlying basis of erythroblastosis fetalis is the free passage of antibodies from mother through the placenta to the fetus. Presumably fetal red cells reach the maternal circulation during the last trimester of pregnancy, when the cytotrophoblast is no longer present as a barrier, and also during childbirth itself. The mother thus becomes sensitized to the foreign antigen. With ABO incompatibility, there is no need for prior sensitization of the mother, since all persons normally possess antibodies against the antigens that are not found within their own red cells. However, mysteries remain. Why does only 1 in 5 infants exposed to such antigenic differences develop erythroblastosis fetalis? Why is the disease more likely if the mother of, say, a group B fetus is of blood group O rather than of blood group A? And why is ABO hemolytic disease usually relatively mild? The answers to these questions may lie in part in the type of antibody developed in the mother. Normally, group O individuals have isoagglutinins against A and B red cell antigens, but these are largely of the 19S IgM type, too large to cross the placental barrier. For unknown reasons, some mothers develop 7S IgG red cell agglutinins, and these are small enough to cross the placenta and induce hemolytic disease in the newborn. That the same process does not occur as readily in the group A mother with a group B fetus remains unexplained. All that can be said is that some unknown protective factors must be variably operative in cases of ABO incompatibility (Denborough et al., 1969).

Before discussing the pathogenesis of Rh-induced erythroblastosis fetalis, we should recall that there are perhaps 25 factors belonging to the Rh system. Among these, the strongest Rh antigens are designated C, D and E. The presence of any one of these produces an Rh-positive individual. When these dominant antigens are not present, their place is occupied by less potent alleles (c, d and e), designated Hr antigens. The fetus receives three linked, specific Rh or Hr determinants from each parent. The resulting genotype might be, for example: DCe-Dce. An Rh-negative individual has the genotype dce-dce, and she does not harbor antibodies against the DCE antigens unless there has been prior sensitization, as for example from a blood transfusion or from previous pregnancies. It is thought that small numbers of red cells from an Rh-positive fetus leak into the maternal circulation, probably during the last trimester of pregnancy, and evoke such sensitization. Antibody titers high enough to cause significant disease do not commonly develop until the third such pregnancy, but this is variable. Approximately 15 per cent of Caucasians are Rh-negative. Thus, although there is approximately a 12 per cent chance that an Rh-positive man will have a child by an Rh-negative woman, fortunately only about 5 per cent of Rh-negative mothers ever have infants with hemolytic disease. This lower than anticipated incidence depends on many factors, such as whether the father is homozygous or heterozygous, the degree of any prior sensitization of the mother, her immunologic reactivity, the number of previous pregnancies and the possible coexistence of ABO incompatibility. When concomitant ABO antigenic differences exist between mother and fetus, any Rh-positive fetal cells which escape into the maternal circulation are rapidly lysed, thus minimizing Rh sensitization.

Morphology. The anatomic findings with erythroblastosis fetalis depend entirely upon the severity of the hemolytic process. Sometimes these infants are stillborn, with marked anemia and manifestations of edema and congestive heart failure. Live-born infants may succumb promptly, or within several weeks, unless there is exchange transfusion. Immediate postnatal death is usually caused by severe hemolysis and consequent circulatory failure. In infants who survive, the disease manifests itself in several ways. In its mildest form, the child may be only slightly anemic and survive without further complications (**congenital anemia of the newborn**). With more severe hemolysis, the anemia and pallor are accompanied by obvious hyperbilirubinemia (**icterus gravis**). More extreme forms of the disease are characterized by circulatory failure and severe edema in the pattern known as **hydrops fetalis.** In all forms, the bone marrow is hyperactive and extramedullary hematopoiesis is present in the liver, spleen and possibly other tissues, such as the kidneys, lungs and even the heart. The increased hematopoietic activity accounts for the presence in the peripheral circulation of large numbers of immature red cells, including reticulocytes, normoblasts and erythroblasts (hence the name erythroblastosis fetalis).

When hyperbilirubinemia is marked (usually above 20 mg. per 100 ml. in full-term infants, often less in premature babies), the central nervous system may be damaged (**kernicterus**). The circulating unconjugated bilirubin is taken up by the brain tissue, where it apparently exerts a toxic effect. The brain becomes enlarged, edematous and, when sectioned, has a bright yellow pigmentation of the basal ganglia, thalamus, cerebellum, cerebral gray matter and spinal cord. This pigmentation is evanescent and fades within 24 hours, despite prompt fixation. It is of interest that adults are protected from this effect of hyperbilirubinemia by the blood-brain barrier.

Clinical Course. As was indicated, the clinical patterns of erythroblastosis fetalis vary from lethal disease (stillborn infants) to the mildest degrees of anemia in otherwise healthy children. Kernicterus may manifest itself by apathy and poor feeding, and later by various indications of cerebral irritability, extrapyramidal signs and cranial nerve palsies. It has been postulated that more subtle evidences of motor and mental retardation may result from lower levels of bilirubin (Boggs et al., 1967). With the most severe form of erythroblastosis fetalis (fetal hydrops), the anemia and kernicterus are accompanied by congestive heart failure and generalized edema.

Since severe erythroblastosis fetalis is readily treated by exchange transfusions, early recognition of the disorder is imperative. That which results from Rh incompatibility may be more or less accurately predicted, since it correlates well with rapidly rising Rh antibody titers in the mother during pregnancy. The initial Rh sensitization can be prevented or at least reduced by the administration of anti-D gamma globulin to the vulnerable mother promptly after the birth of an Rh-positive infant. All antigenically challenging fetal red cells are thus eliminated, and since childbirth itself involves the peak period of sensitization, considerable protection is conferred.

Group ABO erythroblastosis fetalis is more difficult to predict, but it is readily monitored by awareness of the blood incompatibility between mother and father, and by hemoglobin and bilirubin determinations on the vulnerable newborn infant.

MALARIA

It has been estimated that 15 to 20 million persons suffer from this infectious disease, hence it is one of the most widespread afflictions of mankind. The fact that the eradication of malaria is theoretically feasible makes its prevalence even more unfortunate (Editorial, 1974*b*). Malaria is caused by one of four types of protozoa: *Plasmodium vivax* causes benign tertian malaria; *Plasmodium malariae* causes quartan malaria, another benign form; *Plasmodium ovale* causes ovale malaria, a relatively uncommon and benign form similar to vivax malaria; and *Plasmodium falciparum* causes malignant tertian, estivo-autumnal or falciparum malaria, which has a high fatality rate. All are transmitted only by the bite of female anopheline mosquitoes, and man is the only natural reservoir.

Etiology and Pathogenesis. The life cycle of the plasmodia is a well understood but complex process, which may require review. Briefly, it consists of two phases: (1) asexual reproduction, or schizogony, which occurs in man, and (2) sexual reproduction, or sporogony, which occurs in the mosquito. When the parasites are introduced into the blood of man by the mosquito, they circulate only briefly, then invade the liver cells (preerythrocytic cycle). This represents the incubation period of malaria. For **P. vivax** and **P. ovale**, it is about 14 days; for **P. malariae**, 24 days; and for **P. falciparum**, 8 to 20 days. Within the liver, the parasites develop into schizonts, which rupture the liver cells and yield free cryptozoites that in turn enter the red cells. During the erythrocytic cycle, further development of the parasites occurs, yielding trophozoites, which are somewhat distinctive for each of the four forms of malaria. Thus, the specific form of malaria can be recognized in appropriately stained thick smears of the peripheral blood. For details on such parasitology, reference should be made to specialized texts. When the trophozoites are fully grown within the red cells, they divide into merozoites, which rupture the erythrocytes and may then reenter other red cells, where they develop into gametocytes that infect the next hungry mosquito.

The distinctive clinical and anatomic features of malaria are related to the following: (1) Showers of new merozoites are released from the red cells at intervals of approximately 48 hours for *P. vivax*, 72 hours for *P. malariae* and 36 hours for *P. falciparum*. The recurrent clinical spikes of fever and chills are timed with this release. (2) The parasites destroy large numbers of red cells and thus cause a hemolytic anemia. (3) A characteristic brown malarial pigment, probably a derivative of hemoglobin that is identical to hematin, is released from the ruptured red cells along with the merozoites, discoloring principally the spleen, but also the liver, lymph nodes and bone marrow. (4) Activation of the phagocytic defense mechanisms of the host leads to marked RE hyperplasia throughout the body, reflected in splenomegaly, hepatomegaly, lymphadenopathy and increased phagocytic activity of the bone marrow.

Morphology. The anatomic changes within the various parts of the body have been best studied with **P. falciparum,** since it is most lethal. The **spleen** is markedly enlarged, up to 1000 grams or more, and is brown as a result of the accumulation of malarial pigment. In the early stages, the capsule is thin, predisposing to rupture, but later fibrosis produces a toughened, thick capsule. In the well-developed case, the histologic appearance is of extreme congestion of the splenic sinuses, with marked hypertrophy and hyperplasia of phagocytic cells. Parasites are seen within the red cells. The phagocytes contain malarial pigment, which in small amounts appears yellow-brown and finely divided, but later, after accumulation, becomes brown-black and clumped. Accompanying the phagocytosis of pigment is engulfment of parasites, leukocytic debris and red cell debris. As a result, the entire spleen eventually becomes transformed into a mass of phagocytic cells, with markedly thickened fibrous trabeculae and capsule, and with considerable compression and narrowing of the vascular sinusoids.

The **liver** is also enlarged, principally because of hypertrophy and hyperplasia of the Kupffer cells. Like the splenic phagocytes, these become heavily laden with malarial pigment, parasites and debris. The changes in the **bone marrow** and **lymph nodes** are of a similar nature. With the other forms of malaria, the morphology is essentially the same, although less severe.

With malignant falciparum malaria, the **brain** is often prominently involved. Parasites abound within the red cells in the vessels. Minute thromboses are seen in these vessels surrounded by ring hemorrhages in the brain tissue. The thromboses are possibly related to disseminated intravascular coagulation (DIC) (see p. 363), and the hemorrhage to the resulting local anoxia. Focal inflammatory reactions **(malarial granulomas)** may occur about these vessels, consisting of a small focus of ischemic necrosis surrounded by a glial reaction. The development of DIC is a serious and fairly frequent complication of falciparum malaria. It has been suggested that a complement-mediated antigen-antibody reaction contributes to the injury of red cells and platelets, which in turn leads to DIC (Sprichaikul et al., 1975).

Clinical Course. Benign malaria is characterized by recurrent paroxysms of shaking chills, high fever and drenching sweats, correlated with the release of merozoites from the ruptured red cells. Occasionally jaundice is evident. There is progressive hepatosplenomegaly, particularly in those long-standing, smoldering cases associated with partial immunity. In the usual course of events, spontaneous recovery ensues or the patient is dramatically benefited by antimalarial drugs. For unknown reasons, however, relapses are frequent with *P. vivax* and *P. malariae.* Indeed, about 30 per cent of patients with vivax malaria have relapses, sometimes as long as 30 years after the initial infection. Whether these cases are associated with persistence of exoerythrocytic forms or imply a continuation of the erythrocytic cycles at low levels is not known.

Fatal falciparum malaria may begin suddenly or slowly, but it is rapidly progressive, with the development of high fever, chills, convulsions, shock and death, usually within days to weeks. In other cases, falciparum malaria may pursue a more chronic course, but may be punctuated at any time by a dramatic complication known as *blackwater fever.* This syndrome is characterized by the sudden onset of severe chills, fever, jaundice, vomiting and the passage of dark red to black urine. The trigger for this complication is obscure, but it is associated with massive hemolysis, leading to jaundice, hemoglobinemia and hemoglobinuria. As has been mentioned, DIC may be a factor in this form of malaria. With adequate treatment, the prognosis with malaria is good.

NUTRITIONAL ANEMIAS

In this category are included those anemias caused by an inadequate supply to the bone marrow of some substance necessary for hematopoiesis. The most common deficiencies are those of iron, folic acid or vitamin B_{12}, and these will be discussed individually. Infrequently, there is a *pyridoxine-responsive anemia* or a *thiamine-dependent anemia.* Although all these deficiencies may stem from dietary inadequacies, they may also result from defective absorption or abnormal losses of the substance, or—in some cases—from a drug antagonism to it.

IRON DEFICIENCY ANEMIA

This is without question the most common of the anemias. It is characterized by the absence of stainable iron in the bone marrow, with impaired hemoglobin synthesis, which results in a microcytic, hypochromic anemia. Although this disorder occurs in all parts of the world and affects both sexes, women during reproductive years are especially vulnerable as a result of their losses of iron through menstruation.

Etiology and Pathogenesis. Normal iron metabolism involves a very limited iron turnover. It will be remembered that the balance between normal losses and absorption of iron is precarious.

Iron deficiency may result from either inadequate absorption of iron or excess loss of iron. Inadequate absorption can be caused not only by an inadequate diet deficient in eggs, meat, liver and vegetables, but also from malabsorption of an adequate diet, such as may occur when inhibitory factors are included in the diet or in association with one of the malabsorption syndromes (page 488).

Losses of iron in excess of normal daily intake are almost always caused by external bleeding. *In males and in nonmenstruating females this necessarily implies pathologic bleeding.* In women of child-bearing age, however, iron deficiency is often the consequence of physiologic losses. Both the menstruating and the pregnant female lose approximately twice as much iron as the male. Marginal iron stores are extremely common in young women, even in those who are not actually anemic.

Morphology. Except in unusual circumstances, iron deficiency anemia is relatively mild. The red cells are microcytic and hypochromic, reflecting the reduced mean corpuscular volume (MCV) and mean corpuscular hemoglobin concentration (MCHC). Although the bone marrow is hyperplastic, particularly at the level of the normoblasts, the active marrow is usually only slightly increased in volume. Extramedullary hematopoiesis is uncommon. Hemosiderosis is, of course, absent.

The skin and mucous membranes of these patients are pale, and the nails may become spoon-shaped and have longitudinal ridges. In some cases, atrophic glossitis is present, giving the tongue a smooth glazed appearance. When this is accompanied by dysphagia and esophageal webs, it comprises the **Plummer-Vinson syndrome** (see page 466).

Clinical Course. In most instances, iron deficiency anemia is asymptomatic. Nonspecific indications, such as weakness, listlessness and pallor, may be present in severe cases. The red cell count is usually only moderately depressed, between 3,000,000 and 4,000,000 cells per mm.³ It must be remembered, however, that the hemoglobin level is reduced below that commensurate with the red cell count, because the cells are microcytic and hypochromic. Deaths from iron deficiency anemia alone are rare.

FOLIC ACID DEFICIENCY ANEMIA

Deficiency of folic acid is associated with a macrocytic megaloblastic anemia. Like iron deficiency, it is an extremely common cause of anemia. In one study, serum folate levels were below normal in up to 47 per cent of patients admitted to a municipal hospital (Leevy et al., 1965). Folic acid deficiency is even more frequent among alcoholics (Herbert, 1963). Together, folic acid deficiency and vitamin B_{12} deficiency are responsible for more than 95 per cent of the megaloblastic anemias, with the former being far more common than the latter (Sullivan, 1970).

Etiology and Pathogenesis. Most often, folate deficiency is simply the result of an inadequate diet, deficient in such foods as green vegetables, citrus fruits and liver. Such a diet is especially likely among alcoholics. Moreover, it has been shown that alcohol itself directly suppresses the response of the marrow to minimum doses of dietary folic acid (Editorial, 1969c). Women in late pregnancy have a sixfold increase in their requirement for folic acid, and so they may develop a folate deficiency anemia on this basis. Many of the malabsorption syndromes (see p. 488), particularly those caused by disease of the proximal small intestine, result in folate deficiency.

A large variety of drugs may interfere with the absorption or utilization of folic acid and thus produce an anemia in the face of normal amounts of folic acid in the diet. These drugs include: (1) Folate antagonists, such as methotrexate, which inhibit the intracellular dihydrofolate reductase necessary for the conversion of folic acid to metabolically active forms; (2) purine analogues, such as 6-mercaptopurine, and pyrimidine analogues, such as 5-fluorouracil; and (3) drugs which impair absorption of dietary folate, such as diphenylhydantoin and some of the oral contraceptives. These act presumably by blocking the intestinal conjugases that split the polyglutamate moieties of folic acid to monoglutamates (Kahn, 1970).

It will be remembered that folic acid as a single carbon donor is necessary for the synthesis of purine and pyrimidine bases. Since these bases are components of DNA, it follows that folic acid deficiency impairs the formation of DNA. Thus, it is not just a hematopoietic disorder but a systemic one. However, because of the rapid turnover of the hematopoietic cells, defective DNA synthesis within the marrow could be expected to slow markedly the rate of cell division. It is postulated that the longer intermitotic interval provides time for these immature erythroid cells to become abnormally large (*megaloblasts*). Normoblasts are not produced fast enough to maintain normal levels of red cells in the peripheral blood. Such red cells as are produced are abnormally large (*macrocytes*). Similar changes affect the granulocytes, which become enlarged (*macropolymorphonuclear cells*) and hypersegmented. With severe folate deficiency anemia, leukopenia and thrombocytopenia may also be present. Iron utilization is impaired and, unless there is a concomitant iron deficiency, increased stores of iron are deposited diffusely within the marrow, and serum iron levels rise.

Morphology. The principal anatomic changes are seen in the bone marrow and blood, with secondary alterations referable to the anemia in severe cases. The bone marrow is markedly hypercellular and extends into areas formerly occupied by inactive fatty marrow. Occasionally there is extramedullary hematopoiesis in the spleen and liver. The hypercellularity results predominantly from increased numbers of megaloblasts, that is, abnormal erythroblasts. These cells are larger than erythroblasts and have a delicate, finely reticulated nuclear chromatin and a strikingly basophilic cytoplasm. Normoblasts are, by comparison, few in number and there is a notable absence of maturing red cells, suggesting a maturation arrest at the megaloblastic level. Stainable iron is present diffusely throughout the marrow rather than in discrete patches, as in normal bone marrow.

In the peripheral blood, the earliest change is usually the appearance of hypersegmented granulocytes. These appear even before the onset of anemia. While the average number of lobes in a granulocyte nucleus is two to three (2.8 ± 0.4), with the megaloblastic anemias this may be markedly increased (Kahn, 1970). Macrocytosis of the red cells may also be present before the development of anemia. Such erythrocytes are oval in shape and are obviously enlarged, with a mean corpuscular volume (MCV) usually ranging between 120 and 150 μm.^{3} (normal, 87 ± 5μm.^{3}). In a minority of patients, however, the MCV remains normal. Although macrocytes appear hyperchromic because of their large size, in reality the mean corpuscular hemoglobin concentration (MCHC) is normal (34 ± 2 per cent).

Clinical Course. Typically patients with folate deficiency anemia are rather sick and present a complex clinical picture, since the malnutrition that is responsible for folic acid deficiency produces other deficiencies as well. In most cases, a clearly inadequate diet is discovered by history, and the patient may appear obviously malnourished. The onset of the anemia is insidious. Eventually it may become profound and cause weakness, dyspnea, syncope and angina pectoris. Although neurologic manifestations are not characteristic of folate deficiency itself, such patients may demonstrate a peripheral neuropathy on the basis of an associated thiamine deficiency. Obvious protein-calorie deficiency may also be present. Many of these patients have hepatosplenomegaly.

The diagnosis of a megaloblastic anemia is readily made from examination of a peripheral smear and the bone marrow. Of importance is the differentiation of the anemia of folate deficiency from that of vitamin B_{12} deficiency. The most direct and accurate means of so doing is by assays for serum folate and vitamin B_{12}. Normal serum folate levels are between 7 and 20 nanograms (ng.) per ml.; levels below 4 ng. clearly are low and at least contribute to any anemia. Although the presence of free gastric acid rules out vitamin B_{12} deficiency caused by true pernicious anemia, it does not rule out normochlorhydric forms of vitamin B_{12} deficiency.

VITAMIN B_{12} (COBALAMIN) DEFICIENCY ANEMIA—PERNICIOUS ANEMIA

Deficiencies of vitamin B_{12} produce a megaloblastic macrocytic anemia very similar in almost all respects to that of folate deficiency. The most common cause of vitamin B_{12} deficiency is *atrophic gastritis*, which is a fundamental component of *pernicious anemia (PA)*. The etiology and pathogenesis of this diffuse and total atrophy of the gastric mucosa are discussed on page 473. Suffice it to say here that PA is not a common disorder, since it affects only 0.1 per cent of the population. Although the classic case occurs in an elderly individual, either male or female, of Scandinavian descent, it has been described in young people and in blacks.

Etiology and Pathogenesis. While PA is the most common cause of impaired absorption of vitamin B_{12}, inadequate intake of this vitamin may also be seen with many of the malabsorption syndromes (see p. 488), particularly those involving the ileum, where vitamin B_{12} is absorbed. Rarely is vitamin B_{12} deficiency caused by simple dietary deficiency—such a diet would have to be bizarre indeed, almost totally devoid of animal protein products.

It is pointed out in the discussion of atrophic gastritis that diffuse and total atrophy of the gastric mucosa with histamine-fast achlorhydria is a component of PA. Since intrinsic factor (IF) is not produced, vitamin B_{12} cannot be absorbed. Pernicious anemia most probably represents an autoimmune derangement, since these patients have circulating autoantibodies against gastric parietal cells. The controversy over whether PA is *ever* associated with the presence of free gastric acid is largely semantic, depending on exactly how one defines the disease. Certainly, there is little disagreement that PA in the adult is virtually always associated with achlorhydria. However, it is often said that, in children, PA may be present without achlorhydria. One juvenile form of PA is characterized by typical diffuse atrophic gastritis, achlorhydria and circulating autoantibodies against IF. However, in other instances, vitamin B_{12} deficiency anemia in children is associated with normal gastric acid. This results from one of the following disorders: (1) a congenital defect in the synthesis of IF (sometimes termed "congenital pernicious anemia"), with a normal gastric acid secretion and without autoantibodies, or (2) the *Grasbeck-Imerslung syndrome*, characterized by defective absorption in the distal ileum of IF-vitamin B_{12} complex (Roitt and Doniach, 1969).

It is not known precisely how a deficiency of vitamin B_{12} leads to megaloblastic erythropoiesis or to the associated neurologic abnormalities which are often present. Quite possibly the hematologic and central nervous system derangements are caused by different mechanisms (Chanarin, 1973). The only known metabolic roles for vitamin B_{12} are in the conversion of methylmalonyl CoA to succinyl CoA and of homocysteine to methionine. The latter reaction is coupled to the conversion of 5-methyltetrahydrofolate to tetrahydrofolate. For some time it was thought that a deficiency of vitamin B_{12} caused the accumulation of 5-methyltetrahydrofolate at the expense of tetrahydrofolate, the active form of folic acid (*methylfolate-trap hypothesis*). Although there is now considerable doubt as to the validity of this hypothesis, it is probable that some interaction between vitamin B_{12} and folic acid underlies the anemia of vitamin B_{12} deficiency (Editorial, 1975a). It has been suggested that vitamin B_{12} may be required for the transport of 5-methyltetrahydrofolate into the cells (Chanarin et al., 1974). In support of this theory is the fact that with vitamin B_{12} deficiency, serum folate levels are usually somewhat high, whereas the folate content of the erythrocytes is low. The issue remains controversial.

Whatever the precise metabolic role of vitamin B_{12}, the result of its deficiency would seem to be diminished DNA synthesis, analogous to that seen with folate deficiency. This affects those cells throughout the body that are the most actively dividing, principally those in the bone marrow and gastrointestinal tract. In addition, for poorly understood reasons, deficiencies of vitamin B_{12}, unlike folate deficiency, lead to characteristic neurologic abnormalities.

Morphology. The appearance of the bone marrow is similar to that described with folate deficiency anemia. It is soft, red, jelly-like and extremely hypercellular, with extension into the formerly inactive areas. A maturation arrest at the megaloblastic level is seen, with nests of megaloblasts and relatively few normoblasts and maturing red cells (Fig. 11–2). Diffuse stainable iron is present.

The peripheral blood picture is also closely similar to that of folate deficiency anemia, with macrocytes and hypersegmented granulocytes as the hallmarks. In general, the MCV is perhaps higher than with folate deficiency; it is very rarely normal.

The atrophic gastritis characteristic of pernicious anemia will be described on page 473. In addition, atrophic glossitis may be present in these patients. The tongue is beefy red, slightly swollen and has a glazed appearance. Histologically, there is nonspecific submucosal chronic inflammation, with atrophy of the overlying epidermis and

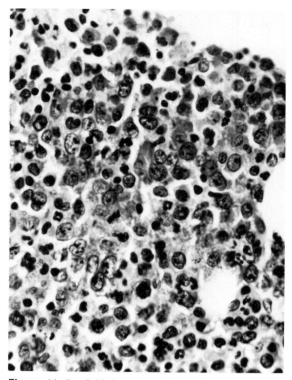

Figure 11–2. A high power detail of bone marrow in pernicious anemia. The center field contains numerous large megaloblasts, identifiable by their vesicular nuclei containing prominent nucleoli. Some of the cells in the periphery are "hypersegmented" neutrophils.

papillae. The neurologic lesions associated with PA (subacute combined degeneration of the spinal cord) are described on page 675.

The elevated levels of unconjugated bilirubin and of serum lactic dehydrogenase (LDH) seen in these patients have been attributed to the intramedullary hemolysis of defective hematopoietic cells. In addition, there is a very slightly shortened survival time of circulating red blood cells (Kahn, 1970). This element of hemolysis contributes to the hemosiderosis that is frequently seen within the liver, spleen and bone marrow. Hepatosplenomegaly, however, is at most minimal. A distinctive lemon-yellow hue is seen in the skin of these patients, but this is not related to the hyperbilirubinemia.

Clinical Course. In general, these patients are less sick than those with folate deficiency anemia. Nonspecific indications of severe anemia include weakness, dyspnea and syncope. Since most of these patients are elderly, the anemia and hypervolemia (which is present for obscure reasons) often lead to angina pectoris, palpitations and high output cardiac failure. As has been mentioned, a distinctive lemon-yellow hue of the skin is classical.

Once a megaloblastic anemia has been diagnosed, the most direct and sensitive method for establishing that it is due to vitamin B_{12} deficiency is by assaying serum vitamin B_{12} levels. The normal range is between 200 and 1000 picograms (pg.) per ml.; under 100 pg. is definitely low. The increased levels of methylmalonyl CoA (MMA-CoA) which occur with vitamin B_{12} deficiency are excreted in the urine, and provide one of the most sensitive and early laboratory tests for vitamin B_{12} deficiency. Of great value is the fact that this test is negative with folate deficiency anemia. Whether or not the vitamin B_{12} deficiency is due to pernicious anemia can be determined directly by IF assay or indirectly by the Schilling test. In these cases, there is histamine-fast achlorhydria. Serum LDH levels are higher than with any other disorder. Like folate deficiency anemia, that due to vitamin B_{12} deficiency responds dramatically and rapidly to the appropriate therapy, with reticulocytosis within 72 hours and clear elevations in red blood cell count within a week. The deranged DNA synthesis characteristic of this form of anemia affects all rapidly metabolizing cells, particularly those in the gastric mucosa. Patients with protracted pernicious anemia have a significantly increased incidence of gastric carcinoma. Perhaps the inhibition of DNA synthesis blocks mitotic division and potentiates nuclear abnormality, which leads in time to cancerous change.

BONE MARROW SUPPRESSION (APLASTIC ANEMIA, AGRANULOCYTOSIS, THROMBOCYTOPENIA AND PANCYTOPENIA)

Suppression of bone marrow function occurs in a wide variety of clinical settings. Most often, all three cell lines are affected, producing a *pancytopenia*. In some cases, however, there is deficient production only of red cells (*aplastic anemia*), of white cells (*agranulocytosis*) or of platelets (*thrombocytopenia*). Thrombocytopenia will be discussed separately in a later section.

Etiology and Pathogenesis. Pancytopenia and aplastic anemia usually occur mysteriously as *idiopathic* disorders. In some of these cases they are associated with lesions of the thymus, particularly thymomas. Less often, marrow failure is clearly the result of exposure to known *myelotoxins*, such as radiant energy, benzene and the wide variety of alkylating agents and antimetabolites used in the treatment of malignant disease. Here the possibility of inducing pancytopenia may be a calculated risk. In addition, a group of *drugs* which are not consistently myelotoxic may, in isolated instances and for mysterious reasons, cause pancytopenia. The chief offenders among these drugs are chloramphenicol and phenylbutazone. Others include the sulfonamides, methylphenylethylhydantoin, gold, mepazine, chlorpromazine and oral hypoglycemic agents. Chemical solvents and insecticides may also cause pancytopenia. When the patient has an identical twin, transfusion of syngeneic marrow cells leads to prompt recovery. This suggests that the disorder involves the injury or destruction of marrow stem cells in a single sweep, without lasting effects on the marrow (Editorial, 1975*b*).

A special form of marrow failure is caused by space-occupying lesions that destroy significant amounts of bone marrow. This is known as *myelophthisic anemia* (perhaps more correctly termed *myelophthisic pancytopenia*), and is most commonly associated with metastatic cancer arising from a primary lesion in the breast, lung, prostate, thyroid or adrenals. Multiple myeloma, leukemia, osteosclerosis, the lymphomas and the reticuloendothelioses are less commonly implicated. Myelophthisic anemia is also seen with a diffuse fibrosis of the marrow, known as *myelofibrosis*. However, this is probably best considered as a myeloproliferative disorder, encompassing proliferation of the stromal fibroblasts (see p. 362).

Milder forms of marrow suppression are seen with *renal diseases*, both acute and chronic, in which there is a normocytic normochromic anemia, probably on the basis of erythropoietin deficiency; *liver diseases*, in which the anemia may be either normocytic or macrocytic; certain *endocrine disorders*, particularly myxedema, which is associated with either a normocytic or macrocytic anemia; *chronic infections;* and *advanced malignant disease.*

Morphology. As was mentioned earlier, the bone marrow may appear hypocellular, normocellular or hypercellular. But we must remember not to equate hypercellularity with increased function. Even **hyper**cellular marrows may be **hypo**functional. In all cases, however, there is failure to produce or release formed elements. Thus, it is obviously impossible from examination of the bone marrow to establish its functional adequacy. **In most cases, the marrow is hypocellular, with an increase in the amount of fat.** Sometimes the more primitive myeloid cells persist, with an apparent failure to form the mature elements. At other times, only the white cell series or only the red cell series may be deficient. Occasionally, there is depletion of megakaryocytes. The marrow in these hypocellular cases becomes sparsely infiltrated with lymphocytes and plasma cells.

Although extramedullary hematopoiesis may be seen in some severe cases, it is usually insignificant, and hepatosplenomegaly is at most minimal.

Secondary morphologic changes depend on which cell lines are affected. With severe anemia, fatty changes may be present in the heart, liver and kidneys.

Thrombocytopenia leads to a characteristic bleeding diathesis (p. 366). Fulminant bacterial infections are common when there is agranulocytosis with a total white cell count of 1000 cells or less per cubic millimeter. With agranulocytosis there is relative lymphocytosis, since the lymphocytes are not affected by the underlying process. The secondary infections take a rather characteristic pattern. Ulcerating necrotizing lesions of the gingiva, floor of the mouth, buccal mucosa, pharynx or anywhere within the oral cavity (agranulocytic angina) are typical. These ulcers are usually deep, undermined and covered by gray to green-black necrotic membranes, from which enormous numbers of bacteria can be isolated. Similar ulcerations may occur in the skin, vagina, anus or gastrointestinal tract. The bacterial growth is massive because of the inadequate leukocytic response. In many instances, the bacteria grow in colony formation (botryomycotic), as though they were cultured on nutrient media.

Clinical Course. Pancytopenia may occur at any age and in both sexes. Usually the onset is gradual, but in some cases the disorder strikes with suddenness and great severity. The initial manifestations vary somewhat depending on the cell line predominantly affected. Anemia may cause the progressive onset of weakness, pallor and dyspnea. Petechiae and ecchymoses may herald thrombocytopenia. Granulocytopenia may manifest itself only by frequent and persistent minor infections or by the sudden onset of chills, fever and prostration. Typically, the red cells are normocytic and normochromic, although occasionally slight macrocytosis is present; reticulocytosis is absent.

Bone marrow biopsy is of aid only when the marrow is hypocellular, or when attempting to exclude myelophthisic anemia. When pancytopenia is secondary to a toxic factor or to some other disorder, the prognosis may be good if the toxin is removed or if the underlying disease is corrected. The idiopathic form of marrow suppression has a bleaker prognosis. Sometimes there is spontaneous remission, but many patients deteriorate rapidly and die within months to a year. Although syngeneic marrow transplantation leads to recovery, allogeneic transplantation is fraught with difficulties, in particular the development of graft-versus-host disease.

POLYCYTHEMIA VERA (PRIMARY POLYCYTHEMIA, VAQUEZ-OSLER DISEASE, ERYTHREMIA)

Polycythemia vera refers to marked increases in the number of red cells without a known physiologic cause. It should be distinguished from *secondary polycythemia*, in which the red cell proliferation occurs as a physiologic response to tissue hypoxia (as in chronic lung disease, right-to-left cardiac shunts and exposure to high altitudes) or to increased levels of erythropoietin (as in certain renal diseases and some malignant tumors).

Polycythemia vera appears insidiously, usually in late middle age. Males are affected somewhat more often than are females, and whites are more vulnerable than blacks.

Etiology and Pathogenesis. The etiology is unknown. No defects in the oxygen absorptive powers of the hemoglobin nor in the oxygen saturation of the marrow can be found. Although a few reports cite excessive levels of erythropoietin, this is most unusual. The disorder is thus considered by many as a neoplastic process analogous to the leukemias (Dameshek, 1951). *Indeed, some experts refer to it as a myeloproliferative disorder because of the fact that in many patients it ultimately becomes transformed into either myelofibrosis or myelogenous leukemia* (pp. 350 and 362). Moreover, even early polycythemia vera typically involves some elevation of white blood cell and platelet levels, as well as the more marked red cell proliferation.

Whatever the underlying cause, the increased red cell mass leads to many secondary alterations, which bear on the morphologic and clinical manifestations. There is a marked increase in total blood volume, sometimes two- or threefold, which may lead to hypertension. This, along with an increase in blood viscosity, places a heavy burden on the heart. A thrombotic tendency can be attributed to the increased viscosity as well as to elevated platelet levels. Paradoxically, these patients simultaneously have an increased bleeding tendency, possibly related to the general plethora.

Morphology. Plethoric congestion of all tissues and organs is characteristic of polycythemia vera. The liver is enlarged and frequently contains foci of myeloid metaplasia. The spleen is also slightly enlarged, up to 250 to 300 gm., and quite firm. The splenic sinuses are packed with red cells, as are all the vessels within the spleen. Occasionally, hematopoiesis can be seen within the red pulp. The major blood vessels are uniformly distended with thick, usually incompletely oxygenated blood.

Thromboses with resultant infarctions are common, affecting most often the heart, spleen and kidneys. For obscure reasons, hemorrhages occur in about a third of these patients, usually in the gastrointestinal tract, oropharynx or brain. Although these hemorrhages are said on occasion to be spontaneous, more often they follow some minor trauma or surgical procedure. Peptic ulceration has been described in about a fifth of these patients.

The basic changes occur in the bone marrow. The erythron is markedly enlarged as the fatty marrow is replaced by dark red, succulent, active marrow. Histologically, striking proliferation of all the erythroid forms is seen, particularly the normoblasts. There is usually some concomitant increase in white cell and platelet formation. This augmented hematopoiesis not only occurs at the expense of the fatty marrow, but may also encroach on the cancellous bone and cortical shafts. If the disease changes its course, the marrow reflects this alteration and thus may become fibrotic or leukemic.

Clinical Course. Patients with polycythemia vera classically are plethoric and often somewhat cyanotic. There may be an intense pruritus. Other complaints are referable to the thrombotic and hemorrhagic tendencies and to hypertension. Headache, dizziness, gastrointestinal symptoms, hematemesis and melena are common. Splenic or renal infarction may produce abdominal pain. Hypertension and the increased blood viscosity may lead to heart failure. Transformation to leukemia is an ominous turn of events. Myelofibrosis is heralded by the reversal from a plethora of blood cells to pancytopenia. It is ironic that these patients, who may once have had to undergo repeated therapeutic phlebotomies, now require blood transfusions.

The diagnosis is usually made in the laboratory. Red cell counts range from 6,000,000 to 10,000,000 per mm.³, with corresponding elevations in hemoglobin and hematocrit values. The white cell count may be as high as 80,000 per mm.³ Classically, granulocyte alkaline phosphatase levels are correspondingly above normal.

About 30 per cent of patients with polycythemia vera die from some thrombotic complication, affecting usually the brain or the heart, 15 per cent from leukemia, an additional 10 to 15 per cent from some hemorrhagic complication and the remainder from a miscellany of causes, sometimes unrelated to this disease (Wasserman, 1954).

A similar but less common entity should be mentioned here—*erythroleukemia*, better known as *Di Guglielmo's disease*. While it also involves an apparently neoplastic proliferation of erythroid cells, the cells are immature erythroblasts rather than mature red blood cells. These nonfunctional cells flood the peripheral circulation and result in a paradoxic anemia. Di Guglielmo's disease is thought to be a variant of acute myelogenous leukemia, discussed on page 350.

WHITE CELL DISORDERS

The most important of the white cell disorders are the malignant proliferative diseases. This category embraces the *lymphomas*, which are characterized by proliferation of native cells within lymphoid tissue; the *leukemias*, which involve flooding of the blood and bone marrow by white cells; and the *dysproteinoses* (or *plasma cell dyscrasias*), which are manifested by the expansion of a single clone of antibody-producing cells. In addition, *Hodgkin's disease*, at one time considered a form of lymphoma, is now classified separately and will be discussed in this section. There are other, less frequent malignant white cell disorders. Some of these can be considered intergradations of the above-mentioned major entities. For example, Waldenström's macroglobulinemia has features of all three—the lymphomas, the leukemias and the dysproteinoses. Together, malignant diseases of the white cells cause about 10 per cent of all cancer deaths. In children under the age of 15 years, they are responsible for a staggering 44 per cent of deaths from cancer.

Few other areas of medicine have enjoyed the attention given to white cell disorders in the past few years. The proliferation of facts and theories has been astounding. Much of the fascination and controversy surrounding white cell disease stems from the growing appreciation of the normal function of the immune system, particularly in protecting against neoplasia. When this system itself becomes the victim of malignant disease and at the same time presumably reacts against it, the picture becomes very complicated. For example, it has become clear that it may not be possible to distinguish a malignant lymphocyte from one transformed in the line of duty by an antigenic stimulus. Before discussing the more fundamental issues being raised, it may be well to review briefly some of the relevant features of the cells of the normal immune system, particularly of the lymphocytes. You will recall that there are two populations of lymphocytes, the T-cells (thymus-dependent), which are necessary for cell-mediated immunity, and the B-cells, which carry immunoglobulins on their surface and are capable of differentiating into immunoglobulin-secreting plasma cells. In postnatal life both T-cells and B-cells are derived from common stem cells within the bone marrow. The same stem cells also give rise to monocytes, granulocytes, red blood cells and platelets. Whether the precursors destined to become lymphocytes are already committed to either the T-cell or B-cell line at the time they leave the bone marrow is unknown. What can be said is that the development of immunologic competence by T-cells requires that they take up temporary residence in the thymus or are, at least, exposed to the thymic hormone, thymosin. Thereafter, the T-cells become dispersed in certain sites throughout the body. In the lymph nodes they are found scattered throughout the deep cortex (paracortex), and in the spleen they occupy the perivascular areas of the white pulp. They are also found in small foci within the GI tract. About 70 per cent of lymphocytes within the circulating blood are T-cells. The B-cells are found in somewhat different, although overlapping, locations. In both the lymph nodes and the white pulp of the spleen, they are concentrated primarily within the lymphoid follicles. They are also scattered throughout the lamina propria of the GI tract and within the bone marrow. About 20 per cent of the circulating lymphocytes are B-cells. Although T-cells and B-cells are identical under the light microscope, they can be distinguished on the basis of receptors or "markers" they carry on their surfaces. Thus, T-cells can be identified by a mysterious ability to bind sheep erythrocytes to their surface to form a rosette pattern ("E rosettes"); by their capacity to undergo transformation in vitro when exposed to the nonspecific mitogen, phytohemagglutinin (PTH); and by their reaction with specific antisera against a theta-like antigen found only in T-cells. B-cells can be distinguished by different (and better understood) marker systems. As you will recall, B-cells have immunoglobulin molecules associated with their cell membranes. These can be demonstrated by immunofluorescent techniques. B-cells also carry surface receptors for the third component of complement (C′3) and for the Fc portion of the IgG molecule. The C′3 receptors have the capacity to bind erythrocytes (E) coated with IgM antibody (A) and complement (C) to form rosettes ("IgM-EAC rosettes"). The Fc receptor can be demonstrated with fluorescein labeled aggregated IgG. Since monocytes may be difficult to differentiate from lymphocytes morphologically, specific markers for them are also of value. Like B-cells, they carry membrane receptors for C′3 and Fc and are capable of forming IgM-EAC rosettes. However, monocytes differ in that they also are capable of forming rosettes

with erythrocytes (E) coated with an IgG antibody (A) in the *absence* of complement ("IgG-EA rosettes"). These marker systems are summarized in Table 11–1.

Recently, scanning electron microscopy has revealed apparently distinguishing morphologic features of T-cells, B-cells and monocytes. In general, T-cells are seen to have a fairly smooth surface, whereas B-cells have multiple tiny villi on their surfaces and monocytes are covered by delicate wavy ruffles. Whether these are truly distinguishing features remains in some dispute. Moreover, in some cells the morphologic characteristics may leave room for doubt; ruffled villi may merge with villous ruffles, and satisfy little but aesthetic tastes.

In contrast to granulocytes, mature lymphocytes are not end-stage cells. When exposed to nonspecific mitogens (such as PTH or pokeweed) or to an antigen to which they are sensitive, they begin active synthesis of nucleic acids and proteins, enlarge and divide—that is, they undergo transformation. Culturing lymphocytes with allogeneic lymphocytes (*mixed lymphocyte culture, MLC*) also induces transformation. When the lymphocytes transform, they undergo a profound change in morphology and are then often termed *immunoblasts.* These cells may be very difficult to differentiate from monocytes (or histiocytes). Moreover, such cells may be mistakenly identified as primitive undifferentiated cells.

Most of the facts just presented have only recently been discovered, and their implications to the study of malignant disease of white cells are only beginning to emerge—and not very neatly, at that. Nevertheless, a great deal of effort is now being directed towards elucidating the origin of malignant white cells by applying our new knowledge of normal white cells and their markers. In this way it is hoped that classifications of white cell diseases which have been primarily morphologic may be refined by information about function. As will be seen, this effort has yielded some interesting results. Along with other studies, it has also raised a number of important questions. Most of these questions will be addressed later in this section. Here we intend only to give you some idea of their nature and range. They include: (1) The validity of the morphologic distinction among immunoblasts, histiocytes (often termed reticulum cells) and undifferentiated cells, and (2) the question of whether lymphomas, leukemias and the dysproteinoses can be sharply differentiated, or whether all three are instead heterogeneous, overlapping sets of disorders. In addition, the very existence of "malignant proliferative" diseases of white cells has been questioned. Some workers believe that many of these

TABLE 11–1. MARKERS FOR LYMPHOID CELLS

	T-Cells	B-Cells	Monocytes
E rosettes	Yes	No	No
Transformation in vitro with PTH	Yes	No	No
Reaction with antiserum against T-cells	Yes	No	No
Reaction with antisera against immunoglobulins	No	Yes	No
Reaction with aggregated IgG	No	Yes	Yes
IgM-EAC rosettes	No	Yes	Yes
IgG-EA rosettes	No	No	Yes

disorders are not malignant, but rather result from a defect in external controls on the cellular proliferation and transformation which characterize an essentially normal immune response. However, this theory is still conjectural. Even if these disorders do represent "malignant diseases," it is established that at least some don't involve increased proliferation at all, but rather are the consequences of a maturation defect with the accumulation of long-lived, immature cells. Thus, even the basic nature of these diseases has become an issue. A good deal of light has been shed on many of these questions in recent years, as will be seen in the later discussions of the individual entities. However, certain cautions should be remembered in accepting the new results. This is particularly true of information based on the identification of cells by markers. It is perfectly possible that markers valid for normal cells may be misleading for abnormal ones. If we recall that, say, lung cancers may produce all manner of ectopic hormones, it should not be difficult to conceive of cancerous T-cells producing surface immunoglobulins and thus masquerading as B-cells (Seligmann, 1974; Nowell et al., 1975; Fialkow, 1974).

Because of all the unanswered questions and because our concepts are undergoing such rapid change, it seems to us wisest to retain the established, largely morphologic classifications of malignant white cell diseases. In particular, we shall classify the lymphomas according to Rappaport (1966). The morphologic classifications have the advantages of widespread use, reasonable simplicity and a fairly good correlation with prognosis. At our present state of knowledge it is premature to attempt a comprehensive classification on the basis of whether the disorders are of stem cell, monocytic, T-cell or B-cell origin. However, we do offer Table 11–2 to show the *probable* origins of some of the malignant white cell disorders, and in the text we shall indicate where this information threatens to modify the older concepts. With this background to fortify us, we may now turn to a discussion of the individual disorders.

THE LYMPHOMAS

The lymphomas are characterized by the proliferation or accumulation of cells native to lymphoid tissue, i.e., lymphocytes, histiocytes or reticular stem cells. Since the lymphomas share the clinical significance of all malignant disease, it will be appreciated that the term "lymphoma," while hallowed by long usage, is actually a misnomer. However, because the more appropriate term, "lymphosarcoma," was once applied to a specific type of lymphoma, use of this term is merely confusing. Lymphomas arise in lymphoid tissue anywhere in the body, usually within lymph nodes, and in most cases they do not diffusely involve the bone marrow or flood the peripheral blood. They cause about 30 per cent of deaths from malignant white cell disease. Although they may develop at any age, they are most frequent between the ages of 50 and 70 years. Men are affected somewhat more often than are women (Silverberg and Holleb, 1975). Certain situations are known to be associated with a greatly increased risk of developing a lymphoma. These include renal transplantation, therapy with immunosuppressive drugs, congenital immune deficiencies and autoimmune diseases, such as SLE. The way in which these conditions predispose to the development of a lymphoma is of great interest, and will be discussed in our consideration of the etiology and pathogenesis of lymphomas. However, because an appreciation of the morphology of lymphomas is helpful in understanding theories about their causation, the morphology will be presented first.

Morphology. The fundamental anatomic changes occur first in the lymph nodes. As the disease advances there is involvement of the liver, spleen and other viscera. In a large series of cases, the cervical lymph nodes were the initial site of involvement in about 40 per cent of cases, and the axillary nodes in 20 per cent. Following them in importance were the inguinal, femoral, iliac and mediastinal nodes (Banfi et al., 1968). Grossly, the affected nodes are enlarged in all forms, and vary in consistency from soft to moderately firm, depending on the amount of fibrous tissue present. In the less aggressive processes, the nodes remain

TABLE 11–2. PROBABLE ORIGINS OF MALIGNANT WHITE CELL DISEASES (CLASSIFIED BY FUNCTIONAL MARKERS)*

I. *Stem Cell Origin*
    Acute lymphocytic leukemia
    Acute myelogenous leukemia
    Chronic myelogenous leukemia
II. *T-Cell Origin*
    Sézary's syndrome
    Some cases of acute lymphocytic leukemia
    Rare cases of chronic lymphocytic leukemia
    ?Hodgkin's disease
    ?Mycosis fungoides
III. *B-Cell Origin*
    Chronic lymphocytic leukemia
    Most lymphomas, including Burkitt's lymphoma
    Waldenström's macroglobulinemia
    Heavy chain disease
    Multiple myeloma
IV. *Monocytic Origin*
    ?"Hairy-cell" leukemia

*Drawn from Hansen and Good (1974) and from Lukes and Collins (1974).

TABLE 11-3. CLASSIFICATION OF LYMPHOMAS*

1. Lymphocytic, well differentiated (WD)
2. Lymphocytic, poorly differentiated (PD)
3. Stem cell (undifferentiated), including Burkitt's
4. Histiocytic
5. Mixed lymphocytic and histiocytic (L & H)

*All may occur in either nodular or diffuse patterns.

discrete and freely moveable, but in other instances, invasion of the capsule and extension into the pericapsular tissues may lead to interadherence and fixation of the nodes, resulting in a matted, irregularly nodular mass of lymphoid tissue. The cut surface is usually fairly homogeneous, yellow-white to pearl gray. Foci of hemorrhage and necrosis may be present with the more aggressive forms.

Table 11—3 presents the histologic classification of Rappaport (1966). This system divides the lymphomas according to whether they are composed chiefly of lymphocytes, of histiocytes or of undifferentiated stem cells. The lymphocytic lymphomas are in turn subdivided according to the apparent differentiation of the cells. **In addition, all forms of lymphoma are thought to occur in either a nodular or a diffuse pattern.** Regardless of cell type, the nodular pattern in general carries a better prognosis, although in some cases it is thought to undergo transition to the more ominous diffuse pattern. An exception to this general rule is the well differentiated lymphocytic lymphoma, which almost always occurs in a diffuse pattern, yet carries a relatively good prognosis. Histologic examination of a lymphomatous node reveals the underlying architecture to be either partially or totally obliterated by neoplastic cells. The sinuses and normal lymphoid follicles are thus flooded by aggregates of neoplastic cells (in the nodular pattern), or by a sea of these cells (in the diffuse pattern). The characteristics of the neoplastic cells themselves are given below for each form of lymphoma.

Lymphocytic Lymphoma, Well Differentiated. In this form, the proliferation is of small to medium-sized, apparently mature lymphocytes, which tend to be of uniform size and configuration. Mitoses are rare. Although nodular distributions may be encountered, the pattern of involvement is usually diffuse, with the monotony of the lymphocytes unbroken by the presence of other cell types (Fig. 11—3). With diffuse involvement, the picture is indistinguishable from that of chronic lymphocytic leukemia. Indeed, well differentiated lymphocytic lymphoma may represent the lymph node origin of chronic lymphocytic leukemia.

Lymphocytic Lymphoma, Poorly Differentiated. The cells are larger than mature lymphocytes and smaller than histiocytes. They are characterized primarily by the marked variability in the size and configuration of their nuclei. The nuclei may be round, elongated or irregular, with amitotic cleavage planes. The nuclear membrane is dis-

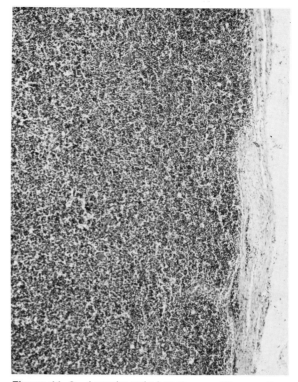

Figure 11-3. Lymphocytic lymphoma, diffuse pattern of involvement. The capsule of the node is on the right. The architecture of the node is obliterated by the monotonous cells, which have obscured the sinusoids.

tinct and the chromatin structure coarse. There is a single nucleolus. Mitoses may be present. This form of lymphoma usually takes a nodular histologic pattern (Fig. 11—4). Occasionally these more anaplastic lymphoid cells display a great deal more aggressiveness and spread beyond the nodes, to produce a localized, large, soft tissue sarcomatous mass, designated by some as a lymphosarcoma in deference to its resemblance to other mesenchymal sarcomas. The term lymphosarcoma has therefore come to be used ambiguously, by some as a generic name for the lymphomas, by others to designate a sarcomatous growth composed of lymphoid cells. The latter usage is preferred and coincides well with the irregular anaplasia of the component cells.

Stem Cell (Undifferentiated) Lymphoma. The stem cells are relatively large, from 15 to 35 μm. in diameter, with large nuclei and pale, scanty cytoplasm. Cell borders are indistinct. The nuclei are round to oval and contain a single small nucleolus and finely divided chromatin. Usually the histologic pattern is diffuse. Interspersed among the stem cells are often large phagocytic histiocytes with abundant cytoplasm, containing phagocytized debris. Against the darker background of neoplastic cells, these create the so-called "starry sky" appearance. Most probably, the histiocytes are benign reactive cells; however, their presence

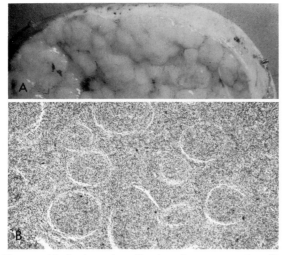

Figure 11–4. Lymphocytic lymphoma, poorly differentiated form, nodular pattern. *A,* A view of the cut surface of an involved lymph node. *B,* A low power microscopic field showing the prominent nodules.

carries a poor prognosis (Oels, 1968). The histologic description just given conforms to that usually accorded the Burkitt lymphoma, to be described later in this chapter. There is therefore much uncertainty about the justification for considering the Burkitt lymphoma as a distinctive variant, but the evidence in support of its viral causation and its peculiar epidemiology warrant this stand, at least for the present.

Histiocytic Lymphoma. The histiocytes show a wide range of variation, depending upon their degree of differentiation. Particularly variable are the amount of cytoplasm and the nuclear size and configuration. With progressive differentiation, the cytoplasm tends to become more abundant, with distinct cell borders. The nucleus is large, often bean or kidney shaped, but frequently quite pleomorphic. Occasionally, these pleomorphic cells are binucleate or multinucleate, and may be very difficult to distinguish from the **Reed-Sternberg cells** of Hodgkin's disease, which will be described later. The nucleolus is usually rather large and prominent, and the chromatin is coarser than in stem cells. Reticulin fibers are usually present in sufficient abundance within the stroma of the node to enclose individual cells. The histologic pattern is either diffuse or nodular. This form of lymphoma was once termed a **reticulum cell sarcoma,** but this term is no longer widely used.

Mixed (L&H) Lymphoma. The very existence of this as a distinct entity is in considerable doubt. Presumably this form of lymphoma involves the simultaneous proliferation of two distinct cell forms, poorly differentiated lymphocytes and histiocytes. However, this interpretation is by no means established since what appear to be histiocytes may simply be transformed lymphocytes. Perhaps it is best to consider this form a variation of the lymphocytic (PD) lymphoma.

The histologic classification given here has come into serious question by several groups of workers (Lukes and Collins, 1974). **Recent evidence suggests that all nodular lymphomas (and probably some of the diffuse ones, as well) are disorders of the B-cells which reside in the germinal centers of the lymphoid follicles (follicular center cells, FCC).** These are the cells which are normally in the process of transformation in response to an appropriate signal. Based on the evidence of an FCC origin for the nodular lymphomas, the objections to Rappaport's histologic classification are twofold: **First, it seems likely that what were considered varying degrees of differentiation may in fact represent stages of transformation.** Thus, cells thought to be primitive may actually be at the opposite end of the spectrum, that is, immunologically quite advanced. **Second, what were termed histiocytes in the older classification may actually be fully transformed B-cells (immunoblasts).** The implications of these possibilities will be more fully explored in the section dealing with the etiology and pathogenesis of the lymphomas.

Whatever the histologic form, with progression, lymph node involvement tends to become more generalized, and the disease often spreads to the spleen, liver and bones, as well as to any other organ. This secondary involvement occurs with the following frequency: liver, 61 per cent; spleen, 54 per cent; bone, 4 to 20 per cent; gastrointestinal tract, 20 per cent; genitourinary tract, 25 per cent; and nervous system, 12 per cent (Jacobs, 1968). In the liver, spleen and bone marrow, the involvement may be diffuse or nodular, or may take the form of a large tumor mass. In the gastrointestinal tract, in which about 5 per cent of lymphomas are said to arise (Jacobs, 1968), the lesions usually take the form of discrete, often polypoid, tumors which may ulcerate, bleed or perforate. Compression of the spinal cord may be caused by extension of paravertebral tumors into the epidural space via the intervertebral foramina or through the vertebrae. In most organs (the kidneys, for example), lymphomatous involvement is predominantly interstitial. The normal parenchymatous elements may thus be widely separated, but their architecture and function are usually preserved.

Etiology and Pathogenesis. Although both the etiology and pathogenesis of the lymphomas are unknown, a number of plausible theories concerning the pathogenesis in turn suggest certain etiologies. Therefore, we shall continue to look at the lymphomas backwards by considering the pathogenesis before the etiology.

There is much evidence for a "two-hit" theory of the development of a lymphoma. *According to this view, some immune stimulus is a necessary first step, followed only later by a neoplastic change.* As mentioned earlier, it has been proposed that most lymphomas arise from follicular center cells (FCC). You will recall that FCC are B-cells which have received some signal to transform—that is, they have been subjected to an antigenic stimulus. In responding to the antigenic stimulus, they normally pass through several stages of transformation, leading to the fully developed immunoblast. Thus, small "virginal" lymphocytes which reach the germinal center undergo a series of morphologic changes, ranging from small to medium-sized "cleaved" cells (cells with an indented nucleus) through medium-sized to large "noncleaved" cells (cells with an oval nucleus) (Editorial, 1974c). The latter are the immunoblasts which are capable of continued proliferation in the presence of a sustained antigenic stimulus. According to Lukes, the development of a lymphoma may involve a block in the transformation of FCC cells (Lukes and Collins, 1974). This may constitute the second event in the two-hit hypothesis. Depending on the level of the block in transformation, the resultant lymphoma may assume any of the morphologic forms described earlier. For example, if transformation is blocked at the small "cleaved cell" stage, the lymphoma might be classified as a stem cell lymphoma. Those lymphomas described as histiocytic would in most cases actually be immunoblastic, since they would involve more or less fully transformed B-cells rather than histiocytes.

Salmon and Seligmann in a provocative hypothesis have similarly related a broader spectrum of white cell disorders to normal stages of B-cell function (Salmon and Seligmann, 1974). They consider normal B-cell function as follows:

1. B_0-cell (stem cell): immunologically uncommitted.
2. B_1-cell (virgin lymphocyte): immunologically committed, but unexposed to antigen.
3. B_2-cell (immunoblast): transformed B-cell.
4. B_3-cell (memory cell): B-cell with previous exposure to antigen but reverted to appearance of virgin lymphocyte.
5. B_4-cell (plasmacytoid lymphocyte): IgM-secreting cell.
6. B_5-cell (plasma cell): immunoglobulin-secreting cell.

According to these workers, B-cells at different stages in their development may be peculiarly vulnerable to certain neoplastic influences. In any given case, the result may be a fairly homogeneous population of white cells arrested at some stage of their development. For example, well differentiated lymphocytic lymphomas may involve proliferation of B_1-cells, whereas "histiocytic" lymphomas may consist of B_2-cells. As we shall see, this hypothesis also would imply that Waldenström's macroglobulinemia develops from B_4-cells and the plasma cell dyscrasias from B_5-cells. Thus, "the proliferating B-cells seem to be 'frozen' at a point along the normal pathway of lymphoid differentiation" (Salmon and Seligmann, 1974). It should be emphasized, however, that the stage of maturation arrest or block in transformation does not necessarily identify the developmental stage of the cell which originally underwent neoplastic change. There is a great deal of evidence that the neoplastic event affects a single cell, the progeny of which may undergo some degree of further maturation. Thus, the neoplastic change may well have occurred in a cell type less mature than those found within the lymphomatous tumor tissue.

Some clues as to the pathogenesis of lymphomas may be gained from a consideration of the known risk factors—renal transplantation, immunosuppressive therapy, congenital immune deficiencies and autoimmune diseases. What are the associations among immune deficiency states (whether congenital or therapeutic), autoimmune diseases and lymphomas? At one time it was thought that the fundamental abnormality was the immune deficiency. According to this view, immune surveillance is so impaired that forbidden clones, which would be destroyed in normal individuals, are able to survive. These forbidden clones may be lymphocytes which react against "self" antigens to produce autoimmune disease, or they may be neoplastic cells which are not recognized as "foreign." Such a hypothesis explains the increased incidence of cancer in patients with immune deficiencies. What it does *not* explain is the selective predisposition to lymphomas as opposed to other tumors. In kidney transplant recipients receiving immunosuppressive drugs, the risk of developing a lymphoma is about 35 times greater than that of the control population, whereas the risk of developing other cancers is only about twice that of normal individuals (Hoover and Fraumeni, 1973). Thus, the forbidden clone hypothesis, although it may explain the slightly increased incidence of cancer in general, does not account for the extreme vulnerability to lymphomas. Clearly, other factors are involved. *It has been suggested that these other factors have in common some interference with the normal negative feedback control of lymphoproliferation.* In normal individuals, negative feedback control of lymphoproliferation is thought to depend on two influences: inhibition by "suppressor" T-cells, and inhibition by antibody of the clone of B-cells which produced it. If either of these feedback mechanisms is impaired, then lymphocyte proliferation and transformation continue unchecked. Thus, certain immune deficiency states may predispose to lymphomas (as opposed to other cancers) by impairment of suppressor T-cell function. It is of interest in this regard that an inbred strain of New Zealand black mice (NZB mice) consistently develops in adulthood an autoimmune disease similar to human SLE, as well as striking lymphoproliferation, often with a subsequent lymphoma. The disease of NZB mice is probably related to a vertically transmitted virus which may produce an immune deficiency state, particularly a defect in "suppressor" T-cells (Gershwin and Steinberg, 1973; Melief et al., 1974). It is intriguing that some of the components of the disease of NZB mice parallel those which predispose to the development of lymphomas in humans. Sustained lymphoproliferation may also result from an inexhaustible supply of antigen, such as occurs with autoimmune disease or with a renal homograft. Thus, kidney transplant recipients may be doubly vulnerable—both through drug-induced depression of suppressor T-cells and through the presence of a continuous source of foreign antigen—that is, the new kidney. In addition to depression of suppressor T-cell function, there are other ways in which negative feedback may be impaired. For example, a block at any point in normal B-cell differentiation may result in failure to produce secretory B-cells capable of elaborating the antibody necessary to inhibit continued expansion of that line of cells. Earlier we discussed the evidence for a block in B-cell maturation or transformation in the lymphomas. We can now appreciate how such a block may be related to excessive lymphoproliferation.

Having discussed ways in which sustained lymphoproliferation may be induced, we come to a highly important issue. What is the relationship between sustained lymphoproliferation and a lymphoma? Is it possible that lymphomatous cells are essentially normal cells devoid of external regulatory controls, or do they at some point undergo internal changes which render them insusceptible to controls? As will be seen, this controversial issue remains unresolved and lurks in the background of much of our consideration of white cell disorders. Most workers would agree, however, that lymphoproliferation provides a fertile soil for the growth of a lymphoma, and that the borderline separating these two conditions is not as clear as we might wish.

Here it is relevant to digress for a moment to describe a newly recognized disorder known as *immunoblastic lymphadenopathy* or *angioimmunoblastic lymphadenopathy with dysproteinemia*. This disorder is of importance because it may represent an intergradation between reactive lymphoproliferation and a lymphoma. It occurs primarily in elderly individuals following chronic antigenic stimulation and is characterized clinically by generalized lymphadenopathy, hepatosplenomegaly, a skin rash and constitutional symptoms (Rappaport and Moran, 1975). Microscopically, there is proliferation of virtually the whole range of B-cells, including mature lymphocytes, immunoblasts, plasmacytoid cells and plasma cells. High levels of serum immunoglobulins are characteristic (Editorial, 1975c). This disorder is clinically fascinating because it may follow one of two entirely different pathways. In some cases, the disease is completely benign and self-limited. In others, however, it behaves as a rapidly progressive malignant disease, leading to death within a few months. The malignant form is sometimes referred to as *immunoblastic sarcoma*. It is thought that treatment with cytotoxic drugs or irradiation may actually contribute to a more malignant outcome. Since immunoblastic lymphadenopathy has only recently been described as a distinct entity, its position among malignant white cell disease is still in considerable doubt. However, at this time it is of great theoretic interest as a possible example of reactive lymphoproliferation run amok.

With this view of the pathogenesis of lymphomas, what can we say of the etiology? A host of viral agents, including the Gross, Graffi, Moloney and Rauscher viruses, have been shown to produce lymphomatous diseases in a variety of experimental animals. In particular, RNA C-type oncogenic viruses (oncornaviruses) can cause leukemia and lymphomas in birds, mice and cats. Recently, oncornaviruses have been implicated in lymphomatous disease of subhuman primates (Gallo et al., 1974). Not unreasonably, then, viruses are suspected of being involved in human lymphomas, although as yet there is no definite proof on this score. Certainly, the suspicion is amply justified by analogy with the diseases of experimental animals. Just what the role of viruses might be, whether causative or merely contributory, is more controversial. The simplest explanation is that viruses are directly causative. This is certainly true of a number of animal viruses, which can transform and establish permanent cell lines *in vitro* and may produce tumors when reinoculated into susceptible hosts.

Alternatively, the role of viruses in the production of lymphomas may be considerably more complicated. There is much speculation that, in humans, latent oncogenic viruses may be activated by a number of influences, such as irradiation, chemicals or other viruses. As discussed in Chapter 3, it has been suggested that the viral genome ("virogene") of oncornaviruses is incorporated into the DNA of all normal cells. According to this theory, the genetic information within the virogene required for malignant transformation ("oncogene") is ordinarily repressed. However, immunoproliferation from any antigenic stimulus may provide an opportunity for derepression of either the virogene or oncogene. Thus, an immune response may activate latent oncogenic viruses (Melief et al., 1974). Support for this concept comes from experiments with the graft-versus-host reaction in mice. It is known that mice subjected to this immunologic reaction frequently develop lymphomas from which oncornaviruses can be recovered. Yet viruses cannot be identified in the lymphocytes of mice of either the recipient or donor strains not undergoing an immunologic reaction (Schwartz, 1972). Other workers believe that the mere expression of latent viruses is not enough to produce disease, but that in addition there must be some genetic alteration of the virus—for example, recombination of DNA during mitosis (Temin, 1974). Still another theory invokes two or more viruses in the production of a lymphoma. The first virus might merely provide the initial immunologic stimulus which is necessary for the possible activation of a latent oncogenic virus. In some cases, the first virus may also act to dampen T-cell suppression of lymphoproliferation, and thus increase the statistical likelihood of a neoplastic event taking place.

None of these theories concerning the possible role of viruses in causing human lymphomas has yet been proved. Since they are not mutally exclusive, it is perfectly possible that more than one may be correct. As we shall see, the evidence for a viral etiology of Burkitt's lymphoma is particularly compelling, and for some of the leukemias is only somewhat less so. However, viruses may not be necessary for the induction of a lymphoma. It is quite possible that latent viruses are only incidentally released during malignant transformation from some other cause. Nevertheless, the consensus is that, at least in some lymphomas, viruses play an important role (Deinhardt, 1974).

Clinical Course. Most lymphoma patients first present as otherwise healthy individuals with painless enlargement of a single node or group of nodes, usually in the cervical chain. At this early stage, the peripheral blood appears entirely normal and bone marrow aspiration is usually normal. Biopsy of the node is required for diagnosis. Occasionally, evidence of extranodal involvement is already present, and indeed symptoms referable to hepatosplenomegaly are the initial complaint in about 25 per cent of patients. With more advanced disease, systemic manifestations occur, including fever, weight loss, weakness and anemia. Lymphadenopathy becomes generalized. The anemia is usually hemolytic, often Coombs positive. Myelophthisic pancytopenia is rare unless there is leukemic transformation, which occurs in about 10 per cent of cases. When leukemic transformation occurs, there is flooding of the blood and bone marrow by the particular lymphomatous cell type. It has been suggested that this is related to a progressive loss of cohesion of the malignant cells. With some of the lymphomas, the association with a corresponding leukemia is much stronger than with others. As mentioned, well differentiated lymphocytic lymphoma is thought simply to represent the tissue expression of chronic lymphocytic leukemia, into which it regularly evolves. In contrast, poorly differentiated lymphocytic lymphoma rarely gives rise to a leukemia. Table 11–4 shows the type of leukemia corresponding to each lymphoma, and indicates the strength of the association (adapted from Lukes, 1968).

As would be expected, the manifestations of advanced widespread disease are truly protean. Involvement of the gastrointestinal tract may produce diarrhea, sometimes with a full-blown malabsorption syndrome (see p. 488), abdominal pain or even complete intestinal obstruction. When the bones are involved, multiple osteolytic defects develop, with resultant pain and pathologic fractures. Enlargement of the kidneys may result from direct lymphomatous infiltration or from obstruction to the lower urinary tract by retroperitoneal tumor tissue. Nervous system involvement can create a bewildering array of central and peripheral findings.

Overall five-year survival with the lymphomas is about 25 per cent (Silverberg and Holleb, 1975). However, in the individual case

TABLE 11–4.

LYMPHOMA	LEUKEMIA	ASSOCIATION
Lymphocytic, well differentiated	Chronic lymphocytic leukemia	++++
Lymphocytic, poorly differentiated	—	—
Stem cell	Acute lymphocytic leukemia	++
Histiocytic	Histiocytic leukemia (Schilling's monocytic)	++

this figure has very little meaning, since the outlook varies widely according to the form of lymphoma, the histologic pattern (whether diffuse or nodular) and the extent of the involvement at the time of diagnosis. A method for staging the extent of involvement with Hodgkin's disease was devised by Peters; this system subsequently was modified and is also applicable to the lymphomas. The modification of Kaplan is given below:

Stage 0: No detectable disease (surgical excision of involved node).

Stage I: Localization to a single node or adjacent group of nodes.

Stage II: Involvement of more than one region, but on only one side of the diaphragm.
   A. Without general symptoms.
   B. With general symptoms, i.e., fever, night sweats, generalized pruritus or marked weight loss.

Stage III: Disease present on both sides of the diaphragm. (This may include the liver or spleen.)
   A. Without general symptoms.
   B. With general symptoms.

Stage IV: Generalized disease demonstrable in bone, lungs, gastrointestinal tract (secondary), skin or kidneys.

(Peters and Middlemiss, 1958; Kaplan, 1962). The extent of lymphomatous disease at the time of diagnosis is by no means independent of the histology, but rather may be considered an expression of it. Thus, the less aggressive histologic patterns tend to be still localized (Stage I) when the patient comes to medical attention. With Stage I disease, five-year survival rate is about 70 per cent (Peters et al., 1968). The best prognosis is offered by the well differentiated lymphocytic lymphoma. Within any one form of lymphoma, the nodular histologic pattern is more benign than the diffuse pattern. Transition to leukemia is an ominous development. Radiotherapy and chemotherapy have considerably altered the natural course of the lymphomas in recent years, and in some instances, with Burkitt's lymphoma for example, apparent cures have taken place.

BURKITT'S LYMPHOMA

This very interesting form of lymphoma was first described by Burkitt in 1958. Although it has the histologic features of the *stem cell lymphoma*, described earlier, its peculiar anatomic distribution, as well as certain epidemiologic features, warrants a separate discussion. *More important, this is the first human cancer that has been strongly linked to a specific virus.*

Burkitt's lymphoma was first described as occurring in a geographic belt extending across Central Africa, where it is the most common type of cancer in children. Subsequently, sporadic cases have been described in other areas, including the United States. In Africa, the disease almost always occurs between the ages of 2 and 14 years, with a median age of 5 years. Most often it manifests itself as a large osteolytic lesion in the jaw (the alveolar process of either the maxilla or mandible) (Fig. 11–5). Of the remaining cases, most present with an abdominal mass. Unlike the other lymphomas, there is usually no significant generalized lymphadenopathy, nor does leukemic transformation usually occur. Without treatment, the disease takes a fulminating course, with death within a year of onset.

In 1964, Epstein and his colleagues described a herpes-like virus which they had isolated from cultures of cells derived from Burkitt's lymphoma tissue. This virus has subsequently become known as the *Epstein-Barr virus* or *EBV*. As we shall see on page 367, it is almost certainly the cause of infectious mon-

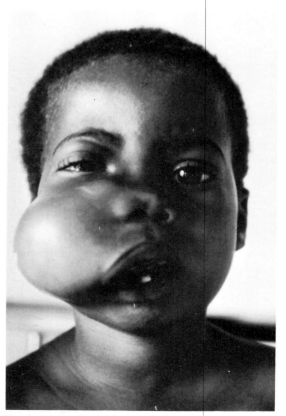

Figure 11–5. Burkitt's lymphoma in a 9 year old child. The maxillary tumor mass is a characteristic presentation of this disease.

onucleosis. Although the evidence that EBV also causes the African form of Burkitt's lymphoma is not conclusive, it is very convincing. Specific antibodies against EBV are found in high titers in all patients with Burkitt's lymphoma. In addition, viral DNA has been demonstrated in the tumor cells by nucleic acid hybridization techniques, and an EBV-determined antigen is present on the cell membranes (Magrath et al., 1975). Most importantly, lymphomas have been induced in nonhuman primates by the inoculation of either EBV-transformed cells or cell-free EBV (Shope et al., 1973; Epstein et al., 1973). In addition, it is a remarkable fact that in order to establish a continuous human lymphoblastoid line *in vitro*, EBV must be present or added to the culture! (Epstein and Achong, 1973). In contrast to the African form of Burkitt's lymphoma, those sporadic cases in the United States do not seem related to EBV (Pagano et al., 1973). Since antibodies against EBV are present in 50 to 80 per cent of the world's adult population, this is obviously a very common virus which, although it may be harbored indefinitely, rarely produces disease (Epstein and Achong, 1973; Hirshaut et al., 1973). Clearly, then, its mere presence is not sufficient to produce a Burkitt's lymphoma. It would seem that in Africa, where Burkitt's lymphoma is endemic, some cofactor must be operative. There is much speculation that this cofactor is the malarial parasite which is endemic in the same geographic regions as is Burkitt's lymphoma. Although malaria is a strong stimulator of the lymphoid system, it also tends to suppress the production of antibodies. This might disrupt the normal negative feedback on lymphoproliferation, as described earlier, and the large population of reactive cells might be vulnerable to malignant transformation by EBV (Epstein and Achong, 1973). Alternatively, chromosomal anomalies (usually a translocation involving chromosome 14) are reported to be present in all Burkitt's lymphomas. Could these anomalies be necessary for EBV oncogenesis (Klein, 1975)? In any case, many studies have indicated that the tumor evolves from the transformation of just one cell and not from a population of cells (Fialkow, 1974). Whatever the causation, the patient's immune response to the tumor seems to play a major role with Burkitt's lymphoma. These patients show a remarkable sensitivity to chemotherapy, and cure is possible in over 50 per cent of African patients with the disease (Burchenal, 1973). This has been correlated not only with pretreatment antibody titers, but also with the development during remission of positive skin tests against autologous tumor extracts.

LEUKEMIA

Leukemia is characterized by diffuse replacement of the bone marrow by more or less immature white cells, which usually also appear in large numbers in the circulating blood. These cells may infiltrate the liver, spleen, lymph nodes and other tissues, thus spreading to organs and tissues throughout the body. Leukemia causes about 45 per cent of deaths from malignant white cell disease, and therefore is the single most important of these disorders. It is particularly devastating to children. For children under the age of 15 years, not only is it by far the most important of the malignant white cell disorders but it also causes fully 33 per cent of *all* cancer deaths.

Leukemia is classified into four major types each of roughly ·equal incidence: (1) acute lymphocytic (sometimes termed lymphoblastic) leukemia, (2) chronic lymphocytic leukemia, (3) acute myelogenous leukemia, and (4) chronic myelogenous leukemia. Table 11–5 shows some of the important distinguishing features of each of these types. However, such a classification is somewhat simplistic, and probably each type is itself heterogeneous. Acute myelogenous leukemia is particularly variable, since any of the cells derived from the myeloblast may be involved. Thus, acute myelogenous leukemia may be further subdivided into myeloblastic, promyelocytic and myelomonocytic forms, as well as erythroleukemia (*Di Guglielmo's disease*). In addition, a monocytic leukemia is recognized. In most cases this is probably of myelogenous origin and may be considered a variant of myelomonocytic leukemia (*Naegeli's leukemia*). However, in a small number of instances, monocytic leukemia may in fact represent true histiocytic leukemia of lymphoid origin (*Schilling's leukemia*). Recently much attention has been given to what may be a distinct form of leukemia, termed "*hairy-cell*" *leukemia* or *leukemic reticuloendotheliosis*. This involves a cell which, with the scanning electron microscope, shows features of both a monocyte and a B-cell. More will be said about this strange disorder later.

Since all leukemias produce similar morphologic changes, they will be discussed together. However, the differences among them will be indicated where relevant, particularly in the discussions of their causation and clinical course.

Etiology and Pathogenesis. Not only is the cause of leukemia unknown, but in some cases the site and cellular origins are in doubt. For example, it is possible that lymphocytic leukemia may arise from clusters of lymphocytes within the bone marrow, from stem cells or

TABLE 11–5

FORM OF LEUKEMIA	AGE	SEX	ENLARGE-MENT OF SPLEEN	ENLARGE-MENT OF LYMPH NODES	ENLARGE-MENT OF LIVER	PROGNOSIS
Acute lymphocytic (~ 20%)	Children	M > F	+	+++	++	4 mo. untreated; 3–6 yr. with therapy
Chronic lymphocytic (~ 30%)	Elderly	M > F	+++	++++	++++	3–4 yr.; may be >10 yr.
Acute myelogenous (~ 25%)	All ages	M > F	++	±	+	6–12 mo.
Chronic myelogenous (~ 25%)	Middle age	M = F	++++	+	++	3–4 yr.

from lymphoid tissue elsewhere in the body. Several studies have been done to determine the origins of leukemic cells by studying their cell "markers," which have yielded interesting results. These will be presented, along with what is known about the causation, for each of the four major types of leukemia. It should be remembered, however, that many workers question the validity of using markers to determine the origins of presumably malignant cells.

Acute Lymphocytic (Lymphoblastic) Leukemia (ALL). The leukemic cells of about 75 per cent of patients with ALL do not have markers associated with either T- or B-cells. These are often termed *"null" cells.* Another 25 per cent have T-cell markers, and a very rare case involves apparent B-cells. Patients with T-cell ALL seem to form a clinically distinct group. They often have thymic masses, and it has been speculated that their disease is more closely related to a form of lymphoma than to null-cell ALL (Sen and Borella, 1975). In contrast, null-cell ALL may represent a disease of marrow stem cells or of lymphoid precursors which have not reached the thymus (Lukes and Collins, 1974). As with the lymphomas, there is much speculation but no proof of a viral etiology. Evidence of recent infection with the Epstein-Barr virus in first-degree relatives of patients with ALL, as well as recent reports of ALL following infectious mononucleosis, has suggested that this virus may play some role. One hypothesis is that the EBV, perhaps through depression of cell-mediated immunity, contributes to activation of a latent RNA tumor virus (Zorbala-Mallios and Sutton, 1974). The possibility that a transmissible agent is involved is supported by reports that in two patients with ALL who received bone marrow transplants the *donor* cells became leukemic (Fialkow, 1974). An alternative interpretation of these reports is that ALL may involve essentially normal cells subjected to an abnormal environment, which somehow results in their proliferation and failure to mature.

Chronic Lymphocytic Leukemia (CLL). Almost all cases of this form of leukemia involve B-cells, with only rare cases of T-cell or null-cell disease (Dickler et al., 1973). As mentioned earlier, the only apparent distinction between CLL and well-differentiated lymphocytic lymphoma is the lack of cohesiveness of the leukemic cells, which permits them to flood the blood and bone marrow. Perhaps CLL and lymphocytic lymphoma (WD) differ merely in their sites of origin or are different stages of the same disease. Therefore, reference should be made to the discussion of the etiology and pathogenesis of the lymphomas on page 344. A fascinating aspect of CLL is the accumulating evidence that it is not a proliferative disorder at all. On the contrary, it seems to involve the accumulation of nonproliferating, immunologically incompetent lymphocytes (Perera and Pegrum, 1974). It is thought that in almost all cases these cells represent the progeny of one deviant cell. Their surface immunoglobulins are monoclonal with one light chain (Fialkow, 1974).

Acute Myelogenous Leukemia (AML). As might be expected, the cells of AML lack both T- and B-cell markers. There are indications that AML is a stem cell disease, since the erythroid line may also be involved (Blackstock and Garson, 1974). Interestingly, the proliferating pool within the bone marrow appears to be decreased rather than increased. Thus, as with CLL, the accumulation of immature cells may be more important in the pathogenesis than is proliferation (Hillen et al., 1975).

Probably we have more clues about the etiology of AML than about any other type of leukemia. In particular, there is exciting new evidence linking AML to an RNA type C tumor virus. Gallo and his colleagues have found "reverse transcriptase" in the leukemic cells of several patients with AML, which was neutralized by antibodies prepared against two nonhuman primate RNA type C tumor viruses. Antibodies against feline, murine and avian RNA type C viruses did *not* inhibit the human enzyme to nearly the same degree (Gallo et al., 1974). More recently, the same group of workers has observed within leukemic cells budding virus particles in cultures of such cells from a patient with AML. In addition, they have shown that the viral particles have the identical sedimentation coefficient of type C RNA virus particles. However, it has not yet been possible to pass the particles serially in any cell culture system, so their oncogenicity remains unestablished. Nonetheless, hybridization studies indicate that this virus is very closely related to the viruses known to cause leukemia and lymphomas in nonhuman primates (Gallagher and Gallo, 1975). This would seem to be the nearest we have come to proving a viral etiology of at least some cases of one type of leukemia (Editorial, 1975*d*). A reported association between the presence of the Epstein-Barr virus and the subsequent development of AML has led to speculation that EBV may cause the activation of an oncogenic RNA tumor virus (Lai et al., 1974).

In addition to viruses, other influences are known to be associated with the development of AML. The experience of the Japanese survivors of the atomic bombs demonstrated only too convincingly the increased risk of AML in individuals subjected to large doses of ionizing radiation. AML may also follow prolonged therapy with alkylating agents for unrelated disorders, and it sometimes terminates other myeloid disorders, such as myeloid metaplasia, aplastic anemia, polycythemia vera or *chronic* myelogenous leukemia (Cardamone et al., 1974).

Regardless of the etiology, the induction of mutations may be an important pathogenetic pathway. Chromosome abnormalities are discernible in 30 to 50 per cent of patients with AML (Blackstock and Garson, 1974). In one study, these consistently took the form of trisomy of chromosome 9, sometimes along with variable changes in chromosome 21 and deletions of chromosome 8 (Ford and Pittman, 1974). However, the data on this subject are not consistent from study to study, and a host of chromosomal abnormalities have been described.

Chronic Myelogenous Leukemia (CML).

This form of leukemia involves granulocytes, which in 90 per cent of patients contain a specific chromosomal abnormality known as the "*Philadelphia chromosome*" (*Ph*[1]-*chromosome*). The Ph[1] chromosome is actually a rearrangement of chromosomes involving a shift of about half of chromosome 22 with translocation to chromosome 9 (Rowley, 1973). Patients who are Ph[1] negative show clinical differences as well, and probably their disease can be considered a distinct entity. In Ph[1] positive patients, all or nearly all of the marrow cells contain the Ph[1] chromosome, including erythroblasts and megakaryoblasts, as well as myeloblasts. Therefore, we can infer that CML is a stem cell disease. Moreover, there is evidence that the affected cells are derived from just one deviant stem cell (Fialkow, 1974). It is of interest in this regard that circulating lymphocytes do not contain the Ph[1] chromosome. However, most patients with CML eventually develop a "blast crisis," in which the relatively mature granulocytes of CML are replaced by blast forms. There is evidence that in some cases these cells are lymphoblasts rather than myeloblasts, yet they also contain the Ph[1] chromosome (Gallo, 1975). There seems to be little doubt that the Ph[1] chromosome is involved in the pathogenesis of CML. Indeed, its presence may precede the clinical onset of CML by years. However, the etiology of this chromosomal rearrangement is completely mysterious. One could invoke radiation or chemical injuries, conceivably in conjunction with a genetic predisposition, or fall back on a nearby virus. At this stage of our knowledge, however, all explanations are equally conjectural.

Morphology. The anatomic alterations of leukemia may be separated into primary changes, attributed directly to the abnormal overgrowth or accumulation of white cells, and secondary changes, caused both by the destructive effects of masses of these cells and by their relative ineffectiveness in protecting against infection. In the **chronic form of lymphocytic leukemia,** the neoplastic cells closely resemble mature lymphocytes, although usually some immature elements can also be found in the peripheral blood. In contrast, **acute lymphocytic leukemia** involves markedly immature forms (lymphoblasts) and sometimes cells indistinguishable from stem cells. In the latter cases, the disorder may be termed a **stem cell leukemia.** The **chronic form of myelogenous leukemia** involves cells which closely resemble normal granulocytes. However, many immature, poorly granulated cells are usually admixed with the normal appearing ones. **Acute myelogenous leukemia,** on the other hand, is characterized by the accumulation of very immature granulocytes (myeloblasts or promyelocytes). In fact, as with ALL, they may be so undifferentiated that the disorder warrants the designation stem cell leukemia. In the myelomonocytic variant, hybrid forms which combine characteristics of both monocytes and granulocytes occasionally are seen. In other cases, the leukemic cells are fairly uniformly monocytic (Naegeli's leukemia). When the erythroid line is predominantly affected, the accumulating cells are red blood cell precursors (Di Guglielmo's disease). The mysterious cells of "hairy-cell" leukemia are about 12 to 20 μm. in diameter, with a round to oval nucleus and abundant cytoplasm. On smears and by phase microscopy, fine hair-like projections are seen at the cell periphery. By scanning electron microscopy the cells are variously described as ruffled or villous (Case records of the Massachusetts General Hospital, 1975).

Although the leukemic cells may infiltrate any tissue or organ of the body, the most striking changes are seen in the bone marrow, spleen, lymph nodes and liver. In the full-blown case, the **bone marrow** develops a muddy, red-brown to gray-white color as the normal marrow is diffusely replaced by masses of white cells (Fig. 11–6). Sometimes these infiltrates extend into previously fatty marrow and encroach upon and erode the cancellous and cortical bone. The bones thus become thinned and radiolucent and may undergo pathologic fractures. With myelogenous leukemia, bony infiltrates may take the form of tumorous masses, termed **chloromas.** These masses may arise within the bone or subperiosteally in any portion of the skeleton, but most often they affect the skull. When first examined, they are a distinctive evanescent green; this color rapidly fades as the unknown

pigment oxidizes. Chloromas are not seen with lymphocytic leukemia.

Massive **splenomegaly** is characteristic of CML. Splenic weights of 5000 gm. or more are not unusual. Such spleens may virtually fill the abdominal cavity and extend into the pelvis. With CLL, enlargement of the spleen is less striking, and the weight of the spleen rarely exceeds 2500 gm. The acute forms of leukemia produce only moderate splenomegaly, usually between 500 and 1000 gm. Like CML, hairy-cell leukemia also produces massive splenomegaly, with diffuse infiltration of the red pulp by the hairy cells. In all forms of splenomegaly the capsule becomes somewhat thickened and frequently adheres to surrounding structures. On sectioning, the parenchyma is firm and muddy gray in color. When the splenomegaly is massive, as is most characteristic of CML, numerous areas of pale infarction may appear throughout the substance. In minimally enlarged spleens, the histologic appearance may be of focal leukemic infiltrates, with a background of fairly well preserved normal architecture. In the lymphocytic forms the white pulp is primarily involved. With more severe involvement the infiltrates become more diffuse. Ultimately the underlying architecture is obliterated, being replaced by a sea of homogeneous leukemic cells. Areas of ischemic necrosis account for the grossly visible pale foci.

Whereas splenomegaly is more prominent with myelogenous than with lymphocytic leukemia, extreme **lymph node enlargement** is more characteristic of the lymphocytic forms (Fig. 11–7). Nevertheless, some degree of lymph node involvement is commonly present with all forms of leukemia, although it may be quite subtle with the myelogenous forms of leukemia, particularly AML. Not all nodes are uniformly affected; the distribution of lymphadenopathy is in fact quite variable from one case to another. The affected nodes remain discrete, rubbery and homogeneous. The cut section is soft and gray-white, and tends to bulge above the level of the capsule. On histologic examination, severely involved nodes are seen to be diffusely flooded by the neoplastic cells. The underlying architecture is obliterated, and sometimes the leukemic cells invade the capsule of the node and flood out into the surrounding tissues. With CLL, the histologic picture is identical to that of a well differentiated lymphocytic lymphoma. With minimal involvement in the myelogenous leukemias, the underlying architecture may be largely preserved. Peripheral lymphadenopathy is conspicuously absent with hairy-cell leukemia.

Enlargement of the liver is somewhat more prominent with lymphocytic than with myelogenous leukemia. Histologically, the lymphocytic infiltrates are characteristically confined to the portal areas, where they may produce a fine mottling, which is apparent grossly on the cut surface. Sometimes there are larger foci of gray-white tumor infiltration which may simulate metastatic disease from

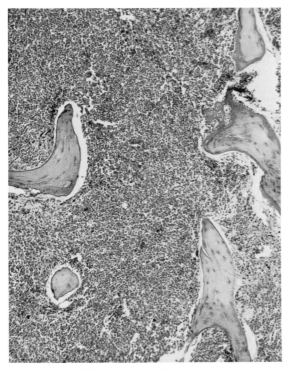

Figure 11–6. Myelogenous leukemia. Low power view of bone marrow to document the flooding by cells of myeloid origin.

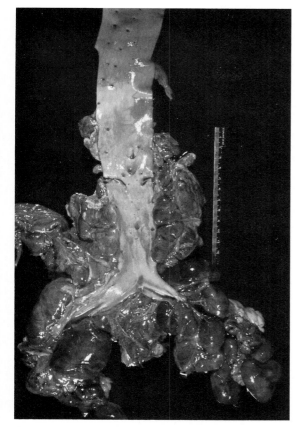

Figure 11–7. Lymphocytic leukemia. Periaortic and periiliac lymph nodes. The marked lymphadenopathy compresses the vessels.

other forms of cancer. The infiltrates of myelogenous leukemia are not well defined and are present within the sinusoids throughout the lobule. Some aggregates of cells may be found in the portal triads but, in addition, cells are dispersed along the liver cords subjacent to the vascular sinusoidal walls.

In addition to the principal sites of involvement, other tissues and organs may be affected. Leukemic infiltrates are frequently found in the kidneys, where they begin as small perivascular aggregates which progressively diffuse throughout the stroma. Similar changes may occur in the adrenals, thyroid, myocardium and indeed any tissue. In all these organs, as well as in the liver, the infiltrates are largely confined to the interstitial connective tissue, with relative preservation of the parenchyma, and for this reason function is seldom seriously impaired. **Infiltrates in the gingiva are particularly characteristic of monocytic leukemia.** These patients have swelling and hypertrophy of the gingival margins, often with secondary infections.

The **secondary changes of all forms of leukemia** derive in large part from the myelophthisic pancytopenia which results from leukemic replacement of the bone marrow. Anemia and thrombocytopenia are characteristic. Many times, the bleeding diathesis caused by the thrombocytopenia is the most striking clinical and anatomic feature of the disease. Petechiae and ecchymoses are seen in the skin. Hemorrhages also occur into the serosal linings of the body cavities and into the serosal coverings of the viscera, particularly of the heart and lungs. Mucosal hemorrhages into the gingivae and urinary tract are common. Intraparenchymal hematomas may develop, most frequently in the brain.

Although the total white blood cell count is usually markedly elevated, the defensive capacity of these abnormal cells is considerably less than normal. This is especially true of the acute forms. There is, then, a **functional** leukopenia with a resultant increased susceptibility to bacterial infection. These infections are particularly common in the oral cavity, skin, lungs, kidneys, urinary bladder and colon.

Clinical Course. While AML affects all age groups roughly equally, ALL is predominantly a disease of children. Both forms of chronic leukemia occur most frequently in older adults. Whatever the age, the clinical manifestations of the acute forms tend to be similar to each other, and those of the chronic forms also parallel each other. Thus, the acute forms usually have an abrupt, stormy onset, manifested by fever, profound weakness and malaise. Typically the hepatosplenomegaly and lymphadenopathy are not sufficiently advanced in these acute cases to be noticeable to the patient or his family. In children, especially, bony infiltration may give rise to bone and joint pain. Within a few weeks to months, recurrent hemorrhages and bacterial infections make their appearance. Disseminated intravascular coagulation (DIC) is a frequent occurrence with the promyelocytic form.

The peripheral white cell count with acute leukemia is typically moderately elevated—between 30,000 to 100,000 cells per mm.[3] In some instances, however, fewer than normal numbers of leukocytes are present in the peripheral circulation, although infiltration of the soft tissues and bones resembles that of the more typical case. This variant is referred to as *aleukemic* or *leukopenic leukemia.* Even in these cases, at least some of the white cells in the blood are abnormally immature and suggest the diagnosis. When acute leukemia involves extremely immature cells, it may be very difficult to differentiate ALL from AML on examination of the peripheral blood. Usually, however, sufficient numbers of more mature cells are present to indicate the correct diagnosis.

Chronic leukemia is more insidious in onset. There may be a long period of vague weakness and weight loss. Sometimes, especially with CML, the first indication of disease is the dragging sensation in the abdomen caused by extreme splenomegaly. In other cases, the disease may be discovered in the course of investigating a profound anemia. With CLL, the anemia of marrow replacement is often complicated by an autoimmune hemolytic anemia. Occasionally, unexplained hemorrhages or recurrent intractable infections suggest the diagnosis. Usually, however, these are late developments.

Extreme elevations of the circulating white cell count are found with CLL and CML, sometimes up to 1,000,000 cells per mm.[3] A similar, though less pronounced, elevation of granulocytes (leukemoid reaction) may be seen in a variety of disorders, including many chronic infections, neoplasms and "collagen" diseases. Diagnosis of CML from the peripheral smear or even from the bone marrow may thus not be completely conclusive. Most important are the findings of the *Philadelphia chromosome* and of low levels of *leukocyte alkaline phosphatase. The former is virtually diagnostic.*

The prognosis with leukemia has improved dramatically over the past decade, largely as a result of dogged step-by-step efforts along several fronts. Indeed, the prognosis is changing so rapidly that it is virtually impossible to give figures that are still accurate at the time they are reported. In particular, the outlook for children with ALL is spectacularly improved. Untreated, this disease is fatal within a few months. With intensive chemotherapy, however, a remission can be induced in almost all patients. (A remission is defined as the return of the bone marrow to a completely normal appearance.) Moreover, maintenance chemotherapy, along with prophylactic irradiation and intrathecal chemotherapy for CNS involvement, has prolonged these remissions considerably. Thus, the median survival of children with ALL has increased from about four months to three to six years. It has been suggested that perhaps as many as half of those still in remission at five years are cured, but it is still too early to be certain of this optimistic prediction (Burchenal, 1973). Unfortunately, the prognosis for those with AML has not improved nearly so markedly. A remission is obtained in 65 per cent of patients with AML, but it is usually of short duration and median survival is only about one year. Efforts to stimulate the immune system with BCG or the inoculation of irradiated allogeneic leukemic cells, or both, are thought to have some beneficial effects in prolonging the remissions of patients with both forms of acute leukemia, but this remains controversial (Gutterman et al., 1974).

Although the outlook for patients with the chronic leukemias has also improved, the change is not so dramatic since the chronic forms are naturally more indolent. The median survival with both CLL and CML is about three to four years, as is the median survival with "hairy-cell" leukemia. However, the course of CLL is highly variable, and a subgroup of patients exists who have a remarkably benign course, sometimes permitting survival for many years even without treatment. With CML a true remission is never obtained, in that the bone marrow, no matter how normal it may appear, is still populated by cells with the Ph[1] chromosome. In about two thirds of these patients, the terminal event is the development of a "blast crisis," with sudden transformation of the disease to a form similar to AML. Rarely, the process may "burn out" and take on the characteristics and prognosis of myeloid metaplasia (p. 362). The 10 per cent of patients with CML who do not have the Ph[1] chromosome constitute an atypical group. Usually they are males over the age of 65 years, who have relatively low white blood cell counts and short survival times.

In all forms of leukemia, death is usually the result of hemorrhage, often into the brain, or superimposed bacterial infections.

THE DYSPROTEINOSES (MULTIPLE MYELOMA, WALDENSTRÖM'S MACROGLOBULINEMIA, AND HEAVY CHAIN DISEASE)

The dysproteinoses are a group of disorders which have in common the expansion of a single clone of immunoglobulin-secreting cells with a resultant increase in serum levels of a single homogeneous immunoglobulin or its fragments. On paper electrophoresis the homogeneous immunoglobulin appears as a dark narrow band in the gamma globulin region, often referred to as an *M-component.* In almost all cases, the dysproteinoses behave as malignant diseases, although occasionally M-components are seen in otherwise normal elderly individuals. Collectively these disorders account for about 15 per cent of deaths from malignant white cell disease, and are most common in middle-aged to elderly individuals. Those who have experienced a prolonged antigenic stimulus, such as with chronic cholecystitis, tuberculosis, osteomyelitis or nonspecific pneumonitis, are thought to be especially vulnerable (Baitz and Kyle, 1964). This association has interesting pathogenetic implications, as will soon be pointed out. The dysproteinoses can be divided into three major disorders: (1) multiple myeloma and its variants, (2) Waldenström's macroglobulinemia, and (3) heavy chain disease.

Multiple Myeloma and Its Variants. Multiple myeloma is by far the most frequent of the dysproteinoses. It consists of multifocal erosive plasma cell tumors, usually scattered throughout the skeletal system. Any of the five classes of immunoglobulins may be produced, although IgG is most frequent. In about half the cases, the light chains are produced in considerable excess of the heavy chains. Because of their relatively low molecular weight, the leftover light chains are readily excreted in the urine, where they are termed *Bence Jones proteins.* Rarely, the plasma cells in multiple myeloma produce *only* light chains, in which case Bence Jones proteins are present in the urine but there is no M-component in the serum. *Multiple myeloma is a monoclonal gammopathy; that is, in any one patient only one specific immunoglobulin is produced, and only one type of light chain, either kappa or lambda.*

Three variants of multiple myeloma are recognized, two of which may simply represent early stages of the disease. *Solitary myeloma* refers to the presence of only a single skeletal lesion; *soft tissue plasmacytoma* is an extramedullary plasma cell tumor which usually appears in the oronasopharynx; *plasma cell leukemia* is a rare form of multiple myeloma accompanied by flooding of the circulating blood by the neoplastic cells.

Waldenström's Macroglobulinemia. This disease involves a sparse infiltration of the bone marrow, spleen, liver and lymph nodes by precursors of plasma cells *(plasmacytoid lymphocytes),* which secrete only IgM. Focal destructive skeletal lesions do not develop. The high serum levels of IgM produce an M-component on paper electrophoresis, and occasionally Bence Jones proteinuria is also present.

Heavy Chain Disease. This is a plasma cell dyscrasia in which only heavy chains are produced. They may be of the IgG, IgA or IgM class. Except for the presence of an M-component, the disease in general simulates a lymphoma. However, the precise characteristics depend to some extent on which heavy chain is involved. With IgG heavy chain disease, there is diffuse lymphadenopathy and hepatosplenomegaly. IgA heavy chain disease shows a predilection for the lymphoid tissue of the small intestine and its mesentery. A small proportion of patients with chronic lymphocytic leukemia secrete IgM heavy chains and hence have concurrent heavy chain disease.

Etiology and Pathogenesis. As you will recall from our discussion of the lymphomas, B-cells differentiate into plasma cells through several intermediate forms, including first the immunoblast and then the plasmacytoid lymphocyte. For this reason, many workers consider the dysproteinoses simply to be one end of a spectrum of B-cell disease. According to this concept, multiple myeloma involves fully differentiated B-cells, whereas Waldenström's macroglobulinemia involves cells arrested at an earlier stage. In either case, the cells are sufficiently differentiated to secrete immunoglobulins into the blood. Because of the homogeneity of the immunoglobulin secreted in any one patient, there is little doubt that the dysproteinoses originate from a single primitive B-cell which gives rise to a clone of more or less completely differentiated cells. In the case of multiple myeloma, there is a great deal of evidence that the initial monoclonal expansion is in response to a specific antigenic stimulus. It is postulated that prolonged proliferation of this clone of cells provides the opportunity for spontaneous mutation or the activation of a latent oncogenic virus, either of which might result in the neoplastic growth of a subclone of this population of cells (Salmon and Seligmann, 1974). Thus, according to this hypothesis, multiple myeloma requires two "hits" for its evolution—a prolonged antigenic stimulus and an oncogenic event.

The evidence that a prolonged antigenic stimulus is necessary for the development of multiple myeloma is both experimental and clinical. Multiple myeloma can be induced in mice by the intraperitoneal injection of a variety of irritant substances, including Freund's adjuvant, mineral oil and plastic. At first, these substances evoke a chronic inflammatory reaction which progresses to granulomas and ultimately to lesions considered to be plasma cell tumors (Potter and MacCardle, 1964). The tumors are transplantable and produce M-components or Bence Jones proteins. These animal models are highly strainspecific, which indicates some genetic predisposition. It is of interest that, although the disease can be easily induced in these mice if they are kept in a normal environment, it is virtually impossible to induce multiple myeloma in germ-free mice of the same strain (Salmon and Seligmann, 1974). The importance of an antigenic stimulus in humans is demonstrated by the fact that the immunoglobulin produced may be specific for an identifiable antigen. For example, a patient with recurrent rheumatic fever later developed multiple myeloma involving an M-component which reacted against streptolysin (Seligmann et al., 1968). In summary, it is possible that the dysproteinoses result from persistent reactive inflammatory proliferation, possibly in conjunction with an oncogenic virus, which leads to a somatic mutation in individuals genetically predisposed.

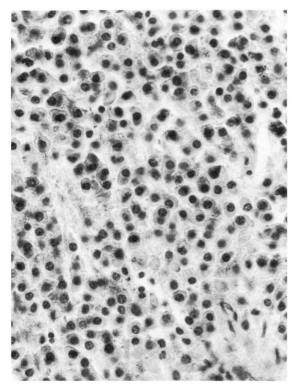

Figure 11–8. Multiple myeloma (plasmacytoma). A high power detail of a lesion in the vertebrae. The entire field is occupied by mature plasma cells with their abundant cytoplasm and eccentric nuclei. Occasionally somewhat atypical cells are seen.

Morphology. Despite the abundance of abnormal biochemical findings, the ultimate diagnosis of multiple myeloma rests on the morphologic identification of abnormal aggregates of plasma cells (Fig. 11–8). In many instances, the neoplastic cells are normal-appearing mature plasma cells, but sometimes more immature forms are found which may even resemble lymphocytes. It may be difficult to identify the neoplastic nature of the well differentiated plasma cell lesions from the cytology of the individual cells; more important is their abnormal aggregation or evidence of their destructive potential in the form of infiltration, invasion and erosion. However, sometimes multinucleated plasma cells are seen in lesions, essentially constituting cancerous giant cells. Electron microscopy has confirmed that the plasma cells have the classic abundant endoplasmic reticulum responsible for the characteristic basophilia and pyroninophilia of the plasma cell cytoplasm. The protein products within the endoplasmic cisternae of these tumor cells have been proved to be gamma globulin. In contrast to the cells of multiple myeloma, the cells of Waldenström's macroglobulinemia are not found in aggregates but rather are diffusely scattered throughout the affected tissues. The cellular composition of the infiltrate tends to be more variable, containing many hybrid forms, ranging from the lymphocyte to the mature plasma cell. The infiltrates of heavy chain disease closely resemble those of Waldenström's macroglobulinemia but, in addition, there is a prominent component of eosinophils and large immunoblastic-type cells.

Multiple myeloma presents as multifocal destructive bone lesions throughout the skeletal system. Although any bone may be affected, the following distribution was found in a large series of cases: vertebral column, 66 per cent; ribs, 44 per cent; skull, 41 per cent; pelvis, 28 per cent; femur, 24 per cent; clavicle, 10 per cent; and scapula, 10 per cent. These focal lesions generally begin in the medullary cavity, erode the cancellous bone and progressively destroy the cortical bone. Pathologic fractures are often produced by the plasma cell lesions; they are most common in the vertebral column, but may affect any of the numerous bones suffering erosion and destruction of their cortical substance. On section, the bony defects are observed to be filled with soft, red, gelatinous tissue. Radiographically, the lesions appear as punched-out defects, usually ranging from 1 to 4 cm. in diameter (Fig. 11–9). In the late stages of multiple myeloma, plasma cell infiltrations of soft tissues may be encountered in the spleen, liver, kidneys, lungs and lymph nodes, or more widely. The individual lesions of the variants of multiple myeloma do not differ significantly from those described above; the difference lies in their distribution at the time of diagnosis.

Renal involvement, generally called myeloma nephrosis, is one of the more distinctive features of multiple myeloma. Grossly, the kidneys may be normal in size or color, slightly enlarged and pale, or shrunken and pale because of interstitial scarring. The most characteristic features are microscopic. Interstitial infiltrates of abnormal plasma cells may be encountered. Even in the absence of these, proteinaceous casts are prominent in the tubules and collecting ducts. Most of these casts are made up of Bence Jones proteins, but some may be only albumin. The epithelial cells within the tubules often become engorged with pale hyaline droplets, presumably protein, or needle-like crystals. Often the cells lining tubules containing casts become necrotic or atrophied, whereas in other instances they apparently fuse to produce highly distinctive, multinucleated epithelial giant cells which encircle or engulf whole casts or fragments of casts. About such tubules, there is often an inflammatory infiltrate of neoplastic cells and mature lymphocytes. Metastatic calcification may be encountered within the kidney because of the hypercalcemia which frequently accompanies multiple myeloma.

Clinical Course. The clinical presentations of the dysproteinoses are varied. Generally, multiple myeloma becomes evident by the progressive development of bone pain, refer-

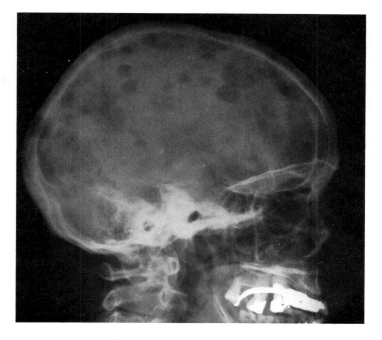

Figure 11–9. Multiple myeloma of the skull (x-ray, lateral view). The sharply punched out bone defects are most obvious in the calvarium.

able to the skeletal lesions. Such pain appears only after a long (possibly as long as 10 to 20 years) asymptomatic period. Commonly associated are anemia, fatigue, coagulation defects with a bleeding diathesis and a predisposition to infections. Coagulation defects are thought to result from some interaction between the myeloma proteins and one of the clotting factors, such as factor V or VII or prothrombin. Vulnerability to bacterial infections apparently reflects an impaired capacity to elaborate normal gamma globulins. Renal insufficiency may also be present. In addition, the neoplastic cells apparently secrete a polypeptide that activates osteoclasts and mobilizes calcium from the bone (Mundy et al., 1974). This may cause the hypercalcemia which often develops with multiple myeloma, and possibly contributes to the bony lesions. Amyloidosis develops in about 5 to 10 per cent of patients with multiple myeloma. The diagnosis of multiple myeloma is often readily made by the characteristic focal, punched out radiologic defects in the bone, especially when these are present in the vertebrae or calvarium. Hypergammaglobulinemia is almost always present. The exact electrophoretic pattern produced by the M-component depends upon the size (molecular weight) and quantity of the specific abnormal protein, and so it may occur across the entire range of the gamma globulins. The abnormal protein can be identified by agar immunoelectrophoresis. Mention has already been made of the identification of Bence Jones protein in the urine. Ultimately, the diagnosis is confirmed by biopsy.

Solitary myeloma may also be brought to attention by skeletal pain but more often is discovered by investigating an unexplained anemia, vulnerability to infections or unexplained proteinuria. The question of soft tissue plasmacytoma should be raised when any neoplasm of the oropharynx and upper respiratory tract is present. The nature of this tumor can sometimes be suspected by identifying the abnormal protein products of the plasma cell, but the diagnosis usually must be made by biopsy. The leukemic pattern is usually a complication of one of the presentations mentioned previously.

With Waldenström's macroglobulinemia, the tissue involvements are complicated by the "hyperviscosity syndrome," caused by the presence in the blood of large amounts of the high-molecular-weight IgM. A multitude of manifestations of this syndrome may be present, including striking RBC rouleaux formation, intravascular coagulation, visual and neurologic disturbances and congestive heart failure. The macroglobulins may be insoluble at cold temperatures, hence they are designated *cryoglobulins*. A bleeding diathesis is particularly prominent with this disease, and may in part result from IgM complexing with certain clotting factors.

The course of the dysproteinoses is extremely variable. Cases are on record in which abnormal gamma globulins have been identified in the serum for years without signs and symptoms of myeloma having developed. In general, patients with multiple myeloma pursue a progressive downhill course and develop multiple bone lesions. This progression is equally true in cases first identified as solitary myeloma and soft tissue plasmacytoma. With multiple myeloma, the most malignant of the dysproteinoses, median survival is only one to two years. Death is usually caused by progressive cachexia (as extraosseous spread occurs), renal failure, infection or hemorrhage.

HODGKIN'S DISEASE

This mysterious disorder is characterized by the presence in lymphoid tissue of distinctive cells known as Reed-Sternberg (R-S) cells, accompanied by a variable leukocytic and connective tissue reaction. Morphologically and clinically, it combines features of a chronic infection with those of a malignant tumor. In this sense, it has much in common with *immunoblastic lymphadenopathy* (p. 346). A valuable point of distinction between the two is the presence of marked hypergammaglobulinemia with immunoblastic lymphadenopathy (Editorial, 1975c). Whether Hodgkin's disease arises as a neoplastic process or whether it becomes transformed into one in the course of time is controversial. In any event, its implications to the patient are those of a malignant tumor. If it is so considered, it accounts for about 10 per cent of malignant white cell disease (Silverberg and Holleb, 1975). Hodgkin's disease affects males and females in a ratio of 3:2, and whites more often than nonwhites. In the United States the age incidence is bimodal, with the first peak between the ages of 15 and 34 years, and the second over the age of 50 years. In less affluent areas of the world, there is no peak in young adulthood, but there are commensurately more childhood cases.

Etiology and Pathogenesis. Like the lymphomas, Hodgkin's disease occurs in several histologic and clinical forms. The hypothesis is widely accepted that the spectrum of Hodgkin's disease represents an interplay between the induction of neoplasia and the host's defensive capabilities (Lukes and Butler, 1966). According to this view, the basic stimulus toward neoplasia affects the Reed-Sternberg cells, and the infiltration of lymphocytes represents the attempts of the host to abort the process. Thus, in the various histologic patterns of this disorder, the numbers of Reed-Sternberg cells and of lymphocytes bear an inverse relationship to each other, and the forms characterized by lymphocytic predominance offer a much more favorable prognosis. In the more aggressive forms, the Reed-Sternberg cells become more numerous and pleomorphic, eventually assuming clearly malignant forms.

There are several theories concerning the precise sequence of events in the development of Hodgkin's disease, but most have in common an element of internecine warfare among the patient's own white cells. One theory postulates a viral infection of a subpopulation of T-cells which alters them antigenically. The remaining T-cells then react against the altered T-cells in an autoimmune response similar to graft-versus-host disease. The resultant disruption of the T-cell system would permit the emergence of malignant cells, the R-S cells. According to this theory, R-S cells are of histiocytic origin (Order and Hellman, 1972). Other theories differ in that the initial event is thought to be the attempted induction of neoplasia, rather than nonneoplastic infection. According to one such hypothesis, the R-S cell itself is of T-cell origin and, as it undergoes malignant transformation from some unknown cause, elicits the formation of antibodies cross-reactive against normal T-cells. Thus, in the defense against malignant disease, the entire T-cell population comes under assault (DeVita, 1973). A variation of this theory suggests an inherent defect in T-cell surveillance, which permits the emergence of malignant immunoblasts (Lukes and Collins, 1974).

Two facts emerge from a consideration of these theories concerning the pathogenesis of Hodgkin's disease. First, the origin of the R-S cell is clearly in dispute, with some workers calling it a histiocyte (Carr, 1975; Kay and Kadin, 1975), some a T-cell (Biniaminov and Ramot, 1974; DeVita, 1973), and others a B-cell (Taylor, 1974). Clearly, the unequivocal determination of its origin would be helpful in understanding the causation of Hodgkin's disease. Second, there is much evidence, incorporated in the pathogenetic theories given, that Hodgkin's disease is basically a T-cell disease. It begins in the thymus or in the thymus-dependent areas of the lymph nodes or spleen (Hellman, 1974). The bulk of the lymphocytes involved have been shown to be T-cells, and probably those cells once thought to be histiocytes are actually transformed lymphocytes (Editorial, 1975e). Scanning electron microscopy shows the R-S cells often surrounded by adherent lymphocytes, which appear to be T-cells (Braylan et al., 1974). In addition, a defect in cell-mediated responses—for example, to a tuberculin or mumps skin test—is a prominent aspect of Hodgkin's disease. Whether such defective T-cell responses occur early in the disease is controversial, but most workers believe that they do (Levy and Kaplan, 1974). Thus, the overwhelming consensus is that Hodgkin's disease involves some derangement in the T-cell system.

The question of a role for a transmissible agent in Hodgkin's disease has intrigued workers in this field for many years. Much epidemiologic work has been done in this area. Evidence of clustering of cases in families and in schools suggests an environmental etiology with some horizontal transmission. It would appear that there is a long incubation period and that healthy individuals can carry the agent (Vianna and Polan, 1973). An increased susceptibility of individuals with HL-A antigens belonging to the 4C system indicates that genetic factors may also be involved (Vianna et al., 1974). However, some workers question the validity of these epidemiologic studies, and certainly any horizontal transmission that may occur bears no resemblance to the infectiousness of, say, measles.

Morphology. As with the lymphomas, no one system of classification of Hodgkin's disease is universally accepted. Here we present that of Lukes and associates, which has now largely replaced the older system of Jackson and Parker (Lukes et al., 1966). The relative incidence of the various patterns of the Lukes classification is also given (Bakemeier, 1970–1971).

The **lymphocyte predominance** form is associated with relatively quiescent disease and long survival times. Affected nodes may be focally or diffusely involved. **Nodular sclerosis** appears to represent a special expression of the disease in the mediastinum, and this form is also associated with a relatively good prognosis. Some believe it to be a distinct disease (Editorial, 1975e). The **mixed pattern** is thought to herald a change in host response, with transition from quiescent to aggressive disease and an intermediate prognosis. This transition may ultimately lead to the **lymphocyte depletion** form, which is associated with aggressive disease and short survival times.

As with the lymphomas, the basic anatomic changes of Hodgkin's disease are in the **lymph nodes.** In the **lymphocyte predominance form,** involvement is usually confined to a single node or group of nodes, usually in the cervical chain. These are discretely enlarged, from 3 to 5 cm., soft to moderately firm and freely moveable. On cut surface, they are tan to gray-white. Typically, the **nodular sclerosing** type involves the anterior superior mediastinum and the scalene, supraclavicular and lower cervical nodes. The gross appearance of these nodes varies with the amount of collagen formation and the degree of cellular infiltration of

TABLE 11–6. PATTERNS OF HODGKIN'S DISEASE

Lymphocyte Predominance	5 per cent
Nodular Sclerosis	52 per cent
Mixed Pattern	37 per cent
Lymphocyte Depletion	6 per cent
Diffuse fibrosis	
Reticular pattern	

the capsules. They are usually firm to hard, and may be either discrete or matted together. The cut surface usually shows yellow-tan nodules separated by gray-white bands. The **mixed** and **lymphocyte depletion** forms are associated with hard, adherent irregular masses of nodes, which may extend in contiguous fashion from the inguinal ligament to the diaphragm along the major vessels, and from the diaphragm to the neck via the mediastinum.

The sine qua non for the histologic diagnosis of Hodgkin's disease is the presence of the Reed-Sternberg cell, first described in 1898 (Reed, 1902). **However, although it is necessary for the diagnosis of Hodgkin's disease, it is not specific, since it has been found in infectious mononucleosis, mycosis fungoides and occasionally lymphomas, as well as in other settings** (Tindle et al., 1972). The Reed-Sternberg cell ranges in size from 15 to 45 μm. in diameter. It is distinguished principally by the presence of multiple nuclear divisions without cytoplasmic division and by large, round, prominent nucleoli. The nuclear divisions may be complete or partial, hence **the Reed-Sternberg cell is either multinucleate or has a multilobed nucleus.** Often the nucleoli are acidophilic and surrounded by a distinctive clear zone, imparting an owl-eyed appearance, the nuclear membrane is distinct. Although the cytoplasm of these cells is variable, it is most often abundant and uniformly pale. Other abnormal cells, which are similar to Reed-Sternberg cells but lack some essential feature, such as the prominent nucleoli, may also be present in Hodgkin's disease. It is probable that these represent intermediate or partially developed Reed-Sternberg cells. Each of the histologic patterns of the Lukes classification will now be described individually.

Lymphocyte Predominance Pattern. This is characterized by the presence of large numbers of lymphocytes, representing the host response to the disease. Cells having the appearance of transformed lymphocytes or possibly histiocytes may also be present, and probably have a similar significance. Characteristic Reed-Sternberg cells are usually extremely difficult to find, although other, similar pleomorphic cells with small nucleoli may be numerous. In the **diffuse** form, the cellular infiltrate is uniform, obliterating the underlying architecture. The **focal** or **nodular** form is characterized by aggregations consisting predominantly of lymphocytes, in the center of which there may be clusters of abnormal pleomorphic cells.

Nodular Sclerosis. In this form, a variable cellular infiltrate is separated into more or less well defined nodules by orderly bands of birefringent collagenous connective tissue (Fig. 11–10). The process may be predominantly cellular or predominantly collagenous. The cellular infiltrate within the nodules is usually mixed. While classic Reed-Sternberg cells are infrequent, a large

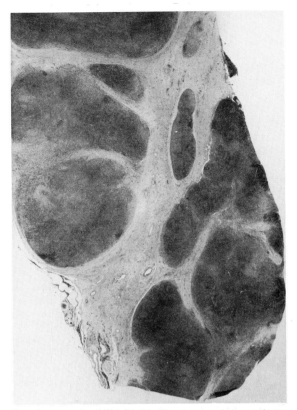

Figure 11–10. Hodgkin's disease, nodular sclerosing pattern. The low power view shows the division of the nodes into well defined nodules by wide, fibrous trabeculae.

variant cell, with abundant pale cytoplasm and small nucleoli, may be present in large numbers. Because of the pallor of the cytoplasm, the centrally placed nucleus often appears to be within a cleared space, hence these forms have been designated "lacunar cells" (Fig. 11–11). The reactive cells within the nodules may be predominantly lymphocytes, although they are often admixed with eosinophils and granulocytes.

Mixed Pattern. The architecture of the node is obliterated by a mixed cellular infiltrate consisting of lymphocytes, histiocytes, neutrophils, eosinophils and plasma cells in varying proportions. Interspersed throughout this heterogeneous infiltrate are Reed-Sternberg cells and other abnormal cells. Some degree of fibrosis typically is present, but it is disorderly and not characterized by collagen formation. Areas of ischemic necrosis sometimes are present (Fig. 11–12).

Lymphocyte Depletion Pattern. This is the pattern most often seen with terminal Hodgkin's disease. It is subdivided into **diffuse fibrosis** and **reticular** forms. There is depletion of all cellular elements except the Reed-Sternberg cells, which are relatively increased in number. Particularly noticeable is the depletion of lymphocytes. In the

form termed diffuse fibrosis the hypocellular node is largely replaced by a proteinaceous, fibrillar material, which represents a disorderly nonbirefringent connective tissue. Whether or not this hypocellularity represents in part the effects of therapy is not clear. With the reticular form the connective tissue element is minimal, and there are instead large numbers of Reed-Sternberg cells. Foci of necrosis are frequent.

It is apparent that Hodgkin's disease spans a wide range of histologic patterns, and that certain forms, with their characteristic fibrosis, eosinophils, neutrophils and plasma cells, come deceptively close to simulating an inflammatory reactive process. The diagnosis, then, of Hodgkin's disease rests solely on the unmistakable identification of the Reed-Sternberg cells, which are found in all forms.

Like the lymphomas, Hodgkin's disease begins in lymph nodes, but in advanced stages, it may involve any tissue or organ. The RE organs are most vulnerable, and the spleen, liver and bone marrow are often studded with metastatic nodules. Such dissemination is more typical of the aggressive lymphocyte depletion pattern but can also be seen with the other patterns.

Clinical Course. The clinical picture of Hodgkin's disease is very similar to that of the

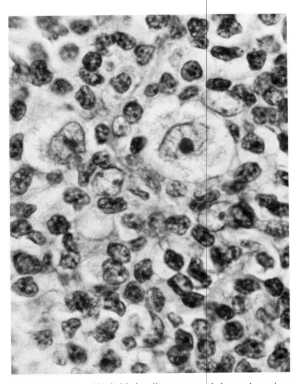

Figure 11–11. Hodgkin's disease, nodular sclerosing pattern. The distinctive "lacunar cell," so called because the nucleus appears to lie within a cleared space, is apparent.

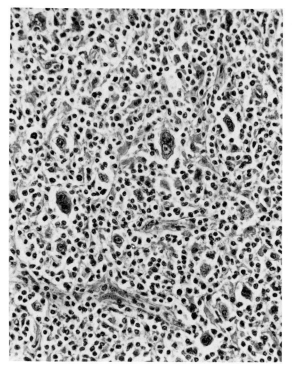

Figure 11–12. Hodgkin's disease, mixed pattern. The background is composed of a mixed cell population, including lymphocytes, plasma cells, histiocytes and neutrophils. Two Reed-Sternberg cells are evident in the midfield. There is a delicate fibrosis in the background.

lymphomas, and a histologic diagnosis is required for their distinction. The process begins with painless enlargement of the involved nodes. Ultimately, there is weight loss, weakness, fever, night sweats, pruritus and anemia. Indications of an immune derangement, such as skin anergy and associated herpes zoster, are often present. A classic Pel-Ebstein fever, characterized by temperature spikes at two to three day intervals, has been described. However, this type of fever is often absent.

The clinical staging system presented in the discussion of the lymphomas was actually devised with reference to Hodgkin's disease (p. 348). For accurate staging, a battery of diagnostic tests is required. One of the more important of these tests is lymphangiography, which reveals any involvement of the retroperitoneal lymph nodes. Laparotomy may also be necessary for accurate staging.

The overall prognosis is about 42 per cent five-year survival, somewhat better than that of the lymphomas (Silverberg and Holleb, 1975). However, here again the prognosis in the individual case is heavily dependent on the histology and the clinical stage, which in

turn are related. This relationship is shown in the following chart, which breaks down each histologic type according to clinical stage at the time of diagnosis (Lukes and Butler, 1966). It should be remembered, however, that, *at any time, a histologic type may become transformed to a more aggressive one, with its more ominous distribution and prognosis.*

Histology	Clinical Stage, Per Cent		
	I	II	III
Lymphocyte Predominance	70	20	10
Nodular Sclerosis	40	40	20
Mixed	35	40	25
Lymphocyte Depletion	15	35	50

Although these values are based on a study too small to have precise statistical significance, it can be seen that the lymphocyte predominance form tends to be Stage I at the time of diagnosis, nodular sclerosis tends to be diagnosed with equal frequency at Stages I and II, the mixed form is most often found at Stage II and the lymphocyte depletion form tends to be discovered at Stage III. The following chart indicates the five-year survival of patients with Hodgkin's disease according to the clinical stage at the time of diagnosis (Kaplan, 1968).

Clinical Stage	Five-Year Survival, Per Cent
I	90
II	70
III	40
IV	20

Hodgkin's disease often responds dramatically to radiotherapy. Survival for more than 10 years without evidence of recurrent disease is considered by many to represent a "cure."

Mycosis Fungoides. The relationship of Hodgkin's disease to a skin disorder known as mycosis fungoides is highly controversial. Some regard the latter as the skin manifestation of Hodgkin's disease, either heralding or following visceral involvement, and have described the presence of Reed-Sternberg cells in the skin lesions (Jacobs, 1968). These lesions begin as poorly defined areas of eczema, followed by the formation of plaques and ultimately of multiple nodules. The dominant histologic feature is a markedly polymorphic dermal infiltrate, consisting of giant cells, histiocytes, lymphocytes and eosinophils. Mitoses are frequent. Those who deny a relationship to Hodgkin's disease have suggested that mycosis fungoides may arise from the mesenchymal cells of the dermis and state that it probably remains confined to the skin (Lukes, 1968). They believe that those cases said to be associated with visceral involvement were actually lymphomas with skin manifestations.

MYELOID METAPLASIA (CHRONIC NONLEUKEMIC MYELOSIS, LEUKOERYTHROBLASTIC ANEMIA, MYELOFIBROSIS)

Myeloid metaplasia is characterized by marked extramedullary hematopoiesis, usually accompanied by fibrous replacement of the bone marrow (*myelofibrosis*). In a sense, it may be considered the pivotal myeloproliferative disorder, since the peripheral blood may show elevations of any of the three marrow cell lines (that is, the red blood cells, the granulocytes and the platelets). It has been suggested that the fundamental disorder is abnormal proliferation of still a fourth marrow cell line, namely, the stromal fibroblasts. Sometimes polycythemia vera and, less often, myelogenous leukemia "burn out," as it were, and terminate in a myelofibrotic pattern. Contrariwise, a patient with apparent myeloid metaplasia may later undergo a polycythemic or leukemic transformation.

Etiology and Pathogenesis. The causation of myeloid metaplasia is unknown. The striking extramedullary hematopoiesis would suggest some type of primary marrow failure, with the consequent resumption of blood formation by the various fetal sites. The presence of myelofibrosis is consistent with this concept. However, no toxic cause for the extensive marrow destruction has been demonstrated, nor is there replacement by, say, leukemic cells. As was mentioned, perhaps the most satisfactory explanation is that the myelofibrosis represents primary overgrowth of a native fibroblastic cell line, analogous to polycythemia vera or myelogenous leukemia.

It should be emphasized here that not all cases of myeloid metaplasia are associated with fibrosis of the marrow. Indeed, bone marrow findings are extremely variable, and the marrow may appear of normal cellularity or even hypercellular. Moreover, in these cases all the formed elements are represented. This would indicate that the extramedullary hematopoiesis is not merely secondary, but probably a basic component of the disease.

Morphology. The principal site of the extramedullary hematopoiesis is the **spleen,** which is usually markedly enlarged, sometimes up to 4000 gm. in weight. On section, it is firm, red to gray and not dissimilar to spleens seen with mye-

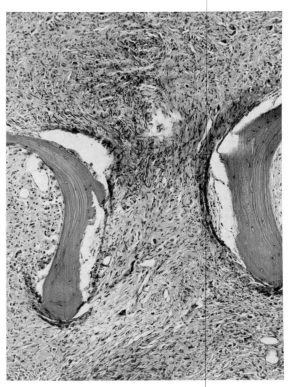

Figure 11–13. Myelofibrosis. The marrow cavity is virtually replaced by fibrous tissue, totally obliterating the normal hematopoietic elements.

logenous leukemia. Histologically, however, the distinction is apparent. There is preservation of the native architecture, as well as orderly hematopoiesis, with relatively normal proportions of maturing red cells, white cells and platelets. **Occasionally, however, disproportional activity of any one of the three major cell lines is seen.**

The **liver** may be moderately enlarged, with foci of extramedullary hematopoiesis. The **lymph nodes** are only rarely the site of blood cell formation and are usually not enlarged. This is an important differential feature, since some degree of lymphadenopathy would be expected with the leukemias.

As was mentioned, the bone marrow findings are variable. While usually it is hypocellular and fibrotic (Fig. 11–13), the marrow may be hypercellular. In any case, none of the three major cell lines shows neoplastic overgrowth, and the marrow is thus distinguishable from that of myelogenous leukemia.

Clinical Course. As was mentioned, myeloid metaplasia is the pivotal myeloproliferative disorder. It may begin with a blood picture suggestive of polycythemia vera or myelogenous leukemia, or it may arise as an apparently primary disease. Its outcome is equally variable. In some instances, a pancytopenia results and repeated blood transfusions are necessary to prolong the lives of these patients. In most, the disease culminates with overgrowth of one of the cell lines, leading to myelogenous leukemia, Di Guglielmo's disease or, rarely, polycythemia. The course and prognosis are then those of the new disorder.

THE HEMORRHAGIC DIATHESES

These disorders are characterized by spontaneous bleeding or excessive bleeding following trauma. Such abnormal hemorrhage may have as its cause:
1. Increased fragility of the vessels
2. Inadequacy of hemostatic responses:
   a. platelet deficiency or dysfunction
   b. derangement in the clotting mechanism

Increased fragility of the vessels occurs with severe *vitamin C deficiency (scurvy)* (p. 257), as well as with a large number of infectious and hypersensitivity *vasculitides.* These include meningococcemia, infective endocarditis, the rickettsial diseases, typhoid and Schönlein-Henoch purpura. Some of these conditions are discussed in other chapters; others are beyond the scope of this book. *A hemorrhagic diathesis purely on the basis of vascular fragility is characterized by: (1) the apparently spontaneous appearance of petechiae and ecchymoses in the skin and mucous membranes (probably on the basis of minor trauma), (2) a positive tourniquet (capillary resistance) test, and (3) a normal platelet count, bleeding time and coagulation time.*

Deficiencies of platelets (thrombocytopenia) are important causes of hemorrhagic disorders. These may occur in a variety of clinical settings, including *marrow suppression* from any cause (see p. 338), an entity known as disseminated intravascular coagulation (DIC), which results in the consumption of platelets (and clotting factors as well) and a primary form termed *idiopathic thrombocytopenic purpura.* In addition, there are disorders in which platelet function is deranged, despite a normal platelet count. Such qualitative defects are seen in uremia, after aspirin ingestion and in von Willebrand's disease. *Thrombocytopenia and platelet dysfunction are similar to increased vascular fragility in that petechiae and ecchymoses are present, as well as easy bruising, nosebleeds, excessive bleeding from minor trauma and menorrhagia. Similarly, the tourniquet test is positive and the coagulation time is normal. However, in contrast to the vascular disorders, the bleeding time is prolonged.*

A bleeding diathesis based purely on a *derangement in the intricate clotting mechanism* differs in several respects from those resulting from defects in the vessel walls or in platelets.

The coagulation time is usually prolonged, while the bleeding time is normal. Petechiae and ecchymoses, as well as other evidences of bleeding from very minor surface trauma, are usually absent. However, massive hemorrhage may follow operative and dental procedures and severe trauma. Moreover, hemorrhages into areas of the body subject to trauma, such as the joints of the lower extremities, are characteristic. In this category is a group of *congenital coagulation disorders.*

One of the most important of the bleeding diatheses, *disseminated intravascular coagulation,* which was already mentioned, involves consumption of both platelets and the clotting factors, hence it presents laboratory and clinical features of both thrombocytopenia and a coagulation disorder. *Von Willebrand's disease* also involves derangements in both modalities. Although *vitamin K deficiency (hypoprothrombinemia)* (p. 254) is theoretically a coagulation disorder, it too may present somewhat mixed features.

In this section the following hemorrhagic disorders will be discussed in this order:
1. DIC—consumption of fibrinogen and platelets
2. Thrombocytopenia—deficiency of platelets
   a. Primary
   b. Secondary
3. Hereditary coagulation disorders (hemophilia)—deficiency in clotting factors

DISSEMINATED INTRAVASCULAR COAGULATION (DIC, CONSUMPTION COAGULOPATHY, DEFIBRINATION SYNDROME)

Disseminated intravascular coagulation is an acute, subacute or chronic disorder characterized by intravascular fibrin deposition, principally within arterioles and capillaries, with a resultant bleeding diathesis from depletion of clotting factors and platelets. It is the human equivalent of the experimentally produced generalized Shwartzman reaction (Brodsky and Siegel, 1970). First described only 20 years ago, this entity is probably a more important cause of pathologic bleeding than all the congenital coagulation disorders, which will be discussed later (McKay, 1965).

Etiology and Pathogenesis. Before presenting the specific disorders associated with DIC, we shall first discuss in a general way the pathogenetic mechanisms by which intravascular clotting can occur. Reference to the earlier comments on normal blood coagulation (p. 219) may be helpful at this point. It suffices here to recall that clotting may be initiated by either of two pathways: the *extrinsic pathway,* which is triggered by the release of tissue thromboplastin into the circulation; and the *intrinsic pathway,* which involves the activation within the blood of factor XII by surface contact, collagen or other negatively charged substances. Both pathways lead to the generation of thrombin. *Clot inhibiting influences* include the rapid clearance of activated clotting factors by the RE system or by the liver (factors X and XI) and activation of fibrinolysis. From this brief review, we can deduce that intravascular coagulation may result from any of the following (Bachmann, 1969):

1. Release of tissue thromboplastin into the circulation (extrinsic pathway).
2. Activation of the intrinsic pathway.
3. Stasis.
4. Defective clearing of activated clotting factors (RE or liver derangements).
5. Defective fibrinolysis (rare).

In actual clinical practice, DIC probably most often results from activation of either the extrinsic or intrinsic coagulation system, with the other influences listed above being only of occasional importance. How is such abnormal initiation of clotting triggered? A variety of mechanisms may be operative, corresponding to the large number of clinical settings in which DIC occurs. Some of these mechanisms are fairly straightforward; others are complicated and poorly understood. Perhaps the simplest involves the direct release of tissue thromboplastin into the circulation—for example, from the placenta in obstetric complications, or from neoplastic cells or necrotic tissue in cancer. Whereas the red blood cells contain only relatively small amounts of thromboplastin, *massive* hemolysis may release sufficient amounts to initiate DIC. In still other cases, platelet aggregation and clotting may result from endothelial damage, which in turn may be due to many causes, such as the deposition of antigen-antibody complexes in the vessel wall, direct or endotoxic damage by microorganisms, temperature extremes or vasculitis.

Whatever the pathogenetic mechanism, DIC has two consequences: (1) First, there is widespread fibrin deposition within the microcirculation. This leads to ischemia in the more severely affected or more vulnerable organs,

and to hemolysis as the red blood cells become traumatized while passing through the fibrin strands *(microangiopathic hemolytic anemia).* (2) Second, a bleeding diathesis ensues as the platelets and clotting factors are consumed. This is further aggravated as the widespread clotting activates fibrinolysis. This secondary fibrinolysis yields circulating *fibrin split products* (FSP), which themselves have an inhibitory effect on platelet aggregation and thus tend to render the remaining platelets nonfunctional (Prentice et al., 1969; Marder et al., 1967). The diagram at the bottom of the page illustrates these effects of DIC.

We will now turn our attention to the specific clinical settings in which DIC occurs. About 50 per cent of individuals with DIC are obstetric patients having certain complications of pregnancy (Merskey et al., 1967). Fortunately, however, in this setting the disorder tends to be reversible with delivery of the fetus. Another 33 per cent of patients with DIC have cancer (Straub et al., 1967; Rand et al., 1969). The remaining associated disorders are varied and legion. The following chart lists the major ones and indicates, where possible, the probable pathogenetic mechanism:

A. Direct release of thromboplastin

   1. Obstetric complications
     a. Premature separation of placenta (abruptio placentae)
     b. Amniotic fluid embolism
     c. Retained dead fetus
     d. Toxemia of pregnancy
   2. Cancer (especially carcinoma of the prostate and promyelocytic leukemia; also carcinoma of the lung, breast, stomach, pancreas, cervix and colon)
   3. Tissue damage
     a. Burns and trauma
     b. Transplant rejection
     c. Heart and lung surgery (especially with extracorporeal circulation)
     d. Heat stroke
   4. Hemolysis
     a. Mismatched transfusions
     b. Falciparum malaria
     c. Certain autoimmune disorders

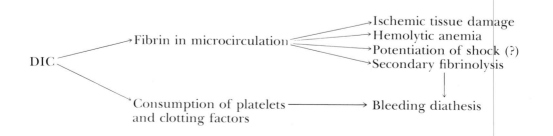

5. Snake bites
6. Fat embolism

B. Pathogenesis uncertain or mixed (e.g., endothelial damage, vasculitis, stasis, hemolysis)

1. Infections (especially gram-negative septicemia, meningococcemia, pneumococcemia)
2. Intravascular antigen-antibody reactions (including SLE, proliferative glomerulonephritis)
3. Thrombocytopenic purpura and the hemolytic uremic syndrome
4. Shock (?)
5. Malignant hypertension (?)
6. Idiopathic pulmonary hypertension (?)

With some of these disorders, DIC is merely a complication, albeit a serious one; with others, there is reason to suspect it has causative significance. It has been suggested, for example, that DIC plays an important role in the pathogenesis of toxemia of pregnancy, although the initial triggering event is unclear. Possibly small fragments of placenta somehow gain access to the maternal circulation and initiate intravascular clotting. Of particular theoretic interest is the postulated intricate association between DIC and a variety of microangiopathies, including the autoimmune and infectious angiitides, the glomerulitides and malignant hypertension. All these entities have in common injury to the vessel walls. Such injury may be produced by the deposition of antigen-antibody complexes, by toxins, or by sustained high blood pressures. It has been postulated that these influences increase the permeability of the vessel wall to all plasma proteins, including fibrinogen (which is then converted to fibrin as the clotting mechanism is activated) (Linton et al., 1969; Paronetto, 1969). As was mentioned, mechanical trauma to passing red blood cells leads to hemolysis, which in turn exacerbates the clotting tendency through the release of thromboplastin. Such a sequence of events would clearly yield a clinical picture in which the roles of the initiating disorder and of DIC were inextricably intertwined. The role of DIC in endotoxic shock is not clear, but it has been suggested that it possibly plays a role in the transition to "irreversible" shock (Hardaway, 1966).

Morphology. The anatomic changes of DIC are related, on the one hand, to the widespread fibrin deposition and, on the other, to hemorrhage. The microthrombi are found principally in the arterioles and capillaries of the kidneys, adrenals, brain and heart. However, no organ is spared, and the lungs, liver and GI mucosa may also be prominently involved. The glomeruli contain small fibrin thrombi, which may evoke only a reactive swelling of the endothelial cells or may be surrounded by a florid focal glomerulitis. The resultant ischemia leads to microinfarcts within the renal cortex. In severe cases, the ischemia may even extend to destroy the entire cortex (**bilateral renal cortical necrosis**—see p. 447). Involvement of the adrenal glands reproduces the picture of the **Waterhouse-Friderichsen syndrome** (see p. 612). Microinfarcts are also commonly encountered in the brain, surrounded by microscopic or gross foci of hemorrhage. These may give rise to bizarre neurologic signs. Similar changes are seen in the heart and often in the anterior pituitary. It has been suggested that DIC may contribute to **Sheehan's postpartum pituitary necrosis** (see p. 596).

When the underlying disorder is toxemia of pregnancy, the placenta is the site of capillary thromboses and occasional florid degeneration of the vessel walls. In addition, as many as 100 per cent of the villi are devoid of syncytiotrophoblast, as opposed to about a third of the villi in a normal placenta at term.

The bleeding tendency associated with DIC is manifested not only by larger than expected hemorrhages near foci of infarction, but also by diffuse petechiae and ecchymoses, which may be found on the skin, serosal linings of the body cavities, epicardium, endocardium, lungs and the mucosal lining of the urinary tract.

Clinical Course. The clinical picture is an apparent paradox, with a bleeding tendency in the face of evidence of widespread coagulation. The onset may be insidious, but more often it is acute or subacute. (The chronic cases are usually associated with cancer or with retention of a dead fetus [Brodsky and Siegel, 1970].) Typically, the abnormal clotting occurs only in the microcirculation, although occasionally large vessels are involved. The manifestations may be minimal, or there may be oliguria with acute renal failure, dyspnea, cyanosis, convulsions and coma. Hypotension is characteristic. When hemolysis is brisk, fever, back pain and jaundice are also present. Only infrequently, usually in the more chronic cases, is there spontaneous massive hemorrhage. Most often, attention is called to the presence of a bleeding diathesis by prolonged bleeding from a venipuncture site or by the presence of petechiae and ecchymoses on the skin. Certainly, in any seriously ill patient, unexplained bleeding from a venipuncture site should raise the possibility of DIC.

The prognosis with DIC is highly variable, depending on the underlying disorder as well as on the degree of intravascular clotting, the activity of the RE system and secondary fibrinolysis. In some cases, it tends to be self-limited; in others, it responds to prompt treatment with heparin. Often it runs a fulminant course, leading to death within days (McKay, 1965).

THROMBOCYTOPENIA

Platelet deficiencies may develop as a primary disorder or secondary to some other derangement. In either case, thrombocytopenia is characterized by a prolonged bleeding time, with a normal coagulation time. In addition, petechiae are often present in the skin, and showers of them suddenly develop distal to the cuff as the blood pressure is taken *(positive tourniquet test).* Platelet counts are, of course, diminished.

Secondary thrombocytopenia may be a component of myelophthisic pancytopenia or of hypersplenism, or it may result from exposure to toxins such as benzol, alkylating agents and antimetabolites. *Thrombotic thrombocytopenia purpura* (TTP) is characterized by the intravascular aggregation of thrombocytes and may be related to DIC.

Primary thrombocytopenia, also known as *idiopathic thrombocytopenia purpura (ITP),* is a mysterious disorder of probable autoimmune origin. Often it develops as a first manifestation of SLE. In most cases, however, ITP occurs as an apparently isolated disorder. Patients are usually children or young adults, and females are affected slightly more often than are males.

An antiplatelet IgG has been identified in the serum of patients with ITP. Administration of this globulin to normal recipients is followed by a reduction in the numbers of circulating platelets (Harrington et al., 1953). The spleen plays an important but poorly understood role in ITP. It is evidently a site of destruction of platelets, presumably coated with IgG. Splenectomized recipients develop less thrombocytopenia when transfused with ITP antiplatelet factor. Moreover, in patients with chronic ITP, splenectomy frequently results in a remission of the disease. There is also some evidence that the spleen is involved in the production of antiplatelet IgG (McMillan et al., 1974). The spleen usually appears remarkably normal, with only minimal — if any — enlargement. Such splenomegaly as may be present is attributable to congestion of the sinusoids and enlargement of the follicles. The marrow is nondiagnostic and may have increased numbers of megakaryocytes, many of which have only a single nucleus and are thought to be young. Indeed, significant findings are confined mostly to the secondary hemorrhages. Hemorrhages may be seen dispersed through-out the body, particularly in the serosal and mucosal linings.

HEREDITARY COAGULATION DISORDERS

Deficiencies of virtually any of the multiple clotting factors have been described, as well as combinations of deficiencies. Most important of these is a heterogeneous group of inherited disorders characterized by low levels of factors VIII or IX (or both), with or without platelet dysfunction. These are the hemophilias, von Willebrand's disease and related entities (Edson, 1970). At one time, the term "hemophilia" was defined simply as a deficiency of factor VIII, but it has become apparent that a clinically indistinguishable disorder can be caused by low levels of factor IX, as well as — rarely — by deficiency in factor XI. Thus, hemophilia is now considered to include: (1) factor VIII deficiency (about 80 per cent), (2) factor IX deficiency (10 to 15 per cent), and (3) factor XI deficiency (about 5 per cent). Von Willebrand's disease is characterized by platelet dysfunction in addition to low factor VIII levels. There is, however, much overlap among these entities, and cases have been described of virtually any combination of derangements in these clotting factors, along with platelet dysfunction. To add to the complexity, although they are usually inherited as sex-linked recessive traits, certain family pedigrees suggest that a second gene locus controlling synthesis of the clotting factors may be located on an autosome and may even be dominant. Only the more important disorders are individually described here.

FACTOR VIII DEFICIENCY (HEMOPHILIA A, CLASSIC HEMOPHILIA)

Factor VIII deficiency is inherited as an X-linked recessive trait, and thus it occurs in males or in homozygous females. However, excessive bleeding has been described in heterozygous females (Editorial, 1973). The clinical syndrome develops only in the presence of severe deficiency. Mild or moderate degrees of deficiency occur but are asymptomatic, although posttraumatic bleeding may be somewhat excessive. In about 10 per cent of cases, factor VIII is actually present in normal amounts but, for some reason, it is functionally abnormal. This subgroup has been designated *hemophilia A+,* while the pure deficiency state is known as *hemophilia A−.* In either case, the clinical result is a tendency toward massive hemorrhage following trauma or operative procedures. In addition, "spontaneous" hemorrhages are frequently encountered in regions of the body normally subject to trauma, particularly into the joints, where they are known as hemarthroses. *Petechiae and ecchymoses are characteristically absent. Although coagulation time is prolonged, bleeding time is normal.* At one time, about 50 per cent of severely affected patients died before the age of five years. However, the recent use of transfusions of factor VIII (or other clotting factors, as needed) has substantially improved the prognosis.

FACTOR IX DEFICIENCY (HEMOPHILIA B, CHRISTMAS DISEASE)

Severe factor IX deficiency is a disorder that is clinically indistinguishable from hemophilia A. Moreover, it is also inherited as an X-linked recessive trait and may occur asymptomatically in mild or moderate degrees. In about 14 per cent of these patients, factor IX is present but nonfunctional and, as with hemophilia A, the disorder is on this basis divided into *hemophilia B+* (or B_M) and the more common *hemophilia B−* (Twomey et al., 1969). *The coagulation time is prolonged; bleeding time is normal.*

VON WILLEBRAND'S DISEASE

Classically, this disease is inherited as an autosomal dominant disorder, characterized by platelet dysfunction, probably on the basis of defective platelet adhesiveness, as well as low levels of factor VIII. The platelet *count* is normal. *These patients may have a prolonged coagulation time, as well as a prolonged bleeding time.* Thus, clinical features of both, including petechiae and ecchymoses, epistaxis, easy bruising, menorrhagia in females and excessive traumatic bleeding, may all be present. It has recently been shown that, as determined by immunoassay, factor VIII consists of both an active component *(procoagulant factor VIII)* and an inactive component *(factor VIII-antigen)* (Zimmerman et al., 1971). *In contrast to patients with hemophilia, who have normal or elevated levels of factor VIII-antigen, those with von Willebrand's disease have lowered levels of both procoagulant factor VIII and factor VIII-antigen.* It has been suggested that the latter may be the mysterious "von Willebrand factor," the serum factor necessary for normal platelet adhesiveness (Snyder, 1974). A "paradoxic" response to factor VIII transfusion—that is, an elevation out of proportion to the amount of factor VIII transfused—is characteristic of von Willebrand's disease. It has been suggested that the factor VIII-antigen present in the transfusion may serve as a precursor in the synthesis of the procoagulant factor VIII (Deykin, 1974). However, many questions remain, and it is possible that the entity known as von Willebrand's disease is actually a heterogeneous group of disorders (Peake et al., 1974).

MISCELLANEOUS DISORDERS

INFECTIOUS MONONUCLEOSIS

This is a benign disease almost certainly caused by the Epstein-Barr virus (EBV), and characterized by fever, generalized lymphadenopathy and the appearance in the peripheral blood of large numbers of atypical lymphocytes. It occurs principally in teenagers and young adults, reaching a peak incidence between the ages of 15 and 19 years. These patients tend to be concentrated in the upper socioeconomic classes, and outbreaks are frequently reported in colleges.

Etiology and Pathogenesis. This disease currently is of great interest for two reasons. First, it is apparently caused by the EBV, the same herpes virus that may cause the malignant Burkitt's lymphoma (p. 348) and which subclinically infects from 50 to 80 per cent of the world's population. The second point of interest is that infectious mononucleosis is an intense lymphoproliferative disorder which, unlike the lymphomas, is self-limited. It is hoped that an understanding of the mechanisms by which infectious mononucleosis is contained might provide some insight into the pathogenesis and control of the lymphomas. Thus, the emphasis in the study of this disease has shifted from the question of what starts it to the question of what stops it (Carter, 1975).

The evidence that the EBV causes infectious mononucleosis is overwhelming. Large epidemiologic studies have shown that only individuals without antibodies against EBV are at risk of developing infectious mononucleosis. The active disease is then associated with the transient appearance of IgM antibodies against EBV, which indicate recent exposure to the virus, in addition to the development of long-lasting IgG antibodies. It is probable that in lower socioeconomic groups exposure to the EBV occurs early in life and is almost always entirely asymptomatic. When such exposure is delayed until adolescence or young adulthood, however, infectious mononucleosis may result in up to two thirds of exposed individuals (Epstein and Achong, 1973). There is much evidence that only the B-cells are actually vulnerable to infection by the EBV, and that most of the "atypical" lymphocytes so characteristic of infectious mononucleosis are T-cells presumably reacting against the infected B-cells (Pattengale et al., 1974). Indeed, these T-cells may represent the effective immune response which means the difference between a fairly trivial disorder and a malignant lymphoma. In this regard, it is of interest that when cultured infectious mononucleosis lymphocytes are transplanted into immunosuppressed experimental animals, they give rise to a malignant lymphoproliferative disorder (Carter, 1975). Moreover, a family has been described in which four members apparently developed infectious mononucleosis which progressed to a malignant lymphoproliferative disease. Most likely the fatal outcome in these cases resulted from a genetically determined defect in immune response (Bar et al., 1974). It would appear, then, that in the spectrum of disease caused by EBV, infectious mononucleosis occupies a position intermediate between that of an infectious disorder and that of a lymphoma. In this respect, it may be considered to have similarities to both immunoblastic lymphadenopathy and Hodgkin's disease, despite its more benign course.

Morphology. The major alterations involve the blood, lymph nodes, spleen, liver, central nervous system and, occasionally, other organs. The **peripheral blood** shows an absolute lymphocytosis with a total white cell count between 12,000 and 18,000 per mm.^{3}, over 60 per cent of which are lymphocytes. These are large, **atypical lymphocytes,** 12 to 16 μm. in diameter, and distinguished primarily by an abundant cytoplasm containing multiple clear vacuolations. These atypical lymphocytes are usually sufficiently distinctive to permit the diagnosis from examination of a peripheral blood smear. In addition, cells indistinguishable from the Reed-Sternberg cells of Hodgkin's disease (p. 358) have been described in infectious mononucleosis.

The **lymph nodes** are typically discretely enlarged throughout the body, principally in the posterior cervical, axillary and groin regions. Histologically, the lymphoid tissue is flooded by atypical lymphocytes, although the underlying architecture is usually preserved. Sometimes the follicles become extremely prominent. When the lymphocytes flood into the medullary portion of the nodes, the histology may simulate that of lymphocytic leukemia. Differentiation then depends on recognition of the atypical lymphocytes. Similar changes commonly occur in the tonsils and lymphoid tissue of the oropharynx.

The **spleen** is enlarged two or three times, weighing between 500 and 1000 gm. It is usually soft and fleshy, with a hyperemic cut surface. The histologic changes are analogous to those of the lymph nodes, showing a heavy infiltration of atypical lymphocytes, which may result either in prominence of the splenic follicles or in some blurring of the architecture. These spleens are especially vulnerable to rupture, possibly in part resulting from infiltration of the trabeculae and capsule by the lymphocytes.

Liver function is almost always transiently impaired to some degree, although hepatomegaly is at most moderate. Histologically, atypical lymphocytes are seen in the portal areas and sinusoids, and scattered, isolated cells or foci of parenchymal necrosis filled with lymphocytes may be present.

The **central nervous system** may show congestion, edema and perivascular mononuclear infiltrates in the leptomeninges. Myelin degeneration and destruction of axis cylinders have been described in the peripheral nerves.

Clinical Course. The clinical presentation and severity of infectious mononucleosis are highly variable. The classic case begins with chills, fever, malaise, painful enlargement of the cervical lymph nodes, and a very severe sore throat. A creamy exudate may be seen over the pharynx and tonsils and, in somewhat less than 50 per cent of cases, small petechiae are present on the palate. A fine macular skin rash resembling rubella develops in 10 to 15 per cent of patients. Splenomegaly is characteristic and may produce left upper quadrant tenderness. Rarely, a patient may have a hepatitis-like syndrome resulting from the liver involvement. The presence of lymphocytosis and the recognition on smear of atypical lymphocytes are crucial to the diagnosis. *In most cases, although not in all, agglutinins to sheep red cells are present (Paul-Bunnell heterophil test).* The prognosis is excellent, with slow but progressive improvement after two to four weeks of febrile illness. Fatalities are rare, and are usually attributable to rupture of the spleen or intercurrent infection.

CAT-SCRATCH DISEASE

This is a benign lesion of unknown (possibly viral) etiology, characterized by a regional lymphadenitis, usually following a cat scratch or thorn puncture. In the usual case, the local injury is trivial, although sometimes it is followed by the development of an erythematous papule or pustule at the site of trauma. One or two weeks later, but occasionally occurring after a delay of several months, the regional nodes of drainage become painfully enlarged, tense and red. They may reach a size of 8 to 10 cm. in diameter, although usually the enlargement is less marked. In about 50 per cent of cases, the nodes suppurate, becoming soft and fluctuant. The histologic reaction is fairly distinctive and can be characterized as "granulomatous abscess formation." When it is full-blown, the lesion consists of an irregular, stellate, round or ovoid abscess containing central debris, with fragmented granulocyte nuclei. This focus is enclosed within a rim of RE cells and fibroblasts, sometimes including giant cells of the foreign body or Langhans type. Plasma cells and lymphocytes frequently surround these granulomas.

Systemic symptoms are common but not invariable. Quite rarely they are severe, with temperatures as high as 105° F. In most instances, however, the disease is mild and subsides spontaneously in weeks to months. Because of the similarity between the histology of cat-scratch disease and that of lymphogranuloma venereum, tularemia, tuberculosis and sarcoidosis, the diagnosis in many cases must be supported by a skin test. This consists essentially of injection into the skin of the suppurative exudate from a known case; a positive test consists of redness and induration 48 hours after intradermal injection.

DERMATOPATHIC LYMPHADENITIS (LIPOMELANOTIC RETICULOENDOTHELIOSIS)

"Dermatopathic lymphadenitis" refers to a distinctive chronic lymphadenitis which affects the lymph nodes draining the sites of chronic dermatologic diseases. It is commonly associated with eczema, psoriasis, exfoliative dermatitis, neurodermatitis and seborrheic dermatitis. The nodes are usually moderately enlarged and characterized by the following: (1) histiocyte hyperplasia in the germinal follicles, (2) hyperplasia of the RE sinusoidal cells, (3) accumulation of melanin and, less prominently, of hemosiderin by the phagocytes within the nodes, and (4) the appearance of finely divided lipid granules in these phagocytic cells. The pathogenesis of these changes appears to lie in the persistent drainage to the involved nodes of melanin pigment and fatty debris from the skin lesion. The condition is of little significance, except for its possible confusion with a lymphoproliferative disorder.

HAND-SCHÜLLER-CHRISTIAN COMPLEX (HISTIOCYTOSIS X)

This disorder with the mysterious synonym is characterized by abnormal proliferation of histiocytes, principally in the RE organs of the body. Sometimes cholesterol accumulates within these lesions as a secondary phenomenon. The etiology is unknown, although an infectious agent is suspected. Three somewhat distinctive clinical and morphologic variants are included within the Hand-Schüller-Christian *complex:* Letterer-Siwe disease, Hand-Schüller-Christian *disease* and eosinophilic granuloma. However, there is still some controversy over whether these entities are actually different stages or expressions of the same basic disorder. Some believe that there is no justification for including them together (Lieberman et al., 1969). Nevertheless, all involve proliferation of histiocytes

and, in the more chronic cases, accumulation of cholesterol within these cells. Whether this accumulation represents increased intracellular synthesis within the abnormal cells, or rather the debris of neighboring necrotic cells, is unknown. In either case it is secondary, and so this complex of disorders should *not* be considered a lipid storage disease.

LETTERER-SIWE DISEASE

This most malignant Hand-Schüller-Christian variant is encountered predominantly in infants of either sex under the age of 1 year. The anatomic involvement is diffuse and the clinical course is usually rapidly fatal. The first findings are a few firm, red to brown skin nodules often thought to be insect bites. Later the skin lesions become generalized in the form of a maculopapular rash or multiple discrete nodules, which may become ulcerated. The spleen, liver, lymph nodes and bones all become involved, with generalized lymphadenopathy, hepatosplenomegaly and a myelophthisic pancytopenia. The histologic change is basically a pure proliferation of histiocytes throughout the involved organs, unrelieved by other histologic features. In a few instances, however, scattered eosinophils, plasma cells, lymphocytes, multinucleate giant cells and lipid-laden foam cells are present.

HAND-SCHULLER-CHRISTIAN DISEASE

This somewhat more benign but also generalized variant tends to affect an older age group and may arise in adults. The median survival is from 10 to 15 years. As with Letterer-Siwe disease, the skin, spleen, liver, lymph nodes and bones are involved, as well as other organs on occasion. *A clinical triad characteristic of this variant comprises diabetes insipidus, exophthalmos and radiolucent bone defects within the skull.* The bony defects are produced by local accumulations of lipid-laden histiocytes, while the exophthalmos and diabetes insipidus are caused by aggregations of the same cells at the base of the skull and orbit, causing pressure on the brain and retro-orbital tissues. Probably only a minority of these patients, however, have the full-blown triad. Histologically, the histiocytosis in this variant takes the form of masses or sheets of lipid-laden foam cells, abundantly interspersed with eosinophils, lymphocytes and plasma cells. Fibrosis may occur in the periphery of these lesions, creating the appearance of a chronic inflammatory granuloma. Central necrosis may heighten this resemblance.

EOSINOPHILIC GRANULOMA

This is the most benign Hand-Schüller-Christian variant and is encountered principally in older children and adults. There is a strong male preponderance. This type is usually confined to one of the bones or rarely to localized skin or visceral involvement. The prognosis is good; long survival is the rule, and sometimes spontaneous remissions occur. The classic radiographic appearance is of a sharply circumscribed focal area of bone destruction simulating a tumor. Sometimes a similar focal lesion is seen in soft tissues. The histologic appearance closely resembles that described for Hand-Schüller-Christian disease, save that eosinophils are more numerous.

SPLENOMEGALY

The spleen is frequently involved in a wide variety of systemic diseases. In virtually all cases, the splenic changes are secondary to disease that is primary elsewhere, and in almost all instances the presentation of the splenic lesion is enlargement. Excessive destruction by the spleen of red cells, leukocytes and platelets may ensue (hypersplenism). Evaluation of splenomegaly is a common clinical problem. It is considerably aided by a knowledge of the usual limits of splenic enlargement caused by the disorders being considered. Obviously, it would be erroneous to attribute enlargement of the spleen into the pelvis to vitamin B_{12} deficiency and equally erroneous to accept as classic a case of hereditary spherocytosis unless there is significant splenomegaly. As an aid to diagnosis, then, we present the following list of disorders, classified according to the degree of splenomegaly characteristically produced:

A. Massive Splenomegaly (over 1000 gm.)
 1. Chronic myelogenous leukemia
 2. Chronic lymphocytic leukemia (less massive)
 3. Lymphomas
 4. Myeloid metaplasia
 5. Malaria
 6. Gaucher's disease
 7. Primary tumors of the spleen (rare)
B. Moderate Splenomegaly (500 to 1000 gm.)
 1. Chronic congestive splenomegaly (portal vein or splenic vein obstruction)
 2. Acute leukemias
 3. Infectious mononucleosis
 4. Early sickle cell anemia
 5. Hereditary spherocytosis
 6. Thalassemia
 7. Autoimmune hemolytic anemia
 8. Idiopathic thrombocytopenic purpura
 9. Niemann-Pick disease
 10. Hand-Schüller-Christian complex
 11. Chronic splenitis (especially with vegetative endocarditis)
 12. Tuberculosis, sarcoidosis, typhoid
 13. Metastatic carcinoma or sarcoma
C. Minimal Splenomegaly (under 500 gm.)
 1. Acute splenitis
 2. Acute splenic congestion
 3. Miscellaneous acute febrile disorders, including septicemia, SLE and intraabdominal infections

REFERENCES

Bachmann, F.: Disseminated intravascular coagulation. DM (Disease-a-Month), Dec., 1969.

Baitz, T., and Kyle, R. A.: Solitary myeloma in chronic osteomyelitis. Arch. Int. Med., 113:872, 1964.

Bakemeier, R. F.: Malignant lymphoma. In Rubin, P. (ed.): Clinical Oncology for Medical Students and Physicians, 3rd ed. Rochester, N. Y., American Cancer Society, 1970–71, p. 332.

Bakemeier, R. F., and Miller, D. R.: The leukemias. In Rubin, P. (ed.): Clinical Oncology for Medical Students and Physicians, 3rd ed. Rochester, N. Y., American Cancer Society, 1970–71, p. 360.

Banfi, A., et al.: Preferential sites of involvement and spread in malignant lymphomas. Europ. J. Cancer, 4:319, 1968.

Bar, R. S., et al.: Fatal infectious mononucleosis in a family. New Eng. J. Med., 290:363, 1974.

Biniaminov, M., and Ramot, B.: Possible T-lymphocyte origin of Reed-Sternberg cells. Lancet, 1:368, 1974.

Blackstein, A. M., and Garson, O. M.: Direct evidence for involvement of erythroid cells in acute myeloblastic leukemia. Lancet, 2:1178, 1974.

Blajchman, M. A., et al.: Immunoglobulins in warm-type autoimmune hemolytic anemia, 1:340, 1969.

Boender, C. A., and Verloop, M. C.: Iron absorption, iron loss and iron retention in man. Brit. J. Haemat., 17:45, 1960.

Boggs, T. R., et al.: Correlation of neonatal serum total bilirubin concentration on developmental status at age eight months. J. Pediat., 71:553, 1967.

Braylan, R. C. et al.: Surface characteristics of Hodgkin's lymphoma cells. Lancet, 2:1328, 1974.

Brodsky, I., and Siegel, N. H.: The diagnosis and treatment of disseminated intravascular coagulation. Med. Clin. North Amer., 54:555, 1970.

Burchenal, J. H.: Features suggesting curability in lymphomas and leukemia. CA, 23:344, 1973.

Cardamone, J. M., et al.: Development of acute erythroleukemia in B-cell immunoproliferative disorders after prolonged therapy with alkylating drugs. Am. J. Med., 57:836, 1974.

Carr, I.: Ultrastructure of malignant reticulum and Reed-Sternberg cells. Lancet, 1:926, 1975.

Carter, R. L.: Infectious mononucleosis: model for self-limiting lymphoproliferation. Lancet, 1:846, 1975.

Case Records of the Massachusetts General Hospital. New Eng. J. Med., 292:689, 1975.

Chanarin, I.: New light on pernicious anemia. Lancet, 2:538, 1973.

Chanarin, I., et al.: The biochemical lesion in vitamin B_{12} deficiency in man. Lancet, 1:1251, 1974.

Dacie, J. V.: Autoimmune hemolytic anemias. Brit. Med. J., 2:381, 1970.

Dameshek, W.: Some speculations on the myeloproliferative syndrome. Blood, 6:372, 1951.

Deinhardt, F.: Introduction to virus-caused cancer: type C virus. Cancer, 34 (Suppl.):1363, 1974.

Denborough, M. A., et al.: Serum blood group substances and ABO hemolytic disease. Brit. J. Haematol., 16:103, 1969.

DeVita, V. T., Jr.: Lymphocyte reactivity in Hodgkin's disease: a lymphocyte civil war. New Eng. J. Med., 289:801, 1973.

Deykin, D.: Emerging concepts of platelet function. New Eng. J. Med., 290:144, 1974.

Dickler, H. B., et al.: Lymphocyte binding of aggregated IgG and surface Ig staining in chronic lymphocytic leukemia. Clin. Exp. Immunol., 14:97, 1973.

Editorial: Alcohol and the blood. Lancet, 2:675, 1969a.

Editorial: Drug resistant malaria. Lancet, 1:1245, 1969b.

Editorial: Hemophilia in women. Lancet, 2:1305, 1973.

Editorial: Treatment of sickle-cell crises. Lancet, 2:762, 1974a.

Editorial: Conquest of malaria: The art of the feasible. Lancet, 1:607, 1974b.

Editorial: Follicular lymphomas. Lancet, 1:1088, 1974c.

Editorial: The methylfolate-trap hypothesis. Lancet, 1:843, 1975a.

Editorial: Bone marrow grafting for aplastic anemia. Lancet, 1:22, 1975b.

Editorial: Immunoblastic-cell proliferations. Lancet, 1:260, 1975c.

Editorial: A human-leukemia virus? Lancet, 1:671, 1975d.

Editorial: Blind alleys in the Hodgkin's maze. Lancet, 1:556, 1975e.

Edson, J. R.: Hemophilia, von Willebrand's disease and related conditions: A spectrum of laboratory and clinical disorders. Hum. Pathol., 1:387, 1970.

Emerson, C. P.: Influence of the spleen on the osmotic behavior and the longevity of red cells in hereditary spherocytosis: A case study. Boston Med. Quart., 5:65, 1954.

Epstein, M. A., and Achong, B. G.: Various forms of Epstein-Barr virus infection in man: established facts and a general concept. Lancet, 2:836, 1973.

Epstein, M. A., et al.: Pilot experiments with EB virus in owl monkeys (Aotus trivirgatus). Int. J. Cancer, 12:309, 1973.

Fialkow, P. J.: The origin and development of human tumors studied with cell markers. New Eng. J. Med., 291:26, 1974.

Ford, J. H., and Pittman, S. M.: Duplication of 21 or 8/21 translocation in acute leukemia. Lancet, 2:1458, 1974.

Gabuzda, T. G.: Sickle cell disease. Delaware Med. J., 43:124, 1971.

Gallagher, R. E., and Gallo, R. C.: Type C RNA tumor virus isolated from cultured human acute myelogenous leukemia cells. Science, 187:350, 1975.

Gallo, R. C.: Terminal transferase and leukemia. New Eng. J. Med., 292:804, 1975.

Gallo, R. C. et al.: The evidence for involvement of type C RNA tumor viruses in human acute leukemia. Cancer, 34(Suppl.):1398, 1974.

Gershwin, M. E., and Steinberg, A. D.: Loss of suppressor function as a cause of lymphoid malignancy. Lancet, 2:1174, 1973.

Gutterman, J. U., et al.: Chemoimmunotherapy of adult acute leukemia: prolongation of remission in myeloblastic leukemia with B.C.G. Lancet, 2:1405, 1974.

Halbrecht, I.: Icterus praecox; further studies on its frequency, etiology, prognosis and the blood chemistry of the cord blood. J. Pediat., 39:185, 1951.

Hansen, J. A., and Good, R. A.: Malignant disease of the lymphoid system in immunological perspective. Hum. Pathol., 5:567, 1974.

Hardaway, R. M.: Syndrome of Disseminated Intravascular Coagulation with Special Reference to Shock and Hemorrhage. Springfield, Ill., Charles C Thomas, 1966.

Harrington, W. J., et al.: Immunologic mechanisms in idiopathic and neonatal thrombocytopenic purpura. Ann. Intern. Med., 38:433, 1953.

Hellman, S.: What laparotomy has wrought. New Eng. J. Med., 20:894, 1974.

Henle, W., et al.: Epstein-Barr virus specific diagnostic tests in infectious mononucleosis. Hum. Pathol., 5:551, 1974.

Herbert, V.: Correlation of folate deficiency with alcoholism and associated macrocytosis, anemia and liver disease. Ann. Intern. Med., 58:977, 1963.

Hillen, H., et al.: Bone-marrow-proliferation patterns in acute myeloblastic leukemia determined by pulse cytophotometry. Lancet, 1:609, 1975.

Hirshaut, Y., et al.: Epstein-Barr-virus antibodies in American and African Burkitt's lymphoma. Lancet, 2:114, 1973.

Hoover, R., and Fraumeni, J. F., Jr.: Risk of cancer in renal-transplant recipients. Lancet, 2:55, 1973.

Ingram, V. M.: The Hemoglobins in Genetics and Evolution. New York, Columbia University Press, 1963, p. 125.

Ingram, V. M., and Stretton, A. O. W.: Genetic basis of the thalassemia diseases. Nature, 184:1903, 1959.

Jacob, H. S., and Jandl, J. H.: Increased cell membrane permeability in the pathogenesis of hereditary spherocytosis. J. Clin. Endocr., 43:704, 1964.

Jacobs, M.: Malignant lymphomas and their management. In Rentchnick, P. (ed.): Recent Results in Cancer Research Series, Vol. 18. New York, Springer-Verlag, 1968.

Jacobs, P., et al.: Intestinal iron transport: studies using a loop of gut with an artificial circulation. Amer. J. Physiol. 210:694, 1966.

Kahn, S. B.: Recent advances in the nutritional anemias. Med. Clin. North Amer., 54:631, 1970.

Kaplan, H. S.: The radical radiotherapy of regionally localized Hodgkin's disease. Radiology, 78:553, 1962.

Kay, M. M. B., and Kadin, M.: Surface characteristics of Hodgkin's cells. Lancet, 1:748, 1975.

Klein, G.: The Epstein-Barr virus and neoplasia. New Eng. J. Med., 293:1353, 1975.

Lai, P. K., et al.: Aplastic anemia, acute myeloid leukemia and EB-virus. Lancet, 1:756, 1974.

Leevy, C. M., et al.: Incidence and significance of hypovitaminemia in a randomly selected municipal hospital population. Amer. J. Clin. Nutr., 17:259, 1965.

Levy, R., and Kaplan, H. S.: Impaired lymphocyte function in untreated Hodgkin's disease. New Eng. J. Med., 290:181, 1974.

Lieberman, P. H., et al.: A reappraisal of eosinophilic granuloma of bone, Hand-Schüller-Christian syndrome and Letterer-Siwe syndrome. Medicine, 48:375, 1969.

Linton, A. L., et al.: Microangiopathic hemolytic anemia and the pathogenesis of malignant hypertension. Lancet, 1:1277, 1969.

Lukes, R. J.: The pathologic picture of the malignant lymphomas. In Zarafonetis, C. J. D. (ed.): Proceedings of the International Conference on Leukemia-Lymphoma. Philadelphia, Lea & Febiger, 1968, pp. 334–356.

Lukes, R. J., and Butler, J. J.: The pathology and nomenclature of Hodgkin's disease. Cancer Res., 26:1063, 1966.

Lukes, R. J., and Collins, R. D.: Immunologic characterization of human malignant lymphomas. Cancer, 34 (Suppl.):1488, 1974.

Lukes, R. J., et al.: Hodgkin's disease: report of nomenclature committee. Cancer Res., 26:1311, 1966.

Magrath, I., et al.: Antibodies to Epstein-Barr virus antigens before and after the development of Burkitt's lymphoma in a patient treated for Hodgkin's disease. New Eng. J. Med., 292:621, 1975.

Marder, V. J., et al.: The importance of intermediate degradation products of fibrinogen in fibrinolytic hemorrhage. Trans. Assoc. Am. Physicians, 80:156, 1967.

McKay, D. G.: Disseminated Intravascular Coagulation—An Intermediary Mechanism of Disease. New York, Hoeber Medical Division, Harper & Row, 1965.

McMillan, R., et al.: Quantitation of platelet-binding IgG produced in vitro by spleens from patients with idiopathic thrombocytopenic purpura. New Eng. J. Med., 291:812, 1974.

Melief, C. J. M., et al.: Immunologic activation of murine leukemia viruses. Cancer, 34 (Suppl.):1481, 1974.

Merskey, C., et al.: The defibrination syndrome: Clinical features and laboratory diagnosis. Brit. J. Haemat., 13:528, 1967.

Mollison, P. L.: Blood Transfusion in Clinical Medicine, 4th ed. Oxford, Blackwell Scientific Publications, 1967, p. 697.

Mundy, G. R., et al.: Evidence for the secretion of an osteoclast stimulating factor in myeloma. New Eng. J. Med., 291:1041, 1974.

Nowell, P. C., et al.: T-cells in chronic lymphocytic leukemia. Lancet, 1:915, 1975.

Oels, H. C., et al.: Lymphoblastic lymphoma with histiocytic phagocytosis. Cancer, 21:368, 1968.

Order, S., and Hellman, S.: Pathogenesis of Hodgkin's disease. Lancet, 1:571, 1972.

Pagano, J. S., et al.: Absence of Epstein-Barr viral DNA in American Burkitt's lymphoma. New Eng. J. Med., 289:1395, 1973.

Paronetto, F.: Systemic nonsuppurative necrotizing angiitis. In Miescher, P. A., and Mueller-Eberhard, H. J. (eds.): Textbook of Immunopathology. New York, Grune and Stratton, 1969, p. 722.

Pattengale, P. K., et al.: Atypical lymphocytes in acute infectious mononucleosis. New Eng. J. Med., 291:1145, 1974.

Peake, I. R., et al.: Inherited variants of factor-VIII related protein in vonWillebrand's disease. New Eng. J. Med., 291:113, 1974.

Perera, D. J. B., and Pegrum, G. D.: The lymphocyte in chronic lymphatic leukemia. Lancet, 1:1207, 1974.

Peters, M. V., et al.: The natural history of the lymphomas related to the clinical classification. In Zarafonetis, C. J. D. (ed.): Proceedings of the International Conference of Leukemia-Lymphoma. Philadelphia, Lea & Febiger, 1968.

Peters, M. V., and Middlemiss, K. C.: A study of Hodgkin's disease treated by irradiation. Am. J. Roentgenol., 79:114, 1958.

Potter, M., and MacCardle, R. C.: Histology of developing plasma cell neoplasia induced by mineral oil in BALB/c mice. J. Nat. Cancer Inst., 33:497, 1964.

Prentice, C. R. M., et al.: Changes in platelet behavior during arvin therapy. Lancet, 1:644, 1969.

Rand, J. J., et al.: Coagulation defects in acute promyelocytic leukemia. Arch. Int. Med., 123:39, 1969.

Rappaport, H.: Tumors of the hematopoietic system. In Atlas of Tumor Pathology. Washington, D.C., Armed Forces Institute of Pathology, 1966.

Rappaport, H., and Moran, E. M.: Angio-immunoblastic (immunoblastic) lymphadenopathy. New Eng. J. Med., 292:42, 1975.

Reed, D.: On the pathologic changes in Hodgkin's disease with special reference to its relation to tuberculosis. Johns Hopkins Hosp. Rep., 10:133, 1902.

Roitt, I., and Doniach, D.: Gastric autoimmunity. In Miescher, P. A., and Mueller-Eberhard, H. J. (eds.): Textbook of Immunopathology. New York, Grune and Stratton, 1969, p. 534.

Rosenfield, R. E., and Ohno, G.: A-B hemolytic disease of the newborn. Rev. Hemat., 10:231, 1955.

Rowley, J. D.: A new consistent chromosomal abnormality crine fluorescence and giemsa staining. Nature, 243:290, 1973.

Salmon, S. E., and Seligmann, M.: B-cell neoplasia in man. Lancet, 2:1230, 1974.

Schwartz, R. S.: Immunoregulation, oncogenic viruses, and malignant lymphomas. Lancet, 1:1266, 1972.

Seligmann, M.: B-cell and T-cell markers in lymphoid proliferations. New Eng. J. Med., 290:1483, 1974.

Seligmann, M., et al.: IgG myeloma cryoglobin with antistreptolysin activity. Nature, 220:711, 1968.

Sen, L., and Borella, L.: Clinical importance of lymphoblasts with T-markers in childhood acute leukemia. New Eng. J. Med., 292:828, 1975.

Shope, T., et al.: Malignant lymphoma in cottontop marmosets after inoculation with Epstein-Barr virus. Proc. Natl. Acad. Sci., 70:2487, 1973.

Silverberg, E., and Holleb, A. I.: Cancer statistics, 1975. CA, 25:8, 1975.

Snyder, D. S.: Von Willebrand's disease, hemophilia A, and factor VIII. Hum. Pathol., 5:277, 1974.

Sprichaikul, T., et al.: Complement changes and disseminated intravascular coagulation in plasmodium falciparum malaria. Lancet, 1:770, 1975.

Straub, P. W., et al.: Hypofibrinogenemia in metastatic carcinoma of the prostate. J. Clin. Path., 20:152, 1967.

Sullivan, L. W.: Differential diagnosis and management of the patient with megaloblastic anemia. Am. J. Med., 48:609, 1970.

Taylor, C. R.: The nature of Reed-Sternberg cells and other malignant "reticulum" cells. Lancet, 2:802, 1974.

Temin, H. M.: Introduction to virus-caused cancers. Cancer, 34(Suppl.):1347, 1974.

Tindle, B. H., et al.: "Reed-Sternberg cells" in infectious mononucleosis? Am. J. Clin. Path., 58:607, 1972.

Twomey, J. J., et al.: Studies on the inheritance and nature of hemophilia B$_M$. Am. J. Med., 46:372, 1969.

Vianna, N. J., and Polan, A. K.: Epidemiologic evidence for transmission of Hodgkin's disease. New Eng. J. Med., 289:499, 1973.

Vianna, N. J., et al.: Familial Hodgkin's disease: an environmental and genetic disorder. Lancet, 2:854, 1974.

Vigi, V., et al.: The correlation between red-cell survival and excess of alpha-globulin synthesis in beta-thalassemia. Brit. J. Haematol., 16:25, 1969.

Wasserman, L. R.: Polycythemia vera—its course and treatment: Relation to myeloid metaplasia and leukemia. Bull. N. Y. Acad. Med., 30:343, 1954.

Weatherall, D. J., et al.: The pattern of disordered hemoglobin synthesis in homozygous and heterozygous beta-thalassemia. Brit. J. Haematol., 16:251, 1969.

Zimmerman, T. S., et al.: Detection of carriers of classic hemophilia using an immunologic assay for antihemophilic factor (factor 8). J. Clin. Invest., 50:255, 1971.

Zorbala-Mallios, H., and Sutton, R. N. P.: E.B.-virus-specific IgM antibodies in first-degree relatives of children with acute lymphoblastic leukemia. Lancet, 1:119, 1974.

Zuelzer, W. W., et al.: Autoimmune hemolytic anemia. Am. J. Med., 49:80, 1970.

CHAPTER 12

Respiratory System

Respiratory infections are more frequent than infections of any other organ, and range from the relatively trivial acute laryngitis or bronchitis to fulminant lobar pneumonia. Cancer of the lung now kills more people than any other tumor. Along with the incredibly huge volume of air we draw into our lungs during a lifetime come all manner of dusts and fumes and gases. These often produce disease and, as the atmosphere increasingly becomes the wastebasket of human endeavor, such diseases threaten to become more common. And finally, secondary disease of the lungs occurs with almost any terminal illness. *Thus, whatever the primary disease, the immediate cause of death is very often pulmonary embolism or bronchopneumonia or pulmonary edema.* It is indeed rare to find the lungs uninvolved at postmortem examination. Respiratory disease, then, is a major source of morbidity and mortality.

In this chapter, only those diseases of the lung encountered with reasonable frequency in general medical practice will be discussed in detail. Some of the less common entities will be described briefly at the end of the chapter. Systemic disturbances which only secondarily involve the lung receive consideration elsewhere in the book.

The lung and tracheobronchial tree manifest disease in an unusually limited number of ways, which often overlap one another. Regardless of the presence of other symptoms or signs, however, the presence or absence of *cough* creates two almost equally large and very useful categories of lung disease. The group not prominently associated with cough tends to manifest itself by difficult breathing *(dyspnea)*. Hence, the major lung diseases will be discussed under these two headings— "cough" and "dyspnea"—and each group will be further subdivided into those entities with a typically acute presentation and those with more insidious development. The chart below shows the groupings and the diseases to be discussed.

Before proceeding to a discussion of cough, dyspnea and the diseases they characterize, a few words on pain and respiratory disease are necessary.

Pain is not an important early symptom of respiratory disease, since the lung and visceral pleura are insensitive to stimuli that ordinarily cause pain. Only when the exquisitely sensitive parietal pleura is involved—as, for example, with certain types of pneumonia or with pulmonary infarction, or when a lesion, such as an abscess or carcinoma, happens to impinge on the pleura—is severe pain produced. The pain is then of a characteristic type, called *pleuritic pain*, which waxes with inspiration and wanes with expiration. The pleura lining the bony rib cage produces pain directly over the involved area. When the pleura lining the dome and central portion of the diaphragm is involved, however, the pain is referred to the shoulder and neck, reflecting the distribution of the phrenic nerve. On the other hand, when the pleura lining the outer portions of the diaphragm is affected, impulses flow into the lower intercostal nerves, and the pain is referred to the wall of the lower thorax and abdomen.

	DYSPNEA	COUGH
ACUTE	1. Bronchial asthma 2. Atelectasis 3. Hyaline membrane disease 4. Pneumothorax 5. Pulmonary edema 6. Pulmonary embolism	1. Bacterial pneumonias 2. Primary atypical pneumonia 3. Acute laryngotracheo-bronchitis
CHRONIC	1. Pulmonary vascular sclerosis 2. Emphysema 3. Pneumoconioses	1. Chronic bronchitis 2. Bronchiectasis 3. Lung abscess 4. Tuberculosis 5. Deep mycoses 6. Lung tumors 7. Carcinoma of the larynx

COUGH

Cough is a reflex action initiated by irritation of afferent nerve endings located in the laryngeal, tracheal and bronchial mucosa. The nerve fibers are chiefly those of the vagus nerve. Although the irritation may be either mechanical or chemical, it usually stems from the accumulation of excess secretions. As such, the cough may be looked upon as the ultimate defense mechanism for keeping the tracheobronchial tree clear, being invoked only when other defenses, such as the beating of cilia and the steady upward flow of the mucus sheet coating the epithelium, have been overwhelmed. Cough is the most common symptom of early respiratory disease. Of course, when pulmonary disease is severe or widespread enough to impair function, dyspnea, too, will develop. However, among those diseases characterized by cough, the cough typically appears before dyspnea and may even precede it by years. From the mechanism of cough induction, it should be clear that this symptom is most likely with diseases primarily affecting the mucosa of the larger airways. Such diseases include acute laryngotracheobronchitis, chronic bronchitis and bronchiectasis. Second, cough can be expected with any process generating large amounts of secretions and exudation which drain into the tracheobronchial tree, such as the pneumonias. And, finally, cough is usually the earliest symptom of localized processes, such as a lung abscess, tuberculosis or carcinoma, which are likely to erode into bronchioles or bronchi long before they become advanced enough to produce dyspnea. Some of the diseases characterized by cough, including acute laryngotracheobronchitis and the pneumonias, have a sudden onset, often with fever and prostration, and run a rapid course. Others, including chronic bronchitis, bronchiectasis, lung abscess, tuberculosis and carcinoma, first manifest themselves with the more or less insidious onset of cough, and typically run a subacute to chronic course.

DYSPNEA

Dyspnea may be defined as awareness by the patient of unusual breathlessness. Since dyspnea is associated with those conditions which interfere with adequate gas exchange in the lungs, it is tempting to explain it teleologically as the body's attempt to get more oxygen. Indeed, it is almost always accompanied by alterations in the rate and depth of breathing. However, the stimuli and pathways by which these alterations are produced are poorly understood, and the basis for the subjective component of dyspnea is still more mysterious. Presumably two types of stimuli may be involved: chemical and proprioceptive (mechanical).

Chemical stimuli include hypoxemia and hypercapnia, both of which have an excitatory influence on respiratory centers in the brain stem. Hypercapnia probably acts indirectly, through the associated increase in hydrogen ions, which in turn act on the brain stem. In clinical practice, hypoxemia nearly always occurs before hypercapnia, since carbon dioxide is more soluble than oxygen and diffuses more readily through the alveolar membrane. Indeed, in early diffuse lung disease, there is often *hypo*capnia, which results from the hyperventilation triggered by hypoxemia. The later development of hypercapnia, then, indicates severe impairment. It should be remembered that dyspnea may occur on a chemical basis from nonrespiratory causes, e.g., metabolic acidosis or severe anemia.

Proprioceptive stimuli may operate through stretch receptors in the walls of the smaller airways, perhaps within the alveoli themselves. In addition, the length-tension inappropriateness (LTI) theory first proposed by Campbell and Howell adds a new dimension to the explanation of dyspnea (Campbell and Howell, 1963). According to this, the relevant receptors are the muscle spindles (gamma loops) located within the respiratory muscles themselves. If the rate of shortening of the inspiratory muscles is impeded because of increased airway resistance or because of decreased compliance, i.e., increased "stiffness," there is a resultant misalignment between the muscle fibers and the muscle spindles. By unknown pathways, such misalignment produces dyspnea.

Dyspnea, then, occurs whenever ventilatory demand exceeds the ability of the respiratory system to meet that demand, and is present with any generalized lung disease, either obstructive or restrictive. Obviously, it is not characteristic of a focal parenchymal process. When dyspnea is the *presenting* manifestation of respiratory disease, the process should be assumed to be a general one that does not produce early cough. Among diseases of this type with an acute onset are asthma (remitting, rather than acute), atelectasis, hyaline membrane disease, pneumothorax, pulmonary edema and pulmonary embolism. Included among those processes characterized by the *insidious* development of dyspnea are pulmonary vascular sclerosis, primary emphysema and the pneumoconioses.

ACUTE DYSPNEA

BRONCHIAL ASTHMA

Asthma is characterized by intermittent attacks of bronchial obstruction as a result of: (1) bronchospasm, (2) mucosal edema, and (3) hypersecretion of viscid mucus. Typically, the attacks are interspersed with symptom-free intervals. The classic case represents an atopic reaction to a variety of allergens, but in many other cases an allergic component is not clearly demonstrable. Both sexes and all ages are susceptible; however, the disease most commonly has its onset in the early decades of life, and it is an important cause of disability among school-age children.

Etiology and Pathogenesis. Bronchial asthma can be divided into the following three categories: (1) *Extrinsic asthma*, the type found in the minority of patients, whose disease is clearly a response to a known extrinsic allergen. (2) *Intrinsic asthma*. This term applies to a larger group of patients, whose asthmatic attacks seem to be triggered by a number of nonspecific stimuli, including the common cold (to which they seem particularly vulnerable), emotional factors, dust, cold weather and exercise. It has been postulated that the patients whose asthmatic attacks follow upper respiratory infections have developed an allergic response to various infectious agents. Although it has been impossible to demonstrate this by skin testing with the microbial antigen, the frequent development of an asthmatic attack following the skin test lends some clinical support to this theory. (3) *Mixed asthma*. This is the form of asthma afflicting the largest group of patients, and is composed of components of both the intrinsic and the extrinsic forms. Frequently, patients with extrinsic or intrinsic asthma later develop the mixed type.

Within the past few years, the pathogenesis of extrinsic asthma has become considerably clarified with the identification and isolation of reagin, the skin and mucous membrane sensitizing antibody that is involved in atopic reactions. Reagin was identified as being at least in part IgE, which is present in minute amounts (0.025 mg. per cent) in normal serum, but which occurs in markedly elevated levels in the sera of patients with extrinsic asthma, as well as with other atopic diseases, such as hay fever and atopic dermatitis (Ishizaka and Ishizaka, 1967). Reagin has the distinctive property of becoming fixed to cells in certain "shock organs," such as the skin and bronchial mucosa, where it persists for weeks, thus sensitizing the particular organ to the allergen. When the patient is then exposed to the allergen, the allergen-reagin interaction causes the release of a variety of chemical mediators, which are responsible for the manifestations of the asthmatic attacks. The most important of these mediators are histamine, bradykinin and SRS-A (slow reacting substance of anaphylaxis) (Frick, 1969). Histamine is released from mast cells and may also be rapidly formed and released from other cells. It causes contraction of smooth muscle, including that of the bronchi; increased vascular permeability; and increased bronchial secretions. It is probably most important in the first few minutes of an asthmatic attack. Bradykinin is formed from precursors in the blood under the influence of a variety of stimuli, including antigen-antibody reactions. It, too, causes smooth muscle contraction, as well as vasodilatation with increased permeability and leukotaxis. The SRS-A is a chemically ill-defined substance which is released, probably from polymorphonuclear leukocytes, by the allergen-reagin reaction. It causes prolonged bronchial constriction and seems to be the principal mediator after the first few minutes. There is also some recent evidence that the reagin-induced reaction may be followed by a slower precipitin-mediated response of the Arthus type, which may involve a number of antigens (Editorial, 1968). It is important to remember that whereas elevated serum levels of IgE are usually associated with extrinsic asthma rather than with the intrinsic pattern, the correlation is not absolute, and there is much overlap (Kay et al., 1974).

The above concept of the pathogenesis of asthma leaves unexplained a number of characteristics of the disease. For example, these patients are known to be hyperreactors to the chemical mediators, and indeed their heightened response to certain pharmacologic agents may be used as a diagnostic test. Is this hyperreactivity basic to the disease or is it a secondary result of it? One theory proposes that such reactivity is basic and represents a congenital or acquired malfunctioning of the beta-adrenergic receptors in the tracheobronchial tree. It has been postulated that the defect involves cyclic AMP, which is necessary for beta-adrenergic stimulation (Franklin, 1974; Reed, 1974). Since these receptors are necessary for bronchodilatation, their malfunctioning leaves bronchoconstriction unopposed, hence this could account for the greater susceptibility of asthmatics to all bronchoconstrictive stimuli (Szentivanyi, 1966). Such a theory has the advantage of explaining the hyperreactivity of the intrinsic asthmatic to nonspecific stimuli, and thus it is generally applicable to both intrinsic and extrinsic asthma.

Morphology. The anatomic changes of asthma are found in the bronchi and bronchioles down to about 1 mm. in diameter. Secondary changes, such as hyperinflation of the alveoli or focal areas of atelectasis, are frequent accompaniments, but the gross diagnosis rests with the demonstration of tenacious mucus plugs lying within bronchi and bronchioles. These often completely occlude the lumina. The walls of the bronchi may appear slightly thicker than usual, and sometimes there is denudation or sloughing of fragments of epithelium. In uncomplicated asthma, there is no significant suppuration within the airways. When infection is present, most would designate the underlying disease as bronchitis, which may itself involve an element of bronchospasm.

In the case of true asthma, there are many striking histologic changes. These include the finding of characteristic plugs of basophilic mucinous secretion lying within bronchi. Classically, these secretions are PAS positive and they contain, in addition to mucus, large numbers of eosinophils, bronchial epithelial cells, Charcot-Leyden crystals (composed of eosinophilic granules) and "Curschmann's spirals," which are curled mucinous fibers. The underlying epithelium is edematous and shows a striking inflammatory infiltrate, principally of eosinophils and leukocytes. There is thickening of the epithelial basement membrane and hypertrophy of the underlying smooth muscle. The bronchial mucous glands sometimes are hyperplastic (Fig. 12—1). Although the lungs often are overinflated, it is uncommon to find true destructive emphysema (p. 386).

Clinical Course. Most of these patients have a family history of atopic disease, including hay fever, infantile eczema and urticaria, as well as of bronchial asthma. These familial cases often begin at an early age, and in general the earlier the onset of the disease, the more severe the attacks. Early asthma is more likely to be of the purely extrinsic form than is asthma which has its onset later in life. On the basis of the anatomic changes, one can anticipate that an asthma attack is characterized by severe dyspnea with wheezing. Because the tracheobronchial tree widens and lengthens during inspiration, the major difficulty is with expiration. The victim labors to get air into his lungs and then cannot get it out, so that there is progressive hyperinflation of the lungs with air trapped distal to the mucus plugs. The result is characteristic prolonged wheezing expirations. This expiratory difficulty causes the patient to make active muscular efforts to expel air from his lungs. He thus increases transpulmonic pressure, which tends to collapse the airways, worsening his situation and establishing a vicious circle.

In the usual case, attacks last from one to several hours, and subside either spontaneously or with therapy, usually by bronchodilators. Intervals between attacks are characteristically free from respiratory difficulty, although not necessarily completely so. Some functional abnormalities are likely to persist, including a diminished 1-second forced expiratory volume and an increased mean residual volume (Editorial, 1974a). Nevertheless, it is the largely intermittent nature of bronchial

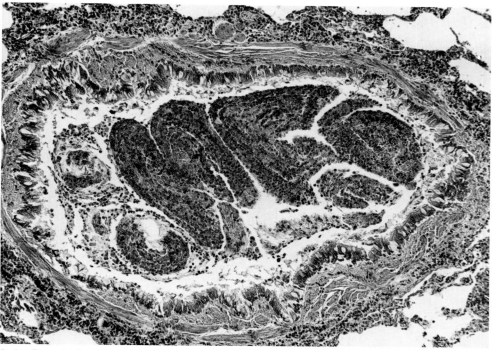

Figure 12–1. Bronchial asthma. A small bronchus containing plugs of mucin secretion, as well as inflammatory cells within the lumen. Note the hypertrophy of mucin-secreting lining cells, the hypertrophy of the smooth muscle, and the peribronchial inflammatory infiltrate.

obstruction, as well as the fact that destructive emphysema rarely occurs with uncomplicated asthma, which distinguishes asthma from chronic obstructive pulmonary disease, which will be discussed later. Occasionally, a severe paroxysm occurs which does not respond to therapy and persists for days and even weeks. This is known as *status asthmaticus.* In these circumstances, the ventilatory function may be so impaired as to result in severe cyanosis and even death. However, in most cases, the disease is more disabling than lethal. When death occurs, it is typically from superimposed infection or from respiratory failure during status asthmaticus.

ATELECTASIS

Atelectasis refers either to incomplete expansion of the lungs at birth (*atelectasis neonatorum*) or to collapse of previously fully aerated alveoli, usually in the adult (*acquired atelectasis*).

ATELECTASIS NEONATORUM

This form may be further subdivided into *primary* and *secondary* patterns. *Primary atelectasis neonatorum* implies that respiration has never been fully established. It is most common in premature infants whose respiratory centers in the brain are not mature and whose respiratory motions are feeble. Precipitating factors include any obstetric complication leading to intrauterine hypoxia during delivery.

The lungs at autopsy are collapsed, red-blue and noncrepitant, flabby and rubbery. Characteristically, these lungs fail to float when immersed in water. Histologically, the alveoli resemble the native fetal lung, with uniformly small alveolar spaces, surrounded by thick septal walls which have a crumpled appearance. A prominent cuboidal epithelium lines the alveolar spaces, and often there is a granular, proteinaceous precipitate mixed with amniotic debris within the air spaces.

Secondary atelectasis neonatorum occurs predominantly in premature infants who have established respiration but whose lungs never become *completely* aerated and who therefore die within the first few days or weeks of postnatal life. Predisposing factors in addition to prematurity include aspiration of secretions or blood during passage through the birth canal and oversedation of the mother. This form of atelectasis is also seen with hyaline membrane disease, to be discussed later.

In contrast to the primary form, the lungs in secondary atelectasis neonatorum are unevenly affected and show areas of collapsed parenchyma alternating with areas of aerated parenchyma. The histologic changes are similar to those described with the primary form alternating with areas of adjacent hyperinflation, sometimes called compensatory emphysema.

ACQUIRED ATELECTASIS

This is also of two major types—*absorption* collapse and *compression* collapse. *Absorption atelectasis* occurs whenever an airway is fully obstructed, so that air cannot enter the distal parenchyma. The air already present in the affected alveoli is gradually absorbed into the blood, and the involved area becomes airless and shrunken. In compensation, adjacent areas of the lung become overexpanded. Obviously, the amount of lung substance affected depends upon the level of obstruction. The most frequent cause of absorption collapse is obstruction of a bronchus by a mucus plug. This frequently occurs postoperatively, when anesthesia has stimulated increased bronchial secretions and when postoperative pain leads to shallow breathing and discourages the patient from coughing to clear the secretions. Bronchial asthma, bronchiectasis and acute and chronic bronchitis may also lead to obstruction by mucus plugs. Sometimes obstruction is caused by the aspiration of foreign bodies, particularly in children or during oral surgery or anesthesia. Airways may also be obstructed by tumors, especially bronchogenic carcinoma; enlarged lymph nodes, as from tuberculosis, for example; and vascular aneurysms.

Compression atelectasis most often is associated with accumulations of fluid or air within the pleural cavity, which mechanically cause collapse of the adjacent lung. This is a frequent occurrence with a pleural effusion from any cause, but it is perhaps most commonly associated with hydrothorax from congestive heart failure. As will be seen, pneumothorax, too, leads to compression atelectasis. In bedridden patients and in patients with ascites, basal atelectasis results from the elevated position of the diaphragms.

In a very small number of cases, massive atelectasis of uncertain pathogenesis follows injury to the chest wall.

With idiopathic massive collapse, or with a large pneumothorax, the entire lung may be folded against the mediastinum. Unless there is a **tension pneumothorax** (page 379), the mediastinum shifts toward the side of collapse. Usually, however, collapse does not involve the whole lung and is not complete. With absorption collapse, especially, there is some collateral aeration through the pores of Kohn and some edema fluid is present. Compression atelectasis caused by pleural effusion or elevated diaphragms is usually basal and bilateral. The collapsed lung parenchyma is shrunken below the level of the surrounding lung substance and is red-blue, rubbery and subcrepitant, with a wrinkled overlying pleura. Histologically, the collapsed alveoli are slitlike. Congestion and dilatation of the septal vasculature are usually present, as a result of loss of the compressive force of the air.

Acquired atelectasis may be either acute or chronic. Usually that due to absorption occurs relatively acutely, manifested by the sudden onset of dyspnea. Indeed, the development of acute respiratory distress within 48 hours of a surgical procedure is virtually diagnostic of atelectasis. It is important that atelectasis be diagnosed early and that there be prompt reexpansion of the involved lung, since the collapsed parenchyma is extremely vulnerable to superimposed infection.

HYALINE MEMBRANE DISEASE (IDIOPATHIC RESPIRATORY DISTRESS SYNDROME OF THE NEWBORN)

This is a disorder of unknown cause, which affects primarily premature infants and which is characterized by the following morphologic features: (1) an acidophilic homogeneous membrane lying free within the alveoli or in apposition to the alveolar walls, (2) uneven expansion of the alveoli, (3) variable necrosis of the alveolar lining cells, (4) capillary and venous engorgement and (5) constriction of the small pulmonary arteries and arterioles. In addition, the hypoxia present in these patients may lead to pulmonary edema and diffuse hemorrhages. Hyaline membrane disease is the most important cause of respiratory failure in the newborn.

Classically, these infants breathe spontaneously at birth and have no apparent respiratory difficulty until at least an hour later. At some time during the first day of life, their respirations become labored, with progressive cyanosis and grunting breath sounds, often leading to death from anoxia. Most such infants are premature, but hyaline membrane disease is also seen in full-term infants, particularly in the offspring of diabetic mothers.

Most authorities now believe that the pathogenesis of hyaline membrane disease involves multiple factors operating concurrently. These may include: (1) increased pulmonary vascular resistance at the level of the small pulmonary arteries and arterioles, (2) a deficiency of *surfactant*, a lipoprotein found in the alveolar lining of full-term infants which lowers surface tension, hence reduces the pressure required to expand the alveoli, (3) increased alveolar wall permeability, with transudation into the air spaces of plasma proteins, (4) ischemic necrosis of the alveolar lining cells, (5) amniotic fluid aspiration, and (6) possibly a defective fibrinolysin system. Obviously, many of these factors may be interrelated. The initiating or trigger factor is, however, unknown. It would seem that the hyaline membrane formation and the variable atelectasis are both secondary phenomena (Stahlman et al., 1964). The hyaline membrane seems to represent a mixture of plasma transudate, necrotic cell debris and aspirated amniotic fluid and cells. Although fibrin was once thought to be a regular component of the hyaline membrane, a recent report indicates that it is only rarely present (Lauweryns, 1970). It is of interest that similar membranes may be seen in adult victims of trauma, particularly in those suffering extensive cutaneous burns (Nash et al., 1974). Many believe the basic disturbance to be hypoperfusion of the lung resulting from pulmonary vasoconstriction. Conceivably, this results in hypoxic damage to the alveolar lining cells, with deficient production of surfactant, as well as an increased capillary permeability. Sloughing of the necrotic cells, variable collapse of the air spaces and formation of the hyaline membrane would then follow. However, such a chain of events is still conjectural at this time. Even in the absence of pulmonary vasoconstriction, prematurity itself is associated with absent or deficient levels of surfactant.

On gross examination, the lungs are somewhat firmer and heavier than normal and are a mottled, red-purple color. Histologically, there are alternat-

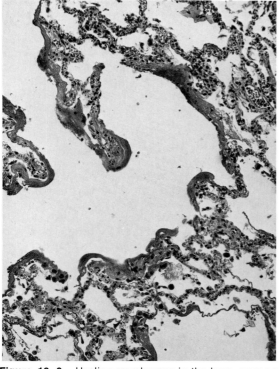

Figure 12–2. Hyaline membranes in the lung, seen as dark staining, acellular coagula lining some of the air spaces.

ing areas of atelectasis and hyperinflation. However, when lung sections are taken immediately after death rather than after a lag of several hours, the lungs are much more evenly aerated (Lauweryns, 1970). Congestion of the alveolar capillaries is marked. The most distinctive morphologic feature is the hyaline membrane which is seen in both the collapsed and the aerated air spaces (Fig. 12–2). Sometimes it appears as a rather thin acidophilic, amorphous coagulum lining the alveolus; in other instances, it virtually fills the air space. Embedded within the hyaline membrane or lying within the alveoli are disintegrating necrotic cells and occasional squamous cells of amniotic origin. Finely granular edema fluid is often present within the alveoli, and red cell extravasation may be seen within the interstitium, as well as in the air spaces.

PNEUMOTHORAX

Pneumothorax refers to the presence of air in the pleural sac. It may occur spontaneously or it may follow trauma, such as puncture of the lung by a fractured rib. The spontaneous type is clinically most important, and it too can be divided into two types—pneumothorax complicating other pulmonary pathology, and (less frequently) idiopathic pneumothorax, which occurs in the absence of demonstrable pulmonary disease. Pneumothorax as a complication of other disease occurs with the rupture of any pulmonary lesion situated close to the pleural surface that allows communication between an alveolus or bronchus and the pleural cavity. Inspired air thus gains access to the pleural space through the defect. Such primary lesions include emphysema, lung abscess, tuberculosis and carcinoma, as well as many other, less common processes. Since these primary diseases are most prevalent over the age of 40, it is apparent that this type of pneumothorax tends to occur in the older age group. In contrast, spontaneous idiopathic pneumothorax characteristically occurs in young, otherwise healthy adults, usually in males. The cause is unknown. Rarely latent tuberculosis underlies these cases, but usually it is not present.

The onset of spontaneous pneumothorax is typically sudden, with dyspnea, tachypnea and pleuritic pain. In severe cases, cyanosis and shock may follow. As the air enters the pleural space, the normally negative pleural pressure tends to become equalized with that of the atmosphere, and the lung collapses to a variable extent, depending on the type of defect. In most cases, the communication between pleura and lung seals itself off as the lung begins to collapse and does not reopen. The air in the pleural cavity is gradually absorbed and the partially collapsed lung reexpands.

This is known as a *closed pneumothorax*. When the communication is large, however, as between a bronchus and the pleural cavity, spontaneous sealing does not take place, and the pressure between the atmosphere and the pleural space is equalized. The lung remains collapsed at end-expiration, and the condition is called an *open pneumothorax*. Occasionally, when the defect is small but does not seal itself off, it acts as a flap valve, permitting air to enter during each inspiration but not allowing it to escape during expiration. The result is a *tension pneumothorax*. The intrapleural pressure in this case can rise well above atmospheric pressure, since enormous amounts of air can be trapped during coughing or on deep inspiration. As a consequence, not only does the lung remain totally collapsed, but the entire mediastinum tends to shift toward the opposite side, compressing the opposite lung. Clearly, then, severe respiratory distress usually accompanies tension pneumothorax, sometimes leading to death by anoxia.

There are several possible complications of pneumothorax. If the lung is not reexpanded within a few weeks, either spontaneously or through medical or surgical intervention, enough scarring may occur so that it can never be fully reexpanded. In these cases, if the tear has sealed and the negative intrapleural pressure has been restored, serous fluid is drawn into the pleural cavity, constituting a *hydrothorax*. With prolonged collapse, the lung becomes vulnerable to infection, as does the pleural cavity when communication between it and the lung persists. *Empyema* is thus an important complication of pneumothorax. Finally, pneumothorax tends to be recurrent. This is understandable when it complicates other pulmonary disease, since the predisposing condition remains. What is more surprising and less readily understood is the fact that idiopathic pneumothorax is also recurrent; the patient recuperating from a small, closed pneumothorax therefore remains at risk.

PULMONARY EDEMA

This entity is discussed along with congestive heart failure in Chapter 10. Suffice it to point out here that pulmonary edema often develops insidiously, manifested by the gradual onset of dyspnea. However, it is very frequently a sudden and dramatic occurrence, and in such cases it constitutes a profound medical emergency.

PULMONARY EMBOLISM

Pulmonary embolism is a major cause of death in hospitalized patients, yet the diagnosis is often unsuspected. The embolus usually arises from thromboses in the deep leg veins, which very frequently produce no symptoms. Any blood clot within the pulmonary arteries is almost certainly of embolic origin, since thrombosis in this location is rare. Significant pulmonary embolism is unusual among healthy ambulatory adults, although some believe that minute, insignificant emboli may be a daily occurrence in all individuals. Whether pregnancy and oral contraceptives are predisposing influences is highly controversial. The latter was discussed on page 240. Far better established is the augmented risk of pulmonary embolism among hospitalized patients. Moreover, those most vulnerable are patients already dangerously ill and therefore least able to withstand the added insult. These patients are usually over the age of 40 years; men and women are affected equally often. The exact incidence of pulmonary embolism is very difficult to determine, and reported incidences vary markedly from study to study. Morrell and Dunnill (1968) performed special examinations of the right lungs in a series of 263 unselected autopsies and found fresh pulmonary emboli in 30 per cent. Of added interest is the fact that older, organizing emboli were found in 20 per cent (either alone or in addition to fresh emboli), although this finding was rarely suggested by the history. It was considered that the emboli had contributed to death in about half those cases in which they were found. In this series, routine examination of the left lungs revealed only 12 per cent to contain emboli. Although pulmonary emboli are slightly more frequent in right lungs, this does not in itself explain the discrepancy. Clearly, the finding of emboli is related to the ardor with which they are sought. In another large series, pulmonary embolism was found in 33 per cent of 2319 autopsies, and in 64 per cent of a specially examined subgroup (Freiman et al., 1965).

Etiology and Pathogenesis. Nearly 95 per cent of pulmonary emboli arise as thrombi in the deep veins of the lower legs (Zimmerman et al., 1949). The factors predisposing to such thromboses and the clinical settings in which thrombosis most often occurs were discussed previously (p. 223).

Morphology. In the lung, the embolus becomes impacted in the vessels of the pulmonary arterial system, the caliber of the vessel depending on the size of the embolus. The significance of the embolus lies in the obstruction it produces. Because of the dual blood supply of the lungs, infarction from an embolus is unusual (occurring in perhaps 5 to 10 per cent of cases), unless there is already impairment of the blood supply, as with congestive heart failure. Only rarely does infarction occur in otherwise healthy individuals, and then only when the occluded vessel is large and the obstruction is not fatal. In any case, pulmonary embolism must not be confused with pulmonary infarction, since the two conditions are by no means synonymous.

Large emboli may impact in the main pulmonary artery or lodge astride the bifurcation, forming a **saddle embolus.** In these cases, sudden death often occurs, either from the blockage of blood flow through the lungs or from acute dilatation of the right side of the heart **(acute cor pulmonale).** Therefore there is no time for significant alterations in the lungs to develop, save perhaps for minimal hemorrhages in the alveoli. Smaller emboli travel out into the more peripheral vessels. The right lung is affected more often than the left, and the lower lobes more often than the upper lobes. Such small emboli in otherwise healthy patients often cause hemorrhages, which vary in size up to 5 to 10 cm. in diameter, depending upon the caliber of the occluded vessel. The hemorrhage may be central in the lung substance, but often it extends to the periphery. Although the underlying pulmonary architecture may be obscured by the suffusion of blood, it is usually preserved by the bronchial circulation, and the normal architecture is restored after resorption of the blood. Only rarely does organization of the hemorrhage yield fibrous scar formation.

Pulmonary emboli cause infarction when the circulation is already barely adequate—namely, in patients with heart disease or chronic lung disorders or in those seriously debilitated from other illness. The infarcts vary in size, from lesions barely visible to the eye to wedge-shaped involvement of large parts of an entire lobe. Characteristically, they extend to the periphery of the lung substance, with the apex pointing toward the hilus of the lung. At first, the infarct is classically hemorrhagic, as has been described earlier (p. 227). In time (i.e., days to weeks), the area becomes red-brown from hemosiderin and is eventually converted into a scar, which is contracted below the level of the surrounding substance.

If the infarct is caused by an infected embolus arising in venous inflammatory disease or from right-sided bacterial endocarditis, the infarct is modified by a more intense inflammatory reaction or may even evolve into an abscess. Such lesions are termed **septic infarcts.**

Clinical Course. Pulmonary emboli may cause sudden death, or they may be totally asymptomatic and trivial, depending on the size and number of emboli and on the condition of the patient. The symptoms evoked are similarly variable. With a massive embolus, death may occur literally in seconds, without any warning signs or symptoms whatsoever. In other cases, there are dyspnea, anxiety, a sensation of substernal pressure and cardiac arrhythmias, all of which may lead to the mistaken diagnosis of myocardial infarction. The diagnosis of a massive pulmonary embolus is supported on chest x-ray by a hyperlucent area representing decreased filling of the pulmonary vessels; the diagnosis is reliably confirmed by pulmonary angiography. As was mentioned earlier, death in these cases is usually from acute anoxia or acute cor pulmonale. Among patients succumbing to massive embolism, 34 per cent die within one hour, another 39 per cent within 24 hours and the remaining 27 per cent in 2 to 5 days (Fowler and Bollinger, 1954).

More often, the emboli are small and the patient survives. In these cases, the symptoms are even more variable, but there is usually some element of dyspnea and tachypnea. Fever is regularly present. In addition, there may be chest pain, characteristically pleuritic in nature, and cough, sometimes with hemoptysis. In other instances, however, showers of emboli may occur on a more or less chronic basis, without any indication of their presence. It is not unusual to find multiple old organized emboli at necropsy in patients who died from other causes and who were not suspected of having pulmonary emboli. Only if infarction occurs are small emboli visible on chest x-ray as areas of consolidation. Without infarction, they are apparent only on lung scan. The problems in prevention and diagnosis are further compounded by the often asymptomatic nature of the deep venous thromboses from which emboli arise. The clinician must always bear in mind the potential for pulmonary emboli in all seriously ill or bedridden patients, and watch for signs of thrombosis in the deep veins of the legs. Such signs include edema, which may be quite subtle, and calf pain on forced dorsiflexion of the foot *(Homan's sign)*, caused by muscular compression of the involved vein.

The significance of a small embolus is that it often presages a larger one. It has been estimated that the patient with a first pulmonary embolus has a 30 per cent chance of a second attack and a 20 per cent chance that this second episode will be fatal. Moreover, multiple small emboli over a period of time may lead to pulmonary vascular sclerosis with pulmonary hypertension and chronic cor pulmonale. For these reasons, anticoagulation or ligation of the veins of the lower extremity or even of the inferior vena cava is commonly recommended in patients who survive their first attack.

CHRONIC DYSPNEA

PULMONARY VASCULAR SCLEROSIS

This term refers to the vascular changes associated with pulmonary hypertension. It is entirely analogous to the vascular changes of systemic hypertension (p. 456). However, in refreshing contrast to systemic hypertension, it is usually possible to discover the cause of pulmonary hypertension. Only rarely must a diagnosis of primary or essential pulmonary hypertension be made, and this is a diagnosis of exclusion.

The known causes of pulmonary hypertension are legion. Many were considered in the discussion of cor pulmonale (p. 309). In addition, left-sided congestive heart failure leads to increased pressure within the pulmonary veins, which may be transmitted back to the pulmonary arterial tree. Long-standing mitral stenosis is a classic cause of pulmonary hypertension with pulmonary vascular sclerosis.

The pathogenesis of *primary pulmonary hypertension* is controversial. Four theories have gained wide acceptance. Drawing on the analogy to systemic essential hypertension, the first theory postulates a vasomotor disturbance, possibly from overactivity of the sympathetic autonomic system, leading to vasoconstriction of the pulmonary vasculature. This functional disturbance only later gives rise to anatomic changes (Kuida et al., 1957). Supporting this concept is the fact that 7 of 23 patients studied in depth by Walcott and his colleagues (1970) gave a history of Raynaud's phenomenon. This would suggest a widespread vasospastic disorder.

The second theory suggests that at least a large proportion of cases of primary pulmonary hypertension are the result of unsuspected miliary pulmonary emboli. This concept gains some support from the facts that asymptomatic emboli are known to occur and that organized blood clots in the smaller pulmonary vessels are a common finding at postmortem examination of patients with primary pulmonary hypertension. Whether these are thrombi which have formed at sites of vascular injury or whether, on the other hand, they are indeed emboli which have excited a vascular reaction is difficult to establish (Blount, 1967; Rosenberg, 1964). The histologic pictures are similar. Primary pulmonary hypertension is also said to be occasionally associated with disseminated intravascular coagulation (see page 363) (Brodsky and Siegel, 1970).

The third hypothesis suggests that primary pulmonary hypertension is a "collagen (or hypersensitivity) disease." The concomitance of Raynaud's phenomenon and DIC, conditions themselves known to be frequently associated with collagen diseases, would support this argument. In addition, some patients have been described with concomitant hypergammaglobulinemia and arthritis (Walcott et al., 1970).

Finally, it has been suggested, perhaps somewhat unimaginatively but nevertheless with sincerity, that primary pulmonary hypertension represents simply a congenital defect in the pulmonary vasculature.

Both sexes and any age group may be affected by *secondary* pulmonary hypertension, depending entirely on the underlying disorder. Although *primary* pulmonary hypertension, too, may occur in either sex and at any age, it is most frequent in young women. Some increased familial incidence has been seen.

Morphology. The vessel changes in both primary and secondary pulmonary vascular sclerosis are basically similar and involve the entire arterial tree, from the main pulmonary artery down to the precapillary arterioles. The lesions in the elastic arteries are confined to atheromatous plaques which, for unknown reasons, are prone to develop with pulmonary hypertension from any cause. This is analogous to the atheromatous diathesis seen with systemic hypertension. However, pulmonary atheromata are rarely as well developed as those in the systemic circuit and are not often calcified or ulcerated. The muscular arteries and the arterioles show concentric medial hypertrophy and intimal fibrosis. Often the internal and external elastic membranes undergo thickening and reduplication. The lumina of the smaller arterioles may be narrowed to pinpoint channels. Although these arterial changes are present in all forms of pulmonary vascular sclerosis, they are most developed in the primary form. As was mentioned earlier, organized thrombi are a common finding in these cases.

Clinical Course. Patients with *secondary* pulmonary vascular sclerosis may present with a mixture of symptoms and signs, attributable both to the underlying disorder and to the secondary pulmonary involvement. In any case, dyspnea ultimately develops, at first on exertion. It may be the first manifestation of mitral stenosis.

Because *primary* pulmonary hypertension usually affects otherwise healthy young women, their disease most often does not come to attention until late in its course. Then, the usual presenting manifestations are dyspnea and fatigue, although occasionally a syncopal attack is the initial complaint. By this time, the changes of pulmonary vascular sclerosis are usually advanced, and right ventricular hypertrophy is present. The prognosis is poor, and death from cor pulmonale usually ensues within two to eight years, although more fulminant cases may cause death within months of the first clinical manifestation. No other entity produces such marked right ventricular hypertrophy (Blount, 1967). Because of the difference in prognoses, it is imperative to recognize all secondary causes of pulmonary hypertension, many of which are remediable.

PNEUMOCONIOSES

The pneumoconioses are a group of diseases caused by the inhalation of mineral or organic dusts. Whether or not a particular dust causes disease depends on four factors: (1) its concentration, (2) the size and shape of the particles, (3) its chemical nature, and (4) the duration of exposure.

Because the natural defense mechanisms of the respiratory tract are so effective, the offending particles must be present in truly overwhelming concentrations to produce clinically overt disease. Under ordinary conditions mucosal ciliary action in the airways removes about 60 per cent of the foreign particles inhaled. Another 30 per cent of particles undergo phagocytosis by the alveolar macrophages, a process requiring a few days. The remaining 10 per cent are removed from the lungs by lymphatic drainage. When the concentration of a dust reaches a critical level, however, these defense mechanisms become overloaded and the particles reach the pulmonary parenchyma in quantities sufficient to cause clinical disease.

The risk from a given dust depends to a large extent on the size and shape of its particles. Particles over 5 μm. in diameter probably never reach the alveoli. Those under 1 μm. in diameter tend to move in and out with the air currents, and very small particles, of the order of 0.02 μm. or less, readily penetrate the alveolar wall and are removed by lymphatic drainage. In general, the most dangerous particles, those that are retained in the alveoli, are between 1 and 5 μm. in diameter.

The manner in which these particles inflict tissue damage is not definitely established, but it is probable that in most cases their action is not direct but rather depends on ingestion by macrophages. If large numbers of macrophages are killed as a result of phagocytizing dust particles, a fibrotic reaction ensues, and it is this fibrosis, with or without granuloma formation, that characterizes the pneumoconioses. The chemical nature of the dust in large part determines the fate of the phagocytes and hence the capacity of the ingested particles to produce disease. Some dusts, such as silica, regularly destroy the macrophages by which they are phagocytized; other dusts are relatively inert.

As the atmosphere becomes increasingly heavily laden with industrial dusts, the number of causative agents increases. *Anthracosis*, caused by the inhalation of soot, is almost universal in urban dwellers. Happily, soot is a relatively harmless dust and does not usually produce significant disease. When it accumulates in large amounts, as in soft coal miners, it may induce chronic bronchitis and centrilobular emphysema or even "black lung" disease. There are many more severe, though fortunately rare, pneumoconioses, including *byssinosis*, caused by cotton dust, *bagassosis*, produced by the fibrous framework of sugar cane, and *ptilosis*, which results from the inhalation of dust from ostrich feathers. Thus, the ostrich, when sticking his head in the sand, may suffer the double jeopardy of ptilosis and silicosis. The more important pneumoconioses are here presented individually.

SILICOSIS

Silica, or silicon dioxide, is the most common constituent of the earth's crust, existing either in its free state or as quartz (the crystalline form), or in its amorphous, colloidal state, present in diatomaceous earth. It is not surprising, then, that silicosis is a hazard in many industries and in virtually all mining, particularly where the quartz content of the rock is high. Gold, tin, copper, coal and iron miners are particularly at risk, as are those employed in the grinding and polishing of metals and stone, or in sandblasting.

Pathogenesis. Particles over 5 μm. in size are, as stated, probably harmless. The particles responsible for silicosis are generally less than 2 μm. in size. The concentration of these smaller particles required to produce silicosis is truly astounding. Up to 5×10^6 particles per ft.^{3} of air is considered within safe limits. On the other hand, the United States Public Health Service has found that prolonged exposure to concentrations of 100×10^6 particles per ft.^{3} inevitably produces silicosis. The uncertain range, between a definitely safe and a definitely pathogenic concentration, represents a factor of 20. In addition to high concentrations, a long duration of exposure is required for the production of silicosis. No well substantiated cases have been observed after exposure for less than two years, and the average time of exposure before development of disease is from 10 to 15 years. For some time, there was considerable controversy surrounding the pathogenesis of silicosis. Experimental evidence now supports the following hypothesis: The particles of silica reaching the alveoli, as with all foreign bodies, are phagocytized by macrophages. The particles are then contained within phagosomes, the structure formed by the engulfing cell membrane as it surrounds the foreign body and is drawn back into the cell and pinched off, coming to lie within the cytoplasm. Ordinarily, the next step is for lysosomes to adhere to the phagosomal wall, discharging their hydrolytic enzymes into the phagosome, thus attempting to destroy the invader without harming the ingesting cell. However, a fine layer of silicic acid present at the surface of the silica particle reacts with the phagosomal membrane, increasing its permeability. Thus, when the lysosomal enzymes are discharged into the phagosome, they escape into the cytoplasm, resulting in the destruction of the macrophage (Allison et al., 1965). The widespread destruction of macrophages, as was mentioned in the general discussion of the pneumoconioses, is a powerful stimulus to fibroblast mobilization and collagen deposition. As the silica particles escape from their dying captors, they are again phagocytized by still other macrophages, which are in turn destroyed, thus completing a vicious circle. Such a sequence of events cannot happen with silicic acid alone, since this agent is not particulate and hence it is not phagocytized. It also cannot happen with diamond dust, for example, because it is inert and remains within the phagosome indefinitely.

Morphology. In the early stages, fine and hard subpleural, peribronchiolar and perivascular nodules give the lung a sandy texture. With progression of the disease, these small nodules increase in size and become scattered throughout the entire lung substance. Coalescence of the nodules then converts the lung into a stony-hard, fibrous tissue, usually gray-black in color because of concomitant anthracosis, with only small intervening areas of compressed or emphysematous lung parenchyma. The tracheobronchial lymph nodes undergo similar changes, becoming transformed into masses of gritty, fibrous tissue. Invariably there is a concomitant pleural reaction, with marked fibrous adhesions between the pleural surfaces, causing total obliteration of the pleural cavity.

The early microscopic changes are rarely observed. From animal experimentation, the initial change is seen to be the accumulation of macrophages within the dust-laden alveolar spaces, with active phagocytosis of the particulate material. Many of the macrophages are killed, while the others become swollen to resemble epithelioid cells. The addition of multinucleated giant cells converts the focus into a granuloma that closely resembles a "hard" tubercle (see p. 50). Progressive fibroblastic proliferation produces a dense collagenous encapsulation, and each nodule eventually becomes a relatively acellular focus of concentric layers of hyaline-appearing connective tissue. Continued layering of this fibrous tissue causes enlargement of these nodules and coalescence of contiguous foci. Between the collagenous lamellae are fine, cleftlike spaces which presumably harbor silica particles. Polariscopic study readily reveals these doubly refractile particles. Scattered aggregates of lymphocytes and plasma cells, trapped masses of anthracotic pigment and secondary bacterial infections may become superimposed on this underlying picture. Coexistent tuberculosis may be distinguished readily or with difficulty, depending upon whether well-formed tubercles with central caseation are present.

Clinical Course. In the early stages of silicosis, the patient is asymptomatic. Frequently the disease is first discovered on a routine chest x-ray; the "snowstorm" appearance of the lungs, characteristic of the phase of fine nodularity, coupled with the occupational history, leads to the diagnosis. As the lungs become progressively fibrous, causing a marked decrease in their compliance and in gas diffusion, the first symptom—dyspnea on exertion—appears. This may not be noticeable until years after the disease has been discovered on chest x-ray. The degree of breathlessness is extremely variable; it may become severe enough to incapacitate the patient, or it may remain relatively mild. Systemic symptoms are unusual with pure silicosis. However, the picture is often complicated by the development of concomitant chronic bronchitis, emphysema or pulmonary tuberculosis, to which these patients are peculiarly vulnerable. In a study of South African miners, it was found that 21 to 24 per cent of those with severe silicosis also had active tuberculosis at the time of death (Chatgidakis, 1963). Other estimates of the frequency of associated tuberculosis are even higher. The onset of active tuberculosis in these patients may be difficult to discern, since respiratory problems are already present and the tubercle bacilli are often not recovered in the sputum. Certainly a high index of suspicion is warranted if systemic signs or symptoms develop.

ASBESTOSIS

This type of pneumoconiosis is caused by the inhalation of asbestos fibers and dust, and is encountered principally among those engaged in the manufacture of insulating and fireproofing materials. Brake linings also contain asbestos. It should be no surprise, then, that minimal degrees of asbestosis have been demonstrated in about 40 per cent of the general population.

Pathogenesis. The duration of heavy exposure necessary to cause disease is extremely variable, ranging from 3 months to 50 years. Even after exposure has ceased, there may be a lag period before the onset of clinical disease. Death from asbestosis has occurred as long as 25 years after the last heavy exposure to asbestos. The crude fibers, ranging from 0.3 to 2 cm. in length, are less damaging than the smaller refined particles, which measure from 20 to 100 μm. in length and are needle-shaped. Because even these smaller particles are considerably larger than those of, say, silica, many of them do not reach the alveoli but tend rather to become impacted in the terminal and respiratory bronchioles. Here they excite a histiocytic and giant cell reaction, which in turn leads to fibrosis. Sometimes the distal airways are obliterated by the fibrotic reaction; in general, there is inflammatory distortion of the distal airways, with hyperplasia of the remaining lining epithelium. Malignant change may occur in this hyperplastic epithelium.

Morphology. The alterations are seen about the bronchioles, principally in the lower lobes. The lung parenchyma in these affected areas may disclose small nodules of diffuse, reticulated fibrous thickening. Large confluent masses of fibrosis, such as are found with silicosis, are rarely observed in asbestosis. There is a marked fibrous pleuritis in the involved regions, with striking thickening of the pleural membrane so that the lung may become encased within a rigid, enclosing fibrous capsule. The pleural space is frequently obliterated by bridging adhesions. Because the asbestos fibers are too large to penetrate the alveolar wall, the involvement rarely extends to the tracheobronchial nodes.

Microscopically, peribronchiolar nodules which extend into the adjacent alveoli are present. The fibrous scarring does not create the dense hyaline nodules of silicosis, but is more cellular and accompanied by a more definite inflammatory mononuclear cell infiltration. Large foreign-body type giant cells are found in these nodules. The pathognomonic feature of the asbestos reaction is the presence of **asbestos bodies,** formed by the deposition of proteins, calcium and iron salts on the long fibrous spicules of asbestos. Because of irregular deposition of these substances, these slender spicules are converted into beaded, segmented structures, which stain yellow to brown and vary in length from 5 to 100 μm. The terminal ends of these asbestos bodies are commonly club-shaped (Fig. 12–3).

Clinical Course. The clinical picture of asbestosis is quite similar to that of silicosis, marked by the insidious onset of dyspnea on exertion. It tends to be more rapidly progressive, however, usually developing in from 5 to 10 years, and occasionally leading to death within one year of the last exposure. Like silicosis, asbestosis predisposes to chronic bronchitis and emphysema. Although there is some increased incidence of tuberculosis among patients with asbestosis, the correlation is not nearly so strong as with silicosis. This relative good fortune of the individual with asbestosis is offset by his increased risk of developing bronchogenic carcinoma or pleural mesothelioma. Bronchogenic carcinoma is said to occur in about 14 per cent of all cases of asbestosis, usually developing about 16 to 18 years after exposure to asbestos (Telischi and Rubenstone, 1961). Pleural mesothelioma was the cause of death in 5 per cent of a series of 325 patients who died from asbestosis, in

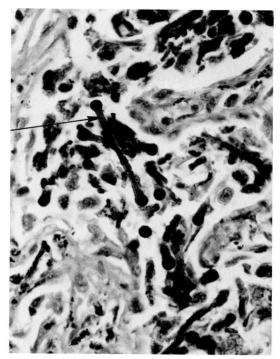

Figure 12–3. Asbestos bodies (arrow), showing the segmentation and terminal clubbed ends.

contrast to the 0.01 per cent incidence of this rare neoplasm in the general population (Selikoff et al., 1967; Belleau and Gaensler, 1968).

BERYLLIOSIS

Berylliosis did not become a significant clinical problem until after World War II, when the industrial use of beryllium first became prevalent. This metal found widespread use after the war as a coating for the inside of fluorescent light tubes, in the radio and television industries, in the construction of guidance system components in the space industry, and in the production of metal alloys. The danger of berylliosis to workers in these fields was not immediately recognized and little or no protection was given them. In 1949 safety precautions were instituted, and the use of beryllium in fluorescent lighting was discontinued. As a consequence, the incidence of berylliosis is finally declining after the sharp upsurge of cases attributable to exposure in the immediate postwar period. Beryllium oxide, finely divided metallic beryllium and its acid salts all apparently are capable of evoking tissue reactions. Depending upon the concentration of the toxic agent and its solubility in tissue fluids, two types of pulmonary involvement may occur: acute berylliosis or, more commonly, chronic berylliosis.

Of the first 271 cases in the Massachusetts General Hospital berylliosis case registry, 56 were of the acute type and 215 were of the chronic type. Exposure to beryllium occurred as follows: 46 per cent worked with fluorescent light tubes; 28 per cent were engaged in the extraction of beryllium from its ore; 16 per cent handled beryllium compounds and 10 per cent merely lived near factories working with beryllium (Hardy, 1961).

Pathogenesis. Individual susceptibility is extremely important and it has been estimated that less than 2 per cent of those at risk actually develop berylliosis. The risk seems to be greater in workers returning to the industry after an absence. For these reasons, it has been speculated that berylliosis may represent a hypersensitivity phenomenon. Supporting this view is the failure to find high levels of beryllium in patients known to have berylliosis. It has been shown that beryllium ions are capable of attaching themselves to protein molecules, hence theoretically they could act as antigens (Aldridge et al., 1949). Moreover, patients with this disease show a positive skin test to beryllium salts. While these facts raise the issue of hypersensitivity as a basis for berylliosis, there is as yet no convincing evidence on this point.

Morphology. Chronic berylliosis, also known as **beryllium granulomatosis**, is characterized by focal granulomas within the alveolar septa, as well as within the alveolar spaces. These granulomas bear a strong resemblance to those of sarcoidosis and tuberculosis, and, indeed, they may sometimes be indistinguishable (Freiman and Hardy, 1970). Classically, they differ from the tubercle in that the necrotic centers contain preserved and degenerating neutrophils. Sometimes, however, these cells become so necrotic as to produce an acellular granular debris that strongly resembles caseous necrosis, making the differentiation from tuberculosis difficult if not impossible. Central necrosis may distinguish these beryllium lesions from sarcoidosis. The degree of granuloma formation is variable from case to case. Sometimes granulomas are difficult to find. Similarly variable is the presence of an accompanying mononuclear interstitial infiltrate. In any case the regional nodes of drainage are commonly affected. Although the pleural surfaces may be thickened and fibrotic, they are usually not involved. With time, the granulomas become progressively fibrotic and lead to large areas of fibrous scarring of the lung.

Accompanying the chronic pulmonary lesions may be granulomatous involvement of the liver, kidney, spleen, lymph nodes and skin. Indeed, chronic persistent ulcerations of the skin may develop at sites of scratches or injuries where beryllium has been introduced.

Acute berylliosis is likely to be caused by beryllium acid salts, which are more soluble and toxic than beryllium oxide or metallic beryllium.

This acute response is reported to have developed within a few hours to days of exposure. Granulomatous reaction is absent, and the pulmonary involvement takes the form of acute, diffuse bronchopneumonia (see p. 392), which usually differs from the bacterial form by the preponderance of mononuclear leukocytes in the inflammatory exudate. It is believed that this acute pneumonitis may resolve without residual scarring.

Clinical Course. There is a latent period usually from weeks to decades between the exposure and the development of clinical signs and symptoms. In some cases, the exposure has been very brief, such as the inhalation of beryllium dust after the accidental breakage of a single fluorescent lamp. After the latent period, the chronic form of the disease manifests itself similarly to the other pneumoconioses, with the insidious onset of dyspnea. Even with lung biopsy, the disease may be indistinguishable from sarcoidosis or healed tuberculosis, and in these cases, the diagnosis depends on epidemiologic and clinical factors, namely, a history of significant exposure, the presence of a diffusion defect and consistent chest x-ray results (Stoeckle et al., 1969). The disease may progress inexorably to death, or it may subside, apparently spontaneously. Steroids have proved beneficial in arresting berylliosis. The prognosis is best when there are well-formed granulomas and a minimal interstitial infiltrate (Freiman and Hardy, 1970). Twenty-four per cent of the 650 cases in the Massachusetts General Hospital case registry, comprising both the acute and chronic types, had died by 1961.

The acute form of berylliosis is manifested by the sudden onset of cough, dyspnea, fever and constitutional symptoms, such as malaise and weakness. Death sometimes occurs within a few weeks, although most of these patients recover (Freiman and Hardy, 1970).

As mentioned, berylliosis, unlike the other pneumoconioses, is not confined to the lungs, but may affect other sites of implantation as well, most noticeably the skin.

EMPHYSEMA

Emphysema is difficult to describe because of the considerable disparity between the clinical usage of the term and the anatomic definition. There is an unfortunate tendency to diagnose emphysema in all patients who manifest a chronic increase in airway resistance (*chronic obstructive pulmonary disease* or *COPD*). In strict usage, however, emphysema is an anatomic entity characterized by an increase in the size of air spaces in the lung distal to the terminal bronchioles. Most American workers, in contrast to their British colleagues, would add to this definition the requirement that there be concomitant destruction of lung tissue (American Thoracic Society, 1962). Whereas these morphologic changes are often present in patients with COPD, they are not an invariable component. Chronic bronchitis may cause similar functional derangements without concomitant emphysema. The interrelationships among emphysema, chronic bronchitis and COPD, then, are complicated. It is helpful to remember that emphysema is an *anatomic* entity and chronic bronchitis is defined as a *clinical* syndrome; both are causes of COPD, which is a *functional* abnormality. Thus, emphysema and chronic bronchitis are not mutually exclusive and, indeed, they very often coexist. Together, in 1973, they were the tenth leading cause of death in the United States.

The definition of emphysema is further complicated by the existence of several morphologic patterns, some of uncertain clinical significance. By far the most important of these patterns are: (1) *panlobular (panacinar) emphysema*, and (2) *centrilobular (centriacinar) emphysema*. These will be discussed in some detail, and less important patterns only briefly described at the end of this section.

Panlobular emphysema is characterized by fairly uniform distention of all air spaces distal to the terminal bronchioles, i.e., the respiratory bronchioles, alveolar ducts, alveolar sacs and alveoli. Alveolar destruction usually is prominent. The changes of centrilobular emphysema, on the other hand, are selective, affecting primarily the respiratory bronchioles, and to a lesser extent adjacent alveoli, with the surrounding parenchyma relatively unaffected. The relative incidences of these two patterns are controversial, largely because of varying criteria used in diagnosing them. A recent review suggests that the centrilobular form is about 20 times as common as the panlobular form (Pratt and Kilburn, 1970). Some measure of the combined impact of these lesions can be gained by the fact that in one unselected postmortem series, some degree of either panlobular or centrilobular emphysema was seen in 50 per cent of patients. The condition caused disability or death in 6.5 per cent of these patients (Thurlbeck, 1963).

Etiology and Pathogenesis. Most often, emphysema accompanies chronic bronchitis, but it may occur as an isolated lesion, and in these cases it is termed *primary emphysema*. The nature of the relationship between chronic bronchitis and emphysema is becoming increasingly controversial. The oldest hypothesis held that chronic bronchitis may lead to emphysema, specifically the centrilobular pattern. It was postulated that chronic inflammation produced airway obstruction, either by permitting collapse of the weakened bronchial walls on expiration or by the presence of mucus plugs or inflammatory stenosis (Leopold and Gough, 1957; Spain and Kaufman, 1953; McLean, 1958). This hypothesis has recently been somewhat modified to restrict the initial inflammation to the small airways, that is, to suggest that the primary event is a bronchiolitis rather than a bronchitis. This is strongly supported by accumulating evidence that the development of either overt chronic bronchitis or emphysema is preceded by long-standing subtle disease of the small airways, at the level of the respiratory bronchioles (Thurlbeck, 1973; McFadden et al., 1974). How would inflammatory obstruction of the respiratory bronchioles lead to air-trapping and tissue destruction? McLean proposed that during inspiration air continues to enter the obstructed units from adjacent acini through the pores of Kohn. On expiration, however, these collateral pathways are closed as the lung recoils and air becomes trapped distal to the obstructed respiratory bronchioles. The pressure of the trapped air disrupts the alveolar walls, and a larger "common pool" results (McLean, 1958). However, this postulated sequence of events has been questioned. A second hypothesis is that the primary event is destruction of the alveolar walls, as a result of some unknown mechanism, and that chronic bronchitis is merely secondary, following because of the consequent impairment of normal defense mechanisms, such as tussive force. According to this view, the known deleterious influence of heavy cigarette smoking on emphysema can be explained by its role in intensifying the bronchitic component and thus further imperiling an already diseased respiratory system. As a third alternative, it is conceivable that the concurrence of chronic bronchitis and emphysema is merely coincidental, and that they simply tend to unmask each other, and are in turn unmasked by cigarette smoking.

The pattern of emphysema associated with chronic bronchitis is not necessarily centrilobular. Increasingly, the panlobular form is being described in these cases, and it is thought by some to represent the end-stage of progressive centrilobular emphysema, with involvement extending to the entire lung. Others believe that there is no such relationship between the two patterns of emphysema, and that neither can be exclusively correlated with a single clinical picture (Reid, 1967).

Nevertheless, in the midst of so much uncertainty, it can be said that of the small group of patients with *primary emphysema* virtually all have panlobular emphysema at necropsy and present a fairly homogeneous clinical picture. This form of emphysema is characterized by the insidious development of increased airway resistance in patients without clinical evidence of chronic bronchitis. In England, primary emphysema accounts for fewer than 6 per cent of cases of COPD. The remainder of cases of COPD are associated with chronic bronchitis, which is discussed on page 395, with or without concomitant emphysema. In the United States, *primary emphysema* is probably relatively more important than in England because of the somewhat lower incidence of clinical chronic bronchitis. Unlike chronic bronchitis, primary emphysema affects women as often as men and has its onset relatively early, usually in the fourth or fifth decade of life.

The cause of primary emphysema is unknown and may be multiple. A familial form has recently been discovered, which is associated with a deficiency in serum α_1-trypsin inhibitor (α_1-antitrypsin). The mode of inheritance was originally thought to be autosomal recessive. However, it has recently become apparent that the inheritance and expression of α_1-antitrypsin deficiency are much more complicated than originally believed. At least 23 different codominant alleles are involved in the formation of α_1-antitrypsin (Editorial, 1975), and deficiencies range from near absolute to near normal levels. Thus, there is a polymorphic spectrum of antitrypsin deficiency. This genetic system is often referred to as the *proteinase inhibitor system (Pi)*, and derangements may affect the liver as well as the lung. In a screening study of a large population, markedly low levels of α_1-antitrypsin, assumed to result from homozygosity, were rare (Morse et al., 1975). It is generally agreed that most of these individuals develop symptomatic COPD by age 40. Whether the much more common heterozygous state, characterized by intermediate levels of α_1-antitrypsin deficiency, is also associated with an increased incidence of emphysema is controversial (Kueppers, 1969; Morse et al., 1975). Conceivably, environmental insults, such as cigarette smoking, may tip the balance in these individuals (Mittman et al., 1971). While α_1-antitrypsin deficiency is undoubtedly a contributor to primary emphysema, it by no means explains all cases. Probably not more than 10 per cent of all patients with primary emphysema are homozygous for α_1-antitrypsin deficiency (Lieberman, 1969). Other factors contributing to this disease are less well established. In general, it is felt that the basic derangement is in the alveolar walls. It has been suggested that a primary "alveolitis," perhaps of microbial causation, may lead to alveolar destruction (Colp et al., 1967). Alternatively, a qualitative defect of connective tissue, principally involving the collagen and the elastic fibers of the alveolar septa, has been postulated (Ebert and Pierce, 1963). In any case, there is diffuse atrophy and destruction of the alveoli. This results in diminished elastic recoil of the lungs, as well as loss of structural support for the bronchioles and bronchi. The diminished pulmonary recoil leads to forced expiration, which in turn aggravates the tendency of the airways to collapse from loss of support. In this manner, airway obstruction eventually occurs, although the primary derangement was loss of lung tissue with a resultant diffusion defect. Whatever its origin, primary emphysema, as was mentioned earlier, is of the panlobular pattern.

Morphology. Whether panlobular or centrilobular in form, it is extremely difficult to appreciate the anatomic changes of emphysema either grossly or by examination of the usual thin histologic sections. Indeed, the recent advances in our knowledge of these entities have derived in considerable part from the use of whole lung thick sections and by using methods that fix and inflate the lungs (Heard, 1960). To the naked eye, both major forms of emphysema usually, although not invariably, produce voluminous lungs that often overlap the mediastinum when the anterior chest wall is removed. With panlobular emphysema, the basal portions of the lungs tend to be most severely affected. The lungs are hypercrepitant and pillowy to palpation. The involved areas are pale, owing to compression of the blood supply. As was mentioned, **panlobular** emphysema uniformly involves the air spaces distal to the terminal bronchioles. Histologically, the walls of these air spaces are seen to be extremely thin, attenuated, fibrotic and bloodless. The distended alveolar pores or fenestrated septa create the appearance of coalescence of air spaces. These distended air spaces extend peripherally to the pleural surface. On thick sections, the lung has a uniformly honey combed appearance (Fig. 12–4).

With centrilobular emphysema, it is generally the upper regions of the lobes that are most affected—i.e., the apices of the upper lobes, as well as the upper portions of the lower lobes.

The involvement is near the center of the lobules, affecting the respiratory bronchioles and extending toward, but not reaching, the periphery of the lobule. There is usually a rim of peripheral, unaffected lung substance. The respiratory bronchioles are the prime site of involvement. These become irregularly enlarged, cystic and confluent, creating abnormal air spaces that can be seen in adequate preparations by hand lens or with the dissecting microscope (Fig. 12–5). It is generally possible to find evidence of old inflammatory changes in the form of collagenization in and about the walls of the respiratory bronchioles, with narrowing of the lumina of the small vessels contained within the walls of the affected bronchioles. The individual bronchioles are unevenly affected, so that there is

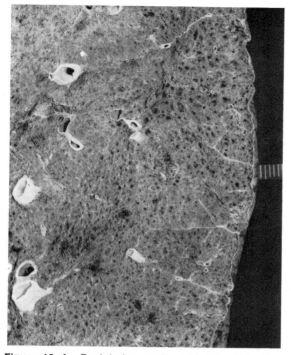

Figure 12–4. Panlobular emphysema. The distention of the air spaces is characteristically uniform in its distribution throughout the lung. Alveoli and alveolar ducts are dilated, with focal areas of parenchymal destruction.

low, flattened diaphragms. Functionally, there is impairment of diffusion as well as ventilatory insufficiency from increased airway resistance. However, ventilation and perfusion remain fairly well balanced, so that blood gas derangements typically occur only late in the course of the disease. The following list of clinical characteristics of the typical patient with primary emphysema should be compared with that given in the discussion of chronic bronchitis (Nash et al., 1965; Ogilvie, 1959).

1. Minimal, nonproductive cough.
2. Relatively early dyspnea.
3. Minimal ventilation-perfusion imbalance.
4. Relatively late cor pulmonale.
5. Relatively late secondary polycythemia.
6. Thin body habitus.
7. Increased total lung capacity, with large, hyperlucent lungs.

Two relatively insignificant forms of emphysema remain.

Paratractional emphysema occurs as a result of scarring from some other lung disease, such as tuberculosis. With scar formation, there is consequent distortion of the lung architecture as some areas of the parenchyma lose their support and others become overdistended. The distribution of the emphysematous

considerable variation in the size of the distended air spaces. Active bronchiolitis may be found. The alveolar spaces appear to be fenestrated and incomplete, but it must be remembered that to a considerable extent, this represents the mouths of alveolar sacs and alveoli arising from the alveolar ducts. Unquestionably, however, perforation of some septa occurs with centrilobular emphysema.

Clinical Course. Most cases of emphysema are not of the primary type, but rather are associated with chronic bronchitis. In these cases, the contribution of each to the clinical picture is unclear. Reference should be made to the discussion of chronic bronchitis on page 395.

The clinical hallmark of primary emphysema is the insidious development of dyspnea without significant cough. Later, secondary chronic bronchitis and cough frequently develop and may obscure the basic nature of the process. Thus it is important to establish through the history which came first—dyspnea or cough. The dyspnea, which is fixed, becomes increasingly severe and may ultimately be present even at rest. Patients with such advanced disease are characteristically wasted in appearance, conceivably because they are simply too breathless to eat. Chest x-ray usually shows large, translucent lungs, with

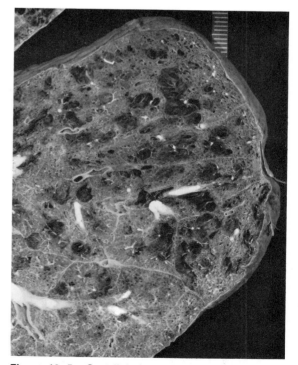

Figure 12–5. Centrilobular emphysema. The distended air spaces are seen in relation to a small arteriole (here shown filled with white radiopaque material) in the center of the primary lung lobules. The parenchyma about the centrilobular lesions is normal.

changes, then, is haphazard, depending on the pattern of the primary disease.

Bullous emphysema applies to any dilatation of air spaces over 1 cm. in diameter. Although such bullae usually are associated with one of the patterns of emphysema already described, they are sometimes encountered in young patients who do not have any underlying pulmonary changes. Under such circumstances, the bullae do not cause pulmonary dysfunction but nonetheless do constitute clinical hazards, since their rupture may be one of the mechanisms leading to spontaneous pneumothorax in the young.

Formerly, an additional type of emphysema, known as *senile emphysema*, was commonly described. However, studies have shown that most of these elderly patients do not develop significant impairment of respiratory function, and it is therefore preferable not to term such senile changes emphysema. The condition is thought to occur in a large number of elderly people. It is believed that the postural changes of aging and the deterioration in the elastic and reticulin fibers of the lung, with resultant loss of elastic recoil of the pulmonary parenchyma, lead to progressive generalized distention of air spaces. Some workers describe accompanying destructive changes.

ACUTE COUGH

BACTERIAL PNEUMONIAS

Normally, the lower respiratory tree is sterile. Bacteria inhaled during inspiration, including potential pathogens, are cleared by the normal defense mechanisms. Among these clearing mechanisms two are of major importance: an intact ciliated epithelium, over which a continual mucus sheet moves upward, and the presence of competent alveolar macrophages. Obviously, anything interfering with normal defense mechanisms predisposes to bacterial pneumonia. Such factors include irritant gases and dusts, viruses, alterations in the consistency of the bronchial mucus, cold and alcohol. Indeed, it has been suggested that most cases of bacterial pneumonia are preceded by virus infection.

Before the antibiotic era, pneumonia was the third leading cause of death, accounting for 7.6 per cent of mortalities in 1937. Although we are perhaps rightfully accustomed to thinking of this scourge as tamed by the introduction of antibiotics, we should remember that it remains an important killer. In 1973, it was the fifth leading cause of death. Undoubtedly, however, a larger proportion of deaths from pneumonia in the antibiotic era occur in elderly patients who are already debilitated by chronic illness. For these patients pneumonia may in some cases be looked upon as a release. Often such terminal pneumonia involves relatively avirulent organisms which gain a foothold either after prolonged therapy with broad-spectrum antibiotics has altered the normal microbial balance or during therapy with immunosuppressant agents.

Bacterial invasion of the lung evokes a solid exudative reaction (consolidation), in which the alveoli are filled with inflammatory cells. When the consolidation occurs in patches throughout a lobe or lung, the anatomic pattern is known as *bronchopneumonia*. When it involves an entire lobe, it is known as *lobar pneumonia*.

LOBAR PNEUMONIA

Involvement of an entire lobe or a large portion of it is usually caused by a relatively virulent organism. Approximately 90 per cent of these cases are caused by pneumococci, most commonly Types I, III, VII or II. However, in a significant minority of cases, the causative agent is *Klebsiella pneumoniae* (Friedländer's bacillus) or *Staphylococcus aureus*. Occasionally the streptococci, *Hemophilus influenzae* or some of the other gram-negative organisms are responsible for this pattern of pneumonia. As pneumococcal pneumonia declines in importance, these less common etiologic types are encountered increasingly frequently. The morphology of lobar pneumonia will be presented in a general way and followed by a short clinical discussion of each of the major etiologic types.

Morphology. Four anatomic stages of lobar pneumonia have classically been described: congestion, red hepatization, gray hepatization and resolution. Effective therapy frequently telescopes or halts progression through these stages, so that at autopsy the anatomic changes do not conform to the older, classic stages.

The first stage, that of **congestion**, consists of rapid proliferation of the bacteria, with vascular engorgement and serous exudation. The alveolar spaces thus contain proteinaceous edema fluid, scattered neutrophils and numerous bacteria. The alveolar architecture is readily apparent.

The stage of **red hepatization**, named for its gross resemblance to the liver, is characterized by the solid packing of the alveolar spaces with neutrophils, extravasated red cells and precipitated fibrin. Fibrin strands may stream from one alveolus through the pores of Kohn into the adjacent alveolus. The underlying pulmonary architecture is thus obscured. An overlying fibrinous or fibrinosuppurative pleuritis is almost invariably present.

The stage of **gray hepatization** involves the

progressive disintegration of leukocytes and red cells along with the continued accumulation of fibrin within the alveoli. The fibrin now appears clumped and amorphous, and classically it contracts somewhat to yield a clear zone adjacent to the alveolar walls, disclosing the preserved native architecture. The pleural reaction at this stage is most intense.

The final stage, that of **resolution,** follows in uncomplicated cases. The consolidative exudate within the alveolar spaces is enzymatically digested, and is either resorbed or removed by coughing. The lung parenchyma is restored to its normal state. The pleural reaction may similarly resolve or undergo organization, leaving fibrous thickenings or permanent adhesions.

This process may involve one or several lobes unilaterally or bilaterally. With pneumococcal pneumonia, the lower lobes, on either or both sides, are typically involved (Fig. 12–6). Pneumonia caused by *Klebsiella pneumoniae* involves only the right lung in 75 per cent of cases (Spencer, 1968), and usually begins as a lobular

process, affecting most often the posterior segment of the upper lobe, ultimately extending to include the entire lobe.

Grossly, during the stage of congestion, the affected lobe is heavy, red and subcrepitant, and on sectioning it yields a free ooze of bloody serous fluid. As red hepatization develops, the lobe becomes a heavy, solid, "plaster cast" of the pleural space. The cut surface at this stage is red, dry and granular, similar to liver tissue, hence the term "hepatization." There is now a yellow, granular, fibrinous exudate layered over the pleura. With the stage of gray hepatization, the cut surface becomes pale gray-brown, although it is still liver-like in texture. The pleural reaction continues to be well developed. As resolution ensues, the lung again becomes wet, soggy and subcrepitant, and again fluid, now turbid, oozes freely on sectioning. The pleural exudate is less well defined, but often there appears on the pleural surface the beginning fibrous shagginess of organization. Frequently there are interlobular adhesions at this stage, and occasionally loculated pockets of pus are found in the interlobular fissures.

This classic evolution may be complicated in the following ways: (1) Tissue destruction and necrosis may lead to abscess formation within the otherwise solidified lung substance, (2) suppurative material may accumulate in the pleural cavity, producing an **empyema,** (3) organization of the exudate may convert areas of the lung into solid fibrous tissue, and (4) bacteremic dissemination may lead to meningitis, arthritis or infective endocarditis.

Clinical Course. *Pneumococcal pneumonia* usually occurs in otherwise healthy adults between the ages of 30 and 50 years, although Type III is more common in elderly individuals and in those already debilitated. Characteristically, the onset is sudden, marked by malaise, violent shaking chills and high fever. The accompanying cough is at first dry or productive of only thin watery sputum; with the stage of red hepatization, the sputum becomes thick, purulent and hemorrhagic, known as "rusty sputum." Type III pneumococcus typically produces a tenacious mucinous sputum, which can also be seen on cut sections of the lung. The pleuritis manifests itself by pleuritic pain and a friction rub; often there is a pleural effusion. Blood cultures are positive in about 65 per cent of cases before antibiotic treatment is instituted (Spencer, 1968). Physical findings vary with the histologic stage. The moist rales heard early and late in the disease disappear during the height of the consolidation. With effective treatment, the patient is often afebrile and feels well within 48 hours, although x-ray changes may be apparent for up to 4 weeks. With therapy, the prognosis is excellent. However, complications may occur, such as meningitis, arthritis

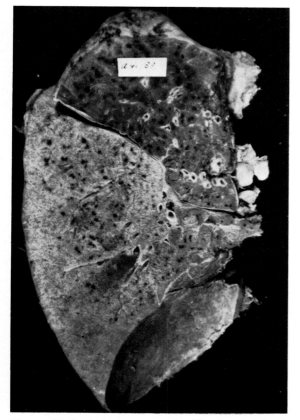

Figure 12–6. Lobar pneumonia. The lower lobe is uniformly consolidated, while the upper lobe is relatively unaffected. Note the "plaster-cast" impression of the dome of the diaphragm preserved in the bottom of the lower lobe, and the fibrinous exudate (pleuritis) layering this diaphragmatic surface.

or infective endocarditis. Later, such residuals as incomplete resolution or empyema may remain. Abscesses are rare.

Klebsiella pneumonia occurs in a slightly older age group than does pneumococcal pneumonia, and it is more frequent among debilitated and malnourished individuals, particularly chronic alcoholics. The onset is similar to that of pneumococcal pneumonia, although prostration is perhaps more severe. The sputum is characteristically extremely thick and gelatinous, so that the patient may have difficulty in bringing it up. Even with treatment, the mortality is considerably higher than with pneumococcal pneumonia, and complete resolution is less frequent. Abscesses are common, as well as areas of fibrosis and bronchiectasis.

Staphylococcal pneumonia is gaining increasing importance, particularly as the most frequent form of pneumonia complicating influenza and as a common occurrence in debilitated hospitalized patients. Most often, it takes the form of a bronchopneumonia with multiple abscess formation, but occasionally it presents as a lobar pneumonia, particularly in infants.

BRONCHOPNEUMONIA (LOBULAR PNEUMONIA)

This patchy pneumonic consolidation usually follows a bronchitis or bronchiolitis. It is a threat chiefly to the vulnerable—infants, the aged, and those suffering from chronic debilitating illness or taking immunosuppressive drugs. Whooping cough and measles are important antecedents in children; in the adult, influenza, chronic bronchitis, alcoholism, malnutrition and carcinomatosis are all predisposing conditions. The patient with pulmonary edema from cardiac failure is particularly vulnerable. Other predisposing factors include long-term therapy with antibiotics, corticosteroids or antimetabolites.

Although virtually any organism may cause bronchopneumonia, it is noteworthy that the organisms involved are often commensals or relatively avirulent. In these instances, the disease is known as an "opportunistic infection." Among the etiologic agents are the staphylococci, the streptococci, pneumococci, *H. influenzae*, *Proteus*, *Pseudomonas aeruginosa*, and the coliforms. The importance of anaerobic organisms as causes of bronchopneumonia is becoming increasingly appreciated. Because of difficulties in obtaining uncontaminated specimens and in culturing these agents, their role has until recently been underestimated. It is now thought that they are responsible for about one third of all cases of bronchopneumonia (Ries et al., 1974). Most important

among the anaerobes are *Fusobacterium nucleatum*, *Bacteroides melaninogenicus* and the peptostreptococci—all constituents of the normal flora of the mouth. (Gorbach and Bartlett, 1974.) Fungi such as Monilia, Aspergillus and Mucor may also cause bronchopneumonia. Because it so frequently occurs as the terminal event in those already mortally ill, it is a very common finding in postmortem examinations.

A special type of bronchopneumonia occurs in patients who have aspirated their gastric contents while unconscious or during repeated vomiting or because of a depressed cough reflex. The resultant pneumonia is partly chemical, owing to the extremely irritating effect of the gastric acid, and partly bacterial. Here the key role is played by a mixed flora of anaerobic and microaerophilic organisms normally present in the oral cavity (Bartlett et al., 1974). In addition, coliform bacteria which under certain circumstances are present in the stomach contents may also play a role. This type of pneumonia may be extremely fulminant and is a frequent cause of death in patients predisposed to aspiration.

Morphology. Bronchopneumonia is characterized by foci of inflammatory consolidation distributed patchily throughout one or several lobes. It is frequently bilateral and basal because of the tendency for secretions to gravitate into the lower lobes. Well developed lesions are slightly elevated, dry, granular, gray-red to yellow and poorly delimited at their margins. They vary in size up to 3 to 4 cm. in diameter. Confluence of these foci occurs in the more florid instances, producing the appearance of total lobular consolidation. When caused by such abscess producers as the staphylococci, central areas of necrosis often appear. The lung substance immediately surrounding areas of consolidation is usually slightly hyperemic and edematous, but the large intervening areas are generally normal. A fibrinous or suppurative pleuritis will develop if the inflammatory focus is in contact with the pleura; however, this is not common. With subsidence, the consolidation may resolve if there has been no abscess formation, or it may become organized, leaving residual foci of fibrosis.

Histologically, the reaction comprises a suppurative exudate that fills the bronchi, bronchioles and adjacent alveolar spaces (Fig. 12—7). Neutrophils are dominant in this exudation, and usually only small amounts of fibrin are present. This standard pattern of reaction may be modified by a number of variables. Any disorder that impairs white cell function, such as leukemia, agranulocytosis or pancytopenia, or any disease that suppresses the immune response, such as hypo- or agammaglobulinemia, steroid therapy or immunosuppressive drugs, may render the patient particularly vulnerable to bacterial or mycotic growth and permit vir-

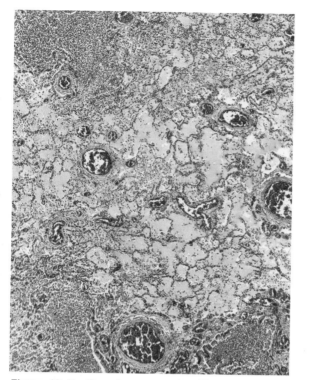

Figure 12–7. Bronchopneumonia. The low power view reveals two foci of pneumonic consolidation on the left. At the lower right, a bronchus is filled with exudate. The intervening alveoli contain edema fluid and occasional white cells. There is an overall intense vascular congestion.

tual colony formation within the areas of exudation **(botryomycosis).**

Particularly in infancy but occasionally in adulthood, the bronchopneumonia may remain interstitial, within the alveolar septa, producing an inflammatory reaction confined to the alveolar walls, with little exudate in the air spaces. *Escherichia coli* is the most common basis for such a reaction pattern in infancy.

Clinical Course. The clinical picture of bronchopneumonia is seldom as well defined as that of lobar pneumonia, in large part because it is frequently overshadowed by the predisposing condition. Moreover, the many etiologic agents have a considerable range of virulence, and the patients vary in vulnerability. In general, the onset is somewhat insidious, often appearing as a nonspecific worsening of the patient's prior condition, with relatively low-grade fever and cough productive of purulent sputum. Respiratory difficulty is typically not prominent. The course is irregular, but resolution usually occurs if treatment is appropriate and the patient is not severely debilitated. Complications are more frequent than with pneumococcal pneumonia,

with abscess formation being especially common.

PRIMARY ATYPICAL PNEUMONIA (PAP)

This rather curious name refers to all those pneumonias not caused by bacteria or fungi. They are unified morphologically by the fact that the inflammatory reaction is largely confined to the interstitium. In only about 50 per cent of cases is an etiologic agent identified (Armstrong, 1969). The agent responsible for the largest group of cases of *known* etiology is *Mycoplasma pneumoniae*, a pleuropneumonia-like organism (PPLO), also known as the *Eaton agent*. It has been speculated that these organisms are simply protoplasts of streptococci, since about 10 per cent of patients with this disease have antistreptococcal MG agglutinins in their serum. *M. pneumoniae* is endemic and causes from 10 to 33 per cent of lower respiratory infections (acute bronchitis and pneumonia) in adults. Disease caused by this organism is uncommon in children under the age of 6 years. Under conditions of unusual crowding, epidemics of *M. pneumoniae* may occur, and this organism has been found responsible for 67 per cent of all cases of pneumonia in military barracks.

Various types of viruses cause most of the remaining cases of PAP of known etiology. Chief among these are the following myxoviruses: influenza types A and B, causing 10 to 14 per cent of adult lower respiratory infections; parainfluenza, principally type 3, accounting for about 4 per cent of these involvements; and the respiratory syncytial group (RSV), which is responsible for a large fraction of acute bronchitis and also occasionally pneumonia. Among infants, RSV is the most common single cause of pneumonia, as well as of bronchiolitis, accounting for 18 to 30 per cent of cases (Loda et al., 1968). Other organisms which may be associated with PAP are the Coxsackie and ECHO viruses, some of the Rickettsiae, and, occasionally, the rubeola and varicella viruses. Infection with most of these viruses does not necessarily produce pneumonia; under favorable clinical circumstances, they may cause only mild upper respiratory infections.

Morphology. Most of these patients recover, and so our understanding of the anatomic changes is necessarily based upon the more severe involvements. Regardless of etiology, the morphologic patterns are similar. The process may be quite patchy, or it may involve whole lobes bilaterally or unilaterally. The affected areas are red-blue, congested and subcrepitant. The weight of the lungs is only moderately increased, in the range of 800 gm. each. Since most of the reaction is intersti-

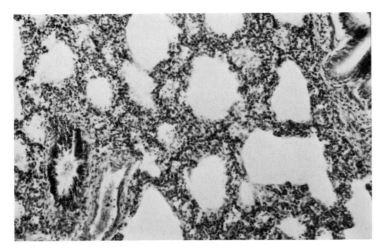

Figure 12–8. Viral pneumonitis. The thickening of the alveolar walls results from an interstitial inflammatory reaction. Although the alveolar spaces are free, the changes would cause serious impairment of gaseous exchange.

tial, little of the inflammatory exudate escapes on sectioning of the lung. There may be a slight oozing of red, frothy fluid. In contrast to lobar pneumonia, consolidation does not occur. With the light microscope, the inflammatory reaction is seen to be virtually confined within the walls of the alveoli (Fig. 12–8). The alveolar spaces themselves are remarkably free of exudate and contain only a scattered pink precipitate of edema fluid, in which are occasional mononuclear cells. The septa are widened and edematous, and usually contain a mononuclear inflammatory infiltrate of lymphocytes, histiocytes and, occasionally, plasma cells. In very acute cases, neutrophils may also be present. Sometimes transudation of fibrin through the walls of severely affected alveolar septa produces a pink hyaline membrane lining the alveolar wall. In fulminant cases of influenza pneumonia, fibrin thrombi are found within the alveolar capillaries, as well as small areas of necrosis of the alveolar wall. In less severe, uncomplicated cases, subsidence of the disease is followed by reconstitution of the native architecture. Often, however, superimposed bacterial infection occurs, resulting in a mixed histologic picture.

Clinical Course. The clinical course is extremely varied, even among cases caused by the same etiologic agent. Often, primary atypical pneumonia masquerades as a severe upper respiratory infection or "chest cold," and presumably many of these go undiagnosed. In contrast, some cases are fulminant and cause death within 48 hours. The onset is usually that of an acute, nonspecific febrile illness, characterized by fever, headache and malaise. Only later do localizing symptoms appear. Typically there is a hacking cough, which, in contrast to that of the bacterial pneumonias, tends to be unproductive of sputum. This is because the inflammatory reaction is largely interstitial. Chest x-rays usually show transient, ill-defined patches, mainly in the lower lobes. Physical findings are charac-

teristically minimal. Because the edema and exudation are both in a strategic position to cause an alveolocapillary block, there may be respiratory distress seemingly out of proportion to the physical and radiologic findings.

Cold agglutinins are found in elevated titer in about 40 per cent of patients whose disease is caused by *M. pneumoniae*. This test is often used to differentiate the viral atypical pneumonias from those caused by *M. pneumoniae*. However, elevated cold agglutinins are also present in 20 per cent of adenovirus infections.

The prognosis is generally good, with complete recovery the rule. However, certain of the atypical pneumonias are noted for their virulence. Thus, varicella pneumonia, which develops in 16 to 30 per cent of adults hospitalized with chickenpox, is characteristically severe. During influenza epidemics, primary influenza pneumonia, while less frequent than secondary staphylococcal pneumonia, often runs a fulminant course, leading to death within a day or two. The mortality in these cases has been reported as high as 80 per cent.

ACUTE LARYNGOTRACHEOBRONCHITIS

Acute inflammation of the larynx and tracheobronchial tree may be caused by viral or bacterial infections, by allergic reactions or by the inhalation of irritating substances. Because of the prevalence of atmospheric pollutants, minor degrees of laryngotracheobronchitis are extremely common. More severe involvement occurs when any of these inciting agents overwhelms the normal defense mechanisms. It is theorized that the initial stage in the development of tracheitis or bronchitis is the elaboration of excessive mucinous secretion in response to focal superficial inflammation. These excessive secretions cannot be cleared by ciliary or peristaltic activity, and reflex coughing follows. With persistent coughing, there may be further trauma to the cilia and even denudation of the tracheal or bronchial mucosa. As a consequence, the physiology of the air passages is deranged, and the initial irritation progresses to clinical disease. If bacterial invasion was not the initial event, it frequently occurs at this point as a secondary infection. The bacteria most commonly involved are *Staphylococcus aureus*, the streptococci, *Hemophilus influenzae*, *Diplococcus pneumoniae* and, rarely, *Corynebacterium diphtheriae*. Of equal importance as etiologic agents are a large group of adenoviruses and some of the ECHO and influenza viruses. Often acute laryngotracheobronchitis follows a bout of the common cold, which in turn may be caused by a multitude of ubiquitous viruses. Infants are more vulnerable than adults, probably because of their shorter and relatively wider tracheobronchial trees and the absence of mucus secreting cells in their small bronchi and bronchioles. Secondary invasion by *H. influenzae* is a frequent occurrence in these children. Whereas acute laryngotracheobronchitis is usually a mild illness in adults, characterized by low-grade fever, malaise, hoarseness and productive cough, it may be life-threatening in infants. Because of the small size of the infant larynx, the airway may be totally obstructed by edema and inflammatory exudate, constituting a pediatric emergency. In addition, *H. influenzae* may give rise to an acute edematous epiglottitis that can produce sudden, marked respiratory difficulty.

The gross morphologic changes may involve the mucosa uniformly or in patches; commonly, the lower portion of the trachea and the main-stem bronchi are involved. The affected mucosa is edematous and hyperemic. The light microscope shows an outpouring of inflammatory exudate on the mucosal surface. When this exudate is chiefly a stringy, basophilic mucus only scantily mixed with leukocytes, the process is called a **catarrhal** laryngotracheobronchitis. If there is a significant element of leukocytic infiltration, it is referred to as **suppurative**. When the inflammatory reaction is more intense, with necrosis of the mucosa in areas, it constitutes an **ulcerative** form. Diphtheria evokes a necrotizing fibrinosuppurative exudate characterized by a coagulum on the surface, designated as **membranous**. Large numbers of eosinophils may be present in the inflammatory exudate, particularly in those instances caused by allergic reactions.

With the control of acute inflammation, these inflammatory changes may subside, the epithelium may regenerate and the normal architecture may be restored. On the other hand, particularly with continued exposure to an irritant, the acute reaction may persist and progress to chronic bronchitis.

CHRONIC COUGH

CHRONIC BRONCHITIS

The definition of chronic bronchitis is primarily a clinical one, based on *the presence of a productive cough for at least three months of the year over at least two consecutive years* (without other specific cause) (American Thoracic Society, 1962). It is a common malady, particularly in cigarette smokers, and is not nearly so trivial as was once thought. When persistent for years, chronic bronchitis may: (1) cause significantly increased airway resistance (COPD), as discussed on page 386, with or without concomitant emphysema, (2) lead to cor pulmonale and right-sided heart failure, and (3) cause atypical metaplasia and dysplasia of the respiratory epithelium, providing a possible soil for cancerous transformation. Accompanying the cough which defines chronic bronchitis are certain histologic changes, principally hypertrophy and hyperplasia of the mucous glands of the tracheobronchial tree, resulting in excessive mucus production. Usually there are concomitant epithelial changes, including hyperplasia, squamous metaplasia and even, as mentioned, dysplasia. While the disease occurs in both sexes and at any age, it is most frequent in middle-aged men. In the northern industrialized countries, chronic bronchitis is a major health problem. In a British survey (Chronic bronchitis in Great Britain, 1961), it was found in 17 per cent of males and 8 per cent of females. In the United States, it is probably somewhat less common.

Etiology and Pathogenesis. Chronic bronchitis probably represents the response of the tracheobronchial tree to chronic irritation by inhaled substances, principally cigarette smoke but also atmospheric pollutants. Several investigators have shown that heavy cigarette smoking alone will induce excessive mucus secretion, lead to squamous metaplasia and dysplasia of the respiratory epithelium and inhibit the normal protective function of the alveolar macrophages (Thurlbeck and Angus, 1964; Auerbach et al., 1962; Green and Carolin, 1967). Even young smokers without clinical evidence of bronchitis show inflammatory changes within their respiratory bronchioles (Niewoehner et al., 1974). Other inhaled substances play a lesser role in the causation of chronic bronchitis. Epidemiologic studies have shown that the death rate from this disease parallels several other factors, including the population density, the degree of industrialization of an area, the sulphur dioxide content of the air and the amount of fog.

The role of infection in chronic bronchitis is not entirely clear. Certainly, as the normal ciliated columnar epithelium is replaced by squamous epithelium and as macrophage function becomes less efficient, important protective mechanisms are lost and the patient becomes more vulnerable to recurrent secondary infections. Further, the capacity to remove mucus is overwhelmed, and accumulated mucus plugs offer haven for microbial invaders. Whether chronic bronchitis always implies *chronic* infection, however, is doubtful. Culture results from large groups of patients have varied. One study has implicated either *D. pneumoniae* or *H. influenzae* in most cases of chronic bronchitis (Buckley et al., 1957). Other studies have found that most cultures are free of bacteria, and still others report as many as 80 to 90 per cent of persons with chronic bronchitis infected with *H. influenzae*. Despite the variable results, it would appear safe to say that bacterial infection is frequent and that the offending organism is usually either *H. influenzae* or *D. pneumoniae*. Viral infection is also common in patients with chronic bronchitis, and it has been reported that about 50 per cent of the recurrent infections that are so typical of this disease are caused by viruses, especially those of the respiratory syncytial group. By the time chronic bronchitis is diagnosed, the disease involves the larger airways. However, there is much evidence that the early changes affect predominantly the small airways, principally the respiratory bronchioles (Thurlbeck, 1973). The centrilobular emphysema often associated with chronic bronchitis may in turn be caused by the inflammatory obstruction of these small airways, as described on page 387 (Niewoehner et al., 1974). At the level of the respiratory bronchioles the damage is largely silent, producing little cough and only subtle evidence of COPD. Thus, by the time the typical manifestations of chronic bronchitis appear, the disease may be extensive.

Morphology. With advanced disease the entire tracheobronchial tree or any portion of it may be affected, although the alterations are ultimately most severe in the lower portion of the trachea, in the main-stem bronchi and at bifurcations. The gross changes are similar to those of acute bronchitis, with hyperemia, swelling and bogginess of the mucous membranes, which are covered with excessive mucinous to mucopurulent secretions. Sometimes heavy casts of secretion and pus fill the bronchi or bronchioles. Sharply defined ulcerations may be present. Occasionally, in contrast to the usual picture, the mucosal lining appears extremely dry, glazed, atrophic and shiny, described as **atrophic chronic bronchitis**. In this form, large tracts of mucosa may desquamate to denude entire segments of the tracheobronchial tree. The basis for such variation in the response to a chronic inflammation is unknown.

As can be anticipated, the light microscope shows an inflammatory response consisting of a mixture of mononuclear cells, usually macrophages, with large numbers of lymphocytes and plasma cells and some neutrophils. Occasionally the lymphocytes are aggregated within the subepithelial and deeper submucosal tissues into large collections, sometimes with the formation of true lymphoid follicles. The mucosa may show all degrees of reactive changes, ranging from simple hyperplasia to squamous metaplasia to dysplasia. Hypertrophy and hyperplasia of the mucous glands are characteristic. Old scarring frequently deforms the smaller airways, leading to multiple stenoses or even obliteration. **Bronchiolitis fibrosa obliterans** occurs when the exudate within the airways organizes to fill the lumen with granulation tissue.

Clinical Course. By definition, patients with chronic bronchitis have a chronic cough, characteristically productive of purulent sputum. The cough usually precedes by years the onset of noticeable functional impairment. Eventually, however, dyspnea on exertion, usually of a peculiar fluctuating nature, develops. Functionally, there is increased airway resistance and, in advanced cases, there is also a markedly distorted ventilation-perfusion relationship, leading to hypoxemia and hypercapnia. Because both chronic bronchitis and primary emphysema (see p. 386) involve an increase in airway resistance, they are often lumped together as "chronic obstructive pulmonary disease" *(COPD)* or "chronic obstructive lung disease" *(COLD)*. Long-standing, severe chronic bronchitis commonly leads to cor pulmonale. When this stage is reached, death usually follows within a few years, either from right-sided heart failure or from respiratory failure, often precipitated by an acute intercurrent infection (Vandenbergh et al., 1973). At necropsy, emphysema is often, although not necessarily, present.

Some interesting studies have revealed several clinical parameters by which the patient with chronic bronchitis may be distinguished from the patient with primary emphysema (Nash et al., 1965; Ogilvie, 1959). Those features that were found to be characteristic of the typical patient with chronic bronchitis are:

1. Marked productive cough.
2. Relatively late dyspnea.
3. Marked ventilation-perfusion imbalance.
4. Relatively early cor pulmonale.

5. Relatively early secondary polycythemia.
6. Normal body habitus.
7. Normal total lung capacity with normal chest x-rays.

A contrasting list, describing the typical patient with primary emphysema, is presented on page 389. It is important to remember that although these entities are separable, they often coexist in the same patient. Moreover, the picture may be further obscured by the presence in these individuals of an element of reversible bronchospasm, a characteristic of still a third disease, asthma.

BRONCHIECTASIS

Bronchiectasis is an abnormal dilatation of medium-sized bronchi and bronchioles (about the fourth to ninth generations), associated with a chronic necrotizing infection within these passages. Most often it represents a complication of some other process, either congenital or acquired, which has altered normal structure. All age groups and both sexes may be affected, and it is frequent in children.

Etiology and Pathogenesis. About 60 per cent of these cases are preceded by an acute respiratory infection (Spencer, 1968), usually bronchopneumonia but frequently, especially in children, whooping cough or measles, with severe secondary bronchitis (Laurenzi, 1969). The infection destroys segments of bronchial mucosa, which are replaced by fibrous scar tissue. Because this fibrotic tissue lacks resilience, the affected bronchi become permanently deformed and dilated under the stresses of respiration. These pouches, denuded of their normal epithelium, ultimately become targets for a variety of organisms, which establish chronic smoldering infection.

Other conditions which predispose to bronchiectasis include obstruction of a bronchus by a neoplasm, a tuberculous lymph node or a foreign body, with stasis of infected secretions distal to the point of obstruction; atelectasis, which deforms the bronchi as their supporting framework collapses; and chronic bronchitis, with its destruction and loss of normal defenses. Bronchiectasis is also seen in association with mucoviscidosis and with congenital malformations of the bronchi. It is a component of *Kartagener's syndrome* (sinusitis, bronchiectasis and situs inversus). Many workers have pointed to a frequent association of sinusitis with bronchiectasis, although a causal relationship, if any, is not clear.

Any of a variety of organisms may be involved. Staphylococci, streptococci, pneumococci, *H. influenzae* and several enteric organisms are commonly isolated. In addition, anaerobic and microaerophilic organisms which normally inhabit the mouth are frequently present in these infections. Whether they are of etiologic significance or simply represent secondary saprophytic invaders is a controversial issue.

Morphology. The involvement may be unilateral or bilateral. The lower lobes—especially the left lower lobe—are most vulnerable, but the right middle lobe and the lingula are also frequently affected. The most severe involvements are found in the smaller bronchi and bronchioles. These airways are dilated, sometimes up to four times normal size, and so they often can be followed virtually out to the pleural surface. The dilated segments may be long and tubelike (cylindroid), or they may be fusiform or saccular in shape. The anatomic changes are best brought out by sectioning the lung at right angles to the long axis of the affected airways. The cut surface of the lung may show an almost cystic pattern, created by the widely dilated bronchioles, with compression of the intervening lung parenchyma. Sometimes this honeycombed appearance is mistaken for bronchogenic congenital cysts. The lumina of the affected bronchi are characteristically filled with a suppurative, yellow-green, sometimes hemorrhagic exudate, which, when removed, exposes a red-green or black, necrotic, edematous, frequently ulcerated mucosa. When the infection extends to the pleura, as it often does, it evokes a fibrinous or suppurative pleuritis.

The histologic findings vary with the activity and chronicity of the disease. In the full-blown, active case, there is an intense acute and chronic inflammatory exudate within the walls of the affected airways, associated with desquamation of the lining epithelium and extensive areas of necrotizing ulceration. There may be squamous metaplasia of the remaining epithelium. In some instances, the necrosis extends down to the smooth muscle and may even completely destroy the wall, so that the infective process is in direct continuity with the lung parenchyma, creating a lung abscess. In the more chronic cases, fibrosis of the bronchial wall and peribronchial fibrosis develop.

When healing occurs, there may be complete regeneration of the lining epithelium. However, usually dilatation and scarring persist.

Clinical Course. The classic patient presents with a chronic cough beginning months to years after an episode of pneumonia. The cough is typically paroxysmal and often violent. Paroxysms tend to occur with changes in position, especially upon arising in the morning, and also during the night. With changes in position, there is drainage of the collected pools of pus into unaffected portions of the bronchi, and this stimulates coughing. The patient raises copious amounts of mucoid to mucopurulent sputum, often of the order of a half-cup per day. Although chronic cough is the most frequent presentation, occasionally an otherwise asymptomatic patient experiences the sudden onset of hemoptysis, which may be quite massive if a large vessel has been eroded. Clubbing of the fingers and toes occurs in 25 per cent of cases (p. 624).

The prognosis with bronchiectasis varies widely. Many, if not most, patients are asymptomatic. Minor degrees of bronchiectasis are found in many postmortem examinations when it is not expected on clinical grounds. In other patients, the condition is symptomatic and partially disabling because of chronic cough and fatigue, but probably it does not materially shorten the life span. Among some patients, however, bronchiectasis represents a profoundly crippling and even life-threatening disease. These patients may develop severe constitutional manifestations, including fever, weight loss and malaise. With widespread involvement, dyspnea and cyanosis may occur, and recurrent bouts of pneumonia are common. The more severe cases are usually associated with early onset. Few childhood bronchiectatics live beyond 40 years of age, unless they are adequately treated, either medically or surgically. These patients with an early onset usually develop one of several complications, such as a lung abscess, septic emboli to the brain, extension of the process to the pleural space, with resultant empyema, or pneumonia. When the disease is widespread and fibrosis encroaches on the pulmonary vascular bed, cor pulmonale may develop. Amyloidosis is an occasional complication in long-standing cases. Death most often results from intercurrent pneumonia.

LUNG ABSCESS

Lung abscess refers to a localized area of suppurative necrosis within the pulmonary parenchyma. The causative organism may be introduced into the lung by any of the following mechanisms: (1) Aspiration of infective material, which may involve material from carious teeth or from infected sinuses or tonsils, and which is particularly likely during oral surgery, anesthesia, coma, alcoholic intoxication, and in debilitated patients with depressed cough reflexes. Aspiration of gastric contents may also lead to lung abscesses. (2) As a complication of pneumonia. As was mentioned earlier, abscess formation is an occasional complication of pneumonia, particularly that caused by *Staphylococcus aureus*, *Klebsiella pneumoniae* and Type III pneumococcus. Mycotic infections and bronchiectasis may also lead to lung abscesses. (3) Bronchial obstruction. This is particularly likely with bronchogenic carcinoma obstructing a bronchus or

bronchiole. Impaired drainage, distal atelectasis and aspiration of blood and tumor fragments all contribute to the development of sepsis. Even more commonly, the abscess forms within an excavated necrotic portion of the tumor itself. (4) Septic embolism, which most frequently is secondary to septic thrombophlebitis, but which may also come from infective endocarditis of the right side of the heart. Infrequent causes of a lung abscess include trauma, with direct introduction of bacteria by penetration of the lung; transdiaphragmatic spread from the peritoneum, e.g., from an amoebic hepatic abscess; and infected hydatid cysts. When all these pathogenetic pathways are excluded, there are still a large number of cases of mysterious origin. These are referred to as "primary cryptogenic lung abscesses."

With so many possible pathways for development, it is not surprising that lung abscesses occur at any age and in either sex. Certain pathways are more common in certain age groups — e.g., a pulmonary abscess associated with bronchogenic carcinoma is most likely over the age of 45. The multiplicity of pathways also explains the large number of possible etiologic organisms. The most commonly isolated aerobic organisms are, in order of frequency, *Streptococcus viridans*, *Staphylococcus aureus*, beta hemolytic streptococci, the pneumococci and a wide variety of gram-negative organisms (Schweppe et al., 1961). Very often there is a mixed infection. Anaerobic bacteria are also present in almost all cases, sometimes in vast numbers. Recently they have been reported to be the *exclusive* isolates in 16 of 26 consecutive cases of primary lung abscess (Bartlett et al., 1974). The most frequently encountered anaerobes were commensals normally found in the oral cavity, principally *Fusobacterium nucleatum*, *Bacteroides melaninogenicus*, peptostreptococci, peptococci and eubacteria. At one time a pathogenic role for these commensals was considered highly doubtful. However, the fact that in this study they were the exclusive isolates in most cases of lung abscess would indicate that they are indeed important pathogens in the lungs.

Morphology. Abscesses vary in diameter from a few millimeters to large cavities of 5 to 6 cm. The localization and number of abscesses are in large part dependent upon their mode of development. Pulmonary abscesses resulting from the aspiration of infective material are much more common on the right side than on the left, and most often are single. Presumably the more frequent involvement of the right lung results, at least in part, from the more vertical course of the right main bronchus. Within the right lung, the most frequent locations for solitary pulmonary abscesses are in the subapical and axillary portions of the upper lobe and in the apical portion of the lower lobe. These locations reflect the likely course of aspirated material when the patient is lying on his right side or on his back, respectively. Abscesses which develop in the course of pneumonia or bronchiectasis are commonly multiple, basal and diffusely scattered. Septic emboli and pyemic abscesses, by the very haphazard nature of their genesis, are commonly multiple and may affect any region of the lungs.

Abscesses begin as a focus of hyperemia, followed in time by central necrosis. At first the enclosing wall is poorly defined, but with time and progressive fibrosis, it becomes more discrete. Rupture through this containing wall may create grapelike multiloculations. At the time of examination, the cavity may be filled with suppurative debris. However, in many cases, the abscess erodes into a bronchus, allowing for partial drainage of the contents. Air, in turn, enters the cavity, and an air-fluid level is apparent on x-ray. Eventually the abscess appears as a rapidly expanding, green-black, multilocular cavity with poor margination. The exudation and edema compress the blood supply, adding an element of ischemic necrosis to the preexisting infection. In such cases, the entire process is termed **gangrene of the lung.** Occasionally, abscesses rupture into the pleural cavity, producing bronchopleural fistulas, often with consequent pneumothorax or with empyema.

The histologic appearance of a lung abscess is that of a nonspecific inflammatory reaction with suppurative destruction of the lung parenchyma within the central area of cavitation. In chronic cases, considerable fibroblastic proliferation produces a containing wall. There is often inflammatory pneumonic consolidation in the immediately adjacent alveoli. Clearly, the healing of such destructive lesions yields a permanent fibrous scar.

Clinical Course. The manifestations of a lung abscess are much like those of bronchiectasis. There is a prominent cough, which usually yields copious amounts of foul-smelling purulent or sanguinous sputum. Occasionally gross hemoptysis occurs. Characteristically, changes in position evoke paroxysms of coughing because of the sudden drainage from the abscess. However, if there is no avenue for drainage—or, sometimes, early in the course—sputum may be minimal. Along with the cough, there is spiking fever and malaise, and, if the abscess extends to the overlying pleura, there may be pleuritic pain. Dyspnea is characteristically absent. Clubbing of the fingers, of uncertain pathogenesis, may become apparent within a few weeks. With chronicity, weight loss and anemia ensue.

Chest x-rays show an air-fluid level if there is communication with an airway; otherwise the density is homogeneous. Since cavitation of a neoplasm may also result in an air-fluid

level, bronchoscopy is necessary to rule out an underlying carcinoma.

The course of an untreated pulmonary abscess is variable. If drainage is good and there is no obstruction, spontaneous healing may occur. However, most cases run a subacute to chronic course, with increasing debilitation of the patient. Complications include brain abscesses or meningitis from septic emboli. Rarely, a patient may develop secondary amyloidosis.

TUBERCULOSIS

Tuberculosis is an acute or chronic communicable disease, caused by *Mycobacterium tuberculosis,* which usually involves the lung but which may also affect any other organ or tissue in the body. Although in North America and Europe the incidence and mortality of this disease have markedly declined since the beginning of the twentieth century, tuberculosis remains one of the leading worldwide causes of death. Along with malaria, it is certainly one of the most important of the infectious diseases.

Incidence. In 1900, tuberculosis was the leading cause of death in the United States, accounting for approximately 200 deaths per 100,000 population. Some appreciation of its awesome impact at that time can be gained by noting that this was a higher death rate than the present death rate from all forms of cancer combined (168 per 100,000 in 1973). Since the turn of the century, the death rate from tuberculosis has plummeted to only 1.8 per 100,000 population in 1973. Along with the reduction in mortality, there has been an accompanying decline in incidence, as better methods of detection and therapy facilitate identification and cure of the asymptomatic carrier before he has spread his disease widely. Heartening as these trends are, it should be remembered that the large city slums represent pockets in which tuberculosis remains a major problem and which continue to act as depots of infection.

Tuberculosis is a disease to which man, as opposed to, say, the unfortunate guinea pig, has a great deal of natural resistance. Probably no more than 5 per cent of Americans now infected with *M. tuberculosis* will ever develop clinical disease. *Tuberculosis as an infection, then, is quite distinct from tuberculosis as a disease.* The number of asymptomatically infected Americans is declining and presently is of the order of 25,000,000. Among young adults, those infected are now outnumbered by those who have never had contact with *M. tuberculosis* (Mitchell, 1967).

Whereas at one time tuberculosis was primarily a disease of children and young adults, it has now become a disease of the elderly. In 1965, 68 per cent of those who died from tuberculosis were over 55 years of age. Males outnumbered females by 3 to 1. Moreover, no longer is the source of disease usually exogenous—that is, contracted from another person with the disease. Instead, about 75 per cent of today's newly discovered symptomatic cases simply represent activation of old asymptomatic infection (Trauger, 1963).

Since only a small proportion of those infected actually develop clinical disease, what are the factors which tend to lower the human host's naturally high resistance? Patients already suffering from certain chronic lung diseases, such as silicosis, are especially vulnerable. Moreover, systemic debilitating disorders, including diabetes mellitus and congenital heart disease, predispose to the development of tuberculosis. Children of preschool age, too, have a heightened susceptibility. And finally, since massive infection is more likely to result in disease than is exposure to smaller numbers of bacilli, those in the health professions who, often unknowingly, come into contact with patients with active tuberculosis have an increased risk of developing the disease. From an epidemiologic point of view, the most important single factor is poverty, with its attendant overcrowding and malnutrition. There is a higher incidence of tuberculosis among blacks than among whites, but it is difficult to ascertain whether this is indeed a racial difference or whether it simply reflects socioeconomic factors. For unknown reasons, natural resistance seems to vary also from individual to individual.

Etiology. The mycobacteria comprise a very large group of gram-positive, acid-fast rods that include both pathogenic and saprophytic organisms. Principal among the pathogenic organisms is *Mycobacterium tuberculosis*. *Mycobacterium tuberculosis* is further subdivided into five strains: human, bovine, avian, murine and piscine. Only the human and bovine strains are pathogenic to man. In addition, there are a number of *unclassified mycobacteria* (also known as *atypical* or *anonymous mycobacteria*), which are increasingly responsible for a disease in man that is clinically indistinguishable from tuberculosis. These will be discussed in a later section.

Mycobacterium tuberculosis is a slender, curved rod averaging 4 μm. in length and less than 1 μm. in diameter. Along with the other mycobacteria, it has the unique property that, once stained, it resists decolorization with acid alcohol. This distinctive staining property is termed acid-fastness. It is probably related to the waxy lipid components of the bacillary bodies. The degree of acid-fastness is quite variable among the mycobacteria. In general, pathogens are more acid-fast than the saprophytes, and the greater the virulence of the pathogen, the greater the resistance to decolorization. The tubercle bacillus has other special characteristics, knowledge of which, as will be seen later, contributes to an understanding of the disease. It is a strict aerobe and grows slowly even in special culture media. The lipid content of these bacilli is unusually high, constituting approximately 50 per cent of the organism. This lipid fraction includes neutral fats, phosphatides and many long-chain waxes. The high lipid content renders these organisms hydrophobic and they tend to grow in clumps which are poorly penetrated by aqueous bactericidal agents. Moreover, they are highly resistant to drying and can survive for long periods of time in desiccated sputum. Other important characteristics of the tubercle bacillus include its inability to grow either at an acid pH or in the presence of aliphatic fatty acids, especially the shorter chain members of the series.

Spread of tuberculosis is usually direct, from person to person, by inhalation of airborne bacilli that have been coughed or sneezed into the atmosphere. Only organisms deposited in the small airways produce infection; hence they must be contained in a spray of fine droplets, less than 10 μm. in diameter. Because of this requirement, it is presently thought that the infectiousness of pulmonary tuberculosis is much lower than formerly supposed. Although dishes, clothing and other articles of daily use may be laden with bacilli, transmission by this route is probably rare (Bates and Stead, 1974). The gastrointestinal tract is the usual portal of entry for the bovine strain, since this is transmitted through contaminated milk. With widespread pasteurization of milk and detection of diseased cattle, bovine tuberculosis is becoming very infrequent and probably accounts for less than 5 per cent of tuberculosis in the United States. Other possible but rare portals of entry include the lymphoid tissue of the oropharynx and open skin lesions.

Pathogenesis. *The destructiveness of the tubercle bacillus derives not from any inherent toxicity, but rather from its distinctive capacity to induce hypersensitivity in its host.* The organism produces no recognizable endotoxins or exotoxins and is virtually innocuous when first introduced into a host. It excites a minimal inflammatory response, much as would inert particulate matter of similar size. After one to two weeks, however, the character of the host reaction abruptly changes, as cell-mediated hypersensitivity to the tubercle bacillus develops (p. 000). An intense proliferative and destructive tissue reaction ensues, which will be described in detail later. Concurrent with the appearance of hypersensitivity is the development of a heightened *resistance* to the disease, based on an acquired capacity of the mononuclear phagocytes to destroy phagocytized bacilli. Because both hypersensitivity and this partial immunity develop, it should be clear that second exposures to this organism will have very different consequences than did the first exposure. *This difference is the basis for considering the disease as comprising two forms: primary tuberculosis, occurring from initial contact with the bacillus; and secondary tuberculosis, resulting either from repeated exposure or from reactivation of a primary focus.*

An allergic response to the injection of tuberculoprotein means that the individual has been infected with the tubercle bacillus. This is the basis for the widely used *Mantoux test,* which involves the intracutaneous inoculation of a measured amount of tuberculoprotein, either O.T. (old tuberculin) or P.P.D. (purified protein derivative). A positive response consists of induration at the injection site (p. 176). The weight of evidence now favors the view that most people who are reactors harbor viable bacilli, but, as was pointed out earlier, disease seldom develops. In most cases, the bacilli in these tuberculin reactors remain sealed off and quiescent, and are not communicable. These are the 25,000,000 Americans referred to earlier as being infected with tuberculosis but not having the disease. The significance of tuberculin testing as a tool is apparent. A positive tuberculin test implies either (1) the presence of active tuberculosis, or (2) previous exposure, hence the risk of developing endogenous disease. The test loses its reliability in situations producing skin anergy. Such situations are severe illnesses, *including overwhelming tuberculosis,* acute illnesses, such as measles, extreme old age or debility, steroid and other immunosuppressive treatment, sarcoidosis and Hodgkin's disease. In general, there is no problem in recognizing these conditions.

The characteristic tissue reaction of both primary and secondary tuberculosis, known as the *tubercle,* was described earlier, on page 49. Basically, as was pointed out, the tubercle is a microscopic granuloma, the center of which is occupied either by a nest of plump, rounded mononuclear cells that vaguely resemble epithelial cells and are therefore designated *epithelioid cells,* or by central caseous necrosis (creating a "soft tubercle").

PRIMARY TUBERCULOSIS

With primary tuberculosis, the source of the organism must always be exogenous. Inhaled tubercle bacilli become implanted upon the alveolar surfaces of the lung parenchyma, most often in the lower part of the upper lobe or upper part of the lower lobe, and usually toward the periphery of one lung. As was mentioned earlier, during the first week to two weeks, there is very little tissue response and the patient is tuberculin negative. Although tubercle bacilli are phagocytized by macrophages, these bacilli continue to grow within the phagocytes and apparently achieve a happy symbiosis. Lymphatic drainage of the bacilli, either within phagocytes or as free agents, is unimpeded, and regional lymph nodes are therefore invariably involved. During the course of the second week of infection, two changes occur: First, sensitivity develops and results in the formation of soft tubercles both at the point of initial infection and within the regional lymph nodes; and second, the phagocytes acquire the capacity to inhibit the growth of ingested bacilli and no longer harbor them as privileged passengers. In the vast majority of cases, arrest of the infection occurs at this point. Progressive fibrosis walls off the focus, and often the necrotic center becomes calcified or ossified. The primary lesion in the lung periphery is known as a *Ghon focus,* and the combination of this lesion and the lymph node involvement is termed a *Ghon complex.* The regular and easy arrest of the process is probably attributable to a number of factors, including the development of hypersensitivity and partial immunity. In addition, cellular destruction within the inflammatory focus leads progressively to an environment unfavorable for the survival of the bacilli. Lipases act upon neutral fats to release fatty acids, and there is the development of a progressive local anaerobiosis and acidosis. The only residuum, then, of tuberculosis infection is the presence of a fibrotic, sometimes calcified, Ghon complex which may, however, harbor still viable organisms. A calcified Ghon complex is a frequent incidental finding on routine chest x-rays of healthy individuals.

In occasional instances, particularly among preschool children, primary infection does not run such a benign course. Several possible complications may develop. In some cases, the tubercle erodes into a bronchus, into which it discharges the contents of its necrotic center. An air-filled cavity then results, and oxygen is thus supplied to the quiescent aerobic bacilli lining its walls. Such *cavitation* restores vigor to the tuberculous process and enables bronchogenic dissemination to occur. The process is then essentially identical in clinical consequences to secondary tuberculosis, to be discussed later. When bronchogenic dissemination is widespread, multiple patchy areas of involvement or large consolidations known as *tuberculous pneumonia* may develop.

In other instances, dissemination occurs via the lymphatic system. The bacilli may then gain entrance to the bloodstream through the thoracic duct. Sometimes there is direct seeding of the blood, when a tubercle erodes into a nearby vessel. It is important to remember that either bronchogenic dissemination or hematogenous dissemination may occur early or after many years of latency. When bloodstream invasion is massive, *acute miliary tuberculosis* ensues, so named because of the resemblance of the multiple tiny lesions to millet seeds. This is often accompanied by *tuberculous meningitis.* These grave complications were once invariably fatal. The pattern of miliary involvement depends both on the route of access to the bloodstream and on the native resistance of exposed organs. With lymphatic dissemination, the bacilli reach the right side of the heart, then return to the lungs, where most are filtered out in the alveolar capillary bed. Miliary tuberculosis in these cases is confined to the lungs. When a tuberculous lesion erodes directly into a pulmonary artery, only the localized area of lung supplied by this single vessel may be involved. When a pulmonary vein is invaded, the miliary lesions seed the entire body or strangely only one organ. The pattern of organ involvement depends on poorly understood factors of natural resistance. The lungs, bones, joints, kidneys, meninges, adrenals, liver, spleen, fallopian tubes and epididymides show little resistance and are commonly involved. In contrast, certain organs, including striated voluntary muscles, the heart, pancreas, stomach, thyroid and testes, are seldom involved in disseminated disease.

Morphology. The parenchymal lesion is usually subpleural, either just above or just below the interlobar fissure between the upper and lower lobes. This takes the form of a small, 1 to 2 cm. in diameter focus of yellow-white caseation. The lesion is rarely cavitated and classically is well delimited from the surrounding substance. Parallel changes occur in the regional tracheobronchial lymph nodes, which become enlarged and caseous. These two foci of tuberculous involvement constitute the Ghon complex (Fig. 12–9). Histologically, primary tuberculosis is characterized by an initial aggregation of neutrophils, which are replaced within 24 to 48 hours predominantly by lymphocytes and histiocytes. During the ensuing week, there is a continued accumulation of lymphocytes and histiocytes, some of which remain viable, whereas others undergo necrosis. The characteristic tubercle usually develops in the second week. As the tubercles enlarge, often with coalescence of adjacent lesions, central caseation evolves. It is to be emphasized that individual tubercles are of mi-

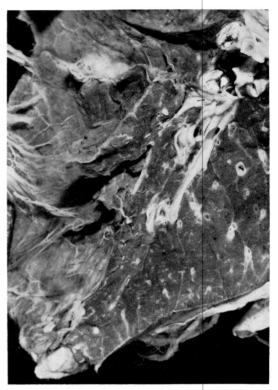

Figure 12–9. Primary pulmonary tuberculosis. The parenchymal focus is present in the lower left subpleural location. Lymph nodes with caseation are visible in the upper right.

croscopic size and it is only when multiple tubercles coalesce or a single tubercle considerably enlarges that they become macroscopic. Variations in host response may be defined in terms of the relative degree of proliferation versus exudation in the tubercles. When the response is largely proliferative, the lesion is characterized by adequate defensive walling off, with progressive scarring, usually accompanied by calcification. In contrast, lesions in the more vulnerable host may be largely exudative in nature, i.e., with extensive inflammatory exudation, caseation and poor localization. In general, the proliferative activity is less adequate in the lymph nodes, and persistent foci of caseation may remain for months or years.

With bronchogenic dissemination and coalescence of lesions in the highly susceptible individual, the infection may spread rapidly throughout large areas of lung parenchyma. Either a diffuse bronchopneumonia or a lobar consolidation, once referred to as "galloping consumption," results. The lobar pattern is characterized by conversion of the affected lobe or lung into a solid, noncrepitant mass of gray-white cheesy material. Such a picture is descriptively known as **pneumonia alba.** Histologically, the alveoli in tuberculous pneumonia are filled with an exudate composed of mononuclear phagocytes trapped within granular fibrinoproteinous material. In the course of time, these areas may undergo total caseous necrosis, with destruction of the underlying parenchyma, whereas in other areas recognizable or abortive tubercles may form and eventually yield confluent areas of fibrocaseous involvement. Usually, however, the patient does not survive long enough to develop an adequate proliferative response. In the absence of well developed tubercles, it may indeed be difficult to establish the nature of the pneumonic process. However, numerous tubercle bacilli are usually present in such exudates, and their identification yields the diagnosis. Death, although usual, is not inevitable in such florid disease, and resolution of the exudate may occur, with considerable restoration of previous architecture. Areas where the underlying structures have been destroyed become scarred, and fibrocalcific residues are therefore the rule. Inevitably, with tuberculous pneumonia, the infection extends into the pleural cavity.

When miliary tuberculosis occurs, it may be confined to the lungs or it may involve other organs as well. In any case, there are numerous tiny lesions scattered throughout the parenchyma of the involved organ. These lesions vary from one to several millimeters in diameter and are distinct yellow-white, firm areas of consolidation, usually without grossly visible caseous necrosis or cavitation. Histologically, however, they show the characteristic pattern of individual or multiple confluent tubercles, with microscopic central caseation.

Clinical Course.
In the overwhelming majority of cases, primary tuberculous infection is an asymptomatic process. Occasionally, serial skin tests reveal its presence by a conversion from tuberculin negative to tuberculin positive results. Subsequent chest x-rays may show a calcified Ghon complex. Among the relatively small number of patients whose initial infection is not arrested, the manifestations of the disease are quite variable, depending on the pattern and extent of involvement.

Progressive pulmonary tuberculosis may develop directly from the primary lesion, without a period of latency, and follow a course identical to that of secondary tuberculosis, which will be discussed later. Sometimes primary tuberculosis presents as a *pleural effusion*, which develops silently but which may, when large, ultimately produce dyspnea. Although a chest x-ray may appear normal after thoracentesis, the effusion nevertheless resulted from direct extension or lymphatic spread to the pleura of underlying microscopic pulmonary tuberculosis. *Tuberculous pneumonia* presents as a febrile debilitating illness, with localizing respiratory symptoms, such as cough, dyspnea and hemoptysis. Dissemination of tuberculosis results either in *isolated organ involvement* or in *acute miliary tuberculosis.*

When the kidneys are the site of metastatic involvement, hematuria may develop. If the infection then descends from the kidneys to the lower urinary tract, manifestations of bladder irritability, such as dysuria and frequency, ensue. Diarrhea and malabsorption usually herald involvement of the gastrointestinal tract, which is commonly confined to the ileocecal region. Tuberculosis is an infrequent but occasional cause of osteitis and monoarticular arthritis. In a minority of instances, Addison's disease results from tuberculous destruction of the adrenal glands. Certainly any of the above signs and symptoms, when occurring in the presence of pulmonary disease, should immediately suggest the diagnosis of tuberculosis.

Acute miliary tuberculosis may have a sudden violent onset, or it may develop over the course of a few weeks. In any case, there is profound prostration and high fever. When there is widespread involvement of the lungs, cough and dyspnea may also be present. Hepatosplenomegaly is common and indicates spread to these organs. Meningeal symptoms and signs indicate the concurrent presence of meningitis. With the advent of effective chemotherapy, there has been a marked improvement in prognosis, and survival is usual in all but the most advanced cases.

SECONDARY TUBERCULOSIS (ADULT, REINFECTION, POSTPRIMARY TUBERCULOSIS)

Although the morbidity of secondary tuberculosis is greater than that of primary tuberculosis, surprisingly the risk of developing it is appreciably lower. This seeming paradox may be attributed to the fact that, whereas the development of partial immunity and hypersensitivity are temporally related, they have very different clinical consequences. Whereas partial immunity establishes some resistance and reduces the chances of infection, the concurrent hypersensitivity implies a more florid tissue response. In one respect, however, this heightened tissue response is beneficial to the patient, since it assists in localizing the infection. Even so, partial immunity and hypersensitivity may be looked upon as opposite sides of the same coin, if it is remembered that such a simile necessarily involves some oversimplification.

Secondary pulmonary tuberculosis is almost invariably localized to the apices of one or both upper lobes. Less frequently, the lesions may be located in the apical segments of the lower lobes. The reason for this usual apical localization is obscure. Because of the preexistence of hypersensitivity, the bacilli excite a prompt and marked tissue response, which tends to wall off the focus. As a result of this localization, the regional lymph nodes are less prominently involved and lymphohematogenous dissemination is less frequent than with primary tuberculosis. On the other hand, cavitation occurs readily with the secondary form, resulting in bronchogenic dissemination. Indeed, *cavitation may be considered the anatomic hallmark of secondary tuberculosis.*

The course of secondary tuberculosis is variable, depending on many factors of host resistance and bacterial virulence, as well as on such accidental factors as the likelihood of erosion into a bronchus. Under the most favorable circumstances, when cavitation does not occur, the minimal pulmonary lesion consists of a 1 to 3 cm. focal area of caseous consolidation, which is frequently self-limited. Healing occurs slowly by fibrosis and calcification. When cavitation occurs, as it frequently does, a number of complications may ensue. Extension either by contiguity or by aspiration of infective material through the bronchi spreads the infection to other portions of both lungs. The sputum becomes infective, a condition known as "open tuberculosis," and when swallowed, it may give rise to intestinal tuberculosis. Any portion of the tracheobronchial tree may also be contaminated by sputum, resulting in endotracheal or endobronchial tuberculosis, or in laryngeal tuberculosis. Commonly, secondary lesions extend to the pleura to produce pleural fibrosis, focal pleural adhesions, inflammatory pleural effusions, or, by direct extension of the bacilli into the pleural cavity, a tuberculous empyema.

The greater resistance of the individual who has had a primary infection is the basis of the BCG (*bacille Calmette Guérin*) vaccine, which is widely used in some countries. This vaccine consists of an attenuated bovine strain of the tubercle bacillus and confers upon the recipient hypersensitivity and partial immunity to the human strain, just as would a primary infection. As a result, there is increased resistance to tuberculosis. When the disease does develop in such vaccinated individuals, it is of the secondary form. Because BCG vaccine renders the individual tuberculin positive, the value of the skin test as an indicator of exposure to the tubercle bacillus is lost. The BCG vaccine is not in general use in the United States, where it is felt that the threat of tuberculosis is not so great as to warrant widespread vaccination with the attendant loss of tuberculin testing as a valuable monitor. The issue is controversial, however. Perhaps the most reasonable course is to reserve the BCG vaccine for populations at high risk.

Morphology. The initial lesion is usually a small focus of consolidation, less than 3 cm. in diameter, located within 1 to 2 cm. of the apical pleura. Such foci are fairly sharply circumscribed, firm, gray-white to yellow areas that have a greater or lesser component of central caseation and peripheral fibrous induration. The regional lymph nodes usually develop foci of similar tuberculous activity. In favorable cases, the initial parenchymal focus develops a small area of caseation necrosis that does not cavitate because it fails to communicate with a bronchus or bronchiole. The subsequent course may be one of progressive fibrous encapsulation, leaving only fibrocalcific scars that depress and pucker the pleural surface and cause focal pleural adhesions. Sometimes these fibrocalcific scars become secondarily blackened by anthracotic pigment. In many instances, a dense, collagenous, fibrous wall may totally enclose inspissated, caseous debris that never resolves and remains as a granular lesion at postmortem examination. Histologically, the active lesions show characteristic coalescent tubercles, usually with some central caseation. In the late lesions, the multinucleate giant cells tend to disappear. While tubercle bacilli can be demonstrated by appropriate methods in the early exudative

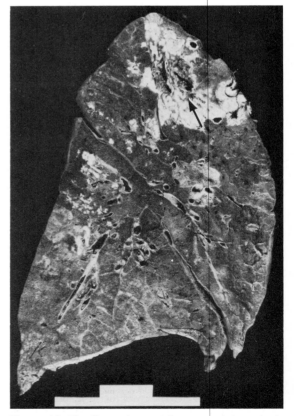

Figure 12–10. Secondary pulmonary tuberculosis. The cut section of the lung discloses massive caseation and cavitation (arrow) in the apex. Scattered foci of caseation as well as areas of pneumonic consolidation are present in both lobes.

and caseous phases, it is usually impossible to find them in the late fibrocalcific stages. However, it cannot be assumed that their absence in histologic sections implies their total destruction, since in many of these instances the presence of the organism can be demonstrated by inoculation into the ever unfortunate guinea pig.

If cavitation occurs, the disease follows a more ominous course (Fig. 12–10). Under these conditions, a ragged, irregular cavity is produced that may progressively increase in size, sometimes to occupy virtually the entire apex of the lung. The cavity is lined by a yellow-gray caseous material and is more or less walled off by fibrous tissue, depending upon the resistance of the host and the age of the lesion. Not uncommonly, thrombosed arteries traverse these cavities to produce apparent fibrous, bridging bands. This tendency for tuberculosis to incite thrombosis is a beneficial one, since it prevents the hematogenous dissemination of bacilli and the erosion of large vessels. On the other hand, many times thrombosis does not occur, and this accounts for the hemoptysis associated with open cases.

With bronchogenic dissemination, advanced fibrocaseous tuberculosis with cavitation occurs. This may affect one, many or all lobes of both lungs. In many cases that have ended in death, postmortem examination reveals the lung converted to a mass of honeycombed cavities, separated only by scant areas of scarring, compressed atelectatic, or compensatorily emphysematous lung parenchyma. In some instances, the cavities coalesce to produce giant, irregular spaces up to 10 or even 15 cm. in diameter. With widespread disease, lesions at all stages of development may coexist.

With progressive secondary tuberculosis, the pleura is inevitably involved and, depending upon the chronicity of the disease, serous pleural effusions, frank tuberculous empyema, or massive obliterative fibrous pleuritis may be found. Usually, by the time the process has extended to multiple cavitations, the pleural reaction has reached the stage of dense fibrosis that virtually blocks removal of the lungs from the chest cavity.

Endotracheal and endobronchial tuberculosis occur when in the course of advanced disease bacilli become implanted on the mucosal linings of the large air passages. These lesions may later become ulcerated, producing irregular, ragged, necrotic ulcers. Laryngeal involvement occurs less frequently. Intestinal tuberculosis is found in about 50 to 80 per cent of patients who die of far advanced disease.

Both isolated organ and miliary tuberculosis were discussed earlier as possible complications of primary tuberculosis. These may also occur with the advanced secondary form.

Clinical Course. The onset of secondary tuberculosis is usually insidious, with the gradual development of both systemic and localizing symptoms. The basis for systemic symptoms is not clear, but they often appear early in the course and include malaise, anorexia, weight loss and fever. Commonly the fever is low-grade and remittent (appearing late each afternoon and then subsiding), with the production of night sweats. With progressive pulmonary involvement, localizing symptoms appear. One of the earliest of these symptoms is a cough which gradually becomes more distressing and yields increasing amounts of sputum, at first mucoid and later becoming purulent. When cavitation is present, the sputum contains tubercle bacilli. Some degree of hemoptysis is present in about half of all cases of pulmonary tuberculosis. Pleuritic pain may also be the first manifestation of the disease, resulting either from spontaneous pneumothorax or from extension of the infection to the pleural surfaces. Certainly the diagnosis of pulmonary tuberculosis should always be entertained whenever there is chronic cough along with constitutional symptoms, or when hemoptysis or spontaneous pneumothorax occurs. The diagnosis is based in part on the history and the physical and radiologic findings of consolidation or cavitation in the apices of the lungs. Ultimately, however, tubercle bacilli must be identified. Acid-fast smears of the sputum, as well as cultures and animal inoculation, should be done. When sputum is unobtainable, gastric washings should be similarly examined. Currently, chemotherapy is usually highly effective except in advanced cases. The prognosis is generally good, but death results in up to 16 per cent of advanced cases. Amyloidosis develops in about 25 per cent of far-advanced cases of tuberculosis, and may contribute to death in a small percentage of these individuals.

ATYPICAL MYCOBACTERIA (UNCLASSIFIED, ANONYMOUS MYCOBACTERIA)

These mycobacteria are being identified with increasing frequency as the etiologic agents in disease clinically and anatomically indistinguishable from that caused by *M. tuberculosis*. They are separated into the following groups according to the color reactions of their colonies: (1) photochromogens (*M. kansasii*), whose colonies are orange-yellow only after exposure to light, (2) scotochromogens, whose colonies are orange-yellow even without light, and (3) nonchromogens (colorless colonies). Although these organisms probably reach the respiratory tree through inhalation, person-to-person contact does not seem to be the usual mode of transmission, as evidenced by the fact that family contacts of these patients do not show a higher rate of the disease. Patients with other chronic lung disease are especially vulnerable to the atypical mycobacteria. Disease caused by photochromogens is most common in urban areas, whereas that produced by the nonchromogens usually prevails in rural areas. The scotochromogens show a predilection for involvement of the cervical lymph nodes. Since there is a weak cross-reaction to standard tuberculin tests, these are of little value in the diagnosis, and the nature of the disease can be established only through culture of the organism. Most of the atypical mycobacteria, particularly the nonchromogens, show some resistance to the usual antituberculosis chemotherapy. Sometimes the lesions will respond to unusually high doses of these drugs, but often surgery is necessary (Corpe et al., 1963).

THE DEEP MYCOSES

Many fungi which are pathogenic to man virtually limit their activities to the skin. Those that also involve the deeper structures are of greater importance. The deep structures most frequently affected are the lungs. In many instances, the guilty fungi are saprophytes which become pathogenic only under special circumstances, such as when the patient is debilitated by chronic illness, when he is receiving cancer chemotherapy or total body irradiation, when he is undergoing prolonged treatment with broad-spectrum antibiotics, or when he is receiving immunosuppressive treatment following organ transplantation. The pattern of disease produced by the deep mycoses is extremely variable. Clinically, it ranges from an acute pneumonitis to a smoldering, chronic process resembling tuberculosis. In general, it can be said that the fungi are weak antigens, produce no toxins and cause tissue damage primarily by virtue of a hypersensitivity reaction by the host against the parasitic proteins. This is particularly true of *Histoplasma capsulatum, Coccidioides immitis, Blastomyces dermatitidis* and *Cryptococcus neoformans.* Filtrates from the laboratory growth of these organisms, termed histoplasmin, coccidioidin, blastomycin and cryptococcin, respectively, are used for skin tests which have a significance exactly analogous to that of the tuberculin test. A positive result (dermal induration at 48 to 72 hours) indicates prior contact with the specific fungus. Unfortunately, however, cross reactions may occur among *H. capsulatum, C. immitis* and *B. dermatitidis* (Salvin, 1968). Only the more important fungi which may involve the lung are described briefly here.

CANDIDIASIS (MONILIASIS)

Candida albicans is an extremely common inhabitant of the oral cavity and skin of normal individuals. Under predisposing circumstances, it may produce an infection of the moist cutaneous areas of the body, such as the mouth, vagina, urinary tract, nails and skin folds.

In these areas, the infection appears as confluent white patches upon a moist reddened surface. The term "thrush" refers to candidiasis in the mouth. Rarely, there is esophagitis, pneumonitis, or endocarditis. Pulmonary candidiasis is usually an acute to subacute process which simulates a bacterial pneumonia (Lurie and Duma, 1970). However, the sputum is not purulent, but rather mucoid or gelatinous. The histologic reaction varies from a nonspecific acute inflammatory response with the formation of microabscesses to a granulomatous pattern which simulates that of tuberculosis. The organisms appear as pale blue, oval, yeast-like bodies, about 3 to 6 μm in length. Many show small buds. On surfaces, such as the bronchial mucosa, abundant hyphae may be seen among the clusters of spores.

A positive skin test is of little diagnostic significance, since so many normal individuals harbor this fungus.

NOCARDIOSIS

Pulmonary nocardiosis is caused by *Nocardia (Actinomyces) asteroides,* which some believe to be an occasional normal inhabitant of the oral cavity. Others, however, maintain that its presence is always of pathogenic significance. Clinically, nocardiosis usually takes the form of an acute bronchopneumonia with abscess formation, although it may occasionally simulate tuberculosis. Sometimes there is an associated empyema.

The gross appearance of the lesion resembles that of a pyogenic bronchopneumonia. Usually a fibrinous pleuritis is apparent. Histologically, there is nonspecific abscess formation. These abscesses may coalesce to produce cavities. The organisms appear as gram-positive, slender, branching filaments, about 1 μm. in thickness. They are partially acid-fast, and when fragmented may resemble mycobacteria.

ASPERGILLOSIS

Aspergillus fumigatus gives rise to one of five patterns of involvement:

(1) A preexisting cavity in the lung, caused by tuberculosis, a lung abscess or bronchiectasis, may become virtually packed with this fungus, creating an **aspergilloma** or "fungus ball." This lesion is purely secondary and not in itself harmful, although on x-ray it may give the appearance of an alarming "coin lesion," requiring differentiation from a carcinoma. (2) The fungus may cause multiple foci of tissue necrosis within the lung, simulating a pulmonary infarction. Histologically, there is coagulative necrosis, with only a minimal inflammatory response. Nearby blood vessels are often

thrombosed and invaded by hyphae of the fungus. Whether the thrombosis or the pulmonary necrosis is primary is unclear. (3) In some instances, there is a hemorrhagic necrotizing pneumonitis, simulating lobar or bronchopneumonia. Consolidation and abscess formation are present, along with invasion of the vessels, with resultant hemorrhagic necrosis. (4) Infrequently aspergillosis takes the form of a chronic granulomatous process, simulating tuberculosis. (5) Also rare is a pseudomembranous tracheobronchitis caused by **A. fumigatus.** This pattern is characterized by ulcerations of the trachea or bronchi, covered by a pseudomembrane of amorphous necrotic debris in which the fungus is embedded. **In all five patterns, the morphology of the causative organism is constant.** The fungi appear as branching, septate hyphae less than 5 μm. in thickness. With special stains, they are seen to be extremely abundant.

HISTOPLASMOSIS

Histoplasma capsulatum is endemic in the east-central part of the United States. Its clinical expressions are varied and include asymptomatic infection, an acute benign respiratory illness, diffuse pneumonitis, lethal disseminated miliary involvement and a smoldering cavitary process simulating secondary tuberculosis. In most residents of endemic areas, infection is asymptomatic or, at most, very mild. Hilar lymphadenopathy and peripheral calcifications identical to those of the Ghon complex are characteristic of histoplasmosis. When this picture is seen in a tuberculin-negative individual, it should suggest prior contact with *H. capsulatum.* In a survey of Tennessee children, 97 per cent of those with pulmonary calcifications had positive histoplasmin skin tests, whereas only 19 per cent had positive tuberculin tests (Christie and Peterson, 1945). Hypersensitivity to histoplasmin becomes manifest within 2 to 3 weeks of infection, and appears to confer protection against subsequent disease. Whether this hypersensitivity, which lasts for years, implies the continued presence within the body of dormant fungi is not clear.

When histoplasmosis takes the form of a diffuse pneumonitis, the alveoli become filled with a mixed inflammatory infiltrate consisting primarily of histiocytes. This infiltrate tends to undergo organization. The miliary and cavitary forms consist of granuloma formation, with or without central caseation. Langhans' giant cells may be present. The fungi are seen as round to oval bodies, about 1 to 3 μm. in diameter, **within the cytoplasm** of the histiocytes or giant cells. Occasionally histoplasmosis becomes disseminated to involve the entire reticuloendothelial system. In these cases, there are hepatosplenomegaly, diffuse lymphadenopathy and multiple ulcerative lesions within the lymphoid tissue of the gastrointestinal tract.

COCCIDIOIDOMYCOSIS

This disease, caused by *Coccidioides immitis*, is similar in many respects to histoplasmosis. It is endemic in the southwestern United States, particularly in the San Joaquin Valley of California, where up to 90 per cent of long-time residents have positive skin tests with coccidioidin. As with histoplasmosis, this hypersensitivity develops within a few weeks of infection and confers protection. Although infection is usually asymptomatic, it may manifest itself as a transient, benign, acute respiratory infection, as a pneumonitis, or as a tuberculosis-like chronic process. In a minority of patients the disease is confined to the development of focal skin lesions at the site of some previous injury. Rarely, the fungus becomes disseminated throughout the body and, in these instances, the disease is highly fatal.

Anatomically, the lesions may take the form of nonspecific abscesses or of granulomas, often replete with central caseation and giant cells. The fungi are found within the liquid exudate or within histiocytes or giant cells. They appear as large, thick-walled, spherical bodies, from 10 to 80 μm. in diameter. They reproduce by endosporulation, and as many as 100 to 200 small endospores between 2 and 5 μm. in diameter may be seen within one parent organism.

NORTH AMERICAN BLASTOMYCOSIS

This disease is caused by *Blastomyces dermatitidis.* It usually affects the lungs primarily but from there may become disseminated to the skin and bones (Salvin, 1968). Sometimes, however, the skin is the primary site of involvement, and in these cases it is assumed that the organisms initially became established in a previous wound. The infection is seen most often in the southeastern United States. Like histoplasmosis and coccidioidomycosis, pulmonary blastomycosis may be asymptomatic or it may manifest itself as an acute, self-limited pneumonitis, or it may lead to life-threatening disseminated disease (Sarosi et al., 1974).

Morphologically, the more severe pulmonary involvements appear as multiple minute abscesses or as tubercle-like granulomas. In the skin, the lesion begins as a small papule which progressively enlarges, sometimes over the course of years. The margins become raised, are red to violet in color and are studded with microabscesses. The central depressed area represents old scarring. Histologically, the skin lesions appear as microabscesses within the dermis, surrounded by an acute and chronic inflammatory reaction. Small granulomatous foci may also be present. The causative organism is a round to oval thick walled body, from 5 to 15 μm. in diameter, which reproduces by budding. The fungi may be found free or within histiocytes or giant cells.

CRYPTOCOCCOSIS

This disease tends to be extremely indolent, evoking very little tissue response. It derives its importance primarily from its predilection for the central nervous system (see p. 664), although the lungs may also be involved. The causative organism, *Cryptococcus neoformans*, although pathogenic, is remarkably inert. Pulmonary involvement may be entirely asymptomatic, or it may produce low-grade fever and cough, reminiscent of carcinoma or tuberculosis.

Histologically, the alveoli may be filled with fungi, and yet there is no inflammatory response. In other instances, there is a granulomatous response, simulating tuberculosis. Only rarely is there an acute inflammatory reaction. The organisms have a distinctive appearance. They are pale, round to oval bodies, from 5 to 10 μm. in diameter, which reproduce by budding. Although their walls are thin, they are surrounded by a thick gelatinous capsule, which appears as a striking clear halo on staining. India ink staining demonstrates this particularly dramatically. The organisms may lie free, or they may be seen within histiocytes or giant cells.

LUNG TUMORS

Most primary lung tumors are malignant and, of these, the overwhelming majority are bronchogenic carcinomas. The following outline shows the approximate incidences of the various types of lung cancer (Galofré et al., 1964). Only bronchogenic carcinoma will be discussed in detail. The other forms of lung cancer will be described briefly at the end of this section.

		Per Cent
A.	Bronchogenic carcinoma	**90**
	1. Squamous cell carcinoma	63
	2. Adenocarcinoma	9
	3. Undifferentiated carcinoma	18
	a. Large cell pattern	11
	b. "Oat cell" pattern	7
B.	Alveolar cell carcinoma	**2**
C.	Bronchial adenoma	**5**
D.	Mesenchymal tumors	**1.4**
E.	Miscellaneous	**1.5**

BRONCHOGENIC CARCINOMA

No other tumor has shown such an alarming increase in incidence as has bronchogenic carcinoma. Whereas it was a rare disease before World War II, it is now the leading cause of death from cancer. Moreover, there are no indications that the incidence of this disease has stopped increasing. Just in the decade of 1963 to 1973, while the total death rate actu-

ally declined somewhat, the death rate from bronchogenic carcinoma has increased by 50 per cent. By 1973, cancer of the lung, predominantly bronchogenic carcinoma, was responsible for 4 per cent of all deaths and 21 per cent of all deaths from cancer (31 per cent in men and 10 per cent in women) (Vital Statistics of the United States, 1974).

Bronchogenic carcinoma affects principally middle-aged men, reaching a peak incidence between the ages of 50 and 60. About four times as many males as females die from this disease. *Bronchogenic carcinoma is uncommon in nonsmokers,* and in these individuals it usually assumes a different histologic pattern from the bulk of neoplasms encountered in smokers.

Etiology and Pathogenesis. The etiology and pathogenesis of this disease partake of the mystery of carcinogenesis in general. Since carcinogenesis has already been discussed, only a few brief remarks will be made concerning the etiology of this particular form of carcinoma. As seems to be the case with all cancers, there is probably no single etiologic agent responsible for bronchogenic carcinoma. Rather, the causation is most likely multifactorial. However, overwhelming evidence indicts cigarette smoking as the single most important etiologic factor known at this time. Whether it ever acts alone or must always act synergistically with other, unknown influences is not clear. In either case, the statistical correlation between cigarette smoking and bronchogenic carcinoma is so strong that this disease—which, as has been pointed out, is the leading form of cancer—is actually rare among nonsmokers. Among cigarette smokers, the danger is proportional to the number of cigarettes smoked daily, the duration of the habit, and the tendency to inhale. The risk in those who smoke over one pack of cigarettes daily is about 46 times that for nonsmokers (Hammond and Horn, 1958). Cigar and pipe smokers, as well as those who have broken the cigarette smoking habit, occupy an intermediate position in terms of risk.

Despite the clear association of cigarette smoking with bronchogenic carcinoma, the precise manner in which the two are linked is unknown. Unfortunately, there is no good experimental model of lung cancer produced by cigarette smoking. Animals other than man apparently are too fastidious to inhale cigarette smoke through the mouth. By inflicting it on them through the nose or through a tracheostomy it is possible to demonstrate some increased incidence of lung cancer, particularly in genetic strains which tend to develop lung tumors spontaneously (Editorial, 1974*b*). However, these cancers are in many respects different from the typical squamous cell bronchogenic carcinoma of man. This fact, along with the inability to duplicate the human habit, raises doubts about such findings.

In the absence of clear-cut evidence, what theories do we have about the carcinogenic effect of cigarette smoke on the lungs? It has been postulated that the hydrocarbons contained within cigarette smoke may not themselves be carcinogenic, but may be metabolized to carcinogenic intermediates by mixed-function oxidases. One such mixed-function oxidase, aryl hydrocarbon hydroxylase (AHH), apparently is induced in cells in varying amounts by cigarette smoke, depending on the presence of two alleles at a single gene locus. Thus, the human population can be divided into three groups, having low, intermediate and high AHH inducibility (the intermediate position reflecting heterozygosity). It has recently been found that in the normal population the frequencies of these three groups are 44.7 per cent, 45.9 per cent and 9.4 per cent, respectively, whereas among a group of patients with bronchogenic carcinoma, the frequencies were 4.0 per cent, 66.0 per cent and 30.0 per cent (Kellermann et al., 1973). Thus, it would seem that the genetically determined capacity to generate high levels of this enzyme is correlated with bronchogenic carcinoma. However, this conclusion, along with the implication that the cancer is caused by metabolites of the hydrocarbon constituents of cigarette smoke, must be evaluated with caution. It is risky to compare patients who already have cancer with those who do not, since the disease itself may have far-ranging effects on cellular function (Rao, 1974). It is conceivable that the high AHH inducibility in lung cancer patients was not present all along, but rather arose in these patients as a result of the tumor (Editorial, 1974c).

An alternative view of the role of cigarette smoking is that it acts as a nonspecific irritant or as a promoting influence. Results of studies of the mucosal lining of the tracheobronchial tree of cigarette smokers demonstrated that smokers were likely to show changes ranging from hyperplasia to squamous cell metaplasia to cellular atypia indistinguishable from carcinoma in situ. Such changes are most likely to occur at the carina and bronchial bifurcations. Interestingly, these same epithelial changes occur in patients with chronic bronchitis, and it has been speculated that the relationship between bronchogenic carcinoma and cigarette smoking is indirect, and that the tumor in fact parallels the incidence of chronic bronchitis, which in turn is more likely with cigarette smoking. Indeed, cigarette smokers who develop bronchogenic carcinoma are twice as likely to have chronic bronchitis as those who do not (Spencer, 1968). It should be pointed out that whereas not all smokers have chronic bronchitis *as clinically defined*, some degree of subclinical bronchiolitis is probably inevitable. An anatomic study of young smokers who died suddenly while not hospitalized showed that all had respiratory bronchiolitis, even though seven had no history of "smoker's cough." It is of interest in this regard that raised serum levels of carcinoembryonic antigen (CEA) are found in about 14 per cent of heavy cigarette smokers, compared to about 2 per cent of nonsmokers (Stevens and Mackay, 1973). It will be remembered that this fetal protein is a marker for a number of malignant tumors, as well as for several inflammatory and regenerative disorders, including chronic bronchitis (Laurence et al., 1972). Whether its appearance in cigarette smokers simply reflects bronchitis or whether it indicates precancerous changes is uncertain.

If cigarette smoking acts merely as an irritant to promote cancer, what then is the initiating factor? Not surprisingly, the possibility of a viral etiology is much discussed. However, attempts to demonstrate that viruses and cigarette smoke act in concert have been largely inconclusive (Editorial, 1974b).

In concluding this consideration of the causation of lung cancer, it is well to remember that cigarette smoking is not the only known epidemiologic correlate. Exposure to certain dusts and ores also increases the risk of developing lung cancer. As pointed out earlier, bronchogenic carcinoma is relatively frequent in patients with asbestosis. Miners involved with radioactive ores show a markedly increased vulnerability. Atmospheric pollution probably plays some role, since there is a slightly higher incidence of lung cancer in urban dwellers than in rural dwellers. In the overall picture, however, the importance of these other factors becomes trivial compared to that of cigarette smoking. Regardless of the mysteries that remain concerning this most important of cancers, one thing appears certain: *lung cancer is in most cases somehow related to cigarette smoking, and therefore, can be considered a largely preventable disease.*

Morphology. It is believed that all the patterns of bronchogenic carcinoma develop from one precursor, the multipotential basal resting cell of the bronchial epithelium. Presumably, under the irritant effects of such agents as tobacco smoke, atypical metaplasia provides a site of origin for the squamous cell tumors. The resting cells are also generally postulated as the site of origin of the adenocarcinomas, but the submucosal mucous glands cannot be excluded as an alternative possibility.

In general, bronchogenic carcinomas arise most

often in and about the hilus of the lung. About 75 per cent of these lesions originate from the bifurcation of the trachea and the first, second and third order bronchi (Fig. 12–11). A small percentage have a more peripheral origin, but these still are not located far out near the pleura. The tumor begins as an area of in situ cytologic atypia within the bronchial mucosa which, over an unknown period of time, then yields a small area of thickening or piling up of the bronchial mucosa. With progression, this small focus, usually less than 1 cm. in diameter, assumes the appearance of an irregular, warty excrescence that elevates or erodes the lining epithelium. The tumor may then follow one of a variety of paths. It may continue to fungate into the bronchial lumen to produce an intraluminal mass. In other cases, it penetrates the wall of the bronchus to infiltrate along the peribronchial tissue into the adjacent region of the carina and mediastinum. It may extend in this fash-

ion into or about the pericardium. In other instances, the tumor grows along a broad front to produce a cauliflower-like intraparenchymal mass that appears to push lung substance ahead of it. Quite rarely, the tumor permeates the pulmonary parenchyma, apparently without obliterating the native architecture, producing a form of pneumonic consolidation. In almost all patterns, the neoplastic tissue is gray-white and firm to hard. Especially when the tumors are bulky, focal areas of hemorrhage or necrosis produce yellow-white mottling and softening. Sometimes these necrotic foci cavitate. Extension may occur to the pleural surface and then within the pleural cavity. In most instances, spread to the tracheobronchial and mediastinal nodes can be found. The frequency of such nodal involvement varies with the stage of the disease and also with the histologic pattern, but by the time the tumor is diagnosed the local nodes are involved in most cases. The scalene nodes are also affected in about 50 per cent of cases, and are readily biopsied as a diagnostic procedure.

More distant spread of bronchogenic carcinoma occurs through both lymphatic and hematogenous pathways. Metastases are characteristically early and widespread. Often a metastasis, frequently in the brain or bones, presents as the first manifestation of underlying bronchogenic carcinoma. While no organ is spared in the spread of these lesions, the adrenals, for obscure reasons, are involved in over 50 per cent of cases. The liver (30 per cent), brain (20 per cent), bone (20 per cent) and the kidneys (15 per cent) are other favored sites for metastases.

The several histologic types of bronchogenic carcinoma shown in the outline on page 408 may occur in pure form; however, they often grow in mixed patterns, making any classification arbitrary. Nevertheless, there are certain distinct features that make a separate consideration of some value.

Squamous cell carcinoma is the form most closely correlated with cigarette smoking, and it is the rising incidence of this form that accounts for the increased frequency of bronchogenic carcinoma in general. Microscopic features are familiar in the well differentiated forms, but many less well differentiated squamous cell tumors are encountered which begin to merge with the undifferentiated large cell pattern (Fig. 12–12). This tumor tends to metastasize locally and somewhat later than the other patterns, but its rate of growth in its site of origin is usually more rapid than that of the other types. It has been estimated that it takes about nine years for these lesions to achieve a mass of 2 cm. in diameter.

The **adenocarcinoma** occurs about equally frequently in males and females. There is no clear correlation between cigarette smoking and the occurrence of this pattern of bronchogenic carcinoma, and there has been no significant increase in

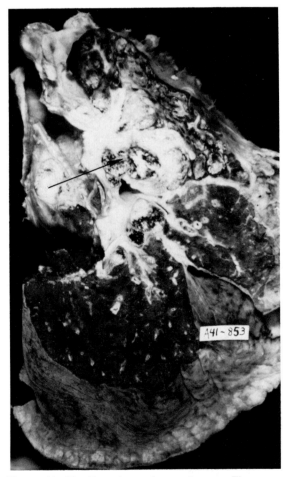

Figure 12–11. Bronchogenic carcinoma. The gray-white tumor tissue is seen infiltrating the lung substance. It has encircled and partially replaced two spottily anthracotic lymph nodes (arrow).

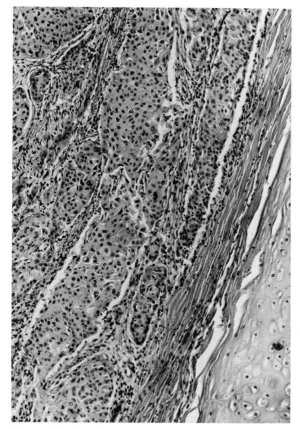

Figure 12–12. Bronchogenic carcinoma, squamous cell type. The bronchial cartilage is seen lower right. The neoplasm has replaced the mucosa and is growing into the lumen.

appear that defy clear-cut differentiation. Some of these cells assume a "spindle cell" appearance that mimics sarcomas. These are the most rapidly growing of all forms of bronchogenic carcinoma and have the poorest prognosis.

A uniform system for staging cancer according to its anatomic extent at the time of diagnosis is extremely useful for many reasons, chiefly for comparing treatment results from different centers. Despite some lack of agreement on a staging system for lung cancer, the following TNM classification has widest acceptance.

Tumor. TX: Demonstrable only by cytology of bronchopulmonary secretions

T1: 3 cm. diameter distal to lobar bronchus

T2: Any size extending to hilar region, or >3 cm. diameter

T3: Any size within 2 cm. of the carina or invading adjacent structures, e.g., the mediastinum or diaphragm

Nodes. N0: None *Metastases.* M0: None

N1: Ipsilateral hilar nodes M1: Distant metastases including to scalene nodes or contralateral hilar nodes

N2: Mediastinal nodes

the frequency of this pattern over the past several years. For these reasons, some suspect that it is a biologically separate disease. These tumors are usually relatively peripheral in location and are characterized by the formation of glands with or without mucinous secretion. It has been suggested that about 25 years is required for the adenocarcinoma to reach a size of 2 cm. Occasionally this pattern arises in an area of scarring, suggesting that the local chronic inflammatory changes have triggered its development.

The **undifferentiated carcinomas** are by default those in which no squamous or adenomatous patterns can be defined. Some produce large anaplastic tumor cells bordering on giant cells, whereas others produce small, closely packed "oat cells." Mitotic figures and tumor necrosis tend to be common in these lesions. There are no significant clinical differences in behavior between the small and large cell varieties, and often intergradations

These data are combined to describe lung cancer as follows:

Occult: Bronchopulmonary secretions contain malignant cells, but there is no other evidence of lung cancer (TX N0 M0).

Stage I: A tumor classified as T1 with or without involvement of the ipsilateral hilar nodes, or a tumor classified as T2 without any nodal involvement (T1 N0 M0, or T1 N1 M0, or T2 N0 M0).

Stage II: A tumor classified as T2 with involvement of the ipsilateral hilar nodes (T2 N1 M0).

Stage III: Any tumor with involvement of the mediastinal nodes or with distant metastases, or any tumor more extensive than T2 (N2 with any T or M, or M1 with any T or N, or T3 with any N or M).

Clinical Course. Many of the clinical features of bronchogenic carcinoma are illustrated in the case history given at the end of this general consideration. The patient to be described was, however, somewhat unusual in that his initial complaint was pain. Most often the tumor is first manifested by the insidious development of cough. However, since the disease frequently occurs in patients who already have chronic bronchitis and hence a cough, the patient may not seek medical attention until there is an accompanying weight loss and anorexia. By this time, the disease is usually widespread. When the pleural surfaces are involved, the first symptoms may be pleuritic pain or dyspnea from the accumulation of a large pleural effusion. Occasionally, blood-streaking of the sputum or frank hemoptysis is the first indication of the disease. In many instances, metastases produce symptoms before the primary tumor is discovered.

Because of the location of these neoplasms near large airways, varying degrees of airway obstruction are common and produce complications in the distal portions of the lung. Such complications include focal emphysema, when there is partial bronchial obstruction, and atelectasis, with total obstruction. The impaired drainage of the involved airway often leads to a pulmonary abscess or bronchiectasis distal to the obstruction. When necrosis and cavitation of the tumor occur, an abscess may develop within the cavity. Compression or invasion of the superior vena cava leads to marked venous congestion or to the full-blown superior vena caval syndrome (see p. 279). The latter occurs in about 5 per cent of cases. Bronchogenic carcinomas, particularly the oat cell tumors, are known to produce on occasion virtually any of the polypeptide hormones, such as ACTH or parathormone. Consequently, these tumors may appear in the guise of an endocrinopathy. Other possible distant effects of bronchogenic carcinoma include the development of pulmonary osteoarthropathy (p. 624) and of peripheral neuropathy (p. 675).

The prognosis with bronchogenic carcinoma is extremely poor, and the disease tends to follow a rapid, inexorable downhill course, leading to death within a year. At the time of diagnosis, only about half the patients are considered able to benefit from surgical exploration. Of these, only half (one quarter of the original group) are found to have resectable lesions. Thus, about three quarters of patients with bronchogenic carcinoma have more or less extensive disease at the time of diagnosis. The overall five-year survival rate is a disappointing 9 per cent (Silverberg and Holleb, 1975). In the following table, drawn from a cooperative study of over 2000 patients

with bronchogenic carcinoma, the two-year survival rate is broken down according to the histologic type and stage of the tumor:

HISTOLOGIC TYPE	PER CENT		
	Stage I	Stage II	Stage III
Squamous cell	46.6	39.8	11.5
Adenocarcinoma	45.9	14.3	7.9
Undifferentiated large cell	42.8	12.9	12.9
Undifferentiated oat cell	6.0	5.0	3.8

OTHER TYPES OF LUNG CANCER

Alveolar cell carcinoma (terminal bronchiolar carcinoma) is a rare form of lung cancer, arising either from the lining cells of the alveoli or from those of the terminal bronchioles. These tumors occur in patients of all ages and both sexes.

They almost always are found in the peripheral portions of the lung. Histologically, they are characterized by distinctive cuboidal to columnar epithelial cells, which line up along the alveolar septa and project into the alveolar spaces, without destroying the native architecture.

Despite the fact that these tumors are histologically more benign and appear to metastasize later than does bronchogenic carcinoma, the overall five-year survival rate is only about 5 per cent.

Bronchial adenomas are malignant neoplasms of low aggressiveness, hence they are misnamed. They affect adults of either sex under the age of 40. Approximately 90 per cent of bronchial adenomas are *carcinoid tumors* similar to those occurring within the gastrointestinal tract (p. 504). These may elaborate 5-hydroxytryptamine and produce the carcinoid syndrome. The remainder of the bronchial adenomas are tumors similar to those of the salivary glands.

Both types tend to grow as fingerlike projections into the lumen of a main-stem bronchus and are usually covered by an intact mucosa. Metastases are infrequent, and these tumors follow a relatively benign course.

Surgical resection is usually successful.

Other tumors of the lung include sarcomas and benign mesenchymal tumors, which are like their counterparts in any other site. *It should be remembered, finally, that the lung is more often affected by metastatic disease than it is by primary tumors.*

To emphasize the features of bronchogenic carcinoma, the following case history is presented.

CASE HISTORY OF BRONCHOGENIC CARCINOMA

Chief Complaint: Pain in the chest of 10 days' duration.

Present Illness: M.S., a 42 year old married male, sought medical attention for relief of pain in the right anterior chest. He stated that about four weeks ago he had caught a cold and developed a cough productive of a thick, yellowish sputum. He had not been febrile and the cold had not kept him from work. The cough seemed to lessen a few days after the onset of his cold, but then worsened again to persist up to the present time. He had never noted any blood in his sputum. He noted the onset of chest pain, principally on coughing, about two weeks ago. The pain was localized chiefly to the anterior chest, on the right, in the region of the fifth and sixth ribs, close to the sternal margin. He attributed this pain at first to having "strained a muscle" while coughing. But, over the past few days, despite the fact that the cough was no more severe, the pain became more pronounced and was sharp and lancelike every time he coughed. In the intervals he was aware of a vague discomfort in the same region. He volunteered that he dreaded sneezing because this provoked sharp, distressing pain. He stated he had often developed a severe cough with any respiratory infection, and that within the past few years he had increasing difficulty "shaking the cough" following acute infection. He denied ever having had blood in his sputum with any of these respiratory ailments. There had been no weight loss nor loss of appetite and, save for the pain and cough, he stated that he felt well and had continued to work. He had smoked one and a half to two packs of cigarettes a day and had done so for approximately 20 years. However, he had given up smoking soon after developing the recent cold.

Past History: The patient had two sons, aged 12 and 9. His wife, children and parents were all living and well. There was no history of tuberculosis in the family. He had always been subject to colds and usually had attacks of "severe bronchitis" with every cold. About two years ago, following one of his respiratory illnesses, he developed a persistent, chronic cough and wheezing and had sought medical attention because he feared he was developing asthma. At that time, he was told he had chronic bronchitis and should give up smoking. A chest film was taken at that time which he stated showed only "chronic bronchitis." Save for military service about 10 years ago, he had always worked as a photographer's assistant in Boston, Massachusetts. He noted that he had been examined before induction and that no disease had been found at that time. The only exposure to unusual air pollutants of which he was aware was in the mixing of photographic developing and printing solutions, and most of these came in fluid form. He doubted that there was any air-borne contamination. [So far as is known, none of the chemicals ordinarily used in photography has been implicated in the causation of carcinoma of the lung.]

Physical Examination: The patient was a well-developed, well-nourished male with no obvious signs of weight loss. Temperature was normal, as was respiration. Examination of the head and neck were entirely negative. There was no adenopathy in the neck or in the supraclavicular or axillary regions. The chest was bilaterally symmetric and moved symmetrically on inspiration. There was no palpable mass or tenderness over either the anterior or posterior chest. Tenderness could not be elicited by pressure over the fifth to sixth rib interspace, where the pain had been localized, nor could it be elicited even with deep inspiration and pressure. However, the patient stated that the pain was still present on coughing. The lungs were normal to percussion bilaterally. On auscultation, some coarse, moist rales were heard on deep inspiration anteriorly and posteriorly over the right upper lobe. These cleared with coughing. Despite the coughing, the patient could produce no sputum for inspection. The mediastinum did not appear widened by percussion, nor was there any deviation of the trachea. There were no signs of pleural fluid nor pleural friction rub. The heart was entirely normal. The results of the remainder of the physical examination were entirely within normal limits. There was no evidence of liver enlargement, nor were any masses present in the abdomen. No adenopathy could be found. There was no sign of clubbing of the fingertips, nor any evidence of cyanosis.

Laboratory Examination: Findings from the examination of the blood and urine were entirely negative. There was no evidence of an anemia, nor of leukocytosis. A tuberculin test was performed and was negative. Chest film disclosed bilateral basal increased bronchovascular markings but there was no evidence of parenchymal disease and no evidence of hilar adenopathy, nor tumor masses. The bronchovascular markings appeared to be bilaterally symmetric. An expectorant cough medication was prescribed, and the patient was advised to return in a week if the symptoms did not abate.

Return Visit—One Week: The patient stated that after taking the cough medicine for several days, his cough became productive of a cloudy white sputum that contained occasional flecks of blood. The pain persisted in the right anterior chest but was perhaps a little less severe. A cytologic smear was prepared from the sputum and cultures were obtained for microbiologic examination. The smear was returned as Class IV (moderately anaplastic cells strongly suggestive but not diagnostic of cancer). The microbiologic examination revealed a variety of nonpathogenic organisms, as well as a few colonies of nonhemolytic staphylococci. Because of the long history of recurrent bronchitis and the recent past episode of respiratory infection, a repeat cytologic examination was advised. On repeat, the cytology report indicated a Class V smear, indicative of cancer. Large anaplastic cells were seen, with an abnormal nuclear to cytoplasmic ratio in the range of 1:1. The nuclei were deeply chromatic and contained prominent nucleoli. [The reliability of a bronchial cytology smear varies somewhat with the laboratory involved. It is generally conceded that even in highly competent hands, a false negative error of approximately 20 to 25 per cent must be anticipated, but the false positive error should not exceed 5 per cent]. On these grounds, the patient was advised to enter the hospital for more thorough investigation.

First Hospital Admission: The patient entered the hospital five days later. The physical examination had not changed from that given above. The pain had not remitted, nor had it worsened. It was still provoked by coughing, but the patient was free of symptoms when not coughing. A detailed radiographic survey of the lungs was performed, involving various oblique, lateral and laminographic views. The radiologic report now suggested that there might be some increased prominence of the right upper lobe bronchi. There was no definite parenchymal disease, nor was there any evidence of mediastinal enlargement. A third cytologic examination was again interpreted as Class V. On the fifth hospital day, bronchoscopy was performed. The thoracic surgeon reported that there was increased mucinous secretion throughout the trachea and some apparent slight reddening and granularity of the tracheal mucosa. At the branching off of the right upper primary bronchus, the reddening and granularity of the lining mucosa were significantly increased. The surgeon also believed that there was some blood staining of the secretions in this region, but he could not be certain that it might not be related to the trauma of bronchoscopy. A biopsy was taken of this region, as well as of the primary bronchus to the right lower lobe, because of some slight roughening of the mucosa in that region as well.

The biopsy of the mucosa at the origin of the primary bronchus to the right upper lobe disclosed an intact bronchial mucosa which, however, had undergone some squamous cell metaplasia, with some mild dysplasia. The normal columnar epithelium had been replaced by a mucosa containing three to four layers of dysplastic squamous cells. The cells were slightly variable in size and shape and slightly increased in their chromaticity, but there was no evidence of tumor giant cells, frank anaplasia or mitotic activity. The basement membrane was intact. Underlying the mucosal epithelium was a moderate chronic inflammatory infiltrate, principally of lymphocytes and histiocytes. In the deep levels of the submucosal connective tissue, there were several nests of unmistakable anaplastic carcinomatous cells, showing definite squamous cell differentiation. No mucosal origin for these cells could be identified in the biopsy. [These findings are consistent with the probability that the carcinoma arose at a locus somewhat remote from the biopsy site.] The biopsy from the primary bronchus to the right lower lobe disclosed dysplastic and metaplastic epithelial changes and inflammatory changes, but no evidence of cancer.

Five days later, a right lung resection was performed. At the time of surgery, there was obvious gray-white tumor tissue encircling the primary bronchus to the right upper lobe and extending proximally along the right mainstem bronchus. This tissue appeared to be confined to an infiltrate collar closely applied to the airways. It did not produce a definite tumorous mass in the parenchymal substance of the lung. However, it appeared at surgery to extend distally. There was an area of slightly increased consistency immediately subjacent to the pleura in the parenchyma of the right upper lobe, anteriorly and midway between the apex and the interlobar fissure. This region was not incised at surgery, and the extent of involvement could not be determined. It appeared at the time of surgery that the lesion did not extend proximally beyond the line of resection of the right main stem bronchus, and that the trachea was not involved. The tracheobronchial nodes appeared somewhat anthracotic, but they were not enlarged. All the nodes that could be seen about the right main-stem bronchus and tracheobronchial region were removed.

Pathologic examination of the specimen confirmed most of the observations made at surgery. A gray-white, firm tumor tissue was found encircling the primary bronchus to the right upper lobe, extending proximally almost to the line of resection of the main-stem bronchus. Similar tumor tissue was found extending peripherally about the second and third order bronchi as far as they could be dissected into the periphery of the lung substance. On opening the airways, a small area of granular, gray-red mucosal thickening was identified at the very origin of the primary bronchus to the right upper lobe. The mucosal lesion did not cover more than 2.0 × 0.5 cm. on surface view. There was no obvious mucosal extension of the lesion into the right main-stem bronchus, nor into any of the more distal branches. The bronchi in this region contained a turbid white tenacious sputum, some of which was blood stained, and the mucosa was reddened. The remainder of the bronchial tree in the middle and lower lobes appeared unremarkable save for some slight congestion. In the region of increased consistency, palpated surgically, the lung parenchyma appeared to be somewhat firmer, but no obvious tumor mass could be identified. The pleural surface appeared to be free of tumor and was gray, smooth and glistening. Seven lymph nodes were excised, all of which appeared somewhat anthracotic and apparently free of tumor upon macroscopic examination. There was no evidence of abscess formation or of suppuration within any of the lobes, and the entire lung appeared to be well aerated.

Microscopic examination revealed the tumor to be a moderately well differentiated squamous cell carcinoma. At the site of the apparent primary mucosal lesion, the normal columnar mucus secreting cells were replaced by masses and nests of anaplastic cancer cells, with considerably increased chromaticity, and occasional tumor giant cells. Mitoses were moderate in number. In places, the tumor cells showed definite squamous differentiation, and occasionally they contained tiny pink nodules of keratohyalin, From this mucosal origin, the tumor penetrated about the bronchial cartilages into the peribronchial tissue. Here it followed the peribronchial stroma back along the right main-stem bronchus all the way to the line of resection of the right main-stem bronchus. The cancer also extended peripherally out to the second and third order bronchioles. This extension continued to the pleura of the anterior right upper lobe in the interalveolar fibrous septa, and tumor nests could be identified in the subpleural connective tissue, as well as within the lymphatics in this region. There was no evidence of extension of the tumor into the alveolar spaces of the lung parenchyma in any section of the lung examined. There was a moderately severe, diffuse chronic bronchitis and patchy foci of squamous cell metaplasia in the right main-stem bronchus and first order bronchi of the right middle and right lower lobes. This metaplasia was in many places somewhat atypical but not frankly cancerous.

Three of the lymph nodes removed from the region of the tracheal bifurcation contained minute foci of metastatic cancer resembling that in the primary site.

Postoperatively, the patient made a relatively uneventful recovery save for an exacerbation of bronchitis in the left lung. This was accompanied by considerable respiratory difficulty, which was successfully alleviated by oxygen and appropriate therapy. The patient was discharged from the hospital on the eighteenth postoperative day.

Follow-up: Two months after surgery, the patient returned for a checkup. He appeared suntanned and healthy and stated that he felt well. The wound was well healed and there was no evidence of abnormality either in the wound or in the examination of the chest. He stated that he was now free of pain and had returned to work. He was seen again four months later, at which time he had no complaints and was feeling quite well and active. He was instructed to return for a chest film six months later. However, about four weeks prior to his anticipated visit (i.e., about five months after the six-month follow-up), the patient returned with a complaint that he had been feeling ill. There were no specific symptoms, but he felt weak and listless. He complained of lack of appetite and stated that he had lost about 10 pounds. On physical examination, no abnormalities were found. Fluid was not present in the right pleural cavity, and there were no changes in the left lung field nor evidence of peripheral adenopathy. Chest x-ray at this time, however, disclosed some widening of the mediastinum. Laboratory examination revealed a hematocrit of 36 per cent. Because of the widening of the mediastinum, a presumptive diagnosis was made of extension of the tumor into the mediastinal nodes and tissues. Radiation was advised as a desperation measure. The radiotherapy produced a considerable amount of debilitation and provoked a chronic cough, but on repeat chest x-ray, there appeared to be some diminution in the widening of the mediastinum. When the cough appeared during radiotherapy, the patient became quite despondent and was certain that he was going to die. The depression was extremely difficult to control, despite liberal use of tranquilizing and mood elevating drugs. He complained of great weakness and did not return to work. He remained at home for an additional six months, following a progressively downhill course, with increasing weight loss, loss of appetite and weakness. Hospitalization became necessary because of the apppearance of severe nausea and vomiting. It was presumed that the tumor had spread about the esophagus.

Hospital Readmission: The patient reentered the hospital approximately six months after his radiotherapy. He exhibited obvious weight loss, debilitation and severe depression. Enlargement of the supra- and infraclavicular nodes on the right was evident. The right pleural cavity contained no obvious signs of fluid. Scattered, moist rales were heard over the left lung field, principally about the hilar region. The abdomen was not distended, and bowel sounds were normal. The liver, however, was enlarged, extending to 3 cm. below the right costal margin. There were no other abnormal findings. In the hope that the tumor might prove to be responsive to chemotherapy, a course of nitrogen mustard therapy was instituted. The patient tolerated the chemotherapy poorly, and developed a severe bone marrow depression, with a white count of 2600 cells per mm.[3] and a hematocrit value of 28. Platelets were reduced to 60,000 per mm.[3] and small petechial hemorrhages appeared in the skin. At the same time, the chronic cough that had been present since radiotherapy became more pronounced and now contained yellow pus, from which *Staphylococcus aureus* was cultured. At this time, auscultation of the lung revealed fine and moist rales throughout the left lower lobe. The patient became febrile, developed progressive respiratory difficulty and died on the sixteenth hospital day.

Postmortem Examination: At autopsy, the body was that of a wasted adult male with numerous small skin petechiae, principally over the trunk and upper extremities. The major anatomic findings were confined to the chest. The entire mediastinum was markedly enlarged and appeared to be replaced by a gray-white tumor. Traces of buried anthracotic nodes could be found within the tissue. The tumor extended about the tracheal bifurcation and encased the middle and lower thirds of the esophagus. It did not extend through the esophageal wall and did not appear on the mucosal surface. This mediastinal cancerous mass could be traced through the diaphragm into the lymph nodes along the lesser curvature of the stomach. The tumor had penetrated the pleura into the right pleural cavity principally along the mediastinum and posterior pleural wall. It also extended into the hilus of the left lung. In addition to this tumorous extension, the left lung contained foci of well developed, moderately advanced bronchopneumonic consolidation, principally in the lower lobe. There was no obvious extension of the tumor into the left pleural cavity, but there was a fine, granular, fibrinous pleuritis overlying the left lower lobe. White tumor tissue could be found in the supra- and infraclavicular nodes, bilat-

erally. The liver was enlarged and contained obvious metastatic nodules of tumor ranging up to 4 cm. in diameter. Both adrenals were enlarged to approximately three times normal size and were replaced by white tumor. The para-aortic nodes contained foci of tumor down to the level of the renal arteries. Numerous white, apparently metastatic deposits up to 3 cm. in diameter were found in the vertebral bodies of the thoracic and lumbar vertebrae. Microscopic examination confirmed the gross findings. Throughout its many sites of spread, the cancer appeared as a moderately well differentiated squamous cell carcinoma. The only other pertinent finding revealed by microscopic examination was evidence of hypocellularity in the bone marrow, apparently as a residual of the chemotherapy.

Final Anatomic Diagnosis:

1. Status post resection of right lung for bronchogenic carcinoma of right upper lobe (17 months prior to death).

2. Recurrent squamous cell bronchogenic carcinoma involving:

a. Mediastinum with encasement of trachea and esophagus.

b. Extension into hilar region of the left lung.

c. Diffuse metastatic involvement of liver, adrenals (bilaterally), thoracic and lumbar vertebrae, supra- and infraclavicular nodes (bilaterally), para-aortic nodes and lymph nodes along the lesser curvature of the stomach.

3. Bronchopneumonia (staphylococcal), left lower lobe, with minimal fibrinous pleuritis.

4. Hypocellularity of bone marrow (postchemotherapy?).

5. Cachexia.

Comment: The most predictable feature of this case is the long history of cigarette smoking. For approximately 20 years the patient had smoked one and a half to two packs of cigarettes per day. Also pertinent in the past history are recurrent episodes of so-called chronic bronchitis. What role cigarette smoking played in these attacks is not certain, but undoubtedly it adds an irritant and therefore augmenting influence to any underlying respiratory disorder.

The insidious growth of this tumor is by no means unusual. It will be recalled that on initial examination of the patient, there was no clearly defined tumor mass seen by x-ray. Indeed, at later surgical resection, the tumor was confined to a peribronchial infiltrate. No parenchymal lesion ever developed. Moreover, this infiltration had extended quite far along the second and third order bronchi, as well as back toward the origin of the right main-stem bronchus. A significant number of bronchogenic carcinomas behave in such a fashion. However, most, as they evolve into clinically manifest lesions, leave the peribronchial location and extend into the lung substance to produce more overt masses, readily detectable by x-ray. In this case, the patient's dominant symptom was chest pain provoked by coughing. This very likely may be attributed to the permeation of the tumor out to the pleural surface of the anterior aspect of the upper lobe.

CARCINOMA OF THE LARYNX

Compared to bronchogenic carcinoma, cancer of the larynx is uncommon, accounting for only 1 per cent of deaths from cancer. It usually develops after the age of 40 years and affects men about 7 times as often as women. Environmental influences, particularly chronic irritation, are probably of great importance in its etiology. Supporting this contention is the fact that neighboring areas of mucosa often show the stratified squamous epithelium to be thickened and hyperkeratotic, with foci of dysplastic epithelial changes. An increased incidence of asbestos exposure has been found in these patients (Stell and McGill, 1973).

About 95 per cent of laryngeal carcinomas are typical squamous cell lesions. Rarely, adenocarcinomas are seen, arising presumably from mucous glands. The tumor usually develops directly on the vocal cords, but it may arise above or below the cords, on the epiglottis or aryepiglottic folds, or in the piriform sinuses. Those confined within the larynx proper are termed intrinsic, while those that arise or extend outside the larynx are designated extrinsic. Squamous cell carcinomas of the larynx follow the growth pattern of all squamous cell carcinomas (described on p. 117). They begin as in situ lesions which later appear as pearly gray, wrinkled plaques on the mucosal surface, ultimately ulcerating and fungating. The degree of anaplasia of these laryngeal tumors is markedly variable. Sometimes massive tumor giant cells and multiple bizarre mitotic figures are seen.

Carcinoma of the larynx manifests itself clinically by persistent hoarseness. It differs in this respect from lung cancer, which usually announces itself by the development of a chronic cough. Later, laryngeal tumors may produce pain, dysphagia and hemoptysis. Patients with this condition are extremely vulnerable to secondary infection of the ulcerating lesion. With irradiation (sometimes with laryngectomy) the prognosis is relatively good. Five-year survival is over 50 per cent (Silverberg and Holleb, 1975). Death often occurs from infection of the distal respiratory passages, along with widespread metastases and cachexia.

Before ending this subject, it might be well to say a few words about two benign lesions of the larynx, the polyp and the papilloma, which also produce hoarseness and must be differentiated from carcinoma. *Polyps* of the larynx are sessile or pedunculated nodules, rarely exceeding 1 cm. in diameter, found on the true vocal cords. Microscopically, they are composed of a core of connective tissue covered by stratified squamous epithelium. There is much evidence to suggest that they are caused by chronic irritation, and some believe that they represent simple inflammatory overgrowth rather than true neoplasms. These lesions are particularly frequent in singers, hence are sometimes called "singer's nodes." The *papilloma* is definitely a neoplasm. It, too, is usually found on the true vocal cords, where it appears as a soft, friable mass with fine finger-like projections. On histologic inspection, the papillae contain a core of fibrous tissue covered by fairly regular stratified squamous epithelium. Sometimes the epithelium shows varying degrees of dysplasia, and for this reason it is believed that papillomas have the potential of undergoing malignant transformation. Multiple papillomas of the larynx, probably of viral etiology, are occasionally found in children.

LESS FREQUENT DISEASES OF THE LUNGS

IDIOPATHIC INTERSTITIAL FIBROSIS (CHRONIC INTERSTITIAL PNEUMONIA, FIBROSING ALVEOLITIS, HAMMAN-RICH SYNDROME)

These terms refer to an increasingly common acute to chronic disease characterized histologically by a diffuse interstitial pneumonitis, progressing to widespread interstitial fibrosis. The initial change seems to be edema of the alveolar walls. Later there is marked hyperplasia and hypertrophy of the cells lining the alveolar septa. The lower lung fields, bilaterally, are usually first affected; ultimately, the process may spread to involve the entire lungs.

The acute form was first described less than 40 years ago as the Hamman-Rich syndrome. Since then, it has become apparent that *chronic* idiopathic interstitial fibrosis is even more common. Males are affected slightly more often than females, and the disease may occur at any age, although most patients are between 30 and 50 years of age. The etiology is unknown, but it is likely that this disease represents a common response to any of multiple etiologies. Sometimes it may represent an unsuspected pneumoconiosis (Miller et al., 1975). Similar changes may occur with some of the collagen diseases, including rheumatoid arthritis and scleroderma. Indeed, rheumatoid factor has been reported in 27 per cent of these cases (Turner-Warwick and Doniach, 1965). The prognosis is variable, although in general the outlook is poor. In most cases, death occurs in about two years. However, the variation in length of survival is great, and occasionally the disease remits spontaneously (Livingstone et al. 1964).

DESQUAMATIVE INTERSTITIAL PNEUMONIA (DIP)

Formerly cases of DIP were considered to represent idiopathic interstitial fibrosis. Only recently has this disease been accepted as a distinct entity, largely because of its clearly better prognosis. It, too, may be acute or chronic. Histologically, the early lesion shows proliferation of the alveolar lining cells and the accumulation within the alveoli of large round cells with an eosinophilic cytoplasm containing yellow-brown granules. Presumably these cells are desquamated from the alveolar walls. Later, interstitial fibrosis occurs, and the disease becomes indistinguishable histologically from idiopathic interstitial fibrosis. This disease often follows respiratory infections, and the question of a viral etiology has been raised. The lesion may clear spontaneously or remain static, and often it responds dramatically to steroids (Goff et al., 1967).

LOEFFLER'S SYNDROME

This was originally described as a benign, self-limited disease characterized by peripheral eosinophilia and irregular pulmonary infiltrates. It now seems, however, that it represents a continuum of disorders, ranging from benign to lethal, which are probably of multiple etiologies. The uniting pathogenetic mechanism in all these disorders is thought to be a hypersensitivity reaction of the Arthus type (Spencer, 1968). Several conditions are known to produce Loeffler's syndrome, but no one of these is regularly associated with it. Such conditions include various parasitic infections, most notably with *Ascaris* larvae, and drug reactions.

At the most benign end of the continuum there are peripheral eosinophilia and foci of exudation into the alveolar spaces in the pattern of a bronchopneumonia. There may also be areas of interstitial edema and septal thickening, with an infiltration of mononuclear leukocytes. Such changes may be entirely asymptomatic and last no more than a month. With more chronic persistence and involvement of other organs, the character of the disease changes, and it is often referred to as *disseminated eosinophilic collagenosis, allergic granulomatosis* or *eosinophilic leukemia*. The lesions include tissue infiltration by eosinophils and focal granulomas with central fibrinoid deposits. At the most severe end of the continuum of Loeffler's syndrome, a necrotizing angiitis is added. These more severe changes are suggestive of polyarteritis nodosa. Indeed, both polyarteritis nodosa and Wegener's granulomatosis, which is discussed below, are considered by many to be closely related to Loeffler's syndrome. With the more severe manifestations, the prognosis is poor (Lecks and Kravis, 1969).

WEGENER'S GRANULOMATOSIS

This is a rare disorder characterized by: (1) focal acute necrotizing vasculitis, affecting virtually any vessel in any organ of the body, but showing a predilection for the respiratory tract, kidneys and spleen; (2) acute granulomatous necrotizing lesions of the respiratory tract, including the nasal and oral cavities, paranasal sinuses, larynx, tracheobronchial tree and lung parenchyma; (3) necrotizing focal or diffuse proliferative glomerulonephritis (see p. 436). The vascular lesions are almost identical to those of polyarteritis nodosa, with fibrinoid necrosis of the vessel wall and diffuse polymorphonuclear and eosinophilic infiltrations. The granulomatous lesions in the respiratory tract show some resemblance to very acute tubercles. The etiology is unknown, but it is considered to represent a hypersensitivity reaction closely related to Loeffler's syndrome. Immunofluorescent studies have demonstrated immunoglobulins and complement in the renal lesions (Roback et al., 1969; Castleman and McNeely, 1969). Moreover, subepithelial glomerular deposits which are thought to represent antigen-antibody complexes have been seen by electron microscopy (Norton et al., 1968). Most of these patients present with the insidious development of purulent rhinorrhea, epistaxis and a picture often interpreted as chronic sinusitis. At one time the usual outcome was death from renal failure within a few months. In recent years, however, the use of cytotoxic drugs has dramatically altered the prognosis, and remission can now be expected in most cases (Editorial, 1972).

GOODPASTURE'S SYNDROME

This unusual syndrome is characterized clinically by hemoptysis followed by acute renal failure. It commonly occurs in males in the second and third decades of life. Histologically, there is acute focal necrosis of the alveolar walls, associated with intra-alveolar hemorrhage, proliferation of the alveolar lining cells, and organization of blood in the alveolar spaces. Hemosiderin-laden macrophages are found in the air spaces, presumably derived from the proliferating septal lining cells. The lesions in the kidneys are those of a necrotizing rapidly progressive glomerulonephritis (see p. 438). It is now known that the pathogenesis involves the development of antibodies cross reactive to the alveolar and the glomerular basement membranes. However, the nature and source of the inciting antigen are not known (see p. 432). Patients usually present first with recurrent episodes of hemoptysis, followed later by renal failure. This disease is thought to be virtually uniformly fatal but, since diagnosis is highly dependent upon postmortem examination, milder, undiagnosed forms may exist. Death may be from massive hemoptysis or from uremia. There have been reports of patients whose pulmonary lesions have resolved following bilateral nephrectomy (with long-term dialysis or renal transplantation) (Pollak and Mendoza, 1971).

IDIOPATHIC PULMONARY HEMOSIDEROSIS

Although there is no renal involvement with this disease, the similarity between the lung lesions of idiopathic hemosiderosis and those of Goodpasture's syndrome will be readily apparent, and it is thought that these two processes are related. The histologic manifestations of idiopathic pulmonary hemosiderosis include proliferation of the septal lining cells, intra-alveolar hemorrhage and interstitial as well as intra-alveolar hemosiderosis. Hemosiderin-laden macrophages are found within the alveoli. This disease is characterized clinically by recurrent episodes of hemoptysis and dyspnea, usually in children under the age of 10 years. The prognosis is better than that of Goodpasture's syndrome and, after a period of years, many of these patients recover spontaneously.

ALVEOLAR PROTEINOSIS

The diagnosis of this disease is a histologic one, based on the presence in the alveoli of a homogeneous, granular, PAS-positive paste. There is no definitive clinical picture. Patients with the lesion may be asymptomatic, or symptoms may be variable, ranging from mild cough and dyspnea to recurrent febrile episodes similar to bacterial pneumonia. The etiology and pathogenesis are controversial. The pathogenesis involves the proliferation of alveolar lining cells, which are desquamated as macrophages into the air spaces. These cells then rapidly undergo degeneration, yielding a lipid-laden proteinaceous paste which fills the alveolar spaces. Failure to clear this debris may reflect an enzymatic or lipoprotein abnormality and may constitute a necessary component of the pathogenesis of this disease. It has been possible to produce a lesion identical to alveolar proteinosis in experimental animals by exposing them to high concentrations of quartz dust. There is no evidence that this is of etiologic significance in man. Rather, it seems probable that there exist multiple etiologies, which, when combined with a defective clearing mechanism, may trigger the disease (Gross and de Treville, 1968). About 33 per cent of these patients die from their disease; the lesion resolves in the remaining 67 per cent.

LIPID PNEUMONIA

Aspiration of oils may lead to patchy or diffuse consolidation of the lungs. This occurs most commonly in infants and the aged, in whom there is impairment of the swallowing reflex, and in adults following the protracted use of oily laxatives or nose drops. Rarely, lipid pneumonia follows the diagnostic use of relatively nonirritating radiopaque oils in x-ray evaluation of the respiratory tree. In general, the more unsaturated the oil, the greater its irritant effect. This lesion is an uncommon cause of clinical disease, and it is usually discovered as an incidental finding on autopsy. When extensive, however, it may presumably lead to embarrassment of pulmonary function.

Grossly, foci of lipid pneumonia are gray to yellow, fairly sharply demarcated and slightly elevated above the surrounding lung surface. The size is variable, often from 1 to 3 cm. in diameter. Because the texture of these lesions is quite firm and granular, they may be confused with tuberculous or neoplastic involvements. Histologically, early lipid pneumonia is characterized by the phagocytosis of emulsified oil in the alveoli by macrophages. Large numbers of macrophages thus accumulate in the alveoli. These phagocytes become distended by large, spherical, intracytoplasmic vacuoles, or by multiple vacuoles. Several such macrophages may coalesce to form giant cells. The alveolar septa characteristically show marked congestion and some widening, but remarkably little leukocytic reaction. With progression of the lesion, fibroblasts migrate into the alveoli to organize the phagocytic exudate. Sometimes the actively growing fibroblastic tissue and foreign body multinucleate giant cells form granulomas which resemble those of tuberculosis or sarcoidosis. Although there may be some resorption of oil with resolution of the exudate, permanent fibrous scarring usually ensues.

CYTOMEGALIC INCLUSION DISEASE

This is a viral disorder characterized morphologically by gigantism of isolated cells and their nuclei, with distinctive intranuclear inclusions. Since the lesions are widespread and the lung is only one of many organs which may be affected, the disorder is included in this chapter somewhat arbitrarily. Overt cytomegalic inclusion disease is seen principally in infants and in severely debilitated adults. A large number of normal adults harbor the virus without experiencing disease (Stern and Elek, 1965).

Cytomegalic inclusion disease is often acquired *in utero*. Such intrauterine infection may manifest itself only much later in life. It is increasingly speculated that this may be an important cause of isolated mental retardation. In other cases, however, the infant disease is only too apparent, widespread and severe. The organs most often affected, in order of frequency, are the salivary glands, kidneys, liver, lungs, pancreas, thyroid, adrenals and brain. Grossly, the anatomic changes are minimal, consisting chiefly of slight enlargement of the involved organs. The brain is often smaller than normal (microcephaly) and may show foci of calcification. Histologically, the characteristic cellular changes can be appreciated. In the glandular organs, it is the parenchymal epithelial cells that are affected, in the brain the ganglion cells, in the lungs the alveolar lining cells and in the kidneys the tubular epithelial cells. The involved cells are strikingly enlarged, often to a diameter of 40 μm., hyperchromatic, and show a marked cellular and nuclear polymorphism. Prominent intranuclear inclusions are present, which may measure 17 μm. in diameter, and are usually set off from the nuclear membrane by a clear halo. Within the cytoplasm of these cells, smaller basophilic inclusions may also be seen. An interstitial pneumonitis may be present, as well as focal necroses within the liver and adrenals. The affected ganglion cells within the brain are often surrounded by a glial reaction, sometimes with calcification. Clinically, these infants are profoundly ill. The cardinal manifestations are jaundice and a bleeding diathesis from an accompanying thrombocytopenia. Those infants who survive usually bear permanent residual effects, including mental retardation and a variety of neurologic impairments.

In the debilitated adult, cytomegalic inclusion disease may represent a newly acquired infection or an activated latent process. Localization to the lungs is much more common in these cases. The morphologic changes are similar to those in the infant, with cytomegaly and intranuclear inclusions affecting the alveolar lining cells, along with an accompanying interstitial pneumonitis. The clinical effects of this infection are often obscured by the underlying predisposing disease. Some respiratory distress may be attributable to cytomegalic inclusion disease, but this is debatable.

SARCOIDOSIS (BOECK'S SARCOID)

Sarcoidosis is a disease of unknown etiology characterized anatomically by the formation of noncaseating epithelioid granulomas in any tissue or organ of the body. It is included in this chapter because the lungs are a favored site of involvement. However, the distribution of the lesions is highly variable, as is the clinical course. The peak incidence is between the ages of 20 and 50 years. Marked geographic and ethnic differences are seen in the frequency of sarcoidosis. For example, in Sweden, the disease occurs about 30 times more often than in the United States. In America it is said to be about 10 times more common in blacks than in whites.

Etiology and Pathogenesis. As mentioned, the causation of sarcoidosis is unknown. Perhaps the most widely accepted hypothesis is that the disorder represents an abnormal immunologic response, possibly to a variety of nonspecific irritants or antigens. Supporting the concept of an immunologic pathogenesis is the transformation and depletion of T-cells with concomitant proliferation of B-cells. Thus, these patients usually show depression of cell-based immunity, as manifested by a negative tuberculin test, along with an increase in circulating immunoglobulin levels. It has been suggested that the inciting antigen responsible for sarcoidosis may be linked to T-cells and altered by them into a complex antigen responsible for the granuloma formation and B-cell proliferation (Iwai and Hosoda, 1974).

Recently it has been pointed out that every one of 131 patients with sarcoidosis had high titers of antibodies against the herpes-like EB virus, first regularly associated with Burkitt's lymphoma cells (see p. 348) (Hirshaut et al., 1970). This contrasts with a 76 per cent prevalence of the antibody in considerably lower titers in a control population. Sarcoidosis is thus the fourth disease known to be regularly associated with high titers of this antibody.

The other three are Burkitt's lymphoma, carcinoma of the posterior nasal space and infectious mononucleosis. Clearly, as this virus becomes associated with more disorders, its etiologic significance in any of them becomes more doubtful. It is most likely that the presence of high titers of EBV antibodies in sarcoidosis simply represents the tendency of these patients to overproduce antibodies against a ubiquitous and ordinarily weak antigen. However, an etiologic role for EBV cannot be ruled out.

Efforts to isolate an infectious agent as a cause of sarcoidosis have been unavailing. The experiments of Mitchell and Rees (1969), however, would appear to implicate a transmissible agent, although it has not been isolated and identified. These workers found that the footpads of mice injected with lymph node homogenates from patients with sarcoidosis developed the characteristic granulomas. Moreover, after injection the mice often showed positive Kveim test results. This is the diagnostic skin test for sarcoidosis and involves a granulomatous response to inoculation of tissue from a patient known to have sarcoidosis. Interestingly, there was little difference between the responses of normal animals and those rendered immunologically deficient by thymectomy and whole-body irradiation (Mitchell and Rees, 1969).

Morphology.
The distinctive, although not diagnostic, morphologic feature of sarcoidosis in all sites is the noncaseating granuloma (Fig. 12–13). This is a "hard tubercle" of epithelioid cells, commonly containing giant cells of either the foreign body or Langhans type. In 80 to 90 per cent of these granulomas, laminated concretions of calcium and proteins, known as **Schaumann's bodies**, can occasionally be found within giant cells. In addition, stellate inclusions, termed **asteroid bodies**, are seen within giant cells in approximately 60 per cent of the granulomas. None of these changes, however, is pathognomonic. Similar hard tubercles are seen with berylliosis, the deep mycoses and syphilis. With long-standing sarcoidosis, the granulomas undergo progressive collagenous fibrosis and ultimately are totally replaced by scar tissue or are hyalinized.

As was mentioned, any tissue or organ of the body may be affected. Only the most common involvements are described here. The **lungs** are often affected. Grossly, they may appear normal, diffusely fibrotic or finely nodular, owing to coalescence of granulomas. Histologically, the granulomas are dispersed more or less evenly throughout the parenchyma of both lungs. These lesions show a marked tendency toward fibrosis and hyalinization, resulting in diffuse pulmonary scarring. The **lymph nodes** are involved in most cases. Lymphadenopathy is classically most marked in the peri-

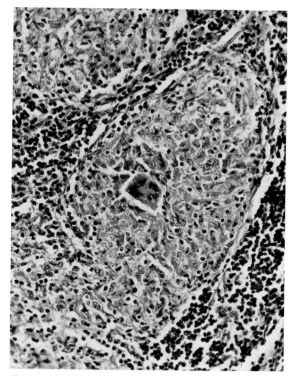

Figure 12–13. Sarcoidosis. A characteristic noncaseating granuloma with a central multinucleated giant cell.

bronchial and hilar regions and may produce a dramatic enlargement visible on chest x-ray. The nodes are soft, gray-red and discrete. On sectioning they may appear normal or contain foci of fibrosis. With the light microscope, typical granulomas can be seen throughout the involved node. The **spleen** is affected in about 75 per cent of patients. Although splenomegaly may be marked, the organ is usually grossly normal and the capsule is unaffected. Histologically, granulomas in various stages of fibrosis are seen dispersed throughout the pulp. The **liver** is involved slightly less often than the spleen. It, too, may be enlarged or grossly normal, and here again the granulomas are scattered throughout the parenchyma, showing no predilection for any specific localization. **Bone** lesions are identified on x-ray in about 20 per cent of these patients. Classically, the short bones of the hands and feet are involved. On x-ray, the changes appear as small circumscribed areas of bone resorption or as a diffuse reticulated pattern throughout the marrow cavity, with widening of the bony shafts and oftentimes new bone formation on the outer surfaces. Histologically, numerous granulomas are present in the marrow cavity. **Skin** lesions are present in about 50 per cent of patients. These are variable, and include nodules resembling erythema nodosum, elevated erythematous plaques and scaling flat lesions similar to those of lupus erythematosus. Granulomas are seen with the light microscope. Involvements of the **eyes** and the **salivary glands** occur in a minority of patients. Unilateral or bilateral inflammation of any part of the eyeball and of the lacrimal glands may be present. Combined uveitis and parotitis due to sarcoidosis is known as the **Mikulicz syndrome.**

Clinical Course. From the widespread distribution of the lesions, it can be anticipated that the clinical manifestations of sarcoidosis are protean. In about 75 per cent of cases, the disease is entirely asymptomatic and is found only incidentally at autopsy. Sometimes attention is called to the disease by the presence of bilateral hilar adenopathy on routine chest x-ray. Occasionally, the pulmonary lesions and subsequent fibrosis produce patchy densities in the lungs which are seen on x-ray. The appearance of erythema nodosum may in other instances herald the disease. An iritis or uveitis with loss of lacrimation sometimes appears and may cause impaired vision. Most symptomatic cases present with vague constitutional signs and symptoms, including fever, weakness and weight loss. The Kveim test is important in establishing the diagnosis. *Only in a minority of well developed cases does one see the classical syndrome of bilateral hilar adenopathy, uveoparotitis, osseous lesions in the short bones of the hands and feet, erythema nodosum, hypergammaglobulinemia, hypercalcemia and hypercalciuria.* Sarcoidosis follows a rather unpredictable course, characterized usually by chronicity or by spontaneous remissions that are sometimes permanent. In only a few instances do the patients pursue a downhill course, to die of intercurrent infections or of cor pulmonale resulting from the diffuse lung fibrosis.

PLEURAL EFFUSION AND HEMOPTYSIS

The evaluations of the patient with hemoptysis and of the patient with fluid in the pleural cavity constitute two of the most frequently encountered clinical problems in medicine. Often both entities occur in the same individual.

When the pleural fluid is a *transudate* that has accumulated passively in the pleural cavity, as with congestive heart failure or severe hypoproteinemia, the condition is termed *hydrothorax.* Hydrothorax from congestive heart failure is probably the most frequent cause of fluid in the pleural cavity. Upon aspiration, such a transudate can be differentiated from an exudate by its low specific gravity (less than 1.012), its low protein content (often less than 1 gm. per 100 cc.) and the presence in the fluid of only a few scattered lymphocytes and mesothelial cells.

There are four major causes of *exudative* fluid in the pleural cavity. These are: (1) malignant disease, either bronchogenic carcinoma or metastatic disease to the lung, often from a primary tumor in the breast, (2) tuberculosis, (3) pulmonary infarction, and (4) pneumonia. The vast majority of patients with an exudative pleural effusion will have one of these four diseases. It is noteworthy that any of these diseases may also produce hemoptysis. Exudative effusions are most often serous to serofibrinous. Occasionally they are serosanguinous. Suppurative effusions are termed *empyema.* All these have a specific gravity above 1.018 and a protein content usually above 3 gm. per 100 ml. The cellular content of the fluid varies with the cause.

Cancer should be suspected as the underlying cause of an exudative effusion in any patient over the age of 40 years, particularly when there is no febrile illness, no pain and a negative tuberculin test. These effusions characteristically are large and frequently serosanguinous. Cytology may reveal the presence of malignant cells. Otherwise, a pleural biopsy may be helpful in the diagnosis.

The most likely cause for an exudative pleural effusion in a patient under the age of 40 years—unless tuberculin test results are negative—is tuberculosis. A history of weight loss, fatigue and low-grade fever supports this diagnosis. These effusions contain relatively few cells, chiefly lymphocytes. The absence of grossly visible pulmonary lesions on chest x-ray following thoracentesis does not exclude this diagnosis. In some cases, it is impossible to isolate tubercle bacilli either from the sputum or from the effusion. In these cases, the diagnosis may be made by pleural biopsy.

The pleural effusion associated with pulmonary infarction frequently is grossly bloody, and may contain many inflammatory cells, both polymorphonuclear and mononuclear. The clinical story of sudden dyspnea and pleuritic pain, along with findings consistent with thrombophlebitis, confirms the diagnosis.

Pneumonic effusions are usually associated with pneumococcal pneumonia and are serous. Although the fluid is commonly sterile, it contains large numbers of polymorphonuclear leukocytes. Clinically apparent pneumococcal pneumonia almost always precedes by a few days the accumulation of such an effusion.

As was mentioned, the four diseases cited frequently produce hemoptysis as well as a pleural effusion. Hemoptysis may also occur from extrapulmonary processes, chiefly congestive heart failure and mitral stenosis, and in association with a bleeding diathesis from any cause. The hemoptysis produced by heart failure is characteristically pink and frothy. That associated with pneumococcal pneumonia is mixed with purulent material and is rusty in color. Grossly bloody hemoptysis may occur with bronchiectasis and, to a lesser degree, with acute or chronic bronchitis. Pleural effusion in these cases is seldom present. Rare causes of hemoptysis include Goodpasture's syndrome and pulmonary hemosiderosis.

REFERENCES

Aldridge, W. N., et al.: Experimental beryllium poisoning. Brit. J. Exp. Path., *30*:375, 1949.

Allison, A. C., et al.: Observations on the cytotoxic action of silica on macrophages. *In* Davis, C. N. (ed.): Inhaled Particles and Vapours. Oxford, Pergamon Press, 1965, p. 121.

American Thoracic Society: Definitions and classifications of chronic bronchitis, asthma and pulmonary emphysema. Am. Rev. Resp. Dis., *85*:762, 1962.

Armstrong, D.: Virus and mycoplasma respiratory infections. Adv. Cardiopulm. Dis., *4*:175, 1969.

Auerbach, O., et al.: Changes in bronchial epithelium in relation to sex, age, residence, smoking and pneumonia. New Engl. J. Med., *267*:111, 1962.

Auerbach, O., et al.: Bronchial epithelium in former smokers. New Eng. J. Med., *267*:119, 1962.

Bartlett, J. G., et al.: The bacteriology of aspiration pneumonia. Am. J. Med., *56*:202, 1974.

Bates, J. H., and Stead, W. W.: Effect of chemotherapy on infectiousness of tuberculosis. New Eng. J. Med., *290*:459, 1974.

Belleau, R., and Gaensler, E. A.: Mesothelioma and asbestosis. Respiration, *25*:67, 1968.

Blount, S. G., Primary pulmonary hypertension. Mod. Concepts Cardiovasc. Dis., *36*:67, 1967.

Brodsky, I., and Siegel, N. H.: The diagnosis and treatment of disseminated intravascular coagulation. Med. Clin. North Amer., *54*:555, 1970.

Buckley, A. R., et al.: Adult chronic bronchitis — the infective factor and its treatment. Brit. Med. J., *2*:259, 1957.

Campbell, E. J. M., and Howell, J. B. L.: The sensation of breathlessness. Brit. Med. Bull., *19*:36, 1963.

Castleman, B., and McNeely, B. U.: Case records of the Massachusetts General Hospital. Weekly clinicopathologic exercises. New Eng. J. Med., *280*:828, 1969.

Chatgidakis, C. B.: Silicone in South African white gold miners: A comparative study of the disease in its different stages. Med. Proc., *9*:383, 1963.

Christie, A., and Peterson, J. C.: Pulmonary calcification in negative reactors to tuberculin. Amer. J. Public Health, *35*:1131, 1945.

Chronic bronchitis in Great Britain. A national survey carried out by the Respiratory Diseases Study Group of the College of General Practitioners. Brit. Med. J., *2*:973, 1961.

Colp, C., et al.: Diffuse emphysema as a result of nonobstructive interstitial pulmonary disease. Am. Rev. Resp. Dis., *96*:788, 1967.

Corpe, R. F., et al.: Status of disease due to unclassified mycobacteria. Am. Rev. Resp. Dis., *87*:459, 1963.

Ebert, R. V., and Pierce, J. A.: Pathogenesis of pulmonary emphysema. Arch. Int. Med., *111*:34, 1963.

Editorial: Progress in asthma. Lancet, *2*:160, 1968.

Editorial: Wegener's granulomatosis. Lancet, *2*:519, 1972.

Editorial: Reversibility of asthma. Lancet, *1*:1327, 1974*a*.

Editorial: Lung tumors in mice exposed to tobacco smoke. Lancet, *2*:506, 1974*b*.

Editorial: Aryl hydrocarbon hydroxylase inducibility and lung cancer. Lancet, *1*:910, 1974*c*.

Editorial: α_1-antitrypsin deficiency — a defect of secretion. New Eng. J. Med., *292*:205, 1975.

Fowler, E. F., and Bollinger, J. A.: Pulmonary embolism: Clinical study of 97 fatal cases. Surgery, *36*:650, 1954.

Franklin, W.: Treatment of severe asthma. New Engl. J. Med., *290*:1469, 1974.

Freiman, D. G., et al.: Frequency of pulmonary thromboembolism in man. New Engl. J. Med., *272*:1278, 1965.

Freiman, D. G., and Hardy, H. L.: Beryllium disease. Hum. Pathol., *1*:25, 1970.

Frick, O. L.: Mediators of atopic and anaphylactic reactions. Ped. Clin. North Amer., *16*:95, 1969.

Galofré, M., et al.: Pathologic classification and surgical treatment of bronchogenic carcinoma. Surg. Gynec. Obstet., *119*:51, 1964.

Goff, A. M.: Desquamative interstitial pneumonia. Med. Thorac., *24*:317, 1967.

Gorbach, S. L., and Bartlett, J. G.: Anaerobic infections. New Eng. J. Med., *290*:1237, 1974.

Green, G. M., and Carolin, D.: The depressant effect of cigarette smoke on the in vitro antibacterial activity of alveolar macrophages. New Eng. J. Med., *276*:422, 1967.

Gross, P., and de Treville, R. T. P.: Alveolar proteinosis. Arch. Path., *86*:255, 1968.

Hammond, E. C., and Horn, D.: Smoking and deathrates: Report on forty-four months of follow-up of 187,783 men. I, II. J.A.M.A., *166*:1159, 1294, 1958.

Hardy, H. L.: Beryllium disease: A continuing diagnostic problem. Amer. J. Med. Sci., *242*:150, 1961.

Heard, B. E.: Pathology of pulmonary emphysema, method of studies. Am. Rev. Resp. Dis., *82*:792, 1960.

Hirshaut, Y., et al.: Sarcoidosis, another disease associated with serologic evidence for herpes-like virus infection. New Eng. J. Med., *283*:502, 1970.

Ishizaka, K., and Ishizaka, T.: Identification of IgE antibodies as a carrier of reaginic activity. J. Immun., *99*:1187, 1967.

Iwai, K., and Hosoda, Y. (eds.): Proceedings of the Sixth International Conference on Sarcoidosis. Tokyo, University of Tokyo Press, 1974, p. 666.

Kay, A. B., et al.: Complement components and IgE in bronchial asthma. Lancet, *2*:916, 1974.

Kellermann, G., et al.: Aryl hydrocarbon hydroxylase inducibility and bronchogenic carcinoma. New Eng. J. Med., *289*:934, 1973.

Kueppers, F.: Obstructive lung disease and alpha-1-antitrypsin deficiency gene heterozygosity. Science, *165*:899, 1969.

Kuida, H., et al.: Primary pulmonary hypertension. Amer. J. Med., *23*:166, 1957.

Laurence, D. J. R., et al.: Role of plasma carcinoembryonic antigen in diagnosis of gastrointestinal, mammary and bronchial carcinoma. Brit. Med. J., *3*:605, 1972.

Laurenzi, G. A.: Suppurative disease of the lung. Adv. Cardiopulm. Dis., *4*:198, 1969.

Lauweryns, J. M.: Hyaline membrane disease in newborn infants. Hum. Pathol. *1*:175, 1970.

Lecks, H. I., and Kravis, L. P.: The allergist and the eosinophil. Ped. Clin. North Amer. *16*:125, 1969.

Leopold, T. G., and Gough, J.: The centrilobular form of emphysema and its relation to chronic bronchitis. Thorax, *12*:219, 1957.

Lieberman, J.: Heterozygous and homozygous alpha-1-antitrypsin deficiency in patients with pulmonary emphysema. New Eng. J Med., *281*:279, 1969.

Livingstone, J. L., et al.: Diffuse interstitial pulmonary fibrosis. Quart. J. Med., *33*:71, 1964.

Loda, F. A., et al.: Lower respiratory tract infection in children. J. Ped., *72*:161, 1968.

Lurie, H. I., and Duma, R. J.: Opportunistic infections of the lungs. Hum. Pathol., *1*:233, 1970.

McFadden, E. R., et al.: Small airway disease. Am. J. Med., *57*:171, 1974.

McLean, K. H.: The pathogenesis of pulmonary emphysema. Am. J. Med., *25*:62, 1958.

Miller, A., et al.: "Nonspecific" interstitial pulmonary fibrosis. New Eng. J. Med., 292:91, 1975.

Mitchell, D. N., and Rees, R. J. W.: A transmissible agent from sarcoid tissue. Lancet, 2:81, 1969.

Mitchell, R. S.: Control of tuberculosis. New Eng. J. Med., 276:842, 905, 1967.

Mittman, C., et al.: Smoking and chronic obstructive lung disease in alpha-1-antitrypsin deficiency. Chest, 60:214, 1971.

Morrell, M. T., and Dunnill, M. S.: The postmortem incidence of pulmonary embolism in a hospital population. Brit. J. Surg., 55:347, 1968.

Morse, J. O., et al.: A community study of the relation of alpha-1-antitrypsin levels to obstructive lung diseases. New Eng. J. Med., 292:278, 1975.

Nash, E. S., et al.: The relationship between clinical and physiological findings in chronic obstructive disease of the lungs. Med. Thorac., 22:305, 1965.

Nash, G., et al.: Pulmonary interstitial edema and hyaline membranes in adult burn patients. Hum. Pathol., 5:149, 1974.

Niewoehner, D. E., et al.: Pathologic changes in the peripheral airways of young cigarette smokers. New Eng. J. Med., 291:755, 1974.

Norton, W. L., et al.: Combined corticosteroid and azathioprine therapy in 2 patients with Wegener's granulomatosis. Arch. Int. Med., 121:554, 1968.

Ogilvie, C.: Patterns of disturbed lung function in patients with chronic obstructive vesicular emphysema. Thorax, 14:113, 1959.

Pollak, V. E., and Mendoza, N.: Rapidly progressive glomerulonephritis. Med. Clin. North Amer., 55:1397, 1971.

Pratt, P. C., and Kilburn, K. H.: A modern concept of the emphysemas based on correlations of structure and function. Hum. Pathol., 1:443, 1970.

Rao, L. G. S.: A.H.H. inducibility and lung cancer. Lancet, 1:1228, 1974.

Reed, C. E.: The pathogenesis of asthma. Med. Clin. North Amer., 58:55, 1974.

Reid, L.: The Pathology of Emphysema. London, Lloyd-Luke, Ltd., 1967.

Ries, K., et al.: Transtracheal aspiration in pulmonary infection. Arch. Int. Med., 133:453, 1974.

Roback, S. A., et al.: Wegener's granulomatosis in a child. Observations on pathogenesis and treatment. Am. J. Dis. Child., 118:608, 1969.

Rosenberg, F. A.: Study of etiologic basis of primary pulmonary hypertension. Am. Heart J., 68:484, 1964.

Salvin, S. B.: Allergic reactions to pathogenic fungi. In Miescher, P., and Muller-Eberhard, H. (eds.): Textbook of Immunopathology. New York, Grune and Stratton, 1968, p. 323.

Sarosi, G. A., et al.: Clinical features of acute pulmonary blastomycosis. New Eng. J. Med., 290:540, 1974.

Schweppe, H. I., et al.: Lung abscess, an analysis of the Massachusetts General Hospital cases from 1943 through 1956. New Eng. J. Med., 265:1039, 1961.

Selikoff, I. J., et al.: Asbestosis and neoplasia [editorial]. Am. J. Med., 42:487, 1967.

Silverberg, E., and Holleb, A. I.: Cancer statistics, 1975. CA, 25:1, 1975.

Spain, D. N., and Kaufman, G.: The basic lesion in chronic pulmonary emphysema. Amer. Rev. Tuberc., 68:24, 1953.

Spencer, H.: Pathology of the Lung. 2nd ed. Oxford, Pergamon Press, 1968.

Stahlman, M., et al.: Pathophysiology of respiratory distress in newborn lambs. Dis. Child., 108:375, 1964.

Stell, P. M., and McGill, T.: Asbestos and laryngeal carcinoma. Lancet, 2:416, 1973.

Stern, H., and Elek, S. D.: The incidence of infection with cytomegalovirus in a normal population. J. Hyg., 63:79, 1965.

Stevens, D. P., and Mackay, I. R.: Increased carcinoembryonic antigen in heavy cigarette smokers. Lancet, 2:1238, 1973.

Stoeckle, J. D., et al.: Chronic beryllium disease. Amer. J. Med., 46:545, 1969.

Szentivanyi, A.: The beta-adrenergic theory of the atopic abnormality in bronchial asthma. Ann. Allerg., 24:253, 1966.

Telischi, M., and Rubenstone, A. I.: Pulmonary asbestosis. Arch. Path., 72:234, 1961.

Thurlbeck, W. M.: Small airways disease. Hum. Pathol., 4:150, 1973.

Thurlbeck, W. M.: The incidence of pulmonary emphysema. Am. Rev. Resp. Dis., 87:206, 1963.

Thurlbeck, W. M., and Angus, G. E.: A distribution curve for bronchitis. Thorax, 19:436, 1964.

Trauger, D. A.: A note on tuberculosis epidemiology. Am. Rev. Resp. Dis., 87:582, 1963.

Turner-Warwick, J., and Doniach, D.: Auto-antibody studies in interstitial pulmonary fibrosis. Brit. Med. J., 1:886, 1965.

Vandenbergh, E., et al.: Course and prognosis of patients with advanced chronic obstructive pulmonary disease. Am. J. Med., 55:736, 1973.

Vital Statistics of the United States, Monthly Vital Statistics Report, Annual Summary for 1973, HRA 74–1120, Vol. 22, No. 13, 1974.

Walcott, G., et al.: Primary pulmonary hypertension. Am. J. Med., 49:70, 1970.

Zimmerman, L. M., et al.: Pulmonary embolism—its incidence, significance and relation to antecedent vein disease. Surg. Gynec. Obstet., 88:373, 1949.

CHAPTER 13

The Kidney and Its Collecting System

Many students find the kidney and its pathology a difficult subject. Much of the difficulty stems from the rather complex histology of the glomerulus, and for this reason we offer a brief review of the ultrastructure of the normal glomerulus before going on to discuss renal disease. As you will recall, the glomerulus is a spherical mass of tangled capillaries derived from multiple divisions of an afferent arteriole which unite to form an efferent arteriole. Except for the stalk containing the afferent and efferent arterioles, the glomerulus is completely enveloped by *Bowman's capsule*, the cup-shaped beginning of the proximal convoluted tubule. The glomerular capillaries are lined by a unique *fenestrated endothelium* perforated by pores about 100 nm. in diameter. These endothelial cells rest on a *basement membrane* which forms a continuous sheet not completely encircling each capillary since it is reflected onto the adjacent capillary. There is, therefore, a narrow zone of the capillary wall that is devoid of basement membrane. The defect is filled either by the endothelial cells themselves or by deeper, underlying cells, the *mesangial cells*. External to the basement membrane are the *visceral epithelial cells* of Bowman's capsule *(podocytes)*. Each of these cells may be likened to an octopus with only the extended tentacles *(foot processes)* reaching out to contact the basement membrane. In any cross section the foot processes are separated by filtration slits of the order of 20 to 50 nm. in width. It is evident, then, that in places where an endothelial cell pore is directly apposed to an epithelial cell filtration slit, the only certain filtration barrier is the glomerular basement membrane. Thus, the functional integrity of the glomerular basement membrane is of immense importance. Possibly, thin diaphragms bridge the epithelial slits and are also of importance. The entire glomerular tuft is supported by mesangial cells lying between the capillaries. Basement membrane-like mesangial matrix forms a meshwork through which the mesangial cells are scattered. These cells are presumably of mesenchymal origin and are closely related to

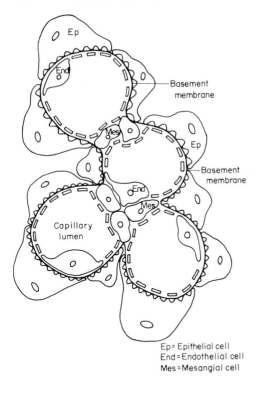

Ep = Epithelial cell
End = Endothelial cell
Mes = Mesangial cell

Figure 13–1. Schematic representation of the structure of glomerular lobule. (From Robbins, S. L.: Pathologic Basis of Disease. Philadelphia, W. B. Saunders Co., 1974.)

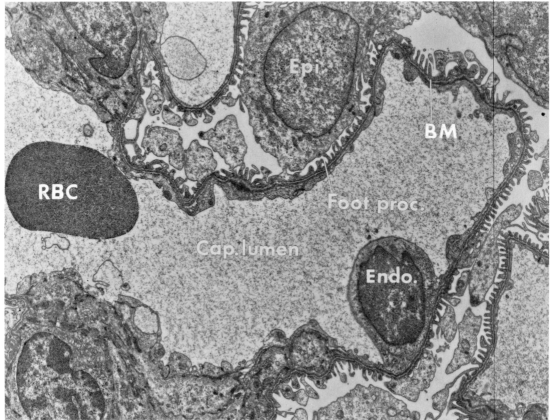

Figure 13–2. Normal rabbit kidney. BM, basement membrane. Endo., endothelial cell. Epi., epithelial cell. Cap. lumen, capillary lumen. RBC, red blood cell. Foot proc., foot processes. × 12,200. (Electron micrograph courtesy of Alan S. Cohen, M.D., Department of Medicine, Boston University School of Medicine. From Robbins, S. L.: Pathologic Basis of Disease. Philadelphia, W. B. Saunders Co., 1974.)

pericytes. They are also phagocytic and capable of laying down both matrix and collagen fibers. Mesangial matrix and glomerular basement membrane develop a rose-purple color with the periodic acid-Schiff (PAS) stain. This property is of great value in studying these structures under the light microscope. In the ordinary H&E stain, it is almost impossible to discern the glomerular basement membrane, sandwiched as it is between endothelial cells and podocytes. The morphologic details described here are shown schematically in Figure 13–1 and on an electron micrograph in Figure 13–2. Figure 13–3 shows a normal glomerulus for later comparison with damaged glomeruli. With this review of the normal glomerulus, we may turn our attention to a few of the general characteristics of renal disease.

Relatively early signs and symptoms of renal disease may include: hematuria, oliguria, generalized edema, pain and palpably enlarged kidneys. Infrequently, there is sudden and dramatic renal failure. Although, as we shall see, such presentations provide valuable information as to the nature of the underlying process, very often there are no such obvious expressions of disease and the first evidence of a kidney disorder is the gradual appearance of renal failure. *Indeed, the great bulk of fatal renal disease is produced by two entities, chronic glomerulonephritis and chronic pyelonephritis, both of which characteristically manifest themselves by the insidious onset of renal failure, often developing over a period of many years.* Although typically there are subtle indications of disease during the pre-failure period, such as nocturia attributable to loss of renal concentrating mechanisms, these usually are not sufficiently alarming to bring the patient to a physician. These patients frequently come to attention only when renal failure is far advanced. At this stage, the anatomic damage to the kidney is extensive, involving all four basic morphologic components—the glomeruli, tubules, blood vessels and interstitium—and it is therefore exceedingly difficult to differentiate one disease entity from another or to discern which morphologic component was first affected. *This tendency for the anatomic pathology of chronic renal disease to merge into a single pattern gives rise to the term "end stage kidneys."* The functional reserve of the kidneys

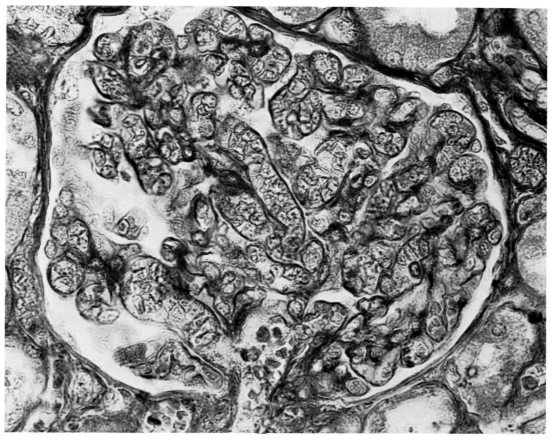

Figure 13–3. Normal glomerulus for comparison with damaged glomeruli. (From Robbins, S. L.: Pathologic Basis of Disease. Philadelphia, W. B. Saunders Co., 1974.)

is great, so that 90 per cent of the nephrons must be destroyed before there is significant functional impairment. *For this reason, the morphologic appearance of "end stage kidneys" may be present for some time before the clinical disease becomes terminal.*

Sometimes a clue to the underlying renal pathology may be gained from x-ray determinations of the size and symmetry of the kidneys. It is apparent that kidneys which are larger than normal must contain some added substances or structures to account for the greater volume, such as excessive amounts of blood or fluid, accumulations of fat, or hypertrophied nephrons. It can also be said that kidneys that are larger than normal cannot reasonably be the seat of pure chronic inflammatory processes, which inevitably produce scarring, atrophy and loss of substance. The distribution of such scarring—whether diffuse or focal, symmetric or asymmetric, bilateral or unilateral—suggests whether the process is a generalized derangement affecting both kidneys symmetrically or is a disease characterized by haphazard involvement.

RENAL FAILURE

It is appropriate here to discuss the manifestations of renal failure, since this may be the outcome with nearly any serious renal disease. First, the terminology must be clarified. The term *azotemia* refers to the retention of nitrogenous wastes, either through inability of the kidney to excrete them or through their failure to be delivered to the kidneys, as in circulatory failure from any cause. This is reflected in an elevated blood urea nitrogen (BUN) and is usually accompanied by other biochemical abnormalities referable to inadequate renal function. When azotemia becomes symptomatic, it is termed *uremia. Uremia is a complex syndrome characterized by a variable and inconstant group of biochemical and clinical changes.* These changes are best understood by a consideration of the principal functions of the kidneys: (1) volume regulation, (2) acid-base balance, (3) electrolyte balance, (4) excretion of waste products, and (5) endocrine functions, including the elaboration of renin, erythropoietin and the active form of vitamin D.

When there is derangement in *volume regulation*, the patient either becomes dehydrated, or he tends to retain salt and water and becomes edematous. With much chronic renal disease, the former occurs early in the course, when there is impairment of concentrating ability, and the latter occurs later, when the glomeruli become hyalinized and plasma can no longer be filtered through to the tubules. Fluid overload may lead to *congestive heart failure* (p. 289), with *pulmonary congestion.* This is particularly likely to occur when there is *hypertension,* which, as we shall see, is a characteristic concomitant of several types of renal disease.

Failure of renal regulation of *acid-base balance* leads to progressive *metabolic acidosis.* The shortness of breath accompanying pulmonary congestion may therefore be compounded by that resulting from acidosis.

Uremia includes multiple *electrolyte derangements,* the most important of which are *hyperkalemia* and *hypocalcemia.* These may both cause dangerous *cardiac arrhythmias,* as well as alterations in myocardial contractility. Furthermore, they tend to produce generalized *muscle weakness* and an increase in *neuromuscular excitability.* The latter leads to the muscle twitching and cramping so often seen with uremia.

Retention of *nitrogenous wastes* is reflected in the *elevated BUN.* Whereas the BUN is customarily taken as an index of renal function, it is not in itself directly responsible for uremic symptoms. However, it is postulated that the liberation of ammonia from the urea of the saliva and intestinal fluid by the action of "urea-splitting" bacteria may be responsible for *inflammatory lesions of the gastrointestinal mucosa.* Patients with advanced uremia frequently have a nonspecific stomatitis, esophagitis, gastritis, enteritis or colitis, and may develop massive gastrointestinal bleeding.

Among the more troublesome components of uremia are the bone lesions, known collectively as *renal osteodystrophy.* These take the form of osteomalacia (p. 251), often accompanied by osteitis fibrosa cystica (p. 615). Both are related to a deficiency of the active form of vitamin D $(1,25-[OH]_2D_3)$ and secondary hyperparathyroidism, although other factors, such as phosphate retention and acidosis, are probably involved (Johnson et al., 1974). Reference should be made to page 251 for a discussion of vitamin D metabolism. Suffice it to say here that the active form of vitamin D may be considered a hormone elaborated by the kidney in response to a tropic hormone, parathyroid hormone (PTH), or to a decrease in serum inorganic phosphate (Reynolds, 1974). With destruction of the renal parenchyma, this endocrine function is lost and the manifestations of vitamin D deficiency ensue. The elaboration of renin by the kidney may also be affected by renal disease. The function of renin and the effect of renal disease on its elaboration are discussed later, in the section dealing with hypertension.

Uremic patients may also develop a variety

of other abnormalities. A diffuse fibrinous *pericarditis* (see p. 310) is present in many patients with uremia. The cause of the pericardial inflammatory reaction is not clear; it has been attributed to the accumulation of either phenols or nitrogenous products in the pericardial sac. However, neither of these postulates has been established. The pericarditis usually is not very severe, does not cause pain and rarely leads to any significant impairment of cardiac function. The *skin* often has a peculiar sallow coloration. This in part results from the accumulation of urinary pigments, principally urochrome, which normally gives urine its characteristic color. The skin color, however, is also materially influenced by a persistent *anemia*, which is present with renal failure. The anemia is characteristically normochromic, normocytic and refractory to any therapy. Although it is considered to be largely the result of impaired renal production of erythropoietin, there is also a shortened life span for the erythrocytes.

Most of the other components of the uremic syndrome are of more or less mysterious pathogenesis. These include *anorexia, nausea and vomiting,* which are almost invariably present and occur relatively early, usually before any of the gastrointestinal inflammatory lesions previously mentioned are evident. Also prominent among the symptoms associated with uremia are profound *disturbances in central nervous system function.* There is usually marked apathy, with impaired concentration; later, convulsions, delirium or coma may develop. It is possible that these abnormalities are based upon the deficiency of ionized calcium in the spinal fluid in addition to the retention of potassium and phosphates, which are antagonists of calcium. However, unquestionably many of the neurologic manifestations are in part referable to the terminal hypertensive crises commonly encountered in these patients. Disturbances in volume regulation which lead to the development of cerebral as well as generalized edema or dehydration undoubtedly also contribute to the neurologic changes. Often a *peripheral neuropathy* is present, with altered tendon reflexes, muscular weaknesses and peroneal palsy manifested by foot drop. Occasionally in uremic patients, there is a *hemorrhagic diathesis* accompanied by purpuric manifestations. Despite the fact that platelets are present in normal numbers, they are qualitatively defective and become relatively ineffective in hemostasis.

This, then, is the syndrome that is termed "uremia." Not all components are present in every patient, and the dominant features may vary from patient to patient. However, it should be emphasized that virtually all the lesions subsequently to be discussed may eventually produce uremia.

GLOMERULAR DISEASES

Understanding the several glomerular diseases is difficult but satisfying. A large part of the difficulty lies in the advanced state of our own ignorance. Although in recent years there has been a rapid influx of new information on this subject, at least as many questions have been raised as have been answered. We owe in great measure our new information as well as our new quandaries to the widespread use of three diagnostic tools: percutaneous renal biopsy, electron microscopy and immunofluorescent staining. As we shall see, the use of these three modalities has resulted in important changes in our concepts of glomerular diseases.

Without going into detail here, we can say that the basic difficulty in understanding glomerular diseases is that the histology seems to bear little relationship to the pathogenesis. There is a slightly better correlation between the histology and the clinical picture. Obviously, there must be reasons for such inconsistencies, but we do not know them. Even more mysterious is the etiology (or etiologies) of the vast bulk of glomerular diseases. As writers, then, we have a problem: shall we consider glomerular diseases according to clinical presentation, to histology or to pathogenesis? The best solution, we believe, is to address ourselves briefly to each of these elements in this introductory material, pointing out which correlations can be made with some justification and which are pure wishful thinking. Against this background, the glomerular diseases will be divided into three groups according to their major clinical presentations. Then, within each of these three groups, the individual disorders are subdivided according to their histology. As will be made clear later, however, there is much overlap among these groups. For example, two usually distinct clinical syndromes may be present simultaneously in the same patient.

The three clinical syndromes we shall consider are: (1) *the nephrotic syndrome,* characterized by massive proteinuria, with consequent hypoalbuminemia and generalized edema, (2) *the nephritic syndrome,* characterized by hematuria (with red cell casts in the urine) and a diminished glomerular filtration rate, usually with some degree of consequent oliguria, azotemia and hypertension, and (3) the insidious development of *uremia* secondary to glomerular disease.

In general, the *nephrotic syndrome* can be

correlated with diseases of the glomerular basement membrane (GBM). You will recall that, because the endothelium is fenestrated, the GBM remains by default the barrier which normally prevents the passage of large amounts of protein into the urine. In many cases of the nephrotic syndrome, light microscopy merely shows thickening of the GBM. By electron microscopy and immunofluorescent studies this apparent thickening of the GBM is often seen to be due to the deposition of foreign materials, such as immunoglobulins, immune complexes or fibrin, on either its endothelial or its epithelial side. Sometimes there is interposition of mesangial matrix between the endothelium and the GBM. In addition, an increased amount of the GBM substance itself may be present. In other cases of the nephrotic syndrome, however, there is no apparent abnormality of the GBM, even on electron microscopy, and some physicochemical derangement must be inferred. The only constant feature in *all* cases is loss of the foot processes of the visceral epithelial cells (podocytes). This is most likely a secondary phenomenon, related to compensatory reabsorption by these cells of some of the escaping protein.

The *nephritic syndrome*, in contrast, is usually caused by those diseases which evoke a proliferative response within the glomeruli. The proliferation may involve endothelial, mesangial or epithelial cells. It is characteristic of inflammatory disorders within the glomerulus. In some but not all cases, there may be, in addition, an infiltration of neutrophils within the capillary lumina, in Bowman's space and sometimes in the periglomerular interstitial tissue. Although the term *glomerulonephritis* was once used indiscriminately to embrace all glomerular diseases, it is best reserved for those acute inflammatory disorders which produce the nephritic syndrome.

When glomerular disease leads to the *insidious onset of uremia*, the dominant histologic feature is hyalinization of the glomeruli, and the lesion is termed chronic glomerulonephritis. This is a misnomer, since there is seldom any evidence of an inflammatory origin. Hyalinization refers to the accumulation within the glomerular tufts of a homogeneous eosinophilic material which resembles GBM substance or mesangial matrix. In the course of hyalinization, the glomerular capillaries are narrowed or obliterated, and the structural detail of the glomeruli is lost. When severe or widespread, all that may remain of the glomeruli under the light microscope are pink hyalinized smudges.

Having briefly characterized the major clinical and histologic presentations of glomerular diseases, what can we say of the etiology and pathogenesis? The known etiologies of glomerular diseases are legion; they include sensitivity reactions to a number of microorganisms and several drugs, as well as serum sickness from any cause. In addition, glomerular involvement is a frequent accompaniment of a variety of systemic disorders, including diabetes mellitus, amyloidosis, the collagen-vascular diseases, such as SLE and systemic sclerosis, and the idiopathic vasculitides, such as polyarteritis nodosa and Henoch-Schönlein purpura. *Nevertheless, despite the plethora of possible origins, the fact remains that in many cases of glomerular disease, no etiology can be found.*

A consideration of the pathogenesis of glomerular diseases is simpler—perhaps too simple, as we shall see. It would seem that most primary glomerular diseases are based on an immune pathogenesis which follows one of only two pathways. *By far the most common of these pathways involves the deposition of circulating immune complexes in the glomeruli (immune complex disease).* In these cases the antigens are not of glomerular origin. *In contrast, the second immunopathogenic mechanism involves the formation of antibodies against the GBM itself (anti-GBM disease).* These two mechanisms will be described separately here, before going on to a detailed consideration of the three clinical syndromes and the individual lesions which cause them. It should be remembered that both pathogenetic mechanisms may produce lesions that are identical under the light microscope, and both may lead to any of the clinical syndromes. Only by electron microscopy and immunofluorescent studies can they be differentiated.

With immune complex disease, the kidney may be considered an "innocent bystander" in that it does not incite the reaction. The antigen is not of renal origin. It may be an endogenous antigen, as in the case of the glomerulopathy associated with SLE, or it may be exogenous, as with the glomerulonephritis which follows a streptococcal infection. A number of other antigens have recently been implicated, including the surface antigen of the hepatitis B virus (HBsAg); various tumor antigens, such as carcinoembryonic antigen (CEA); *Treponema pallidum, Plasmodium falciparum;* and several viruses. However, in most cases the inciting antigen is unknown. Whatever the antigen may be, the immune complexes are formed in the circulation and are then mechanically trapped in the glomeruli, where they produce injury, probably in large part through the binding of complement, although there are indications that complement-independent injury may also occur. In those cases in which complement is bound, neutrophils are attracted to the area and phagocytize the immune complexes. With phagocytosis, some cells die and lysosomal enzymes are released, damaging the endothelial cells and the GBM. As a response to injury, the endothelial and mesangial cells proliferate, and later there may be epithelial cell proliferation as well. Platelet clumping releases vasoactive amines, which further increase the permeability of the capillaries, resulting in increased filtration of plasma proteins (Cochrane and Dixon, 1968). The plasma proteins, as well as fibrin, may be secondarily deposited in the glomerular capillary lumina (intravascular coagulation) and filter into the mesangium and beneath the endothelium (Stiehm and Trygstad, 1969). Electron microscopy reveals the immune complexes as granular deposits or "humps" which lie either in the mesangium and between the endothelial cells and the GBM *(subendothelial deposits)*, or between the outer surface of the GBM and the podocytes *(subepithelial deposits)*. The precise location probably depends on a number of factors, including the type, quantity, timing and duration of exposure to the antigen (Cameron, 1972). It is probable that very small, soluble immune complexes form subepithelial deposits, while larger, less soluble complexes are deposited in the mesangium and beneath the endothelium (Case Records of the Massachusetts General Hospital, 1974).

Why does immune complex disease not occur whenever there is an antigen-antibody reaction? Some light is thrown on this subject through the study of experimental serum sickness in animals, which can be considered the experimental counterpart of immune complex disease in man. When rabbits are immunized daily with heterologous serum albumin, they may respond in one of three ways (Christian, 1969). About one third of the animals are tolerant, and there is very slow and gradual clearing of the antigen without antibody formation. In contrast, over half of the rabbits are good antibody producers; they rapidly develop a large antibody excess, which forms precipitating complexes with the antigen. These complexes are rapidly cleared by the reticuloendothelial system. Although an acute glomerulonephritis may occur in these cases, it is always benign and self-limited. The third group of animals, comprising 10 to 20 per cent of the animals, may be considered poor antibody formers. Although antibody is produced, it is specific for only a few of the large number of possible determinants on the antigen molecule, and this fact limits the degree of "latticework" possible between antigen

and antibody (Pincus et al., 1968). Moreover, there is a sustained antigen excess. As a result, the complexes formed are of relatively small size, and hence are soluble. They are too small for clearance by the RE system and therefore circulate for hours in antigen excess. When this happens, the animals develop a progressive form of glomerular disease and die with uremia.

How do these facts relate to the human disease? Can an exact parallel be drawn with the experimental model? If so, why should some individuals fail to clear the offending antigen? In the case of SLE, the answer seems, at least in part, relatively straightforward. Because the antigens are endogenous, there is a continuing source of antigen excess. In the case of an exogenous antigen, such as the streptococcus, however, the answer is unknown. Many hypotheses have been offered. Conceivably, those strains of streptococci which are capable of causing glomerulonephritis ("nephritogenic" streptococci) evoke antibodies which are cross-reactive, albeit not entirely specific for some autologous antigen; such a postulation has the advantage of explaining not only the continuing source of antigen but also the only partial specificity between antibody to a foreign agent and autologous antigen. It is of interest in this connection that whereas several other antigens sometimes associated with glomerular disease, such as the surface antigen of the hepatitis B virus (HBsAg) and carcinoembryonic antigen, have been eluted from the glomerular lesion, streptococcal antigens have never been positively identified within the diseased glomeruli. It has been observed that all nephritogenic strains of streptococci happen to be those sensitive to bacteriophage. Conceivably, it is these viruses rather than the streptococci which evoke the immunologic response, and which continue to persist in some form in their new host. Supporting such a concept is the fact that all spontaneously occurring forms of glomerular disease in animals are of the immune complex type and attributable to chronic viral infections. All of these speculations focus on the nature of the antigen. An alternative suggestion is that the critical factor in the development of immune complex disease is not the nature of the antigen, but rather the immunologic status of the host. Defective clearing of antigen might occur with a number of disorders—for example, with a hereditary deficiency of complement or with a derangement in T-cell function. A number of studies are in progress to investigate these possibilities (Peters and Lachmann, 1974).

The second and less frequent immunopathogenetic mechanism in the production of primary glomerular disease involves the formation of anti-GBM antibodies (Lerner, 1967). It has its experimental prototype in the nephritis of rabbits called *Masugi nephritis* or *nephrotoxic serum nephritis* (Chase, 1967). This is produced by injecting rabbits with rat kidney. When the rabbit builds antibodies to the rat kidney, they are cross-reactive with his own kidney. Indeed, because vascular basement membrane is antigenically similar everywhere, these antibodies may in some instances react with any basement membrane to which they are exposed. The GBM is, of course, particularly vulnerable because the endothelial fenestrations leave it readily accessible to circulating antibodies. Characteristically, in lesions involving anti-GBM antibodies, the immune deposits are not discernible either by light microscopy or by electron microscopy. Only by immunofluorescent microscopy are the anti-GBM antibodies and complement revealed as a smooth linear fluorescence following the line of the GBM. *This linear pattern of anti-GBM disease, then, contrasts strikingly with the granular pattern of immune complex disease (often termed, with admirable scientific precision, the "lumpy-bumpy" pattern).* As with immune complex disease, in anti-GBM disease complement is sometimes bound to the GBM, and attracts neutrophils. Ultimately, it is the lysosomal enzymes of these white cells which mediate the damage. However, complement-independent pathways have also been suggested (Couser et al., 1973).

What is the source of the inciting GBM antigen in human anti-GBM disease? Recently it has been shown that autologous GBM antigen is present in normal human urine. Moreover, this has been proved nephritogenic when injected into animals. It has been postulated that this may be the source of the original antigen in human anti-GBM disease. According to this theory, lymphoid cells exposed to normal urine, particularly when drawn to the kidney by an infectious agent, might then be stimulated to form antibodies against the autologous GBM antigen present in the urine (Dixon, 1968). Alternatively, the GBM antigens may be slightly modified by a biologic agent, such as a virus, which renders them foreign to the immune system and thus provokes an immune response directed against the GBM. So far these are only plausible speculations; there is as yet little experimental evidence to support them.

With this discussion of the immunopathogenetic mechanisms involved in glomerular diseases, we turn our attention to the three clinical syndromes described earlier and the individual entities which produce them. These

are summarized in Table 13–2 at the end of this section (p. 441).

THE NEPHROTIC SYNDROME

The nephrotic syndrome refers to a clinical complex comprising the following findings: (1) generalized edema, the most obvious clinical manifestation, (2) massive proteinuria, with the daily loss in the urine of 4 gm. or more of protein, (3) hypoalbuminemia, with plasma albumin levels less than 2.5 gm. per 100 ml., and (4) hyperlipidemia and hyperlipiduria. At the outset there is little or no azotemia, hematuria or hypertension. The components of the nephrotic syndrome bear a logical relationship to one another. The initial event is a derangement in the basement membrane of the glomeruli, resulting in an increased permeability to the plasma proteins. It will be remembered from the discussion of the normal kidney that the basement membrane acts as the only unfenestrated barrier through which the glomerular filtrate must pass. Any increased permeability of the GBM, then, allows protein to escape from the plasma into the glomerular filtrate, first the smaller albumin molecules and then, if it is sufficiently permeable, the larger globulins. Massive proteinuria may result. With longstanding or extremely heavy proteinuria, the serum albumin tends to become depleted, resulting in hypoalbuminemia and a reversed albumin-globulin ratio. The generalized edema of the nephrotic syndrome is in turn largely a consequence of the drop in osmotic pressure produced by hypoalbuminemia. As fluid escapes from the vascular tree into the tissues, there is a concomitant drop in plasma volume, with diminished glomerular filtration. Compensatory secretion of aldosterone, along with the reduced GFR, promotes retention of salt and water by the kidneys, thus further aggravating the edema. By repetition of this chain of events, quite massive amounts of edema (termed *anasarca*) may accumulate. The genesis of the hyperlipidemia is more obscure. One hypothesis proposes that the loss of albumin reduces the capacity for serum transport of lipids, thus retarding their normal metabolism and producing hyperlipidemia. This concept, however, is purely speculative. There is no verified explanation for the hyperlipidemia and hypercholesterolemia characteristic of the nephrotic syndrome. Hyperlipiduria simply reflects the hyperlipidemia and increased GBM permeability.

The relative frequencies of the several causes of the nephrotic syndrome vary somewhat from study to study. All agree, however, that the age range of the population under study is of great importance. In children

TABLE 13-1. CAUSES OF THE NEPHROTIC SYNDROME

	CHILDREN (PER CENT)	ADULTS (PER CENT)
Primary Renal Disease	95	75
1. Minimal change disease	65	25
2. Membranous nephropathy	5	30
3. Focal glomerulosclerosis	?	?
4. Membranoproliferative glomerulonephritis	?	?
5. Proliferative glomerulonephritis	20	15
Secondary Causes (most often SLE, diabetes mellitus and amyloid)	5	25

under the age of 15 years, for example, the nephrotic syndrome is almost always caused by a lesion primary to the kidney, while among adults it may often be associated with a systemic disease. Table 13-1 represents a composite derived from several studies of the causes of the nephrotic syndrome, and is therefore only approximate. As the table indicates, the most frequent *systemic* causes of the nephrotic syndrome are SLE, diabetes and amyloid (Seymour et al., 1971). The renal lesions produced by these disorders have been described elsewhere in this text. It is evident that the most important of the *primary* glomerular lesions which characteristically lead to the nephrotic syndrome are *minimal change disease* and *membranous nephropathy*. The former is most important in children; the latter in adults. Two other primary lesions, *focal glomerulosclerosis* and *membranoproliferative glomerulonephritis*, also produce the nephrotic syndrome but are of relatively minor importance. These four lesions will be discussed individually. A fifth primary cause of the nephrotic syndrome, *proliferative glomerulonephritis (PGN)*, will not be considered in this section. While it is obviously an important cause of the nephrotic syndrome, this very common lesion is far more likely to produce the *nephritic* syndrome and so will be discussed later.

MINIMAL CHANGE DISEASE (LIPOID NEPHROSIS)

This relatively benign disorder is the most frequent single cause of the nephrotic syndrome. It is also the most mysterious, since even with the electron microscope no morphologic changes can be discerned which would explain the clinical findings. Moreover, it is unique among the primary glomerular diseases in that there is no evidence for either an immune complex or an anti-GBM pathogenesis. Thus, the strange name is apposite. Although minimal change disease may develop at any age, it is most common in chil-

dren between the ages of 1 and 5 years, and affects boys more often than girls. It has been said that most patients have a history of a nonspecific respiratory illness or of an immunization, but so do many normal children in this age group (Kashgarian et al., 1974). As stated, the etiology and pathogenesis are completely unknown. Since antibodies have been exonerated in this disease, cynics will not be surprised to learn that it is now suspected of being a T-cell disorder (Shalhoub 1974; Krueger and Bulla, 1974). In one study, lymphocytotoxins were found in 5 of 8 patients with minimal change disease, but their relationship to the renal disease is purely speculative (Ooi et al., 1974).

Morphology. The presence of the nephrotic syndrome implies that the kidneys are large and pale, since all tissues of the body are edematous. With the light microscope the glomeruli appear entirely normal. The cells of the proximal convoluted tubules are often heavily laden with lipids, but this is secondary to tubular reabsorption of the lipoproteins passing through the diseased glomeruli. This appearance of the proximal convoluted tubules is the basis for the older term for this disorder, "lipoid nephrosis." Even with the electron microscope, the GBM appears perfectly normal. However, the very presence of the nephrotic syndrome would indicate some alteration in the GBM, presumably at a physicochemical level, beyond the range of the electron microscope. **The only obvious glomerular abnormality is fusion of the foot processes of the podocytes.** The cytoplasm of the podocytes is thus smeared over the external aspect of the GBM, obliterating the network of arcades between the podocytes and the GBM. This change, however, is thought to be secondary to the proteinuria and related to compensatory reabsorption by these cells of some of the escaping protein. In support of this interpretation is the fact that during remissions of the disease, when the proteinuria abates, the podocytes resume their normal architecture.

Clinical Course. The disease first manifests itself by the insidious development of the nephrotic syndrome in an otherwise healthy individual. The protein loss is typically confined only to the smaller serum proteins, chiefly albumin (*selective proteinuria*). This selectivity can be a valuable clue in distinguishing minimal change disease from other causes of the nephrotic syndrome. The prognosis with this disorder is good. Even without therapy, spontaneous remissions are common. It was once thought that minimal change disease may in some cases evolve into another, more ominous lesion, but the newer evidence is against this. Most likely minimal change disease does not progress to renal failure, and the small number of patients who do die succumb to secondary effects of the nephrotic syndrome. These include infections, presumably on the basis of chronic loss of antibodies and thromboembolism related to a hypercoagulability state. Among the many remarkable features of minimal change disease is the fact that those patients who do not experience a spontaneous remission usually respond very well to corticosteroids or cyclophosphamide or both. Most patients can be expected to enter a prolonged remission with such therapy, and in many cases therapy can be withdrawn without relapse. Because of its responsiveness to therapy, particularly early in the course, it is very important that minimal change disease be differentiated from the other causes of the nephrotic syndrome. The ten-year survival is over 90 per cent (Cameron, 1972).

MEMBRANOUS NEPHROPATHY (EPIMEMBRANOUS NEPHROPATHY, MEMBRANOUS GLOMERULONEPHRITIS)

This is a slowly progressive disease of young adulthood and middle age, characterized morphologically by well-defined alterations in the GBM. The pathogenesis involves the deposition of immune complexes on the epithelial side of the GBM. *Hence, membranous nephropathy is a form of immune complex disease.* The reasons for the subepithelial localization of the deposits and for the distinctive response of the GBM to them are not clear. This location may result because the formed complexes are relatively small and filter through the membrane (Case Records of the Massachusetts General Hospital, 1974). In most cases the inciting antigen cannot be identified. However, a number of known antigens are apparently responsib e for a minority of cases. These include several tumor antigens, such as carcinoembryonic antigen, in patients with cancer. Indeed, it is becoming apparent that there is a frequent association between membranous nephropathy and cancer. Sometimes the renal disease is the first indication of an occult malignancy. Possibly oncogenic viruses may also evoke immune complexes (Couser, 1974). Another recently appreciated association is that between membranous nephropathy and the presence of circulating hepatitis B surface antigen (HBsAg), often without clinical evidence of liver disease. Immune complexes containing HBsAg have been eluted from the glomeruli in such cases. It has been pointed out that their presence may be secondary to the chronic renal disease rather than causative, in view of the known vulnerability of patients with any long-standing renal disease to subclinical hepatitis B (see p. 515). This controversy remains unresolved. Glomerular disease is a very common complication of SLE, and in a minority of patients takes the form of membranous nephropathy. In these instances, DNA antigen-antibody complexes have been eluted from the glomeruli. Treponemal antigen has been identified in the glomeruli of patients with membranous nephropathy and secondary syphilis. Drug reactions may evoke a lesion indistinguishable from membranous nephropathy. Offending agents include gold, mercury and penicillamine. It was once thought that renal vein thrombosis in some mysterious fashion leads to membranous nephropathy. However, most workers now believe that the thrombosis is secondary rather than causative, and related to the hypercoagulable state induced by the renal disease (Cameron, 1972). In summary, it would seem that a multitude of possible etiologies may be responsible for membranous nephropathy, most or all of which operate through a single pathogenetic pathway, but in the majority of cases no clearly defined etiology is evident.

Morphology. As with minimal change disease, the kidneys are large and pale, secondary to the generalized edema. Under the light microscope the basic change appears to be a diffuse thickening of the GBM. The cells of the proximal convoluted tubules contain lipid droplets but, as pointed out in the description of minimal change disease, this is a secondary change which occurs with any lesion producing the nephrotic syndrome. With silver methenamine staining of the GBM, it can be seen that the apparent thickening is due in part to subepithelial deposits which nestle against the GBM and are separated from each other by small spike-like protrusions of GBM matrix ("spike and dome" pattern). As the disease progresses, these "spikes" close over the deposits, thus incorporating them into the GBM. Silver staining at this stage reveals a spongy "moth-eaten" texture which reflects the incorporation of the immune deposits. With the electron microscope, the "spike and dome" pattern is confirmed. With progression of the disease, the incorporated deposits are catabolized and eventually disappear, leaving for a time cavities within the GBM. These are later filled in, with a progressive deposition of GBM matrix (Kashgarian et al., 1974). In addition, the podocytes lose their foot processes. This change is most likely secondary to the leakage of large amounts of protein, as mentioned earlier in the discussion of minimal change disease. The consequent close apposition of the podocytes to the GBM probably contributes to the appearance of GBM thickening under the light microscope. The nature of the subepithelial and intramembranous deposits is elucidated by immunofluorescent microscopy. In most cases the deposits contain IgG and complement, but complement may not be present, particularly after the early stage of the disease. It has been suggested that the GBM injury may be independent of complement and neutrophils (Kashgarian et al. 1974). Certainly, there is little or no proliferative response or neutrophilic infiltrate, as one might expect with complement-mediated injury.

Clinical Course. The clinical onset of membranous nephropathy is indistinguishable from that of minimal change disease. It is characterized by the insidious development of the nephrotic syndrome, usually without any antecedent illness. However, proteinuria may be present without the full-blown nephrotic syndrome. In contrast to minimal change disease, the proteinuria is nonselective. Globulins are lost in the urine, as well as the smaller albumin molecules. Membranous nephropathy follows a notoriously indolent course. Despite frequent spontaneous remissions, it is in general slowly progressive, leading eventually to some degree of renal insufficiency. When this occurs, the glomeruli usually become completely hyalinized and the histologic picture thus merges with that of chronic GN, to be discussed later. In one prospective study of patients with membranous nephropathy, involving follow-up periods of 2 to 13 years, some degree of renal insufficiency developed in 35 per cent of patients, another 25 per cent underwent spontaneous remission and in 40 per cent the disease was stable (Erwin et al., 1973). Overall 10-year survival for adults is about 40 per cent. In children the disease is apparently more benign, and permits a 90 per cent 10-year survival (Cameron, 1972). There is no evidence that corticosteroid or cyclophosphamide therapy modifies the course.

FOCAL GLOMERULOSCLEROSIS

This interesting lesion was once thought to evolve from minimal change disease in a small percentage of cases. However, the dominant view today is that it is a discrete entity (Jenis et al., 1974; Cameron, 1972). It is most common in adolescents, and produces a steroid-resistant nephrotic syndrome, with nonselective proteinuria.

The disease first affects the juxtamedullary glomeruli, hence the term **focal**. If juxtamedullary glomeruli are not included in a percutaneous renal biopsy, the diagnosis may be missed. It is probably for this reason that early cases were once diagnosed as minimal change disease. Histologically, focal glomerulosclerosis is characterized by mesangial hyalinization of some glomerular tufts, with sparing of others, a distribution termed **segmental**. In affected glomeruli, immunofluorescent microscopy reveals deposits of immunoglobulins, usually IgM, and complement in the mesangium.

Focal glomerulosclerosis is usually slowly but relentlessly progressive, with the lesion extending ultimately to involve the glomeruli diffusely. Ten-year survival is about 50 per cent (Cameron, 1972).

MEMBRANOPROLIFERATIVE GLOMERULONEPHRITIS (MPGN) (MESANGIOCAPILLARY GN, CHRONIC HYPOCOMPLEMENTEMIC GN)

MPGN is an infrequent disorder which is of particular interest for two reasons. First, although it usually results in the nephrotic syndrome, it may instead cause the nephritic syndrome. Often elements of both are present simultaneously. Second, membranoproliferative GN is associated with chronic low serum levels of the complement components $C'3$ to $C'9$, with normal levels of $C'1$, $C'4$ and $C'2$. Apparently there is some serum factor which activates complement via the alternate or properdin pathway. Whether the hypocomplementemia is of pathogenetic significance is unknown.

Membranoproliferative GN is most common in older children and adolescents. The most frequent presentation is the nephrotic syndrome accompanied by hematuria.

The morphology of the lesion is consistent with the mixed clinical picture — that is, there are both GBM changes and glomerular cellular proliferation. By light microscopy, one can see that the GBM is thickened and there is diffuse proliferation of mesangial cells, with an increase in mesangial matrix. Silver methenamine stains show the GBM to be split into layers owing to interposition of mesangial matrix ("tram-track appearance"). Immunofluorescent microscopy shows variable findings. Usually $C'3$ can be found deposited within the mesangium and GBM. In addition, there may be deposits of immunoglobulins, particularly IgG, within the mesangium and beneath the endothelium.

The disease is slowly progressive, with a 10-year survival of about 40 per cent (Cameron, 1972).

THE NEPHRITIC SYNDROME

This is a clinical complex, usually of acute onset, characterized by (1) hematuria with red cell and hemoglobin casts in the urine, (2) some degree of oliguria and azotemia, and (3) hypertension. While there may also be some proteinuria and even edema, these are usually not sufficiently marked to cause the nephrotic syndrome. As with the nephrotic syndrome, the elements of the nephritic syndrome can be related to the anatomic changes. The lesions which cause the nephritic syndrome have in common an inflammatory proliferation of the cells within the glomeruli, often accompanied by a neutrophilic infiltrate. This inflammatory reaction injures the capillary walls, permitting the escape of red cells into the urine. It also encroaches on the capillary lumina, thus leading to a reduction in the glomerular filtration rate. The reduced glomerular filtration rate is manifested clinically by oliguria with reciprocal fluid retention and azotemia. Hypertension is probably a result of both the fluid retention and some augmented renin release from the ischemic kidneys.

Three basic lesions may produce the nephritic syndrome: *diffuse proliferative glomerulonephritis, focal (proliferative) glomerulonephritis* and *rapidly progressive glomerulonephritis.* As we shall see, each is quite variable and probably represents a heterogeneous group of disorders and of stages of disorders. It is likely that all three are associated with either an immune complex or an anti-GBM pathogenesis.

DIFFUSE PROLIFERATIVE GLOMERULONEPHRITIS (DIFFUSE PGN)

This is probably the most frequent of all the glomerular lesions. It is usually an immune complex disease, although occasionally it may be associated with anti-GBM antibodies. Sometimes there is no discernible immune mechanism (Hinglais et al., 1974). Possibly in some of these cases the biopsy was taken after the immune complexes had already been cleared. The inciting antigen may be either exogenous or endogenous. The prototype of diffuse PGN caused by an *exogenous* antigen is *poststreptococcal GN*, while that produced by an *endogenous* antigen is *lupus nephritis*, found with SLE. Each of these forms will be described separately in some detail. It is important to remember, however, that diffuse PGN may occur in a variety of other clinical settings, and is very often idiopathic. For example, infections with organisms other than the streptococci may be associated with diffuse PGN. These include certain staphylococcal infections, as well as a number of common viral diseases, such as mumps, measles and chickenpox. The lesion may also be associated with infective endocarditis and with a number of systemic vasculitides, including polyarteritis nodosa, Henoch-Schönlein purpura and Wegener's granulomatosis. More often, however, these disorders involve a focal GN, to be described later.

The classic case of poststreptococcal GN develops in a child 1 to 4 weeks following recovery from a streptococcal infection elsewhere in the body. Only certain "nephritogenic" strains of the beta hemolytic streptococci are capable of evoking glomerular disease. At one time the initial infection was most likely to be a pharyngitis caused by streptococci Types 12, 4 or 1, but it is probable that skin sepsis with Types 49 or 57 is now a more important antecedent (Cameron, 1972). Sometimes the disease occurs in epidemics. As mentioned earlier, whereas poststreptococcal GN is clearly an immune complex disease, it has not been proven that the antigen is entirely derived from the bacteria. The onset of the kidney disease is usually abrupt, heralded by malaise, a slight fever, nausea and the nephritic syndrome. However, biopsy studies have indicated that subclinical disease may be frequent (Freedman et al., 1966). In the usual case, oliguria, azotemia and hypertension are only mild to moderate. Characteristically, there is gross hematuria, with the urine appearing smoky brown rather than bright red. Presumably the hemoglobin released by the hemolysis of red cells undergoes transformation to hematin in the relatively acid urine, and it is the hematin which imparts the brown color to the urine. Occasionally, however, the urine is bright red. Some degree of proteinuria is a constant feature of the disease and, as mentioned earlier, may occasionally be severe enough to produce the nephrotic syndrome. *Valuable clues to the diagnosis include a transient depression of serum complement levels, lasting for about a month, and elevations in serum antistreptolysin O and antistreptokinase titers.*

Grossly, the kidneys may appear entirely normal or they may be moderately enlarged, perhaps up to 180 gm. each. The cortical surface is smooth and free of scarring, as would be anticipated during the acute phase of any inflammation. Fine, punctate petechiae, produced by the acute inflammatory rupture of glomerular capillaries, may be scattered over the cortical surface. With the light microscope, the most characteristic change is a fairly uniform increased cellularity of the glomerular tufts affecting nearly all glomeruli, hence the term **diffuse.** The increased cellularity is due both to proliferation and swelling of endothelial and mesangial cells and to a variable neutrophilic infiltrate. Sometimes there are thrombi within the capillary lumina and necrosis of the capillary walls. In the more severe cases, there may in addition be proliferation of the parietal epithelial cells, forming epithelial "crescents" around Bowman's capsule. In general, these have ominous significance. When they involve the majority of the glomeruli, the pattern merges with that of rapidly progressive GN, to be discussed. In the early stages of the disease, the electron microscope shows the immune complexes arrayed as subepithelial "humps" nestled against the GBM (Fig. 13–4). These deposits are usually cleared over a period of about 2 months. Immunofluorescent studies reveal IgG and complement within the deposits.

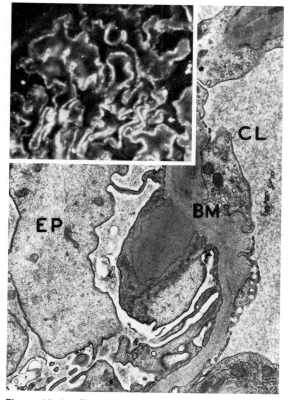

Figure 13–4. Electron micrographic detail of the basement membrane (BM) of the glomerulus in the "immune complex" form of diffuse PGN. A lumpy immune complex deposit is attached to the epithelial surface of the basement membrane just to the left of the symbol BM. It is enclosed within a cytoplasmic process of the epithelial cell (EP). (CL, capillary lumen.) The inset at upper left is a detail of an immunofluorescent stain of the glomerulus in this disease. Seen are the irregular, luminescent, lumpy deposits arrayed about the margins of the glomerular capillaries.

Oddly enough, the prognosis with such a common disease is still in some dispute. Nearly all workers agree that complete recovery occurs in the vast majority of patients, particularly in epidemic cases. Whether this lesion ever leads to rapidly progressive GN or to chronic GN is the source of the controversy. This issue will be resolved only by long-term prospective biopsy studies. The present evidence indicates that recovery occurs in about 95 per cent of cases, sometimes only after years of persistent urinary abnormalities. A small percentage of patients, however, probably do develop more serious lesions, which lead ultimately to renal failure.

Glomerular disease is a common occurrence in patients with SLE (p. 184). As mentioned earlier, diffuse PGN associated with SLE is the prototype of immune complex disease caused by endogenous antigens. Serum complement is low, and DNA antigen and anti-DNA antibodies have been identified in the glomeruli.

The gross and light microscopic changes in the kidneys are identical to those of any other form of diffuse PGN, and involve proliferation of the endothelial and mesangial cells. However, with the electron microscope an important difference can be discerned. **You will recall that the immune deposits of poststreptococcal GN are subepithelial. In contrast, those of SLE are principally subendothelial and mesangial.** Immunofluorescent staining indicates that the deposits in SLE contain complement and a variable profile of immunoglobulins, most notably IgA and IgM, as well as IgG. It has been suggested that the larger immunoglobulins may form relatively large insoluble complexes which are unable to penetrate the GBM, hence remain in a subendothelial location (Case Records of the Massachusetts General Hospital, 1974).

FOCAL (PROLIFERATIVE) GLOMERULONEPHRITIS (FOCAL GN)

This is a histologic diagnosis, based on the presence of changes, usually proliferative, in only some of the glomeruli (*focal involvement*). The lesion may also affect only isolated tufts within any one glomerulus (*segmental involvement*). Most cases of focal GN are secondary to one of a number of systemic diseases. The most frequent of the systemic diseases leading to focal GN are Henoch-Schönlein purpura, in children, and polyarteritis nodosa (particularly the microscopic form), in adults (Cameron, 1972). Other causes include infective endocarditis, SLE, Wegener's granulomatosis and the early stages of Goodpasture's syndrome. Like diffuse PGN, this is usually an immune complex disease. It differs in that the immune complexes are largely localized to the mesangium of most glomeruli. At one time this lesion was referred to as focal embolic GN and thought to be caused by septic emboli released from a focus of infective endocarditis. It is now clear, however, that even with infective endocarditis, the renal lesion represents an immune complex disease; moreover, it has become apparent that other disorders are more common as antecedents of focal GN.

Occasionally focal GN occurs as an isolated disorder. In these cases it is usually associated with a syndrome known as *benign recurrent hematuria* or *Berger's disease* (Editorial, 1975a). This syndrome usually affects children, and begins as an episode of gross hematuria occurring within a day or two of a nonspecific upper respiratory infection. Typically, the hematuria lasts for several days, then subsides, only to recur every few months. In the majority of cases, these recurrent episodes of hematuria eventually cease, and the disorder is entirely benign. *Although the etiology of Berger's disease is unknown, the pathogenetic hallmark is the deposition of IgA in the mesangium.* Some have considered Berger's disease to be a variant of Henoch-Schönlein purpura, a lesion also associated with IgA deposition in the mesangium (Tsai et al., 1975). In contrast to Berger's disease, however, Henoch-Schönlein purpura is a systemic syndrome involving the skin (purpuric rash), GI tract (abdominal pain) and joints (arthritis), as well as the kidneys.

Before describing the morphology of focal GN, it should be pointed out that *many of the diseases associated with this lesion may also produce diffuse GN.* This has given rise to speculation that focal GN may simply represent an early stage of diffuse PGN (Ginzler et al., 1974). This is a very controversial issue which remains unresolved. In the case of SLE, for example, the prognosis is very different for those patients with the focal lesion as opposed to diffuse PGN. Some studies indicate that these two lesions are discrete entities and remain so throughout their course (Mery et al., 1975).

Grossly, the kidneys are usually of normal size and color but often have irregularly scattered petechial hemorrhages over their surface. Microscopically, randomly scattered glomeruli are involved, often with sparing of several tufts within an affected glomerulus. There is typically proliferation of the mesangial cells, sometimes accompanied by endothelial cell proliferation. Usually the proliferation is adjacent to a focus of necrosis within the affected glomerular tuft. However, sometimes there is very little proliferation, and the necrotic component dominates the histologic appearance. Fibrin deposition and capillary thromboses are common in the foci of glomerular necrosis. In severe cases, there may be epithelial cell proliferation with "crescent" formation, to be described later. Late in the development of the lesion, the involved areas undergo fibrosis with obliteration of a segment of the glomerulus. By immunofluorescent microscopy, the presence and location of immune deposits varies with the underlying disorder. Sometimes none can be demonstrated.

It is of interest that in three of the disorders associated with focal GN, there is deposition of relatively large amounts of IgA in the mesangium. These disorders are Henoch-Schönlein purpura, Berger's disease and SLE. All have a very good prognosis, and it has been suggested that this reflects the ready accessibility of the offending immune complexes to the mesangial cells, which are phagocytic (Leathem, 1975). In general, when focal GN occurs as an isolated lesion, the prognosis is excellent. However, when the lesion is a component of a systemic disorder, the prognosis is variable and, as might be expected, depends on the primary disease.

RAPIDLY PROGRESSIVE GLOMERULONEPHRITIS (RPGN) (EXTRACAPILLARY PGN)

This is both a histologic and a clinical diagnosis. The diagnostic histologic change is the formation of epithelial "crescents" in over 70 per cent of the glomeruli. These are produced by marked proliferation of the parietal epithelial cells of Bowman's capsule, with the formation of crescentic clusters of cells filling Bowman's space. Clinically, RPGN is associated with severe oliguria and, in the absence of chronic hemodialysis or renal transplantation, death from renal failure within weeks to months. Clearly, then, this is the most lethal of the glomerular diseases.

It would seem that nearly any cause of diffuse or focal PGN may on occasion lead to RPGN. Rarely, even poststreptococcal GN shows such progression (Case Records of the Massachusetts General Hospital, 1975). Low serum complement levels help to identify patients whose disease has progressed from poststreptococcal GN. However, most often RPGN develops suddenly, without any history of renal disease. In some of these patients, it is associated with lesions in the lung and with hemoptysis, a picture known as *Goodpasture's syndrome* (presented on p. 418). This has long been the prototype of glomerular disease associated with an anti-GBM pathogenesis. It is thought that the antibodies react not only with the GBM but also with the basement membrane in the alveoli of the lung, since vascular basement membrane is everywhere antigenically similar. *It has recently become apparent that anti-GBM RPGN may also occur without associated lung lesions and that, indeed, this is probably the most common pathogenetic pathway of RPGN.* Less frequently, immune complexes are found.

Morphology. The kidneys are enlarged and pale, often with petechial hemorrhages on the cortical surface. Early in the course, the microscopic changes may be similar to those of diffuse PGN, marked only by endothelial and mesangial proliferation. However, the histologic picture is soon dominated by a striking proliferation of the epithelial cells to form crescents. These eventually obliterate Bowman's space and compress the glomeruli (Fig. 13–5). Renal biopsies have indicated that the crescents may form extremely rapidly, within a few days of the onset of the disease. **Fibrin strands are prominent between the cellular layers in the crescents, and it is currently believed that it is**

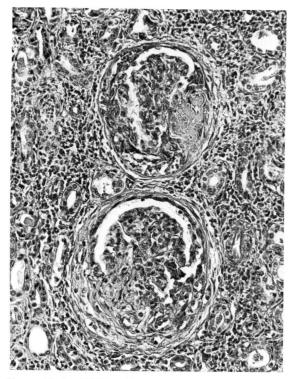

Figure 13–5. RPGN, with extensive obliteration of the glomerular spaces by masses of epithelial cells. The periglomerular interstitial tissue contains a heavy infiltrate of white cells, causing widening of the intertubular spaces.

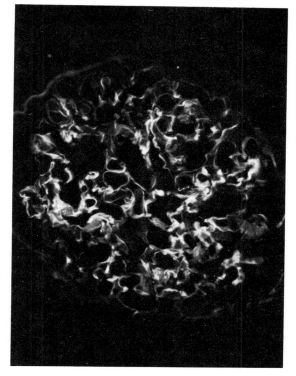

Figure 13–6. The linear immunofluorescent pattern of RPGN produced by anti-GBM antibodies.

the escape of fibrin into Bowman's space which incites the epithelial proliferation (Morita et al., 1973). Necrosis of portions of the glomerular tufts is common. Electron microscopy may, as mentioned, disclose subepithelial deposits, but more often the GBM appears normal. On immunofluorescent microscopy, however, it can be seen that this "normal" GBM contains a linear deposit of IgG, complement and fibrinogen (Fig. 13–6). If the patient survives long enough, the crescents tend to become organized, with eventual total hyalinization of the glomeruli. Rarely, the crescents disappear and the patient recovers (Case Records of the Massachusetts General Hospital, 1975).

Clinical Course. The onset of RPGN is much like that of diffuse PGN, except that the oliguria and azotemia are more pronounced. Some patients begin with a classic history of poststreptococcal GN which fails to resolve within a month or two and progressively worsens over the following weeks. Eventually, nearly all patients become virtually anephric. As mentioned in the discussion of Goodpasture's syndrome, the pulmonary lesions may resolve following bilateral nephrectomy with chronic hemodialysis or renal transplantation.

THE INSIDIOUS ONSET OF UREMIA— CHRONIC GLOMERULONEPHRITIS (CHRONIC GN)

As mentioned in the introductory material to this chapter, in the great majority of cases, life-threatening renal disease does not produce obvious symptoms early in its course, but rather manifests itself by the insidious onset of uremia. Two lesions, *chronic glomerulonephritis* and *chronic pyelonephritis,* are most often responsible. Indeed, it has been reported that approximately 60 per cent of all patients requiring chronic hemodialysis or renal transplantation have the diagnosis of chronic glomerulonephritis. Chronic pyelonephritis is not a glomerular disease, hence will be discussed in a later section.

By the time chronic GN is discovered, the glomerular changes are so far advanced that it is very difficult to discern the nature of the original lesion. Probably it represents the end-stage of a variety of entities. It has been estimated that perhaps 20 per cent of cases of chronic GN stem from diffuse PGN, 30 per cent follow membranous nephropathy and as many as 50 per cent arise totally mysteriously as an apparently primary disease in patients with no history of other renal involvement. Although chronic GN may develop at any age, it is usually first noted in young and middle-aged adults. As might be expected from such diverse etiologies, immunofluorescent studies may show the immune complex pattern of immunoglobulin deposition in some cases and the anti-GBM pattern in others, but in most there are no immune deposits. Whether they were once present and ultimately cleared or whether they were never present is not known.

Morphology. Classically, the kidneys are symmetrically contracted, and their surface is red-brown and diffusely granular, closely resembling advanced BNS (p. 459). Such kidneys weigh about 80 to 90 gm. each. On sectioning, the cortex may be markedly thinned, to 0.5 cm. or less, and the demarcation between cortex and medulla may be largely obliterated.

Microscopically, the feature common to all cases is fibrous scarring of the glomerulus and Bowman's space, sometimes to the point of complete replacement or "hyalinization" of the glomeruli (Fig. 13–7). This obliteration of the glomeruli is the end-point of all cases, and it is impossible to ascertain from such kidneys the nature of the earlier lesion. In some cases, however, particularly with previous biopsies, it is possible to distinguish examples of primary proliferative involvement from the membranous form. Often, there are mixed stigmata, with proliferating endothelial and epithelial cells trapped in reduplicated and exaggerated basement membrane-like material.

The obstruction to blood flow between afferent and efferent arterioles secondary to glomerular damage must of necessity have an impact upon the other elements of the kidney. There is, then, marked interstitial fibrosis, associated with atrophy and replacement of many of the tubules in the cortex. The small and medium-sized arteries are frequently thick-walled, with narrowed lumina, secondary to hypertension as well as to atrophic alterations. Lymphocytic and, rarely, plasma cell infiltrates are present in the interstitial tissue. As damage to all structures progresses it may become difficult to ascertain whether the primary lesion was glomerular, vascular or interstitial. For this reason, such markedly damaged kidneys are designated "end stage kidneys."

Clinical Course. Most often chronic GN develops insidiously and is discovered only late in its course, after the onset of renal insufficiency. Very frequently, renal disease is first suspected with the discovery of proteinuria, hypertension or azotemia on routine medical examination. In some patients the course is punctuated by transient episodes of either the nephritic or the nephrotic syndrome. Some of these may seek medical attention for their edema. As the glomeruli become obliterated, the avenue for protein loss is progressively closed and the nephrotic syndrome thus becomes less common with more advanced disease. Some degree of proteinuria, however, is constant in all cases. Hypertension is very common and, when severe, augurs a poor prognosis. Although microscopic hematuria is usually present, grossly bloody urine is infrequent.

The prognosis is poor, with relentless progression to uremia and death the rule. The rate of progression is extremely variable, however, and 10 years or more may elapse between onset of the first symptoms and death. As mentioned, an overview of the glomerular diseases is presented in Table 13–2.

INTERSTITIAL NEPHRITIS (PYELONEPHRITIS)

Interstitial nephritis refers to inflammatory disease of the kidneys which is most prominent in the interstitium and tubules. The glomeruli may be spared altogether, or secondarily affected only very late in the course. In

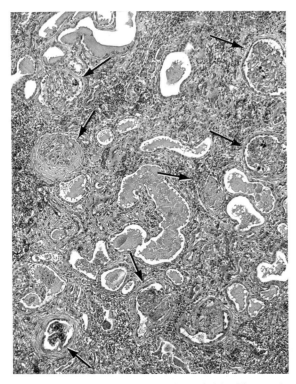

Figure 13–7. Chronic glomerulonephritis. The markedly damaged glomeruli (arrows) show varying stages of obliteration, to the point at which they are difficult to distinguish from the background interstitial fibrosis. There is marked tubular atrophy and distortion, and many tubules contain heavy protein casts.

TABLE 13–2. GLOMERULAR DISEASES

CLINICAL PRESENTATION	LESION	ETIOLOGY	IMMUNOLOGY	HISTOPATHOLOGY	PROGNOSIS
Nephrotic Syndrome	Minimal Change Disease	?	None known	Loss of foot processes	Excellent; 10-year survival over 90%
	Membranous Nephropathy	Idiopathic; tumor antigens; SLE; drugs; hepatitis B; other viruses	Immune complex disease; epi- and intramembranous deposits IgG and C′	Thickening of GBM with "spike and dome" pattern of immune deposits	Fair; 10-year survival in adults 40%, in children 90%
	Focal Glomerulosclerosis	?	Variable; often IgM and C′ in mesangium	Focal and segmental hyalinization of glomerular tufts	Fair; 10-year survival about 50%
	Membranoproliferative GN (Hypocomplementemic)	?	Variable; C′3 in mesangium and GBM; sometimes immunoglobulins	Proliferation of mesangial cells with interposition of mesangial matrix in GBM ("tram-track" appearance)	Fair; 10-year survival about 40%
Nephritic Syndrome	Diffuse PGN	Nephritogenic streptococci; SLE; viruses; infective endocarditis; polyarteritis nodosa; idiopathic	Usually immune complex disease; subepithelial or subendothelial deposits; IgG, IgA, IgM, C′	Proliferation of mesangial and endothelial cells; neutrophilic infiltrate	Variable; depending on cause; 10-year survival range 50 to 95%.
	Focal GN	Berger's disease; Henoch-Schönlein purpura; polyarteritis; infective endocarditis; Wegener's granulomatosis; idiopathic	Usually immune complex disease; IgA in mesangium	Focal and segmental proliferation of mesangial cells, sometimes endothelial cells	Variable, depending on cause; usually excellent
	RPGN	Idiopathic; Goodpasture's syndrome; progression of diffuse PGN	Usually anti-GBM disease; linear IgG, C′ and fibrinogen; sometimes immune complex disease	Epithelial "crescents" in 70% of glomeruli; proliferation all elements; fibrin deposition	Poor; death in weeks to months, unless dialysis or transplantation
Insidious Onset of Uremia	Chronic GN	Idiopathic; progression of membranous nephropathy or diffuse PGN	Variable; sometimes immune complex or anti-GBM disease	Hyalinization of all glomeruli	Fair to poor; may be survival for several years

most cases of interstitial nephritis, the renal pelvis is prominently involved, hence the more descriptive term *pyelonephritis* (pyelo = pelvis). However, a confusing situation has arisen in which the term pyelonephritis is often applied only to those cases of bacterial origin, while the term interstitial nephritis is reserved for the others. This usage seems to us ill-advised for two reasons: first, in a great many instances, it is not known whether the disease is bacterial or not; and second, it carries the implication that lesions not caused by bacteria do not involve the renal pelves. As we shall see in the discussion of analgesic abuse, this clearly is not the case. Therefore, in this chapter we shall speak of pyelonephritis as an anatomic entity which may have a number of causes.

Pyelonephritis may be either acute or chronic. The acute form is relatively benign. It almost always represents a bacterial infection, although viral etiologies have been proposed (Editorial, 1974a). Chronic pyelonephritis, on the other hand, is one of the more treacherous of renal diseases in that it often leads to renal failure without producing any symptoms until renal function is markedly impaired. The role of bacteria as a cause of chronic pyelonephritis is controversial; however, most would agree that there are a significant number of cases which may not be bacterial.

ACUTE PYELONEPHRITIS

Acute pyelonephritis is an extremely common, usually benign, suppurative inflammation of one or both kidneys, usually caused by bacteria. Among clinically significant infections, it is second in frequency only to the respiratory infections (Kleeman et al., 1960). Moreover, it seems likely that an additional large number of cases go unrecognized, manifested only by asymptomatic bacteriuria. (Bacteriuria is considered "significant" when there are more than 10^5 bacteria per milliliter of urine; numbers below this are likely to represent contamination of the specimen.)

Etiology and Pathogenesis. Infection of the kidney is usually caused by bacteria ascending from the lower urinary tract or adjacent lymph nodes (Vivaldi et al., 1959). However, acute pyelonephritis may occasionally result from bacteremia with seeding of the kidneys. This is particularly likely when there is some ureteral obstruction, such as a renal stone. The principal causative organisms are the enteric gram-negative rods. By far the most common etiologic agent is *Escherichia coli.* Other important organisms when there is obstruction are *Proteus vulgaris, Pseudomonas aeruginosa, Klebsiella pneumoniae,* the enterococci and the hemolytic staphylococci. Ordinarily, bladder urine is sterile, despite the presence of bacteria in the distal urethra, and tends to remain so because of antimicrobial properties of the bladder mucosa, principally its elaboration of IgA. The periodic emptying of the bladder also serves to eliminate bacteria as well as to bring any remaining organisms into contact with the hostile bladder mucosa. However, the urine itself represents an excellent culture medium. Thus, *the inadvertent introduction into the bladder of large numbers of organisms during catheterization or other urinary tract instrumentation may overwhelm the natural defense mechanisms.* In addition, partial urinary obstruction with stasis of urine is an important predisposing factor. When stasis occurs bacteria may multiply in peace, without being unceremoniously flushed out or destroyed by the bladder wall. Accordingly, acute pyelonephritis is particularly frequent among patients with some degree of urinary tract obstruction, such as may occur with benign prostatic hypertrophy or in pregnancy. It is also common in young women, in whom partial obstruction may result from urethral edema secondary to trauma, the basis for the so-called "honeymoon cystitis." There is some controversy over whether urinary stasis or obstruction is a necessary factor or merely a contributory one in so-called "ascending" pyelonephritis. Certainly not all cases of acute pyelonephritis involve mechanical obstruction. Perhaps functional obstruction, e.g., incompetence of the physiologic sphincter at the ureterovesical junction with consequent reflux

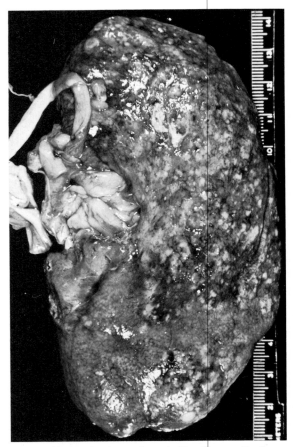

Figure 13–8. Acute pyelonephritis. The cortical surface is studded with focal pale abscesses, more numerous in the upper pole and midregion of the kidney; the lower pole is relatively unaffected. Between the abscesses there is dark congestion of the renal substance.

(*vesicoureteric reflux, VUR*), may be present. More will be said about this important subject in the discussion of chronic pyelonephritis.

Morphology. The affected kidney or kidneys may be normal in size or somewhat enlarged. **Characteristically, discrete, yellowish, raised abscesses are grossly apparent on the renal surface** (Fig. 13–8). They may be widely scattered or limited to one region of the kidney, or they may coalesce, to form a single large area of suppuration. Rarely, the entire kidney is converted into one large suppurative mass. In the usual presentation, the abscesses are most prominent in the cortex. In the typical case, renal pelvic changes are not marked. However, hyperemia, granularity of the pelvic mucosa or even suppuration is occasionally present.

The pathognomonic histologic feature of acute pyelonephritis is suppurative necrosis or abscess formation within the renal substance. In the early stages, the suppurative infiltrate is limited to the interstitial tissue, but later, abscess formation causes tubular destruction. Large masses of neutrophils frequently extend along involved nephrons into the collecting ducts, giving rise to the characteristic white cell casts found in the urine. Typically, the glomeruli appear to be rather resistant to the infection, and often abscesses surround glomeruli without actually invading them.

When the element of obstruction is prominent, particularly when the obstruction is high in the urinary tract, the suppurative exudate may be unable to drain and thus fills the renal pelvis, calyces and ureter, producing **pyonephrosis.** Not only is the infection, then, more serious, but renal damage from hydronephrosis also occurs (see p. 455).

A second and, fortunately, infrequent special form of pyelonephritic involvement is necrosis of the renal papillae, known as **necrotizing papillitis.** This is particularly common among diabetics who develop acute pyelonephritis, and also with the chronic interstitial nephritis associated with analgesic abuse (p. 444). It may also complicate acute pyelonephritis when there is significant urinary tract obstruction. This lesion consists of a combination of ischemic and suppurative necrosis of the tips of the renal pyramids (renal papillae). It is thought that this peculiar pattern of pyelonephritis is based on acute inflammatory, edematous embarrassment of the blood supply to the papillae. **The pathognomonic gross feature of necrotizing papillitis is gray-white to yellow necrosis of the apical two-thirds of the pyramids.** This is usually sharply defined from the preserved basal portion by a narrow zone of hyperemia. One, several or all papillae may be affected. Microscopically, the papillary tips show characteristic coagulative necrosis. There is no inflammatory infiltrate within the necrotic tips, and the leukocytic response is limited to the junction between preserved and destroyed tissue. Large masses of proliferating bacteria are sometimes found within the acellular necrotic foci.

When the bladder is involved in a urinary tract infection, as it often is, **acute** or **chronic cystitis** results. In long-standing cases associated with obstruction, the bladder may be grossly hypertrophied, with trabeculation of its walls, or it may be thinned and markedly distended from retention of urine. In the early stages, the mucosal wall is merely hyperemic. Later, the normal velvety mucosa is replaced by a friable, granular and hemorrhagic surface which may contain many shallow ulcers filled with suppurative exudate. Severe progressive infection may lead to sloughing of large areas of the mucosa. Perforation through the bladder wall with extension to perivesical structures occasionally occurs. The histologic changes are those expected of a nonspecific acute or chronic inflammation. The inflammatory infiltrate is usually but not necessarily confined to the tunica propria of the mucosa. With chronicity, fibrous thickening and rigidity of the bladder wall commonly develop.

Clinical Course. When uncomplicated acute pyelonephritis is clinically apparent, the onset is usually sudden, with pain at the costovertebral angle and systemic evidence of infection, such as chills, fever and malaise. Urinary findings include pyuria and bacteriuria. In addition, there are usually indications of bladder and urethral irritation, i.e., dysuria, frequency and urgency. Functional abnormalities are typically slight and transient, although anuria may occur in severe cases. Even without antibiotic treatment, the disease tends to be benign and self-limited. The symptomatic phase of the disease usually lasts no longer than a week, although bacteriuria may persist much longer (Bailey et al., 1969). Nevertheless, single episodes of uncomplicated acute pyelonephritis have been known to produce irreversible renal damage, and in cases involving predisposing influences, the disease may become recurrent or chronic, leading eventually to serious chronic pyelonephritis.

The development of necrotizing papillitis greatly worsens the prognosis. These patients show evidence of overwhelming sepsis. When the involvement is unilateral, nephrectomy may be necessary. Bilateral necrotizing papillitis is usually, but not invariably, fatal.

The significance of *asymptomatic* significant bacteriuria is controversial. Although this is very uncommon in males, it is present in 3 to 5 per cent of females. The prevalence rises with age, being about 1 per cent at the age of 5 years. During pregnancy, the prevalence may be as high as 13 per cent (Norden and Kass, 1968). Many believe that in the absence of obstruction, asymptomatic bacteriuria in nonpregnant women may be entirely benign (Asscher, 1974; Editorial, 1974b). However, in childhood it may signify important disease. Pregnant women with bacteriuria have been reported to have an increased frequency of premature births and their infants have been said to show a higher rate of perinatal mortality. These findings are difficult to evaluate, particularly in view of the known influence of socioeconomic factors on both the prevalence of bacteriuria and of perinatal mortality. What can be said with some assurance is that about 20 per cent of pregnant women with asymptomatic bacteriuria develop symptomatic acute pyelonephritis later during the pregnancy, and that eradication of the bacteriuria prevents this (Asscher, 1974).

CHRONIC PYELONEPHRITIS (CHRONIC PN)

The constellation of changes known as chronic PN is second only to chronic glomerulonephritis as a cause of death from renal failure. This form of chronic renal disease is more often encountered in patients suffering from some form of urinary tract obstruction, as with prostatic enlargement or renal stones, and in this setting it is referred to as obstructive chronic pyelonephritis. The condition may also occur in patients free of obstructive disease (nonobstructive chronic pyelonephritis). The obstructive pattern usually represents a persistent or recurrent bacterial infection, having its origin in an earlier attack of acute pyelonephritis. The etiology of the nonobstructive variant is more controversial. Most probably it represents a heterogeneous group of disorders, as discussed below.

Etiology and Pathogenesis. Until recently, it was assumed that nonobstructive chronic PN simply represented smoldering bacterial infection of one or both kidneys. This is no longer accepted dogma, and the issue now is controversial. The basis for the controversy is the extremely poor correlation between demonstrable past or present bacterial infection and the anatomic lesion known as chronic PN (Angell et al., 1968). Although this may in part reflect the fact that the anatomic diagnosis must be based on a composite of nonspecific changes and may often be made too loosely, misdiagnosis does not alone account for the lack of bacteriologic findings. Three explanations have been offered. The first suggests that the bacterial infection is recurrent rather than continuous, and that renal damage occurs stepwise over a long period of time, during which random urine cultures may be negative for bacteria. A second theory postulates that an earlier bacterial infection may *indirectly* lead to chronic PN through persistence of bacterial antigen or through conversion of the causative organisms to protoplasts, which theoretically could survive indefinitely in the hyperosmolar milieu of the renal medulla. Using immunofluorescent techniques, Aoki and his colleagues (1969) reported the presence of bacterial antigen in most cases of "abacterial" as well as known bacterial chronic PN. However, other workers have been unable to confirm these findings (Schwartz and Cotran, 1973). Moreover, experimental studies with animals would suggest that antigen persisting after eradication of infection is not associated with progressive disease and, indeed, is gradually cleared (Cotran, 1963). Finally, it has recently been hypothesized that in a significant number of instances the disease arises, without antecedent infection, from unknown *nonbacterial* causes. Since virus is readily recoverable from the urine in a number of viral diseases, it has been suggested that repeated or recurrent viral infection may underlie some cases of chronic

PN. However, although logical, this is merely speculative (Editorial, 1974a).

One well-established nonbacterial cause of chronic PN is the long-term ingestion of large doses of certain analgesics (*analgesic nephropathy*). This drug-associated lesion probably begins in the papillae and is usually accompanied by necrotizing papillitis (see p. 443), although this is not an invariable or distinguishing feature. Since most patients who develop this lesion have taken mixtures of both phenacetin and aspirin, there is still some disagreement as to which drug is the culprit. Animal studies indicate that aspirin is probably the major offender (Nanra and Kincaid-Smith, 1970), but most agree that drug mixtures are more dangerous than either drug alone (Editorial, 1973a). In a large study of analgesic nephropathy, it was found that 84 of 86 patients had taken a mixture of phenacetin and aspirin; the remaining two had taken only aspirin. The total dose required to produce disease was enormous, ranging from 2 to 51 kg of phenacetin plus 2 to 69 kg of aspirin, ingested over a period averaging 16 years (Murray, 1971).

In recent years it has become evident that nonobstructive chronic PN is also often associated with a functional derangement of the vesicoureteric junction which results in reflux of urine toward the kidney (*vesicoureteric reflux, VUR*) (Hodson and Wilson, 1965). This form of chronic PN is thought to begin in early childhood, when there may be actual reflux within the kidney itself. The lesion in these cases is sometimes termed *reflux nephropathy*, but it is indistinguishable from chronic PN. It has been suggested that this back pressure may produce scarring of the kidney in the absence of infection (Editorial, 1974c). However, there is frequently accompanying bacteriuria, and it is difficult to say whether the infection is of secondary or primary importance in producing the lesion.

Morphology. One or both kidneys may be involved, either diffusely or patchily. When the involvement is diffuse, an irregularly contracted or sometimes a fairly uniformly small, granular kidney is produced. **Even when involvement is bilateral, the kidneys are not equally damaged and therefore are not equally contracted. This uneven scarring is useful in differentiating chronic PN from the causes of more symmetrically contracted kidneys, namely, BNS and chronic GN.** Moreover, pyelonephritic kidneys may weigh less than 50 gm. each, and such extreme reduction in renal weight is rarely caused by the other two lesions. With these severely shrunken kidneys there is atrophy or blunting of the papillae and a marked increase of peripelvic fat, replacing the atrophic parenchyma.

As mentioned earlier, the microscopic changes are largely nonspecific, and many similar alterations may be seen with other disorders, such as hypokalemia or ischemia from any cause. The term "pyelonephritis" means, literally, inflammation of the kidney and its pelvis, and the presence of inflammatory changes in the pelvic wall with papillary atrophy and blunting is a sine qua non for the diagnosis and the differentiation of chronic pyelonephritis from other forms of chronic renal disease. Heptinstall (1969) has emphasized the diagnostic importance of finding such fibrosis in the calyceal fornices, blunting or atrophy of the papillae and a layer of chronic inflammatory cells beneath the papillary epithelium. In addition, the parenchyma shows: (1) Uneven interstitial fibrosis and an inflammatory infiltrate of lymphocytes, plasma cells and occasionally neutrophils. The presence of large numbers of neutrophils distinguishes the "active" disease from the "inactive" or "healed" form, but it is doubtful whether this distinction is clinically useful. (2) Dilatation or contraction of tubules, with atrophy of the lining epithelium. Many of the dilated tubules contain pink to blue glassy-appearing casts known as "colloid casts," which suggest the appearance of thyroid tissue, hence the descriptive term "thyroidization" of the kidney. Often neutrophils are seen within the tubules. (3) Concentric fibrosis about the parietal layer of Bowman's capsule, termed periglomerular fibrosis. (4) Vascular changes similar to those of benign or malignant arteriolosclerosis (Fig. 13–9).

Clinical Course. Most patients with chronic pyelonephritis come to medical attention relatively late in the course of their disease because of the gradual onset of renal insufficiency or because signs of kidney disease are noticed on routine laboratory tests. Often the renal disease is first heralded by the development of hypertension. Mild proteinuria is typical, but proteinuria sufficient to be associated with the nephrotic syndrome is rare. With analgesic nephropathy, there may be sudden pain and hematuria due to impaction of sloughed necrotic papillae within a ureter (Editorial, 1973a). Pyelograms are characteristic and therefore are important in confirming the diagnosis; they show the affected kidney to be asymmetrically contracted, with some degree of blunting and deformity of the calyceal system (caliectasis). The presence or absence of significant bacteriuria is not particularly helpful diagnostically. Its absence should certainly not be taken to rule out chronic pyelonephritis. If the disease is bilateral and progressive, tubular dysfunction occurs early, followed ultimately by glomerular damage, with consequent azotemia. Death usually results from uremia. When the lesion is associated with analgesic abuse, cessation of

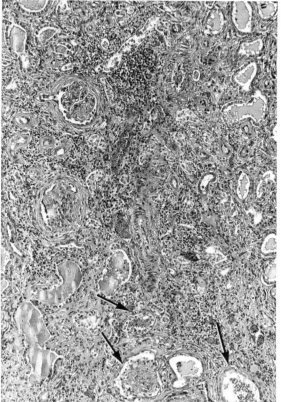

Figure 13–9. Chronic pyelonephritis, with marked distortion of the renal architecture. The two glomeruli on the left show extensive periglomerular fibrosis. There is an intense interstitial, mixed leukocyte infiltrate and several of the tubules (arrows) contain white cell and protein casts. Other tubules contain "colloid casts."

the drugs is usually but not always followed by considerable improvement in renal function (Murray et al., 1971).

ACUTE RENAL FAILURE

The three lesions discussed below (acute tubular necrosis, renal cortical necrosis and the hepatorenal syndrome) invariably produce acute renal failure. Acute tubular necrosis (ATN) and cortical necrosis typically follow some other profound medical crisis, such as septicemia, shock or a widespread burn. The hepatorenal syndrome is associated with hepatic failure. Although renal failure may in rare instances be very transient and self-limited, it usually represents a perilous medical situation, persisting after successful treatment of the precipitating event. However, with ATN, appropriate treatment permits full recovery.

For the first few days, the only indication of

renal failure may be oliguria, defined as a daily urine output of less than 400 ml. During this time, the clinical picture is usually dominated by the insult which precipitated the renal lesion. This is not always the case, however. Not infrequently, ATN occurs in patients who seem to be only mildly ill and who have not had any dramatic precipitating event. In either case, the inability of the kidneys to carry out their functions becomes manifest in two or three days; the signs and symptoms of uremia develop rapidly, in hours to days, rather than over the course of months to years, as is characteristic of chronic renal failure.

Cortical necrosis, unlike ATN, is irreversible, hence its implications are far more grave. However, both conditions may represent different degrees of response to essentially the same type of injury. As will be seen below, in neither case is the pathogenesis clear, but the initial insult to the kidneys is probably ischemia, possibly from vascular shunting, possibly as a result of microthrombi formation in the small vessels.

As was mentioned previously, acute diffuse PGN, RPGN and occasionally acute pyelonephritis may also cause acute renal failure. With these lesions, the functional impairment of the kidney stems from the presence of an acute inflammatory reaction with edema.

ACUTE TUBULAR NECROSIS (ATN)

Acute tubular necrosis is a reversible renal lesion which arises in a variety of diverse clinical settings and causes acute renal failure. The great majority of these clinical settings, ranging from severe trauma to acute pancreatitis to septicemia, have in common a period of inadequate blood flow to the peripheral organs, usually accompanied by marked hypotension. A virtually identical lesion may be produced by certain poisons, massive hemolytic crises (e.g., transfusion reactions) and crushing injuries. Recently it has been observed that methoxyflurane (Penthrane), commonly used as an anesthetic, may cause ATN (Hollenberg et al., 1972). Because of the many precipitating factors, ATN occurs very frequently. Moreover, its reversibility gives it added clinical importance, since proper management means the difference between full recovery and virtually certain death.

Pathogenesis. Regardless of the fact that nearly any medical, surgical or obstetric calamity may produce ATN, there are probably only two basic pathogenetic pathways, each of which in turn results in severe damage to the tubular epithelium. The first and most important of these pathways involves diminished renal blood flow secondary to a generalized drop in blood pressure or decrease in the effective circulating blood volume which induces the clinical syndrome known as shock (p. 213). Because the epithelial cells of the renal tubules, particularly those in the proximal segments, are exquisitely vulnerable to ischemia, they are damaged to a variable extent, while the remainder of the kidney is apparently unchanged. When ATN is produced by the ingestion of poisons, such as mercury or carbon tetrachloride, the pathogenetic pathway is slightly different. In these cases, the effect on the tubular epithelium is direct, produced by contact with the poison as it is excreted in the urine, rather than being mediated through hypoperfusion. In either case, the major damage is to the tubular epithelium. The manner in which such tubular damage produces acute renal failure, persisting even after the return to normal of the blood pressure, is unclear. One theory postulates mechanical obstruction of the tubules, with a concomitant impairment of glomerular filtration caused by the back pressure. Such mechanical obstruction is thought to result from several factors. It has been hypothesized that escape of urine through the damaged tubular epithelium into the interstitium elevates intrarenal pressure and causes collapse of the tubules. In addition, swelling of tubular cells, along with plugging of the tubules by casts of necrotic epithelial cells and debris, may contribute to obstruction of the lumina. Supporting the concept of such tubular obstruction is the frequent association of ATN with hemoglobinuria and myoglobinuria. However, even in these cases, the hemoglobin or myoglobin casts are found only in scattered tubules. If mechanical obstruction were indeed the only explanation for the acute renal failure, one would expect to find casts uniformly throughout the kidneys, as well as an increase in intrarenal pressure. Experiments have shown that, contrary to expectations, there is no rise in interstitial pressure; if anything, there is a decrease in such pressure. More recently, attention has been focused on a selective decrease in renal cortical blood flow which occurs during ATN. This probably reflects an intrarenal vasomotor abnormality. It has been suggested that there is intense vasoconstriction of the afferent arterioles, perhaps mediated by the renin-angiotensin system (p. 457). In addition, intravascular coagulation within the glomeruli has been described and may contribute to the decreased glomerular filtration (Clarkson et al., 1970). It must be emphasized that despite a plethora of attractive theories, the pathophysiology of the renal failure of ATN is obscure. Most likely, the full-blown disorder results from the operation of several synergistic factors rather than just one (Harrington and Cohen, 1975).

Morphology. The morphologic changes in the hypotensive form of ATN were described on page 216. The major features include the following: Microscopically, the most striking finding is the presence of patchily distributed hemoglobin pigment casts in the tubules. These casts are usually granular and amorphous, but occasionally they take on a densely coagulated appearance. With routine stains, they usually appear orange to red-brown. Special stains reveal the presence of hemoglobin. When crushing injuries have induced ATN, the casts are composed of myoglobin, indistinguishable from hemoglobin in tissue sections. The epithelial cells surrounding the casts may show necrosis or degeneration. An interstitial inflammatory reaction composed of polymorphonuclear leukocytes, lymphocytes and plasma cells often appears in these areas. In addition, there is usually a generalized interstitial edema.

The basic ischemic tubular changes, which are thought to represent the initial alterations, vary from patient to patient and also within the same organ. They run the gamut of cloudy swelling, fatty change, frank necrosis and even complete disruption of the tubule with its basement membrane, referred to as **tubulorrhexis**. These changes show a haphazard distribution, which is thought to reflect the unpredictable patterns of vasoconstrictive ischemia. Two features differentiate nephrotoxic ATN from the ischemic pattern: the tubular basement membranes are preserved, and generally the distal tubular segments of the nephron are spared.

If the patient survives for a week, epithelial regeneration becomes apparent in the form of mitotic activity in the persisting tubular epithelial cells. Except where the basement membrane is destroyed, regeneration is total and complete. Morphologic examination after recovery shows no evidence of previous nephropathy.

Clinical Course. The clinical course of ATN from the time of the precipitating event may be divided into four phases. The initial phase, lasting for about 36 hours, is usually dominated by the inciting medical, surgical or obstetric event. Although hypotension or frank shock is often a part of the picture at this stage, many patients with no apparent drop in blood pressure go on to develop ATN. Whether these patients have had transient episodes of hypotension that escaped notice is not clear. Conceivably, intrarenal shunting of the blood flow to the kidneys had occurred. The only indication of renal involvement during this initial phase is a decline in urine output with a rise in BUN. At this point, oliguria could be explained on the basis of a transient decrease in blood flow to the kidneys.

The second and most important phase begins anywhere from the second to the sixth day. Urine output falls dramatically, usually to between 50 and 400 ml. per day. Sometimes it declines to only a few milliliters per day, but complete anuria is rare. Oliguria may last only a few days, or it may persist as long as three weeks. The usual length of this phase is about 10 days. Since blood pressure is by now normal or high, the scanty urine output cannot be explained on a hemodynamic basis. The clinical picture is dominated by the signs and symptoms of uremia and fluid overload. In the absence of careful supportive treatment and dialysis, most patients can be expected to die during this phase. With good care, however, survival is the rule.

The third or diuretic phase is ushered in by a steady increase in urine volume, reaching up to about 3 liters per day over the course of a few days. Because tubular function is still deranged, serious electrolyte imbalances may occur during this phase. There also appears to be an increased vulnerability to infections. For these reasons, about 25 per cent of deaths from ATN occur during the diuretic phase.

During the fourth and final phase, there is a progressive return of the patient's well-being. Urine volume returns to normal. However, subtle functional impairment of the kidneys, particularly of the tubules, may persist for months. With modern methods of care, patients who do not succumb to the underlying precipitating problem have a 90 to 95 per cent chance of recovering from ATN.

DIFFUSE CORTICAL NECROSIS

This is an infrequent lesion which in about 50 per cent of cases follows the obstetric emergency, premature separation of the placenta (abruptio placentae). Another 30 per cent of cases occur as a complication of septic shock (Matlin and Gary, 1974). In addition, diffuse cortical necrosis may occur in the setting of nearly any medical, surgical or obstetric calamity, and in this respect, it is similar to ATN. In sharp contrast to ATN, however, cortical necrosis is irreversible. At one time, this condition was thought to be invariably fatal, but recently it has been appreciated that patchy involvement of the cortices may occur, and this is compatible with survival.

Pathogenesis. The same etiologic factors that cause ischemic ATN may also lead to cortical necrosis, and it is possible that in these instances both result from varying degrees of renal ischemia. With relatively mild ischemia, only the tubular cells are affected, and ATN ensues. On the other hand, with severe or long-standing ischemia, not only the tubular cells but all elements of the more vulnerable cortex are affected, and diffuse coagulative necrosis of the cortices occurs. Intermediate reductions in renal blood flow may lead to patchy cortical necrosis. The primary cause of impaired blood flow to the renal cortices is not clear, and it may vary from case to case. In many instances, renal ischemia is simply the result of generalized hypotension. In addition, however, intravascular coagulation within the interlobular and afferent arterioles is a necessary component of cortical necrosis (Matlin and Gary, 1974). This is most marked when the underlying disorder is an obstetric complication. Possibly the intravascular coagulation results from hypotension and stasis; in other instances, it may be primary and may itself lead to ischemia. (Reference should be made to the discussion of disseminated intravascular coagulation [DIC] on page 363.) Local vasoconstriction or intrarenal shunting may play a role in cortical necrosis. Experimental models of this lesion can be produced by all these methods. Conceivably these pathogenetic pathways are simultaneously operative when cortical necrosis follows premature separation of the placenta, since there is an especially marked association between this obstetric emergency and cortical necrosis.

Morphology. The gross alterations of massive ischemic infarction of the parenchyma are sharply limited to the cortex. On external examination, the kidney is usually enlarged and the surface has a variegated color of marked congestion and hemorrhage, interspersed with pale, yellow-white, irregular areas of infarction. On sectioning, these changes are seen to be limited to the cortex and more or less completely spare the medulla.

The histologic appearance is that of acute ischemic infarction. Rarely, there may be areas of apparently better preserved cortex. At the deeper levels, the areas in contact with the preserved medulla, there is usually a massive leukocytic infiltration. Intravascular thromboses may be prominent, and occasionally acute necroses of small arterioles and capillaries are present. Hemorrhages occur into the glomeruli, together with precipitation of fibrinoid material. In the uncommon instances of survival, calcification of necrotic areas occurs, along with scarring and shrinkage of the kidney.

Clinical Course. The onset of cortical necrosis is similar to that of ATN. Urine output falls, reaching oliguric levels within a day or two. In contrast to ATN, cortical necrosis frequently is characterized by complete anuria (Hamburger and Walsh, 1968). However, more often urine output is in the range of 50 to 100 ml. daily. The clinical picture is that of uremia, and unless the patient is dialyzed, death ensues within days. With dialysis, life may be prolonged for months, but since the lesion is irreversible, recovery cannot be expected. Occasionally, when the involvement is patchy, renal function returns and the patient survives. In these cases, the kidney is scarred, with areas of necrosis visible on x-ray as spotty calcifications.

HEPATORENAL SYNDROME

Until recently, the very existence of the hepatorenal syndrome as a distinct entity was questioned, with many workers insisting that it was simply ATN occurring in a patient with hepatic failure. However, it now seems clear that the hepatorenal syndrome is a specific cause of acute renal failure, which must be distinguished from ATN and cortical necrosis. In contrast to the latter two lesions, this syndrome is a clinical and not a morphologic diagnosis (Koppel et al., 1969). The kidneys appear entirely normal, and the renal shutdown is on a purely functional basis. In part, therefore, the diagnosis is one of exclusion and can be made with certainty only when acute renal failure occurs in a patient with liver disease and with histologically normal kidneys.

The pathogenesis of the renal involvement in the hepatorenal syndrome is unclear, but it seems to be related to the development of shunts within the kidneys, causing blood to bypass the cortices. Such vasospastic changes have been demonstrated by angiography (Epstein et al., 1970). Possibly the inability of the failing liver to clear endotoxins from the portal circulation plays a causative role, since endotoxin has known vasoconstrictor properties (Wilkinson et al., 1974). Alternatively, it has been suggested that an imbalance between the hepatic supply of angiotensinogen (renin substrate) and the renal release of renin may underlie the derangement (Iwatsuki et al., 1973). In any case, the onset of the hepatorenal syndrome is often triggered by sudden hemodynamic changes, such as those brought about by paracentesis or gastrointestinal bleeding. The onset is sudden, marked by oliguria with a rapidly rising BUN. The prognosis is extremely poor. Recovery is rare and occurs only with improvement of hepatic function. The kidneys remain morphologically normal and have been shown to be suitable for use as donor organs in renal transplantation.

TUMORS

Many types of benign and malignant tumors occur in the urinary tract. In general, benign tumors such as small (rarely over 2.5 cm. in diameter) cortical adenomas or medullary fibromas (interstitial cell tumors) are trivial and without clinical significance. The most common malignant tumor of the kidney is the renal cell carcinoma, followed in frequency by Wilms' tumors and by primary tumors of the calyces and pelves. Other types of renal cancer are extremely rare and need not be discussed here. Tumors of the lower urinary tract are about twice as common as renal cell carcinomas, and are described at the end of this section.

RENAL CELL CARCINOMA

Renal cell carcinoma is the type of neoplasm usually meant by the term "cancer of the kidney." It represents 80 to 90 per cent of all malignant tumors of the kidney and 2 per cent of all cancers. These lesions are most common in late middle age, from the fifth to seventh decades, and males are affected twice as often as females. Although no neoplasm has an absolutely predictable course, *the renal cell carcinoma distinguishes itself by being especially variable in its behavior.* Because of a histologic similarity between the cells of this tumor and normal adrenal cells, it was once thought that the renal cell carcinoma arose from adrenal rests within the kidney, hence the well entrenched misnomer "hypernephroma." However, this view has been discarded.

Morphology. These cancers are usually large by the time they are discovered, and appear as spherical masses 3 to 15 cm. in diameter. Usually they occupy one pole of the kidney, most often the upper one. The cut surface is yellow-gray-white, with prominent areas of cystic softening or of hemorrhage, either fresh or old (Fig. 13—10). The margins of the tumor are well defined, giving a false impression of encapsulation. This appearance results from its characteristic expansile type of growth, which compresses the renal parenchyma rather than infiltrating it. However, at times small processes project into the surrounding parenchyma, and small satellite nodules are found in the surrounding substance, providing clear evidence of the aggressiveness of these lesions. As the tumor enlarges, it may fungate through the walls of the collecting system, extending through the calyces and pelvis as far as the ureter. Even more frequently, the tumor invades the renal vein and grows as a solid column within this vessel, sometimes extending in snakelike fashion as far as the inferior vena cava and even into the right side of the heart. Occasionally there is direct invasion into the perinephric fat and adrenal gland.

It has been the practice to classify renal cell carcinomas histologically either on the basis of the degree of cell vacuolation or on the basis of the arrangement of the cells. Thus, depending on the amount of lipid they contain, the cells may appear almost totally vacuolated, or they may be solid. The classic vacuolated (lipid-laden) or "**clear cells**" are demarcated only by their cell membranes; the nuclei are usually pushed basally and are small and somewhat pyknotic (Fig. 13—11). At the other extreme are the **solid cells**, resembling the tubular epithelium, which have round, small, regular nuclei enclosed within granular pink cytoplasm. These cells may show great regularity of cytologic detail. Some, however, exhibit marked degrees of anaplasia with numerous mitotic figures, and giant cells. Between the extremes of clear cells and solid cells, all intergradations may be found. Cellular arrangement, too, varies widely; the cells may form abortive tubules or papillary

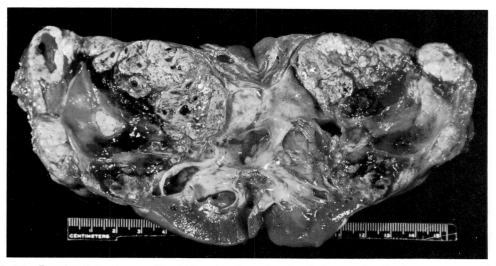

Figure 13—10. Renal cell carcinoma. The kidney has been hemisected, exposing the tumor mass, which totally replaces and expands the upper pole of the kidney. Prominently shown are the areas of necrosis, hemorrhage and cystic softening of the tumor. Only the lower pole of the kidney is recognizable below.

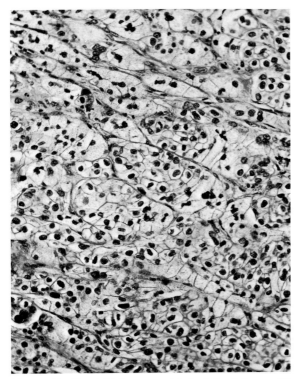

Figure 13–11. A high power detail of the "clear cell" pattern of a renal cell carcinoma.

patterns, or they may cluster in cords or disorganized masses. The stroma is usually scanty but highly vascularized. Despite the existence of distinct cell types and arrangements, classifying tumors on these bases is at best arbitrary and may be misleading, since the tumors in question tend not to be homogeneous, and all variations may be present in any one tumor.

There is no TNM system in widespread use for evaluating the extent of a renal cell carcinoma at diagnosis. It has been suggested that the tumor be classified according to the following stages: (Rubin, 1968).

Stage I: The tumor is entirely intrarenal without invasion of the capsule.

Stage II: There is invasion of the perinephric fat and microscopic evidence of venous and lymphatic involvement.

Stage III: There is gross invasion of the renal vein and the lymph nodes.

Stage IV: Distant metastases are present.

Clinical Course. Renal cell carcinomas have a number of peculiar clinical characteristics that create especially difficult but challenging diagnostic problems. The symptoms vary, but *the most frequent presenting manifestation is hematuria, occurring in somewhat over 50 per cent of cases.* Macroscopic hematuria tends to be intermittent and fleeting, superimposed on a steady microscopic hematuria. In

other patients, the tumor may declare itself simply by virtue of its size, when it has grown large enough to produce flank pain and a palpable mass. By the time this occurs, however, there are usually other extrarenal clues. Among these extrarenal effects are fever and polycythemia, both of which may be associated with a renal cell carcinoma but which, because they are nonspecific, may be misinterpreted for some time before their true significance is appreciated. Fever is present in about 15 per cent of these patients. If symptoms specifically referable to the kidney are not present, the patient may be considered to have a "fever of unknown origin" (FUO). The basis for this pyrexia is unknown. Polycythemia is an interesting but less frequent accompaniment of renal cell carcinoma, affecting about 3 per cent of patients with this disease. It is assumed that the polycythemia results from elaboration of erythropoietin by the renal tumor, but this has not been definitely proved. In a significant number of patients, the primary tumor remains silent and is discovered only after its metastases have evoked symptoms. This tendency for metastases to be discovered before the primary tumor is one of the common characteristics of renal cell carcinoma. The favored locations for metastases are the lungs and the bones, followed by the regional lymph nodes, the liver, the adrenal glands and the brain. In 10 to 15 per cent of cases, the tumor metastasizes to the opposite kidney. It must be apparent that renal cell carcinoma presents with many faces, some quite devious, but *the triad of painless hematuria, long-standing fever and dull flank pain is virtually pathognomonic.*

The overall five-year survival rate is about 37 per cent, but it varies with the size of the tumor on discovery and the presence of local extension or invasion of the renal vein. With Stage I and II disease, five-year survival is nearly 50 per cent; with Stage III and IV disease, on the other hand, it is no better than 10 per cent. Moreover, the five-year survival is a relatively poor indicator of cure with these tumors, because of their extremely bizarre behavior. There are many known cases of metastases lying dormant and unsuspected for up to 20 years after an apparently curative nephrectomy, then suddenly becoming clinically aggressive. Conversely, there are occasional reports of spontaneous disappearance of known metastases after removal of the primary tumor. Not infrequently, when there is only one known metastasis, removal of both the primary tumor and the metastasis produces an apparent cure. In the face of such unpredictability, it is not surprising that these tumors give rise to many diagnostic and prognostic errors.

WILMS' TUMOR

Although Wilms' tumor occurs infrequently in adults, it is the third most common organ cancer in children under the age of 10. Only the lymphoproliferative disorders and the central nervous system tumors cause more cancer deaths in children (Silverberg and Holleb, 1974). These tumors contain a variety of cell and tissue components, all derived from the mesoderm. There is evidence that the vulnerability to Wilms' tumor is in many cases inherited, in the sense that one of the mutations required for its expression is vertically transmitted (Knudson and Strong, 1972).

By the time they are discovered, Wilms' tumors are usually huge spherical masses, dwarfing the kidney. On sectioning, they have a variegated surface, dependent upon the tissue types present. Myxomatous soft fish-flesh areas, solid gray hyaline cartilaginous tissue and areas of hemorrhagic necrosis are the usual components. The aggressive nature of these neoplasms is manifested by their propensity to rupture through the renal capsule and extend locally into the perirenal tissues. Involvement of the other kidney occurs in about 20 per cent of cases.

Histologically, **the characteristic features are primitive or abortive glomeruli, with poorly formed Bowman spaces, and abortive tubules, all enclosed in a spindle cell stroma.** This combination of mesenchymal spindle cells and tubules has caused these tumors to be called adenosarcomas or carcinosarcomas. In addition, striated muscle, smooth muscle, collagenous fibrous tissue, cartilage, bone, fat cells and areas of necrotic tissue containing cholesterol crystals and lipid macrophages may all be seen. The most consistent of these various elements are the striated muscle cells. **The histologic diagnosis rests upon identification of the primitive glomeruli and tubules as well as the strongly supportive evidence of striated muscle fibers.**

Patients usually present with complaints referable to the tumor's enormous size. Commonly there is a readily palpable abdominal mass, which may extend across the midline and down into the pelvis. Less often, the patient presents with fever and abdominal pain, with hematuria or, occasionally, with intestinal obstruction as a result of pressure from the tumor. Until recently, the outlook for these patients was bleak. Now, however, excellent results are obtained with a combination of radiotherapy, nephrectomy and chemotherapy. Two-year survival rates have increased from 40 to as high as 90 per cent in one series, and survival for two years usually implies a cure. These results are all the more remarkable since in many of these patients, pulmonary metastases, present at diagnosis, disappear under the therapeutic regimen.

TUMORS OF THE URINARY COLLECTING SYSTEM (RENAL CALYCES, PELVIS, URETER, BLADDER, AND URETHRA)

Since the entire urinary collecting system from renal pelvis to urethra is lined with transitional epithelium, its epithelial tumors assume similar morphologic patterns. Tumors in the collecting system above the bladder are relatively uncommon; those in the bladder, however, are even more frequent as a cause of death than are kidney tumors. Nevertheless, in the individual case, a small lesion in the ureter, for example, may cause urinary outflow obstruction and have greater clinical significance than a much larger mass in the capacious bladder. We shall consider first the range of anatomic patterns, followed by their clinical implications.

Tumors arising in the collecting system of the urinary tract range from small benign papillomas to large invasive cancers. The papillomas are usually fragile, small (0.2 to 1.0 cm.) frondlike structures, having a delicate fibrovascular axial core covered by multilayered, well differentiated, transitional epithelium. In some of these lesions, the covering epithelium appears as normal as the mucosal surface whence these tumors arise; such lesions are almost invariably noninvasive and benign, and do not recur once removed. Larger papillomas may develop, usually in the bladder, ranging from 1 to 2 cm. in diameter. In these, the epithelium is generally somewhat atypical, with some variability in cell and nuclear size and some disarray in the cells' normal relationships to one another. It is this pattern that is called by some an "atypical transitional cell papilloma," while others call it a transitional cell carcinoma, Grade I. These lesions are rarely invasive, but may recur after removal. Whether the regrowth is a true recurrence or a second primary growth is uncertain. Progressive degrees of cellular atypia and anaplasia are encountered in papillary exophytic growths, accompanied by increase in size of the lesion and evidence of invasion of the submucosal or muscular layers. These tumors are unequivocally transitional cell carcinomas, Grade II or Grade III, depending on the degree of anaplasia and invasiveness. As these cancers approach the Grade III pattern they tend to be flatter than the benign papillomatous forms, to cover larger areas of the mucosal surface, to invade more deeply and to have a shaggier necrotic surface (Fig. 13–12). Some are so anaplastic as to merit the description of undifferentiated carcinoma.

An additional morphologic variation may also appear. Some of the Grades II and III transitional cell carcinomas may develop areas of squamous cell metaplastic differentiation. These lesions too should be classified as Grade II or III transitional cell carcinoma with areas of squamous differentiation. Some prefer to call all such tumors with areas

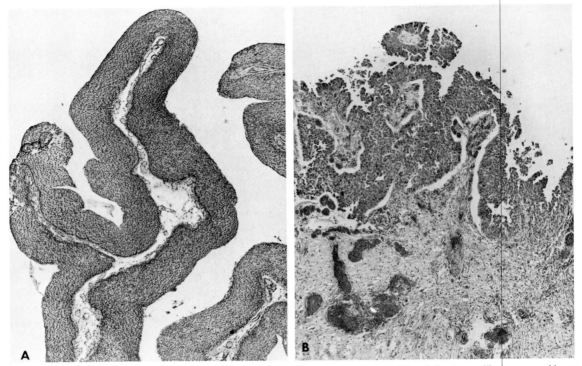

Figure 13–12. *A,* A grade I papillary transitional cell carcinoma of the bladder. The delicate papilla is covered by orderly transitional epithelium. *B,* A grade III transitional cell carcinoma showing the disorderly anaplastic epithelium with superficial invasion of the underlying connective tissue.*

of squamous differentiation squamous or epidermoid cancers, and others reserve these designations for those cancers composed wholly of squamous cells. Whatever the practice, foci of squamous metaplasia within a transitional cell carcinoma do not worsen the prognosis. Indeed, well differentiated pure squamous cell carcinomas have the same biologic behavior as do well differentiated transitional cell carcinomas. Carcinomas of Grades II and III infiltrate surrounding structures, spread to regional nodes and on occasion metastasize widely.

The depth of penetration of invasive lesions constitutes the most important determinant of the chances of successful resection. In particular, those which have invaded the deep musculature of the bladder wall have a very much worse prognosis than do those which have extended only to the superficial musculature. Accordingly, tumors of the bladder are staged by depth of penetration. The most widely used system is that of Jewett and Strong (1946):

Stage O: Carcinoma in situ.
Stage A: Subepithelial infiltration.
Stage B1: Invasion of superficial muscle.
Stage B2: Invasion of deep muscle.
Stage C: Invasion of perivesical fat.
Stage D1: Involvement of regional lymph nodes.
Stage D2: Involvement of periaortic lymph nodes.

From the clinical standpoint, *whatever the level of origin and degree of anaplasia, painless hematuria is the dominant clinical presentation of all of these tumors.* Since most arise in the bladder we shall consider these first. They affect men about twice as frequently as women, and usually develop between the ages of 50 and 70 years. Although the great majority occur in individuals without a known history of exposure to industrial solvents, bladder tumors are 50 times more frequent in those exposed to beta naphthylamine (p. 90). Cigarette smoking, chronic cystitis and schistosomiasis of the bladder are also believed to induce higher attack rates. *The clinical significance of bladder tumors depends on several factors: obviously, on their benign or malignant nature, on their location within the bladder and — most importantly — on the depth of invasion of the lesion.* Save for the clearly benign papillomas, all tend stubbornly to recur after removal, and indeed often become more aggressive with each recurrence. Lesions that invade the ureteral or urethral orifices pose special problems, since they may cause urinary tract obstruction. In general, with shallow lesions, the prognosis after removal is good, but when deep penetration of the bladder wall has occurred, whatever the histologic pattern, the five-year survival rate is less than 20 per cent. Overall five-year survival is 57 per cent (Silverberg and Holleb, 1975).

Although papillary and cancerous neoplasms of the lining epithelium of the collecting system occur much less frequently in the renal pelvis than in the bladder, they nonetheless make up 5 to 10 per cent of primary renal tumors. Painless hematuria is the most characteristic feature of these lesions, but in their critical location they produce costovertebral angle pain as hydronephrosis develops. Infiltration of the walls of the pelvis, calyces and renal vein worsens the prognosis. Despite removal of the tumor by nephrectomy, less than 50 per cent of patients survive for five years. Cancer of the ureter is, fortunately, the rarest of the tumors of the collecting system. Five-year survival is less than 10 per cent (Frank, 1970–71).

URINARY OUTFLOW OBSTRUCTION

Under this heading we discuss three disparate entities which have in common some degree of obstruction to the outflow of urine at some level of the kidney or collecting system. *Urolithiasis* refers to stone formation within the kidney or collecting system. Most uroliths form within the kidney and produce their most serious consequences when they move into the ureter and cause obstruction. *Polycystic kidney disease* is a hereditable anomaly which may be associated with more or less complete intrarenal blockage of outflow from the kidney. In milder cases, however, the principal effect of the disease is destruction of the renal parenchyma rather than obstruction. The third entity discussed under this heading is *hydronephrosis*. By definition, this refers to obstruction at some level of the collecting system, with resultant increased pressures within the kidney.

UROLITHIASIS

Urolithiasis refers to calculus formation at any level within the urinary collecting system, but most commonly within the kidney. It is a frequent disorder, as evidenced by the finding of stones in about 1 per cent of all autopsies. Symptomatic urolithiasis is most common in males. A familial tendency toward stone formation has long been recognized.

Etiology and Pathogenesis. About 65 per cent of renal stones are composed of either calcium oxalate or calcium oxalate mixed with calcium phosphate. Another 15 per cent are composed of magnesium ammonium phosphate, and 10 per cent are either uric acid or cystine stones (Williams, 1974). In all cases, there is almost invariably an organic matrix of mucoprotein making up about 2.5 per cent of the stone by weight.

The cause of stone formation is obscure, particularly in most cases of calcium-containing stones. Probably urolithiasis usually depends on a confluence of predisposing conditions. *The most important is almost certainly an increased urine concentration of the stone's constituents.* Some of the other predisposing conditions will be mentioned later in the discussion. Most patients with calcium stones have hypercalciuria. In a third of them there is hypercalcemia or another discernible cause of hypercalciuria (Coe and Kavalach, 1974). These cases include hyperparathyroidism, Cushing's syndrome, diffuse bone disease, immobilization, vitamin D intoxication, sarcoidosis, the milk-alkali syndrome and renal tubular acidosis. *However, most cases of calcium stones are associated with idiopathic hypercalciuria.* In these cases, there are probably at least two pathways by which hypercalciuria develops, both of unknown etiology. The first involves hyperabsorption of calcium from the intestine, promptly offset by an increased renal output; the second involves an impairment in renal tubular reabsorption of calcium. Despite the hypercalciuria, hypercalcemia is not present. In a small group of patients with idiopathic calcium stones, there is neither hypercalcemia nor hypercalciuria (Pak et al., 1975). Infrequently, hyperoxaluria is present, usually as a result of hyperabsorption of dietary oxalate, which, for some reason, may accompany steatorrhea.

The causes of the other types of renal stones are better understood. *Magnesium ammonium phosphate stones almost always occur in patients with a persistently alkaline urine due to recurrent urinary tract infections* (Williams, 1974). In particular, the urea splitting bacteria, such as *Proteus vulgaris* and the staphylococci, predispose toward urolithiasis. Moreover, bacteria may serve as particulate nidi for the formation of any kind of stone. In avitaminosis A, desquamated squames from the metaplastic epithelium of the collecting system act as nidi.

Gout and diseases involving rapid cell turnover, such as the leukemias, lead to high uric acid levels in the urine and the possibility of *uric acid stones. Cystine stones* are almost invariably associated with a genetically determined defect in the renal transport of certain amino acids, including cystine. In contrast to magnesium ammonium phosphate stones, *both uric acid and cystine stones are more likely when the urine is relatively acidic.*

In addition to factors already mentioned, such as urine pH and the presence of bacteria, urolithiasis may be influenced by other, less certain factors. Changes in the urinary content of the mucoproteins which form the organic matrix of uroliths may be important. Urinary stasis predisposes to infection and to increased reabsorption of water, thus concentrating the urine. Stasis, then, favors stone formation. Oliguria from any cause (for example, dehydration) similarly increases the concentration of all urinary solutes. Finally, since even in normal individuals calcium and phosphate are present in the urine in amounts that exceed their solubility product, it is possible that urolithiasis may result from the lack of influences which normally inhibit precipitation. Inhibitors of crystal formation in urine include pyrophosphate, mucopolysaccharides, diphosphonates, small polypeptides, urea, citrate, magnesium, certain amino acids and trace metals. Despite this lengthy list, no deficiency of any of these substances has been consistently demonstrated in patients with urolithiasis (Williams, 1974).

Morphology. Stones are unilateral in about 80 per cent of patients. Often, many stones are found within one kidney. They tend to remain small, having an average diameter of 2 to 3 mm., and may be smooth or jagged. Occasionally, progressive accretion of salts leads to the development of branching structures known as **staghorn calculi,** which create a cast of the renal pelvic and calyceal system.

Clinical Course. Stones may be present without producing either symptoms or significant renal damage. This is particularly true with large stones lodged in the renal pelvis. Smaller stones may pass into the ureter, producing a typical intense pain known as renal or ureteral colic and characterized by paroxysms of flank pain radiating toward the groin. Often at this time there is gross hematuria. The clinical significance of stones lies in their capacity to obstruct urinary flow or to produce sufficient trauma to cause ulceration and bleeding. In either case, they predispose to bacterial infection.

NEPHROCALCINOSIS

Nephrocalcinosis refers to the presence of calcium deposits within the renal parenchyma, rather than in the collecting system, as in urolithiasis. It is an infrequent disorder, occurring about one-tenth as often as urolithiasis. Commonly, the deposits are found within the various renal basement membranes and in the epithelial cells, as well as in the lumina of the tubules. Such diffuse calcification presents a dramatic picture on x-ray.

Nephrocalcinosis may occur with a variety of disorders, including hypercalcemia from any cause, renal tubular acidosis and renal parenchymal disease, which serves as a site for "dystrophic" calcification (see p. 24). Obviously, it is frequently associated with urolithiasis, since many of the predisposing conditions are the same. The course depends largely on the etiology. Sometimes it is rather benign; in other cases, it may contribute to uremia and death.

POLYCYSTIC KIDNEY DISEASE

This is a hereditary disease characterized by expanding multiple cysts of both kidneys, which ultimately destroy the intervening parenchyma. It is seen in approximately 1 in 400 to 500 autopsies. Often there is accompanying cystic involvement of other organs, principally the liver and pancreas. Many classifications of renal cystic disease have been proposed. The most definitive is that given by Osathanondh and Potter (1964). Two clinical forms are most common: *polycystic disease of the newborn* and *adult polycystic disease.* The former is characterized by the presence of full-blown cysts at birth, a large proportion of which are blind pouches into which the glomerular filtrate flows *(closed cysts).* Children with this condition do not survive beyond infancy. At postmortem examination, the kidneys are several times normal size and totally cystic.

The cysts in the adult form, by contrast, are usually only potential at birth and develop slowly throughout subsequent years, rarely producing symptoms before the age of 15 years. Moreover, most of the cysts are in continuity with functioning nephrons *(open cysts).* Inheritance of this form is through a dominant autosomal gene of variable penetrance.

Morphology. The kidneys in the adult form may achieve enormous sizes, and weights up to 4 kg. for each kidney have been recorded (Fig. 13–13). These very large kidneys are readily palpable abdominally as masses extending into the pelvis. On gross examination, the kidney seems to be composed solely of a mass of cysts of varying sizes up to 3 or 4 cm. in diameter, with no intervening parenchyma. The cysts are filled with fluid, which may be clear, turbid or hemorrhagic.

Microscopic examination reveals some normal parenchyma dispersed among the cysts. The cysts themselves may arise at any level of the nephron, from tubules to collecting ducts, and therefore have a variable, often atrophic lining. Occasionally, Bowman's capsules are involved in the cyst formation, and in these cases, glomerular tufts may be seen within the cystic space. The pressure of the expanding cysts leads to ischemic atrophy of the intervening renal substance. Evidence of superimposed hypertension or infection is common.

Clinical Course. Polycystic kidney disease in the adult usually does not produce symptoms until the fourth decade. By this time, the kidneys are quite large. The most common complaint of the patient is flank pain or at least a heavy, dragging sensation. Acute distention of a cyst, either by intracystic hemor-

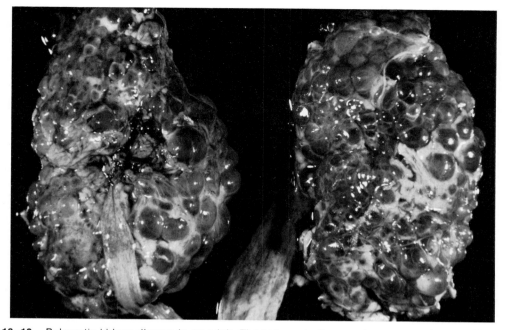

Figure 13–13. Polycystic kidney disease in an adult. The kidneys both comprise masses of cysts with no grossly apparent intervening normal parenchyma. The ureters are also malformed and are abnormally dilated.

rhage or by obstruction, may cause excruciating pain. Sometimes attention is first drawn to the lesion by palpation of an abdominal mass. Intermittent gross hematuria commonly occurs. The most important complications, because of their deleterious effect on already marginal renal function, are hypertension and urinary tract infection. Hypertension of varying severity develops in about 75 per cent of patients. When severe, it markedly worsens the prognosis. Urinary tract infections following instrumentation are frequent and unusually resistant to eradication.

While this disease is ultimately fatal, the outlook is in general better than with most chronic renal diseases. The condition tends to be relatively stable and progresses only very slowly, even after the development of marked azotemia. Although death usually occurs at about age 50, there is wide variation in the course of this renal disorder, and nearly normal life spans are reported. Death usually results from uremia or hypertensive complications.

HYDRONEPHROSIS

Hydronephrosis refers to the dilatation of the renal pelvis and calyces, with accompanying atrophy of the parenchyma, caused by obstruction to the outflow or urine. The obstruction may be sudden or insidious, and it may occur at any level of the urinary tract, from the urethra to the renal pelvis. The following list cites the most common causes:

A. Congenital: Atresia of the urethra, valve formations in either ureter or urethra, aberrant renal artery compressing the ureter, renal ptosis with torsion or kinking of ureter
B. Acquired:
   1. Foreign bodies: Calculi, necrotic papillae
   2. Tumors: Benign prostatic hypertrophy (BPH), carcinoma of the prostate, bladder tumors (papilloma and carcinoma), contiguous malignant disease (retroperitoneal lymphoma, carcinoma of the cervix or uterus)
   3. Inflammation: Prostatitis, ureteritis, urethritis, retroperitoneal fibrosis
   4. Neurogenic: Spinal cord damage with paralysis of the bladder
   5. Normal pregnancy: Mild and reversible

Bilateral hydronephrosis occurs only when the obstruction is below the level of the ureters. If blockage is at the ureters or above, the lesion is unilateral. Sometimes obstruction is complete, allowing no urine to pass; usually it is only partial.

It has been shown that even with complete obstruction, glomerular filtration persists for some time, and the filtrate subsequently diffuses back into the renal interstitium and perirenal spaces, whence it ultimately returns to the lymphatic and venous systems. Because of this continued filtration, the affected calyces and pelvis become dilated, often markedly so. The unusually high pressure thus generated in the renal pelvis, as well as that transmitted back through the collecting ducts, causes compression of the renal vasculature. Both arterial insufficiency and venous stasis result, although the latter is probably more important. The most severe effects are seen in the papillae, since they are subjected to the greatest increases in pressure. Damage becomes progressively less marked toward the cortex. Accordingly, the initial functional disturbances are largely tubular, manifested primarily by impaired concentrating ability. Only later does glomerular filtration begin to diminish. Experimental studies indicate that serious irreversible damage occurs in about three weeks with complete obstruction, and in three months with incomplete obstruction (Hamburger and Walsh, 1968).

Morphology. **Bilateral** hydronephrosis (as well as unilateral hydronephrosis when the other kidney is already damaged or absent) leads to renal failure, and the onset of uremia tends to abort the natural course of the lesion. In contrast, **unilateral** involvements display the full range of morphologic changes, which vary with the degree and the speed of obstruction. With subtotal or intermittent obstruction, the kidney may be massively enlarged, with lengths in the range of 20 cm., and the organ may consist almost entirely of the greatly distended pelvicalyceal system. The renal parenchyma itself is compressed and atrophied, with obliteration of the papillae and flattening of the pyramids. On the other hand, **when obstruction is sudden and complete, glomerular filtration is compromised relatively early, and as a consequence, renal function may cease while dilatation is still comparatively slight.** Depending on the level of the obstruction, one or both ureters may also be dilated **(hydroureter).**

Microscopically, the early lesions show tubular dilatation, followed by atrophy and fibrous replacement of the tubular epithelium, with relative sparing of the glomeruli. Eventually, in severe cases, the glomeruli, too, become atrophic and disappear, converting the entire kidney into a thin shell of fibrotic tissue. With sudden and complete obstruction, there may be coagulative necrosis of the renal papillae, similar to the changes of necrotizing papillitis (p. 443). In uncomplicated cases, the accompanying inflammatory reaction is minimal. Complicating pyelonephritis, however, is common. Thus, pregnant women, who normally have minimal degrees of physiologic hydronephrosis, are vulnerable to urinary tract infections.

Clinical Course. *Bilateral* complete obstruction produces anuria, which is soon brought to medical attention. When the obstruction is below the bladder, the dominant symptoms are those of bladder distention. Paradoxically, incomplete obstruction causes polyuria rather than oliguria, as a result of defects in tubular concentrating mechanisms, and this may obscure the true nature of the disturbance. Unfortunately, *unilateral* hydronephrosis may remain completely silent for long periods of time, unless the other kidney is for some reason nonfunctioning. Often the enlarged kidney is discovered on routine physical examination. Sometimes the basic cause of the hydronephrosis, such as renal calculi or a constricting tumor, produces symptoms which indirectly draw attention to the hydronephrosis. Removal of obstruction within a few weeks usually permits full return of function. However, with time, the changes become irreversible.

HYPERTENSION

Elevated blood pressure is a staggering health problem for three reasons: it is very common, its effects are sometimes devastating and it remains asymptomatic until very late in its course. Because of the intimate relationship between the kidneys and blood pressure, we have chosen to discuss hypertension in this chapter. However, its effects are widespread and no organ is spared. Hypertension has been identified as the single most important risk factor in both coronary heart disease (p. 292) and cerebrovascular accidents (p. 646), it may also lead directly to congestive heart failure (hypertensive heart disease, p. 308) and to renal failure. There is no magic threshold of blood pressure above which an individual is considered hypertensive and below which he is safe. Rather, the detrimental effects of blood pressure increase continuously as the pressure increases. Hypertension, then, must be defined somewhat arbitrarily. Most would agree that a sustained diastolic pressure above 90 mm. Hg is an essential feature. It has been customary to consider a sustained systolic pressure above 140 mm. Hg as also constituting hypertension, but when this exists without diastolic hypertension, the consequences are minimal and the clinical significance very different. Using a diastolic pressure above 90 mm. Hg as a standard, then, about 20 to 30 per cent of the adult population of the United States is hypertensive (Davis, 1973). The prevalence increases with age, although when present in young adults it tends to be more severe. Blacks are affected about twice as often as whites and apparently are more vulnerable to its complications. Although females are hypertensive more often than males, this sex preponderance is limited to the older age groups in which the disease is likely to be relatively benign. Under the age of 50 years, hypertension is more common in males (Lew, 1973).

About 90 per cent of hypertension is idiopathic and apparently primary (essential hypertension). Of the remaining 10 per cent, most is secondary to renal disease or, less often, to narrowing of the renal artery, usually by an atheromatous plaque (renovascular hypertension). Only relatively infrequently is secondary hypertension the result of adrenal disorders, such as primary aldosteronism, Cushing's syndrome and pheochromocytoma. *Both essential and secondary hypertension may be either benign or malignant, according to the clinical course.* In most cases hypertension remains fairly stable over years to decades and, unless a myocardial infarction or cerebrovascular accident supervenes, is compatible with a long life. This form of the disorder is termed *benign hypertension* and produces a renal lesion known as *benign nephrosclerosis.* Whereas a benign course is most characteristic of idiopathic or essential hypertension, it may also be seen with the secondary disorder. In contrast, about 5 per cent of hypertensives show a rapidly rising blood pressure which, untreated, leads to death within a year or two. Appropriately enough, this is called *accelerated* or *malignant hypertension,* and the corresponding renal lesion *malignant nephrosclerosis.* The full-blown clinical syndrome of malignant hypertension includes severe hypertension (a diastolic pressure over 120 mm. Hg), renal failure and bilateral retinal hemorrhages and exudates, with or without papilledema. This form of hypertension may develop in previously normotensive individuals, or it may be superimposed upon preexisting benign hypertension, either essential or secondary. In its pure form, malignant hypertension usually affects younger individuals than does benign hypertension. Typically, it develops in the fourth decade.

The morphology and clinical course of the two renal lesions, benign and malignant nephrosclerosis, will be considered separately later. First we shall discuss what is known of the etiology and pathogenesis of hypertension in general.

Etiology and Pathogenesis. Although the cause of the bulk of cases of hypertension is unknown, speculations abound, and the subject is a source of lively controversy. In our consideration, a reasonable starting point is the observation that "all hypertension involves increased volume relative to arteriolar capacity" (Laragh, 1973). Thus, hypertension may reflect one or both of two conditions: an increased plasma volume ("volume hypertension"), or increased vasoconstriction (resistance) ("vasoconstrictor hypertension"). Probably mixtures of both are most common (Laragh, 1975). Because we know more about secondary hypertension than about essential hypertension, we shall first consider how these conditions might arise in the secondary disorder. It has long been recognized that manipulation of the kidneys in experimental animals would occasionally produce sustained hypertension, but until 1934 the results were sporadic and not always reproducible. A breakthrough came in that year, when Goldblatt in his now famous experiment showed that hypertension could consistently be produced in animals by partially constricting a renal artery. He proposed that renal ischemia somehow led to hypertension. It is presently thought that this is mediated through the *renin-angiotensin-aldosterone (RAA) system.* The normal function of this system will be briefly reviewed before relating it to pathologic states.

Renin is released into the bloodstream by the juxtaglomerular apparatus of the kidney as a response to a number of stimuli. These stimuli probably include hypoxia, a decrease in volume or pulse pressure of the afferent arteriole, stimulation of the renal nerves and a decreased sodium concentration in the distal tubule (perceived by the macula densa) (Oparil and Haber, 1974). Although renin itself has no pressor activity, it acts as a proteolytic enzyme which hydrolyzes angiotensinogen, an alpha-2-globulin produced by the liver, to yield angiotensin I. Angiotensin I is a decapeptide, also without pressor activity. It in turn is split by a plasma enzyme to yield the octapeptide, angiotensin II, the most potent pressor known. This pressor acts directly on the arterioles, producing vasoconstriction, and is also a strong stimulus to aldosterone production. It is inactivated in about 15 minutes by the enzyme angiotensinase, found in many tissues of the body, including the kidney. Angiotensin II exerts a negative feedback control on renin release, both directly and indirectly through its effects on blood volume, blood pressure and sodium balance (Oparil and Haber, 1974). The important and complicated role of sodium on blood pressure homeostasis is worthy of particular note, since the dietary intake of salt is so variable. In general, sodium stores are inversely related to renin release. When blood pressure rises for any reason, there is normally an increase in the urinary output of sodium and water (natriuresis), which tends to lower blood pressure by diminishing plasma volume. On the other hand, if salt intake is markedly reduced, the RAA system is activated to defend the blood pressure (Thompson and Dickinson, 1973). Thus, there is a delicate balance between sodium retention, which tends to produce "volume hypertension," and renin release, which tends to produce "vasoconstrictor hypertension." There is some evidence that the relationship between blood pressure and the kidney may not be confined to the variable elaboration of renin and excretion of sodium. Some workers have proposed that the kidney plays a role in preventing hypertension through the elaboration of some *hypo*tensive agent, and that renal disease interferes with this function, producing hypertension by default, or "renoprival hypertension." The validity of renoprival hypertension remains very uncertain, but the presence of vasodilating prostaglandins in the renal medulla lends credence to such a hypothesis. With this brief review of blood pressure homeostasis, we may turn our attention to secondary hypertension.

It is now well appreciated that hypertension may accompany almost any chronic disease of the renal parenchyma and it is also present regularly with acute lesions which produce the nephritic syndrome (see p. 435). In addition, hypertension is frequently seen with polycystic kidneys, hydronephrosis and systemic arteritis when it involves the kidneys. Renovascular hypertension occurs when either the renal artery or the aorta proximal to the kidneys is partially obstructed. Such obstruction is usually produced by an atheromatous plaque, but in a minority of cases it is caused by fibromuscular hyperplasia of the renal artery. A human counterpart of the Goldblatt kidney is thus produced. *In both humans and experimental animals with renovascular hypertension, there are usually markedly elevated levels of renin in the renal vein serving the ischemic kidney. Clearly, in these cases there is activation of the RAA system.* When vascular reconstruction or nephrectomy is performed, the hypertension may be abolished, particularly when it is of recent onset. The procedure is less successful with long-standing hypertension, because the hypertension eventually affects the contralateral kidney, causing it, too, to elaborate increased amounts of renin. With bilateral renal *parenchymal* disease, the situation is less clear and probably a good deal more complicated. Some of these patients do elaborate markedly increased amounts of renin, and the pathogenesis of the hypertension may be analogous to that of renovascular hypertension. In these cases bilateral nephrectomy with hemodialysis may lead to alleviation of the hypertension. *However, more often the hypertension associated with bilateral renal disease seems related to an inability to excrete sodium and water* (Editorial, 1975*b*). This is probably frequently compounded by inappropriate renin release in the face of the increased volume. As the parenchyma of the kidneys is destroyed, an element of renoprival hypertension may also be added. Thus, renal disease would seem to be associated with varying mixtures of volume and vasoconstrictor hypertension.

Secondary hypertension due to adrenal dysfunction usually involves the hypersecretion of one of the mineralocorticoids. Primary aldosteronism (Conn's disease) is the best established of these disorders and is discussed on page 609. In addition, other mineralocorticoids, such as deoxycorticosterone (DOC) and 18-OH-DOC, have been identified as causes of adrenal hypertension. *Hypertension associated with primary mineralocorticoid excess contrasts with renal and renovascular hypertension in that renin levels are depressed rather than elevated.* This reflects the negative feedback effects of the mineralocorticoids on renin release. Thus, the elevated blood pressure can be considered to reflect hypervolemia rather than vasoconstriction.

Having discussed the RAA system in secondary hypertension, what can we say of its role in essential hypertension? Here we enter an area of intense debate. On the one hand, there are investigators who contend that essential hypertension is a heterogeneous group of disorders which can be separated according to renin levels (Laragh, 1974). In about 57 per cent of patients with essential hypertension, renin levels are within the normal range; 25 per cent have subnormal renin levels which do not respond to stimulatory measures such as salt depletion; and 18 per cent have elevated renin release. Whereas the pathogenesis of all three forms is unknown, these workers believe that low-renin essential hypertension carries an inherently better prognosis. Moreover, it would seem to call for therapy directed toward reducing plasma volume rather than toward relieving vasoconstriction. Other workers deny the existence of low-renin essential hypertension as a discrete entity. They contend that renin release tends to fall with age both in normal individuals and in those with long-standing benign hypertension. Thus, the low-renin group simply represents older patients who have had their disease longer (Padfield et al., 1975; Lebel et al., 1974).

If essential hypertension is considered as a homogeneous group, what can be said of the pathogenesis? There are several theories, but none has been proved. One postulates that there is some disturbance in the normal negative feedback of blood pressure on renin release. According to this view, all hypertensives *should* have low renin levels. The fact that most have normal renin levels is taken to indicate an *inappropriate* renin release (Lucas et al., 1974). Others suggest an alteration in the relationship between blood pressure and natriuresis such that natriuresis occurs only at higher than normal pressures (Brown et al., 1974).

It should be noted that these theories pertain only to the pathogenesis. The etiology of essential hypertension remains even more mysterious. It has been suggested that sustained hypertension is preceded by a period of vasomotor lability which may last for years. During this period patients show marked fluctuations in blood pressure. It seems likely that this vasomotor lability is mediated through the autonomic nervous system in response to various stimuli, including stress. Whether such a derangement in autonomic function continues to be operative when sustained hypertension develops is questionable. Nevertheless, it may in some way set up the conditions for the development of hypertension. In this regard it should be pointed out that environmental influences materially affect the likelihood of developing hypertension. This is illustrated by the lower incidence of hypertension in Chinese people living in their native country as compared to the Chinese living in the United States. Heredity is also important as a predisposing factor. When both parents are hypertensive, about 50 per cent of their offspring will themselves develop elevated levels of blood pressure.

Malignant hypertension, as pointed out earlier, is far less common than benign hypertension, occurring in only about 5 per cent of patients with elevated blood pressure. The basis for the development of malignant hypertension is controversial. Even the answer to so fundamental a question as whether the hypertension causes the renal lesion or the renal lesion produces the hypertension is not yet firmly established. However, extensive recent investigation has begun to yield some answers—as well as new questions. From this work, the following picture of this mysterious disease has begun to unfold: The initial event appears to be some form of vascular damage to the kidneys. This may result from long-standing benign hypertension, with eventual injury to the arteriolar walls, or it may spring from arteritis of some form without elevated blood pressure. In either case, the result is increased permeability of the small vessels to fibrinogen as well as to other plasma proteins. This is considered by many to be the decisive event in the genesis of malignant hypertension. (Giese, 1973; Gerber and Paronetto,

1974). In some cases IgG and complement have been identified in the renal arteriolar walls, suggesting an immune complex disease (Paronetto, 1965). Be this as it may, fibrinogen is deposited in the arteriolar walls, and the clotting mechanism is activated. Microthrombi thus form in the vessels. The combination of these two changes presents the appearance of fibrinoid necrosis of arterioles and small arteries. This intramural and intravascular clotting, along with a resultant hyperplasia of the intima, causes the lumina of the arterioles to become narrowed and shaggy. The striking hyperplastic response of the intima is known as "onion-skinning" because of the appearance of concentric layers of intimal cells. Mechanical trauma to red cells coursing through these damaged vessels produces hemolysis and anemia, known as *microangiopathic hemolytic anemia*. With disruption of the red cells, there is further stimulus to the clotting mechanism as well as some inhibition of fibrinolysis. The vicious circle is now complete, and the deposition of fibrin continues. Patients with this condition have elevated serum levels of fibrin split products (FSP), which is clear evidence of intravascular coagulation (see p. 363). The kidneys become markedly ischemic. With severe involvement of the renal afferent arterioles, the renin-angiotensin system (p. 457) receives a powerful stimulus, and indeed *patients with malignant hypertension have markedly elevated levels of plasma renin.* Renin itself increases vascular permeability and so contributes to fibrinoid deposition. As with hypertension secondary to renal disease, the normal relationship between renin and natriuresis no longer obtains, and so the hypertension may have a hypervolemic component superimposed on a vasoconstrictive pathogenesis (Lebel et al., 1974; Editorial, 1973b). Apparently, this is a particularly ominous combination, and from this point of view it is not surprising that malignant hypertension often accompanies chronic renal disease.

BENIGN NEPHROSCLEROSIS (BNS)

Benign nephrosclerosis refers to the renal lesion associated with, and presumably caused by, the arteriolar narrowing secondary to benign essential hypertension. The same lesion may also be seen in very elderly normotensive individuals and in patients with diabetes mellitus. However, it is most consistently associated with hypertension. This renal lesion is a frequent form of anatomic nephropathy if one includes the high proportion of minimal involvements. It is, therefore, a frequent incidental autopsy finding in individuals over the age of 60 years. Males are affected more

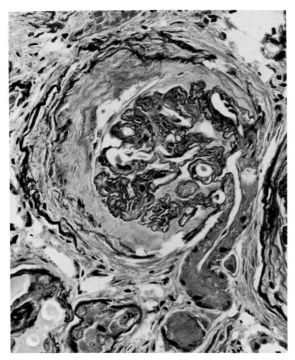

Figure 13–14. Benign nephrosclerosis. Microscopic detail of a glomerulus and its afferent arteriole sectioned obliquely. The arteriole has hyaline, thickened walls and a narrowed lumen. The glomerulus is obsolescent and has marked fibrous thickening of the parietal layer of Bowman's capsule.

often than females, despite the fact that hypertension is more common in the latter.

The kidneys are symmetrically atrophied, each weighing 110 to 130 gm., with a diffuse, fine surface granularity, which resembles grain leather. They are somewhat pale and gray, reflecting the ischemic nature of the process.

Microscopically, the basic anatomic change is thickening of the walls of the small arteries and arterioles, known as **hyaline arteriolosclerosis.** This appears as a homogeneous, pink hyaline thickening, at the expense of the vessel lumina, with loss of underlying cellular detail. Electron microscopic studies indicate that the hyaline material arises by intramural deposition of plasma proteins and reduplication of the intimal basement membrane. Similar vascular changes are seen with benign hypertension in other organs of the body. The narrowing of the lumina results in a markedly decreased blood flow through the affected vessels, and thus produces ischemia in the organ served. Renal ischemic parenchymal changes, along with the vascular alterations, are necessary for the diagnosis of BNS. All structures of the kidney show ischemic atrophy. The glomeruli develop axial thickening and fibrosis, and sometimes there is fibrotic replacement of Bowman's spaces (Fig. 13–14). The axial thickening, designated **diffuse glo-**

merulosclerosis, results largely from increased numbers of mesangial cells, increased matrix and basement membrane thickening. This diffuse pattern should not be confused with the **nodular glomerulosclerosis** of the diabetic, which was discussed previously (p. 136). In far advanced cases of BNS, the glomerular tufts may become obliterated by this homogeneous hyalinization. Diffuse tubular atrophy and interstitial fibrosis are present. Often there is a scant interstitial lymphocytic infiltrate.

It should be remembered that many renal diseases cause hypertension, which in turn may lead to BNS. Thus, this renal lesion is often seen superimposed on other, primary kidney diseases. In these cases, the histologic features may be very difficult to interpret.

Because this renal lesion alone rarely causes severe damage to the kidney, it very infrequently leads to uremia and death. Nonetheless, there is usually some functional impairment, such as loss of concentrating ability or a variably diminished glomerular filtration rate. A mild degree of proteinuria is a constant finding. Usually these patients die from hypertensive heart disease, from cerebrovascular accidents or from causes unrelated to their hypertension.

MALIGNANT NEPHROSCLEROSIS (MNS)

In pure MNS, the gross alterations may be quite minimal. Commonly, vascular congestion produces a slight increase in kidney size. A frequent pattern is that of irregular congestive mottling. Because of the extremely rapid course of the disease, ending in death, there is no time for scarring and contraction to develop. Small petechial hemorrhages often appear on the cortical surface as the result of rupture of arterioles or capillaries. On sectioning, the kidneys are quite normal in appearance, with the possible exception of cortical petechiae.

Microscopically, the most important changes are seen in the interlobular and afferent arterioles (Fig. 13–15). The basic lesion is a fibrinoid deposit interpreted as a necrotizing arteriolitis of the vessel walls. This is manifested by thickening of the intima and media, which assume a homogeneous acidophilic appearance as a result of the deposition of fibrin and plasma proteins. Often there is disruption or fragmentation of the vessel walls, with disappearance of cell nuclei. Noteworthy is the scantiness of the inflammatory infiltrate. Much more dramatic in appearance is the accompanying hyperplasia of the intima. New cells, of uncertain origin, proliferate in progressively tighter concentric rings at the expense of the vessel lumen, which eventually may be all but obliterated. As was mentioned, the origin of these cells is controversial. They have been thought to be derived from smooth muscle cells within the intima or, alternatively,

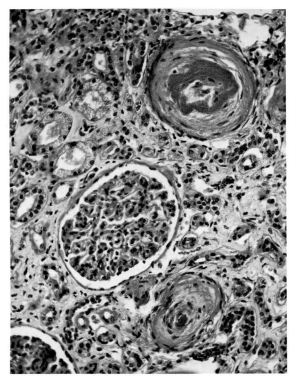

Figure 13–15. Malignant nephrosclerosis. Two markedly thickened vessels are seen above and below the glomerulus. The vessel above contains a heavy deposit of fibrinoid and demonstrates necrotizing arteriolitis.

from fibroblasts. It is not uncommon to see small thrombi within the lumina of the vessels. Glomeruli are not primarily attacked. Occasionally they may be patchily affected by extension of the afferent arteriole lesion into the glomerulus. Moreover, capillary and arteriolar lesions may secondarily produce severe ischemic alterations in the glomeruli, taking the form of segmental necrosis and endocapillary and extracapillary proliferation, often with an inflammatory infiltrate. The proximal convoluted tubules, which are particularly sensitive to ischemia, may show such degenerative changes as granularity of the cytoplasm or fatty change. Rupture of glomerular capillaries causes hemorrhage into the glomerular space, leading to petechial markings on the cortical surface and to hematuria.

The onset of malignant hypertension, whether primary or secondary, is sudden and initially dominated by cerebral and cardiovascular manifestations, although it may be ushered in by a transient episode of macroscopic hematuria. Proteinuria becomes pronounced, and microscopic hematuria is constant, punctuated by intermittent bouts of gross hematuria. The patient complains of headache, nausea, vomiting and visual derangements, particularly the development of scotomata or blurring. Examination of the eyes usually but not invariably reveals hemorrhages and exudates, and often papilledema is seen. There may be impaired consciousness and even convulsions. Congestive heart failure is frequent, particularly in older patients. Later, renal failure dominates the picture.

Among untreated individuals, five-year survival is extremely rare, and most patients die within a year. The cause of death is usually uremia, although occasionally the patient succumbs to a cerebrovascular accident or to heart failure. With treatment, the outlook is much better. The two-year survival rate is about 70 per cent, five-year survival about 50 per cent. The chances for long-term survival are largely dependent on early treatment, before significant renal insufficiency has developed.

In concluding this chapter on diseases of the kidney, we may state that the justification for the frequently used clinical term "cardiovascular-renal disease" should now be apparent. Hypertension may arise from extrarenal causes and have significant effects on the kidney when it causes renal arterial and arteriolar narrowing, as exemplified by benign nephrosclerosis. Conversely, hypertension may be renal in origin and secondarily have serious effects on the heart, brain and arterial system, leading to hypertensive heart disease, cerebral hemorrhages and augmented atherosclerosis. Moreover, all the destructive kidney diseases have generalized consequences, inducing the uremic syndrome described in the early pages of this chapter. Thus, the kidney and its afflictions occupy a central role in many forms of systemic disease, all of which are of grave clinical significance.

REFERENCES

Angell, M. E., et al.: "Active" chronic pyelonephritis without evidence of bacterial infection. New Eng. J. Med., *278*:1303, 1968.

Aoki, S., et al.: "Abacterial" and bacterial pyelonephritis. New Eng. J. Med., *281*:1375, 1969.

Asscher, A. W.: Urinary tract infection. Lancet, *2*:1365, 1974.

Bailey, R. R., et al.: Renal damage after acute pyelonephritis. Brit. Med. J., *1*:550, 1969.

Blaker, F., et al.: Membranous nephropathy and hepatitis-B antigen. Lancet, *2*:955, 1974.

Brown, C. B., et al.: Combined immunosuppression and anticoagulation in rapidly progressive glomerulonephritis. Lancet, *2*:1166, 1974.

Brown, J. J., et al.: Renal abnormality of essential hypertension. Lancet, *2*:320, 1974.

Brzosko, W. J., et al.: Glomerulonephritis associated with hepatitis-B surface antigen immune complexes in children. Lancet, *2*:477, 1974.

Cameron, J. S.: The natural history of glomerulonephritis. *In* Black, D. A. K. (ed.): Renal Disease. Oxford, England, Blackwell Scientific Publications, 1972, p. 195.

Case Records of the Massachusetts General Hospital:

Weekly clinicopathological exercises. New Eng. J. Med., *290*:1365, 1974.

Case Records of the Massachusetts General Hospital: Weekly clinicopathological exercises. New Eng. J. Med., *292*:307, 1975.

Chase, W. H.: Pathogenesis of glomerulonephritis: Review of three types of experimental nephritis. Can. Med. Ass. J., *97*:852, 1967.

Christian, C. L.: Immune-complex disease. New Eng. J. Med., *280*:878, 1969.

Clarkson, A. R., et al.: Glomerular coagulation in acute ischaemic renal failure. Quart. J. Med., *39*:585, 1970.

Cochrane, C. G., and Dixon, F. J.: Cell and tissue damage through antigen-antibody complexes. *In* Miescher, P. A., and Mueller-Eberhard, H. J. (eds.): Textbook of Immunopathology. New York, Grune and Stratton, 1968, p. 94.

Coe, R. L., and Kavalach, A. G.: Hypercalciuria and hyperuricosuria in patients with calcium nephrolithiasis. New Eng. J. Med., *291*:1344, 1974.

Costanza, M. E., et al.: Carcinoembryonic antigen-antibody complexes in a patient with colonic carcinoma and nephrotic syndrome. New Eng. J. Med., *289*:520, 1973.

Cotran, R. S.: Retrograde proteus pyelonephritis in rats. Localization of antigen-antibody in treated sterile pyelonephritic kidneys. J. Exp. Med., *117*:813, 1963.

Couser, W. G., et al.: Experimental glomerulonephritis in the guinea pig. Lab. Invest., *29*:236, 1973.

Couser, W. G., et al.: Glomerular deposition of tumor antigen in membranous nephropathy associated with colonic carcinoma. Am. J. Med., *57*:962, 1974.

Davis, J. O.: The control of renin release. Am. J. Med., *55*:333, 1973.

Dixon, F. J.: The pathogenesis of glomerulonephritis. Amer. J. Med., *44*:493, 1968.

Editorial: The wages of analgesics. Lancet, *2*:1484, 1973*a*.

Editorial: Sodium and the pressor role of angiotensin. Lancet, *2*:1065, 1973*b*.

Editorial: Virus infection of the kidney and urinary tract. Lancet, *1*:19, 1974*a*.

Editorial: Urinary-tract infection in general practice. Lancet, *1*:83, 1974*b*.

Editorial: V. U. R. + I. R. R. = C. P. N. Lancet, *2*:1120, 1974*c*.

Editorial: Recurrent hematuria in children and young adults. Lancet, *2*:114, 1975*a*.

Editorial: When to measure renin. Lancet, *1*:783, 1975*b*.

Epstein, M., et al.: Renal failure in the patient with cirrhosis. Am. J. Med., *49*:175, 1970.

Erwin, D. T., et al.: The clinical course of idiopathic membranous nephropathy. Mayo Clin. Proc., *48*:697, 1973.

Evans, D. J.: Pathogenesis of membranous glomerulonephritis. Lancet, *1*:1143, 1974.

Finlayson, G., et al.: Immunoglobulin A glomerulonephritis. Lab. Invest., *32*:140, 1975.

Frank, I. N.: Urologic and male genital cancers. *In* Rubin, P. (ed.): Clinical Oncology for Medical Students and Physicians, 3rd. ed. Rochester, N. Y., American Cancer Society, 1970–1971, p. 190.

Freedman, P. et al.: Subclinical renal response to streptococcal infection. New Eng. J. Med., *275*:795, 1966.

Fry, J.: Natural history of hypertension. Lancet, *2*:431, 1974.

Gamble, C. N., and Reardan, J. B.: Immunopathogenesis of syphilitic glomerulonephritis. New Eng. J. Med., *292*:449, 1975.

Gerber, M. A., and Paronetto, F.: New patterns of immunoglobulin deposition in the lesions of malignant nephrosclerosis, with special reference to IgE. Am. J. Path., *65*:535, 1971.

Giese, J.: Renin, angiotensin and hypertensive vascular damage: a review . Am. J. Med., *55*:315, 1973.

Ginzler, E. M., et al.: Progression of mesangial and focal

to diffuse lupus nephritis. New Eng. J. Med., *291*:693, 1974.

Hamburger, J., and Walsh, A.: Nephrology. Philadelphia, W. B. Saunders Co., 1968, pp. 661, 1183.

Harrington, J. T., and Cohen, J. J.: Current concepts. Acute oliguria. New Eng. J. Med., *292*:89, 1975.

Heptinstall, R. H.: The enigma of chronic pyelonephritis. J. Infect. Dis., *120*:104, 1969.

Hinglais, N., et al.: Long-term prognosis in acute glomerulonephritis. Am. J. Med., *56*:52, 1974.

Hodson, C. J., and Wilson, S.: Natural history of chronic pyelonephritic scarring. Brit. Med. J., *2*:191, 1965.

Hollenberg, N. K., et al.: Irreversible acute oliguric renal failure. A complication of methoxyflurane anesthesia. New Eng. J. Med., *286*:877, 1972.

Iwatsuki, S., et al.: Recovery from "hepatorenal syndrome" after orthotopic liver transplantation. New Eng. J. Med., *289*:1155, 1973.

Jenis, E. H., et al.: Focal segmental glomerulosclerosis. Am. J. Med., *57*:695, 1974.

Jewett, J. H., and Strong, G. H.: Infiltrating carcinoma of the bladder. Relation of depth penetration of the bladder wall to incidence, local extension and metastases. J. Urol., *55*:366, 1946.

Johnson, W. J., et al.: Prevention and reversal of progressive secondary hyperparathyroidism in patients maintained by hemodialysis. Am. J. Med., *56*:827, 1974.

Kashgarian, M., et al.: Renal Disease. Universities Associated for Research and Education in Pathology, Inc. Kalamazoo, Michigan, The Upjohn Company, 1974.

Kleeman, C. R., et al.: Pyelonephritis. Medicine, *39*:3, 1960.

Koppel, M. H., et al.: Transplantation of cadaveric kidneys from patients with hepatorenal syndrome. New Eng. J. Med., *280*:1367, 1969.

Knudson, A. G., and Strong, L. C.: Mutation and cancer: a model for Wilms' tumor of the kidney. J. Nat. Cancer Inst., *48*:313, 1972.

Krueger, G. R. F., and Bulla, M.: Cellular immunity in minimal-lesion nephrosis. Lancet, *2*:1023, 1974.

Laragh, J. H.: Vasoconstriction-volume analysis for understanding and treating hypertension: The use of renin and aldosterone profiles. Am. J. Med., *55*:261, 1973.

Laragh, J. H.: An approach to the classification of hypertensive states. Hospital Practice, January, 1974, p. 61.

Laragh, J. H.: Angiotensin blockade: new pharmacologic tools for understanding and treating hypertension. New Eng. J. Med., *292*:695, 1975.

Leathem, A.: Mesangial and Kupffer cells. Lancet, *1*:277, 1975.

Lebel, M., et al.: Sodium and the renin-angiotensin system in essential hypertension and mineralocorticoid excess. Lancet, *2*:308, 1974.

Lerner, R. A.: Role of anti-glomerular basement membrane antibody in the pathogenesis of human glomerulonephritis. J. Exp. Med., *126*:989, 1967.

Lew, E. A.: High blood pressure, other risk factors and longevity: the insurance viewpoint. Am. J. Med., *55*:281, 1973.

Lucas, C. P., et al.: Disturbed relationship of plasma-renin to blood pressure in hypertension. Lancet, *2*:1337, 1974.

Matlin, R. A., and Gary, N. E.: Acute cortical necrosis. Am. J. Med., *56*:110, 1974.

McCoy, R. C., et al.: IgA nephropathy. Am. J. Path., *76*:123, 1974.

Merrill, J. P.: Glomerulonephritis. New Eng. J. Med., *290*:313, 394, 1974.

Mery, J. P., et al.: Glomerulonephritis in SLE. New Eng. J. Med., *292*:480, 1975.

Morita, T., et al.: Structure and development of the glomerular crescent. Am. J. Path., *72*:349, 1973.

Murray, R. M., et al.: Analgesic nephropathy: clinical syndrome and prognosis. Brit. Med. J., *1*:479, 1971.

Nanra, R. S., and Kincaid-Smith, P.: Papillary necrosis in rats caused by aspirin and aspirin-containing mixtures. Brit. Med. J., *3*:559, 1970.

Norden, C. W., and Kass, E. H.: Bacteriuria of pregnancy: a critical appraisal. Ann. Rev. Med., *19*:431, 1968.

Ooi, B. S., et al.: Lymphocytotoxins in primary renal disease. Lancet, *2*:1348, 1974.

Oparil, S., and Haber, E.: The renin-angiotensin system. New Eng. J. Med., *291*:389, 446, 1974.

Osathanondh, V., and Potter, E. L.: Pathogenesis of polycystic kidneys. Type, I, due to hyperplasia of intestinal portions of collecting tubules. Type 2, due to inhibition of ampullary activity. Type 3, due to multiple abnormalities of development. Arch. Path., *77*:466, 474, 485, 1964.

Padfield, P. L., et al.: Is low-renin hypertension a stage in the development of essential hypertension or a diagnostic entity? Lancet, *1*:548, 1975.

Pak, C. Y. C., et al.: A simple test for the diagnosis of absorptive, resorptive and renal hypercalciurias. New Eng. J. Med., *292*:497, 1975.

Paronetto, F.: Immunocytochemical observations on the vascular necrosis and renal glomerular lesions of malignant nephrosclerosis, Amer. J. Path., *46*:901, 1965.

Pedreira, J., et al.: HBsAg subtype and chronic glomerulonephritis. Lancet, *2*:1513, 1974.

Peters, D. K., and Lachmann, P. J.: Immunity deficiency in pathogenesis of glomerulonephritis. Lancet, *1*:58, 1974.

Pincus, T., et al.: Experimental chronic glomerulitis. J. Exp. Med., *127*:819, 1968.

Reynolds, J. J.: The role of 1,25-dihydroxycholecalciferol in bone metabolism. Biochem. Soc. Spec. Publ., *3*:91, 1974.

Rubin, P.: Cancer of the urogenital tract: kidney, current concepts in cancer. J.A.M.A., *204*:603, 1968.

Schwartz, M. M., and Cotran, R. S.: Common enterobacterial antigen in human chronic pyelonephritis and interstitial nephritis. New Eng. J. Med., *289*:830, 1973.

Seymour, A. E., et al.: Contributions of renal biopsy studies to the understanding of disease. Am. J. Path., *65*:550, 1971.

Shalhoub, R. J.: Pathogenesis of lipoid nephrosis: a disorder of T-cell function. Lancet, *2*:556, 1974.

Silverberg, E., and Holleb, A. I.: Cancer statistics, 1974 — worldwide epidemiology. CA, *24*:2, 1974.

Silverberg, E., and Holleb, A. I.: Cancer statistics, 1975. CA, *25*:8, 1975.

Spear, G. S., et al.: Idiopathic hematuria of childhood. Hum. Pathol., *4*:349, 1973.

Stiehm, E. R., and Trygstad, C. W.: Split products of fibrin in human renal disease. Amer. J. Med., *46*:774, 1969.

Thompson, J. M. A., and Dickinson, C. J.: Relation between pressure and sodium excretion in perfused kidneys from rabbits with experimental hypertension. Lancet, *2*:1362, 1973.

Tsai, C. C., et al.: Dermal IgA deposits in Henoch-Schönlein purpura and Berger's nephritis. Lancet, *1*:342, 1975.

Vivaldi, E., et al.: Ascending infection as a mechanism in pathogenesis of experimental non-obstructive pyelonephritis. Proc. Soc. Exper. Biol. Med., *102*:242, 1959.

Wilkinson, S. P., et al.: Relation of renal impairment and hemorrhagic diathesis to endotoxemia in fulminant hepatic failure. Lancet, *1*:521, 1974.

Williams, H. E.: Nephrolithiasis. New Eng. J. Med., *290*:33, 1974.

CHAPTER 14

The Gastrointestinal System

The disorders considered in this chapter comprise a multitude of entities occurring at every level of the gastrointestinal tract, from the oral cavity to the rectum. Here they are classified according to the dominant sign or symptom evoked, including *dysphagia, hematemesis, pain, anorexia, diarrhea* and *melena*. It should be recognized that many, if not most, disorders of the gastrointestinal tract produce more than one of these manifestations. In these cases, we have chosen to categorize them according to the earliest or most specific clinical manifestation. At the end of the chapter are grouped miscellaneous and relatively unimportant entities which stubbornly defy such efforts to impose order.

DYSPHAGIA

Dysphagia refers to difficulty in swallowing, resulting either from mechanical obstruction or from neuromuscular dysfunction. The patient typically describes it as a sensation of food sticking somewhere on the way to the stomach. It should be distinguished from *odynophagia* (painful swallowing), with which it may or may not be associated.

The most important causes of dysphagia are *carcinoma of the esophagus, achalasia* and certain concomitants of *hiatus hernia*, including *esophagitis* with spasm or fibrous strictures (Hawkins, 1967). (In general, however, hiatus hernia and esophagitis are more prominently characterized by pain than by dysphagia and are discussed under the former heading.) Recently, it has been suggested that the mysterious mucosal webs known as *lower esophageal rings* may in fact be the single most common cause of dysphagia (Goyal et al., 1970). Other, less frequent causes of dysphagia include *pharyngoesophageal diverticula (Zenker's diverticula)*, the *Plummer-Vinson syndrome, scleroderma*

(p. 194) and *gastric carcinoma* (p. 483), as well as an obstructive foreign body in the esophagus.

Severe feeding difficulties in the newborn may be caused by congenital malformations of the esophagus. Most common is *esophageal atresia*. In this disorder, a segment of the esophagus is represented by only a thin non-canalized cord, with the resultant formation of a blind upper pouch connecting with the pharynx and a lower pouch leading to the stomach. In most of these cases, the lower pouch communicates through a fistulous tract with the trachea, as may the upper pouch. Less frequent is congenital *esophageal stenosis*, manifested by fibrotic thickening of a portion of the esophageal wall. Total *agenesis* of the esophagus also occurs, but this is uncommon.

In addition, a variety of neurologic derangements, such as cerebrovascular accidents and botulism, may produce dysphagia. It must be remembered, too, that compression of the esophagus with resultant dysphagia may be caused by such extragastrointestinal lesions as goiters, enlarged lymph nodes and aortic aneurysms. Last to be considered in any evaluation of dysphagia is the psychologic disorder *globus hystericus*.

Here we shall discuss four of the more important causes of dysphagia: achalasia, diverticula, esophageal webs (rings) and esophageal carcinoma.

ACHALASIA (CARDIOSPASM)

Achalasia is a disorder of uncertain origin characterized by ineffectual peristalsis of the esophagus with consequent functional obstruction. The pathogenetic mechanism probably involves either a structural or a functional derangement in the parasympathetic innervation of Auerbach's myenteric plexus. Remaining neuromuscular activity is uncoordinated and purposeless. The body of the esophagus shows diminished tone and motility, while the esophagogastric sphincter (lower esophageal sphincter) remains perpetually contracted. Traditionally it has been thought that the sphincter remains contracted because it does not receive the normal stimulus to relax in anticipation of a peristaltic wave. It has recently been suggested that there may be an abnormal sensitivity to the constricting effect of gastrin, which is important in maintaining the tone of the lower esophageal sphincter (Cohen et al., 1971). At any rate, the fundamental cause of the functional disorganization is unknown. It has been variously attributed to a congenital abnormality, to nutritional deficiencies and to emotional factors.

Morphology. A variety of anatomic changes have been described. The body of the esophagus is in general flaccid and often greatly distended **(megaesophagus)**, whereas the esophagogastric junction is contracted. In many patients, the ganglion cells of Auerbach's plexus are absent or reduced in number. Whether this represents a fundamental congenital abnormality or whether it merely reflects degenerative changes acquired with long-standing dysfunction is controversial. In other instances, no anatomic defects are apparent, and it is assumed that there is a functional block at the synapses between the vagal fibers and Auerbach's plexus.

With long-standing achalasia, stasis of food and secretions occurs proximal to the contracted esophagogastric junction, with consequent superimposed chronic esophagitis. Nonspecific ulceroinflammatory lesions and fibrotic thickening of the mucosa may therefore be present (see p. 471).

Clinical Course. Although achalasia may manifest itself at any age, it most commonly has its onset between the ages of 30 and 50 years. Males and females are affected equally frequently. The predominant symptom is dysphagia, which often has an abrupt onset during a period of emotional stress. The patient initially complains of a sensation of sticking of food, along with a dull ache beneath the lower sternum. These paroxysms become more frequent, and eventually regurgitation of undigested food occurs, particularly when the patient is in a horizontal position. Complete obstruction may ensue. In some instances, achalasia is complicated by concomitant *megacolon* or *megaureter*. Congenital megacolon, also known as *Hirschsprung's disease*, is analogous to achalasia in that it involves an absence of the ganglion cells of the myenteric plexus. Usually the rectum and rectosigmoid are affected, producing a functional obstruction at this level, with massive dilatation and hypertrophy proximal to it. This disorder most often manifests itself clinically as constipation and abdominal distention.

About 80 per cent of patients with achalasia obtain relief by a muscle-splitting dilatation of the esophagogastric junction, and most of the remainder can be benefitted temporarily. Because achalasia causes stasis of food and chronic irritation, it predisposes to the development of carcinoma just proximal to the point of functional obstruction at the esophagogastric junction. A pulsion diverticulum may also develop at this site (see next section).

DIVERTICULA OF THE ESOPHAGUS

Diverticula of the esophagus may be of two types—*pulsion* or *traction*. Pulsion diverticula are caused by weaknesses in the esophageal musculature, by local increases in intraluminal pressure, or by both. Traction diverticula result from the pull of inflammatory adhesions on the external aspect of the esophageal wall.

Commonly, diverticula are solitary and occur at one of three locations in the esophagus: (1) at the pharyngoesophageal junction, (2) in midesophagus, or (3) near the esophagogastric junction.

Pulsion diverticula at the pharyngoesophageal junction *(Zenker's diverticula)* are the most important type. They arise at the posterior wall, where the intrinsic musculature is weak and depends for support on the encircling fibers of the cricopharyngeus muscle. Between these fibers, a diverticular pouch may protrude and eventually become quite large. Dysphagia occurs eventually, with regurgitation of undigested food. Stasis of food within the diverticulum may lead to esophagitis and ulceration.

Epiphrenic diverticula are pulsion diverticula occurring in the distal esophagus, often in association with a hiatus hernia or with achalasia. Symptoms attributable to the diverticulum are rare.

Traction diverticula usually develop at midesophagus, near the bifurcation of the trachea, where tuberculous tracheobronchial lymph nodes become adherent to the external aspect of the esophageal wall. Other nearby inflammatory lesions may also lead to traction diverticula. Usually these outpouchings are small and only rarely are they symptomatic.

ESOPHAGEAL WEBS (RINGS)

A horizontal fold of mucosa projecting into the esophageal lumen may be one of two types. The most common type usually occurs at the squamocolumnar junction, often in association with a hiatus hernia (see p. 471), and is variously known as a *"lower esophageal ring,"* *"Schatzki ring"* (Schatzki and Gary, 1956) or *"Ingelfinger ring"* (Ingelfinger and Kramer, 1953). Less commonly, an esophageal web is seen in the upper esophagus as a component of the *Plummer-Vinson syndrome* (also known as the *Paterson-Kelly syndrome).* This syndrome is usually seen in women with iron deficiency anemia, and is characterized by the triad of anemia, atrophic glossitis and dysphagia. There may be an associated atrophic esophagitis. The esophageal web in the Plummer-Vinson syndrome typically develops at the level of the cricoid cartilage.

LOWER ESOPHAGEAL RING

Narrowings of this type are now thought to be extremely common lesions and possibly they are the most frequent cause of dysphagia. Their reported incidence varies. In Schatzki and Gary's original series, reported in 1956, a lower esophageal ring was found in 4.6 per cent of individuals who were given barium meals, although it was symptomatic in only 0.5 per cent. More recent studies indicate that it is present in about 10 per cent of patients who are given routine barium meals.

The etiology and pathogenesis are unknown. Although a lower esophageal ring is present in about 15 per cent of patients with hiatus hernia, the relationship, if any, is not clear. Histologic evidence of esophagitis is usually conspicuously absent, as is a history of substernal pain (Goyal et al., 1970).

Grossly, the lower esophageal ring appears as a smooth mucosal ledge, 2 to 4 mm. thick, ringing the circumference of the esophagus, about 4 to 5.5 cm. above the diaphragm. As was mentioned, most lie at the squamocolumnar junction (just above the esophagogastric sphincter) and, histologically, are covered by squamous epithelium on their upper surface and columnar epithelium on their lower aspect. Between the surfaces lies lamina propria, occasionally containing a few central muscle fibers. Although mild inflammatory changes are sometimes present, the mucosa typically is quite normal.

When the central opening of a lower esophageal ring is less than 13 mm. in diameter, dysphagia ensues. Patients who have symptoms rarely are under the age of 40 years, and may be of either sex. At first, dysphagia is episodic, occurring usually during a hurried meal, and separated by long symptom-free intervals. Gradually, the episodes become more frequent, and may be elicited even by soft foods. In many instances, however, the condition remains stable for years or, more often, is entirely asymptomatic. Schatzki found that of 66 lower esophageal rings, 46 remained unchanged for five years, 19 progressively encroached on the esophageal lumen, and one actually regressed.

CARCINOMA OF THE ESOPHAGUS

About 2 per cent of all cancer deaths in the United States are caused by this particularly cruel and deadly form of cancer. The disease rarely occurs before middle age, and affects men about three times as frequently as women. Roughly 90 per cent of these lesions are typical squamous cell carcinomas; the remainder are adenocarcinomas, which presumably arise from ectopic cardiac glands or from esophageal mucous glands. These relative incidences are somewhat controversial, however, depending upon whether carcinoma arising at the esophagogastric junction is regarded as esophageal or gastric in origin.

Etiology and Pathogenesis. There are four points on which there is general agreement:

1. Environmental influences weigh heavily in the development of esophageal carcinoma—even more so than in the case of gastric cancer (Alvarez and Colbert, 1963; Boyd et al., 1964; Adler, 1963a; Wynder and Bross, 1961; Editorial, 1974c). In contrast, there is little evidence for genetic predisposition. To some degree, then, esophageal carcinoma is a preventable disease. The importance of environmental factors is underscored by the tremendous geographic variation, at least 200-fold, in the incidence of this form of cancer (Editorial, 1973). Regions of the world in which there is an extraordinarily high incidence of esophageal cancer include: (1) eastern and southern Africa, (2) the Caribbean island of Curaçao, and (3) parts of a vast belt extending from the Middle East through central Asia to northern China. The search for a possible etiologic agent common to these areas has been unrewarding. Quite possibly such a single agent does not exist, but rather in each high-risk area a different carcinogenic influence is operative.

2. Any influence producing a disturbance in esophageal structure or physiology such that food and drink remain in contact with the mucosa longer than is normal tends to predispose to carcinoma, particularly squamous cell carcinoma, proximal to the derangement. Such a disturbance may result from partial obstruction or from a decrease in eosphageal motility (Adler, 1963a; Calkins, 1964). Underlying disorders include achalasia, lye strictures, esophageal diverticula and the Plummer-Vinson syndrome. In cases of achalasia, the incidence of subsequent carcinoma is about 4 per cent—13 times higher than in the general population. About the same percentage of patients with lye stricture as with achalasia can be expected to develop cancer 25 to 40 years after lye ingestion; and 10 per cent of those with esophageal diverticula eventually develop a neoplasm. The Plummer-Vinson syndrome seems to carry an especially high risk, probably as a result of the partial obstruction produced by mucosal webs in conjunction with the regenerative efforts of the abnormal epithelium. About 16 per cent of patients with the Plummer-Vinson syndrome develop carcinoma of the oropharynx or upper third of the esophagus, proximal to the webs, and, conversely 70 per cent of patients with cancer of the oropharynx and upper esophagus demonstrate some of the findings of the Plummer-Vinson syndrome.

3. An incompetent esophagogastric sphincter mechanism, with resultant reflux esophagitis, exposes the individual to a greater than normal risk of carcinoma, particularly adenocarcinoma, of the distal esophagus and cardia (Stemmer and Adams, 1960; Adler, 1963a; Calkins, 1964; Dawson, 1964). Underlying disorders may be present, including a congenitally short esophagus, prolonged vomiting or hiatus hernia. Since most of these tumors develop near the esophagogastric junction, some believe that they are merely extensions from carcinoma arising in the stomach and should properly be considered gastric. On the other hand, the dominant view is that most of these adenocarcinomas actually do arise in the esophagus. Certainly this is possible in patients with the so-called "Barrett esophagus." In these individuals the normal squamous epithelium of the distal esophagus becomes replaced by columnar epithelium, probably originating in ectopic cardiac glands. This phenomenon is thought to represent an adaptive response to chronic acid-pepsin irritation in individuals with recurrent reflux esophagitis. Be that as it may, the "Barrett esophagus" does provide a focus for the origin of adenocarcinoma within the esophagus.

4. There is a positive correlation between the incidence of esophageal cancer in general, on the one hand, and alcoholism and tobacco smoking, on the other (Boyd et al., 1964). The frequency of esophageal cancer among heavy drinkers is about 25 times that among controls (Wynder and Bross, 1961). The carcinogenic influence is probably not alcohol itself, but rather one of the many contaminants in alcoholic drinks, including heavy metals and nitrosamines (Editorial, 1974c). There is also a correlation, though less marked, between smoking and esophageal carcinoma. In contrast to bronchogenic carcinoma, esophageal carcinoma is more frequent in heavy smokers of pipes and cigars than in cigarette smokers.

Morphology. Esophageal carcinoma tends to occur at one of three locations in the esophagus: near the esophagogastric junction (distal third of the esophagus)—40 to 50 per cent of all esophageal carcinoma; at the level of the aortic arch (middle third)—30 to 40 per cent; and at the level of the cricoid cartilage (upper third)—10 to 30 per cent. Early lesions are usually discovered incidentally and appear as small, gray-white plaques on the mucosa. Ultimately, in months to years, these encircle the circumference of the esophagus and simultaneously invade the submucosa. From this point, one of three gross morphologic patterns may evolve. The most common is a necrotic **ulcerating** lesion, which excavates deeply into surrounding structures and may erode into the respiratory tree, aorta, mediastinum or pericardium. The second pattern is that of a fungating **polypoid** mass, which protrudes into the lumen. The third variant is a diffuse **infiltrative** tumor that tends to spread within the wall of the esophagus, causing thickening, rigidity and narrowing of the lumen, with linear irregular ulcerations of the mucosa. As was mentioned, most of these tumors are histologically typical squamous cell carcinomas; the remainder are adenocarcinomas.

Not until esophageal carcinoma has undergone considerable local extension does metastatic disease develop. The pattern of spread depends on the location of the lesion within the esophagus. Lesions of the middle and upper thirds tend to remain confined within the thorax, involving the regional lymph nodes, larynx, trachea, thyroid and recurrent laryngeal nerves. Those tumors of the lower third are more likely to involve lymph nodes below the diaphgram as well as the mediastinal nodes. In addition, direct spread to the pericardium may occur in these cases.

Carcinoma of the esophagus has been staged as follows (Morton, 1970—71):

Stage I: Limited to esophagus; less than 5 cm. in length.

Stage II: Limited to esophagus, greater than 5 cm. in length, with resectable nodes.

Stage III: Lesion greater than 10 cm. in length; extension through esophagus into adjacent structures; inoperable nodes or inoperable lesion.

Stage IV: Lesion as in Stage III; evidence of perforation, fistula or distant metastases.

Clinical Course. Dysphagia is almost always the first symptom, but this characteristically does not develop until the lesion has spread at least halfway around the circumference of the esophagus. Weight loss is extreme because of the effects of the dysphagia added to the general anorexia characteristic of most malignant tumors. Depending somewhat on the exact location of the tumor, other manifestations of esophageal carcinoma include intractable hiccoughs or hoarseness, caused by involvement of the phrenic or recurrent laryngeal nerves, respectively; cough, as a result of invasion of the respiratory tree; and hemorrhage, when a large vessel is eroded. Superimposed infection is frequent. Occasionally, the first indication of the tumor is the dramatic aspiration of food through a tracheoesophageal fistula. Such fistulas are almost always caused by carcinoma of the esophagus, since bronchogenic carcinoma rarely invades the esophagus.

The insidious nature of this disease, as well as certain technical difficulties associated with surgical resection of the upper and middle esophagus, keep overall five-year survival rate below 5 per cent. Most lesions are Stage III or IV when first diagnosed. The outlook is best for those with lesions near the esophagogastric junction.

HEMATEMESIS

Hematemesis, or the vomiting of blood, is one of the most dramatic and frightening of all presentations of illness. It is also one of the most serious, carrying with it a mortality rate of over 10 per cent (Zollinger and Nick, 1970). The major causes of hematemesis vary in their relative frequencies from study to study, depending largely on the population group under consideration. Overall, the most important lesions causing hematemesis and their approximate frequencies are as follows (Mendeloff et al., 1966):

	Per Cent
Peptic ulcer	65
Gastritis	11
Gastric carcinoma	2
Hiatus hernia	2
Miscellaneous, including esophageal varices and lacerations	10
Unknown	10

However, among alcoholics the picture is somewhat different. As will be seen, these patients are especially vulnerable to acute gastritis and, when they have Laennec's cirrhosis, to esophageal varices. The following frequencies of causes of hematemesis among 158 patients with Laennec's cirrhosis demonstrate the altered pattern among this population (Merigan et al., 1960):

	Per Cent
Esophageal varices	53
Gastritis	22
Peptic ulcer (duodenal 14, gastric 6)	20
Unknown	5

Only three disorders causing hematemesis are discussed under this heading: *esophageal varices, esophageal lacerations (the Mallory-Weiss syndrome),* and *acute stress ulcers.* These *first* manifest themselves by hematemesis. In contrast, the other lesions which may produce upper gastrointestinal bleeding, while perhaps more common, usually have already called attention to themselves in other ways. For example, although up to 10 per cent of peptic ulcers may present with hematemesis, most have been associated with a long history of pain before the onset of any bleeding. It should be remembered, then, that despite this classification, most cases of hematemesis are caused by peptic ulcer disease or by gastritis.

ESOPHAGEAL VARICES

Dilatation of the esophageal venous plexus occurs whenever portal hypertension reverses the flow of blood in the portal vein and diverts it through the coronary and esophageal veins into the azygos system (p. 523). The most common underlying disorder is Laennec's (alcoholic) cirrhosis of the liver; other forms of cirrhosis as well may be responsible. Conversely, about two thirds of all cirrhotic patients have esophageal varices. Rarely, the portal hypertension results from portal vein thrombosis, pylephlebitis or compression or invasion of major portal radicles by a tumor. Whatever the underlying cause, esophageal varices draw their momentous clinical import from their vulnerability to rupture, with massive, usually fatal, hemorrhage. *Indeed, ruptured esophageal varix is probably the most common cause of* fatal *upper gastrointestinal hemorrhage* (Orloff et al., 1967).

Morphology. In surgical or postmortem specimens, esophageal varices may be difficult to demonstrate because of their collapse following transection, with drainage of the contained blood. When not collapsed, they appear as bluish, submucosal, serpentine ridges, running in the long axis of the distal esophagus and bulging into the lumen. Although the overlying mucosa may be normal, it is often somewhat eroded and inflamed because of its exposed position, and these secondary changes enhance the likelihood of rupture. If rupture has occurred in the past, thrombosis or marked inflammation may be seen.

Clinical Course. Esophageal varices are characteristically silent until rupture occurs. The ensuing clinical picture is then catastrophic, with the sudden onset of massive, painless hematemesis. Among patients with cirrhosis of the liver, varices are, of course, a frequent cause of hematemesis, but it should be remembered that these patients are also more vulnerable to other causes of hematemesis, such as acute gastritis. Differentiation between a bleeding esophageal varix and gastric causes of hematemesis is often difficult, sometimes depending on history, x-ray studies and esophagogastroscopy.

The prognosis with a ruptured esophageal varix is remarkably poor. About 70 per cent of patients succumb during their first episode of bleeding (Orloff et al., 1967; Merigan et al., 1960). There is some evidence that the outlook is improved by surgery, either varix ligation or portacaval shunt.

ESOPHAGEAL LACERATIONS (MALLORY-WEISS SYNDROME)

Infrequently, small mucosal tears occur near the esophagogastric junction following repeated vomiting, usually in an alcoholic. However, not all such patients are alcoholics and, rarely, there is no history of antecedent vomiting. It has been speculated that the lacerations are related to a failure of normal reflex relaxation of the esophageal musculature during the vigorous antiperistaltic contractions of vomiting. Others believe that such lacerations always imply an associated hiatus hernia (see p. 471) with consequent inadequate diaphragmatic support for the distal esophagus.

The lacerations, varying in length from a few millimeters to several centimeters, lie in the long axis of the distal esophagus or astride the esophagogastric junction. Only the mucosa may be involved, or the lacerations may perforate the entire esophageal wall. The histology is of a nonspecific traumatic defect, followed, if the patient survives, by an inflammatory response.

Hematemesis is usually sudden and massive. Not infrequently, the hemorrhage is fatal.

ACUTE STRESS ULCERS (CURLING'S ULCERS)

These superficial mucosal lesions develop in the stomach, duodenum or both, within hours to two weeks following any extreme stress. They are particularly common after severe burns, trauma, sepsis and shock from any cause. Those associated with burns are known as *Curling's ulcers.* The pathogenesis of these lesions is unknown, but it is thought to involve local ischemia (Czaja et al., 1974). There is no increase in gastric acidity (Eiseman and Heyman, 1970). Following head injury or intracranial surgery, similar lesions, known as *Cushing's ulcers,* may develop. In contrast to other stress ulcers, these often penetrate the full thickness of the mucosa and are associated with marked hypersecretion of gastric acid, perhaps due to an increased release of gastrin (Silen, 1974).

Clinically, stress ulcers manifest themselves by the sudden onset of upper gastrointestinal bleeding. Other indications of their presence, such as pain, are absent or are masked by the underlying disorder. In about 50 per cent of cases, bleeding can be controlled by conservative measures, but recurrences are frequent.

Morphology. Acute stress ulcers may be single or multiple, and affect the stomach, duodenum or both, in that order. The individual defect tends to be circular and small, less than 1 cm. in diameter, and characteristically it does not penetrate the muscularis but involves only the superficial mucosa. The margins are poorly defined, without significant hyperemic reaction, and the rugal pattern is undisturbed. Acid digestion of blood frequently stains the ulcer base a dark brown color. Sometimes stress ulcers are poorly circumscribed, appearing only as a diffuse erosion of the gastric mucosa. As will be seen, in these cases the anatomic picture merges with that of acute gastritis with hemorrhage.

Depending upon the duration of the lesion, the histologic changes are those of a more or less well defined acute inflammatory infiltration in the ulcer margins and base. However, unlike chronic peptic ulcers, to be discussed later, acute stress ulcers are not associated with fibrous scarring or with thickening of the underlying blood vessel walls.

PAIN

Abdominal pain is the most common symptom of gastrointestinal disease. It may also be caused by pancreatic, biliary, renal and female genital tract disease, as well as by certain systemic and extra-abdominal disorders. Such pain often heralds a major abdominal crisis demanding surgical intervention. Clearly, then, the evaluation of abdominal pain is one of the most challenging and important tasks confronting the clinician. Although a detailed discussion of the differential diagnosis of abdominal pain is beyond the scope of this book, perhaps the following few comments on the subject will aid the reader in better correlating the major gastrointestinal diseases with their clinical presentations.

Obviously, the *location* of pain within the abdomen is of diagnostic importance, as are its character and concomitant physical findings. Vomiting is so frequently an accompaniment of abdominal pain from virtually any cause as to have little differential value.

Upper abdominal pain of gastrointestinal origin may be caused by lesions of the stomach and proximal small bowel. Although esophageal disorders may also produce epigastric pain, they are more commonly associated with substernal discomfort. *Nevertheless, certain esophageal lesions are included under this heading for convenience.* Thus, the pain of hiatus hernia, esophagitis, gastritis and peptic ulcer disease is either substernal or in the upper abdomen. It should not be forgotten that pancreatic, biliary and renal diseases are also typically associated with upper abdominal pain. Of equal importance is the fact that pain from thoracic lesions, such as myocardial infarction and pneumonia, may be referred to the upper abdomen.

Midabdominal pain is characteristically caused by disorders of the small intestine. Among these are infectious diseases of the small bowel, Crohn's disease and Meckel's diverticulum. Acute appendicitis typically presents early as midabdominal discomfort and later as right lower quadrant pain.

Lower abdominal pain is characteristic of lesions of the colon, including infectious diseases and ulcerative colitis. As was mentioned, right lower quadrant pain is characteristic of late appendicitis and, often, of Crohn's disease. Left lower quadrant pain occurs with diverticular disease.

The *severity* of the pain of gastrointestinal disease ranges from the vague and extremely mild discomfort which may be associated with atrophic gastritis to the agonizing pain of a perforated peptic ulcer. *Severe abdominal pain which requires immediate evaluation to determine whether an emergency laparotomy should be performed is known in medical jargon as an "acute abdomen."* Usually, but not necessarily, local or generalized peritonitis is present in these patients. Local peritonitis is characterized by guarding, muscular spasm and rebound tenderness referred to the involved area; with generalized peritonitis, there is often board-like rigidity of the entire abdominal wall. Bowel sounds are absent.

Peritonitis — local or generalized — may be caused either by bacterial infection or by chemical irritation. Bacterial soiling from penetration or perforation of an inflamed viscus is the most common etiology. In this manner, acute appendicitis, acute cholecystitis, pelvic inflammatory disease (PID), diverticulitis, ulcerative colitis and Crohn's disease may all cause an acute abdomen with peritonitis. Acute appendicitis is the most frequent cause of an acute abdomen, with or without peritonitis, followed in frequency by acute cholecystitis. *Chemical peritonitis results from the presence in the peritoneum of hydrochloric acid, pancreatic enzymes, blood or bile.* Common causes include perforation of a peptic ulcer, acute pancreatitis, a ruptured tubal pregnancy and perforation of the gallbladder.

An acute abdomen *without* peritonitis may occur with obstruction of a hollow viscus or early in the course of a vascular calamity, such as a mesenteric occlusion. Obstruction differs from peritonitis in that bowel sounds are hyperactive rather than absent, and the pain is of a characteristic colicky nature. The intensity of the pain is roughly inversely proportional to the size of the lumen of the obstructed viscus. Thus, there is decreasingly severe pain associated with obstruction of the ureters, bile ducts, and small and large intestines in that order.

It must be remembered that a variety of systemic metabolic disorders may simulate an acute abdomen. These include the porphyrias, sickle cell anemia, uremia and diabetic ketosis.

Infectious diseases of the bowel, Crohn's disease and ulcerative colitis, all of which have just been mentioned in the brief survey of abdominal pain, are discussed in detail under the heading *diarrhea*, since, when diarrhea is present, it is a somewhat more specific manifestation of gastrointestinal disease.

HIATUS HERNIA

Hiatus hernia refers to an upward herniation of the stomach through the esophageal hiatus, such that a portion of the stomach comes to lie above the diaphragm. Two anatomic variants are recognized. The more common one, comprising about 90 per cent of cases, is known as a *sliding hiatus hernia.* This is associated with a shortened esophagus; the esophagogastric junction as well as a portion of the stomach lies above the diaphragm. The less common variant is the *paraesophageal hiatus hernia,* characterized by a defect or weakening of the hiatus such that a portion of the gastric fundus rolls up alongside the esophagus into the thorax. The esophagogastric junction remains in its normal position. Coexistence of these two variants occurs.

The reported incidence of hiatus hernias varies markedly from study to study, in part because many mild ones are totally asymptomatic and are demonstrable only by careful x-ray studies. Most would agree that sliding hiatus hernias are extremely frequent, occurring in from 7 to 40 per cent of otherwise normal individuals (Editorial, 1969b). They are thought to be more common with obesity and advancing age, and to affect women more often than men. However, one study, in which sliding hiatus hernias were found in 33 per cent of symptom-free individuals, yielded no correlation with age, sex or obesity (Dyer and Pridie, 1968).

Etiology and Pathogenesis. The cause of hiatus hernias is unknown. Doubtless some cases of the sliding type result from a congenitally short esophagus, but this explanation is not satisfactory for all cases. While it is speculated that the esophagus may in other instances become shortened because of chronic inflammation with fibrotic retraction, this is probably a result rather than a cause of hiatus hernia.

Morphology. After death, when relaxation of the gastrointestinal tract allows the stomach to slip back into the abdominal cavity, only the largest hiatus hernias are grossly demonstrable. Nor are there diagnostic histologic changes in an uncomplicated hiatus hernia. However, very frequently an associated reflux esophagitis (p. 471), an esophageal ring or stricture (p. 466) or, rarely, a "Barrett esophagus" (distal esophagus lined by columnar epithelium) (p. 467) may arouse suspicion of an underlying hiatus hernia.

Clinical Course. The clinical significance—if any—of a *sliding* hiatus hernia has been debated for years. The traditional view is that a sliding hiatus hernia necessarily implies incompetence of the esophagogastric sphincter with consequent reflux of gastric

juices. The classical symptoms, then, are retrosternal pain ("heartburn") due to reflux esophagitis, and occasional reflux of gastric juices into the mouth. The symptoms are more pronounced when reflux is most likely, e.g., while lying supine or when bending forward. *However, the correlation between hiatus hernia, demonstrable reflux of gastric contents and symptoms is, in general, poor.* About 50 per cent of all patients with hiatus hernia have no symptoms at all, and of the remainder, only about 9 per cent have the classical symptoms (Palmer, 1968). In many patients reflux cannot be demonstrated. Pointing to this poor correlation among presumably related phenomena, a few heretics have recently suggested that the esophagogastric sphincter is quite capable of functioning adequately without any support from the surrounding diaphragm, that is, even when it is located in the thorax. According to this view, the competence of the sphincter is almost entirely dependent on hormones, principally gastrin. Thus, the presence of a hiatus hernia would by no means imply reflux esophagitis (Salter, 1974; Cohen and Harris, 1971). Nevertheless, at least some patients with a hiatus hernia do have symptoms. It has been suggested that the retrosternal pain of hiatus hernia may, at least in some cases, be caused by disturbances in esophageal motility rather than by reflux. The issue remains unsettled.

Dysphagia may be associated with a hiatus hernia when there is a complicating esophageal stricture or mucosal ring.

The *paraesophageal* form of hiatus hernia manifests itself somewhat differently. Rather than exhibiting burning pain and reflux, these patients usually complain of postprandial bloating and belching. Rarely, twisting and strangulation of the herniated portion of the stomach occurs.

Patients with hiatus hernia usually lead a fairly normal life with, at most, only occasional episodes of discomfort. Serious complications, principally chronic peptic esophagitis with stricture formation, may develop, but these are relatively infrequent. Hiatus hernias are said to be associated with a slightly increased risk of developing esophageal carcinoma.

ESOPHAGITIS

Inflammation of the esophagus is seen in a variety of circumstances. Often it represents an agonal change. The following list indicates some of the more important clinical settings associated with esophagitis:

1. Recurrent reflux of gastric juice ("reflux" or "peptic esophagitis"), thought by most to be related to a hiatus hernia.

2. Repeated ingestion of irritant foods,

such as alcohol or very hot liquids; or the accidental or suicidal ingestion of corrosive agents, such as lye, other strong alkalies or acids.

3. Nonspecific bacterial infection, with hematogenous seeding of the esophagus or direct spread from, say, a mediastinitis or pericarditis.

4. Uncommon localization of tuberculosis, syphilis, or fungal infection; monilial esophagitis is becoming increasingly common as survival of debilitated patients is prolonged.

5. Prolonged gastric intubation.

6. Uremia.

7. Plummer-Vinson syndrome (see p. 466).

Morphology. As might be expected, the anatomic changes of esophagitis depend upon the cause, the duration and the severity of the process. With mild involvement, hyperemia may be the only alteration. More severe degrees of injury result in mucosal edema and inflammation, with areas of superficial necrosis, sometimes with pseudomembrane formation, ulceration and sloughing of the esophageal lining. Typically, moniliasis produces large gray-white inflammatory pseudomembranes teeming with the causative fungus. With chronicity or following a single profound insult, such as lye ingestion, progressive fibrous scarring may develop. Occasionally, such scarring leads to the formation of an annular stricture. These are most often associated with long-standing reflux esophagitis.

Histologically, the inflammatory infiltrate of esophagitis is usually nonspecific. Depending on whether the process is acute or chronic, polymorphonuclear or mononuclear leukocytes may predominate. However, with esophagitis caused by tuberculosis, syphilis or mycosis, the characteristic tissue reactions of these processes are produced. With reflux esophagitis, a "Barrett esophagus" may be present (see p. 467), and any ulcerations in the columnar epithelium, then, closely resemble peptic ulcers of the stomach. Annular strictures caused by reflux esophagitis usually develop at the squamocolumnar junction, which in the Barrett esophagus may be as high as the middle third of the esophagus.

Sometimes esophageal erosions or ulcers occur agonally or even after death. They are seen as shallow, irregular ulcers, having brown digested blood in their bases. These lesions are not associated with inflammatory changes. In order to differentiate them from true esophagitis with ulceration, they are termed **esophagomalacia.**

Clinical Course. The clinical picture depends somewhat on the cause of the esophagitis. For example, agonal, uremic or bacteremic esophagitis may be either asymptomatic or completely overshadowed by the more serious, underlying disease. Reflux esophagitis, as was mentioned in the discus-

sion of hiatus hernia, is characterized by recurrent burning substernal pain and reflux of gastric juice into the mouth. The development of a stricture is heralded by the insidious onset of dysphagia. However, dysphagia in these cases is almost always preceded by a history of long-standing, characteristic pain. Certain types of esophagitis, such as that of the Plummer-Vinson syndrome and that following lye ingestion, predispose to the later development of cancer. Bleeding may occur with severe esophagitis, but only rarely is it sufficiently profuse to cause hematemesis or overtly bloody stools.

GASTRITIS

Laymen and physicians alike are guilty of using this term as a "wastebasket" diagnosis for all manner of nonspecific transient complaints—in particular, for any vague epigastric discomfort or vomiting. In reality, the designation gastritis should be reserved for several specific gastric derangements which can be diagnosed with certainty only by gastroscopy and biopsy. The two most important types of gastritis—*acute* and *atrophic*—are probably quite unrelated, and have in common only some degree of shedding of the gastric surface epithelium and a variable inflammatory infiltrate (Croft, 1967). These will be discussed separately.

ACUTE GASTRITIS

This lesion probably occurs almost as frequently as it is diagnosed, but because of its usually benign and transient nature, its presence is rarely confirmed histologically. *Acute gastritis represents the response of the stomach to local irritants.* As such, its severity is highly variable, depending on the etiologic circumstances.

Etiology and Pathogenesis. *The most frequent causes of acute gastritis are alcohol, salicylates and staphylococcal endotoxin.* Often patients take aspirin as an antidote for alcohol, as indeed for nearly anything, thus exposing their hapless gastric mucosa to a pair of offenders thought by some to potentiate each other (Editorial, 1970c).

Slight occult bleeding occurs in about 70 per cent of patients who take aspirin regularly for, say, rheumatoid arthritis. In about 15 per cent of these patients, blood loss is over 10 ml. daily, and iron deficiency anemia develops. Individual vulnerability to aspirin is highly variable. Less common etiologic agents include digitalis, iodine, tetracycline, caffeine, cinchophen and phenylbutazone. *Very severe gastritis occurs with the accidental or suicidal ingestion of mercury, strong acids or alkalies.* Unproved but possible factors in mild acute gastritis are very spicy foods and excessively hot or cold foods.

Morphology. Even under normal circumstances, the mucus-secreting columnar cells of the gastric surface epithelium lead a precarious existence, surviving only 2 to 4 days. When exposed to any unusual irritant, they are shed and replaced even more rapidly. In this sense, very mild acute gastritis, defined as unusually rapid turnover of the gastric epithelium, constitutes a heightened physiologic response. With more severe insults, there may be hyperemia, edema and denudation of the superficial layer of the mucosa. Only rarely are the deeper levels involved. After removal of the causative agent, regeneration of the sloughed epithelium is usually complete within a few days.

When exposure to the irritant is intense or long-standing, hemorrhagic erosions of the gastric mucosa may ensue. Such erosions merge, on the one hand, with focal acute stress ulcers, and on the other, with diffuse destruction of the entire mucosa, as when strong corrosives are swallowed. **Diffuse hemorrhagic erosive gastritis** is also known to occur with both heavy alcohol use and aspirin ingestion, either separately or together. A similar lesion, of uncertain pathogenesis, is often seen as a component of uremia.

Clinical Course. Depending on the causative agent and the severity of the lesion, acute gastritis may be entirely asymptomatic, may cause variable degrees of epigastric pain, nausea and vomiting, or may produce massive hematemesis and melena. Mild cases, such as those resulting from ingestion of certain of the drugs and caffeine, commonly cause little or no discomfort. Acute gastritis from staphylococcal endotoxin is associated with the sudden onset, about 5 hours after eating contaminated food, of intense epigastric distress and vomiting, but it is transient and self-limited. A similar picture following overenthusiastic intake of alcohol is perhaps even more familiar. Aspirin use is associated with a variety of rather vague complaints, such as "sour stomach" and "heartburn." Sometimes, patients with acute gastritis caused by aspirin ingestion may remain entirely unaware of any problem until the sudden onset of hematemesis or melena. So widespread and indiscriminate is the use of this drug that it has been estimated that 25 per cent of all cases of hematemesis and melena in the London area are triggered by aspirin ingestion (Valman et al., 1968). Similarly, alcohol may without warning cause sudden hemorrhagic erosive gastritis. While bleeding in these cases may be severe, it usually ceases spontaneously within 36 hours. Because of the relative safety of conservative management, x-ray and gastroscopic differentiation from other causes of hematemesis is important.

ATROPHIC GASTRITIS

This most common form of *chronic* gastritis is characterized by progressive and irreversible atrophy of the glandular epithelium of the stomach, with loss of the acid-secreting parietal cells and the pepsin-secreting chief cells. Elaboration of intrinsic factor (IF) is also impaired. The process may be focal or diffuse, partial or total. *Diffuse total atrophy, resulting in histamine-fast achlorhydria, is a component of pernicious anemia (PA).* However, atrophic gastritis may also be seen in individuals without impairment of vitamin B_{12} absorption.

Atrophic gastritis is a very common lesion, having been found in about 10 per cent of the general population (Isokoski et al., 1969). The incidence increases markedly with age. There is some familial predisposition, as well as an association with a number of other pathologic entities, principally autoimmune disease of the thyroid. Heavy alcohol intake and tobacco smoking also seem to predispose to atrophic gastritis.

Etiology and Pathogenesis. The cause of atrophic gastritis is unknown. Many workers now believe that there are two distinct forms of this disorder: (1) *autoimmune (type A) atrophic gastritis,* which progresses to PA in about 20 per cent of cases and is often associated with other autoimmune disorders, and (2) *simple (type B) atrophic gastritis,* which occurs as an isolated lesion, particularly in elderly individuals, and is not associated with impairment of vitamin B_{12} absorption. Simple atrophic gastritis is at least three times as frequent as the autoimmune form. It should be emphasized that there appears to be some overlap of these forms, and in occasional patients the distinction between them is very difficult.

In general, autoimmune atrophic gastritis is separated from simple atrophic gastritis by the presence of circulating antibodies against gastric parietal cells. In addition the lesion tends to involve the corpus of the stomach diffusely, causing severe impairment of acid-pepsin secretion, while sparing the antrum. These patients and their first-degree relatives have a greater than expected incidence of thyroid disease, Addison's disease of the adrenals, and diabetes mellitus, as well as of antibodies against gastric and thyroid antigens. As mentioned, PA eventually develops in about 20 per cent of patients with autoimmune atrophic gastritis. Prospective studies have shown that this progression may take from 1 to 18 years after the diagnosis of atrophic gastritis (Irvine et al., 1974; Strickland and Mackay, 1973).

Many patients with autoimmune atrophic gastritis have serum antibodies against IF, as well as those against gastric parietal cells.

These are of two types. The most frequent is a blocking antibody (type 1), which couples with IF in such a way as to prevent its combining with vitamin B$_{12}$; the other (type 2) is a binding antibody, which attaches elsewhere on the IF molecule and may therefore react with the IF-B$_{12}$ complex. The significance of antibodies against IF is uncertain. Their presence in the serum does not seem to determine which patients with autoimmune atrophic gastritis later develop PA (Irvine et al., 1974; Strickland and Mackay, 1973; Rose et al., 1970.) However, IF antibodies may also be found in the gastric juice, and these may be of more significance in contributing to the development of PA (Rose et al., 1970). The presence within the gastric mucosa of a prominent lymphoid infiltrate, sometimes with the formation of germinal follicles, suggests that a cell-based immunologic process may also be involved in the pathogenesis of autoimmune atrophic gastritis. Quite possibly the primary mechanism is a mucosal cell-based immune reaction and the serum antibodies are merely incidental.

Simple atrophic gastritis differs from the autoimmune form in several respects. First, autoantibodies are usually not present with simple atrophic gastritis. The atrophic changes tend to be focal, with only moderate impairment of acid-pepsin secretion. The antrum is involved as well as the fundus. Patients with simple atrophic gastritis are in general not at risk of developing PA, although rare cases have been described. Those who retain some capacity for acid secretion are, however, at risk of developing gastric peptic ulcers. It has been suggested that dysfunction of the pyloric sphincter, by exposing the stomach to regurgitation of duodenal fluid, may underlie the development of atrophic gastritis, which in turn predisposes to ulceration (Strickland and Mackay, 1973). The causation of simple atrophic gastritis is far from settled, however, and the absence of serum antibodies against gastric parietal cells does not exclude a role for cell-based immune mechanisms.

Morphology. The stomach wall loses its rugal folds and becomes flattened, glazed and red. Submucosal vessels can usually be discerned through the thinned mucosa. Occasionally, superficial hemorrhagic erosions occur.

Three characteristic histologic changes are present:

(1) **Atrophy of the glandular epithelium of the gastric fundus:** The glands are shortened and may be cystically dilated. Many become totally atrophic. **The most important feature is loss of the parietal cells and, to a lesser extent, the chief cells, which are replaced by mucus-secreting cells.** These changes may be focal or diffuse. Even in affected areas, the loss of parietal and chief cells may be complete or only partial. Interglandular connective tissue becomes scanty.

(2) **Abnormalities of the surface epithelium:** There is an increased turnover of the surface epithelial cells, which become stunted and deformed. Villus-like projections may form and, coupled with loss of specialized secretory cells, may cause the gastric mucosa to resemble that of the intestine (intestinal metaplasia, intestinalization).

(3) **Interstitial infiltration of the mucosa by lymphocytes, plasma cells, eosinophils and occasionally neutrophils.** In long-standing cases, lymphoid follicles may be prominent in the lamina propria.

Clinical Course. Atrophic gastritis may be asymptomatic, or it may be associated with vague abdominal complaints, such as epigastric discomfort and occasionally nausea and vomiting. Histamine-fast achlorhydria is present with PA, but in other cases variable gastric acidity may remain. Infrequently, hemorrhagic erosions of the atrophied epithelium produce significant bleeding, with hematemesis and melena.

The clinical importance of atrophic gastritis lies almost solely in its relationship to other, more serious disorders—namely, PA, of which it is a component; gastric peptic ulcer; gastric carcinoma; and iron deficiency anemia. The hematologic aspects of PA have been discussed in Chapter 11.

Perhaps more than 50 per cent of patients with a gastric peptic ulcer have an associated atrophic gastritis, and it is thought that the latter condition antedates and predisposes to the ulceration. *Of greater import is the fact that approximately 10 to 15 per cent of patients with atrophic gastritis eventually develop gastric carcinoma.* There would seem to be a prolonged premalignant phase, as evidenced by an interval of 10 to 20 years between the development of atrophic gastritis and the appearance of overt carcinoma (Siurala et al., 1966; Cheli et al., 1973). Because of its greater prevalence, simple atrophic gastritis is a more important precursor of cancer than is the autoimmune form. Whether or not one form of atrophic gastritis carries an *inherently* greater risk of cancer than the other is controversial. For mysterious reasons, patients with atrophic gastritis are also vulnerable to recurrent iron deficiency anemia. Whether this can be attributed to loss of iron in the rapidly shed gastric epithelial cells is not clear. There is some evidence that a minimum level of gastric acidity is required for the efficient absorption of iron in the intestine.

PEPTIC ULCERS (CHRONIC ULCERS)

These are chronic, usually solitary ulcerations, which may occur at any site in the gastrointestinal tract that is exposed to acid-pep-sin secretion. By definition, peptic ulcers do not occur in patients with achlorhydria, although they may develop with varying degrees of hypochlorhydria. Peptic ulcers may be found in any of the following six sites, listed in order of descending frequency: (1) duodenum, (2) stomach, (3) esophagus, when there is reflux, (4) at the margins of a gastroenterostomy (stomal ulcer), (5) in the jejunum near the ligament of Treitz in patients with the Zollinger-Ellison syndrome (see p. 544), and (6) in a Meckel's diverticulum that contains ectopic gastric mucosa. *About 98 per cent of peptic ulcers occur either in the duodenum or the stomach, and it is with those that we are here principally concerned.*

At present, it is estimated that about 10 per cent of the population of the United States has or will have a peptic ulcer. Duodenal ulcers are 5 to 10 times more common then gastric ulcers. Duodenal ulcers may develop at any age, and are quite frequent in early adulthood. Men are affected about four times as often as women. Gastric ulcers tend to affect an older age group, and show a male preponderance of about 2 to 1.

Etiology and Pathogenesis. Despite the importance of peptic ulcers, concepts related to their pathogenesis remain largely speculative and, while they are reasonable, they are not very satisfactory when applied to the individual case. *It is generally accepted that peptic ulceration reflects an imbalance between the levels of acid-pepsin secretion and the normal defenses of the neighboring mucosa.* In rare instances, one or the other of these factors is overwhelming and the development of an ulcer can be readily explained on this basis. For example, with the Zollinger-Ellison syndrome, which is caused by a gastrin secreting tumor of the pancreas, gastric acid secretion is so high as to make eventual ulceration inevitable, regardless of the defensive forces. With perhaps somewhat less justification, a stomal ulcer may be considered to result almost entirely from inadequate mucosal defenses at the traumatized margins of the gastroenterostomy, since these patients necessarily have a reduced acid output. Such clear-cut instances, however, represent only a very small proportion of peptic ulcers. *In the overwhelming majority of cases of duodenal and gastric ulcers, the relative contribution to ulcerogenesis of aggressive and defensive factors is murky, at best.* While patients with duodenal ulcers have, on the average, higher than normal levels of acid secretion, and those with gastric ulcers have, on the average, lower than normal acid secretion, there is much overlapping, not only between each of these groups and the intermediate normal population, but also between the two groups themselves. *Nevertheless, in a*

general way it might be said that duodenal ulcers tend to reflect increased acid-pepsin secretion, whereas gastric ulcers are more likely to result from decreased resistance.

What causes the increased acid-pepsin secretion sometimes associated with duodenal ulcers? In general, fasting plasma gastrin levels are normal in these patients. However, there is some evidence that gastrin release *in response to food* may be augmented (Reeder et al., 1970; McGuigan and Trudeau, 1973). When it is recalled that high acid levels normally exert a negative feedback on gastrin release, even normal gastrin levels become surprising (Wesdorp and Fischer, 1974). Conceivably, there is some sort of upward readjustment of the balance between gastrin release and acid secretion. In a very small percentage of patients with a duodenal ulcer, fasting gastrin levels are markedly elevated. Hyperplasia of the gastrin-containing cells (G-cells) of the pyloric antrum has been demonstrated in some of these cases. Confusingly, this unusual cause of duodenal ulcers has been referred to as the Zollinger-Ellison syndrome type I, even though there is no lesion of the pancreas (Ganguli et al., 1974).

As can be seen, very little is known about the variably elevated levels of acid-pepsin secretion sometimes associated with a duodenal ulcer. What of the decreased resistance associated with gastric ulcers? Among the factors which normally defend the mucosa against acid-pepsin digestion are an abundant mucus secretion and an adequate blood flow. No doubt, other and as yet undefined protective factors are operative. In this context, the association between gastric ulcers and atrophic gastritis is of interest. *As was already mentioned, about 50 per cent of patients with gastric ulcers also have atrophic gastritis, and hence have an abnormal mucosa.* Although a deficiency of mucus secretion in these patients has been hypothesized, it has not been clearly demonstrated.

The importance of a normal blood flow in the prevention of peptic ulcer has long been recognized. Perhaps the increased vulnerability of the elderly to gastric ulcers reflects primarily the arteriosclerotic changes in the vessels of the gastric mucosa. It is known that the walls of underlying vessels in the region of peptic ulceration are often extremely thickened, but it is unknown whether these changes precede the ulceration or merely result from a secondary inflammatory response.

Even less completely understood than the imbalance between acid-pepsin secretion and normal mucosal defenses are the hereditary and environmental factors which may operate to create these imbalances. For example, peptic ulcer disease is largely confined to "civilized" areas of the world, and it is widely suspected to develop more frequently in stress-prone individuals. A positive correlation with cigarette smoking is of some interest in this regard (Friedman et al., 1974). Less ill defined is the fact that premenopausal women have a much lower incidence of peptic ulcer than do postmenopausal women, raising the possibility that estrogens may act in some protective way. In contrast, some believe adrenal corticosteroids to be ulcerogenic, although their mechanism of action is obscure.

It has been suggested that delayed emptying of the stomach from any cause, such as an imbalance in the gastrointestinal hormones or duodenal scarring, predisposes to the development of gastric ulcers. Of some support to this theory is the fact that 25 to 33 per cent of gastric ulcers occur in patients who have had a previous duodenal ulcer. A hereditary factor in the genesis of peptic ulcers is apparent in the known greater than chance association of duodenal ulcers with blood group O and of gastric ulcers with blood group A (Menguy, 1970).

Clearly, then, there is no one simple cause of peptic ulcer disease. A multitude of influences, many as yet unknown, may operate not only in different patients but also within any one patient.

Morphology. The salient macroscopic features of duodenal and gastric ulcers can be considered according to site, size and appearance.

Site. The favored locations are, in order of frequency, the anterior wall of the first portion of the duodenum, the posterior wall of the first portion, the second portion of the duodenum, and the lesser curvature of the pyloric antrum (Fig. 14–1). Gastric ulcers, however, may occur anywhere in the stomach, and as many as 14 per cent occur on the greater curvature, classically the site of ulcerating carcinomas. It should be noted that all of the principal sites, while located just "downstream" from the source of acid secretion, do not themselves involve acid secreting mucosa.

Size. Benign peptic ulcers in general are smaller than ulcerating carcinomas. About 50 per cent of peptic ulcers are less than 2 cm. in diameter, 75 per cent are less than 3 cm. and only 10 per cent are larger than 4 cm. in diameter. In contrast, about 50 per cent of ulcerating carcinomas are over 4 cm. in diameter. Obviously, the overlap is so great as to make size alone useless in distinguishing a benign from a malignant lesion.

Appearance. Of greater importance in distinguishing between benign and malignant forms is the gross appearance of the crater itself. **The classic peptic ulcer is a sharply punched-out, round to oval defect, with well defined perpendicular walls and a smooth, clean base. The mucosal margins are virtually level with the surrounding mucosa and overhang only slightly on the upstream portion of the circumference. Contrast this appearance with that of the heaped-up, shaggy margins and necrotic base of an ulcerating carcinoma (see p. 484).**

The crater of a benign ulcer may penetrate only the superficial mucosa, or it may extend into the muscularis (Fig. 14–2). Occasionally, penetration of the entire wall occurs, and in these cases the base of the ulcer may be formed by the adjacent pancreas, omental fat or adherent liver. With most chronic peptic ulcers, underlying scarring causes puckering of the mucosa so that mucosal folds radiate out from the crater in spokelike fashion. Such a mucosal pattern provides a valuable clue to the location of the lesion for surgeon, pathologist and radiologist alike.

The histologic appearance varies with the activity, chronicity and degree of healing. During the active phase, four zones are classically demonstrable: (1) The base and margins have a superficial

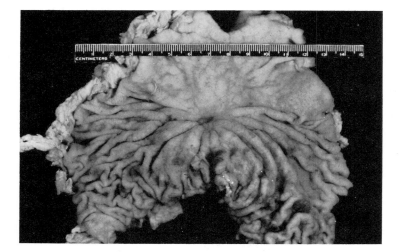

Figure 14–1. Gastric ulcer. The stomach has been opened along the greater curvature. Centrally placed is an oval ulcer crater positioned along the lesser curvature. Note the radiating rugal folds.

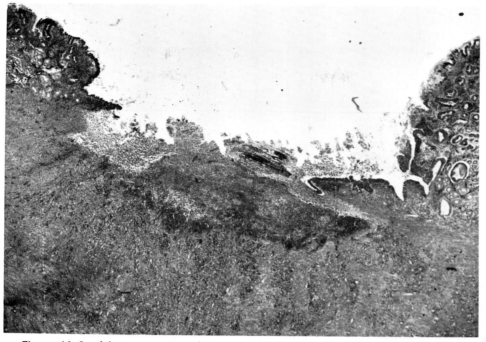

Figure 14–2. A low power view of a peptic ulcer to illustrate the depth of the lesion.

thin layer of necrotic fibrinoid debris, which is not visible to the naked eye. (2) Beneath this layer is a zone of active, nonspecific cellular infiltrate, with neutrophils predominating. (3) In the deeper layers, especially in the base, there is active granulation tissue infiltrated with mononuclear leukocytes. (4) The granulation tissue rests on a more solid fibrous or collagenous scar, which fans out widely toward the serosal surface. The vessel walls within the scarred area are characteristically thickened and occasionally are thrombosed. More or less complete healing may occur. When the crater is superficial and scarring minimal, reepithelialization may leave no residual trace of the defect. With deeper chronic lesions, regeneration is less perfect, presumably because of impaired blood supply, and varying degrees of scarring and deformity ensue.

Clinical Course. Episodic pain is the most common manifestation of peptic ulcer, although over 10 per cent of patients are entirely asymptomatic until complications arise. The location, character and intensity of the pain are highly variable. Usually pain is centered in the epigastrium, but it may be referred to the back, particularly with posterior penetrating lesions, or it may be substernal. While the pain is classically described as gnawing, its character may instead be aching, burning or pressing. Intensity varies from mild to severe. *The single most important aspect of peptic ulcer pain is its episodic nature, both over a single day and over the longer course of the patient's life.* Months may pass during which the individual is entirely asymptomatic, only to have a recrudescence of his symptoms for several weeks, followed again by a quiescent period. During the symptomatic intervals, persons with a duodenal ulcer commonly experience their greatest discomfort when they are hungry, about 2 to 3 hours after the last meal. The pain is then steady and continues until it is relieved by food or antacids. These patients may also be awakened by the pain in the early morning, about 2 A.M., and require food before they can return to sleep.

With a gastric ulcer, the pain typically occurs almost immediately after eating. While this difference in timing between duodenal and gastric ulcer pain is of some distinguishing value, there is sufficient variability to make it not altogether reliable in the individual case. Another criterion of limited usefulness is the more frequent association of nausea and vomiting with a gastric ulcer.

Complications of peptic ulcer disease include: (1) bleeding, (2) perforation, with peritonitis, (3) obstruction from edema or from scarring of the duodenum, and (4) intractable pain. *Malignant transformation is unknown with duodenal ulcers, but it is a small though important risk with gastric ulcers.* About 1 per cent of gastric peptic ulcers undergo malignant transformation.

Bleeding is the most frequent complication of a peptic ulcer. From 25 to 33 per cent of these patients bleed (Chandler, 1967), sometimes massively. Nearly 10 per cent are entirely asymptomatic until the sudden onset of hematemesis or melena. Such massive bleeding implies the erosion of a major vessel in the base of the ulcer crater. The mortality rate in these patients ranges from 3 to 10 per cent (Balasegaram, 1968), and this represents about 25 per cent of the total deaths attributable to peptic ulcer disease.

Perforation of the ulcer through the wall of the stomach or duodenum occurs in only about 5 per cent of patients, but it is responsible for about 65 per cent of deaths from peptic ulcer disease (Fig. 14–3). These patients experience sudden excruciating epigastric pain, and within minutes develop a chemical peritonitis with a boardlike abdomen as a result of the escape of hydrochloric acid into the peritoneum. Perforation, like bleeding, may occur without prior symptoms.

Some degree of narrowing of the duodenum occurs with most peptic ulcers at this site, either from edema during the active inflammatory phase or from later scarring. Infrequently, deformity of the duodenum is sufficiently severe to produce total obstruction of the lumen, with intractable vomiting. Obstruction rarely is a problem with gastric ulcers, except for those that straddle the pylorus.

Diagnosis of peptic ulcer disease is usually made on the basis of barium x-ray studies and sometimes by gastroscopy. Radiographic studies are about 90 per cent accurate in diagnosing duodenal ulcers and 70 per cent accurate with gastric ulcers.

Peptic ulcer disease is rarely fatal, but it is a serious diathesis, and its sufferer is chained to a glass of milk and a bottle of antacid. Those with a duodenal ulcer can usually struggle through bouts of active disease in this fashion with their entrails intact. Because of the danger of carcinoma masquerading as a benign gastric ulcer, patients with a gastric lesion are more likely to come to surgery.

APPENDICITIS

Acute appendicitis is one of the most common of gastrointestinal diseases. Although it may occur at any age, it is most frequent in young adults. The sexes are affected approximately equally.

Etiology and Pathogenesis. Despite its frequency, the etiology of acute appendicitis is only incompletely understood. Most probably the usual inciting event is obstruction of the appendiceal lumen by a fecalith, although other causes of intraluminal obstruction (tumors, pinworms) may occasionally be operative. In any case, with obstruction, the outflow of mucus secretion is blocked and the appendix becomes distended. Possibly this distention compromises the blood flow within the wall of the appendix, thereby rendering it vulnerable to invasion by ordinarily harmless native bacteria. Indeed, cultures of acutely inflamed appendices most commonly yield local organisms, such as *E. coli* or the enterococci. After inflammation and bacterial invasion have ensued, the process is usually irreversible, even when the fecalith is spontaneously dislodged.

Morphology. In **early acute appendicitis,** there is a scant neutrophilic exudation throughout the mucosa, submucosa and muscularis. The subserosal vessels are congested and are often surrounded by a neutrophilic emigration. The congestion transforms the normally glistening serosal covering into a reddened, dull, granular membrane. As the process develops, the neutrophilic exudate becomes more marked, and the serosa is covered by a fibrinopurulent material (Fig. 14—4). Foci of suppurative necrosis develop within the wall of the appendix, and at this stage the process may be termed **acute suppurative appendicitis.**

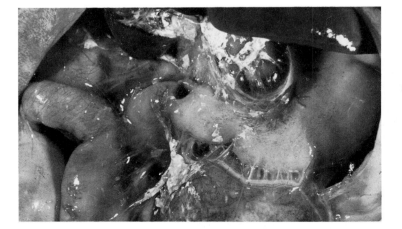

Figure 14–3. A perforated duodenal ulcer. The circular defect is evident on the superior aspect of the first portion of the duodenum. The white deposits comprise spilled gastric contents and fat necrosis.

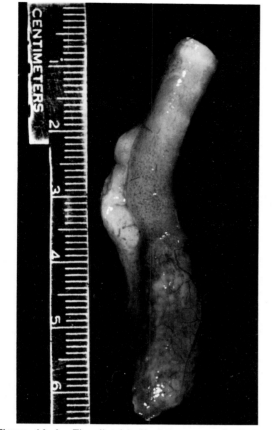

Figure 14–4. The distal half of the appendix (below) is swollen and darker in color because of inflammatory congestion, and the serosa is layered by a fibrinopurulent exudate.

Eventually, the inflammatory edema compromises the blood supply, and gangrenous necrosis is superimposed on this picture, resulting in large areas of greenish hemorrhagic ulceration of the mucosa and green-black foci of necrosis extending throughout the wall to the serosa. This stage, **acute gangrenous appendicitis,** immediately precedes rupture of the appendix. At surgery, a fecalith is commonly but not invariably found within the lumen.

The histologic picture during these stages of acute appendicitis is entirely nonspecific and follows the typical patterns of acute inflammation, suppuration and gangrenous necrosis in any tissue. Since some degree of superficial inflammation may follow drainage of exudate into the appendix from a more proximal lesion, such as ileitis, the histologic diagnosis of acute appendicitis requires some involvement of the muscularis.

The entity of **chronic** appendicitis is a subject of some controversy. Involved is the issue of whether recurrent acute attacks which spontaneously sub-side should be termed chronic disease. Truly persistent, smoldering chronic inflammation of the appendix does occur, but it is rare. It is characterized grossly by a thickened fibrotic appendix. Histologically, there is a mononuclear leukocytic infiltrate throughout the wall, principally in the subserosa, sometimes aggregated into large lymphoid follicles.

Clinical Course. The classical case of acute appendicitis, which develops over the course of a day or two, begins with a mild periumbilical discomfort, followed by anorexia, nausea and vomiting. As the appendix becomes distended, the discomfort begins to localize in the right lower quadrant of the abdomen and becomes a deep, constant ache, accompanied by tenderness to palpation. Later, when the inflammation becomes well advanced, bacteria are able to permeate the damaged wall, even before actual perforation has occurred. Involvement of the overlying parietal peritoneum results, causing severe pain and rebound tenderness. Fever and leukocytosis are present at this stage.

When surgical removal of the appendix is delayed beyond this point, the following complications may ensue: (1) generalized peritonitis, (2) periappendiceal abscess formation, (3) pylephlebitis, with thrombosis of the portal venous drainage, (4) hepatic abscess formation, or (5) septicemia. Generalized peritonitis may or may not imply actual rupture of the appendix. Ironically, rupture is sometimes accompanied by a temporary dramatic relief of pain.

The diagnosis of even the classic case described above presents many problems. The following disorders may have a similar or even identical clinical presentation: (1) mesenteric lymphadenitis, occurring in children in response to a generalized systemic infection that produces enlargement and tenderness of all nodes, particularly the mesenteric, (2) pelvic inflammatory disease (PID) (p. 573), (3) intraperitoneal hemorrhage from any cause, e.g., a ruptured ectopic pregnancy or a ruptured ovarian follicle (mittelschmerz), (4) Crohn's disease (see p. 499), and (5) Meckel's diverticulitis (p. 480). *To further complicate matters, deviations from the classic clinical pattern abound, particularly in infants and very aged individuals.* This cannot be emphasized too strongly. In these atypical cases, surgery must often be performed without a clear-cut diagnosis, simply because the penalty for delay is too great. In one analysis of 5800 cases of appendicitis, the correct diagnosis was made preoperatively in 82 per cent, and the mortality rate for those patients who came to surgery before gangrene had developed was only 0.1 per cent. In contrast, when surgery was delayed until the appendix had ruptured, providing a clear diagnosis, the mortality rate was 13 per cent (Barnes et al., 1962).

MECKEL'S DIVERTICULUM

Persistence of a vestigial remnant of the omphalomesenteric duct may give rise to a solitary diverticulum of the small intestine, usually within 12 inches of the ileocecal valve. Rarely, it occurs in a more proximal location, sometimes up to 3 feet from the ileocecal valve.

Meckel's diverticula vary in size and structure from a fibrotic cord to a pouch having a lumen larger than that of the ileum and a length up to 6 cm. The histology of the wall is basically similar to that of the small bowel, but in about one half of cases, there are also heterotopic islands of functioning gastric mucosa. Peptic ulceration in the adjacent mucosa may give rise to symptoms resembling an acute appendicitis or to mysterious intestinal bleeding (Fig. 14–5). Rarely, perforation occurs, or the inflammatory disease causes adhesion to nearby loops of bowel, with resultant intestinal obstruction. Pancreatic rests may occur in Meckel's diverticula, but they are infrequent.

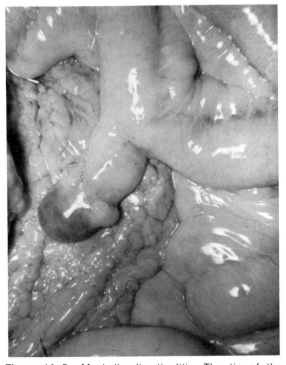

Figure 14–5. Meckel's diverticulitis. The tip of the diverticulum is reddened because of peptic ulceration of a contained rest of gastric epithelium.

MESENTERIC VASCULAR OCCLUSION

Occlusion of either the arterial supply or venous drainage of the small bowel leads, within 18 hours, to infarction of the segment of gut served by the affected vessel. Approximately 60 per cent of these cases are caused by arterial occlusion, usually as a result of heart disease with embolism or of local atherosclerotic disease with in situ thrombosis (*mesenteric thrombosis*) (Fig. 14–6). The remaining 40 per cent result from propagating retrograde venous thrombosis, usually following upper abdominal surgery (such as a gastrectomy) (Whittaker and Pemberton, 1938). Clearly, on the basis of the predisposing factors, mesenteric *arterial* occlusion is most likely in elderly individuals, particularly in diabetics. Men are affected somewhat more often than are women.

Morphology. Regardless of whether the occlusion is arterial or venous, the infarction always appears grossly hemorrhagic. This is because of the rich anastomotic arcades of the arterial supply of the mesentery which bring in blood from the margins of the lesion. Initially, the affected segment of bowel is dusky purple-red, owing to the intense congestion. Later, the wall becomes edematous, rubbery and hemorrhagic. With arterial occlusion, the demarcation from adjacent normal bowel is fairly sharply defined; venous occlusion results in relatively ill defined margins. The lumen at this stage contains blood or bloody mucus. Ecchymotic discoloration or hemorrhage in the mesentery accompanies the bowel changes. In about 24 hours, a fibrinous or fibrinosuppurative exudate appears on the serosa, rendering it dull and granular. Mucosal ulceration and secondary bacterial invasion with perforation of the wall occur within a few days. The causative vascular occlusion should be sought, but it is often difficult to find.

The histologic changes depend on how long the patient has survived; most do not live long enough to develop ulcerations and perforations. The early lesions are characterized by marked congestion of the vessels, chiefly those of the submucosa, followed by hemorrhagic infarction of the entire wall. Later, a nonspecific inflammatory infiltrate is seen, followed ultimately by ulcerations and perforations. If death occurs within 24 hours, there may be little inflammatory reaction.

Clinical Course. Like other vascular calamities (e.g., dissecting aneurysm) within the abdomen, mesenteric occlusion is often characterized by the sudden onset of excruciating pain in the absence of positive physical findings. There may be associated nausea, vomiting or bloody diarrhea. At this stage, it may be extremely difficult to distinguish mesenteric vascular occlusion from more common causes of an acute abdomen, especially a perforated

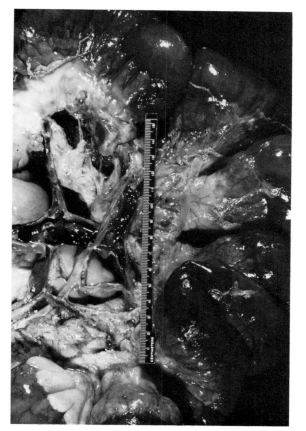

Figure 14–6. Mesenteric thrombosis. The open veins contain a dark thrombus, and the involved loops of small intestine are darkened by the venous infarction.

peptic ulcer or acute pancreatitis. Some clue to the correct diagnosis may be offered, however, by the unusual tendency of vascular calamities to produce *severe* pain significantly before physical findings develop. Unless mesenteric vascular occlusion is recognized and treated early, these patients follow an extremely fulminating course, leading to death within 48 hours from shock, perforation and sepsis, or hemorrhage.

In recent years, it has become increasingly appreciated that mesenteric occlusion may in many instances be only partial, and may produce a clinical syndrome known as *intestinal angina*. This syndrome is characterized by postprandial periumbilical pain and diarrhea, sometimes associated with steatorrhea. In an attempt to avoid pain, the patient may reduce his food intake and consequently lose weight. Intestinal angina is thought to be based on functional disturbances in intestinal motility and absorption caused by relative ischemia. It is important not only as a cause of debility in its own right, but because it may presage total mesenteric vascular occlusion.

ACUTE HEMORRHAGIC ENTEROPATHY (GASTROINTESTINAL HEMORRHAGIC NECROSIS)

This not infrequent disorder is characterized by patchy or diffuse hemorrhagic destruction of the mucosa and submucosa anywhere in the gastrointestinal tract, from the stomach to the rectum. *The sparing of the deeper layers, i.e., the muscularis and serosa, differentiates this lesion from the infarction just described.*

The pathogenesis is not known with certainty, but it is thought to be related to extreme splanchnic vasoconstriction in states of low cardiac ouptut. Thus, the disorder is commonly seen with shock, severe cardiac failure or arrhythmias. It is described in the consideration of shock on page 217.

DIVERTICULAR DISEASE

Diverticula of the colon are small herniations of the mucosa and submucosa through defects in the muscularis. They are usually multiple, and are most abundant in the sigmoid colon (95 per cent). Diverticula become increasingly common with age. After the age of 50 years, they are present in about 10 per cent of the population, both men and women.

Until recently, *diverticulosis* (the presence of multiple diverticula) was, on clinical grounds, sharply distinguished from acute and chronic *diverticulitis* (inflammation of the diverticula). As will be seen, except perhaps in the case of acute diverticulitis, such a distinction is probably no longer tenable.

Etiology and Pathogenesis. While congenital foci of weakness in the bowel wall may render certain individuals vulnerable to the later development of diverticula, environmental influences are probably the decisive factor. Paramount among these influences would seem to be the low-residue diet consumed in the industrialized countries. Indeed, diverticulosis is almost unknown in underdeveloped areas where food is, as yet, "unrefined." In contrast, where life and food are softer, the disorder is becoming more frequent and is being seen at an ever younger age. Experimentally, rats on a low-residue diet have been shown to develop diverticulosis, whereas a high-residue diet conferred protection (Carlson and Hoelzel, 1949).

What is the mechanism, then, by which diet influences the development of diverticula? Painter has suggested that the abnormally soft fecal stream in patients on a low-residue diet requires excessive contraction of the sigmoid colon in exercising its normal function of controlling fecal access to the rectum. This excessive contraction is segmental and leads to the development of high pressures within each segment. The pulsion force thus generated causes first thickening of the sigmoid musculature, and later creation of diverticula at points of relative weakness (Painter, 1969).

Morphology. Diverticula usually appear as multiple, flask-shaped sacs, about 0.5 to 1.0 cm. in greatest diameter, aligned along the margins of the taenia coli. The mouths of these sacs may be very difficult to see on the mucosal surface. Although diverticula occur principally in the sigmoid colon, they may extend proximally and eventually involve nearly the entire colon. Occasionally a solitary, large diverticulum occurs in the cecum.

On histologic examination, the muscularis at these outpouchings is either absent or markedly attenuated, so that the diverticular wall is composed essentially of mucosa, subserosal fat and serosa (Fig. 14–7). There is striking hypertrophy of the musculature of the intervening colon, both the taenia coli and the circular muscles.

Secondary inflammation, or diverticulitis, is thought to develop when feces become impacted within the diverticula. A nonspecific acute or chronic inflammatory reaction ensues, and eventually involves the entire thickness of the diverticular wall. The intervening hypertrophied wall also is af-

fected and, with chronicity, becomes fibrotic as well as thickened. The resultant irregular stenosis may on x-ray or gross examination closely resemble that of colonic carcinoma. Bacterial cultures usually yield a mixed flora, with *E. coli* predominating. Permeation of the infection or perforation of a diverticulum leads to pericolic abscesses or, less frequently, to generalized peritonitis. Sometimes sinus tracts or fistulous communications with neighboring viscera develop.

Clinical Course. Many, if not most, patients with diverticular disease remain asymptomatic. Of those who seek medical attention, about 80 per cent present with a characteristic colicky, left lower quadrant pain. Concomitant changes in bowel habits, including either constipation or recurrent diarrhea, are often but not invariably present. Bloody stools or melena occurs in about 22 per cent of symptomatic patients (Editorial, 1970*b*). *Attempts to correlate clinical and radiologic findings with anatomic changes have demonstrated the futility of distinguishing on clinical grounds between diverticulosis and chronic diverticulitis.* The typical colicky pain, which was earlier thought to indicate inflammatory narrowing of the lumen, with partial obstruction, may also result from excessive segmental contraction of the colon with functional obstruction. Indeed, in one series, only one third of surgical specimens removed for "diverticulitis" showed sufficient inflammation to account for the symptoms (Morson, 1963). The remaining specimens merely showed diverticula and hypertrophy of the bowel wall. Such hypertrophy may even be present and symptomatic in the absence of diverticula. On barium enema, thickening of the bowel wall as a result of inflammation may be difficult to differentiate from that resulting from hypertrophy.

The development of a pericolic abscess, sinus or fistulous tract, or peritonitis implies acute diverticulitis, which is usually clinically distinct from chronic diverticular disease. In addition to systemic indications of sepsis, a tender mass is often palpable in the lower abdomen. Occasionally, these patients first seek medical attention because of an acute abdomen.

Most patients with diverticular disease can be managed conservatively and lead a relatively normal life. However, when acute diverticulitis extends outside the bowel, or when severe hemorrhage or obstruction occurs, surgical intervention may be necessary.

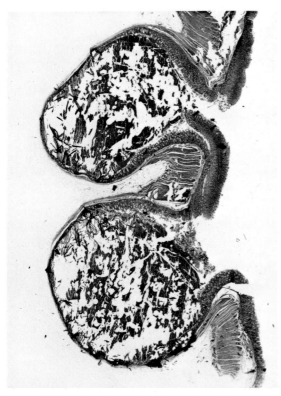

Figure 14–7. Diverticulosis of the colon. A low power microscopic view of two diverticula showing their thin walls and absence of muscular coats. There is no evidence of inflammation, but they are stuffed with fecal matter.

INTESTINAL OBSTRUCTION

A large variety of disorders may produce obstruction to the free flow of gastrointestinal contents. Only the most important will be presented here. In one large series of cases, 44 per cent were caused by *hernias*, 30 per cent by *adhesions*, 10 per cent by *neoplasms*, 5 per cent by *intussusception*, 4 per cent by *volvulus*, and the remaining 7 per cent by a multitude of miscellaneous disorders (McIver, 1933).

HERNIAS

Hernia refers to the protrusion of a serosa-lined pouch through any weakness or defect in the wall of the peritoneal cavity. The principal sites of such weakness are the inguinal and femoral canals, the umbilicus and old surgical scars. The significance of hernias lies in the propensity for segments of viscera to become trapped in them. Most commonly and of greatest import is entrapment of the small bowel, but the large bowel, omentum or any other viscus, such as the ovary, may be involved. If the neck of the defect is sufficiently narrow, the venous drainage of the protruding viscus is impaired. The resultant congestion and edema may produce so much swelling that the viscus is permanently trapped or *incarcerated.* Moreover, this swelling may lead to further pressure on the vasculature and possibly may encroach on the arterial supply, thus resulting in ischemic necrosis of the trapped viscus, or a *strangulated hernia.* When the small bowel is involved, the anatomic picture is identical to that produced by a mesenteric vascular occlusion (p. 480).

INTESTINAL ADHESIONS

Fibrous bands may develop from organ to organ or from organ to peritoneal wall in the course of a healing peritonitis or following any abdominal surgery. These adhesions can create closed loops through which other viscera may slide and eventually become trapped, just as in a hernial sac. Partial or complete intestinal obstruction ensues, sometimes with infarction of the involved viscus.

INTUSSUSCEPTION

In this disorder, one segment of small intestine, constricted by a wave of peristalsis, suddenly invaginates into the immediately distal segment of bowel. Once trapped, the invaginated segment is propelled by peristalsis further into the distal segment, pulling its mesentery along behind it. Intussusception is more common in infants and children than in adults, and in this age group it usually occurs apparently spontaneously in otherwise healthy bowels. In these cases, reduction can frequently be accomplished by the administration of an enema. In adults, however, an intussusception most often implies some intraluminal mass or lesion that serves as a point of traction, and pulls the base of attachment and segment of gut along with it. Surgical exploration is necessary not only to determine the underlying cause but also to reduce the intussusception. Otherwise, intestinal obstruction may be followed in time by infarction, as the mesenteric blood supply becomes progressively compressed.

VOLVULUS

Volvulus refers to complete twisting of a loop of bowel about its mesenteric base of attachment. It is seen most commonly in the small intestine, but large redundant loops of sigmoid may sometimes be involved. Obstruction and infarction are common in these cases.

PYLORIC STENOSIS

Since pyloric stenosis is an important cause of dramatic total intestinal obstruction in newborn infants, this congenital disorder is also presented at this time. Males are affected four times as often as females. These children usually have persistent projectile vomiting after each feeding. Anatomically, the pylorus is thick and firm, about 2 to 3 cm. in length and 1 to 2 cm. in thickness. The enlargement is due entirely to hypertrophy and spasm of the muscular coat; the mucosal lining is normal. The disorder can usually be corrected by simple splitting of the hypertrophied muscle, without entering the lumen. As was mentioned earlier, peptic ulcers may be a cause of *acquired* pyloric stenosis with obstruction.

ANOREXIA

Although loss of appetite occurs with many pathologic states and particularly with cancer, it is usually preceded by some other, albeit possibly overlooked, manifestation of disease. Among the gastrointestinal disorders, gastric carcinoma is perhaps unique, then, in that anorexia is the most characteristic *first* indication of the lesion.

GASTRIC CANCER

Although cancer of the stomach is an infrequent form of malignant disease, it is unusually lethal and on this account, it is the seventh most important cause of death from cancer in the United States. Forty years ago, it had the dubious honor of leading this list, but, whereas the incidence of many other forms of cancer has increased or remained static, that of gastric cancer has shown an absolute decline.

By far the most important type of gastric neoplasm is the carcinoma, and our discussion here will be confined to this form. Occasionally, however, relatively trivial adenomas (polyps), intramural leiomyomas and neurofibromas are found in the stomach, and, infrequently, mesenchymal cancers occur in this organ, including the fibrosarcoma, leiomyosarcoma, endothelial sarcoma and the lymphomas.

Gastric carcinoma is principally a disease of the elderly, although it may occur at any age, and it affects males about one and a half times as frequently as females.

Etiology and Pathogenesis. Both hereditary and environmental factors seem to influence the development of gastric carcinoma, although the latter are probably somewhat more important (Dawson, 1967). Possibly both underlie the wide geographic variations in the importance of this form of cancer. Gastric carcinoma is far more frequent in certain countries (e.g., Japan, Iceland, Finland and Chile) than it is in the United States. In Japan it is responsible for over half of all male cancer deaths. Although the exact reasons for these discrepancies are unknown, they have been attributed to differences in diet and food preparation, particularly to the heavy use of smoked foods in high risk areas, as well as to genetic traits. Japanese immigrants to the United States show an incidence of gastric carcinoma intermediate between those of their native and adopted countries. Besides these regional and ethnic variations, a familial tendency toward gastric carcinoma is well established. The lesion is also known to occur more often in individuals with blood group A than in those with other blood groups. At present it is suspected that the presence of nitrites in some foods may increase the risk of gastric cancer.

In addition to environmental and hereditary factors, certain pathologic conditions are well known to carry with them a high risk of associated gastric carcinoma. These include: (1) the three related disorders, pernicious anemia, atrophic gastritis and achlorhydria, and (2) gastric adenomas (polyps).

As was mentioned in the discussion of atrophic gastritis, the risk of carcinoma developing among these patients, particularly where there is intestinal metaplasia, is considerably greater than among the normal population. With atrophic gastritis, the incidence of subsequent development of gastric carcinoma is between 10 and 15 per cent. Whether this results from the increased turnover of surface epithelium cells in these patients or is somehow related to the associated achlorhydria is not known. Conceivably, normal acid secretion in some way protects against the development of carcinoma. It is of interest that only 25 per cent of patients with gastric carcinoma have normal levels of acid secretions; most of the remainder have varying degrees of hypochlorhydria.

Focal malignant changes are found in 10 to 20 per cent of gastric adenomas, indicating that these otherwise benign polypoid tumors can be precursors of cancer. It cannot be assumed, however, that all polypoid cancers have arisen from benign adenomas, since some cancers may assume this form from the outset.

A most controversial issue has been the risk of malignant transformation of gastric peptic ulcers. Some have suggested that true malignant transformation occurs in perhaps 10 per cent of gastric peptic ulcers (Dawson, 1967). However, most would place the risk at 1 per cent or even less. Perhaps the higher figure can be attributed to the frequent initial misdiagnosis of an ulcerating carcinoma as a benign peptic ulcer.

Studies have shown that gastric cancers in general tend to arise over rather large areas of the mucosal surface rather than in a solitary deviant gland or cell. Indeed, differing histologic patterns of cancer may arise in adjacent loci and eventually coalesce to produce a morphologically heterogeneous tumor. This would indicate that, whatever the nature of the predisposing influences, they usually operate over a large area of the stomach.

Morphology. Over 50 per cent of gastric carcinomas originate in the pyloric antrum. Their gross morphology usually takes one of three forms:

	Per Cent
Ulcerative	28
Polypoid	23
Infiltrative (linitis plastica)	13

The remaining third are so advanced at the time of diagnosis as to be unclassifiable.

The **ulcerative form** appears as a crater with raised, beaded, overhanging margins and a shaggy necrotic base (Fig. 14—8). In many cases, the crater is found in the center of an elevated mucosal plaque, which suggests that the lesion was originally a solid plateau that underwent ischemic necrosis and ulceration at its center. Gross characteristics which tend to distinguish an ulcerative carcinoma from a benign peptic ulcer include its tendency to affect the greater curvature of the stomach, its raised, beaded margins, its necrotic shaggy base and its greater size. However, there is much overlapping and absolute reliance must not be placed on these criteria in any given case. These factors were considered in the discussion of peptic ulcers.

The **polypoid carcinoma** appears as a large, fungating, cauliflower-like mass which protrudes into the gastric lumen, usually from a broad base.

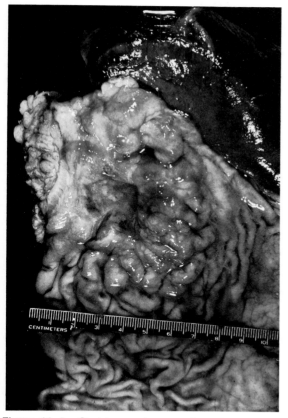

Figure 14–8. Gastric carcinoma, ulcerative pattern. The irregular ulcer crater is situated high in the fundus and has penetrated into the adjacent spleen, which can be seen above it. Note the beaded margins of the ulcer crater and the irregular base.

These vary in size from rather small masses of 3 to 4 cm. to tumors that virtually fill the lumen (Fig. 14–9). Whether they can in general be assumed to arise from preexisting benign adenomas is controversial.

The **infiltrative carcinoma** either may grow superficially over the surface of the mucosa or may permeate the entire thickness of the wall. Superficial spread produces a large, plaque-like lesion which smooths out the mucosa and flattens the rugal folds. More often, infiltrative carcinoma permeates the entire wall, producing a pattern known as **linitis plastica.** The wall of the stomach in these cases is strikingly thickened, up to 3 cm., and assumes a cartilaginous rigidity. On sectioning, gritty white tumor can be seen permeating the wall, particularly the submucosa and subserosa, and spreading apart the layers of the stomach. The mucosa becomes atrophic, flattened, and fused to the underlying wall. Shallow ulcerations are often present, and seeding of the serosal surface is frequently apparent.

It is probable that, in general, gastric carcinoma

arises as an in situ lesion which remains confined to the glandular epithelium without involving even the lamina propria of the mucosa. The time required for these lesions to evolve into invasive carcinomas is unknown; that such evolution occurs is well documented by the frequent presence of persistent in situ changes at the margins of frank carcinomas. In any case, these lesions ultimately become typical invasive cancers. **Whatever the gross appearance of the tumor, the histologic pattern is usually that of a well differentiated adenocarcinoma.** Although they tend to be fairly well differentiated, some gastric carcinomas, particularly of the infiltrative type, show various degrees of undifferentiation and may even be totally undifferentiated. With linitis plastica, the increased thickness of the wall results not only from tumor, but also from a massive desmoplastic reaction. Indeed, it is sometimes difficult to find the cancer cells amid the fibrous tissue.

Most polypoid carcinomas produce a glandular, sometimes papillary, histologic pattern. Mucin secretion is common in all of the tumor types. The mucin may remain within cells, producing "signet

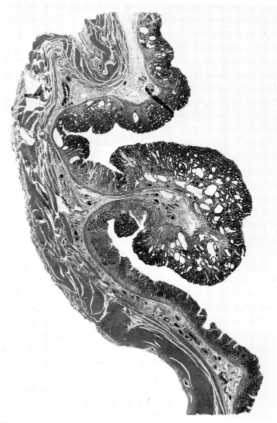

Figure 14–9. Gastric carcinoma, polypoid pattern. A low power microscopic view through a small polypoid cancer in a patient who had pernicious anemia. The lesion is virtually in situ and has not invaded its stalk nor the underlying wall.

ring" cells, or be distributed extracellularly as large accumulations of interstitial or intraglandular basophilic mucin.

In the ulcerative form, neoplastic tissue is found both in the margins and at the base of the crater. The ulcer is, as it were, carved out of tumor. In contrast, when a peptic ulcer becomes malignant, the transformation occurs at the mucosal margins. Very often, if the cancerous change is not too far advanced, the base remains free of tumor infiltration, and these lesions can be distinguished on this basis.

Attempts to devise a system for staging gastric carcinoma according to its extent at the time of diagnosis have not been altogether successful. Recently a rather complicated TNM staging classification has been developed based on the findings at surgical exploration rather than on clinical assessment (Wood, 1968). In addition to TNM evaluation it includes data on the precise location of the tumor within the stomach and the depth to which it penetrates the mucosa. The following, older staging system is simpler and perhaps equally useful (Wynder et al., 1963):

Stage I: Limited to stomach wall without evidence of nodal involvement; operable and resectable.

Stage II: Limited to stomach wall, with microscopic nodal disease; operable and resectable.

Stage III: Extension to adjacent surrounding organs, such as liver, pancreas and transverse colon; sometimes with grossly positive nodes; operable but not usually resectable.

Stage IV: Distant metastases, especially to liver, parietal peritoneum, and ovary; surgery only for diagnosis or palliation.

Clinical Course. Unfortunately, gastric carcinoma usually remains silent until quite late in its course. Even after symptoms arise, they tend to be vague and tolerable to the patient, so that the average lapse of time between their appearance and the patient's seeking medical attention is from 6 months to 1 year. By the time the classical syndrome of anorexia, weight loss and epigastric pain with a palpable mass has developed, the lesion is far advanced. While occult bleeding from the tumor is common, often leading to iron deficiency anemia, hematemesis and melena from this cause are rare. Other atypical presentations are obstruction with vomiting (when the lesion is at the pylorus), and dysphagia (when the cardia is involved). Rarely, a patient presents with peritonitis from perforation of the cancer through the wall of the stomach.

Quite frequently, obvious metastatic disease is the first indication of a gastric carcinoma. Regional lymph nodes and the liver are usually first involved, and the patient may present with hepatomegaly or ascites. Characteristically, there is spreading not only to the regional lymph nodes, but also to the supraclavicular (*Virchow's*) nodes and scalene nodes. Since these are readily accessible to biopsy, their typical involvement is of diagnostic importance. Another peculiarity of gastric carcinoma is its tendency toward widespread intraperitoneal seeding. This seeding is most apparent in the pelvis, where a tumor mass in the peritoneal cul-de-sac may be palpable on rectal examination (*rectal shelf*). *Krukenberg tumors* of the ovaries (see page 579) may result from, among other things, seeding from a gastric carcinoma. Direct spread of the primary tumor through the wall of the stomach to adjacent viscera also is common.

Diagnosis of gastric carcinoma may be made by a variety of techniques, including barium x-ray studies, gastroscopy, cytology and scalene node biopsy. Cytologic examination of gastric secretions is especially important with early in situ lesions and as a routine method for evaluating patients with predisposing disorders, such as atrophic gastritis. When properly done, 70 to 90 per cent of cases can be diagnosed by this method.

The overall five-year survival rate with gastric carcinoma is a disappointing 13 per cent. In individual cases, however, the prognosis is highly variable and depends on several factors:

(1) *The length of the history when diagnosed.* Paradoxically, the longer the history, the better the prognosis, probably because these lesions are inherently less aggressive.

(2) *The extent of the lesion.* As would be expected, in situ lesions offer a much better prognosis (95 per cent five-year survival) than does widespread metastatic disease.

(3) *The morphologic type of lesion.* Polypoid tumors offer a somewhat better prognosis than do the other types, whereas five-year survival with linitis plastica is extremely rare.

(4) *The degree of differentiation.* As with most cancers, poorly differentiated lesions tend to be more aggressive.

DIARRHEA

Diarrhea refers to the frequent passage of loose or watery stools. It may or may not be associated with colicky pain. *Acute* diarrhea is most often caused by any of a wide variety of infectious diseases of the small or large intestine. Among these, only the most important will be described briefly. Intestinal malabsorption, Crohn's disease and ulcerative colitis are the major causes of *chronic* or recurrent diarrhea.

INFECTIOUS DISEASES OF THE GASTROINTESTINAL TRACT

This diverse group of entities usually involves the small or large bowel, or both, and ranges in clinical importance from a trivial gastroenteritis, known as "food poisoning," to fulminant and fatal typhoid fever. Here we will limit ourselves to the most important of these infections: typhoid fever, bacillary dysentery, cholera, amoebic colitis and staphylococcal colitis.

TYPHOID FEVER

Typhoid fever is caused by the gram-negative bacillus *Salmonella typhi* and is characterized by ulcerations of the small intestine and a striking systemic reticuloendothelial hyperplasia. Similar changes occur with *paratyphoid*, caused by *S. paratyphi* and *S. schottmuelleri*. Less virulent salmonellae, such as *S. typhimurium* or *S. enteritidis*, produce a mild gastroenteritis, often called simply "food poisoning," a result of the local effects of endotoxins.

Typhoid fever is transmitted by the fecal contamination of water, food or other articles which reach the mouth. The incubation period is from 10 to 14 days. During this time, the organisms are localized in the lymphoid tissue of the gastrointestinal tract, principally Peyer's patches, where they proliferate and cause marked hypertrophy of the lymphoid masses.

Peyer's patches appear as sharply delineated, elevated plaques up to 8 cm. in diameter. During the second week of the disease, the mucosal coverings of the hypertrophied lymphoid masses tend to slough, presumably as a result of pressure ischemia, producing oval ulcerations running along the axis of the small bowel. Histologically, there are characteristic aggregations of plump RE cells (macrophages), often containing phagocytized bacteria, red cells (through *erythrophagocytosis*) and debris. Although a scattered infiltrate of lymphocytes and plasma cells is present about these foci, polymorphonuclear leukocytes are conspicuously absent. Such aggregations are termed "typhoid nodules."

At the end of the incubation period, the organisms flood the circulating blood and seed the RE system throughout the body. The spleen and liver become enlarged, reflecting their engorgement and hyperplasia of the RE or Kupffer cells. At this time, the patient usually appears severely ill, with fever, prostration, abdominal cramps and occasionally bloody diarrhea. *Bradycardia and leukopenia are characteristic.* During the second week, an erythematous, macular, "rose spot" rash may appear. Bacilli appear in the stools in the sec-

ond or third week. Serum antibody levels become demonstrable during the second week. The most important complications of typhoid fever are profuse intestinal hemorrhage, perforation of the bowel wall and rupture of the spleen. About 2 per cent of those patients who recover become "carriers" and continue to harbor the causative organisms, usually in the biliary tract.

BACILLARY DYSENTERY

This disease is caused by the shigellae, a group of gram-negative bacilli which include *Sh. dysenteriae*, *Sh. flexneri*, *Sh. boydii* and *Sh. sonnei*. Like the salmonellae, these organisms are usually transmitted in contaminated food. *In contrast to the salmonellae, they tend to affect the colon rather than the small bowel, bacteremia usually does not occur and tissue damage remains confined to the gastrointestinal tract.* It is thought that many of the effects of the shigellae can be attributed to release of an endotoxin. Morphologically, the mucosa of the colon becomes hyperemic and edematous, and enlargement of the lymphoid follicles creates small projecting nodules. Within 24 hours, a fibrinosuppurative exudate covers the mucosa and sometimes produces a dirty gray to yellow pseudomembrane. Superficial irregular ulcerations appear in the mucosa and, in severe cases, large tracts of mucosa may be denuded. *Despite their extent, however, these ulcerations tend to remain superficial.* The histologic reaction is predominantly that of a mononuclear leukocytic infiltrate, although a neutrophilic exudate may cover the surfaces of the ulcers. Congestion, edema and thromboses of the small underlying vessels are also present.

Bacillary dysentery has an abrupt onset after an incubation period that may be as short as one day. Crampy abdominal pain and diarrhea precede fever. The stools are characteristically mixed with mucus and blood. Bacteria can be isolated from the stools during the early stages of the disease; antibodies become demonstrable during the second week.

CHOLERA

This important acute diarrheal disease is caused by either *Vibrio cholerae* or *Vibrio El Tor*, which are curved gram-negative bacilli. The vibrios are not themselves invasive, but rather act through the elaboration of a toxin which is intensely irritating to the bowel wall. Although the epithelium remains intact, the underlying vasculature becomes engorged, and there is a massive outpouring of fluid and electrolytes into the lumen of the gut. Clinically, this results in severe vomiting, abdominal cramps and profuse diarrhea, consisting of a slightly yellowish fluid containing flecks of mucus ("rice water stools"). Anatomically, the changes are not marked, consisting essentially of an inflammatory reaction in the lamina propria, characterized by engorgement of the capillaries, dilatation of the central lacteals and a predominantly mononuclear cellular infiltrate. *The significance of cholera lies in the profound dehydration and electrolyte imbalance it causes.* With proper and adequate fluid replacement, it is usually a self-limited disease. However, those most likely to contract cholera—the poor and undernourished and those living under unsanitary conditions—are precisely those least likely to receive adequate medical care. For this reason, about 33 per cent of these patients die of their disease.

AMOEBIC COLITIS

Amoebic colitis is caused by the protozoan *Entamoeba histolytica.* It is an interesting disorder in that, for obscure reasons, infection is not synonymous with disease. Indeed, about 10 per cent of the population of the United States harbors this protozoan, yet suffers no ill effects. In a small percentage of individuals, however, particularly in certain areas of the world, fulminant diarrheal disease may ensue. In still other instances, the disorder may be chronic or remittent, and may appear only after a long period of latency. Some believe that asymptomatic infection involves organisms of smaller size, possibly an entirely different species of amoeba.

Amoebic colitis is transmitted by fecal contamination of water or food. When transmitted, the organism is in the form of a cyst which is up to 20 μm. in diameter and contains one to four nuclei. Only within the bowel are the invasive trophozoites released. These are amoeboid forms, up to 25 μm. in diameter, with a single small nucleus. Within the colon (most often the cecum and ascending colon), the trophozoites invade the crypts of the colonic glands and elaborate strong proteolytic enzymes and hyaluronidases, which permit them to burrow into the epithelium, chemically digesting the tissues in their path. They are ultimately halted by the muscularis mucosae, which seems to constitute a barrier to their further progress. At this level, they fan out to create a characteristic undermined ulceration having a flask shape, i.e., a narrow neck and a broad base. As the undermining progresses, the surface mucosa is deprived of its blood supply and tends to slough. *Histologically, the most important feature of these lesions is the relative absence of inflammatory infiltration.* Only when there is secondary bacterial infection is there a significant local leukocytic response.

Clinically, these patients have mild to severe abdominal cramps, diarrhea and occasionally melena. Constitutional symptoms may be minimal or absent, unless there is secondary bacterial invasion. In about 40 per cent of cases, trophozoites penetrate blood vessels and are drained to the liver, where they produce solitary or multiple abscesses. These are composed of a shaggy fibrin lining, containing a chocolate-colored paste that consists of partially digested debris and blood. Similar abscesses may develop in the lung, either by drainage of parasites through the blood or by direct penetration through the liver capsule and diaphragm. Occasionally the brain and meninges are also secondarily involved.

STAPHYLOCOCCAL COLITIS

This form of colitis occurs in patients whose normal colonic flora is altered by the prolonged use of antibiotics, permitting the overgrowth of antibiotic-resistant *Staphylococcus aureus.* The lesions are entirely nonspecific, consisting of areas of acute suppurative ulceration and focal hemorrhages. Identification of the causative organism is required for the diagnosis.

Closely related to staphylococcal colitis is an entity termed *pseudomembranous colitis.* This is also seen in patients on prolonged antibiotic therapy, although it has not been associated with any one causative organism. Anatomically, it is characterized by ulcerations covered by a sloughing, green-brown to black, necrotic mucosal surface.

INTESTINAL MALABSORPTION

Malabsorption refers to impairment of absorption of any or all constituents of the normal diet, and it occurs with a large variety of disorders. Because *steatorrhea* (presence in the stools of over 6 gm. of fat daily) is commonly a conspicuous component of malabsorption, the terms are often used interchangeably. However, while malabsorption may be limited to faulty fat absorption, it often includes, as well, impaired absorption of proteins, carbohydrates, vitamins and minerals.

As would be expected, the clinical manifestations of malabsorption are protean and highly variable, depending largely on the selectivity with which the various dietary constituents are affected. Common to most of these patients, but not all, are diarrhea, steatorrhea, weight loss, weakness and lassitude. *It is important to note that malabsorption is one of the few disorders which cause weight loss despite an increased appetite.* Steatorrhea is characterized by the frequent passage of bulky, greasy, foul-smelling stools. Necessarily, this malabsorption of fat is accompanied by diminished absorption of the fat-soluble vitamins (A, D, E and K), as well as by deficient calcium absorption. These patients may thus present with a hemorrhagic diathesis due to hypovitaminosis K, or with manifestations of hypovitaminosis D (see Chapter 8) and hypocalcemia, such as tetany, osteomalacia and osteoporosis. When malabsorption is not limited to fats, protein deficiencies ensue and may lead to edema as a result of hypoalbuminemia. Hypoglycemia with a flat glucose-tolerance curve may be present. Megaloblastic anemia results from impaired folic acid and vitamin B_{12} absorption, and interference with iron absorption may cause a microcytic anemia. Any of the vitamin B deficiency states may develop, as well as fluid and electrolyte imbalances.

There are a great many causes of intestinal malabsorption, and these may be classified in a number of ways. Here we shall consider them according to the site of the underlying pathology. Thus, intestinal malabsorption may be of (1) *gastric,* (2) *pancreatic,* (3) *hepatobiliary* or (4) *intestinal (enterogenous)* origin.

Gastric dysfunction may result in unregulated dumping of food into the intestine, with consequent poor mixing with the intestinal juices. Moreover, normal gastric function and acidity are necessary to stimulate fully the release of the pancreatic digestive enzymes. *Probably the most frequent cause of this form of malabsorption is therapeutic gastrectomy for peptic ulcer disease.*

When *pancreatic disease,* such as chronic pancreatitis, interferes with exocrine function, steatorrhea and protein malabsorption ensue, although absorption of carbohydrates, minerals and water soluble vitamins remains unimpaired.

Hepatobiliary disease leads to steatorrhea when the concentration of conjugated bile salts in the small intestine falls below 4 millimoles per liter. Below this level, the number of micelles is insufficient to dissolve a normal dietary lipid load (Badley et al., 1969).

Reference should be made to Chapter 15 for discussion of the specific pancreatic and hepatobiliary diseases that may cause malabsorption.

Malabsorption is most profound and nonselective when it is caused by intrinsic intestinal pathology (*enterogenous malabsorption*). As will be seen, a large number of structural (often iatrogenic), microbial, biochemical and functional disorders are included under this umbrella. Two of the more interesting enterogenous causes of malabsorption—celiac disease and Whipple's disease—will be discussed later in some detail. Many of the other disorders are presented in other chapters. The fact that enterogenous malabsorption is, with few exceptions, nonselective and affects

carbohydrate as well as fat and protein absorption provides a useful diagnostic tool, the d-xylose tolerance test. *Patients with isolated pancreatic or hepatobiliary disease retain their ability to absorb d-xylose, whereas those with intrinsic intestinal disease do not.*

From the foregoing classification of the causes of malabsorption, it should be apparent that there may be a good deal of overlapping among categories. Thus, malabsorption based on gastric dysfunction may also be associated with a consequent reduction of pancreatic digestive function. Moreover, after gastrectomy, a blind duodenal loop may permit overgrowth of an abnormal bacterial flora which somehow alters normal fat and vitamin B_{12} absorption, and so adds an "enterogenous" element to gastric malabsorption. As another example, bile salt deficiencies result not only from hepatobiliary disease but also from intrinsic disease of the ileum, with consequent failure to reabsorb and conserve bile salts. Despite these overlaps, the more important causes of malabsorption and their admittedly crude classification are presented in Table 14–1.

TABLE 14–1. CAUSES OF INTESTINAL MALABSORPTION

I. Gastric
   1. Gastric resection, e.g., for peptic ulcer disease
   2. Pernicious anemia (see page 473)
   3. Zollinger-Ellison syndrome (see page 544)
II. Pancreatic (see Chapter 15)
   1. Chronic pancreatitis
   2. Carcinoma of the pancreas
   3. Cystic fibrosis of the pancreas (mucoviscidosis)
III. Hepatobiliary (see Chapter 15)
   1. Chronic hepatocellular disease, especially biliary cirrhosis
   2. Biliary obstruction, e.g., carcinoma of the common bile duct, choledocholithiasis
IV. Enterogenous
  A. Structural
   1. Celiac disease—biochemical (?)
   2. Crohn's disease (see page 491)
   3. Intestinal resection and bypass
   4. Scleroderma (see page 194)
   5. Amyloid (see page 202)
   6. Lymphoma (see page 342)
  B. Microbial
   1. Whipple's disease
   2. "Blind loop" syndrome
   3. Jejunal diverticula
   4. Parasitic infection
  C. Biochemical
   1. Disaccharidase deficiency
   2. Abetalipoproteinemia (?)
  D. Functional
   1. Acute enteritis
   2. Other causes of rapid transit

CELIAC DISEASE (NONTROPICAL SPRUE, GLUTEN ENTEROPATHY)

Celiac disease is caused by either an immune or a toxic reaction to the gliadin fraction of wheat or rye gluten, and is characterized by marked atrophy of the intestinal villi and microvilli. The disease is most often diagnosed in young to middle-aged adults, although it may appear in children. Until recently, the misconception flourished that adult celiac disease differed from the childhood form, but such a distinction is probably spurious. Indeed, over 50 per cent of patients diagnosed in adulthood recall symptoms dating back to childhood. On the other hand, the distinction between celiac disease and *tropical sprue* is real. The latter is most probably caused by an infectious agent, and is quite unrelated to gluten ingestion. However, morphologically the two entities are indistinguishable.

The mechanism by which gliadin causes celiac disease is not understood. However, the evidence is mounting that celiac disease is a form of hypersensitivity response, perhaps genetically conditioned. Family studies indicate that approximately 10 per cent of first-degree relatives are affected (Robinson et al., 1971). Significant increases in the serum level of IgA have been identified in these patients, as well as decreased levels of IgM and a host of other, more variable immunologic abnormalities (Asquith et al., 1969; Editorial, 1974b). Lymphocytes within the intestinal mucosa of patients with celiac disease are reported to be sensitized to gliadin (Ferguson et al., 1975). The possibility of a genetically determined immunologic derangement is supported by the increased vulnerability of individuals with certain histocompatibility antigens. In particular, individuals with the HL-A8 antigen have a tenfold greater risk of developing celiac disease than does the control population (McDevitt and Bodmer, 1974). However, the case for an immunologic pathogenesis is not yet proved. There are those who believe that the appearance of serum immunoglobulin abnormalities is merely secondary to mucosal damage with increased permeability to gut antigens. Possibly the relevant genetic derangement is not in the immune system but rather in the formation of an abnormal peptidase responsible for gliadin metabolism. This may be directly toxic to the intestinal mucosa, or it may provoke an immune reaction (Yeomans, 1974).

The characteristic anatomic finding in celiac disease is marked atrophy of the villi and microvilli of the jejunum. These become distorted and blunted, and may even disappear. The surface epithelial cells become cuboidal and stain poorly, and their nuclei assume irregular positions within the cells, rather than maintaining the usual basal orientation. Electron microscopy discloses mitochondria of abnormal size and shape, with distortion of

their cristae. Ribonucleoprotein granules are abnormally abundant. There is an increase in depth of the intervillous crypts and a marked chronic inflammatory response in the lamina propria, composed of lymphocytes and plasma cells and occasionally eosinophils.

Clinically, these patients present with an often bewildering array of complaints referable to the nonselective malabsorption described earlier as characteristic of enterogenous malabsorption states. In one study, only eight of 21 patients demonstrated the classic syndrome of diarrhea, weight loss, steatorrhea and malnutrition. The remainder presented first with a variety of miscellaneous findings, including anemia, edema, tetany and bone pain due to hypocalcemia (Mann et al., 1970). It has been assumed that the malabsorption is based on the tremendous decrease in absorptive surface area resulting from loss of the villi and microvilli. However, it is probable that biochemical derangements also contribute to the dysfunction.

A gluten-free diet results in a dramatic and highly gratifying reversal of the anatomic and clinical changes of celiac disease. Within weeks to months, the mucosa returns to an entirely normal appearance, and the symptoms disappear. However, it has been suggested that minimal ultrastructural changes may persist.

The diagnosis of celiac disease depends on the demonstration of malabsorption (including failure to absorb d-xylose), a typical peroral jejunal biopsy and response to a gluten-free diet.

WHIPPLE'S DISEASE

This rare disorder is characterized anatomically by the infiltration of the small intestinal lamina propria with distinctive foamy macrophages, often closely associated with intra- and extracellular bacillary bodies. Similar macrophages may often be found elsewhere in the body, including the lymph nodes, liver, spleen and brain. The disease was first described by Whipple in 1907 and, while much has been learned about it since that time, its etiology has still not been proved. Whipple's disease occurs in the later decades of life, with a male predominance in the ratio of 8:1.

Before we discuss the causation, the morphology of this lesion will be described, since certain aspects of this bear directly on the question of etiology. The small intestine is usually totally involved, with thickening of the wall, dulling of the serosa and some thickening and induration of the mesentery. The thickening of the intestinal villi may produce a remarkable resemblance to a bearskin rug. With the light microscope, the villi are seen to be distended and blunted, owing to the accumulation of masses of macrophages within the lamina propria. These macrophages are characterized by the presence of numerous large, PAS-positive granules within their cytoplasm. In addition, accumulations of fat globules can be seen — within the macrophages, lying free within the lamina propria and within the mucosal and mesenteric lymphatic vessels. The epithelium itself appears relatively normal, although there is some vacuolation and replacement of columnar cells by cuboidal cells. When thick tissue sections are fixed in osmium and embedded in epon, distinctive bacillary bodies are seen in the lamina propria, particularly just beneath the basement membrane. The capillaries near the epithelium are also cuffed by these rod shaped structures. Occasionally, they are seen within the cytoplasm of macrophages (Trier et al., 1965).

With the electron microscope, the nature of these alterations can be better understood. The bacillary structures are seen in abundance just beneath the basement membrane in the upper third of the villi and within macrophages and polymorphonuclear leukocytes. Their length is about 2.5 μm. and their width about 0.3 μm. It is thought most likely that they are indeed bacteria (Adams et al., 1963). The distinctive PAS-positive granules within the macrophages are seen to be irregular structures up to 8 μm. in greatest diameter. They consist of a complex of closely packed membranes, matrix and probable bacteria in varying stages of disintegration. Many polymorphonuclear leukocytes are also seen in the upper lamina propria, some containing phagocytized bacteria. The surface epithelium shows some shortening and irregularity of the microvilli, as well as excessive cytoplasmic fat globules and lysosome-like membranous structures.

From this morphologic description, what can be said of the etiology of Whipple's disease? Although the classic criteria for establishing a bacterial etiology have not been met, there is much in favor of this theory. The bacillary bodies of Whipple's disease have never been described in normal biopsies nor in any other intestinal disease. Moreover, in remissions or during treatment, they tend to disappear, and their return is seen to correlate with a clinical relapse. Nevertheless, it must be emphasized that the organisms have never been cultured, despite repeated attempts using many culture media, nor has the disease been transmitted to animals. Neither is there any indication that Whipple's disease is contagious in man. It has been suggested that the disease is caused by nonspecific organisms in patients with an immunologic deficit, most likely an impairment in cell-based immunity (Maxwell et al., 1968).

Whipple's disease is characterized clinically by severe malabsorption, with diarrhea and steatorrhea, emaciation, fever, joint pains and a gray-brown melanin pigmentation of the skin. Diagnosis depends on finding the characteristic macrophages on jejunal biopsy. Without treatment, these patients usually follow an inexorable downhill course and die within four years of the diagnosis. However, antibiotic treatment, particularly with tetracycline, has resulted in dramatic remissions as well as in apparent cures.

CROHN'S DISEASE (REGIONAL ENTERITIS)

Crohn's disease is a chronic, relapsing, granulomatous inflammatory disorder, which classically affects the terminal ileum, but which may involve any portion of the gastrointestinal tract. In addition, occasionally there are associated extragastrointestinal manifestations, including arthritis, uveitis and a variety of skin lesions.

While Crohn's disease is not common, most clinicians are under the impression that its incidence is increasing (Editorial, 1970a; Miller et al., 1974). It usually develops in young adulthood, and affects males and females about equally frequently. The incidence is greater among Jews than among other whites, and whites as a group are more vulnerable than are blacks. There is some evidence of a familial tendency.

Etiology and Pathogenesis. The etiology of Crohn's disease is unknown. Theories abound, some of them mutually exclusive, and the acceptance of any one hypothesis varies virtually with the season. Perhaps the two most favored theories are: (1) that Crohn's disease is caused by an as yet unidentified infectious agent, and (2) that the disease is based on an abnormal hypersensitivity reaction. Both may, of course, be simultaneously true.

Attempts to isolate an infectious agent have so far been fruitless. Nonetheless, suspicion persists that some elusive microbe — perhaps a virus, protoplast or anaerobic bacterium — underlies Crohn's disease. Mitchell and Rees (1970) offered in support of this concept the production of the characteristic chronic granulomatous tissue reaction of Crohn's disease in the footpads of mice by inoculating them with gut or lymphatic tissue from patients with the disease. Mice inoculated with similar material from normal patients showed no such response. Subsequently, many of the features of Crohn's disease were produced in rabbits by injecting tissue from patients with Crohn's disease directly into the ileum (Cave et al., 1973). However, other workers have failed to reproduce these findings (Bolton et al., 1974).

The concept that Crohn's disease involves

some sort of immune derangement is similarly enticing but inconclusive. The typical granulomatous response of the affected gut and nearby lymph nodes is certainly reminiscent of tuberculosis, mycosis and schistosomiasis, all of which involve an element of hypersensitivity. There is some evidence of impaired T-cell function in these patients (Ramachandar et al., 1974). *No autoantibodies have yet been regularly demonstrated with Crohn's disease* (Perlmann and Broberger, 1968).

The close similarity of the granulomas of Crohn's disease to those of sarcoid has stimulated much conjecture over the relationship between these two disorders. Mitchell and his colleagues (1969) found that 23 of 45 patients with Crohn's disease had a positive Kveim test for sarcoid (granulomatous tissue response to inoculation of tissue from patients with sarcoid). Moreover, many of the mice whose footpads were injected with material from patients with Crohn's disease developed a positive Kveim test, whereas none of the control animals did. Accordingly, it has been suggested that both diseases may involve similar antigens, to which there is cross sensitivity, or that there may be a common etiology.

Of equal interest is the question of a relationship between Crohn's disease and ulcerative colitis. This will be discussed further in the section dealing with ulcerative colitis (p. 493).

From our brief tour of the edifice of speculation built around Crohn's disease, the essential mystery of the disease should be apparent. Whatever the ultimate cause, however, the lesion is thought to begin in the lymphoid tissue and in the adjacent lymph nodes of the affected portions of the gut, with eventual obstruction of the lymphatic channels of drainage. It is proposed that this pathogenetic mechanism then leads to the lymphedema of the gut, with a consequent inflammatory and fibrotic reaction in the intestinal wall.

Morphology. The terminal ileum is involved in approximately 80 per cent of patients. In 40 per cent, the colon is involved, either alone or concomitantly with ileal disease. Crohn's disease of the colon is often termed "granulomatous colitis." Less frequently, other levels of the gastrointestinal tract are affected. In particular, anal lesions may precede by years other manifestations of Crohn's disease. A very characteristic feature of Crohn's disease is the segmental nature of the involvement. Affected segments of intestine are sharply demarcated from adjacent normal areas. When these segments are multiple, separated by normal gut, they are termed "skip lesions."

The first gross alteration in the affected portion of intestine is the insidious development of edematous thickening of the gut wall. Subsequently, the

edema is replaced by fibrous tissue, which produces an abnormally rigid length of intestine, similar in texture to a rubber hose. The lumen is markedly narrowed, and so permits passage of only a thin stream of barium, giving rise to the x-ray "string sign" of Crohn's disease. **The entire thickness of the gut wall is involved,** and the serosal surface appears dull and granular. Parallel edematous thickening with consequent fibrosis affects the mesentery of the involved segment. On cross section of the gut, it can be seen that the fibrosis involves principally the submucosal and subserosal zones. Characteristic long, narrow serpentine ulcers may be seen virtually buried in the long axis of the gut (Fig. 14–10). These may penetrate the entire wall, creating abscesses within the peritoneal cavity or mesenteric fat. When the colon is involved, the changes are essentially the same, although fibrous thickening and stenosis are less pronounced.

The histologic changes, from the mucosal surface outward, include: (1) variable ulceration and destruction of the mucosa, (2) a submucosal inflammatory infiltrate, with marked fibrosis, (3) relative

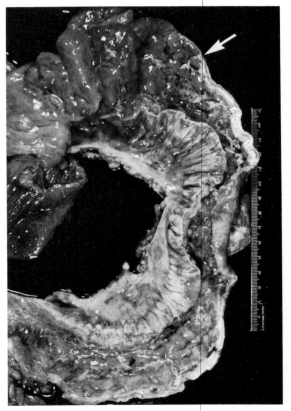

Figure 14–10. Crohn's disease (regional enteritis). The terminal ileum has been opened to disclose (below) the ulcerated mucosa covered by shreds of exudate. The process terminates at the loop seen at the top of the figure. The progressive disappearance of the thickening of the bowel wall is best seen at the arrow.

sparing of the muscularis, and (4) marked sub-serosal inflammation and fibrosis. The mucosal ulcerations show a nonspecific inflammatory response composed of neutrophils, lymphocytes, histiocytes and plasma cells. Between the ulcers, the glands may be distorted and cystically dilated. Within the submucosa and subserosa, the inflammatory infiltrate is largely mononuclear, and often it is aggregated into lymphoid follicles. **In half of the cases, granulomata markedly similar to those of sarcoid are seen within these aggregates.** Multinucleated giant cells, some of which contain Schaumann's bodies (p. 421), are present in the granulomas. Similar chronic granulomatous inflammatory changes may affect the regional lymph nodes.

Before concluding the description of the morphology of Crohn's disease, we should mention a disorder which may produce similar lesions. This is known as **potassium chloride enteropathy,** seen in patients taking potassium chloride tablets. The lesions consist basically of focal hemorrhages, congestion and fibrous thickening of the small bowel mucosa, particularly in the jejunum. Because many of these lesions are sharply segmental, sometimes annular, and produce narrowing of the bowel by progressive fibrosis, they are readily confused with Crohn's disease.

Clinical Course. The clinical presentation and course of Crohn's disease are quite variable. Most often these patients seek medical attention because of chronic intermittent diarrhea with colicky abdominal pain (usually in the right lower quadrant), weight loss and malaise. Low-grade fever is common, and occasionally may be the only manifestation. While some degree of melena is present in about 50 per cent of cases, it is usually slight.

Sometimes the first indications of disease arise from gastrointestinal complications, such as intestinal obstruction, perforation with intra-abdominal abscesses, fistula formation between adherent loops of bowel, hemorrhage, toxic dilatation of the colon, or peritonitis. About 10 per cent of patients with Crohn's disease first come to medical attention because of anal lesions, including perianal abscesses or fistulas. Manifestations of malabsorption, including steatorrhea, protein-wasting and deficiencies of vitamin B_{12}, folic acid and iron, may occur when the disease is extensive. Occasionally, extragastrointestinal manifestations develop before obvious involvement of the gut. Prominent among these are arthritis of the large joints, ankylosing spondylitis, uveitis, erythema nodosum and pyoderma gangrenosum.

About 10 per cent of patients with Crohn's disease, particularly younger individuals, have an acute onset, with severe right lower quadrant pain and tenderness, vomiting, diarrhea, fever and leukocytosis. In these cases, exploratory laparotomy may be necessary to distinguish this disorder from acute appendicitis. With an acute onset, the prognosis is relatively good, with permanent spontaneous remission in about 50 per cent of patients.

With the more insidious form of the disease, spontaneous remissions are less frequent. Most patients have a remitting-relapsing course, often with increasingly short intervals between relapses, until ultimately a progressive phase is reached. In the absence of complications, surgical removal of the involved gut is ill-advised because of the tendency of the lesion to recur in a previously uninvolved segment of the intestine. Despite the extreme inanition and disability often associated with Crohn's disease, fatalities are uncommon. Whether or not patients with granulomatous colitis are especially vulnerable to cancer of the colon is controversial. One recent study indicates a twentyfold increased risk of colonorectal cancer among those who developed granulomatous colitis before the age of 21 years (Weedon et al., 1973).

ULCERATIVE COLITIS

This is a serious and rather common chronic relapsing, remitting disease, characterized by diffuse superficial ulcerations of the colon. Occasionally, the lesions may extend proximally to include a short segment of the distal ileum. Extragastrointestinal manifestations, including arthritis, uveitis, skin lesions, venous thromboses and various liver disorders, occur even more commonly than with Crohn's disease.

While ulcerative colitis may develop at any age, it most frequently has its onset in young adulthood. A second peak in incidence occurs at about 50 years of age (DeDombal et al., 1969).

Etiology and Pathogenesis. Although ulcerative colitis is idiopathic, increasing evidence suggests that an immunologic derangement plays some role either in its causation or in its perpetuation. Specific autoantibodies against a mucopolysaccharide constituent of colonic mucous cells are present in most patients with ulcerative colitis. Autoantibody titers seem unrelated to the duration or severity of the disease or to the presence of extragastrointestinal manifestations, nor are these titers influenced by colectomy. Asymptomatic relatives of patients with ulcerative colitis also show an increased incidence of anticolonic autoantibodies (Perlmann and Broberger, 1968).

It is unlikely that these autoantibodies represent a secondary response to nonspecific damage to the colon mucosa, not only because they occasionally are found in asymptomatic individuals, but also because they are *not* found with other lesions of the colon. What, then, triggers their formation? It is well known that the normal flora of the colon and the colonic mucosa share some common antigens. Conceivably, the mucosa of these patients is abnormally permeable and permits the absorption of unusual amounts of bacterial antigen from the lumen. This antigen might then elicit the formation of antibodies that are cross reactive with the colonic mucosa.

Are the autoantibodies associated with ulcerative colitis cytotoxic? A recent study using immunofluorescent staining showed unusually large numbers of plasma cells containing IgG and IgA, along with the C'3 component of complement, within the rectal mucosa of patients with ulcerative colitis. It was inferred that the antibody was locally produced, that it was probably directed against bacterial antigen, and that the resultant complement-binding antigen-antibody complexes were cytotoxic (Ballard and Shiner, 1974). Others, however, doubt the validity of these inferences (Baklien and Brandtzaeg, 1974).

The possibility that a cell-based immune reaction plays some role in the pathogenesis of ulcerative colitis has also been raised. It has been shown that lymphocytes from these patients are specifically cytotoxic to human colon cells in vitro. In addition, as with Crohn's disease, there is some evidence of a derangement in T-cell function in patients with ulcerative colitis (Ramachandar et al., 1974).

As was mentioned in the discussion of Crohn's disease, the relationship between it and ulcerative colitis, if any, is a controversial point of great interest. For some time, Crohn's disease was thought never to involve the colon, for the simple reason that those instances of colonic involvement were ascribed to ulcerative colitis. When the distinctive histopathology of Crohn's disease of the colon became recognized, a sharp distinction was then drawn between this entity, often known as "granulomatous colitis," and ulcerative colitis. Recently, the distinction between Crohn's disease and ulcerative colitis has again become blurred. Despite the rather clear histopathologic differences, certain epidemiologic and clinical aspects point to some connection between the two disorders. Both show a familial tendency and both are present with more than chance frequency within the same family (Editorial, 1970*d*). Indeed, these disorders often develop in the same patient. Of 676 cases of Crohn's disease, 60 had concomitant ulcerative colitis (Perlmann and Broberger,

1968). *However, although specific autoantibodies to colonic cells have been found in patients with ulcerative colitis, autoantibodies are not known to be present with Crohn's disease.* Nonetheless, certain clinical similarities are striking, particularly the frequent occurrence with both disorders of identical *extragastrointestinal manifestations.* Conceivably, these two disorders simply represent differing tissue responses of anatomically distinct segments of the gut to the same underlying insult.

Morphology. Although occasionally ulcerative colitis may arise in the cecum or right colon, it is, in contrast to Crohn's disease of the colon, more typically a disorder of the left colon. Usually it begins in the rectosigmoid area, whence it may extend to involve progressively larger areas and sometimes the entire colon. In about 33 per cent of patients, the process spreads to the distal ileum.

The histologic features of ulcerative colitis will be presented before the gross alterations, since an understanding of the latter depends to a considerable extent on knowledge of the former.

The earliest lesions are microabscesses in the crypts of the mucosal glands. As these microabscesses increase in size, they undermine the mucosal margins, which eventually slough, creating small, flask shaped ulcerations. A nonspecific inflammatory infiltrate is present at the bases and margins of the ulcers, and sometimes a subjacent acute vasculitis is found. In the acute stages, the ulcers usually remain confined to the mucosa and submucosa. At this level, they tend to enlarge and coalesce, with their undermining margins creating a network of tunnels covered by tenuous mucosal bridges (Fig. 14–11). With long-standing, severe disease, the ulcers may erode into the muscularis and sometimes even penetrate the entire wall. The inflammatory infiltrate in the more chronic lesions becomes mononuclear. Attempts at mucosal regeneration often lead to metaplasia and dysplasia of the epithelium, with cystic dilatation of the glands. Fibrotic scarring may develop, but it is characteristically far less marked than that of Crohn's disease.

Grossly, the changes may be minimal until the subterranean excavation just described becomes quite extensive. Large mucosal defects then become apparent, and, indeed, virtually the entire mucosa may be sloughed. In these advanced cases, islands of surviving epithelium or of epithelialized granulation tissue may appear to be elevated in contrast to the surrounding excavation. Such multiple tiny protrusions, seen in about 15 per cent of cases of ulcerative colitis, are termed **pseudopolyps** (Jalan et al., 1969). Some degree of edematous thickening of the colon is characteristic, and in long-standing cases, minimal to moderate fibrous rigidity of the bowel may develop. In relatively mild cases, virtual restoration of the normal mucosal architecture may occur during remissions.

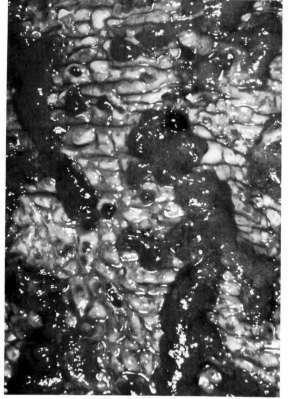

Figure 14–11. Ulcerative colitis. The dark, irregular pattern comprises ulcerations which have in many instances coalesced, leaving virtual islands of residual, paler mucosa. A tendency toward pseudopolyp formation is already evident.

Clinical Course. Most commonly, ulcerative colitis develops insidiously over the course of several months, manifesting itself by diarrhea, often consisting of a mixture of blood, mucus and flecks of feces; tenesmus and colicky lower abdominal pain, relieved by defecation; and variable constitutional signs, including fever and weight loss. Grossly bloody stools are far more common than with Crohn's disease, and blood loss may be considerable.

In a minority of patients, the onset of ulcerative colitis is abrupt and fulminant, with uncontrollable diarrhea, and the rapid development of severe fluid depletion and electrolyte imbalances. The mortality rate in this group is high.

Extragastrointestinal manifestations are even more common with ulcerative colitis than with Crohn's disease, and, when the bowel disturbance is mild, may be the predominant complaint of the patient. Ankylosing spondylitis occurs in about 17 per cent of patients with ulcerative colitis, and arthritis of the large joints affects another 6 per cent. About 11 per cent

have uveitis. Other extragastrointestinal manifestations of ulcerative colitis include a tendency toward venous thromboses, aphthous ulceration of the mouth, oral moniliasis and a variety of skin lesions which may also be seen with Crohn's disease, including erythema nodosum and pyoderma gangrenosum. All these disorders not only may precede the onset of the bowel disease, but also may persist after colectomy, Of great interest is the association of liver disease with ulcerative colitis. The frequency of this association varies from study to study, but probably about 15 per cent of patients with ulcerative colitis have some abnormalities of liver function. Liver biopsies in these patients may show a variety of changes, including fatty change, pericholangitis, and biliary cirrhosis. For some time, it has been suspected that the liver lesions may result from portal bacteremia, but this has not been conclusively demonstrated (Eade and Brooke, 1969).

The course of ulcerative colitis is variable. Most patients follow a chronic relapsing-remitting course, with exacerbations tending to follow any stress, emotional or physical. In some cases, the disease takes a smoldering, continuous course, remaining more or less under control. A variety of gastrointestinal complications may arise. When the onset is acute, and also during severe exacerbations, necrosis of the colon may be so widespread that the bowel ceases to function altogether and virtually disintegrates. This is manifested by sudden cessation of diarrhea and progressive distention of the colon, known as *toxic dilatation* or *toxic megacolon,* and it requires emergency colectomy. Other life-threatening complications include massive hemorrhage and perforation with peritonitis. Strictures of the colon, which produce obstruction and which are easily confused with carcinoma, occur in about 11 per cent of patients. Perianal disease is less common than with Crohn's disease.

Because involvement of the rectosigmoid colon is common, the diagnosis can usually be made on sigmoidoscopy and biopsy. Barium enema may reveal a typically rigid smooth bowel, with rounding of the flexures and loss of the haustra. Specific infectious etiologies must always be ruled out.

The prognosis with ulcerative colitis varies with the clinical pattern of the disease. The mortality is highest in the first months, and improves with chronicity. About 8 per cent of patients die within one year of the onset of their disease, usually of peritonitis, sepsis, hemorrhage or fluid and electrolyte disturbances. With very long-standing disease, however, especially when it is unremitting, the outlook again darkens because of an increasing risk of malignant transformation. This risk increases with duration of the disease and applies almost entirely to patients who have had their disease for longer than 10 years. One study showed that after 10 years the risk of developing colonorectal cancer in patients who had developed ulcerative colitis before the age of 14 years is 20 per cent per decade (Devroede et al., 1971).

The chart at the bottom of the page shows some of the distinguishing characteristics of Crohn's disease, particularly as it affects the colon, and of ulcerative colitis.

MELENA

Melena refers to the passage of tarry black or mahogany red stools caused by the presence in the feces of large amounts of blood and blood pigments. It should be distinguished, on the one hand, from *occult* gastrointestinal bleeding, and, on the other, from bright red rectal bleeding. The causes of melena are legion, and include lesions anywhere in the gastrointestinal tract, from the esophagus to the colon. Among the more important of these lesions, we have already discussed peptic ulcers, gastritis, Meckel's diverticulum, mesenteric vascular occlusion, acute hemorrhagic enteropathy, ulcerative colitis and diverticular disease. Remaining to be considered here are two lesions which often call attention to themselves by producing melena or rectal bleeding: *polyps of the colon* and *carcinoma of the colon*.

POLYPS OF THE COLON

Three patterns of colonic polyps are recognized, each of which has distinctive morphologic and clinical characteristics: (1) the sporadic *pedunculated adenoma*, (2) the *villous adenoma*, and (3) *heredofamilial polyposis*. Some lesions, however, demonstrate mixed features of both the pedunculated adenoma and the villous adenoma.

PEDUNCULATED ADENOMA
(ADENOMATOUS POLYP)

These extemely common polyps are composed of a small spherical head attached to

the colon by a stalk (Fig. 14–12). Since stalks are extemely variable in length and thickness, the diagnosis of pedunculated adenoma is made when the head of the polyp can be moved freely in all directions through a 90 degree arc. Pedunculated adenomas occur in both sexes and in all age groups, although they become increasingly common with advancing age. Estimates of their frequency range from 10 per cent of adults to 50 per cent of those over 30 years of age (Castleman and Krickstein, 1966).

Morphology. Autopsy studies indicate that about 50 per cent of pedunculated adenomas occur in the ascending and transverse colons, and a third in the rectosigmoid. Pedunculated adenomas are solitary in about 50 per cent of patients; the remaining half harbor two or more of these lesions, and about 16 per cent have more than five (Helwig, 1947).

Grossly, they appear as soft, red, raspberry-like spheroids, commonly less than 1 cm. in diameter but occasionally as large as 4 cm., attached to the colon by a stalk of variable length. On histologic examination, a central core of fibrovascular tissue is seen to arise in the submucosa and extend through the center of the stalk into the head. Although the stalk is usually covered by fairly normal colonic epithelium, that of the head is highly variable. It may fit anywhere in the spectrum from normal colonic epithelium through hyperplasia and dysplasia to frank carcinoma in situ. The hyperplastic polyps ("polypoid hyperplasia") are characterized by abnormally tall and sometimes branching glands, with deep crypts. The epithelial cells themselves become tall, lose their capacity to secrete mucin, and have variably located, somewhat hyperchromatic nuclei. Mitoses are common. With increasing atypicality, the cells lose their regular palisade arrangement and become disorganized and heaped up, with the formation of abnormal glandular patterns. The benign nature of the lesion is, however, indicated by the absence of invasion of the central fibrous core. Nonetheless, the line between polypoid hyperplasia and carcinoma in situ becomes very finely drawn indeed. Invasion of the underlying fibrous core is considered to be the most reliable criterion of malignant transformation, although even in these cases, the development of metastatic disease is held by some to be rare.

Crohn's disease	*Ulcerative colitis*
Right sided	Left sided
Segmental	Diffuse
Transmural	Superficial
4+ fibrosis	1+ fibrosis
Chronic granulomatous inflammatory response	Acute to chronic nonspecific inflammatory response

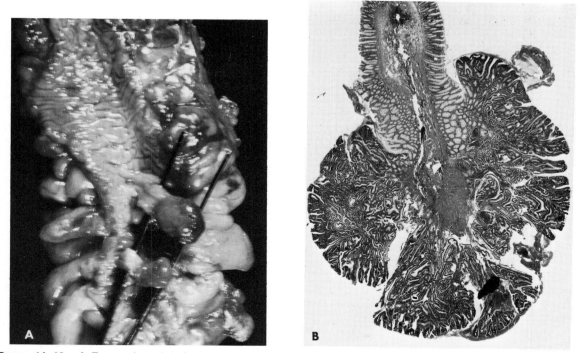

Figure 14–12. *A,* Two pedunculated adenomas of the colon displayed on top of the forceps. The berry-like heads are attached on elongated, slender stalks. *B,* A low power view of one of these lesions, showing the normal mucosa covering the stalk and the polypoid hyperplasia of the epithelium in the head of the polyp.

Clinical Course. Pedunculated adenomas are most often discovered as incidental lesions at autopsy or during routine sigmoidoscopic examinations or barium enemas. Occasionally, however, they become traumatized in their exposed position and are then a source of significant bleeding.

The relationship, if any, of pedunculated adenomas to cancer of the colon is the subject of one of the liveliest controversies in medicine (Ingelfinger et al., 1966). On the one hand are those who believe the risk of malignant tranformation to be as high as 30 per cent; on the other hand are those who contend that these lesions give rise to "biologic" cancer (i.e., capable of invasion and metastases) in less than 0.1 per cent of cases. The arguments on both sides are persuasive, and will be set forth briefly.

Those who see pedunculated adenomas as important threats believe it is unreasonable to suppose that cancer does *not* arise in lesions known to show a spectrum of progressively ominous histologic changes. Moreover, the fact that they may occur in a mixed pattern with villous adenomas, which are universally recognized as having a high malignant potential (as will be discussed next in this chapter), is taken to imply guilt by association. Indeed, it has been suggested that pedunculated aden-

omas and villous adenomas are merely growth variants of the same lesion, with the same potential for malignancy. Furthermore, some studies have suggested a correlation between the presence of pedunculated adenomas and carcinoma of the colon (Baker and Jones, 1966).

In contrast, the prevailing opinion is that pedunculated adenomas are virtually harmless. While acknowledging that transformation to aggressive carcinoma is possible, supporters of this view believe it to be exceedingly rare. They draw a sharp distinction between histologic carcinoma and biologic, or clinically significant, carcinoma. Despite the frequently atypical epithelium of pedunculated adenomas, it is thought that these atypical cells seldom invade more than their stalk and even more rarely metastasize. Any correlation between carcinoma of the colon and polyps is of dubious statistical significance, in view of the very high incidence of polyps in the general population. Certainly, any statistical correlation cannot be absolute, since polyps are so much more common than carcinomas of the colon. Even granting a small statistical correlation between the two lesions, it has been pointed out that their association does not necessarily mean that the carcinoma arises in a polyp (Castleman and Krickstein, 1966).

With apologies for the anticlimax, it should be said in conclusion that the controversy may be of greater academic than practical importance. Since both colonic carcinoma and villous adenomas may occasionally take a pedunculated form, lesions of this nature discovered on barium enema which are beyond the reach of a peranal biopsy must be surgically investigated, regardless of the prevailing philosophy about pedunculated adenomas.

VILLOUS ADENOMA (SESSILE ADENOMA, PAPILLARY ADENOMA)

The villous adenoma is a papillary structure which is attached to the colonic mucosa by a broad base. Rarely, it is pedunculated. Although these lesions occur much less frequently than pedunculated adenomas, it is generally agreed that they present a very substantial risk of containing within them foci of carcinoma. They are found most often in the elderly, and may affect either sex.

Morphology. Villous adenomas are found principally in the rectosigmoid, and occur only infrequently in the right and transverse colons. Grossly, the lesion appears as a fungating, cauliflower-like mass, usually over 5 cm. in diameter by the time it is discovered, but elevated no more than 3 cm. above the surrounding mucosa. Lesions up to 20 cm. in diameter are not uncommon. Often there are foci of hemorrhage or ulceration on their pale gray surfaces. Histologically, these adenomas are composed of small, finger-like villi, sometimes branching and rebranching (Fig. 14–13). The villi have a loose fibrovascular core and are covered by epithelial cells of varying normalcy. In some areas, the epithelial cells may resemble closely those of the colonic mucosa; in others they are obviously anaplastic. The most valuable histologic criteria of malignancy are: (1) piling up of anaplastic cells to form multilayered masses, (2) formation of small atypical gland patterns within these masses, and (3) invasion of the underlying fibrous core.

Clinical Course. Because of their propensity for hemorrhage and ulceration, coupled with their exposed position in the distal colon, villous adenomas often come to attention because of rectal bleeding. In other instances, these lesions secrete copious amounts of mucoid material, and the patients may then complain of the frequent passage of mucus per rectum. Sometimes a profound hypokalemic alkalosis occurs, which is attributable to the loss of potassium in this mucoid material. Because of their location, villous adenomas are usually readily discovered on proctoscopic or sigmoidoscopic examination.

There is little disagreement that the villous adenoma leads to life-threatening carcinoma of the colon in many, if not all, cases. As many as 70 to 80 per cent of villous adenomas contain clearly malignant areas at the time of diagnosis. Some believe that, with painstaking microscopic examination of many serial sections of the lesions, all these tumors will be discovered to

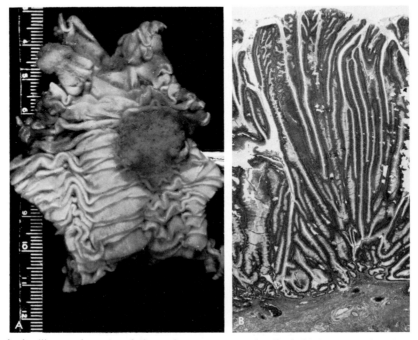

Figure 14–13. *A,* A villous adenoma of the colon, seen grossly. *B,* A high power detail of the long, villous glandular fronds. There is no evidence of cellular atypicality or of carcinoma in the view given.

harbor areas of cancerous change. As was mentioned earlier, rarely villous adenomas are pedunculated, and these are thought by some to be relatively benign. In the individual case, it is perhaps safest to assume that the lesion is cancerous until exhaustive histologic studies disprove the assumption.

HEREDOFAMILIAL POLYPOSIS

Relatively infrequently, multiple polyps occur as a hereditary trait, transmitted predominantly as an autosomal dominant. Four distinct syndromes are of clinical importance: (1) *familial multiple polyposis of the colon*, (2) the *Peutz-Jeghers syndrome*, (3) *Gardner's syndrome*, and (4) *Turcot's syndrome* (autosomal recessive).

Familial multiple polyposis of the colon is characterized by myriads of polyps that are morphologically indistinguishable from small pedunculated adenomas, covering virtually the entire colonic mucosa and sometimes extending into the proximal gastrointestinal tract, including the stomach. Although the disease is congenital, the polyps do not actually appear before the second decade of life. On the other hand, a family member who has not developed polyps by the age of 40 years is probably spared. *There is with this disorder a high incidence of malignant transformation of polyps.* Indeed, unless the colon is removed, it is possible that with time this entity will inevitably give rise to cancer. Whether this results from a concurrent genetic predisposition in these patients, or whether it merely reflects the increased probability of malignant transformation among literally hundreds of polyps, is not clear.

The *Peutz-Jeghers syndrome* includes polyps of the entire gastrointestinal tract, particularly the small intestine, and associated deep melanin pigmentation of the buccal mucosa, lips and digits. *Although the polyps resemble in all anatomic details those of multiple familial polyposis, they rarely give rise to cancer.* Because of this, some believe that the polyps represent hamartomatous overgrowths rather than true neoplasms.

The *Gardner syndrome* refers to the association of colonic polyposis with extracolonic neoplasms. The skin, subcutaneous tissue and bone may be involved.

The *Turcot syndrome* combines polyps of the colon with brain tumors. In contrast to the other entities, it is transmitted as an autosomal recessive.

CANCER OF THE COLON AND RECTUM

In the United States colorectal carcinoma is the second most frequent cause of death from cancer in both men and women. Only lung cancer kills more men, and only breast cancer kills more women. When both sexes are considered together, colorectal carcinoma still remains second to lung cancer. In general this is a tumor of the middle-aged and elderly, reaching a peak incidence between the ages of 50 and 70 years. However, there are many exceptions to this generality, as, for example, when cancer of the colon develops as a complication of ulcerative colitis or of familial multiple polyposis. Colorectal carcinoma is located in the colon probably somewhat more commonly than in the rectum. Men and women are equally vulnerable.

Etiology and Pathogenesis. As is the case with all cancer, the precise cause (or causes) of colorectal carcinoma is unknown. A minority of these tumors develop as complications of other disorders known to carry with them a high risk of cancerous transformation. These include heredofamilial polyposis, villous adenoma, ulcerative colitis, and, perhaps, granulomatous colitis (Crohn's disease of the colon). There is also a slight familial predisposition toward cancer of the colon, with the risk to a first degree relative of a patient being about three times that of the general population. *However, there is ample evidence that in the overwhelming majority of cases of colorectal carcinoma, unknown environmental factors are of paramount importance.* Much of this evidence is epidemiologic. Population studies show colorectal carcinoma to be a disease of affluent industrialized societies, with a very high incidence in North America and Europe and a relatively low incidence in most of Asia, Africa and South America. It is also a disease of modern times, having assumed importance only within this century. Immigrants from low-risk to high-risk areas acquire the risk of their adopted country. Moreover, within relatively low-risk areas, affluent subpopulations or those who have become "Westernized" have a higher incidence of colorectal carcinoma than does the surrounding population (Burkitt, 1973; Editorial, 1974a).

Granting, then, that environmental influences are important, what is their nature? In searching for the cause of colorectal carcinoma, it is only logical to suspect that the fecal material passing through the bowel may play a role. Obviously, this is in turn affected by the diet. It is becoming increasingly appreciated that the diet in modern affluent societies differs greatly from that in traditional or economically poorer societies. The intake of refined carbohydrates, fat and protein (particularly meat) is higher, whereas the intake of fiber is markedly lower. As we shall see, this affects the nature of the bacterial flora of the colon, and the concentration of bile acids and neutral steroids within the feces. Moreover, the transit time of food through the gastrointestinal tract is approximately doubled in affluent societies, from about 35 hours in African villagers to about 70 hours in England (Burkitt, 1973). *It has been hypothesized that the higher incidence of cancer of the colon and rectum in affluent societies, then, reflects the prolonged contact with the bowel wall of compounds produced by the action of intestinal bacteria on biliary and dietary constituents* (Burkitt, 1973; Editorial, 1974a; Hill and Aries, 1971; Editorial, 1974d). This hypothesis is supported by three sets of data: (1) There is a change in the bacterial flora in affluent societies, with relatively large numbers of *Bacteroides* and other anaerobic organisms and relatively small numbers of enterococci and other aerobic bacteria (Hill et al., 1971). (2) The concentration of bile acids and neutral steroids in the feces is higher, perhaps as a result of higher fat intake, and these are more extensively degraded into possible carcinogens (Hill and Aries, 1971). (3) As mentioned, transit time is increased, providing a longer time for bacterial action on fecal constituents and for contact between resulting carcinogens and the bowel wall. As attractive as this hypothesis is, only parts of it have been buttressed with facts and there remains the task of identifying the specific carcinogens involved.

Whatever the etiology, the cancer probably arises from many cells rather than from a single cell, and is preceded by a prolonged period of carcinoma-in-situ (Fialkow, 1974). It is thought that the transformed cells are those on the mucosal surface, which are normally inactive, rather than the proliferating cells in the crypts of Lieberkühn. Apparently, the carcinogenic influence causes these surface cells to resume cell division rather than become senescent and slough off into the bowel lumen (Cole, 1973).

Morphology. Colonorectal carcinoma occurs in a fairly well-defined pattern of distribution: rectum, 50 per cent; sigmoid, 20 per cent; descending colon, 6 per cent; transverse colon and splenic flexure, 8 per cent; cecum and ascending colon, 16 per cent. It is apparent that approximately 70 per cent of colonorectal carcinomas are within reach of the sigmoidoscope (Moertel et al., 1958). However, there is some indication that this distribution has been changing in recent years, with fewer tumors arising in the lower rectum (Editorial, 1974d). Infrequently, multiple carcinomas arise concurrently, most often in patients with heredofamilial polyposis.

These tumors have been classified descriptively in a number of ways, but it suffices from our standpoint to distinguish two patterns: carcinomas of the left side and those of the right. Carcinomas of the left side tend to grow in an annular encircling fashion. They produce a so-called "napkin-ring" constriction of the bowel with early symptoms of obstruction. These lesions may begin as sessile masses, but over the span of one to two years, they grow to infiltrate and encircle the circumference (Fig. 14–14). On the right side, the lesions tend to grow as polypoid fungating masses which extend along one wall of the more capacious cecum and ascending colon. Obstruction is uncommon (Fig. 14–15). Thus, from the standpoint of gross morphology and clinical behavior, most carcinomas of the left and right colon behave as two distinct tumor types.

The early lesion on the left side appears as a small elevated button or as a small polypoid mass. As the tumor grows, it forms a flat plaque which continues to increase in size. It eventually extends circumferentially to encircle the wall. It has been estimated that it takes approximately one to two years for such a lesion totally to encircle the lumen. The deeper layers are invaded only slowly, and for a long time the neoplasm tends to remain superficial. Eventually, the mid-circumference of the ring ulcerates as penetration of the bowel wall en-

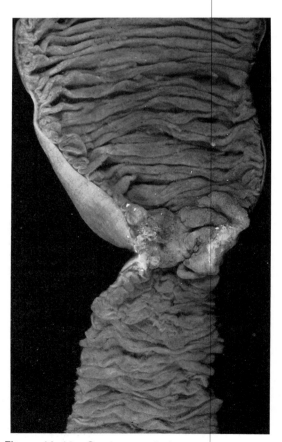

Figure 14–14. Carcinoma of the rectosigmoid. The narrow annular lesion has caused obstructive dilatation of the proximal bowel above.

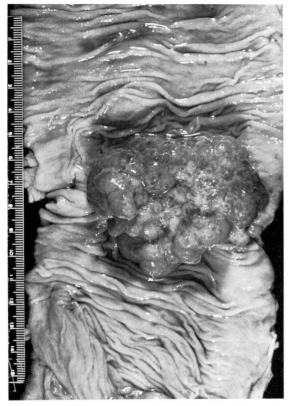

Figure 14–15. Carcinoma of the right colon. The polypoid cancer projects into the lumen, but has not caused obstruction.

croaches on the blood supply. At this time, the annular constriction characteristically shows heaped-up margins with a central ulceration or excavation. Infrequently, left-sided lesions produce little luminal growth but, instead, infiltrate the bowel wall and cause flattening and small ulcerations of the mucosa. Extension of the tumor through the bowel wall into the pericolic fat and regional lymph nodes occurs as the lesion progresses. The penetration of the bowel wall may on occasion produce pericolic abscesses or even peritonitis.

Cancers in the right colon begin as sessile lesions similar to those of the left but progressively assume a polypoid fungating appearance. They frequently become bulky, cauliflower-like masses which protrude into the lumen. Plaque-like or ulcerative lesions of the right side occur, but very infrequently. These right-sided tumors eventually penetrate the wall and extend to the mesentery, regional lymph nodes, liver, and more distant sites. Because they occur in the more capacious cecum and ascending colon, they do not cause obstruction and may remain clinically silent for long periods of time. Quite uncommonly, colonic carcinomas of the right side grow in an invasive infiltrating fashion, with mucosal flattening and ulceration without luminal projections.

Unlike the gross pathology, the microscopic characteristics of right- and left-sided colorectal carcinomas are similar. Ninety-five per cent of all carcinomas of the colon and rectum are adenocarcinomas, many of which produce mucin. Commonly, this mucin is secreted extracellularly, either within gland lumina or within the interstitium of the gut wall. Because this secretion dissects the wall, it aids the extension of the cancer and worsens the prognosis. Occasionally, undifferentiated growth is observed. In the anal region, some of these cancers differentiate as adenoacanthomas.

Clinical Course. It is now appreciated that colonorectal carcinoma is present for a considerable time before it produces clinical manifestations. When signs and symptoms do appear, their nature depends on the location of the lesion. Tumors in the rectum and sigmoid are often associated with spotty bleeding, which coats the surface of the stools. Changes in bowel habits are common, including changes in frequency of defecation and in the consistency of the stools, Because of partial obstruction, patients with left-sided lesions often complain of colicky pain or "gas." Occasionally, acute obstruction occurs. Right-sided colonic cancer is more insidious in its presentation. Bleeding occurs, but it is often occult, and may not be discovered until iron deficiency anemia develops. Sometimes there is a vague discomfort in the right lower quadrant.

All colorectal cancers spread by direct extension into adjacent structures and by metastasis through the lymphatic and venous systems. The pericolic and periaortic nodes are most often first involved. Later, there are metastases to the liver, lungs and bones.

As mentioned, nearly 70 per cent of colonorectal carcinomas can be seen and biopsied through the sigmoidoscope. Right-sided lesions may be revealed by barium enema. In 1965, Gold and Freedman described in patients with carcinomas of the digestive tract high titers of an antigen normally present in embryonic entodermal epithelium. This was termed carcinoembryonic antigen (CEA). It is present in about 75 per cent of patients with colorectal carcinoma. However, early hopes for its use as a screening device were not realized, since it may also be present in high titers in individuals with a host of nonmalignant inflammatory and hyperplastic disorders, as well as in some normal cigarette smokers (Hansen et al., 1974). As we shall see, assays of CEA are now used mainly to evaluate the success of cancer therapy. Recently, an isomer of CEA, termed CEA-S, was isolated. There is some evidence that this isomer is less likely to be present with nonmalignant disease than is CEA, and it may therefore be of value for diagnostic screening (Edgington et al., 1975).

However, these results have not yet been confirmed.

The overall five-year survival rate with the colonorectal carcinoma is about 43 per cent. Because of the relatively early manifestations of left-sided lesions, one might reasonably expect these to have a better prognosis. However, they tend to be more infiltrative, and the prognosis with right-sided lesions is actually somewhat better. The outcome is more influenced by the depth of anatomic spread than by their location within the bowel. On this basis, Dukes separated his patients with rectal carcinoma into three groups, and he and Bussey showed the difference in prognosis (Dukes, 1932; Dukes and Bussey, 1958): (1) Type A: growth confined to the rectum, with no extrarectal spread and no lymphatic metastasis—five-year survival, about 98 per cent; (2) Type B: spread by continuity into extrarectal tissues, no lymphatic metastasis—survival, about 78 per cent; (3) Type C: lymphatic metastasis present—survival, 32 per cent. Unfortunately, at least half of all patients with colonorectal carcinoma fall into Dukes Type C group when first diagnosed (Morton, 1970–71). For those whose disease is still localized, however, medicine and surgery have much to offer, and the prognosis is excellent. Failure of CEA titers to fall after surgery, or reappearance of high titers at a later date, is a reliable sign of a poor prognosis (Mach et al., 1974).

MISCELLANEOUS LESIONS

CANCER OF THE ORAL MUCOUS MEMBRANES

These oral tumors constitute about 5 per cent of all malignant disease, although they are a relatively uncommon cause of death. Approximately 90 per cent are squamous cell carcinomas. The remainder are adenocarcinomas, melanomas and, less frequently, various forms of sarcoma. Only rarely do these tumors occur before middle age, and there is a male predilection of about 9 to 1.

The role of chronic irritation in the pathogenesis of cancer of the oral mucous membranes is uncertain. Although such irritating influences as tobacco smoking and trauma from ill-fitting prosthetic appliances or jagged edges of carious teeth are frequently associated with the development of oral cancer, their ubiquity raises the possibility of mere coincidence. It can be said, however, that oral cancer is often preceded by leukoplakia (see p. 548), a lesion that can more certainly be ascribed to chronic irritation, and it has been shown experimentally that chronic irritation hastens the onset of chemically induced buccal cancer (Renstrup et al., 1962).

The lower lip is the most common site of cancer of the oral mucous membranes. Among the less frequent sites are: the tongue (usually the lateral border or ventral surface), the floor of the mouth, the alveolar mucosa, the palate and the buccal mucosa. Multiple primary tumors occur, either simultaneously or sequentially, in about 19 per cent of all cases (Moertel and Foss, 1958).

Although the clinical presentation and the prognosis are to some extent dependent on the exact site of the lesion, the morphologic picture is in general the same for the group as a whole. Cancer of the oral mucous membranes is first apparent as a small, indurated plaque, nodule or ulcer, which may become fissured and necrotic on the surface. As was mentioned, leukoplakia often precedes or coexists with oral squamous cell carcinoma. With continued growth, the tumor may either project as a large cauliflower-like mass, pushing aside normal structures, or it may appear as an extensive ulcerated crater, eroding and destroying all contiguous structures. Such destructive lesions may penetrate the jaws and cause loss of teeth, and they may even erode through to the face, paranasal sinuses or orbit, producing severe disfigurement.

Histologically, these lesions are almost always typical squamous cell carcinomas, which were described on page 117. Among the less frequent histologic types, the adenocarcinomas are most likely to occur on the hard and soft palates, and the melanomas on the palate and alveolar mucosa. **Macroscopically,** these are indistinguishable from squamous cell lesions.

Regional lymph node involvement is invariable with oral cavity cancers as the disease progresses. With laterally placed lesions, the nodal spread may be unilateral. The metastases tend to remain confined to these regional nodes until very late in the course, when distant metastases to the lungs, liver and bone may occur.

The clinical manifestations of these tumors are, as was mentioned, somewhat dependent on the exact site involved. Overall, however, early growth tends to be asymptomatic, at least until secondary infection supervenes. Lesions in mobile areas, such as the anterior portion of the tongue, the floor of the mouth or the cheek, are more likely to be painful early in their course. The ready visibility of carcinomas of the lower lip and the anterior portion of the tongue, which appear as a slight surface encrustation, a papillary mass, an ulcer or a persistent fissure, coupled with their tendency not to metastasize until quite late in their course, gives them a better prognosis than lesions in other sites. In these relatively happy circumstances, the five-year survival rate is of the order of 95 per cent. In less fortunate cases, death results from sepsis, dehydration, malnutrition, hemorrhage or airway obstruction.

SALIVARY GLAND TUMORS

The salivary glands are affected infrequently by a large variety of tumors, the most common of which is known, probably inappropriately, as the "mixed tumor." The parotids are the most frequently involved of the salivary glands. For every 100 cases of parotid gland tumors, about 10 tumors occur in the submandibular glands, 10 involve minor salivary glands, and one involves the sublingual glands (Editorial, 1969*a*). Over 80 per cent of parotid gland tumors are benign. Although tumors of the other salivary glands are benign in less than 50 per cent of cases, nevertheless their infrequency relative to parotid gland tumors means that, overall, salivary gland tumors are most often benign.

PLEOMORPHIC ADENOMA (MIXED TUMOR) OF THE SALIVARY GLANDS

These tumors embrace a range of biologic behavior, from those that are clearly benign to overtly cancerous lesions. The origin of this most common of the salivary gland tumors is still debated. Although possibly it is derived from both epithelial and mesenchymal elements, the consensus favors its being of purely epithelial origin, and therefore a pleomorphic adenoma. The source of the controversy lies in the frequent presence of islands of chondroid matrix. Does this imply that true chondrocytes are present in addition to epithelial elements, or is the cartilage-like tissue elaborated by metaplastic myoepithelial cells? The latter explanation is considered more likely.

Pleomorphic adenomas of the salivary glands usually occur between the ages of 20 and 40 years, and are almost always benign. Following resection, local recurrence is frequent, but this is thought to result from inadequate excision. In only 2 to 5 per cent of cases does a true cancer arise from a mixed tumor.

Pleomorphic adenomas of the parotid gland appear as ovoid masses, up to the size of a grapefruit, but usually smaller, just anterior to and beneath the ear, obliterating the angle of the jaw. The larger ones may deflect the ear lobe and, rarely, may cause pressure necrosis, with ulceration of the overlying skin. Although these lesions are encapsulated, they frequently penetrate through their own capsules, creating technical difficulties in achieving complete excision.

Histologically, these tumors are extremely pleomorphic, with variations in cellular morphology not only among different tumors but also from focus to focus within the same tumor. The basic neoplastic cells probably arise from the ductal epithelium and comprise both epithelial and myoepithelial elements. These cells range in shape from polyhedral through cuboidal to columnar, and may be arrayed in acinar or ductal arrangements, in strands within a connective tissue stroma, or in solid sheets. Frequently, the malignant forms recapitulate the growth of a basal cell or squamous cell carcinoma, but in most instances the epithelial cells, whatever their array, appear quite mature and normal. The stroma itself is a distinctive part of the histology. Often it consists of interlacing strands or tongues of loose myxoid tissue containing stellate cells. Islands of cartilage-like material are characteristic. The benign variants are usually encapsulated. However, progressive degrees of aggressiveness and anaplasia are encountered, and some of these lesions are obviously invasive and malignant (Fig. 14–16).

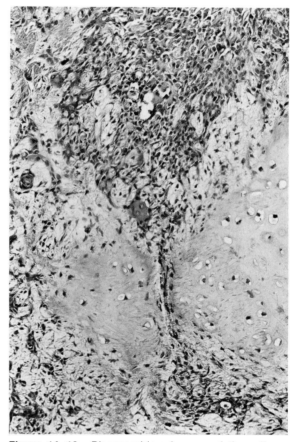

Figure 14–16. Pleomorphic adenoma of the salivary glands. The microscopic field contains areas of epithelial cells (above), two islands of apparent cartilaginous matrix and an abundant myxoid stroma.

Pleomorphic adenomas of the salivary glands manifest themselves as painless, slowly growing masses. Involvement of the facial nerve results in varying degrees of facial palsy, and impingement on the trigeminal nerves produces pain and sometimes the symptoms of tic douloureux. Their biologic behavior is exceedingly difficult to assess from morphologic examination. Often tiny pseudopods of invasiveness are left behind in the removal of an apparently encapsulated neoplasm, producing recurrence. Regrettably, with each recurrence, there is a tendency for increased anaplasia and invasiveness, giving rise to the dictum that "the best chance of removal is the first."

CARCINOID TUMORS (ARGENTAFFINOMAS)

These are curious tumors of low-grade malignancy, which are believed to arise from the Kultchitsky cells of the gastrointestinal glands. Like the normal Kultchitsky cells, the cells of carcinoid tumors show an affinity for silver salts, hence the name *argentaffinoma*. These cells are thought to be part of a system of migrating cells of neuroectodermal origin which are capable of secreting polypeptide hormones. This system, known as the APUD system, is further described on page 617. In one series of 54 carcinoid tumors, 32 arose in the appendix, 11 in the colon or rectum, 8 in the small intestine, one in the stomach and one in the duodenum; one was of unknown origin. Rarely, they originate outside the gastrointestinal tract, in the bronchi, biliary tree or pancreas (Baeza, 1969). Although these patients may be of any age, the lesion is most common in middle age. Carcinoid tumors of the appendix tend to affect a younger age group. The tumors are somewhat more common in females than in males.

Carcinoid tumors are, in general, rare. However, in the small intestine, *any* primary cancer is unusual and in this location the carcinoid tumor is the third most frequent cause of malignant disease. Adenocarcinomas and sarcomas (including lymphomas) of the small intestine are seen only somewhat more frequently (Brookes et al., 1968).

Morphology. Carcinoid tumors usually appear as discrete, firm, submucosal plaques or nodules, up to 5 cm. in diameter. Multiple lesions are seen in about 25 per cent of cases, particularly in the small intestine. Invasion of the underlying muscularis and serosa, with extension into the mesentery, is common. However, the overlying mucosa usually remains intact. On transection, the tissue is classically yellow-tan, although it may be gray-white and grossly indistinguishable from other types of neoplasm.

Histologically, carcinoid tumors are composed of nests, strands or masses of regular polygonal to cuboidal epithelial cells, with uniform oval, deeply chromatic and finely stippled nuclei. Only rarely is this monotonous uniformity broken by mitoses, giant cells or extreme anaplasia. In some instances, gland patterns are produced (Fig. 14–17). Within the cytoplasm are granules of yellow-brown lipochrome pigment, which produce the gross yellowish coloration. Silver impregnation techniques reveal a fine black granularity throughout the cytoplasm. The histologic pattern is faithfully reproduced in sites of metastases, principally the regional lymph nodes, liver, lungs and bones.

Clinical Course. The clinical significance of carcinoid tumors is threefold: (1) They may invade or metastasize but only rarely; (2) they occasionally produce partial or complete gastrointestinal obstruction; and (3) they may elaborate a variety of substances which give rise to a bizarre symptom complex known as the *carcinoid syndrome* and comprising paroxysmal flushing, cyanosis, diarrhea, bronchoconstriction and hypotension. There may also be endocardial thickening in the right side of the heart. Although it is true that many of these tumors, particularly those in the appendix, have been considered to be benign, it should be emphasized that the distinction between benign and malignant carcinoid tumors is very difficult to make on histologic grounds. Probably it is best to consider all as neoplasms of low-grade malignancy. Still, carcinoid tumors of the appendix and rectum rarely metastasize, whereas those of the small intestine frequently do (Morton, 1970–71).

The pathogenesis of the carcinoid syndrome has not been completely elucidated. At one time it was thought to be attributable to release by these tumors of *serotonin* (5-hydroxytryptamine). Only very large lesions or those with multiple metastases were thought to elaborate sufficient serotonin to produce the clinical syndrome. However, when administered alone, serotonin does not reproduce the carcinoid attack, and it is therefore likely that other substances are involved in triggering these paroxysms. One such substance is referred to as VIP (vasoactive intestinal peptide) (Pearse, 1974). In addition to flushing, cyanosis, diarrhea, wheezing and hypotension, patients with the carcinoid syndrome often have heart murmurs from fibrous deformities of the right-sided valves. Possibly the vasomotor activity of the substances elaborated by carcinoid tumors leads to proliferation of fibrous tissue within the heart. Because the lungs are rich in the monoamine oxidases which inactivate these products, the left side of the heart is protected.

It should not be supposed that the carcinoid

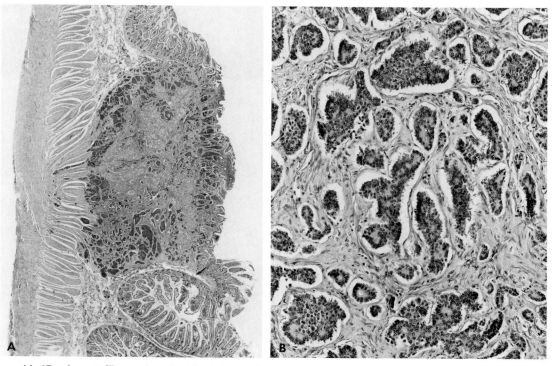

Figure 14–17. Argentaffinoma (carcinoid) of the small intestine. *A,* A low power view of the small lesion. It has expanded into the submucosa and nests of cells are seen penetrating the muscularis. *B,* High power detail indicates the uniformity in size of the cells. Some gland patterns are evident.

syndrome, for all its diagnostic importance, is present in all patients with carcinoid tumors. Indeed, in most cases, these lesions are asymptomatic and come to attention only incidentally. In other cases, they may provoke symptoms of acute appendicitis or lead to partial or complete obstruction of the bowel lumen. The elaboration of serotonin by carcinoid tumors leads to elevated amounts of its excretory breakdown product, *5-hydroxyindole-acetic acid* (5-HIAA), in the urine and provides a valuable diagnostic laboratory test.

MUCOCELE OF THE APPENDIX

Mucocele of the appendix, which may occur in either a benign or a malignant form, refers to the progressive cystic dilatation of the distal appendix by accumulated mucinous material. The benign disease is about 10 times more common than the malignant form.

A **benign mucocele** is caused by obstruction of the proximal appendix, usually by inflammatory scarring or fecaliths. Sterile mucus then accumulates in the distal portion, producing a spherical or fusiform dilatation, sometimes up to 15 cm. in diameter, although usually it is much smaller. The wall is thinned and attenuated, so that the cyst may appear translucent; the contents are clear mucin. The mucosa is atrophied, smooth and shiny, and the wall may consist only of fibrous tissue and attenuated smooth muscle. Only rarely do these lesions rupture and, because usually they are sterile, the resultant inflammatory reaction is mild and localized.

A **malignant mucocele** results from a primary **mucinous cystadenocarcinoma** of the appendix. Similar tumors arise in the ovary, where they are more common (see p. 576 for a more detailed discussion). Suffice it to say here that the appendix becomes progressively distended by proliferating tumor cells, which secrete copious amounts of mucinous material. In about 25 per cent of these cases, the mucocele ruptures, and the surfaces of the peritoneum become seeded with mucus secreting tumor cells. The peritoneal cavity may thus become virtually filled with mucinous, jelly-like material, constituting the entity termed **pseudomyxoma peritonei.** Interestingly, the tumor cells implanted on the peritoneal surfaces rarely invade the underlying wall or viscera.

REFERENCES

Adams, W. R., et al.: Some morphologic characteristics of Whipple's disease. Am. J. Path., *42*:415, 1963.
Adler, R.: Collective review: Hiatal hernia and esophagitis. Inter. Abstr. Surg., *116*:1, 1963*a.*
Adler, R. H.: The lower esophagus lined by columnar

epithelium. Its association with hiatal hernia, ulcer, stricture, and tumor. J. Thorac. Cardiov. Surg., 45:13, 1963b.

Alvarez, A. F., and Colbert, J. G.: Lye stricture of the esophagus complicated by carcinoma. Canad. J. Surg., 6:470, 1963.

Asquith, P., et al.: Serum immunoglobulins in adult celiac disease. Lancet, 2:129, 1969.

Badley, B. W. D., et al.: Intraluminal bile-salt deficiency in the pathogenesis of steatorrhea. Lancet, 2:400, 1969.

Baeza, M. G.: Carcinoid tumors of the gastrointestinal tract. Dis. Colon Rectum, 12:147, 1969.

Baker, J. W., and Jones, H. W.: The malignant potentiality of the colorectal polyp constitutes a major consideration in treatment. In Ingelfinger, F., Relman, A., and Finland, M. (eds.): Controversy in Internal Medicine. Philadelphia, W. B. Saunders Co., 1966, p. 207.

Baklien, K., and Brandtzaeg, P.: Immunohistochemical localization of complement in intestinal mucosa. Lancet, 2:1087, 1974.

Balasegaram, M.: Haematemesis and melaena: A review of 326 cases. Med. J. Austral., 1:485, 1968.

Ballard, J., and Shiner, M.: Evidence of cytotoxicity in ulcerative colitis from immunofluorescent staining of the rectal mucosa. Lancet, 1:1014, 1974.

Barnes, B. A., et al.: Treatment of appendicitis at the Massachusetts General Hospital, 1937–1959. J.A.M.A., 180:122, 1962.

Bolton, P. M., et al.: Aetiology of Crohn's disease. Lancet, 2:951, 1974.

Boyd, J., et al.: The epidemiology of gastrointestinal cancer with special reference to causation. Gut, 5:196, 1964.

Brookes, V. S., et al.: Malignant lesions of the small intestine. Brit. J. Surg., 55:405, 1968.

Burkitt, D. P.: Some diseases characteristic of modern Western civilization. Brit. Med. J., 1:274, 1973.

Calkins, W. G.: Premalignant gastrointestinal lesions. Geriatrics, 19:707, 1964.

Carlson, A. J., and Hoelzel, F.: Relation of diet to diverticulosis of the colon in rats. Gastroenterology, 12:108, 1949.

Castleman, B., and Krickstein, H.: Carcinoma arising in adenomatous polyps of the colon is greatly exaggerated. In Ingelfinger, F., Relman, A., and Finland, M. (eds.): Controversy in Internal Medicine. Philadelphia, W. B. Saunders Co., 1966, p. 220.

Cave, D. R., et al.: Further animal evidence of a transmissable agent in Crohn's disease. Lancet, 2:1119, 1973.

Chandler, G. N.: Bleeding from the upper gastrointestinal tract. Brit. Med. J., 4:723, 1967.

Cheli, R., et al.: A clinical and statistical follow-up of atrophic gastritis. Am. J. Dig. Dis., 18:1061, 1973.

Cohen, S., and Harris, L. D.: Does hiatus hernia affect competence of the gastroesophageal sphincter? New Eng. J. Med., 284:1053, 1971.

Cohen, S., et al.: Role of gastrin supersensitivity in the pathogenesis of lower esophageal sphincter hypertension in achalasia. J. Clin. Invest., 50:1241, 1971.

Cole, J. W.: Carcinogens and carcinogenesis of the colon. Hosp. Prac., September, 1973, p. 123.

Croft, D. N.: Gastritis. Brit. Med. J., 4:164, 1967.

Czaja, A. J.: Acute gastroduodenal disease after thermal injury. New Eng. J. Med., 291:925, 1974.

Dawson, J. L.: Short notes of rare or obscure cases. Adenocarcinoma of the middle oesophagus arising in an oesophagus lined by gastric (parietal) epithelium. Brit. J. Surg., 51:940, 1964.

Dawson, J. L.: Carcinoma of the stomach. Brit. Med. J., 4:533, 1967.

DeDombal, F., et al.: Aetiology of ulcerative colitis. I. A review of past and present hypotheses. Gut, 10:270, 1969.

Devroede, G. J., et al.: Cancer risk and life expectancy of

children with ulcerative colitis. New Eng. J. Med. 285:17, 1971.

Dukes, C. E.: The classification of cancer of the rectum. J. Path. Bact., 35:323, 1932.

Dukes, C. E., and Bussey, H. J. P.: The spread of rectal cancer and its effect on prognosis. Brit. J. Cancer, 12:309, 1958.

Dyer, N. H., and Pridie, R. B.: Incidence of hiatus hernia in asymptomatic subjects. Gut, 9:696, 1968.

Eade, M. N., and Brooke, B. N.: Portal bacteremia in cases of ulcerative colitis submitted to colectomy. Lancet, 1:1008, 1969.

Edgington, T. S., et al.: Association of an isomeric species of carcinoembryonic antigen with neoplasia of the gastrointestinal tract. New Eng. J. Med., 293:103, 1975.

Editorial: Salivary gland tumours. Lancet, 1:655, 1969a.

Editorial: Asymptomatic hiatus hernia. Lancet, 1:870, 1969b.

Editorial: Crohn's disease. Brit. Med. J., 2:65, 1970a.

Editorial: Diverticular disease. Brit. Med. J., 2:126, 1970b.

Editorial: Susceptibility to aspirin bleeding. Brit. Med. J., 2:436, 1970c.

Editorial: Ulcerative colitis and Crohn's disease. Lancet, 1:1326, 1970d.

Editorial: Oesophageal cancer on the Caspian Littoral. Lancet, 2:1365, 1973.

Editorial: Beware of the ox. Lancet, 1:791, 1974a.

Editorial: The coeliac philosophy. Lancet, 2:501, 1974b.

Editorial: Leads in oesophageal cancer. Lancet, 2:504, 1974c.

Editorial: Beyond the examining finger. Lancet, 2:1185, 1974d.

Eiseman, B., and Heyman, R. L.: Current concepts. Stress ulcers—a continuing challenge. New Eng. J. Med., 282:372, 1970.

Ferguson, A., et al.: Cell-mediated immunity to gliadin within the small-intestinal mucosa in coeliac disease. Lancet, 1:895, 1975.

Fialkow, P. J.: The origin and development of human tumors studied with cell markers. New Eng. J. Med., 291:26, 1974.

Friedman, G. D., et al.: Cigarettes, alcohol, coffee and peptic ulcer. New Eng. J. Med., 290:469, 1974.

Ganguli, P. C., et al.: Antral-gastrin-cell hyperplasia in peptic-ulcer disease. Lancet, 1:583, 1974.

Gold, P., and Freedman, S. O.: Specific antigenic similarity between malignant adult and normal fetal tissues of the human digestive system. J. Clin. Invest., 44:1051, 1965.

Goyal, R. K., et al.: Lower esophageal ring. New Eng. J. Med., 282:1298, 1355, 1970.

Hansen, H. J., et al.: Carcinoembryonic antigen (CEA) assay. Hum. Pathol., 5:139, 1974.

Hawkins, C. F.: Disease of the digestive system. Dysphagia. Brit. Med. J., 4:663, 1967.

Helwig, E. B.: Evolution of adenomas of the large intestine and their relation to carcinoma. Surg. Gynec. Obstet., 84:36, 1947.

Hill, M. J., and Aries, V. C.: Faecal steroid composition and its relationship to cancer of the large bowel. J. Pathol., 104:129, 1971.

Hill, M. J., et al.: Bacteria and aetiology of cancer of large bowel. Lancet, 1:95, 1971.

Ingelfinger, F. J., and Kramer, P.: Dysphagia produced by a contractile ring in the lower esophagus. Gastroenterology, 23:419, 1953.

Ingelfinger, F. J., et al. (eds.): Controversy in Internal Medicine. Philadelphia, W. B. Saunders Co., 1966, p. 207.

Irvine, W. J., et al.: Natural history of autoimmune achlorhydric atrophic gastritis. Lancet, 2:482, 1974.

Isokoski, M., et al.: Parietal cell and intrinsic factor antibodies in a Finnish rural population sample. Scand. J. Gastroent., 4:521, 1969.

Jalan, K. N., et al.: Pseudopolyposis in ulcerative colitis. Lancet, 2:555, 1969.

Mach, J. P., et al.: Detection of recurrence of large-bowel carcinoma by radioimmunoassay of circulating carcinoembryonic antigen (C.E.A.). Lancet, 2:535, 1974.

Mann, J. G., et al.: The subtle and variable clinical expression of gluten-induced enteropathy. Am. J. Med., 48:357, 1970.

Maxwell, J. D., et al.: Lymphocytes in Whipple's disease. Lancet, 1:887, 1968.

McDevitt, H. O., and Bodmer, W. F.: Immune-response genes and disease. Lancet, 1:1269, 1974.

McGuigan, J. E., and Trudeau, W. L.: Differences in rates of gastrin release in normal persons and patients with duodenal-ulcer disease. New Eng. J. Med., 288:64, 1973.

McIver, M. A.: Acute intestinal obstruction. Am. J. Surg., 19:163, 1933.

Mendeloff, A. I., et al.: Symposium: Gastrointestinal bleeding. Current Med. Dig., 33:1527, 1966.

Menguy, R.: Pathophysiology of peptic ulcer. Am. J. Surg., 120:282, 1970.

Merigan, T. C., et al.: Gastrointestinal bleeding with cirrhosis. New Eng. J. Med., 263:579, 1960.

Miller, D. S., et al.: Changing patterns in epidemiology of Crohn's disease. Lancet, 2:691, 1974.

Mitchell, D. N., et al.: The Kveim test in Crohn's disease. Lancet, 2:571, 1969.

Mitchell, D. N., and Rees, R. J. W.: Agent transmissible from Crohn's disease. Lancet, 2:168, 1970.

Moertel, C. G., and Foss, E. L.: Multicentric carcinomas of the oral cavity. Surg. Gynec. Obstet., 106:652, 1958.

Moertel, C. G., et al.: Multiple carcinomas of the large intestine: a review of the literature and a study of 261 cases. Gastroenterology, 34:85, 1958.

Morson, B. C.: The muscle abnormality in diverticular disease of the sigmoid colon. Brit. J. Radiol., 36:385, 1963.

Morton, J.: Alimentary tract cancer. In Rubin, P. (ed.): Clinical Oncology for Medical Students and Physicians. 3rd ed. Rochester, N.Y., American Cancer Society, 1970–71, p. 115.

Orloff, M. J., et al.: The UCLA interdepartmental conference. The complications of cirrhosis of the liver. Ann. Int. Med., 66:165, 1967.

Painter, N. S.: Diverticular disease of the colon. Lancet, 2:586, 1969.

Palmer, E. D.: The hiatus hernia-esophagitis-esophageal stricture complex. Twenty year prospective study. Am. J. Med., 44:566, 1968.

Pearse, A. G. E.: The APUD cell concept and its implications in pathology. Pathol. Annu., 9:27, 1974.

Perlmann, P., and Broberger, O.: Lower gastrointestinal system. In Miescher, P., and Mueller-Eberhard, H. (eds.): Textbook of Immunopathology. New York, Grune and Stratton, 1968, p. 551.

Ramachandar, K., et al.: B-lymphocytes in inflammatory bowel disease. Lancet, 2:45, 1974.

Reeder, D. D., et al.: Effect of food on serum gastrin concentrations in duodenal ulcer and control of patients. Surg. Forum, 21:290, 1970.

Renstrup, G., et al.: Effect of chronic mechanical irritation on chemically induced carcinogenesis in the hamster cheek pouch. J.A.D.A., 30:770, 1962.

Robinson, D. C., et al.: Incidence of small intestinal mucosal abnormalities and of clinical coeliac disease in the relatives of children with coeliac disease. Gut, 12:789, 1971.

Rose, M. S., et al.: Intrinsic-factor antibodies in absence of pernicious anemia. Lancet, 2:9, 1970.

Salter, R. H.: Lower esophageal sphincter. Lancet, 1:347, 1974.

Schatzki, R., and Gary, J. E.: The lower esophageal ring. Am. J. Roentgenol., 75:246, 1956.

Silen, W.: Editorial—potpourri dissected. New Eng. J. Med., 291:974, 1974.

Siurala, M., et al.: Studies of patients with atrophic gastritis: a 10–15 year follow-up. Scand. J. Gastroent., 1:40, 1966.

Stemmer, E. A., and Adams, W. E.: The incidence of carcinoma at the esophagogastric junction in short esophagus. Arch. Surg., 81:771, 1960.

Strickland, R. G., and Mackay, I. R.: A reappraisal of the nature and significance of chronic atrophic gastritis. Dig. Dis., 18:426, 1973.

Trier, J. S., et al.: Whipple's disease: Light and electron microscopic correlation of jejunal mucosal histology with antibiotic treatment and clinical status. Gastroenterology, 48:684, 1965.

Valman, H. B., et al.: Lesions associated with gastroduodenal haemorrhage, in relation to aspirin intakes. Brit. Med. J., 4:661, 1968.

Weedon, D. D., et al.: Crohn's disease and cancer. New Eng. J. Med., 289:1099, 1973.

Wesdorp, R. I. C., and Fischer, J. E.: Plasma-gastrin and acid secretion in patients with peptic ulceration. Lancet, 2:857, 1974.

Whipple, G. H.: A hitherto undescribed disease characterized anatomically by deposits of fat and fatty acids in the intestinal and mesenteric lymphatic tissues. Bull. Johns Hopkins Hosp., 18:382, 1907.

Whittaker, L. D., and Pemberton, J. deJ.: Mesenteric vascular occlusion. J.A.M.A., 111:21, 1938.

Wood, D.: TNM System of Classification for Gastrointestinal Cancer. Proceedings of the Sixth National Cancer Conference. Philadelphia, J. B. Lippincott, 1968.

Wynder, E. L., and Bross, I. J.: A study of etiological factors in cancer of the esophagus. Cancer, 14:389, 1961.

Wynder, E. L., et al.: An epidemiological investigation of gastric cancer. Cancer, 16:1461, 1963.

Yeomans, N. D.: Pathogenesis of coeliac sprue. Lancet, 2:843, 1974.

Zollinger, R. M., and Nick, W. V.: Upper gastrointestinal tract hemorrhage. J.A.M.A., 212:2251, 1970.

CHAPTER 15

The Hepatobiliary System and the Pancreas

It is reasonable to consider the liver, biliary tract and pancreas together because of their anatomic proximity, closely interrelated functions and the similarity of the symptom complexes induced by many of their disorders. The liver dominates this group, because it is literally the crossroads of the body. The portal and systemic circulations join here to drain through a common venous outflow. The intermediary metabolism of all foodstuffs occurs here. It is the major locus of synthetic, catabolic and detoxifying activities in the body. Moreover, the liver is crucial in the excretion of heme pigments, and through its Kupffer cells it participates in the immune response. Since it occupies this pivotal role, it is fortunate that the liver has an enormous reserve capacity. It has been shown in the experimental animal that removal of 80 to 90 per cent of the hepatic parenchyma is still compatible with normal liver function. Hepatic disease therefore does not become manifest until it produces widespread damage and, conversely, focal lesions may remain silent even though they are productive of considerable hepatic damage. Diffuse diseases of the liver

may eventually deplete the functional reserve. When such happens, they often cause jaundice and sometimes liver failure. Since these two syndromes are common to so many hepatic disorders, they will be considered first.

JAUNDICE

Jaundice or *icterus* comprises a yellow discoloration of the skin and sclerae produced by accumulations of bilirubin in the tissues and interstitial fluids. Under optimal conditions (daylight), it usually becomes visible when the hyperbilirubinemia exceeds 2 to 3 mg. per 100 ml. of serum. The intensity of the jaundice depends on many factors, including the level of hyperbilirubinemia, the rate of diffusion of bilirubin from the plasma into the interstitial fluid and the binding of this pigment in the tissues.

A consideration of the mechanisms of jaundice involves an understanding of the formation, transportation, metabolism and excretion of bilirubin. Our review can be only brief, but the subject has been well presented by others (Gartner and Arias, 1969; Robinson, 1968). Suffice it to say here that approximately 85 per cent of the bilirubin is derived from the breakdown of red cells that have lived their life span (100 to 120 days), with the conversion of the heme pigment by heme oxygenase to biliverdin and thence to bilirubin. This conversion occurs within reticuloendothelial cells, principally in the spleen. A small amount of bilirubin (15 per cent), often called "shunt bilirubin," is formed directly in the bone marrow, mostly as a by-product of hemoglobin synthesis, and some is formed in the liver from the rapid turnover of hemoproteins such as the cytochromes and catalases (Robinson et al., 1966). Whatever its origin, bilirubin formed outside the liver is bound principally to albumin and transported via the blood to the liver. At this point bilirubin is not soluble in water, nor can the albumin-bilirubin complex be filtered through the glomeruli. The significance of this in distinguishing the various forms of jaundice will become apparent later. In some mysterious fashion the albumin-bilirubin complex dissociates at the plasma membrane of the hepatocyte, and the bilirubin enters the liver cell where it is conjugated, chiefly to glucuronide (perhaps some to sulfate) through the intermediation of glucuronyl transferase. In contrast to unconjugated bilirubin, conjugated bilirubin is water soluble and in certain circumstances may be excreted in the urine. In normal circumstances, however, it is entirely secreted into the biliary canaliculi. When the bile reaches the duodenum, the diglucuronide is split, and the bilirubin is converted by bacterial action in the small intestine to urobilinogen. Much of this urobilinogen is reabsorbed in the distal small intestine, some to be recaptured by the liver *(enterohepatic circulation)* and some to be excreted by the kidneys *(urinary urobilinogen).* The nonabsorbed fraction of urobilinogen is further transformed in the gut to *urobilin (stercobilin)* and excreted with the feces.

From this brief review, it can be seen that hyperbilirubinemia differs depending on whether the bilirubin is unconjugated or conjugated. With *unconjugated hyperbilirubinemia,* there is *no bilirubin in the urine* (acholuric jaundice); however, as the liver conjugates and secretes the increased amounts of bilirubin delivered to it, more urobilinogen is formed in the gut, and this is reflected in *increased urinary urobilinogen.* With *conjugated hyperbilirubinemia,* on the other hand, *bilirubin appears in the urine.* Since the disorder responsible for the backup of conjugated bilirubin into the blood implies some derangement in its excretion into the gut, *urinary urobilinogen is usually decreased.* These two forms of hyperbilirubinemia can somewhat more laboriously be distinguished by specific serum tests. Without going into detail, it should be noted that the commonly used van den Bergh test shows a *direct* reaction with conjugated bilirubin and an *indirect* reaction with the unconjugated form. The differences between unconjugated and conjugated hyperbilirubinemia not only are of diagnostic significance, but have direct clinical implications as well. Unconjugated bilirubin is toxic to tissues, particularly nerve tissues, and when high levels are reached, this pigment may cross the blood-brain barrier, especially in the newborn, producing serious brain damage, known as *kernicterus.* Thus, the level of the bilirubin is a major concern in hemolytic disease in the newborn (resulting usually from Rh or ABO incompatibility between mother and child). Conjugated bilirubin, in contrast, is nontoxic.

Having reviewed bilirubin metabolism and presented the types of jaundice in a general way, we turn now to the specific pathophysiologic mechanisms which cause jaundice. *The critical steps in bilirubin metabolism involve (1) its rate of production, (2) its uptake in the liver cells, (3) its conjugation with glucuronic acid, and (4) its secretion into the bile canaliculi and biliary tract.* The pathophysiology of hyperbilirubinemia can be considered, then, under these four headings.

1. *Excess production of bilirubin.* Hemolytic disease (an increased rate of red cell destruction) is the most common cause of excessive bilirubin production. The resultant jaundice is called *hemolytic jaundice.* The hyperbilirubinemia (predominantly unconjugated) rarely exceeds 5 mg. per 100 ml., however active the hemolysis may be, because the normal liver is capable of handling most of the overload. Any damage to the liver, such as intercurrent disease or significant hypoxia, attendant, for example, on the hemolytic process, damages hepatocytes and leads to more severe jaundice, often with a conjugated component. Much less frequently, unconjugated hyperbilirubinemia is encountered in certain forms of essentially nonhemolytic anemia, such as pernicious anemia. Here it is presumed to result from direct synthesis of shunt bilirubin in the bone marrow. On occasion, patients who have had a pulmonary hemorrhage or infarction, or massive hemorrhage in any site in the body, may become icteric, presumably as a result of resorption of the heme pigment of the destroyed red cells. As may be surmised, in all forms of jaundice from excessive production of bilirubin, the urine urobilinogen levels rise, but the patient is acholuric.

2. *Reduced hepatic uptake of bilirubin.* The

precise mechanism of transfer of bilirubin from the plasma to the hepatocyte is poorly understood. All that is clear is that the albumin is dissociated at the plasma membrane and the bilirubin then transferred to acceptor proteins within the hepatocyte. Abnormalities of uptake are principally encountered in some cases of the genetic disorder called *Gilbert's disease* (p. 534). As would be expected, the hyperbilirubinemia results from the accumulation of unconjugated bilirubin and so the urine is acholuric. Inadequate uptake may also be encountered in the recovery phase of viral hepatitis (p. 514).

3. *Impaired conjugation of bilirubin.* Bilirubin is conjugated in or on the membranes of the smooth endoplasmic reticulum of the hepatocytes, through the action of glucuronyl transferase. Two molecules of glucuronic acid derived from uridine diphosphate glucuronic acid are linked to one molecule of bilirubin to produce the bilirubin diglucuronide. Although the transferase is present in other tissues, all or virtually all conjugation occurs in the liver. The *Crigler-Najjar syndrome* is a hereditary disease of man characterized by a complete deficiency of glucuronyl transferase in the liver. These patients have unconjugated hyperbilirubinemia. The Gunn rat, which has a similar defect, provides an excellent laboratory model for study. In some cases of Gilbert's disease, a partial deficiency of glucuronyl transferase is present. *Neonatal jaundice* may, in some part, be due to immaturity of the hepatic conjugating system during the early days of life.

4. *Impaired excretion of conjugated bilirubin (cholestasis).* The secretion or excretion of conjugated bilirubin may be impaired at the level of the liver cell membrane, within the bile canaliculi or at any level within the excretory duct system. Depending on the level of the derangement, disorders of bilirubin secretion or excretion are usually divided into intrahepatic and posthepatic causes of cholestasis. The *Dubin-Johnson* and *Rotor syndromes* are hereditary disorders in which the defect appears to reside in the transfer of bilirubin and other organic anions across the hepatocyte membrane. Various *drugs*, such as anabolic steroids, estrogens and certain contraceptive agents, reduce the capacity of the liver to secrete organic anions and thus may cause intrahepatic cholestasis. Acute viral infection of the liver *(viral hepatitis)* and the various *cirrhoses* may act at several levels. Damage to the liver cell may impair the conjugating or secretory mechanisms, or the swelling and disorganization of liver cells can compress and block the canaliculi or cholangioles. All these disorders are intrahepatic causes of cholestasis.

Posthepatic cholestasis results from obstruction to the extrahepatic bile ducts. Frequent causes include *gallstones* impacted in the common or main hepatic ducts, and *carcinoma* of the extrahepatic bile ducts, ampulla of Vater or head of the pancreas (which may then impinge on the common bile duct). Less common causes for such obstruction exist. Acute infections within the biliary tract *(cholangitis)* may fill the lumina with pus. In the newborn or infant, atresia or agenesis of the extrahepatic bile ducts will lead to posthepatic obstruction. Obviously, strategically localized inflammatory or neoplastic lesions near the porta hepatis may block the major hepatic ducts by enlargement of impinging lymph nodes. Tumors or inflammatory lesions strategically located at the outflow of the hepatic ducts behave as extrahepatic obstructions.

When the blockage to the bile ducts is complete, bile disappears from the stools altogether (acholic stools). Obviously, urinary urobilinogen also disappears. The characteristic brown color of the stools is lost, and they are instead gray and putty-like. Since bile is necessary for the absorption of fats from the small intestine, there is malabsorption of fats and fat-soluble vitamins and minerals. Impaired absorption of vitamin K induces hypoprothrombinemia and thus predisposes to hemorrhage — a particular threat in those who may require surgery, for example, on the biliary tract. In all forms of obstructive jaundice, whether intrahepatic or posthepatic, bile salts as well as bilirubin may be regurgitated into the blood. These produce intense itching, a particularly agonizing symptom to patients with obstructive lesions. Cholestasis is also associated with significant elevations of plasma cholesterol levels and, indeed, these patients may develop localized accumulations of lipophages laden with cholesterol in the skin (xanthomas). *Although cholestasis initially causes fairly pure conjugated hyperbilirubinemia, eventually the retained bile damages the liver cell and reduces its capacity to take up unconjugated bilirubin.* Thus, in most cases of obstructive jaundice, there is eventually some added component of unconjugated hyperbilirubinemia.

A recapitulation of some of these patterns of jaundice is provided in Table 15-1. Overall, the most frequent causes of jaundice in adults are viral hepatitis, cirrhosis, posthepatic biliary obstruction and drug reactions.

HEPATIC FAILURE

The ultimate consequence of many liver diseases is hepatic failure. In one series of 60 cases, *cirrhosis* was the most common cause of

TABLE 15-1. CLINICAL CORRELATIONS OF HYPERBILIRUBINEMIA

POSTULATED MAJOR MECHANISM	CLINICAL SYNDROME	FORM OF BILIRUBIN*	BILE IN URINE	UROBILINOGEN IN URINE
Excessive production: Increased red cell breakdown	Hemolytic disorders	Almost all unconjugated	0	Increased
Direct production in marrow	Shunt bilirubin in hematologic disorders	Almost all unconjugated	0	Increased
Impaired uptake by hepatocyte	Gilbert's syndrome (some cases)	Almost all unconjugated	0	Normal
	? Some forms of drug induced cholestasis	Almost all unconjugated	0	?
Glucuronide conjugation defect	Crigler-Najjar syndrome	Almost all unconjugated	0	Decreased
	Immaturity of liver (jaundice of newborn)	Almost all unconjugated	0	Variable
	Gilbert's syndrome (some cases)	Almost all unconjugated	0	Variable
	? Some forms of drug induced cholestasis	Almost all unconjugated	?	?
Impaired secretion or transport into bile sinusoids (intrahepatic obstruction)	? Dubin-Johnson and Rotor syndromes	60 to 80% unconj.; 20 to 40% unconj.	+	Normal
	Some forms of drug induced cholestasis	20 to 40% unconj.	+	Usually decreased
	Hepatitis	20 to 40% unconj.	+	Usually decreased
	Cirrhosis	20 to 40% unconj.	+	Usually decreased
Posthepatic obstruction	Gallstones, tumors, etc.	20 to 40% unconj.	+	Low to 0

*Unconjugated forms give indirect van den Bergh test results; conjugated forms give direct van den Bergh test results.

hepatic failure, followed in order by *viral hepatitis* and *chemical and drug injury* (Adams and Foley, 1953). As may be suspected, the liver is diffusely involved in these conditions. Focal lesions, as was mentioned earlier, rarely produce hepatic failure, and so it is uncommon with primary or metastatic tumors, focal infections, localized infarcts and trauma to the liver. With diffuse liver disease, the onset of hepatic failure develops in one of several ways. The enormous functional reserve of the liver may be insidiously eroded, it may be depleted in several discrete waves or it may be suddenly and totally overwhelmed. Not infrequently, hepatic failure may be triggered by intercurrent disease, as for example a massive hemorrhage, which imposes new stresses on a marginally compensated liver. *Liver failure manifests itself in a host of clinical dysfunctions.* Disturbance of any one of the hundreds of liver functions may dominate the symptom complex. Certain features are, however, usual.

As may be deduced, *jaundice is an almost invariable finding.* The most common disorders cause increased conjugated bilirubin, but the unconjugated form may also accumulate.

Hepatic failure is frequently characterized by disturbances of consciousness, often termed *metabolic encephalopathy*, ranging from mild lethargy to coma. Personality changes and a variety of neurologic deficits may appear. *Most characteristic is a flapping tremor of the outstretched hands, usually called a "liver flap" but more sedately designated* asterixis. Many investigators relate the metabolic encephalopathy to the elevated blood levels of ammonia which result from the inability of the liver to convert ammonia to urea. However, the issue is controversial and by no means settled. Very few anatomic changes have been identified in the brain in this syndrome. The most noticeable is an increase in the number of astrocytes, principally in the cerebral cortex, thalamus, pontine nuclei, ventricular nuclei and substantia nigra. Alterations in the neurons themselves have not been identified, and it can only be assumed that the glial changes reflect some as yet undetected, more significant CNS change.

Altered hepatic metabolism and excretion

of hormones give rise to a variety of endocrine abnormalities. Hypogonadism and gynecomastia clearly result from imbalances in the androgen-estrogen levels. Palmar erythema (a reflection of local vasodilatation) and "spider" angiomas of the skin have also been attributed to hyperestrinism, but with little proof. The angiomas comprise a central, pulsating, dilated arteriole, from which small vessels radiate.

A characteristic sweet-sour pungent odor known as *fetor hepaticus* has been described in hepatic failure. The odor is also detectable in the urine. The substance or substances responsible for such an odor have not been identified but are thought to be related to the production of mercaptans.

Peptic ulceration is more common in patients with hepatic insufficiency or failure than in the normal population. The association is poorly understood, but it has been attributed to faulty metabolism of either histamine or gastrin.

Acute renal failure is also encountered in some instances of hepatic disease *(the hepatorenal syndrome)*. Strangely, despite the profound functional disturbance, no morphologic changes are apparent in the kidneys. This mysterious disorder was discussed on page 448. The development of the hepatorenal syndrome indicates a very poor prognosis.

A host of other nutritional and metabolic changes occur, including weight loss, muscle wasting and hypoglycemia (presumed to result from inadequate stores of liver glycogen) or, rarely, transient hyperglycemia (from loss of liver cell uptake of blood glucose). Abnormalities in triglyceride metabolism are also encountered. Major synthetic pathways, such as the formation of plasma proteins, including principally albumin, globulin, and prothrombin, are slowed or halted. Hypoprothrombinemia may contribute to a bleeding diathesis in these patients. A hemolytic anemia is also associated with severe liver disease. This is thought to be due to some abnormality in the plasma of patients with liver disease which results in the accumulation of free cholesterol in the cell membranes of the red blood cells. The red blood cells then assume an abnormal configuration *(spur cells)* and undergo hemolysis (Shohet, 1974). As we shall see, when liver failure is accompanied by portal hypertension, the tendency toward hemolysis is further exacerbated by hypersplenism.

The widely used liver function tests represent methods of evaluating some of the more important functions of the liver. Total serum proteins, albumin-globulin ratio and prothrombin level all focus on protein synthetic capacities. The bromsulphalein excretion test assays the uptake of the dye from the blood, its conjugation and then its excretion by the liver cell—a sensitive index of general hepatocyte function. Cephalin flocculation and thymol turbidity are used as additional indicators of hepatocyte injury, but the precise hepatic derangement evaluated by these latter tests is uncertain.

Hepatic insufficiency and failure is often, but not always, irreversible. The hepatocyte is capable of regeneration. If the intercurrent stress can be brought under control or the liver function supported by palliative means, the injured liver may once again be able to cope. In accord with this reasoning, it has been shown that exchange transfusions may, presumably by lowering blood levels of unknown toxic substances, effect remarkable improvement in patients with hepatic failure and, indeed, start the patient on the road to recovery (Berger et al., 1966). Unfortunately, however, severe liver failure more often leads to death.

MAJOR HEPATOBILIARY AND PANCREATIC CLINICAL SYNDROMES

Although hepatobiliary and pancreatic disease may become manifest in any of a bewildering array of ways, certain syndromes are repetitive and embrace the great preponderance of clinical problems. *The major diseases of these organs can therefore reasonably be discussed under the following symptom complexes: (1) silent hepatomegaly, (2) acute malaise and fever, (3) signs and symptoms of portal hypertension, including principally ascites, (4) painless jaundice, (5) pain, usually localized in upper quadrants, and (6) metabolic abnormalities.* Many disorders have variable presentations, and one patient may have pain in the right upper quadrant, for example, while another patient may have as the dominant feature of the same disorder silent hepatomegaly. Some of this variation and overlap will be cited within the following sections. Nevertheless, the categories still have validity for the majority of patients.

SILENT HEPATOMEGALY

The most important cause for the appearance of hepatomegaly without other distinctive signs or symptoms is *fatty change*. Its causes were given earlier on page 18. It will be remembered from this discussion that severe fatty change is seen most often in the chronic alcoholic with or without deficiency of lipotropes, in diabetes mellitus, in obesity and in protein malnutrition, such as occurs in kwashiorkor. The organ may be increased to two or three times its normal weight. Despite the massive accumulations, liver function may be preserved. As was cited earlier, the alteration is reversible, and there is restoration of normal structure if, for example, the alcohol ingestion is stopped or the dietary deficiency is corrected.

Neoplasia in the liver, secondary or primary, is perhaps the second most common cause of marked hepatomegaly. Secondary neoplasia is far more frequent than primary. Since the liver filters the portal blood, it becomes a prime target for all metastatic cancers arising in the gastrointestinal tract. Metastatic tumors may also reach the liver through the systemic circulation and lymphatic drainage. Leukemic infiltrates and lymphomas frequently affect the liver. In most of these neoplastic involvements, widespread seeding results, and the multiple implants create an irregular nodularity of the surface and anterior margin, which is palpable clinically. Weights of over 3500 gm. are not uncommon. On occasion, tumor implantations impinge upon and obstruct a major excretory bile duct. If biliary drainage is impeded sufficiently, obstructive jaundice appears.

Amyloidosis (p. 202) and chronic passive congestion (p. 291) cause less extreme liver enlargements without functional impairment. Rarely, when the amyloid deposits are very heavy, hepatic insufficiency may develop.

PRIMARY TUMORS OF THE LIVER

Tumors of the liver are uncommon; some produce hepatomegaly. Benign tumors are usually incidental and rarely cause hepatomegaly. The most common forms are the *cavernous hemangioma* (1 to 4 cm. in diameter) and the *bile duct adenoma* (up to 3 cm. in diameter). Recently, an association has been reported between benign adenomas of the liver and the use of oral contraceptives. Unfortunately, while histologically benign, these tumors are life-threatening because of a tendency toward hemorrhage (Editorial, 1973c). Malignant tumors may cause rapidly progressive hepatic enlargement, which often is silent. In some, however, pain is a dominant symptom. These tumors may arise from the hepatocyte (*hepatocarcinoma*) or from bile duct epithelium (*cholangiocarcinoma*). Occasionally, mixed forms occur. The hepatocarcinomas, often loosely called *hepatomas*, account for 80 per cent of all primary cancers of the liver. In the United States, most develop in the sixth and seventh decades of life, but there is a small peak in the first decade (Patton and Horn, 1964). The peak in childhood raises the

possibility of some hereditary genetic predisposition, but this is not yet well documented. The sexes are affected about equally (Silverberg and Holleb, 1974).

Etiology and Pathogenesis. There are striking differences in the worldwide incidence of hepatic cancers, which may offer some clues as to their causation. In the United States they are relatively rare, causing fewer than 3 per cent of all deaths from cancer. In certain African and Asian countries, however, cancer of the liver is very much more frequent. Indeed, there are regions of Africa in which primary carcinoma of the liver represents 50 per cent of all cancers in men and 20 per cent of those in women. There are many hints that cancer of the liver is to a large extent an environmental disease. *Among the influences thought to contribute to its development, the most important are: (1) hepatocarcinogens in food, (2) cirrhosis of the liver, (3) persistent viral infection, and (4) parasitic infections of the liver.* Hepatocarcinogens in food include aflatoxins (a product of the mold *Aspergillus flavus*) and cycasin (found in cycad nuts). Their oncogenic potential has been clearly shown in animals. In tropical areas, the *Aspergillus* mold grows readily on most cereals, nuts and vegetables, providing high levels of aflatoxin. Cycad nuts are an item of the diet in these same locales. The possible causal relationship of these experimental hepatocarcinogens to liver cancer in man is certainly not established, but it is of great concern. The importance of cirrhosis as a precursor to hepatic cancer cannot be overestimated. In the United States, about 80 per cent of hepatocarcinomas and 30 per cent of cholangiocarcinomas arise in cirrhotic livers. Among the types of cirrhosis the two most frequently leading to cancer are *postnecrotic scarring (cirrhosis)* (p. 528) and *pigment cirrhosis* (p. 530). Pigment cirrhosis, which is associated with hemochromatosis, and liver cancer are very prevalent in the same areas of Africa. Evidence for persistent viral infection is the relatively high frequency of hepatitis B surface antigen (HBsAg) in the serum of patients with liver cancer, as opposed to that of the normal control population. This association is particularly marked in high incidence areas of the world. In Taiwan, for example, 80 per cent of patients with hepatocarcinoma have serum HBsAg, whereas only about 14 per cent of the control population carries the same antigen (Tong et al., 1971). Parasitism with the liver fluke (*Clonorchis sinensis*) and schistosomiasis are both known to increase the risk of liver cancer.

Morphology. Both the hepatocarcinoma and the cholangiocarcinoma may occur as: (1) a solitary massive tumor, (2) multiple nodules scattered throughout the liver, or (3) a diffuse infiltration of the entire hepatic substance. The hepatocarcinoma may be yellow-white on transection, but classically it has a green hue, imparted by bilirubin pigmentation elaborated by the neoplastic hepatic cells. The cholangiocarcinoma is white and unpigmented, because bile duct epithelium cannot form bile. Obstruction of a major duct by either form of cancer will cause jaundice in the affected non-neoplastic parenchyma. Histologically, the hepatoma presents a varied pattern, ranging from trabeculae and cords reminiscent of the normal hepatic cords to very anaplastic, rapidly growing lesions having huge tumor giant cells. As was mentioned, the hallmark of the hepatocarcinoma is the elaboration of bile by the tumor cells. The cholangiocarcinoma more often takes the form of an adenocarcinoma with an abundant fibrous stroma. Some secrete mucin.

Both forms of cancer tend to remain localized to the liver, but may metastasize to regional nodes, lungs, bone, adrenal glands and other tissues. These cancers (particularly the hepatocarcinoma) also have a strong propensity for invading blood vessels. Thus, this form of neoplasm may obstruct the hepatic vein, producing the **Budd-Chiari syndrome** (p. 533), or it may block the portal vein, producing portal hypertension.

Clinical Course. Although primary carcinomas in the liver may present as silent hepatomegaly, they are often encountered in patients with cirrhosis of the liver who already have symptoms of the underlying disorder. In these circumstances, rapid increase in liver size, sudden worsening of ascites, or the appearance of bloody ascites, fever and pain call attention to the development of a tumor. The fever is attributed to resorption of necrotic tumor products. Jaundice may be absent; if present, it is typically mild.

Within the past several years, a diagnostic test of considerable theoretic interest has been described. An embryonic protein, termed *alpha₁-fetoprotein*, has been found in the serum of about 75 per cent of patients with primary hepatocarcinoma. It does not appear with the cholangiocarcinoma (Abelev, 1968; Smith, 1970). This serum globulin is normally present in the fetus, but it disappears after birth. Presumably its synthesis is repressed in postnatal life. Its appearance in patients with hepatocarcinoma suggests that in the neoplastic transformation, the coding for this protein is derepressed. Occasionally, alpha₁-fetoprotein is found in patients with liver disease other than tumors. It is also found with multipotential tumors (gonadal cancers or teratocarcinomas) arising anywhere in the body. Nevertheless, its presence in high titer in the serum has value as a screening procedure, since elevations in liver diseases other than cancer tend to be low and transient (Kohn and Weaver, 1974). The prognosis with either hepatocarcinoma or cholangiocarcinoma is poor. Although cures have been accomplished by radical partial hepatectomy, they are rare, and overall five-year survival is only about 5 per cent (Silverberg and Holleb, 1974.)

ACUTE MALAISE AND FEVER

Malaise and fever are obviously nonspecific clinical findings, since they are evoked by a great many disorders throughout the body. Relative to the organs now being considered, malaise and fever are most characteristic of those diseases having prominent necrotizing and inflammatory components. Some disorders, such as acute pancreatic necrosis and acute cholecystitis, produce malaise and fever, but pain is the dominant characteristic. To be considered here are the diseases that are manifested principally only by malaise and fever; such pain as may be present is not a very significant part of the syndrome. Fitting this description are viral hepatitis in its various forms, massive liver necrosis, neonatal hepatitis and ascending cholangitis, with its frequent concomitant, liver abscesses.

VIRAL HEPATITIS

Viral hepatitis is one of the most exciting and rapidly unfolding subjects in medicine. Only an overview of present concepts can be given here, and it must be borne in mind that new information will inevitably be forthcoming and require revision of these concepts.

Two forms of viral hepatitis have long been recognized: *hepatitis A*, formerly called "infectious hepatitis," and *hepatitis B*, formerly called "serum hepatitis." Although there are some who maintain that these two forms of hepatitis are really simply different expressions of the same virus, the overwhelming weight of evidence favors their being caused by two distinct viruses. The evidence is both clinical and immunologic. Hepatitis A has a relatively short incubation period, averaging about a month, whereas hepatitis B is characterized by a much longer incubation period, usually from two to three months. The immunologic evidence for distinct viruses is even stronger. Although both hepatitis A and hepatitis B confer protection against reinfection with the same agent, neither protects against the other. Evidence suggests that hepatitis B represents about 40 per cent of acute viral hepatitis (Nielsen et al., 1974). Less is known about the relative frequency of hepatitis A. It should be emphasized at this point that not all cases of viral hepatitis can be neatly divided between these two forms. A significant number of patients with what appears to be viral hepatitis do not show evidence of either hepatitis A or B. In particular, parenterally transmitted hepatitis often may not be caused by either virus (Feinstone et al., 1975). Some have inferred from this the presence of an additional form, caused by a hepatitis C virus, but this is poorly established at this time (Prince et al., 1974).

Over the past decade it has become clear that exposure to the hepatitis viruses, particularly to hepatitis B, is followed by one of three types of expression, covering a broad spectrum:

1. Acute Hepatitis
   a. Overt, with jaundice, fever and malaise
   b. Subclinical (*anicteric hepatitis*)
2. Chronic Hepatitis
   a. Overt (*chronic active hepatitis*)
   b. Subclinical (*chronic persistent hepatitis*)
3. No Liver Damage
   a. Virus cleared, possibly from GI tract, without viremia
   b. *Carrier state* develops

These variations in expression will be considered more fully later. *Suffice it to say here that the term viral hepatitis is usually limited to the acute form of the disease, characterized by moderate liver injury and overt symptoms which generally clear over the span of weeks to months and rarely cause death.* Chronic hepatitis, to be discussed in a later section, may have several sources, including direct progression from acute hepatitis. Anicteric hepatitis is probably at least as important a source of chronic hepatitis as is overt acute hepatitis. Since our knowledge of hepatitis B is considerably more advanced than that of hepatitis A, we shall break loose from the constraints of the alphabet and discuss the causation of hepatitis B first. Following a brief presentation of the little we know of hepatitis A, we shall describe the morphology common to both.

Hepatitis B. Our new knowledge of hepatitis B began with the discovery by Blumberg and associates of an antigen, termed *Australia antigen*, which proved to be a specific marker of hepatitis B (Blumberg et al., 1965). Subsequently Dane and co-workers discovered the presence of a 42 nm. spheroidal particle *(Dane particle)* in the serum of hepatitis patients with Australia antigen (Dane et al., 1970). The Dane particle is separable into an outer coat, and an inner core, about 27 nm. in diameter. It is highly probable that the Dane particle is the complete hepatitis B virus, the outer coat is the protein envelope of the virus,

and the core the nucleocapsid. Excess outer coat, which is present in the serum as 20 nm. particles, proved identical to the Australia antigen, and is best termed the *hepatitis B surface antigen (HBsAg)*. Elongated aggregates of the surface antigen are also found in the serum of patients with hepatitis B. These appear as filamentous tubules, 20 nm. in diameter and up to 250 nm. in length. The core of the Dane particle is termed the *hepatitis B core antigen (HBcAg)*. It has icosahedral symmetry, supporting its identity as a viral nucleocapsid (Skikne and Talbot, 1974). The surface and core antigens are immunologically distinct, and evoke separate antibodies, termed *anti-HBs* and *anti-HBc*, respectively. Although HBsAg is almost certainly not the complete virus, then, it does imply the presence of virus (Gocke, 1974). HBsAg therefore remains an important marker for hepatitis B, since it is readily found in the serum of patients with this disease. It has also been identified in almost every other body fluid, including urine, semen and saliva—an embarrassment of riches. In contrast, the complete Dane particle is more difficult to find in serum, and the naked core is present almost exclusively in the nuclei of infected hepatocytes. As if all this were not enough, we must tell you (with trepidation) that it has become apparent that the HBsAg is itself antigenically heterogeneous. An "a" determinant is common to all HBsAg; two additional determinants, "w" and "r," reflect geographic variation, with "w" being more common in Western countries and "r" more frequent in the Orient. Of greater interest are the "d" and "y" determinants. Although they, too, show geographic variation, in general "d" is more common in drug addicts and in those with chronic disease (Editorial, 1973*a*). A new precipitating antigen termed "e" has recently been described, which seems to be associated with acute hepatitis that is destined to progress to chronic hepatitis or cirrhosis (Nielsen et al., 1974). It should be cautioned, however, that investigations of antigenic subtypes have begun only recently, and their significance is unclear, at best. Perhaps the most interesting information to come from them is the finding that asymptomatic carriers who have migrated in childhood from one geographic area to another show the "r" or "w" determinant of their place of birth. This would indicate that the carrier state is usually developed very early in life.

Hepatitis B was once thought to be transmitted only parenterally, by transfusion of infected blood or by the use of contaminated needles. *It has recently become clear, however, that perhaps as many as 60 per cent of cases of hepatitis B involve nonparenteral transmission* (Vittal et al., 1973). Thus, the hepatitis B virus is a significant cause of sporadic hepatitis. The nonparenteral mode of transmission remains somewhat uncertain. There is some evidence for venereal transmission (Heathcote et al., 1974), but oral transmission through sneezing, coughing or kissing is probably most important (Villarejos et al., 1974).

As listed earlier, there are three expressions of infection with hepatitis B virus:

(1) The patients may develop overt acute hepatitis, to be described later. Late in the incubation period, HBsAg, DNA polymerase and anti-HBc appear in the serum, probably corresponding to the periods of viremia and active viral replication within the liver. The DNA polymerase disappears within a few weeks; the HBsAg is cleared within 12 weeks; and the titer of anti-HBc gradually declines over several years. Anti-HBs doesn't even appear until well after the acute episode (Krugman et al., 1974). Subclinical acute hepatitis occurs in an unknown number of individuals. There is some evidence that it is twice as common as overt hepatitis. It may be simply a milder, anicteric form of acute hepatitis which clears rapidly. However, chronic liver disease may ensue, and, indeed, is thought to be more likely to stem from subclinical infection than from overt acute hepatitis. Subclinical disease which persists is particularly likely in patients with immunologic impairment, such as occurs with lymphomatous disease, chronic renal failure or immunosuppressive drug therapy.

(2) In about 10 per cent of patients with overt acute hepatitis B, chronic disease develops—usually either *chronic persistent hepatitis* or *chronic active hepatitis*, both described more fully later. Progression to chronic disease can be assumed when serum HBsAg fails to clear over a period of 12 weeks. As mentioned, chronic hepatitis is particularly likely when there is an immunologic defect. Chronic persistent hepatitis is also characteristic of neonatal hepatitis transmitted when the mother develops hepatitis near the time of delivery (Schweitzer et al., 1973).

(3) Asymptomatic carriers of HbsAg constitute 0.1 to 0.8 per cent of the normal population in the United States. The incidence is higher among the families of carriers, about 7 per cent (Szmuness et al., 1973). In some parts of the world, particularly in the tropics, the percentage of asymptomatic carriers is much higher than in the United States, comprising up to 20 per cent of the normal population. Those who come in contact with hepatitis B virus very early in life are more likely to become carriers, as are those who are repeatedly exposed to the virus—for example, drug addicts. In most of these cases, there is no evidence of even subclinical liver disease.

Why are there such differences in the response to hepatitis B virus? Probably the answer to this question rests with the host rather than with the virus. In order better to appreciate the possibilities, we must first describe what is known of the pathogenesis of hepatitis B. Immunofluorescence and immune electron microscopic studies indicate that the nucleus of the hepatocyte is the prime site of viral core replication, while the endoplasmic reticulum of the cytoplasm produces aggregates of the protein coat, which appear as long tubular structures. Most likely the protein coat is manufactured in considerable excess (Gyorkey et al., 1974). The mechanism by which cell damage occurs is not known. *However, the dominant opinion is that a cell-mediated response develops, which destroys the infected hepatocytes, thus limiting the disease.* As we know, antibodies also develop, and antigen-antibody complexes may be responsible for some of the distant manifestations which occasionally occur with acute hepatitis, such as arthritis, urticaria and, rarely, glomerulonephritis. In any case, in normal individuals one might expect a vigorous response, with destruction of the infected hepatocytes, albeit at the price of some clinical disease, but with ultimate elimination of the viruses. Rarely, there is fulminant disease and death. At the other extreme are patients with little or no cell-mediated response. In these patients the virus might continue to proliferate, with little cell damage, thus existing in a commensal relationship with the host. One can readily understand such a situation in patients with profound immunologic deficiencies, but what of the many asymptomatic carriers who seem to have an entirely normal immune system in every other way? Why they fail to clear the virus is a mystery. Between these two extremes are situations in which a partial cell-mediated response results in continuous limited growth of the virus, with more or less smoldering liver disease. Such patients would then develop chronic persistent hepatitis or chronic active hepatitis (Javitt et al., 1973). Indeed, as we shall see, there is some evidence for immunologic derangements in patients with these disorders. Clearly, the field of hepatitis B has been well fertilized with new facts, and speculation grows well in such soil.

Hepatitis A. Although possibly more common than hepatitis B, less is known about hepatitis A. This reflects the fact that no serum marker for hepatitis A, analogous to the HBsAg of hepatitis B, has been discovered. Recently, however, Feinstone and his coworkers, using immune electron microscopy, identified in the stools of patients with hepatitis A a 27 nm. virus-like particle—antigenically distinct from HBcAg and HBsAg (Feinstone et al., 1974). Moreover, antibodies against this agent were shown to develop during the course of hepatitis A (Almeida et al., 1974). Whereas the virus-like particle has not been propagated, its transmission to primates has resulted in hepatitis (Dienstag et al., 1975). Thus, we may be nearing an explosion of knowledge concerning hepatitis A similar to that of hepatitis B. At present, however, it remains a relatively mysterious disease. Although classically it is thought to be spread by the oral-fecal route, there is no reason to assume that parenteral transmission could not also occur. As mentioned, the incubation period is shorter than that of hepatitis B, ranging from 2 to 6 weeks. Unlike hepatitis B, hepatitis A frequently occurs in epidemics in closed populations, hence is sometimes termed "epidemic hepatitis." It is also the type of hepatitis typically associated with eating contaminated clams or oysters, or with drinking contaminated water. Whether or not hepatitis A can lead to chronic liver disease is unclear. If so, such progression is probably far less common than with hepatitis B. Most likely it almost always produces an acute, self-limited disease.

Morphology. Grossly and at the level of the light microscope, the morphologic changes encountered in hepatitis A and B are virtually indistinguishable. They range from very subtle alterations in those with mild disease to extensive hepatic necrosis in those with the more severe expressions. During the incubation and prodromal period, liver biopsies reveal only slight diffuse hepatocellular swelling, along with some swelling and hyperplasia of Kupffer cells. A sparse lymphocytic infiltrate, admixed with a few macrophages, can be seen in the portal areas. Sometimes lymphocytes are unusually abundant in the sinusoids. Isolated liver cell necrosis with disappearance of the necrotic cells, sometimes called "cell dropout," may be present but is not prominent and is difficult to detect. At this stage of the disease, the liver would be of normal color and perhaps slightly swollen, hence increased in weight.

With the onset of symptoms, the classic features of viral hepatitis appear. The liver is heavy, swollen and tense, and, depending on the amount of bile stasis, more or less jaundiced. Three major histologic features are evident: (1) liver cell injury and necrosis, (2) regeneration of liver cells, and (3) a reticuloendothelial reaction with portal infiltration of macrophages and lymphocytes.

The liver cell injury ranges from marked swelling of cells to frank necrosis. As the parenchymal cells swell, the cytoplasm appears watery and vacuolated, classically referred to as "ballooning degeneration." These changes are most evident in the centrilobular regions. Isolated liver cell dropout or small focal areas of necrosis now become more prominent, particularly in the centrilobular regions. Some hepatocytes show a pale eosinophilic ground-glass cytoplasm with an eccentrically placed nucleus. Similar anuclear structures are termed "Councilman bodies." Their significance will be considered later. The combination of cellular swelling and liver cell necrosis disrupts the normal liver cords and produces a disarray of the lobule under low power examination. Intrahepatic cholestasis is seen in some cases in the form of small droplets of bile pigment in liver and Kupffer cells, along with inspissated bile within the canaliculi. For unknown reasons, some livers show no evidence of bile stasis.

Concurrent with the hepatocellular damage, evidence of regeneration may be found in the form of occasional mitotic figures and nests of crowded disorganized cells, suggesting proliferative foci.

The reticuloendothelial reaction is quite prominent and takes the form of swelling and reduplication of Kupffer cells. Within the focal areas of liver cell necrosis, nests of lymphocytes and macrophages are present, the latter sometimes containing obvious cell debris. Similar aggregations of cells are found in the portal triads, occasionally accompanied by a sparse infiltrate of eosinophils and, rarely, of neutrophils (Fig. 15–1).

The electron microscope reveals distinctive features in hepatitis B. It can be seen that the eccentric nuclei and ground-glass appearance of the cytoplasm of occasional hepatocytes is caused by marked distention of smooth endoplasmic reticulum. This displaces the nucleus and other organelles to one side. Within the cisternae of the endoplasmic reticulum may be seen long filaments, most likely aggregations of the viral protein coat. Their appearance, of course, depends on the plane of section. Those seen in cross section appear as small circular structures, about 22 nm. in diameter, containing dense central dots (**"owl eye particles"**). Much less frequently, intranuclear particles are found in acute hepatitis B, presumably representing the nucleocapsids. These are also spheroidal structures, about 25 nm. in diameter, but lack the electron dense central dot (Huang et al., 1974).

Although the previous description of gross and light microscopic changes pertains to the typical cases of both forms of viral hepatitis, a great many variations on this theme are encountered. The hepatocellular necrosis may be more extensive and extend from one lobule to another, so-called "bridging" necrosis. The hepatitis may be quite severe and induce massive necrosis, as will be described in a later section of this chapter. In still other patients, the hepatitis may not resolve and may become persistent or chronically active.

Clinical Course. Many of the clinical features of the two forms of viral hepatitis have

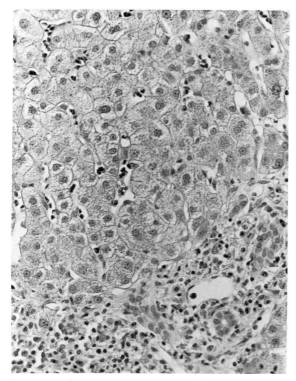

Figure 15–1. Viral hepatitis. The portal tract below is rimmed with a mononuclear infiltrate. The hepatocytes show some loss of normal architecture and vary in size and shape. "Ballooning degeneration" is most evident at the upper left.

already been mentioned. Only the acute disease will be described here. In the United States, the peak incidence of epidemic hepatitis is in autumn and early winter, and it occurs predominantly in children and young adults. Hepatitis B is encountered at any age. Parenteral transmission is most likely in the older age groups, reflecting their greater risk of hospitalization, and in young drug addicts. Malaise, fever, jaundice and abnormal liver function test results are characteristic of the clinically evident cases of both hepatitis A and hepatitis B. The hyperbilirubinemia is both conjugated and unconjugated. Sometimes, as was mentioned, these patients pass through a phase of total cholestasis, at which time stool bilirubin and urine urobilinogen levels almost disappear.

Hepatitis A usually runs a course of four to six weeks and is almost always followed by complete recovery. As discussed earlier, the course of hepatitis B is far more unpredictable. Probably about 85 per cent of patients with clinically overt acute hepatitis B recover completely. About 3 per cent die of fulminant disease (massive liver necrosis). The re-

mainder develop chronic disease, either subclinical or overt.

It would also appear that in some instances cryptogenic cirrhosis (p. 533) and hepatocarcinoma (p. 513) may be related to prior infection with hepatitis B. At least there is some guilt by association, since there are increased frequencies of serum HBsAg in patients with these disorders (Javitt et al., 1973). However, such a progression is not well established. Part of the difficulty in documenting a relationship between hepatitis B infection and chronic liver disease is the fact that progression so often develops from an initially anicteric infection (Dudley et al., 1972).

MASSIVE LIVER NECROSIS

In bygone years, this entity was called *acute yellow atrophy,* but the designation is inappropriate, since the disease is not an atrophic but rather a necrotic process. Massive destruction of the liver may be produced by fulminant viral hepatitis, by mushroom poisoning and by a variety of hepatotoxic agents, including carbon tetrachloride, chloroform, cinchophen, arsenicals, tetracyclines, heavy metals, phosphorus and, of recent interest, the anesthetic halothane. In a current analysis of 150 cases of fulminant hepatic failure, 80 patients were presumed to have a form of viral hepatitis. In an additional 35 patients, the necrosis developed less than three weeks after halothane anesthesia, and 27 of these patients had had multiple exposures to the anesthetic. In some, it should be noted, the liver damage occurred after the first exposure (Trey et al., 1968). It is important, however, to make clear that hundreds of thousands of patients have been anesthetized with halothane, and the hazard, while real, is small. Indeed, the anesthetist might well argue that the risks involved in the use of other anesthetics, including ether, may be greater than the hazard of developing posthalothane liver necrosis. Certain drugs are also suspected of being possible causes of liver necrosis. These include iproniazid and para-aminosalicylic acid, both of which are used in the therapy of tuberculosis. In these cases, however, it has been difficult to rule out clearly the existence of an underlying viral infection (McIntyre and Sherlock, 1965).

The factors that determine the severity of the liver injury are poorly understood. With some of the chemical agents mentioned above, such as chloroform and the inorganic chemicals, the amount of liver damage is related to dosage. However, hypersensitivity may play a role in some patients, as is suspected in drug and halothane induced massive liver necrosis. Lymphocyte transformation, presumed to be an index of immunologic stimulation, has been described in patients with post-halothane hepatitis (Paronetto and Popper, 1970). Others, however, favor direct toxicity even for these agents, and point to the fact that the reaction may occur on first exposure. Host factors such as the nutrition of the patient and alcoholism may be important influences, particularly in viral infections.

The changes found in the liver depend upon the extent of the injury and the duration of survival of the patient. During the first day, with massive necrosis, the liver is enlarged and has a tense capsule. Often large hemorrhagic areas can be seen, both subcapsularly and on transection. The consistency may be normal or more firm than usual, owing to edema. During the next few days, the liver shrinks rapidly in size and develops a wrinkled capsule and a flabby consistency (Fig. 15–2). Variegated areas of hemorrhage, yellow necrosis and bile staining now appear. If the entire liver is involved, death usually occurs at this stage. With less extreme damage, preserved areas of hepatic substance are found, with flabby, shrunken, variegated intervening regions. As the destroyed liver substance is removed, these necrotic areas collapse, and the entire liver may be reduced to as little as 800 gm. in weight. Regeneration in the marginal zones often creates an unusual irregularity to the vital tissue. If the patient survives, the damaged areas become progressively fibrotic, producing what will be described as postnecrotic scarring (p. 528).

Histologically, massive necrosis begins with destruction of the centrilobular zones. Depending on the rapidity of the necrotizing process, some fatty change may be present. More often, the affected hepatocytes undergo progressive coagulative changes. Total lobules are obliterated over a wide area. In time, the margins of these areas, if such exist, develop an acute inflammatory infiltrate. Removal of the necrotic liver cells causes collapse of the framework, and the portal triads now crowd closely together, being separated only by debris and collapsed fibrous framework. It should be noted that usually the portal structures and periportal fibrous tissue survive and apparently are resistant to the hepatotoxic injury. Hemorrhages, bile stasis and Kupffer cell reactions confuse the histologic picture during the still active phase. By the end of the first week, the inflammatory infiltrate is now largely mononuclear, and beginning vascularization and fibroproliferation become evident. The progressive ingrowth of fibrous tissue converts the necrotic areas to the broad scars characteristic of the postnecrotic form of cirrhosis.

The course of fulminant hepatic necrosis may be extremely short, measured in terms of days. In other patients, however, the damage is less extensive, and death may occur weeks after the acute attack. Still other affected persons may survive because of the large reserve capacity of the liver. In all patients, malaise, fever and jaundice are prominent early manifestations. Unexplained fever may, indeed, herald the beginning of the underlying disease. Obviously, all of the liver functions are deranged, and hypoprothrombinemia with a hemorrhagic diathesis, as well as depletion of serum proteins, constitutes a serious problem. The destroyed liver cells release large amounts of intracellular enzymes. Elevated serum levels of GOT and LDH are classic but, it should be noted, do not consistently parallel the severity of the liver damage.

CHRONIC HEPATITIS

Chronic hepatitis is divided into two somewhat distinct forms: *chronic persistent hepatitis* and *chronic active (or aggressive) hepatitis.* Patients with chronic persistent hepatitis show only a mild derangement in their liver function tests, no physical signs of disease, and few

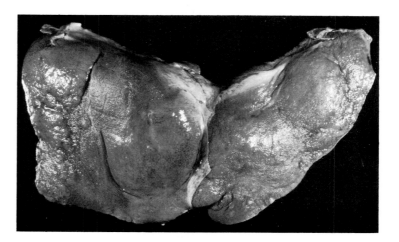

Figure 15–2. Massive hepatic necrosis. The destruction of liver substance has caused irregular collapse and irregular wrinkling of the capsule. The gross lobularity is due to the random areas of preserved hepatic substance.

if any symptoms. In contrast, those with chronic active hepatitis show marked derangements in their liver function tests and have obvious and usually progressive disease, frequently characterized by hepatosplenomegaly and recurrent jaundice, as well as by anorexia, weakness and malaise (Javitt et al., 1973). As might be anticipated, there is some overlap between these two forms and they may in many cases represent progression along a spectrum of liver disease.

The genesis of chronic hepatitis is unknown. As you will recall from the section on viral hepatitis, about 10 per cent of patients with overt acute hepatitis B infection develop chronic hepatitis, which is equally divided between the persistent and active forms (Nielsen et al., 1974). However, such patients who have undergone clear-cut progression from acute to chronic hepatitis probably represent no more than half of all patients with chronic hepatitis (Dudley et al., 1972). Thus, there is a large group of patients whose chronic liver disease would appear to arise *de novo*, possibly from anicteric acute hepatitis. Even among those who have undergone progression from acute viral hepatitis, the question remains as to why a small minority of individuals are unable to eliminate a virus which seems to be readily cleared by most individuals. As we shall see, *many investigators suspect that chronic hepatitis represents an aberrant immune response in genetically susceptible individuals exposed to an inciting agent, such as the hepatitis B virus or a drug.* Indeed, evidence of impaired T-cell function has been demonstrated in a number of these patients (Yeung Laiwah, 1971; Ito et al., 1972). Before exploring this issue further, we shall separately describe first chronic persistent hepatitis, then the more important entity, chronic active hepatitis.

CHRONIC PERSISTENT HEPATITIS

This lesion may be found in five clinical settings which probably overlap considerably: (1) It may represent persistence of acute viral hepatitis, marked by the continued presence of the hepatitis B surface antigen (HBsAg) in the serum, (2) it may be found in a minority of apparently healthy carriers of HBsAg, (3) it may follow anicteric hepatitis, particularly in patients with known immunologic impairment, such as that due to lymphomatous disease or immunosuppressive therapy, (4) it is the typical response of the neonate to hepatitis B infection transmitted from the mother (Schweitzer et al., 1973), (5) it occurs as an altogether mysterious lesion without evidence of hepatitis B infection. This last represents an important category, since several studies indicate that no more than half the patients

with chronic persistent hepatitis have HBsAg in their serum. Conceivably, in these patients, hepatitis B virus was eradicated, but not before it provoked the emergence of some autoimmune response (Javitt et al., 1973).

The morphologic changes with chronic persistent hepatitis are not significantly different from those of mild viral hepatitis (see p. 517). Its hallmark is a chronic mononuclear inflammatory response confined to the portal triads, but with preservation of the portal limiting plate—that is, the hepatocytes encircling the portal canal.

The prognosis with chronic persistent hepatitis is not at all clear. Probably most cases which develop from overt acute viral hepatitis eventually resolve or, at least, do not progress. In some instances, however, the lesion may become increasingly aggressive and lead eventually to chronic active hepatitis or cirrhosis (Dudley et al., 1972).

CHRONIC ACTIVE HEPATITIS (CHRONIC AGGRESSIVE HEPATITIS)

Because this is a clinically overt lesion, and a life-threatening one at that, somewhat more is known about it than about chronic persistent hepatitis. It, too, may be associated with persistence of hepatitis B virus following acute disease, either overt or—perhaps more important—anicteric. However, only a minority of patients with chronic active hepatitis have the marker for hepatitis B virus (that is, HBsAg) in their serum. *Among the remaining patients is a large group who demonstrate various autoimmune phenomena, including a positive LE preparation, ANA antibodies, RA factor, and antibodies against smooth muscle and mitochondria. This form of chronic active hepatitis has been termed* lupoid hepatitis, *although there is no established relationship with SLE.* It is of interest that whereas occasional patients may show evidence of both chronic hepatitis B infection and so-called lupoid hepatitis, these two forms of chronic active hepatitis are in general mutually exclusive. Thus, patients with acute viral hepatitis who are destined to develop chronic active disease may declare themselves in one of two ways—HBsAg persisting in the serum beyond the third month of illness, *or* ANA antibody and a positive LE test presenting shortly after the onset of illness (Vittal et al., 1973). Chronic active hepatitis may also develop after taking certain drugs, such as alpha-methyldopa.

Before discussing the possible pathogenetic mechanisms, we shall briefly describe the morphology of chronic active hepatitis, which is common to all presumed etiologies. In general, the changes are remarkably similar to those of acute viral hepatitis. There is disarray of the liver cords, with some hepatocyte necrosis admixed with evidence of regeneration. The most prominent finding is an intense infiltrate of lymphocytes and plasma cells in the portal areas. Although the portal plate is intact with chronic persistent hepatitis, it is disrupted with chronic active hepatitis, and the inflammation extends into the parenchyma (Javitt et al., 1973). In most instances scarring eventually appears. At first the scarring is more or less random, but eventually it may become widespread, extending in delicate bands bridging portal areas. Thus, chronic active hepatitis merges with cirrhosis, to be discussed later.

As with acute hepatitis B infection, the electron microscope may in some instances reveal nucleocapsid-like particles within the hepatocyte nuclei, and filamentous structures thought to represent viral coat material in the cytoplasm (see p. 517). Indeed, when present, the intranuclear particles are seen in far greater numbers in chronic active hepatitis than in acute hepatitis. Aggregates of these particles may also be seen in the cytoplasm and extracellularly, within the bile canaliculi and in the spaces of Disse. The Dane particles, which

are difficult to demonstrate in acute hepatitis, may also be more readily seen with chronic active hepatitis. In these cases they are found within the cisternae of the endoplasmic reticulum, as well as in the serum. Their appearance is quite distinct. The core is well delineated and separated from the outer fuzzy coat by a narrow clear zone (Huang et al., 1974) (Fig. 15–3).

There is much evidence that chronic active hepatitis is an immunologic disorder, perhaps triggered by many environmental factors, including hepatitis B virus and drugs. The prominence of the lymphocytic and plasma cell response suggests this, as does the beneficial effect of immunosuppressive therapy. Higher frequencies of two histocompatibility antigens, HL-A1 and HL-A8 are found in patients with chronic active hepatitis, particularly the lupoid form (Eddleston and Williams, 1974). The significance of the autoantibodies and of the abnormal immunoglobulin levels which are frequently present

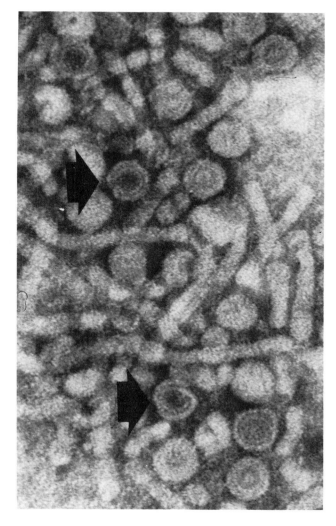

Figure 15–3. Chronic hepatitis. Electron micrograph ($\times$ 220,000) of negatively stained pellet prepared from the serum of a patient with chronic hepatitis. Numerous double-shelled Dane particles (arrows) and 20 nm. tubules are present. (Courtesy of Dr. Michael Gerber, Associate Professor of Pathology, Mount Sinai School of Medicine, New York.)

in patients with chronic active hepatitis is unclear. These autoantibodies are neither organ nor species specific. It has been suggested that they are the result rather than the cause of the liver disease. However, increased frequencies of these antibodies and of abnormal immunoglobulin levels are also found in the families of patients with chronic active hepatitis, suggesting a genetic predisposition (Golding et al., 1973). Be that as it may, most workers believe that the *fundamental* pathogenetic derangement is in cell-mediated rather than humoral immune function, and that the antibodies are incidental. As mentioned, there is in vitro evidence that the T-cells of some patients with chronic active hepatitis fail to transform under appropriate stimuli. Alternatively, it has been suggested that the pathogenesis in patients with lupoid hepatitis is very different from that in patients with continued hepatitis B virus infection. According to this hypothesis, in the former group there is an initial hepatitis B infection which elicits a normal immune response, with elimination of the virus. However, T-cell suppressor function is deficient in these patients, and antibody activity continues unchecked against the altered hepatocyte surface antigens. This, then, leads to chronic liver disease. In contrast, patients with chronic active hepatitis who show continued hepatitis B infection might simply have a defect in antibody response, with failure to clear the virus (Eddleston and Williams, 1974). This ingenious hypothesis, however, remains unproved.

Because progression from acute hepatitis through chronic active hepatitis to cirrhosis has in many cases been well documented, it has been suggested that these disorders may represent a spectrum of autoimmune disease affecting the liver. Autoantibodies of the same type found with some cases of chronic active hepatitis are also present in many patients with primary biliary cirrhosis and with so-called cryptogenic cirrhosis (Golding et al., 1973). Moreover, evidence of persistent hepatitis B virus is present in a significant minority of patients with cryptogenic cirrhosis and, interestingly, with hepatocarcinoma (but not with primary biliary cirrhosis). The relationships, if any, among these liver diseases, then, is a source of intense interest at this time, but little is definitely known.

Clinically, chronic active hepatitis runs a variable course. In many patients progression is remarkably slow. In others, particularly those with the lupoid form, progression is rapid, leading to liver failure and death within a few years. Manifestations include anorexia, weakness and malaise, along with other widespread evidence of impairment in liver func-

tion. Jaundice may or may not be present. Eventually, many of these patients develop cirrhosis, with consequent portal hypertension (p. 523). Remarkable improvement is often obtained with steroids or immunosuppressive drugs.

NEONATAL HEPATITIS

It is probable that the lesion called neonatal hepatitis is not a specific entity, but rather is a reaction pattern of very young hepatocytes to any one of a number of damaging influences. Characteristic of this form of liver disease, which occurs in the early weeks or months of life, is transformation of virtually all hepatocytes to giant cells, many multinucleate and some creating syncytium-like masses of protoplasm harboring dozens of nuclei. Hence, the often-used synonym for this condition is *giant cell hepatitis.* Many viruses, including those of cytomegalic inclusion disease, herpes simplex, rubella and the Coxsackie agents, have been thought to produce this lesion. Is this pattern of reaction related only to age difference, or do the many viral agents mentioned as possible causes of neonatal hepatitis all produce a uniform lesion, distinctive from the usual viral hepatitis? The changes induced by biliary duct atresia or agenesis bear on this question. When total cholestasis is present from birth, the liver undergoes changes virtually indistinguishable from neonatal hepatitis, save perhaps for more prominent bile stasis. Similarly, in congenital syphilis and hemolytic disease of the newborn, giant cells are formed in the liver. The evidence, then, suggests that neonatal hepatitis is an age related reaction pattern, perhaps to many causes of liver injury. An exception would seem to be the pattern of liver disease caused by hepatitis B infection of the neonate. This virus is thought to be readily transmitted from the mother near the time of delivery, and HBsAg was found in four of seven cord bloods tested. In contrast to the neonatal hepatitis described here, however, hepatitis B infection in newborns usually evokes morphologic changes characteristic of chronic persistent hepatitis (p. 520).

Morphologically, the giant cell transformation is accompanied by disarray of the lobular architecture and marked bile stasis within the distorted canaliculi and giant hepatocytes. Although they are hard to find, the bile ducts and portal triads are unaffected. These livers are usually enlarged and deeply green. No early nodularity or fibrosis is present, but either may develop in later stages, creating a form of cirrhosis.

Clinically the acute disease mimics posthepatic obstructive jaundice but later, as the disease persists, signs of portal hypertension appear. About one third of these infants die during the acute phase, one third recover completely and the remainder have progressive liver dysfunction, many to die eventually of the complications of portal hypertension.

CHOLANGITIS AND LIVER ABSCESS

The designation *cholangitis* refers to inflammation of the bile ducts and should be distinguished from *cholangiolitis*, which implies involvement of smaller bile ductules, such as occurs in viral hepatitis. Cholangitis is almost always caused by bacteria, although reflux of pancreatic juice and chemical agents have been suspected as being contributing factors on rare occasions. In the usual case, biliary tract disease and partial or complete obstruction to the outflow of bile underlie the development of the infection. As might be anticipated, the common organisms are *E. coli*, enterococci, other gram-negative rods and the Salmonellae. The flora then is the same as that associated with acute cholecystitis. In the great majority of cases, the cholangitis is associated with cholecystitis and is to be considered an extension of the same inflammatory process. Rarely, cholangitis is found as a primary disorder, and its pathogenesis in this instance is obscure. Conceivably, systemic infection might seed the biliary tract.

The acute stage of the disease is characterized by suppuration within the bile ducts, which ascends into the intrahepatic ramifications. Spread of the infection outside the ducts produces liver abscesses. With persistence of the inflammation, transition to chronic cholangitis occurs and is followed by fibrosis about the ducts. When the process occurs within the intrahepatic ramifications, secondary biliary cirrhosis results (p. 529).

In the usual case, the dominant clinical manifestations are malaise and fever, sometimes hectic in nature. Jaundice may appear, usually in those cases having a prominent obstructive component. Although hepatomegaly may be present, more often it is absent. Sometimes pain may appear, and the liver becomes tender on clinical palpation as a result of tension of the capsule. Whereas *chronic* cholangitis evokes less striking symptoms, it may be more dangerous because biliary cirrhosis sometimes ensues.

Liver abscesses may arise not only as complications of acute cholangitis, but also from seeding via the portal vein, the hepatic artery or the lymphatics. Thus, hepatic abscesses develop following infections within the abdominal cavity, which either drain through lymphatics or invade the portal vein (*pylephlebitis*). The causative bacteria are those already cited in the discussion of cholangitis. The liver may also be seeded by systemic infections, particularly bacterial endocarditis (Sherman and Robbins, 1960).

The lesions vary from microscopic foci to massive areas of suppurative necrosis. In general, they are from 1 to 3 cm. in diameter and are usually multiple. Rupture through the capsule may lead to subhepatic or subdiaphragmatic abscesses and peritonitis. On rare occasion, the infection may trek from the subdiaphragmatic location into the thoracic cavity. Liver abscesses may be totally silent if they are small and few in number. When they evoke symptoms, the clinical disease is usually indistinguishable from acute cholangitis, which, of course, is a frequent accompaniment.

There remain two special forms of liver abscess to be briefly described.

Amoebic abscesses of the liver are one of the most serious complications of amoebic dysentery. The parasites presumably reach the liver through the portal vein. The abscess characteristically contains a brown paste-like exudate rather than pus, but the diagnosis depends upon the histologic identification of the parasites in the wall of the abscess. From the liver, these abscesses may burrow through the subdiaphragmatic space to enter the lungs and occasionally embolize from there to the brain.

Echinococcus granulosus is a small tapeworm of dogs which includes man among its intermediate hosts. In the intermediate host it typically produces cysts of the liver. Although not common in the United States, there are some areas of the world in which these cysts are very common. When severely involved, the liver may contain one to many echinococcus cysts, virtually replacing whole lobes. These large cysts are referred to as "mother cysts." They contain bile-stained fluid in which can be found multiple, small, thin-walled daughter cysts. Histologic examination of the mother cyst discloses its wall to be composed of laminated layers of chitinous material, and prolonged and careful search may reveal the scolices or hooklets of the echinococcus.

ASCITES AND OTHER MANIFESTATIONS OF PORTAL HYPERTENSION

In the human portal vein, the pressure normally varies between 5 and 10 cm. H_2O. This pressure is abnormally elevated in disorders that: (1) obstruct the portal vein before it enters the liver (*prehepatic obstruction*), (2) impair flow through the liver, or (3) hamper the venous outflow from the liver *(posthepatic obstruction)*. The second mechanism is most important and is usually caused by the group of hepatic diseases known as the cirrhoses. Although there are several forms of cirrhosis, which will be discussed presently, all have as a common denominator widespread injury to the liver resulting in diffuse fibrous scarring and nodularity, which distort the connective tissue and vascular framework. Regeneration of injured hepatic cells contributes significantly to the nodularity. While such diffuse damage may produce many symptoms, such as anorexia, jaundice and indeed features indicative of liver insufficiency, the most definitive findings pointing to a diagnosis of cirrhosis stem from the development of portal hypertension. In a series of patients with cirrhosis, it was found that ascites was the presenting complaint in 46 per cent and gastrointestinal bleeding in 23 per cent, both consequences of portal hypertension (Blaisdell and Cohen, 1961).

Prehepatic causes of portal hypertension include portal vein thrombosis or marked narrowing, usually as a result of tumorous involvement, and *posthepatic causes* include hepatic vein thrombosis (Budd-Chiari syndrome, p. 533), constrictive pericarditis (p. 312), compression or obstruction of the inferior vena cava (p. 279) and long-standing severe right ventricular failure (p. 291). Our principal interest here is in the *hepatic causes* of portal hypertension, i.e., the cirrhoses. In passing, it might be noted that acute inflammation with swelling of hepatocytes or fatty change may cause sufficient sinusoidal compression to induce portal hypertension, but this is generally transient and reversible.

Whatever the cause, portal hypertension results in a constellation of clinical findings that is quite characteristic—i.e., ascites, the development of collateral venous channels, and splenomegaly.

Ascites is an intraperitoneal accumulation of watery fluid containing small amounts of protein, in the range of 1 to 2 gm. per 100 cc. Many liters may collect, causing abdominal distention. Although the fluid may contain a scant number of mesothelial cells and lymphocytes, it does not, in the uncomplicated case, contain polymorphonuclear leukocytes or red cells. Solutes such as glucose, sodium and potassium have essentially the same concentrations in the ascitic fluid as in the blood. A considerable amount of sodium and albumin may be lost when large volumes of ascitic fluid are tapped to relieve the abdominal distention.

The genesis of ascitic fluid is complex. Scarring within the liver increases hydrostatic pressure within the portal system, not only through obstruction but also through the creation of arteriovenous communications within the scars. Transudation of plasma into the peritoneum results from the portal hypertension. Cirrhosis also impairs synthesis of albumin and lowers the colloid osmotic pressure of the plasma. Another key factor is retention of sodium and water. With portal hypertension and the resultant sequestration of a large volume of blood within the splanchnic bed, renal blood flow and glomerular filtration rate fall. This in itself leads to sodium retention. In addition, aldosterone and ADH are elaborated, further augmenting salt and water retention. Since these hormones are metabolized in the liver, severe hepatic dysfunction may result in even higher levels. *Thus, although the effective circulating blood volume may be lower than normal, a constellation of influences tends to increase fluid retention within the splanchnic bed and the accumulation of ever larger volumes of ascitic fluid.* The composition of the fluid is not only plasma transudate; an additional factor is increased formation of lymph within the liver and the abdominal viscera (Steigmann et al., 1967). This lymph fluid may leak through the liver capsule, but more importantly, it probably weeps from all peritoneal surfaces within the abdomen. In about 20 per cent of patients, the ascitic fluid passes through transdiaphragmatic lymphatics into the pleural cavities, particularly on the right, to cause *hydrothorax.*

Collateral venous channels might also be referred to as portal vein bypasses. When the pressure rises in the portal vein, collateral vessels are enlarged wherever the systemic and portal circulations share common capillary beds. The most important collateral channels are found in the lower esophageal plexus where the portal and azygous systems intermingle. When portal flow is obstructed, the esophageal plexus becomes engorged, and dilatation of these veins results. Some appear beneath the esophageal mucosa in the form of varices. Once such varices rupture, bleeding is exceedingly difficult to control, and the hematemesis frequently is fatal (p. 468). *These varices occur in about 67 per cent of patients with advanced cirrhosis, cause hematemesis in about 25 per cent of patients and indeed are the principal cause of death in almost this same number.* Varices may also develop in the anal-rectal region, where the superior mesenteric vein of the portal system communicates via the inferior mesenteric system with the hemorrhoidal plexus of the caval system. Thus, a third to a half of patients with cirrhosis develop hemorrhoids. Perhaps because the hemorrhoidal communications are remote from the liver, the pressures in these anal-rectal varices are not as high as those in the esophagus. Serious hemorrhage does not often arise from rupture of hemorrhoids. If the fetal umbilical vein fails to become obliterated, it may communicate with veins about the umbilicus to produce an externally visible vascular pattern called *caput medusae.*

Splenomegaly is readily attributed to the prolonged congestion of the spleen. Such spleens may achieve weights of up to 1000 gm. A variety of hematologic abnormalities may appear secondary to the splenic enlargement, including anemia, leukopenia and thrombocytopenia. All these hematologic alterations are attributed to *hypersplenism* and may be encountered in any form of splenic enlargement. In former years, the combination of hematologic changes and splenomegaly was referred to as *Banti's syndrome.* It is important to remember, however, that liver failure itself may lead to anemia and a bleeding diathesis, quite apart from any associated hypersplenism.

Against this background, we can turn to a consideration of the major causes of portal hypertension—i.e., the various forms of cirrhosis and hepatic and portal vein obstruction.

CIRRHOSIS OF THE LIVER

In the United States, cirrhosis of the liver has recently undergone an appalling increase in frequency, and by 1973 was the seventh most important cause of death (U.S. Vital Statistics, 1974). Although there is some difficulty in defining cirrhosis precisely, it may be thought of as a diffuse trabeculated, sometimes massive, scarring throughout the liver, sufficient to produce disorganization of the lobular architecture and nodularity throughout the liver substance. The nodularity is heightened by the regenerative activity that follows liver cell injury and death (Popper and Zak, 1958).

For many reasons, no universally acceptable classification of cirrhosis exists. The etiology of many forms is poorly understood. The morphology is not always distinctive. And in a considerable number of instances, there are neither etiologic nor morphologic clues to the chain of events leading to the diffuse liver damage. We therefore deal frequently with disease of uncertain genesis producing nondistinctive morphologic change. Nonetheless, a reasonable categorization can be offered as follows. An approximate relative frequency is given as a percentage after each type.

	Per Cent
1. Cirrhosis associated with alcohol abuse	50
2. Postnecrotic scarring	15
3. Biliary cirrhosis (primary and secondary)	10
4. Cirrhosis associated with hemochromatosis (pigment cirrhosis)	5
5. Indeterminate and miscellaneous types	20

CIRRHOSIS ASSOCIATED WITH ALCOHOL ABUSE

In the past, this form of cirrhosis has variously been called Laennec's, portal or nutritional cirrhosis. Some would flatly designate it "alcoholic cirrhosis." The present term is used to indicate that the role of alcohol, as will be seen, is still somewhat controversial. However, the association between prolonged chronic alcohol ingestion and the cirrhosis is unmistakable. In the United States and other affluent societies, the growing menace of alcohol abuse is reflected in an increasing incidence of "alcoholic cirrhosis" (Popper et al., 1969). Although at one time this was almost exclusively a male disorder, changing mores have made it clear that women are just as susceptible. Moreover, this disease does not occur predominantly in the fringes of society. All levels are affected, and indeed, in Great Britain, its highest incidence is among those in the professions.

Pathogenesis. The genesis of this form of cirrhosis is still an area of heated debate. Certain observations are widely accepted. *There is an unmistakable association between its appearance and alcohol abuse.* A history of chronic alcoholism can be obtained in up to 90 per cent of patients. The amount and duration of alcohol intake are significant. It has been suggested by Popper and Orr (1970) that an intake below 80 ml. of ethanol per day rarely leads to significant liver injury, while levels above 160 ml. favor cirrhosis. *The diffuse fibrous scarring is almost invariably preceded by fatty change,* a lesion described on page 17. There is indeed an inverse relationship between the amount of fat and the severity of fibrous scarring. Once we leave these grounds, we are on more shaky footing.

There are two major areas of uncertainty: (1) the precise role of alcohol, and (2) the relationship between the fatty change and the development of fibrosis. Stated simply, the first question asks *whether alcohol is a direct hepatotoxin that destroys liver cells and thus induces scarring or whether it merely substitutes for other sources of calories and so leads to dietary deficiencies.* Abundant evidence has been marshalled for both points of view. As was discussed in an earlier chapter, alcohol abuse in man clearly results in fatty change in the liver (Lieber and

Spritz, 1966). This effect of alcohol is remarkably quick. Young nonalcoholic volunteers developed fatty change in the liver within two days when they consumed 18 to 24 ounces of alcohol per day, despite a concomitant nutritionally adequate diet (Rubin and Lieber, 1968). Smaller amounts of alcohol over a longer time span have the same effect. The mechanisms of accumulation of the fat include: (1) increased transport of fat from the periphery to the liver, (2) reduced fatty acid oxidation in the liver, (3) increased synthesis of triglycerides in the liver to restore NAD reduced to NADH by oxidation of alcohol, and—possibly—(4) impaired mobilization of lipids as lipoproteins as a result of inadequate protein synthesis (Lieber, 1969). Rubin and Lieber believe *increased transport to the liver and decreased oxidative capacity account for most of the fat* (Rubin and Lieber, 1969). Correlated with this decreased oxidative capacity are the mitochondrial alterations observed in these livers by Iseri, Gottlieb, and others (Iseri, 1966).

There is a somewhat more tenuous opinion that alcohol is not a direct hepatotoxin. According to this view, chronic alcoholism leads to nutritional imbalances, particularly a deficiency of the lipotropes (Porta et al., 1970). Proponents of this view point out that a protein deficient diet in rats induces fatty change and the addition of alcohol isocalorically does not enhance the process (Porta and Gomez-Dumm, 1968). In the chronic alcoholic, there may be not only a deficiency of protein but also of the lipotropes choline and methionine.

Until recently most investigators believed that fatty change did not progress to cirrhosis. There were several reasons for this view, perhaps the most important of which was the inability to demonstrate such progression in experimental animals. Moreover, while malnutrition alone in humans produces fatty change, it is known not to lead to cirrhosis in most cases. Fatty change induced by alcohol in volunteers was found to be readily reversible.

Within the past few years, however, new evidence has appeared which indicates both that (1) alcohol alone may be sufficient to cause cirrhosis, and (2) fatty change may progress to cirrhosis. The most important finding leading to these conclusions was the demonstration in baboons that the chronic consumption of alcohol produced a spectrum of liver disease ranging from fatty change through hepatocellular necrosis to cirrhosis (Rubin and Lieber, 1974). Care was taken that these animals were maintained on a nutritionally adequate diet. The link, then, between fatty change and cirrhosis would seem to be a stage of hepatocellular necrosis with reactive inflammation, now known as *alcoholic hepatitis*. In the course of al-

coholic hepatitis, pink hyaline droplets or aggregates (representing accumulations of microfilaments), sometimes termed alcoholic hyalin or *Mallory bodies*, appear within the cytoplasm of some hepatocytes. These are thought to represent an abnormal protein synthesized by the damaged cells. Although they are occasionally seen with other lesions of the liver (for example, with hepatocarcinoma), they are most closely related to alcoholic hepatitis, and their presence is an index of the severity of the lesion (Popper, 1974). With the recognition of the importance of alcoholic hepatitis as the precursor of cirrhosis in experimental animals, many hepatologists have become convinced that alcohol leads to a similar spectrum of changes in man. The mechanism by which alcohol exerts its toxic effect, however, remains unknown. Recently it has been suggested that the actual toxic agent is acetaldehyde, the immediate metabolite of ethanol. Higher blood levels of this metabolite have been found in alcoholics than in a control population given the same amount of alcohol intravenously (Korsten et al., 1975).

Morphology. Early, the liver is markedly fatty and enlarged, perhaps up to 4000 gm. It is soft, yellow, greasy and readily fractured. Only trace amounts of fibrous tissue are present, and therefore there is little induration. The histologic features of fatty change have been described previously (p. 17). With the onset of alcoholic hepatitis, there is variable evidence of hepatocyte damage, ranging from swelling of occasional hepatocytes to focal areas of necrosis. A polymorphonuclear infiltration of these foci is characteristic, as is the alcoholic hyalin previously discussed. This appears under the light microscope as a fine skein of dispersed droplets distributed within the cytoplasm of the cell (Fig. 15–4). The nature of the hyalin is still something of a mystery, but studies by Iseri and Gottlieb (1971) and by Wiggers and his colleagues (1973) disclose a filamentous substructure suggesting an abnormal secretory product of the hepatocytes. Often canalicular and intracellular bile stasis are also present.

Fibrosis is first central and perivenular. **In time the liver shrinks in size, becoming less fatty and more fibrotic** (Fig. 15–5). The scarring begins to appear in the portal triads and eventually bridges them, enclosing single lobules. Lymphocytic infiltration and bile duct reduplication are now more evident in these scars. The liver is still yellow, but it now has a well demarcated, finely nodular external and transected surface. The nodules are small and range from 0.1 to 0.5 cm. in diameter, with the larger nodules presumably resulting from regeneration. The fibrous scarring does not merely represent the collapsed preexisting framework, but also involves active fibroproliferation (Fig. 15–6).

With advance of the disease, the liver is trans-

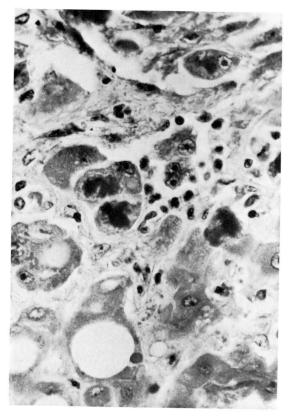

Figure 15–4. So-called "alcoholic hyalin" in the cirrhosis associated with alcohol abuse. The irregular dark configurations within the liver cells in the center field and at the upper right are characteristic of the morphologic appearance of this mysterious substance.

formed into a small, atrophic, indurated organ weighing less than 1500 gm. The fat disappears and the liver becomes brown and markedly nodular. Alcoholic hyalin and cell necrosis now are generally absent. The regenerative reaction has produced considerable variation in the size of the liver cells, as well as in their orientation. The scarring consists of broad bands which surround or divide individual lobules. The scarring may become so marked as to simulate the pattern encountered in postnecrotic scarring. Thus, the end stages of "alcoholic cirrhosis" may be exceedingly difficult to differentiate from other forms of cirrhosis.

Clinical Course. The course of this form of cirrhosis is extremely unpredictable. In many patients, the disease is entirely asymptomatic for long periods of time. Indeed, in a postmortem review of patients with this hepatic disorder, the clinical diagnosis had been made in only about 33 per cent (Stone et al., 1968). Usually the first signs relate to portal hypertension, resulting in the classic picture of a grossly distended abdomen filled with ascitic fluid along with wasted extremities and a

pathetically drawn face. In some cases, the first manifestation is jaundice. The hyperbilirubinemia is of both conjugated and unconjugated forms. The injured liver cell cannot secrete bile, and eventually it loses its capacity to take up unconjugated bilirubin. Not infrequently, the cirrhosis is compensated and the disorder is asymptomatic until some stress upsets the balance. A massive hemorrhage from esophageal varices may be followed by hepatic insufficiency or even hepatic failure. Sometimes such bleeding is the first sign of the submerged cirrhosis. Intercurrent infections may also trigger hepatic decompensation. The host of abnormalities described as hepatic failure then becomes manifest. In some patients, the marginal compensation is eroded by a wave of massive necrosis caused by alcoholic hepatitis. This is thought often to be triggered by an alcoholic spree. Such acute exacerbations may occur at any stage of the development of cirrhosis and may be recurrent. Therefore, it must not be assumed that hepatic insufficiency or failure implies the advanced fibrotic stage of the disease. Each bout of alcoholic hepatitis carries with it a high mortality rate, ranging between 10 and 20 per cent (Rubin and Lieber, 1974).

The long-term outlook for patients with cir-

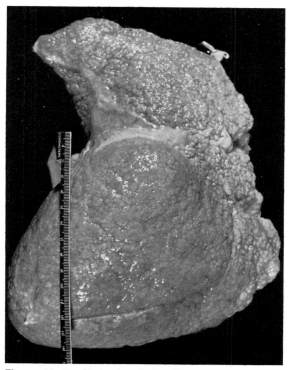

Figure 15–5. Cirrhosis of the liver associated with alcohol abuse, showing the characteristic diffuse nodularity induced by the underlying fibrous scarring.

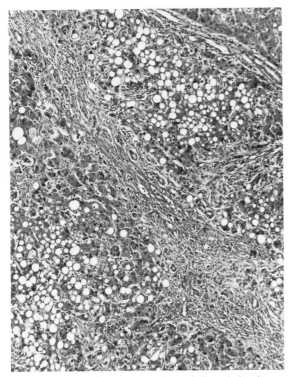

Figure 15–6. A low power view of the cirrhosis associated with alcohol abuse. The fibrous scarring separates islands of hepatocytes, many of which contain fatty vacuoles of varying size.

rhosis is very unpredictable. Numerous reports indicate that the disease can be arrested if the patient will abstain from alcohol (Powell and Klatskin, 1968). Because it is difficult to elicit the patient's cooperation, 80 to 90 per cent die of their disease within five years. The causes of death are predominantly liver failure, intercurrent infections, gastrointestinal hemorrhage and hepatoma, in that order. The source of the fatal hemorrhage is usually esophageal varices, but it may be peptic ulceration or esophageal laceration.

POSTNECROTIC SCARRING (CIRRHOSIS)

Whenever there is *total* destruction of an hepatic lobule, reconstitution is not possible and scarring must result. As is indicated in our discussion of *massive liver necrosis* (p. 518), necrosis of total lobules and indeed whole lobes is encountered in fulminant viral hepatitis and in poisonings from carbon tetrachloride, chloroform, toxic mushrooms, cinchophen, tetracycline, phosphorus, heavy metals and certain drugs. The resultant fibrosis is entirely dependent on the distribution of the necrosis. Some would not include postnecrotic

scarring as a form of cirrhosis; they point out that a single large area or one whole lobe may be affected, producing a wide field of scarring, with the remainder of the liver unaffected. Moreover, the necrosis generally occurs as a single massive assault, and the scarring is an end stage. However, more often the necrosis is patchy and widely distributed, and the scarring is sufficiently diffuse and accompanied by regeneration to create a nodular, distorted liver, which satisfies all the more stringent criteria of cirrhosis.

The morphology of postnecrotic scarring is as varied as the unpredictable distribution of massive necrosis. Sometimes the liver becomes grotesquely misshapen by alternating massive scars and intervening spared areas. Characteristically, the spared areas are entirely normal in color and consistency. A whole lobe may be converted into an atrophic, fibrotic appendage. In other circumstances, the scarring may be quite diffuse, producing irregular lumpiness. The resultant nodules generally are much larger than those encountered in the alcoholic form of cirrhosis. **The diagnostic features of postnecrotic scarring are precisely the large size of the scars and the wide intervening zones of normal hepatic substance.** The overall size of the liver is quite variable, but it is usually reduced, sometimes markedly (Fig. 15–7).

Histologically, the classic features are the combination of broad scars replacing entire liver lobules, interspersed with completely normal hepatic substance (Fig. 15–8). Within the scars, a mononuclear infiltrate and bile duct and ductular proliferation and reduplication are present. Often, closely crowded large ducts and portal triads are seen in scars as residuals left behind in the collapse of the intervening necrotic hepatic substance. Regenerative activity may be found in hepatocytes bordering on the scars. At an earlier stage of the process, necrotic liver cells may persist, along with an acute inflammatory infiltration and vascularized fibroplasia. Fatty change generally is absent, although of course it may be a residual of a preexisting liver injury.

From the clinical standpoint, one would anticipate that these patients would provide, in most instances, a history compatible with massive necrosis of the liver. Although this is sometimes true, in over half the cases no acute episode precedes the development of postnecrotic scarring. It must be assumed that the liver damage occurred insidiously. In all cases, it is obvious that sufficient hepatic parenchyma must be spared to permit survival of the patient. The irregular pattern of scarring may produce a lobularity that is palpable clinically. Signs of portal hypertension may or may not develop, depending upon the distribution and severity of the fibrosis. Theoretically, liver function should stabilize once

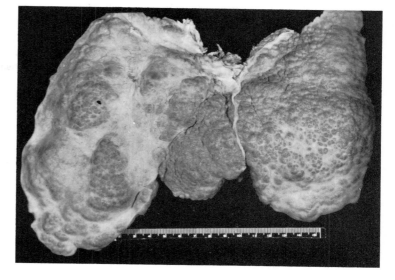

Figure 15–7. Postnecrotic scarring, characterized by irregular random areas of massive fibrosis alternating with other areas of more delicate scarring, producing the finer nodularity. The lobe on the left has been almost totally destroyed.

scarring has developed. However, for obscure reasons, conceivably involving impaired blood supply or continuing liver disease, patients with postnecrotic scarring may suffer progressive deterioration of liver function and die of hepatic failure some years later. Perhaps marginal zones of liver cells, working at full metabolic capacity with barely adequate blood supply, slowly yield to the overload and in this way the functional capacity ebbs and the scarring increases. Most of these patients die within the first year of developing massive necrosis, but a significant number die three to five years later of slowly advancing hepatic insufficiency.

BILIARY CIRRHOSIS

This pattern of cirrhosis implies diffuse injury and scarring distributed throughout the liver in close relationship to the interlobular bile ducts. Whatever the nature of the injury, it appears to be localized at first to the biliary tract, and the scarring thus begins about these ducts and then involves the portal triads. Eventually, the fibrous tissue extends out to interconnect with adjacent portal areas and thus enclose individual lobules. *Several forms of injury have been identified, and biliary cirrhosis has been divided into primary and secondary types.* We can consider the *secondary type* first because its genesis is relatively simple. It is encountered in patients who have had posthepatic obstructive jaundice or biliary tract infections. Complete obstruction to the outflow of bile produces back pressure throughout the entire biliary system. The interlobular bile ducts and cholangioles are damaged by the impacted, inspissated bile, and the injury leads to an inflammatory reaction and scarring. Subtotal obstruction often leads to an ascending cholangitis and cholangiolitis as bacteria ascend within or about the ramifications of the biliary tract. The gram-negative bacilli and enterococci are the common culprits. Inflammation of the portal triads and periportal scarring ensue without striking evidence of inspissation of bile.

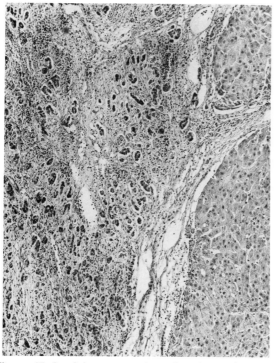

Figure 15–8. A low power view of postnecrotic scarring of the liver. The massive fibrous scar contains many closely crowded bile ducts resulting from the total destruction of whole liver lobules. The islands of preserved liver cells on the right are free of fat.

Primary biliary cirrhosis is less clearly understood. It is almost exclusively a disease of middle-aged women. At one time, it was considered a form of cholangiolitic viral hepatitis leading to cirrhosis. However, hepatitis B surface antigen has been identified in only a few of these patients, and there is no proof of a viral etiology. These patients have a number of abnormal immunologic changes, but it is still not known whether they have causative significance or are merely secondary findings. Immune complexes, containing principally IgM, and transformed lymphocytes and plasma cells have been found in and around bile ducts in this disorder (Fox et al., 1969). As mentioned earlier in the discussion of chronic hepatitis (p. 520), variety of autoantibodies are found in patients with primary biliary cirrhosis. These include antibodies against mitochondria (M-antibody) in nearly all such patients, and smooth muscle antibody, antinuclear antibodies and rheumatoid factor in a significant minority (Golding et al., 1973). The mitochondrial antibodies are neither organ nor species specific. Their presence is valuable in differentiating primary from secondary biliary cirrhosis (M-test). Such autoantibodies are also more frequent in the families of patients with biliary cirrhosis, suggesting a genetic predisposition. Often patients with primary biliary cirrhosis have an associated disease of an autoimmune nature, such as Sjögren's syndrome, rheumatoid arthritis or thyroiditis (Sherlock and Scheuer, 1973).

Morphology. Common to all patterns of biliary cirrhosis is a diffuse, regular and delicate scarring about each lobule, which gives a fine, sandpaper texture to the surface of the liver. The liver may or may not be green, depending on the genesis of the scarring and on the amount of bile stasis. In the secondary forms that have a large obstructive component, bile staining is prominent. In the primary form, bile stasis may or may not be present, depending upon the amount of destruction of the interlobular bile ducts. The liver generally is almost normal or only slightly reduced in size.

Histologically, the principal characteristics of this form of cirrhosis are: (1) regularity of fibrosis, extending out to interconnect portal triads, (2) bile duct and ductular injury, proliferation, regeneration and reduplication within the scars, and (3) a mononuclear infiltration, principally of lymphocytes admixed with plasma cells, in the scars. The fibrous tissue rarely invades the lobules, as it may with alcoholic cirrhosis. Secondary features relate to the particular pathogenetic mechanism. In the form induced by obstruction, bile stasis is prominent. The bile duct, ductules and canaliculi contain inspissated bile. Large accumulations of bile (referred to as **"bile lakes"**) may be present within the hepatic substance. In the disease produced by ascending cholangitis, inflammatory cells, principally polymorphonuclear leukocytes, are scattered within the finer ramifications of the biliary tract. They are also prominent in the periductular fibrous tissue. In the primary form of biliary cirrhosis, plasma cells are prominent in the periductular fibrous tissue. Lymphoid follicles may appear in these areas. In the same location, aggregations of lipid filled macrophages and granulomas resembling those of sarcoid are present. This granulomatous reaction may be a sequel to the death of lipophages within the scars, but it has also been offered as proof of a possible immunologic mechanism. The lipophages are presumed to reflect the hypercholesterolemia that is so characteristic of this form of biliary cirrhosis. As was previously mentioned, immune complexes can be demonstrated in the bile duct epithelium but not within hepatocytes (Paronetto et al., 1967).

Clinical Course. The clinical findings are very variable and depend upon the genesis of the liver disease. Jaundice and itching are prominent, particularly in those with the obstructive form of the disease. Fever, right upper quadrant pain and marked leukocytosis are characteristic of the ascending infectious variety. Primary biliary cirrhosis usually begins with the insidious onset of pruritus, with jaundice developing only later (Sherlock and Scheuer, 1973). For obscure reasons, hypercholesterolemia may be encountered. Indeed, these patients have skin xanthomas and often have florid atherosclerosis, with an increased risk of myocardial infarction (Schaffner, 1969). Because all forms of biliary cirrhosis yield deficient flow of bile into the duodenum, the malabsorption syndrome is more often encountered with this form of cirrhosis than with the others. In most cases of biliary cirrhosis, whatever the pathogenesis, hepatic failure ultimately ensues, but in contrast to the other cirrhoses *portal hypertension is uncommon* until very late in the course.

PIGMENT CIRRHOSIS— HEMOCHROMATOSIS

The most important iron storage disorder, hemochromatosis, is a well-defined clinical syndrome characterized by: (1) a heavily hemosiderotic "portal" cirrhosis known as pigment cirrhosis, (2) pancreatic fibrosis and siderosis, (3) siderosis of other organs and (4) pigmentation of the skin. The combination of features (2) and (4) has given rise to the clinical designation "bronze diabetes" (Marble and Bailey, 1951). Additional characteristics of the usual case are greatly increased body stores of iron of up to 80 g.; elevated levels of plasma iron, in the range of 200 to 250 μg. per 100 ml. of plasma; and excessive saturation of transferrin, of the order of 60 to 70 per cent. Most constant among these various features are the iron overload, systemic siderosis and pigment cirrhosis. Diabetes may be absent in one third of patients, and the pigmentation is so subtle (a summer tan) as to be readily missed or absent in about one half. The classic form of hemochromatosis is preponderantly a male disease, in the ratio of 9 to 1, and it rarely becomes manifest before the age of 40 years. The sex distribution is attributed to the protection against iron overload afforded to women by menstruation and pregnancy, whereas the age range is compatible with the many years required to accumulate the ten- to twenty-fold increases of total body iron. In patients receiving multiple transfusions or having other exogenous sources for their iron overload, there is no sex predilection.

Etiology and Pathogenesis. The nature of the fundamental defect leading to such massive iron overload is unknown. There are two widely held but opposing conceptions: (1) that the disease is a hereditary inborn error of iron metabolism, or (2) that no genetic defect need be invoked, since there are adequate grounds for accepting hemochromatosis as an acquired disorder.

Support for the genetic, metabolic theory is provided by the occasional familial distribution of this disease (Sheldon, 1935; Crosby, 1966). Elevated levels of plasma iron and excessive saturation of transferrin have been identified in immediate relatives of patients with hemochromatosis (Morgan, 1961; Walsh et al., 1964). However, no clear-cut pattern of mendelian inheritance has been established. An increased mucosal uptake and retention of iron has been reported in certain patients with this disorder (Boender et al., 1967). This increased transfer of iron across the mucosal cells is attributed to an enzyme abnormality in intestinal mucosal cells, but the evidence for this is meager (Mazur and Sackler, 1967). Other studies have suggested an increased tissue avidity for iron in the form of excessive synthesis of tissue iron-binding proteins (Goldberg and Smith, 1960). However, this conception also is not well established. A deficiency of a specific gastric inhibitor of iron absorption is offered as another possible genetic defect, but here again the evidence is contradictory (Davis et al., 1966; Smith et al., 1969). If there is a genetic defect, then, its existence and nature have not been clearly elucidated (Powell, 1970; Boender and Verloop, 1969).

The opposing view of the nature of hemochromatosis is that it is an acquired disease which develops from (1) excesses of dietary iron, or (2) prolonged parenteral administration of iron—for example, from repeated transfusions. Emphasis is placed on the known imperfections in mucosal control of iron absorption and on the variation among individuals in the amount of iron absorbed following even relatively normal levels of dietary intake. It has been pointed out that with increasing loads of dietary iron, the absolute amount absorbed also increases. Presumably, South African Bantus, who brew their beer and cook their food in iron utensils, develop systemic hemosiderosis on this basis. Some develop a disorder quite similar to hemochromatosis. A higher than anticipated incidence of hemochromatosis has been observed among wine-drinking populations (MacDonald, 1963). Here it is argued that the alcohol first induces cirrhosis of the liver. For mysterious reasons, cirrhosis from any cause leads to increased iron absorption, and wine contains large amounts of iron. In these cases, then, the hemochromatosis would be secondary to alcoholic cirrhosis. Patients receiving transfusions or iron-containing drugs throughout their life, such as those having some form of chronic anemia, have sometimes developed hemochromatosis. Thus, it is held that a mysterious genetic defect need not be invoked, since the "mucosal block" is not perfect and, in some circumstances, the iron is delivered directly to the body (as in transfusions), bypassing any theoretical block.

These somewhat conflicting theories have been reconciled by postulating two forms of the disease: a primary and a secondary or "exogenous" syndrome. Indeed, it is contended that exogenous hemochromatosis and the primary disease have many dissimilarities (Charlton and Bothwell, 1966). In general, the idiopathic disease is characterized by larger stores of body iron which are more mobilizable and chelatable than the deposits in the exogenous forms (Powell, 1970). Perhaps we are dealing with two separate diseases or the same (or virtually the same) end point of two pathways. Alternatively, it is possible to consider hemochromatosis a genetic disease which requires environmental stress for its clinical expression (Crosby, 1970).

Still another issue remains in the pathogenesis of this controversial disease: Is the iron overload in the tissues responsible for the organ injury? In particular, what is the cause of the pigment cirrhosis of the liver? According to those who believe in a genetic defect, the iron gradually accumulates, causing siderosis and injury of the organs in which the iron is stored (Crosby, 1966). Those who see it as an acquired disease, however, suggest instead that cirrhosis is possibly the fundamental defect and it, in turn, leads to the increased iron absorption and hemosiderosis. In support of this contention is the high incidence of alcoholism in patients with hemochromatosis. Alternatively, the hemosiderosis, whatever its cause, may overload and blockade the RE system with pigment, thus exposing the liver to endotoxins or bacteremias as the cause of the cirrhosis (MacDonald et al., 1968). Since there is so much speculation, it must be apparent that the relationship of the iron overload and pigment to the cellular and organ damage is still obscure.

Morphology. The morphologic changes are characterized principally by systemic hemosiderosis accompanied by cirrhosis of the liver and fibrosis of the pancreas. The most striking involvement is the **pigment cirrhosis.** Classically, the liver is diffusely and finely nodular, chocolate-brown and enlarged up to perhaps 3.0 kg. The nodules vary from several millimeters to 1.0 cm. in diameter and are set apart by fine strands of interlacing connective tissue. The brown pigmentation is produced by massive amounts of hemosiderin deposited within hepatic parenchymal cells, as well as within Kupffer cells and bile duct epithelium and in the areas of scarring (Fig. 15--9). At one time,

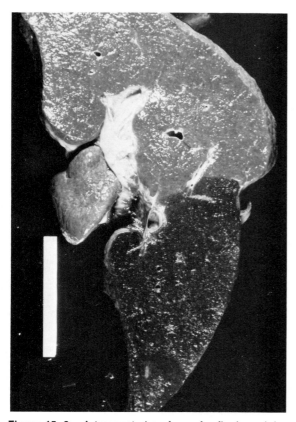

Figure 15–9. A transected surface of a finely nodular liver with pigment cirrhosis. Potassium ferriferrocyanide has been applied to the lower half, and the contained hemosiderin has produced the black discoloration.

much was made of the finding of so-called **hemofuscin,** principally in fibroblasts, bile duct epithelium and the smooth muscle cells of the walls of blood vessels. At present, such hemofuscin is recognized as the common lipofuscin found almost ubiquitously in all forms of cirrhosis, as well as in other forms of tissue injury. It is generally believed that primary hepatocarcinoma is a more frequent complication of pigment cirrhosis than of the other forms of cirrhosis (p. 513) (Warren and Drake, 1951). The incidence of intercurrent liver carcinoma, as cited in the literature, varies from 8 per cent up to the extraordinary level of 42 per cent.

The pancreas is extensively pigmented and often has a diffuse interstitial fibrosis. The hemosiderin is found in both the acinar cells of the exocrine glands and the islet cells. Pigment is also present in the interstitial stroma. There is no clear correlation between the levels of siderosis of the pancreas and the occurrence or severity of diabetes mellitus.

The **reticuloendothelial system** throughout the body is heavily pigmented. Some contend that in the primary idiopathic form of the disease, the RE system is less involved than parenchymal cells, whereas in the secondary, acquired forms of the disease, the RE system is first overloaded, virtually to the point of blockade, and the excess iron is then shunted into the parenchymal cells. In any event, the siderosis is usually sufficiently marked to color the spleen and lymph nodes brown.

The **heart** often has hemosiderin granules within the myocardial fibers. Indeed, in some cases, the pigmentation is sufficiently extensive to cause a striking brown coloration, and these patients may even show signs and symptoms of heart dysfunction.

Virtually any or all of the glandular and epithelial cells of the body may be pigmented, including the thyroid acini, the testicular cells, the cortical cells of the adrenal, the lining epithelial cells of the renal tubules and the cells of the salivary glands.

Mention was made earlier that these patients also have skin pigmentation, hence the designation "bronze diabetes." It is paradoxical that most of this pigmentation results from an increased production of melanin within the basal layer of the epidermis. Some siderosis may be found in fibroblasts in the corium of the skin, chiefly about the dermal appendages.

Clinical Course. The controversy over the role of iron as the ultimate cause of tissue injury is more than academic. If the disease may be acquired, and if excess iron is injurious, then clearly efforts should be made as early as possible to control the dietary intake in vulnerable patients. Moreover, phlebotomy offers a method of draining iron (about 200 to 250 mg. per 500 ml. of blood) from the body. Indeed, repeated phlebotomies in these patients have yielded: (1) reduction in iron deposits in the liver, (2) improvement in liver function, and (3) amelioration of the diabetes. Whether such improvement is related to the depletion of iron or is secondary to better medical care is still uncertain. How effective such treatment will be in altering the usual course of this disease remains to be established. In earlier times, patients usually followed a long, protracted downhill course extending over years. Of a series of patients autopsied at the Boston City Hospital, nearly 50 per cent died of infections, 17 per cent of heart failure, 10 per cent of liver cell carcinoma, 7 per cent of gastrointestinal bleeding, 5 per cent of liver failure, and the remainder of miscellaneous causes (MacDonald and Mallory, 1960).

INDETERMINATE AND MISCELLANEOUS FORMS OF CIRRHOSIS

In any collection of cirrhoses of the liver, as many as 20 per cent will conform to none of the previously described morphologic and pathogenetic categories. The temptation is to discern suggestive findings and thus to assign these cases to one or another of the better characterized entities. However, it is probably wiser to retain a wastebasket designation of *indeterminate* or *cryptogenic cirrhosis* as a reminder of the mysteries shrouding the genesis of scarring of the liver. It is entirely possible that these indeterminate cases reflect multiple causes of liver injury—for example, the concurrence of alcohol abuse and chronic viral hepatitis or other such combinations. It is of interest in this regard that about one fifth of patients with cryptogenic cirrhosis have hepatitis B surface antigen in their serum (Javitt et al., 1973). Another group of approximately equal size has a variety of autoantibodies similar to those often associated with lupoid hepatitis or with primary biliary cirrhosis (Golding et al., 1973). It is entirely possible, then, that cryptogenic cirrhosis may in many cases represent the end stage of chronic active hepatitis or of a lupoid hepatitis. Recently it has become apparent that a genetically determined deficiency of serum α_1-antitrypsin may be associated with cirrhosis as well as with emphysema (see p. 386). Presumably in these cases the liver synthesizes defective α_1-antitrypsin, which it is unable to secrete into the serum, and so the enzyme accumulates within the liver cells (Weiser et al., 1975). Another genetically determined cause of cirrhosis is Wilson's disease, which results from a defect in copper metabolism. Here there is degeneration of the basal ganglia of the brain, as well as cirrhosis (see p. 672).

Here we should describe the entity *posthepatitic cirrhosis*. This is a poorly defined lesion of somewhat obscure origin. Despite the designation posthepatitic, it does not necessarily imply a prior viral infection. However, hepatitis B is known to lead to scarring in some cases and may be one of the origins of this pattern of cirrhosis. As described by Gall (1966), posthepatitic cirrhosis is characterized by a fine trabecular scarring, enclosing single or multiple liver lobules with relative preservation of the intralobular architecture. Such scarring is perfectly compatible with the fibrosis seen in occasional cases of hepatitis B and may represent the end stage of chronic active hepatitis. Possibly this is a morphologic lesion having many origins, the common denominator being diffuse submassive injury to the liver with consequent widely distributed but delicate scarring.

HEPATIC AND PORTAL VEIN THROMBOSIS

Hepatic vein thrombosis (Budd-Chiari syndrome) constitutes a posthepatic cause of portal hypertension. Portal vein thrombosis falls within the prehepatic category. Thrombosis in either of these large venous channels usually results from focal infections or tumors which either invade the walls of the veins directly or compress the lumen from without. The hepatocarcinoma in particular has a predilection for invading the hepatic veins and growing within the radicles into the major outflow channels. In the case of the portal vein, it is usually affected in the region of the porta hepatis. The lymph nodes in this vital area are often secondarily involved by inflammatory and neoplastic processes. On occasion, thromboses beginning within the finer ramifications of the portal drainage system propagate in the direction of blood flow, eventually occluding the main channel. This sequence may follow intra-abdominal surgery, particularly on structures within the upper abdomen, or be triggered by a localized infection within the peritoneal cavity. If the thrombus becomes infected, the extension of the inflammatory process into the portal vein creates what is known as *pylephlebitis*.

The Budd-Chiari syndrome is inevitably followed by rapidly progressive portal hypertension and ascites. Surprisingly, extrahepatic portal vein thrombosis may cause little or no ascites, despite elevation of the pressure within the portal system.

SILENT JAUNDICE

Jaundice appearing in an otherwise asymptomatic patient is quite characteristic of certain disorders of the liver and biliary tract. So insidious may the hyperbilirubinemia be in these patients that not infrequently the jaundice is called to the attention of the patient by family or friends who have noticed yellowing of the sclerae. Genetic disorders in bilirubin metabolism, drug induced cholestasis and carcinoma of the extrahepatic bile ducts are the major causes. It should be emphasized that while some of these conditions make the patient "more yellow than sick," others, such as cancer of the extrahepatic bile ducts, usually are fatal.

HEREDITARY DISORDERS OF BILIRUBIN METABOLISM

The *Gilbert syndrome* is characterized by unconjugated hyperbilirubinemia (Black and Billing, 1969). It is a somewhat poorly defined entity, with multiple causes. Although it is in general considered to be hereditary, some patients have no apparent hereditary background for this condition. The causes of such unconjugated hyperbilirubinemia include: (1) compensated hemolysis, in which active erythropoiesis maintains normal hemoglobin levels despite excessive red cell destruction, (2) excessive bilirubin production in the bone marrow, referred to earlier as "shunt hyperbilirubinemia," and (3) an inherited abnormality of bilirubin uptake into the hepatocytes. As was mentioned earlier, conceivably disorders of the plasma membrane of the hepatocyte might account for the defect in the handling of bilirubin, but this is purely theoretical and has not been demonstrated directly. The hereditary form of the Gilbert syndrome is transmitted as an autosomal dominant. Rarely, a member of such a family has reduced levels of hepatic transferase, perhaps linking this disorder to the Crigler-Najjar syndrome, discussed below.

The *Crigler-Najjar syndrome* is characterized by nonhemolytic, unconjugated hyperbilirubinemia. It occurs in two forms. The more serious type, transmitted as an autosomal recessive, usually becomes manifest in infancy. These infants or children totally lack hepatic glucuronyl transferase and so are unable to conjugate bilirubin. Kernicterus frequently develops during the neonatal period. While most of these infants die of their cerebral disease, a few have survived to adult life. In the less serious form, there is a partial conjugation defect and less severe hyperbilirubinemia. These patients are jaundiced but not sick. The disorder is thought to be transmitted as an autosomal dominant. Although it would seem plausible that the two levels of severity might be manifestations of homozygosity and heterozygosity, no family has been identified in which both forms are present.

No significant hepatic changes have been described.

The *Dubin-Johnson* and *Rotor syndromes* are both characterized principally by conjugated hyperbilirubinemia. These disorders presently are considered to represent reduced hepatic capacity to excrete various organic anions, including conjugated bilirubin. Both are thought to be transmitted as autosomal dominants. Although in both the basic architecture of the liver is preserved, in the Dubin-Johnson syndrome the liver is black. In this form, the hepatocytes contain a finely divided, poorly characterized pigment considered by some to be a form of lipofuscin and by others to be melanin-like. The possible origin of the latter is attributed to impaired biliary excretion of norepinephrine and epinephrine metabolites. Rotor's syndrome, in contrast, does not include pigmentation of the liver. For more details on these interesting familial disorders, reference should be made to Schmid (1966).

DRUG INDUCED CHOLESTASIS

In its broadest interpretation, cholestasis implies obstruction, partial or total, of bile flow. Morphologically, it is manifested by bile plugs in canaliculi and ducts, bile within hepatocytes, and phagocytosis of this pigment by Kupffer cells. Such bile stasis may, of course, be produced by a host of extrahepatic and intrahepatic disorders, which hinder the outflow of the biliary tracts. Cholestasis is obviously a feature of many of the disorders discussed in this chapter. Here we are concerned with those forms not associated with significant liver damage or symptoms other than the appearance of jaundice. It should, however, be pointed out that when cholestasis leads to clinically apparent jaundice, the retained bile salts in the blood often produce itching.

Drug induced cholestasis may be encountered following the use of anabolic steroids, such as methyltestosterone, as well as some of the substitute analogues. It is sometimes encountered in the third trimester of normal pregnancy, in which case it is termed *recurrent jaundice of pregnancy.* Cholestasis has also been reported with the use of contraceptive pills. In all these forms, there is little or no evidence of active inflammation within the liver and, following the pregnancy or discontinuation of the drug, the jaundice abates without sequelae. Another group of drugs, including chlorpromazine, iproniazid (closely related to isoniazid), tetracycline, the sulfonamides, tolbutamide, thiouracil, mercaptopurine and cinchophen, induces not only cholestasis but also liver cell injury, suggesting a possible hypersensitivity reaction. These patients may have other features supporting the concept of some immunogenic reaction, including fever, malaise and skin eruptions typical of many drug sensitivities. When such a reaction is initiated by drugs, it may not be completely reversible, and residual hepatic damage in the form of increased periportal fibrosis has been encountered.

As was discussed earlier, Popper and Schaffner (1970) propose that all forms of cholestasis, even those with such obvious extrahepatic causes as obstruction to the common bile duct, ultimately result in deranged handling of bilirubin by hepatocytes. According to this view, the basic disorder is a disturbance in the secretion of the bile salt micelles, which in turn injures the hepatocytes and impairs cellular bilirubin secretion (p. 510). The hyperbilirubinemia is largely conjugated, but often it has a small unconjugated component.

CARCINOMA OF EXTRAHEPATIC BILE DUCTS INCLUDING AMPULLA OF VATER

While cancers of the pancreas and gallbladder usually evoke pain as a primary or secondary manifestation, those arising in the extrahepatic ducts and ampulla of Vater are extremely insidious and generally produce silent jaundice. The locations of these tumors in descending order of frequency are: (1) the common bile duct, especially its lower end, (2) the junction of the cystic, hepatic and common ducts, (3) the hepatic ducts, (4) the cystic duct, and (5) the duodenal portion of the common bile duct, including the periampullary region. Collectively, these neoplasms are less common than those arising in the gallbladder.

Almost all are extremely small, presumably because, in their strategic locations, they produce posthepatic obstructive jaundice and hepatic decompensation very early. Accordingly, they rarely metastasize widely, but rather infiltrate in the local region and sometimes spread to the lymph nodes of the porta hepatis or to the liver. Some infiltrate the wall of the duct, causing thickening and narrowing of the lumen, whereas others fungate directly into the lumen. Almost all are adenocarcinomas, more or less well differentiated, some with papillary patterns. Mucin secretion is sometimes present. Gallstones are found less frequently in these cancers (in less than one third of patients) than in carcinomas of the gallbladder. One would expect the gallbladder to be enlarged with these tumors, according to **Courvoisier's law.** This law states that neoplasms which obstruct the common bile duct result in enlargement of the gallbladder, whereas obstructing calculi do not, since the gallbladder is too scarred from chronic disease to permit enlargement. However, in practice, Courvoisier's law is not very binding. Indeed, only about a third of cancers of the bile ducts and ampulla of Vater are associated with a palpably enlarged gallbladder (Adams, 1970–71).

The clinical diagnosis is brought to attention by painless obstructive jaundice and pruritus. Roentgenographic and pancreatic secretory studies may help to locate the cause of the jaundice. Subnormal pancreatic secretion following secretin stimulation would indicate a lesion in the ampullary region, affecting the outflow of the pancreatic ducts, while normal pancreatic secretion would suggest a higher level of involvement. Although melena may be produced by periampullary tumors, it is more characteristic of those arising in the head of the pancreas. Worth noting is the possibility of *intermittent* biliary tract obstruction as these lesions ulcerate and permit transient restoration of bile flow (Thorbjarnarson, 1959). Only the periampullary lesions offer hope for cure. If discovered early, they permit a 33 per cent five-year survival (Adams, 1970–71).

PAIN

Vague pain and upper abdominal discomfort may appear with any disorder of the liver, gallbladder or pancreas. Acute severe or disabling pain is a hallmark of certain disorders, i.e., cholelithiasis, cholecystitis and pancreatitis (pancreatic necrosis). Less acute but still severe is the pain evoked by carcinoma of the pancreas and, to a lesser extent, by carcinoma of the gallbladder. In the inflammatory disorders, the pain is often of sudden onset, disabling and sometimes calamitous. The neoplastic processes are characterized rather by the insidious development of pain that progressively intrudes until it dominates the clinical problem.

CHOLELITHIASIS

Gallstones and inflammatory disease of the gallbladder are intimately interrelated, but may occur separately. When they coexist, it is still uncertain as to which precedes. In the United States, about 10 to 20 per cent of the adult population has gallstones. They are rare in the first two decades of life. The four "F's" — fat, female, fertile (multiparous) and forty — characterize the population with the highest incidence. Hemolytic disease also predisposes to stone formation. Recently it has been shown that estrogen-containing drugs are associated with more than twice the normal risk of gallstone formation (Boston Collaborative Drug Surveillance Program, 1974).

Although gallstones may form anywhere in the biliary tract, the great preponderance arise in the gallbladder. In about 80 per cent of cases, **cholesterol** is the chief component of gallstones. Usually these are mixed stones, containing in addition to cholesterol other bile constituents, but occasionally they are pure. As we shall see, cholesterol stones are not related to hypercholesterolemia, but instead depend upon local concentrations of cholesterol in the bile. Cholesterol stones are classically 1 to 5 cm. in diameter, pale yellow, round or oval, and often translucent. On fracture they may reveal spicules radiating from a central point. These stones are also radiolucent. In gallbladders containing such stones, nests of lipophages frequently appear immediately subjacent to the lining epithelium — **cholesterolosis.** Because these nests create yellow-white flecks against the bile-stained surrounding mucosa, the descriptive term "strawberry gallbladder" has been applied. Pigment stones, composed of **calcium bilirubinate,** are next in importance to cholesterol stones. In contrast to cholesterol stones, pigment stones are often fairly pure, in which case they are usually associated with a hemolytic disorder. They are jet-black "jackstones" or, when mixed, spheroids usually under 1 cm. in diameter. They almost never occur singly, and may be present in great numbers. Although calcium carbonate is often a component of mixed stones, pure **calcium carbonate** stones are rare. Conceivably some cause for increased alkalinity of the bile favors the precipitation of calcium carbonate. These stones generally vary in size from sand-like grains to faceted gray-white polyhedral structures up to 2 cm. in diameter.

The genesis of cholesterol stones is something of a mystery (Carey and Small, 1972). Normally, cholesterol is insoluble in an aqueous medium. In bile it is maintained in solution by the formation of micelles having a central core of cholesterol surrounded by a hydrophilic shell made up of bile salts and phospholipids (chiefly lecithin). Thus, the relative proportion of these three constituents is of critical importance. *If the ratio of bile acid plus lecithin to cholesterol falls below a certain level, the bile becomes supersaturated with cholesterol (lithogenic bile), and gallstone formation may occur.* This much is generally agreed upon. More controversial are the nature and cause of a disturbance in this ratio. Is the bile acid-lecithin level abnormally low, or is the cholesterol level abnormally high? Once again, we must summon our courage and equivocate. Most likely both of these situations may occur, and indeed both may be necessary for gallstone formation. Several pathogenetic mechanisms have been proposed:

1. *Elaboration of an abnormal bile by the liver.* The possibility of defective bile acid synthesis by the liver has generated a great deal of interest in recent years (Small, 1972). It has been shown that patients with gallstones have reduced bile acid pools (Vlahcevic et al., 1972). Although in some specific circumstances, such as with disease of the terminal ileum, this may reflect abnormal losses of bile in the feces, in other instances it may reflect diminished hepatic production of bile acids. However, it has recently been shown that patients with reduced bile acid pools tend to compensate through an increased turnover of bile through the enterohepatic cycle (Northfield and Hofmann, 1973).

2. *Increased cholesterol secretion in the bile.* It has been shown that cholesterol production is roughly proportional to total body weight and that this tends to be reflected in increased cholesterol secretion in the bile. Certainly such a mechanism would explain the undoubted increased risk of gallstones among obese individuals.

3. *Local factors within the gallbladder which favor stone formation.* Such factors include stasis, infection and the presence of material to serve as a nidus, such as bacteria or cell debris. At one time these were thought to be the most important predisposing factors; then they were eclipsed by the theory that gallstones result from defective bile formation, that is, from derangements in hepatic metabolism. Recently, local factors have enjoyed a resurgence in their considered importance. In part this resurgence reflects the discovery that even in normal individuals, the bile becomes lithogenic during fasting as bile salts remain sequestered within the gallbladder and cholesterol secretion continues unabated (Grundy, 1973). Such bile stasis may occur in other, pathologic situations, such as with incomplete emptying of the gallbladder. In these cases, the hepatic bile becomes progressively more lithogenic. Mixing within the gallbladder is probably incomplete and diffusion of cholesterol from a nonmicellar to a micellar phase is delayed, favoring stone formation. Other local conditions which may predispose to gallstone formation include inflammation of the gallbladder wall, which causes reabsorption of bile salts by the abnormally permeable gallbladder wall, with a consequent relative increase of cholesterol. In addition, as mentioned, bacteria and cell debris could serve as a nidus for the precipitation of cholesterol.

In summation, it seems more likely that except in extreme situations more than one of these factors must be present for gallstone formation. For example, in an obese individual increased secretion of cholesterol may normally be matched by an increase in bile acid production. If, however, there is some factor limiting such a compensatory response—say, hepatic dysfunction—then gallstone formation would occur.

The clinical significance of gallstones lies in three aspects—their potential for producing obstructive jaundice, their association with cholecystitis and their possible role in the induction of cancer of the gallbladder. Moreover, at any time and without warning, they may pass into the neck of the gallbladder or ducts and produce one of the most severe forms of pain (*biliary colic*) to which man is heir.

CHOLECYSTITIS

Inflammation of the gallbladder may be acute, chronic or acute superimposed on chronic. In the United States, cholecystitis is preceded only by appendicitis as an indication for abdominal surgery. Its distribution in the population closely parallels that of gallstones and indeed stones are present in 80 to 90 per cent of all patients with cholecystitis.

The roles of chemical injury, bacterial infection and gallstones in the initiation of cholecystitis are subjects of contention. The central issues are: Can cholecystitis be caused by chemical injury which predisposes to infection, or is it initiated by bacterial invasion? Could stone formation in the noninflamed gallbladder be the initial event, which is followed by mechanical injury and bacterial invasion?

Bacteria can be cultured from about 80 per cent of all acutely inflamed gallbladders. When only chronic inflammation is present, the incidence falls to about 30 per cent. The most common offenders are *E. coli* and enterococci. On occasion, *Salmonella typhi* localize in the gallbladder following a systemic infection. Bacteria are indisputably absent in some cases. Therefore, it has been proposed that supersaturation or imbalances in the constituents of the bile, such as high levels of bile salts or acids, may induce chemical inflammation. Secondary invasion by bacteria may then ensue. On the other hand, the development of cholecystitis during a systemic bacterial infection suggests an initial bacterial invasion.

Stones could contribute to both mechanisms. If they arise first, they might cause trauma to the wall of the gallbladder and predispose to bacterial invasion. They might also cause obstruction and stasis, and thus favor supersaturation, with resultant chemical injury. Obstruction of the cystic or common ducts would distend the gallbladder and impair the blood supply and lymphatic drainage. Indeed, stones are frequently found in the cystic duct and neck of the gallbladder in acute cholecystitis, but less commonly they are a cause of such obstruction in gallbladders showing only chronic inflammation. In any event, cholelithiasis and cholecystitis are virtually Siamese twins. Pancreatic reflux has also been proposed as a predisposing influence in the induction of inflammation of the gallbladder. Amylases, lipases and proteases can be identified in the bile in many of these cases, and reflux of duodenal juices up the common duct can sometimes be demonstrated. But it must be admitted that such reflux also occurs in some normal individuals as well. Pancreatic secretions may predispose to primary injury, as well as to secondary alterations in the bacterial flora of the bile, but it is doubtful that they contribute significantly to the general causation of cholecystitis. However, we still have no definite answers to these enigmas.

In **acute cholecystitis,** the gallbladder is usually enlarged, tense, edematous, fiery red and often covered with a fibrinosuppurative exudate. Areas of black, gangrenous necrosis may be evident. The wall is characteristically thickened and edematous, and there is generally extensive inflammatory ulceration of the mucosa. As was mentioned, stones are almost invariably present, and not infrequently one is impacted within the neck of the gallbladder, strongly suggesting that it triggered the flareup (Fig. 15–10). The histologic changes are characteristic of any acute inflammatory response. Sometimes the lumen is filled with frank pus, creating **empyema of the gallbladder.**

In **chronic cholecystitis,** the gallbladder may be large, but more often it is contracted. The serosa may be smooth or dulled by subserosal fibrosis. The wall is variably thickened, gray-white and tough. Stones are usually present, as was already mentioned. Mucosal ulcerations are not frequent. The inflammatory reaction is that of a mononuclear infiltrate, and the submucosal and subserosal levels are often fibrosed. Not infrequently the changes of chronic cholecystitis are found with a superimposed acute inflammatory reaction.

On occasion, when a stone has been impacted in the neck of the gallbladder or cystic duct for long periods of time, resorption of the bile solids (excluding the stones) occurs, leaving only a clear, mucinous secretion. This pattern is designated **hydrops of the gallbladder.**

Cholecystitis has many potential consequences. The acute form announces itself loudly with severe, steady, upper abdominal pain, often radiating to the right shoulder. Sometimes, when stones are present in the neck of the gallbladder or in ducts, the pain is colicky. Fever, nausea, leukocytosis and prostration are classic. Slow penetration of the bacteria yields pericholecystic abscesses, or the gangrenous gallbladder may suddenly rupture, producing a violent, acute peritonitis. The bacterial infection may ascend the bile ducts, resulting in intrahepatic ascending cholangitis. Liver abscesses may follow.

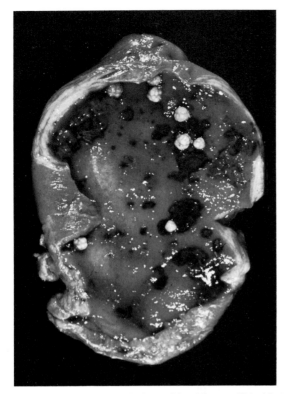

Figure 15–10. Acute cholecystitis. The gallbladder has been opened to show the edematous, thickened wall and glazed, congested mucosa on which rest some small multifaceted gallstones. The dark, irregular patches are areas of mucosal ulceration.

The chronic form of the disease does not have the striking manifestations of the acute form, but is characterized instead by recurrent attacks of either steady or colicky epigastric or right upper quadrant pain. Nausea, vomiting and intolerance of fatty foods are frequent accompaniments. The diagnosis of both the acute and chronic disease often rests on cholecystography (Graham-Cole series) demonstrating malfunctioning of the gallbladder or revealing the presence of stones. It hardly needs to be stated that in the absence of obstructing stones or infection within the common duct, jaundice will not be present.

ACUTE AND CHRONIC PANCREATITIS (ACUTE PANCREATIC NECROSIS; CHRONIC RELAPSING PANCREATITIS)

Acute pancreatitis, also known as *acute hemorrhagic pancreatitis*, is better called *acute pancreatic necrosis*, since it constitutes sudden enzymatic destruction of pancreatic substance by activated lytic pancreatic enzymes. Chronic pancreatitis is more properly referred to as *chronic relapsing pancreatitis*, since it probably represents recurrent miniature attacks of acute pancreatic necrosis. As we shall see, these two forms of pancreatitis are somewhat distinct clinically. Both are most common in middle life; the acute form is somewhat more frequent in females, and the chronic relapsing form is considerably more frequent in males.

Etiology and Pathogenesis. The pathogenesis of pancreatitis is still a mystery. *It is generally agreed that alcoholism and biliary tract disease are both very important contributing factors.* The mechanisms by which these conditions lead to pancreatitis are unknown. It has been observed, however, that the actual attack is very often triggered by an alcoholic debauch or by an excessively large meal. There is also an increased incidence of pancreatitis in patients with hyperparathyroidism. A hereditary form of pancreatitis has been identified, but this accounts for only a very small number of cases (Logan et al., 1968). *There is virtually universal agreement that pancreatic enzymes cause the destruction.* But are they activated within the ducts or instead must the ducts first be ruptured or destroyed, releasing these enzymes prior to activation? Moreover, which of the many pancreatic enzymes are most important? First the question of which are the key enzymes will be examined, followed by a consideration of how these enzymes are activated or released.

Acute pancreatic necrosis is characterized by massive autodigestion of cell proteins and fat. For a long time, trypsin and lipase were considered to be the culprits. As is well known, trypsin is secreted by the pancreas in an inactive form, trypsinogen. A considerable amount of evidence now suggests that trypsin is not a major factor. An endogenous inactivator is present in pancreatic secretion that would neutralize this activated enzyme. Moreover, significant amounts of trypsin have not been detected in either experimental or clinical pancreatitis. However, trace amounts of activated trypsin may participate in a chain reaction, as will be discussed. The observations regarding the role of lipase are more confusing. Some have reported that in the experimental animal lipase is capable of inducing the fat necrosis characteristic of the disorder; others deny this (Elliott et al., 1957). Recently, attention has shifted to two other enzymes, elastase and phospholipase A. Proelastase may be activated by trace amounts of trypsin. It has been identified in the human disease and may be responsible for injury to blood vessels, thus explaining the prominence of hemorrhage in acute pancreatic necrosis. It might also weaken the support of ducts, favoring their rupture (Geokas et al., 1968). Phospholipase A has strong cytotoxicity and damages cell membranes. Injection of this agent produces necrotizing effects in animals and there is evidence that it is operative in man (Creutzfeldt and Schmidt, 1970).

How do these enzymes bring about pancreatic necrosis and how do alcoholism and biliary tract disease fit into these conceptions? Two tentative proposals will be offered. The first might be called the *reflux theory*. Bile and duodenal contents which gained access to the pancreatic ducts might activate intrapancreatic enzymes. Certainly bile acids could liberate minute amounts of active trypsin which would transform proenzymes into phospholipase A and elastase. In turn, phospholipase A could convert the bile lecithin into lysolecithin, a highly toxic substance. However, secretory pressures normally are higher in the pancreatic ducts than in the biliary system, so why would reflux occur? Biliary disease might cause reflux in several ways, the most direct by blockage of the ampulla of Vater by biliary calculi. Such a mechanism would be operative when the main pancreatic duct and the common bile duct form a common channel. In a recent study, gallstones were recovered from the feces of 34 of 36 patients with acute pancreatitis and known gallstones, as opposed to 3 of 36 patients with gallstones but no pancreatic disease. Presumably, the pancreatitis was triggered by transient obstruction of the ampulla by migrating gallstones (Acosta and Ledesma, 1974). Spasm and fibrosis of the sphincter of Oddi have also been invoked as causes of reflux in biliary disease. Duodenal reflux has been a potent mechanism in the induction of pancreatitis in the experimental animal. In this model pancreatitis can be prevented by ligation of the pancreatic ducts. In man, the sphincter of Oddi normally blocks such reflux. Could biliary tract disease or the ingestion of alcohol with duodenal edema alter the sphincteric mechanism?

The second general proposition might be referred to as the *hypersecretion-obstruction theory*. Its proponents propose that rupture of ducts occurs when the pancreas is stimulated to active secretion against partial duct obstruction. The buildup of pressure might rupture small ducts. Alcohol is a potent stimulator of pancreatic secretion. It might also produce duodenal edema, hence impair the outflow of secretions. As was discussed, biliary tract disease or a stone impacted in the common outlet of the biliary and pancreatic systems could also induce obstruction. Unhappily for this theory, pancreatic duct ligation does not evoke massive pancreatic necrosis in experimental animals. However, *total* obstruction might suppress pancreatic secretion altogether and may therefore not be a good

mimic of the clinical problem. Theories abound, but all struggle with the evidence.

Morphology. The morphology of acute pancreatic necrosis stems directly from the action of activated enzymes.

The basic histologic changes are four in number: (1) proteolytic destruction of pancreatic substance, (2) necrosis of blood vessels with subsequent hemorrhage, (3) necrosis of fat by lipolytic enzymes, and (4) an accompanying inflammatory reaction. The extent and contribution of each of these alterations depend upon the duration and severity of the process and vary from one case to the other. In the very early stages, the changes consist only of edema, vascular congestion and a neutrophilic infiltration of the pancreatic interstitium. With progression, there is a focal enzymatic fat necrosis of the exocrine and endocrine cells, with relative preservation of the stroma. This represents the **proteolytic destruction** of the parenchyma. **Hemorrhagic extravasation** may be minimal to extreme. In the milder cases, the interstitium is suffused with red blood cells and fibrin clots; in severe cases, large areas of the pancreatic substance are virtually converted to a mass of blood clot. Perhaps the hallmark of acute pancreatic necrosis is **enzymatic fat necrosis**. This process was described briefly on page 25 and will be recapitulated here. Enzymatic fat necrosis occurs in the peripancreatic fat and in fat depots throughout the abdominal cavity, as well as in the pancreas itself. Liberated lipase enzymatically cleaves the triglycerides stored in the fat cells. Histologically, these cells appear as shadowy outlines of cell membranes filled with pink, granular, opaque precipitate. Presumably, this granular material is derived from the hydrolysis of fat. The liberated glycerol is reabsorbed, and the released fatty acids combine with calcium to form insoluble salts that precipitate in situ. Depending on the amount of calcium deposition, amorphous basophilic precipitates may be visible within the necrotic focus. The **leukocytic reaction** appears between the areas of hemorrhage and necrosis, and in particular rims the foci of fat necrosis. It is less intense than would be anticipated from the amount of tissue damage, highlighting the essential enzymatic rather than inflammatory nature of the destruction (Fig. 15–11). If the patient survives, milder lesions may resolve completely or, when more severe, they may be replaced by fibrosis and calcification. Occasionally, liquefied areas are walled off by fibrous tissue to form cystic spaces, known as **pancreatic pseudocysts**.

Grossly, acute pancreatic necrosis is easily recognized. It is characterized by areas of blue-black hemorrhage interspersed with other areas of gray-white necrotic softening and sprinkled with foci of yellow-white chalky fat necrosis (Fig. 15–12). In individual cases, any one of these three components may dominate. Typically, there are ac-

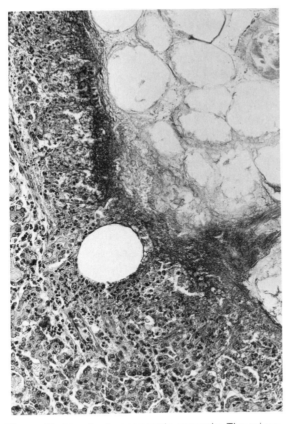

Figure 15–11. Acute pancreatic necrosis. The microscopic field shows a focus of necrosis of the fat cells at upper right, rimmed by an inflammatory hemorrhagic reaction. Preserved pancreatic parenchyma is seen at the bottom left.

companying changes in the remainder of the abdominal cavity. In the majority of instances, the peritoneal cavity contains a serous, slightly turbid, brown-tinged fluid in which globules of oil can be identified (so-called "chicken broth" fluid). The liquid fat globules result from the lipolytic actions of enzymes on adult fat cells. In late cases, this fluid may become secondarily infected, to produce suppurative peritonitis. Additionally, foci of fat necrosis may be found in any of the fat depots, such as the omentum, mesentery of the bowel and properitoneal deposits. **Occasionally, fat necrosis has been described in fat depots outside the abdominal cavity.** This clearly indicates that the released enzymes cause their damage not only by direct escape into the peritoneal cavity, but also, in all probability, by absorption into the blood and lymphatic systems with transport throughout the body. It should be emphasized that the characteristic chalky white foci of fat necrosis and the peritoneal fluid are important findings in establishing the diagnosis of pancreatic necrosis on laparotomy.

As mentioned, attacks of chronic recurrent pan-

creatitis may simply resemble miniature episodes of acute pancreatic necrosis. The morphologic changes are sometimes limited to edema with a minimal interstitial leukocytic infiltrate, but they may include foci of necrosis as described above. **An important point of distinction, however, is the stepwise irreversible destruction of the pancreas which characterizes chronic recurrent pancreatitis.** Eventually such organs become shrunken and fibrotic, with areas of calcification that are readily apparent on x-ray. Pseudocyst formation is common. An occasional pseudocyst may become as large as 20 cm. in diameter, and present as an abdominal mass.

Clinical Course. As might be anticipated, the onset of acute pancreatic necrosis is usually calamitous, manifested by severe abdominal pain, and often followed by shock. Elevated serum levels of lipase and amylase are very important diagnostic findings. The amylase level rises within the first 24 hours, the lipase somewhat later (72 to 96 hours). Both remain elevated during the height of the acute inflammatory necrosis and fall 2 to 5 days after the acute phase passes. It should be cautioned, however, that a variety of other diseases may secondarily affect the pancreas and produce elevation of these serum enzymes (perforated peptic ulcer, carcinoma of the pancreas, intestinal obstruction, peritonitis and indeed any disease that secondarily impinges upon the pancreas). Recently, it has been suggested that an elevated renal clearance of amylase relative to creatinine clear-

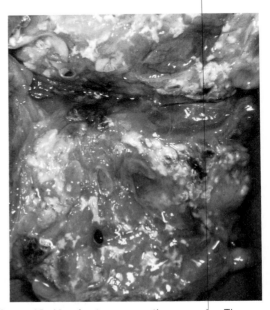

Figure 15–12. Acute pancreatic necrosis. The pancreas has been cross sectioned to disclose the focal areas of pale fat necrosis and darker areas of hemorrhage. Often there is more extensive hemorrhage.

ance is a more specific finding in pancreatitis. Hypocalcemia often develops, presumably because calcium is depleted by binding with fatty acids in the abdomen. Jaundice, hyperglycemia and glycosuria appear in fewer than half of the patients. The mortality rate with acute pancreatic necrosis is high, about 20 to 25 per cent (Editorial, 1975). If the patient survives the acute attack, scarring ensues, and if sufficient destruction of pancreatic substance has occurred, diabetes mellitus and the malabsorption syndrome may be late sequelae. However, such sequelae are more characteristic of the chronic relapsing form of pancreatitis.

Chronic relapsing pancreatitis is less lethal than is the acute disease, but it eventually impairs both the endocrine and exocrine functions of the pancreas. This is the form most closely related to alcoholism. In contrast to the acute disease, chronic relapsing pancreatitis produces recurrent attacks of vague upper abdominal discomfort known to the intern as a "rum belly." Sometimes the pain may be quite severe. The serum levels of pancreatic enzymes are sometimes, but not always, elevated. More often, disturbed islet cell and acinar function are manifested by the development of diabetes mellitus and the malabsorption syndrome. In the latter circumstance deficient pancreatic function can usually be demonstrated by the secretin test.

CARCINOMA OF THE GALLBLADDER

Among the cancers of the biliary tract, carcinoma of the gallbladder is most common. In 60 to 90 per cent of cases, gallstones are also present and, indeed, the incidence of this form of neoplasia follows the pattern of cholelithiasis, affecting females about four times as often as males. Most surgeons believe that gallstones play a causal role in the genesis of cancer by producing chronic irritation of the gallbladder mucosa. In this connection, the close similarity between bile acids and the carcinogen methylcholanthrene raises yet another possibility.

Most cancers of the gallbladder are adenocarcinomas, some mucin secreting. These grow either in an infiltrative pattern, thickening the gallbladder wall, or as exophytic lesions fungating into the lumen. About 5 to 10 per cent are squamous cell carcinomas or adenoacanthomas. Presumably these arise from metaplastic columnar epithelium. All generally spread by local extension. Direct permeation of the liver is characteristic of those arising in the liver bed of the gallbladder. Many situated near the neck of the gallbladder evoke symptoms highly reminiscent of gallstones or cholecystitis. Some grow along the cystic duct, eventually obstructing the common bile duct. Those arising in the fundus of the gallbladder remain silent until their advance impinges upon some structure or function which evokes clinical manifestations. The gallbladder is palpable in about two thirds of patients. Although jaundice eventually develops in most patients, it is relatively mild. Spread to the porta hepatis nodes and liver is frequent. Although widespread metastatic dissemination may occur, it is uncommon.

In a recent series, *right upper quadrant pain was the most common symptom evoked by these lesions* (Warren et al., 1968). Indeed, the symptoms may be indistinguishable from those of cholecystitis or cholelithiasis — symptoms which may be all too familiar to these patients, hence not particularly alarming. More ominous is the appearance of anorexia and weight loss. The five-year survival rate is a tragic 3 per cent.

CARCINOMA OF THE PANCREAS

The term "carcinoma of the pancreas" is meant to imply carcinoma arising in the *exocrine* portion of the gland. (The much less frequent islet tumors will be discussed in the next section.) Carcinoma of the pancreas is now the fourth most frequent cause of death from cancer in the United States. Moreover, its incidence has been steadily and rather rapidly increasing over the years. Unfortunately, the death rate keeps pace, since only rarely is this form of cancer curable. Carcinoma of the pancreas further distinguishes itself by offering virtually no clues as to its etiology or pathogenesis. Males are affected slightly more often than females. The peak incidence occurs at about 60 years of age.

Morphology. Approximately 60 per cent of the cancers of this organ arise in the head of the organ; the remainder are equally divided between the body and tail. Virtually all of these lesions are adenocarcinomas arising in the ductal epithelium. Some may secrete mucin, and many have an abundant fibrous stroma. These desmoplastic lesions therefore present as gritty, gray-white, hard masses. The consistency of these cancers is not too dissimilar from that of a pancreas with chronic inflammatory changes or even of the normal pancreas, a point of importance to the surgeon attempting to identify such lesions by palpation of the organ. The tumor, in its early stages, infiltrates locally and eventually extends into adjacent structures (Figs. 15–13 and 15–14).

With carcinoma of the head of the pancreas, the ampullary region is invaded, obstructing the outflow of bile. In this infiltrative growth, it frequently surrounds and compresses, and less commonly directly invades, the common bile duct or ampulla of Vater. Ulceration of the tumor into the duodenal mucosa may occur. As a consequence of the in-

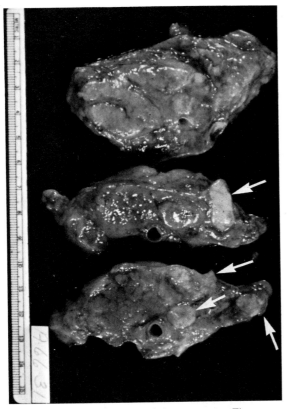

Figure 15–13. Carcinoma of the pancreas. The cross sections of the gland disclose the nodules of pale tumor which virtually replace the entire gland in the top slice, and which are evident as nodules (see arrows) in the lower slices.

volvement of the common bile duct, there is marked distention of the gallbladder in about half of the patients with carcinoma of the head of the pancreas. According to Courvoisier's law, neoplastic obstruction of the biliary outflow tract characteristically induces gallbladder distention, whereas calculous obstruction implies chronic cholecystitis and a fibrotic, undistensible gallbladder. This so-called "law," however, has repeatedly shown itself to be unreliable. Because of the strategic location of carcinomas of the head of the pancreas, patients usually die of hepatobiliary dysfunction while the tumor is still relatively small and not widely disseminated.

In marked contrast, carcinomas of the body and tail of the pancreas remain silent for some time, and may be quite large and widely disseminated by the time they are discovered. They impinge upon the adjacent vertebral column, extend through the retroperitoneal spaces and occasionally invade the adjacent spleen and adrenals. They may extend into the transverse colon or stomach. Peripancreatic, gastric, mesenteric, omental and portahepatic nodes are frequently involved, and the liver is often strikingly seeded with tumor nodules, producing hepatic enlargement of up to two to three times the normal size. Such massive hepatic metastases are quite characteristic of carcinoma of the tail and body of the pancreas, and are attributed to invasion of the splenic vein that courses directly along the margins of the pancreas. Distant metastases occur, principally to the lungs and bones.

Microscopically, there is no difference between carcinomas of the head of the pancreas and those of the body and tail of the pancreas. Most grow in

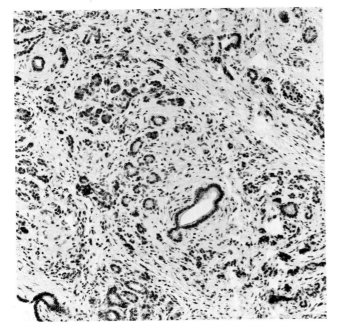

Figure 15–14. Carcinoma of the pancreas. The desmoplastic adenocarcinoma has almost totally replaced the native architecture. Only one normal duct (below center) remains. The cancer grows in small nests and strands of cells scattered in an abundant stroma. Occasionally it reproduces glandlike patterns.

more or less well differentiated glandular patterns. As mentioned, they may be either mucinous or non-mucin secreting. In some cases, the gland patterns are atypical, irregular and small, and lined by anaplastic cuboidal to columnar epithelial cells. Other variants grow in a totally undifferentiated pattern. Rarely, there are adenoacanthomatous patterns, or extremely anaplastic tumors with giant cell formation, numerous mitoses and bizarre pleomorphism.

Clinical Course. From the preceding discussion, it should be evident that carcinomas in the pancreas remain silent until their extension impinges upon some other structure. It is when they erode to the posterior wall of the abdomen and affect nerve fibers that pain appears. There has long been a prevalent misconception that carcinoma of the pancreas is a painless disease. Many large series have clearly documented that pain is usually the first symptom, although unfortunately, by the time pain appears, these cancers have already encroached on adjacent structures. *Those arising in the head of the pancreas eventually cause jaundice, while those of the body and tail remain difficult to diagnose until weight loss and pressure on adjacent organs make evident the cause of the pain.* The pain classically is dull and steady, radiates through to the back, and is exacerbated by reclining and relieved by bending forward. Nausea, vomiting and anorexia, although common, are not helpful diagnostic clues. In some patients, significant weight loss makes evident the seriousness of the problem, but, regrettably, most often the tumor has already metastasized. The patient with a lesion in the head of the pancreas may develop jaundice early enough to permit surgical removal. Eventually jaundice is intense. With lesions that arise in the body and tail, gastric or bowel disturbances, malabsorption, diabetes mellitus or splenomegaly (obstruction of the splenic vein) may be the first localized finding. Spontaneously appearing *phlebothrombosis,* also called *migratory thrombophlebitis,* is sometimes seen with carcinoma of the pancreas, particularly those of the body and tail *(Trousseau's sign).* But, as was mentioned, this syndrome is not pathognomonic of a cancer in this organ (p. 107).

Because of the insidiousness of these lesions, there has long been a search for biochemical tests indicative of their presence. Elevated serum levels of carcinoembryonic antigen (CEA) are found in 91 per cent of patients with carcinoma of the pancreas—a higher percentage of patients than with any other disorder, including carcinoma of the colon (Hansen, et al., 1974). However, the presence of elevated CEA levels with so many disorders, as well as in some normal cigarette smokers, limits its usefulness as a screening procedure. Because of the difficulties in establishing the diagnosis, the final diagnosis is usually made at exploratory laparotomy, by which time the lesion is advanced. Five-year survival is only 2 per cent, and most patients survive less than a year after diagnosis (Silverberg and Holleb, 1974).

METABOLIC PANCREATIC ISLET DISORDERS

Hyperfunctioning of the islets of Langerhans usually produces one of three distinctive syndromes: (1) *hyperinsulinism,* due to beta-cell hyperfunction, (2) the Zollinger-Ellison syndrome, caused by the elaboration of *gastrin* from an islet lesion, and (3) a recently defined *hyperglucagon* syndrome, consisting of diabetes, anemia and a characteristic skin rash, involving tumors of the alpha-2-cells (Mallinson et al., 1974). Very often lesions of the islets produce more than one of these indigenous hormones. In addition, ectopic hormones, such as ACTH, MSH or a secretin-like material, may be produced by carcinomas of the pancreatic islets (Editorial, 1973b). The islet cells are also apparently capable of elaborating a number of other polypeptide hormones, including VIP (vasoactive intestinal peptide), a recently identified substance or group of substances which may be responsible for a watery-diarrhea syndrome, also known as "pancreatic cholera" (Soergel, 1975). This capacity of cells in the pancreatic islets to synthesize a variety of polypeptide hormones places them within the far-flung APUD system of hormone-secreting cells, described on page 617.

The most frequent of the syndromes produced by hyperfunctioning of the islets of Langerhans is hyperinsulinism, followed in importance by the Zollinger-Ellison syndrome. In many cases, the latter is accompanied by dysfunction in other endocrine glands. It is then a component of the disorder known as multiple endocrine adenomatosis (MEA I), discussed on page 617.

All of these syndromes are associated with virtually identical morphologic lesions in the pancreas, and so the anatomic changes can be presented as a group, after which we shall give brief clinical characterizations of hyperinsulinism and the Zollinger-Ellison syndrome. One of three lesions may be present: (1) hyperplasia of the islets, (2) benign adenomas (single or multiple), or (3) carcinoma of the islets. Only rarely are these lesions nonfunctioning. In the hyperplastic form, the islets are diffusely enlarged, two- or threefold, but nonetheless have normal architecture and apparently normal cells. The adenomas are small, encapsulated brown nodules, rarely over 5 cm. in diameter (Fig. 15–15). Multiple adenomas of varying size may be scattered throughout the pancreas. Histologically, these benign tumors look remarkably like giant islets, and there is preservation of the regular cords of islet cells. As will be mentioned shortly, special stains may reveal differences in the cell populations of these tumors in the various syndromes. Surprisingly, the malignant tumors of islet cell origin are composed of virtually normal-appearing cells showing very little anaplasia. Rarely, undifferentiated lesions are encountered. Accordingly, the diagnosis of cancer on histologic grounds is difficult and rests largely on unmistakable evidence of local invasion or, more securely, on metastatic spread to such sites as the regional lymph nodes or the liver. Wider dissemination is uncommon.

Lesions causing **hyperinsulinism** are composed dominantly or completely of beta cells. Analysis of pancreatic islet lesions inducing hyperinsulinism indicates that about 70 per cent are solitary adenomas, approximately 10 per cent are multiple adenomas, 10 per cent are metastasizing tumors that must be interpreted as carcinomas, and the remainder are a mixed group of diffuse hyperplasia of the islets and adenomas occurring in ectopic pancreatic tissue. Diffuse hyperplasia of the islets as a cause of hyperinsulinism is primarily encountered in infants born of diabetic mothers. Here the changes are presumably compensatory to the high blood glucose levels in the fetus.

It is hardly necessary to detail the symptomatology of excess insulin, but it may be of value to point out that the hypoglycemia, particularly in the early morning before breakfast, may be so extreme as to produce coma and even death. Less extreme cases often pass unrecognized for long periods of time, despite such vague complaints as attacks of dizziness, periodic lapses of memory and general weakness. The astute clinician may be able to elicit a definite relationship between these complaints and the intervals between meals.

The *Zollinger-Ellison syndrome* is caused by lesions of other than beta cells (Zollinger and Ellison, 1955). Clinically, it is characterized principally by extraordinary gastric acid hypersecretion (10 to 20 times normal) and consequent multiple, intractable peptic ulcerations, sometimes in unusual locations, such as the jejunum, third and fourth portions of the duodenum, and esophagus. Some patients have diarrhea, malabsorption and hypokalemia. Gastrin (or a gastrin-like secretagogue) has been extracted from some of these tumors and presumably explains most of the clinical features. The cell type responsible for the elaboration of the gastrin is still uncertain. The alpha cell elaborates glucagon, which decreases gastric secretion.

In a review of the Zollinger-Ellison syndrome, 60 per cent of cases were found to be caused by malignant tumors of the islets, 30 per cent were caused by benign adenomas and 10 per cent were associated with diffuse islet hyperplasia (Ellison and Wilson, 1964). Some patients had multiple adenomas in the pancreas, as well as adenomas of the parathyroids and pituitary, and so presumably they had MEA I (p. 617). Recently it has become appreciated that a syndrome indistinguishable from the Zollinger-Ellison syndrome may be produced by hyperplasia of the G-cells within the gastric antrum (see p. 475). In these cases there is no lesion of the pancreatic islets. In what can only be construed as a monumental conspiracy to generate confusion, this is sometimes termed the Zollinger-Ellison syndrome type I, while the originally described syndrome involving a pancreatic lesion is called the Zollinger-Ellison syndrome type II (Ganguli et al., 1974).

REFERENCES

Abelev, G. I.: Production of embryonal serum alpha-globulin by hepatomas: Review of experimental and clinical data. Cancer Res., *28*:1344, 1968.

Acosta, J. M., and Ledesma, C. L.: Gallstone migration as

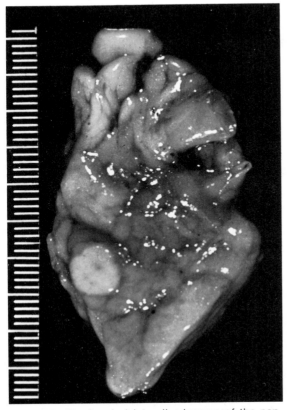

Figure 15–15. A pale islet cell adenoma of the pancreas (lower left). Despite its small size, it produced hyperinsulinism.

a cause of acute pancreatitis. New Eng. J. Med., *290*:484, 1974.

Adams, J. T.: *In* Philip Rubin, ed.: Clinical Oncology for Medical Students and Physicians. 3rd ed. New York, American Cancer Society, 1970–1971, p. 141.

Adams, R. D., and Foley, J. M.: The neurological disorder associated with liver disease in metabolic and toxic disease of the nervous system. Res. Publ. Ass. Nerv. Ment. Dis., *32*:98, 1953.

Almeida, J. D., et al.: Virus-like particles in hepatitis-A positive fecal extracts. Lancet, *2*:1083, 1974.

Berger, R., et al.: Transfusions in the treatment of fulminating hepatitis. New Eng. J. Med., *274*:497, 1966.

Black, M., and Billing, B. H.: Hepatic bilirubin U.D.P.-glucuronyl transferase activity in liver disease and Gilbert's disease. New Eng. J. Med., *280*:1266, 1969.

Blaisdell, F. W., and Cohen, R.: Cirrhosis of the liver. Clinical course in 2,377 patients at the San Francisco General Hospital. Calif. Med., *94*:353, 1961.

Blumberg, B. S., et al.: A new "antigen" in leukemia serum. J.A.M.A., *191*:541, 1965.

Boender, C. A., and Verloop, M. C.: Iron absorption, iron loss and iron retention in man. Studies after oral administration of a tracer dose of $^{59}FeSO_4$ and $^{131}BaSO_4$. Brit. J. Hemat., *17*:45, 1969.

Boender, C. A., et al.: Iron absorption and retention in man. Nature (London), *213*:1237, 1967.

Boston Collaborative Drug Surveillance Program: Surgically confirmed gallbladder disease, venous thromboembolism, and breast tumors in relation to postmenopausal estrogen therapy. New Eng. J. Med., *290*:15, 1974.

Carey, C. M., and Small, D. M.: Micelle formation by bile salts. Arch. Intern. Med., *130*:506, 1972.

Charlton, R. W., and Bothwell, T. H.: Hemochromatosis: dietary and genetic aspects. *In* Brown, E. B., and Moore, C. V. (eds.): Progress in Hematology. New York, Grune and Stratton, 1966, p. 298.

Creutzfeldt, W., and Schmidt, H.: Aetiology and pathogenesis of pancreatitis. Scand. J. Gastroent., Suppl. 6:47, 1970.

Crosby, W. H.: Heredity of hemochromatosis. *In* Ingelfinger, F. J., Relman, A., and Finland, M. (eds.): Controversy in Internal Medicine, Philadelphia, W. B. Saunders Co., 1966, p. 261.

Crosby, W. H.: Iron enrichment. Arch. Intern. Med., *126*:911, 1970.

Dane, D. S., et al.: Virus-like particles in serum of patients with Australia-antigen-associated hepatitis. Lancet, *1*:695, 1970.

Davis, P. S., et al.: Reduction of gastric iron-binding protein in hemochromatosis. Lancet, *2*:1431, 1966.

Dienstag, J. L., et al.: Immune electron microscopy and hepatitis A. Lancet, *1*:102, 1975.

Dudley, F. J., et al.: Natural history of hepatitis-associated antigen-positive chronic liver disease. Lancet, *2*:1388, 1972.

Eddleston, A. L. W. F., and Williams, R.: Inadequate antibody response to HBAg or suppressor T-cell defect in development of active chronic hepatitis. Lancet, *2*:1543, 1974.

Editorial: Acute pancreatitis. Lancet, *1*:205, 1975.

Editorial: Deeper into hepatitis B. Lancet, *2*:887, 1973*a*.

Editorial: Liver tumours and steroid hormones. Lancet, *2*:1481, 1973*c*.

Editorial: Streptozotocin for islet-cell carcinoma. Lancet, *2*:1063, 1973*b*.

Elliott, D. W., et al.: Alterations in pancreatic resistance to bile in the pathogenesis of acute pancreatitis. Ann. Surg., *146*:669, 1957.

Ellison, E. H., and Wilson, S. D.: The Zollinger-Ellison syndrome, reappraisal and evaluation of 260 registered cases. Am. Surg., *160*:512, 1964.

Feinstone, S. M., et al.: Hepatitis A: Detection by immune electron microscopy of viruslike antigen associated with acute illness. Science, *182*:1026, 1974.

Feinstone, S. M., et al.: Transfusion-associated hepatitis not due to viral hepatitis type A or B. New Eng. J. Med., *292*:767, 1975.

Fox, R. A., et al.: Impaired delayed hypersensitivity in primary biliary cirrhosis. Lancet, *1*:959, 1969.

Gall, E. A.: Posthepatitic cirrhosis: fact and fancy. *In* Ingelfinger, F., Relman, A. S., and Finland, M. (eds.): Controversy in Internal Medicine. Philadelphia, W. B. Saunders Co., 1966, p. 244.

Ganguli, P. C., et al.: Antral-gastrin-cell hyperplasia in peptic-ulcer disease. Lancet, *1*:583, 1974.

Gartner, L. M., and Arias, I. M.: The formation, transport, metabolism, and excretion of bilirubin. New Eng. J. Med., *280*:1339, 1969.

Geokas, M. C., et al.: The role of elastase in acute hemorrhagic pancreatitis in man. Lab. Invest., *19*:235, 1968.

Gocke, D. J.: Type B hepatitis—good news and bad. New Eng. J. Med., *291*:1409, 1974.

Goldberg, L., and Smith, J. P.: Iron overloading and hepatic vulnerability. Am. J. Path., *36*:125, 1960.

Golding, P. L., et al.: Multisystem involvement in chronic liver disease. Am. J. Med., *55*:772, 1973.

Grundy, S. M.: Cholesterol-bile acid interactions in gallstone pathogenesis. Hospital Prac., Dec., 1973 p. 57.

Gyorkey, F., et al.: Cytoplasmic localization of hepatitis B surface (viral coat) antigen (HBsAg) by electron microscopy. New Eng. J. Med., *290*:1488, 1974.

Hansen, H. J., et al.: Carcinoembryonic antigen (CEA) assay. Hum. Pathol., *5*:139, 1974.

Heathcote, J., et al.: Hepatitis-B antigen in saliva and semen. Lancet, *1*:71, 1974.

Huang, S. N., et al.: A study of the relationship of viruslike particles and Australia antigen in liver. Hum. Pathol., *5*:209, 1974.

Iseri, O.: Ultrastructure of fatty liver induced by prolonged ethanol ingestion. Am. J. Path., *48*:535, 1966.

Iseri, O., and Gottlieb, L. S.: Alcoholic hyalin and megamitochondria as separate and distinct entities in liver alcoholism. Gastroenterology, *60*:1027, 1971.

Ito, K., et al.: Chronic hepatitis-migration inhibition of leukocytes in the presence of Australia antigen. New Eng. J. Med., *286*:1005, 1972.

Javitt, N. B., et al.: Combined Clinical and Basic Science Seminar. Persistent viral hepatitis. Am. J. Med., *55*:799, 1973.

Kohn, J., and Weaver, P. C.: Serum alpha$_1$-fetoprotein in hepatocellular carcinoma. Lancet, *2*:334, 1974.

Korsten, M. A., et al.: High blood acetaldehyde levels after ethanol administration. New Eng. J. Med., *292*:386, 1975.

Krugman, S., et al.: Viral hepatitis, type B, DNA polymerase activity and antibody to hepatitis B core antigen. New Eng. J. Med., *290*:1331, 1974.

Lieber, C. S., and Spritz, N.: Effects of prolonged ethanol intake in man: Role of dietary, adipose, and endogenously synthesized fatty acids in the pathogenesis of the alcoholic fatty liver. J. Clin. Invest., *45*:1400, 1966.

Lieber, C. S.: Metabolic derangement induced by alcohol. Ann. Rev. Med., *18*:35, 1969.

Logan, A., Jr., et al.: Familial pancreatitis. Amer. J. Surg., *115*:112, 1968.

MacDonald, R. A.: Idiopathic hemochromatosis: genetic or acquired? Arch. Intern. Med., *112*:184, 1963.

MacDonald, R. A., and Mallory, G. K.: Hemochromatosis and hemosiderosis: autopsy study of 211 cases. Arch. Intern. Med., *105*:686, 1960.

MacDonald, R. A., et al.: Studies of experimental hemochromatosis. Disorder of the reticuloendothelial system and excess iron. Arch. Path., *85*:366, 1968.

Mallinson, C. N., et al.: A glucagonoma syndrome. Lancet, *2*:2, 1974.

Marble, A., and Bailey, C. C.: Hemochromatosis. Am. J. Med., *11*:590, 1951.

Mazur, A., and Sackler, M.: Hemochromatosis and hepatic xanthine oxidase. Lancet, *1*:254, 1967.

McIntyre, N., and Sherlock, S. (eds.): Therapeutic Agents and the Liver.. Philadelphia, F. A. Davis, 1965.

Morgan, E. H.: Idiopathic hemochromatosis: a family study. Austr. Ann. Med., *10*:114, 1961.

Nielsen, J. O., et al.: Incidence and meaning of the "e" determinant among hepatitis-B-antigen positive patients with acute and chronic liver diseases. Lancet, 2:913, 1974.

Northfield, T. C., and Hofmann, A. F.: Biliary lipid secretion in gallstone patients. Lancet, *1*:747, 1973.

Paronetto, F., et al.: Antibodies to cytoplasmic antigens in primary biliary cirrhosis and chronic active hepatitis. J. Lab. Clin. Med., *69*:979, 1967.

Paronetto, F., and Popper, H.: Lymphocyte stimulation induced by halothane in patients with post halothane hepatitis. New Eng. J. Med., *282*:277, 1970.

Patton, R. B., and Horn, R. C., Jr.: Primary liver carcinoma. Autopsy study of 60 cases. Cancer, *17*:757, 1964.

Popper, H.: Alcoholic hepatitis—an experimental approach to a conceptual and clinical problem. New Eng. J. Med., *290*:159, 1974.

Popper, H., and Orr, W.: Current concepts in cirrhosis. Scand. J. Gastroent., Suppl. *6*:203, 1970.

Popper, H., and Schaffner, F.: Pathophysiology of cholestasis. Hum. Pathol., *1*:1, 1970.

Popper, H., and Zak, F. G.: Pathologic aspects of cirrhosis. Am. J. Med., *24*:592, 1958.

Popper, H., et al.: The social impact of liver disease. New Eng. J. Med., *281*:1455, 1969.

Porta, E. A., and Gomez-Dumm, C. L. A.: New Experimental Approach in Study of Chronic Alcoholism. Lab. Invest., *18*:352, 365, 379, 1968.

Porta, E. A., et al.: Recent advances in molecular pathology. A review of the effects of alcohol on the liver. Exp. Molec. Path., *12*:104, 1970.

Powell, L. W.: Changing concepts in hemochromatosis. Postgrad. Med. J., *46*:200, 1970.

Powell, W. J., and Klatskin, G.: Duration of survival in patients with Laennec's cirrhosis. Influence of alcohol withdrawal and possible effects of recent changes in general management of the disease. Am. J. Med., *44*:406, 1968.

Prince, A. M., et al.: Long-incubation post-transfusion hepatitis without serological evidence of exposure to hepatitis-B virus. Lancet, 2:241, 1974.

Robinson, S. H., et al.: The sources of biopigment in the rat. Studies of the "early labeled" fraction. J. Clin. Invest., *45*:1569, 1966.

Robinson, S. H.: The origins of bilirubin. New Eng. J. Med., *279*:146, 1968.

Rubin, E., and Lieber, C. S.: Alcohol induced hepatic injury in nonalcoholic volunteers. New Eng. J. Med., *278*:869, 1968.

Rubin, E., and Lieber, C. S.: Current concepts: Alcohol and fatty liver. New Eng. J. Med., *280*:705, 1969.

Rubin, E., and Lieber, C. S.: Fatty liver, alcoholic hepatitis and cirrhosis produced by alcohol in primates. New Eng. J. Med., *290*:128, 1974.

Schaffner, F.: Treatment of primary biliary cirrhosis. Mod. Treat., *6*:205, 1969.

Schmid, R.: Hyperbilirubinemia. *In* Stanbury, J. B., Wyngaarden, J. B., and Fredrickson, D. S. (eds.): The Metabolic Basis of Inherited Disease. 2nd ed. New York, McGraw Hill Book Company, 1966, p. 871.

Schweitzer, I. L., et al.: Viral hepatitis B in neonates and infants Am. J. Med., *55*:762, 1973.

Sheldon, J. H.: Hemochromatosis. London, Oxford University Press, 1935.

Sherlock, S., and Scheuer, P. J.: The presentation and diagnosis of 100 patients with primary biliary cirrhosis. New Eng. J. Med., *289*:674, 1973.

Sherman, J. D., and Robbins, S. L.: Changing trends in the casuistics of hepatic abscess. Am. J. Med., *28*:943, 1960.

Shohet, S. B.: "Acanthocytogenesis"—or how the red cell won its spurs. New Eng. J. Med., *290*:1316, 1974.

Silberberg, E., and Holleb, A. I.: Cancer statistics, 1974—worldwide epidemiology. Ca, *24*:2, 1974.

Skikne, M. I., and Talbot, J. H.: The identification and structural analysis of viral particles in serum hepatitis. Lab. Invest., *31*:246, 1974.

Small, D. M.: Gallstones, diagnosis and treatment. Postgrad. Med., *51*:187, 1972.

Smith, J. B.: Alpha-fetoproteins: Occurrence in certain malignant diseases and review of clinical applications. Med. Clin. N. Am., *54*:797, 1970.

Smith, P. M., et al.: Postulated gastric factor enhancing iron absorption in hemochromatosis. Brit. J. Hemat., *16*:443, 1969.

Soergel, K. H.: Hormonally mediated diarrhea. New Eng. J. Med., *292*:970, 1975.

Steigman, F., et al.: Lymph flow disturbances in intractable ascites in cirrhotic patients. J. Lab. Clin. Med., *70*:893, 1967.

Stone, W. D., et al.: The natural history of cirrhosis. Quart. J. Med. (New Series), *37*:119, 1968.

Sutnick, A. I., et al.: Anicteric hepatitis associated with Australia antigen. Occurrence in patients with Down's syndrome. J.A.M.A., *205*:670, 1968.

Szmuness, W., et al.: Familial clustering of hepatitis B infection. New Eng. J. Med., *289*:1162, 1973.

Thorbjarnarson, B.: Carcinoma of the bile ducts. Cancer, *12*:708, 1959.

Tong, M. J., et al.: Hepatitis-associated antigen and hepatocellular carcinoma in Taiwan. Ann. Intern. Med., *75*:687, 1971.

Trey, C., et al.: Fulminant hepatic failure. Presumable contribution of halothane. New Eng. J. Med., *279*:798, 1968.

U. S. Vital Statistics: Monthly vital statistics report. Annual Summary for 1973, HRA 74-1120, *22*, No. 13, June 27, 1974.

Villarejos, V. M., et al.: Saliva, urine and feces as transmittors of type B hepatitis. New Eng. J. Med., *291*:1375, 1974.

Vittal, S. B. V., et al.: Acute viral hepatitis, course and incidence of progression to chronic hepatitis. Am. J. Med., *55*:757, 1973.

Vlahcevic, Z. R., et al.: Relationship of bile acid pool size to the formation of lithogenic bile in female Indians of the Southwest. Gastroenterology, *62*:73, 1972.

Walsh, R. J., et al.: A genetic study of hemochromatosis. Abstracts of the Tenth Congress of International Society of Hematology, F–16, 1964.

Warren, K. W., et al.: Gallbladder carcinoma. Surg. Gynec. Obstet., *126*:1036, 1968.

Warren, S., and Drake, W. L., Jr.: Primary carcinoma of the liver in hemochromatosis. Amer. J. Path., *27*:573, 1951.

Weiser, M. M., et al.: α_1-antitrypsin deficiency–a defect of secretion. New Eng. J. Med., *292*:205, 1975.

Wiggers, K. D., et al.: The ultrastructure of Mallory body filaments. Lab. Invest., *29*:652, 1973.

Yeung Laiwah, A. A. C.: Lymphocyte transformation by Australia antigen. Lancet, *2*:470, 1971.

Zollinger, R. M., and Ellison, E. H.: Primary peptic ulcerations of the jejunum associated with islet cell tumors of the pancreas. Am. Surg., *142*:709, 1955.

Zuckerman, A. J.: Editorial: New tests for hepatitis B virus. New Eng. J. Med., *290*:1373, 1974.

CHAPTER 16

The Male Genital System

In this chapter the major anatomic subdivisions of the male genital system—the penis, the scrotum and its contents, and the prostate—will be considered individually. Although there is some overlap, diseases tend initially or predominantly to affect only one of these structures. An exception to this anatomic consideration is the grouping of the venereal diseases together at the end of the chapter. Because the pathologic processes are quite similar in both sexes and to facilitate comparison, the effects of venereal disease in the female are also discussed in this section. No derogation of either sex is intended by this arrangement.

PENIS

The principal lesions of the penis are infectious, congenital or neoplastic. In most cases they affect the surface of the penis, and hence are readily visible to the patient. The more important infectious processes are venereally transmitted and discussed at the end of the chapter. Remaining to be described here are the congenital anomalies, *hypospadias, epispadias* and *phimosis*, and a group of tumors, ranging from the benign *papilloma* through the "premalignant" lesions, *leukoplakia* and *Bowen's disease*, to *carcinoma of the penis*.

HYPOSPADIAS AND EPISPADIAS

Among the more frequent congenital anomalies of the penis is termination of the urethra at the ventral surface of the penis *(hypospadias)* or at its dorsal surface *(epispadias)*. Because the abnormal opening is often constricted, partial outflow obstruction, with its attendant risk of urinary infection and hydronephrosis, may result. In addition, these anomalies may be causes of sterility when the abnormal orifice is situated near the base of the penis. Frequently, hypospadias and epispadias are associated with failure of normal descent of the testes and with malformations of the bladder; sometimes they are associated with more serious congenital deformities.

PHIMOSIS

When the orifice of the prepuce is too small to permit its retraction over the glans penis, the condition is designated *phimosis*. This may be a congenital anomaly, or it may be acquired by inflammatory scarring. In either case, phimosis permits the accumulation of secretions and smegma under the prepuce, favoring the development of secondary infection and further scarring. The nonspecific infection of the glans and prepuce which often accompanies phimosis is termed *balanoposthitis.* Forcible retraction of the prepuce may cause constriction, with pain and swelling of the glans penis, a condition known as *paraphimosis.* Urinary retention may develop in severe cases.

PAPILLOMA (CONDYLOMA ACUMINATUM)

This is the only benign tumor of the penis that occurs with sufficient frequency to merit description. It is one of the rare tumors in man known to be caused by a virus. Although the trauma and irritation of coitus may aggravate the lesion, it is not a venereal disease.

Most often, the tumors are seen about the coronal sulcus and inner surface of the prepuce, and range from minute sessile or pedunculated excrescences of 1 mm. in diameter to large, raspberry-like masses several centimeters in diameter. Histologically, there is a villous connective tissue stroma covered by hyperplastic epithelium. The basement membrane is intact, and there is no evidence of invasion of the underlying stroma, nor is malignant transformation known to occur.

"PREMALIGNANT" LESIONS

"Premalignant" lesions of the penis include *leukoplakia* and *Bowen's disease*. Both appear as plaque-like thickenings of the epithelium which microscopically disclose a spectrum from hyperplasia through dysplasia to carcinoma-in-situ. The more benign-appearing hyperplastic or dysplastic lesions are termed leukoplakia, whereas Bowen's disease refers to carcinoma-in-situ. *Neither lesion is specific to the penis, but may occur on any mucosal surface of the body, including the vulva and the oral cavity. Their importance lies in their liability to progress to squamous cell carcinoma.* Somewhat confusingly, Bowen's disease of the penis has also been designated *erythroplasia of Queyrat*.

Leukoplakia, a pearly white plaque, is thought to be related to chronic irritation. It is characterized by thickening of the epidermis, resulting either from an increase in surface keratinization or from hyperplasia of the underlying cells, principally those of the prickle cell layer. Although the orderly transition from basal to surface cell is usually preserved, some variability in nuclear and cell size may be present. Commonly, there is an intense mononuclear leukocytic infiltrate in the dermis. If the epithelial abnormalities are more marked, with bizarre cell types and disordered cellular alignment (anaplasia), the lesion may qualify as carcinoma-in-situ or Bowen's disease.

CARCINOMA OF THE PENIS

In the United States, squamous cell carcinoma of the penis accounts for no more than 0.5 per cent of cancer in the male (Silverberg, 1973). Other forms of cancer of the penis are even more rare. Preventing the retention of smegma by early circumcision confers protection against squamous cell carcinoma of the penis. This lesion is extremely rare among men who were circumcised early in life. On the other hand, phimosis, balanoposthitis, syphilis and chronic irritation are thought to play important predisposing roles. The incidence of carcinoma of the penis increases with age (Eisenberg, 1966). As mentioned, this form of cancer may be preceded by leukoplakia or Bowen's disease.

Morphologically, squamous cell carcinoma of the penis usually initially appears as a small, grayish, crusted papule on the glans or prepuce, near the coronal sulcus. When the plaque reaches about 1 cm. in diameter, the center usually ulcerates and develops a necrotic, secondarily infected base, with ragged, heaped-up margins. Less frequently, the tumor takes a papillary form, resembling the benign papilloma. This form enlarges to produce a cauliflower-like, fungating mass. Both patterns are locally destructive and may cause large necrotizing erosions. Histologically, the appearance is that of squamous cell carcinomas occurring anywhere on the skin or mucosa (see p. 117).

Carcinoma of the penis tends to follow a slow, indolent course. Metastases to the inguinal nodes are present in only 22 per cent of patients at the time of diagnosis. Widespread dissemination is uncommon until late in the course. For all stages, five-year survival is about 70 per cent (Silverberg, 1973).

SCROTUM, TESTIS, EPIDIDYMIS

The more important disorders of the scrotum and its contents involve the testes. *Some of these disorders produce testes that are smaller than normal, and others cause enlargement.* In the first category are congenital abnormalities which result in failure of the testes to develop normally at puberty. These include *cryptorchidism*, to be described later, and *Klinefelter's syndrome*. In addition, a variety of disorders to be cited presently result in atrophy of previously normal sized testes.

A number of diseases cause enlargement of the testes. By far the most important are *testicular tumors*, which are usually associated with insidious painless enlargement. Second in importance are *infections (orchitis)*. These usually produce more rapid, painful swelling. A third, relatively infrequent cause of testicular enlargement is *torsion of the testis*. In this case, violent movement or physical trauma causes twisting of the spermatic cord, with consequent impairment of blood flow to and from the testis. Usually there is some underlying structural abnormality, such as incomplete descent of the testis, absence of the gubernaculum testis or testicular atrophy, which permits excessive mobility of the testis within the tunica vaginalis. Because the thick-walled arteries are less vulnerable to compression than are the veins, there is intense vascular engorgement and, in severe cases, extravasation of blood into the interstitial tissue of the testis and epididymis, with consequent hemorrhagic infarction. There is usually little doubt about the diagnosis, because of the intense pain and rapid swelling, often with bloody discoloration of the scrotum.

It is important to remember that the clinical distinction between enlargement of testicular origin and that due to disorders within the epididymis or scrotum itself is not always easily made. Indeed, swelling due to infection more often originates in the epididymis than in the testis. In addition, abnormal collections of fluid or herniated intestinal loops in the scrotal sac may initially be confused with a testicular mass. While of relatively trivial consequence compared to, say, carcinoma of the testis, these disorders of the scrotum are extremely common. They will be briefly described before discussing testicular tumors and infections in more detail.

A clear serous accumulation within the tunica vaginalis—the serosa-lined sac enclosing the testis and epididymis—is termed a *hydrocele.* It may be a response to neighboring infections or tumors, or it may be a manifestation of generalized edema from any cause. Often, however, it develops slowly and painlessly, without apparent cause. *Hydroceles are frequent and are the most common cause of scrotal enlargement.* They may be differentiated from true testicular masses by transillumination.

Much less frequent are *hematoceles,* that is, blood in the tunica vaginalis as a result of tissue trauma or bleeding diatheses, and *chyloceles,* an accumulation of lymphatic fluid resulting from lymphatic obstruction.

With an *inguinal hernia,* loops of intestine may descend into the tunica vaginalis, causing marked scrotal enlargement. This is easily differentiated from testicular disease by the presence of bowel sounds in the scrotum and by the reduction of the hernia through the widened inguinal ring. This is also a common cause of scrotal enlargement, since inguinal hernias are seen in 1 per cent of the pediatric population (Wang et al., 1970).

CRYPTORCHIDISM

Normally the testes descend from their initial embryonic position in the coelomic cavity to the pelvic brim in the third month of fetal life, a process termed *internal descent.* During the last two months of intrauterine life, *external descent,* or passage of the testes through the inguinal canals to the scrotal sac, takes place. When either process is incomplete, resulting in the malpositioning of the testis anywhere along this pathway, the condition is termed *cryptorchidism.* It is a common condition, seen in about 0.7 per cent of schoolboys (Wang et al., 1970). Sometimes it is hereditary, but usually it occurs as a seemingly random congenital anomaly, often attributable to a short spermatic cord, a narrow inguinal canal, inadequate development of the gubernaculum testis or fibrous adhesions in the pathway of descent.

Cryptorchidism is unilateral in 60 per cent of cases and bilateral in 40 per cent (Dougall et al., 1974). When it is unilateral, the right testis is somewhat more frequently affected than the left. Before puberty, the malpositioned testis is often normal in size and consistency. However, by puberty and sometimes earlier, progressive atrophy ensues, with diminution in size and an increase in consistency as a result of progressive fibrosis. Spermatogenic activity ceases. Microscopically, the tubules become atrophic, outlined by prominent, thickened basement membranes, and eventually they become virtually totally replaced by fibrous tissue. There is an accompanying hyperplasia of the interstitial cells of Leydig as well as of the stroma. Such testicular atrophy is nonspecific, and may be seen in many other conditions, including progressive arteriosclerotic encroachment on testicular blood supply, end-stage orchitis, hypopituitarism, prolonged administration of female sex hormones, cirrhosis of the liver, some forms of malnutrition, obstruction to the outflow of semen and irradiation.

With cryptorchidism, the age at which the atrophic changes become well developed and irreversible is highly variable. They tend to occur earlier in abdominal testes than in those lying in the inguinal canal or lower. In general, surgical placement of the testis within the scrotum (orchidopexy) by the age of 10 years permits normal development and spermatogenesis (Dougall et al. 1974). Untreated cryptorchidism is asymptomatic. Often there is an associated inguinal hernia. When the condition is bilateral, it results in sterility. Although the issue is controversial, most investigators accept the view that undescended testes are more vulnerable to carcinoma than are scrotal testes, but the increased risk is probably slight.

KLINEFELTER'S SYNDROME

This syndrome is characterized by primary failure of the testes to develop at puberty, with resultant eunuchoidism (Fig. 16–1). It is responsible for about 3 per cent of infertility in males (Grumbach et al., 1957). This disorder is described on page 161.

TESTICULAR TUMORS

About 97 per cent of testicular tumors are thought to arise from pluripotent germ cells. Almost all of these are malignant to some degree or another. Most of the remaining 3 per cent originate from the interstitial cells of

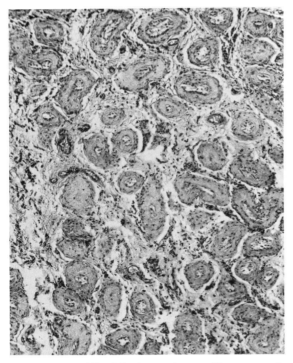

Figure 16–1. Klinefelter's syndrome. The spermatic tubules are totally atrophic and hyalinized, and appear as doughnut-shaped masses of collagenous tissue.

Leydig or the Sertoli cells and are usually benign, although they may elaborate steroids and thus cause endocrinopathies.

Germ cell tumors of the testes are about twice as frequent as carcinoma of the penis, accounting for roughly 1 per cent of cancer in males (Frank, 1970–71). Their peak incidence occurs at about the age of 30 years; then there is a decline in frequency, followed by a smaller peak at about the age of 75 years. During the early peak, it is the most common form of cancer in males. Moreover, in both the United States and Europe, there has been evidence of a marked increase in incidence since World War II, particularly in this early age range. As with other cancers of children or young adults, there is thought to be a congenital component in its causation (Silverberg, 1973). In New York, an ethnic differential was found among young men, with Jews being affected twice as commonly as non-Jews, and Protestants twice as often as Catholics (Editorial, 1968). These tumors are usually manifested by enlargement or palpable hardness of the affected testis, often accompanied by a feeling of heaviness.

Testicular germ cell tumors are of four types: (1) seminoma, (2) embryonal carcinoma, (3) teratoma and teratocarcinoma, and (4) choriocarcinoma (Dixon and Moore, 1953). Mixtures of these types are seen in at least 15 per cent of cases (Frank, 1970–71).

The **seminoma** accounts for approximately 40 per cent of testicular neoplasms, and it is characterized by fairly well differentiated sheets or cords of uniform polygonal cells, with distinct cell membranes, central round nuclei and clear cytoplasm. Typically, there is a variable fibrous stroma, with a

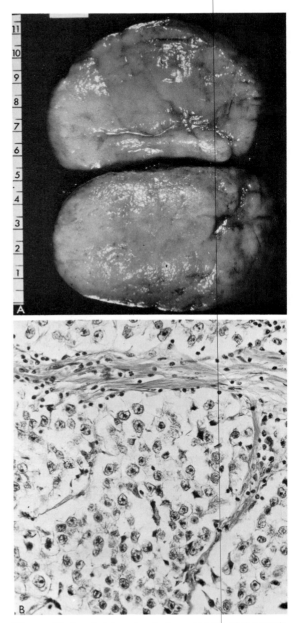

Figure 16–2. *A*, A hemisected seminoma of the testis. The gray-white, fleshy mass totally replaces the testis. Note that its size is approximately 5 × 7 cm. and it has therefore caused testicular enlargement. *B*, A high power detail of a seminoma of the testis, showing sheets of neoplastic cells with clear cytoplasm and regular nuclei. The cell membranes are best seen in the lower left field. The fibrous stroma contains a relatively scant lymphoid infiltrate.

prominent lymphocytic infiltrate and occasional granulomatous formations. These tumors tend to grow rapidly, as large, gray-white, fleshy masses (Fig. 16–2) but remain confined within the tunica albuginea until late in their course.

Clinically, the seminoma characteristically remains localized for a time and then metastasizes to regional and aortic lymph nodes. The tumor is remarkably radiosensitive and, with radiotherapy, about 90 per cent of these patients survive for at least 10 years.

In contrast to the seminoma, *embryonal carcinomas* are poorly differentiated and highly malignant. They represent about 20 per cent of testicular tumors.

Although they are generally smaller than the seminomas, appearing grossly as discrete, gray-white nodules, they are locally invasive and tend to metastasize widely. There are several microscopic patterns, including a form characterized by sheets of cells similar to the seminoma. However, these cells are larger and more pleomorphic, with darker, granular cytoplasm. Moreover, the stroma is minimal, and there is no lymphocytic infiltrate. Other embryonal carcinomas may show irregular acinar or papillary formations (Fig. 16–3). Ten-year survival with these tumors is about 35 per cent.

The *teratoma* and *teratocarcinoma* refer to a spectrum of increasingly poorly differentiated tumors characterized by the presence of a

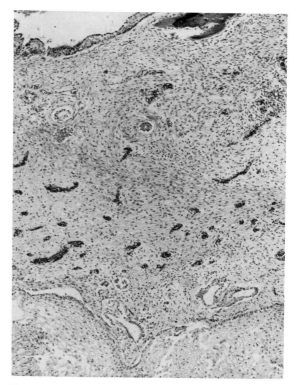

Figure 16–4. Histologic detail of a testicular teratoma. A spicule of bone (top center) is immediately to the right of a cystic space lined by columnar, respiratory-looking epithelium. The center of the field shows areas resembling white matter of the brain, in which small glands are scattered. At the bottom is a large nest of stratified squamous epithelium.

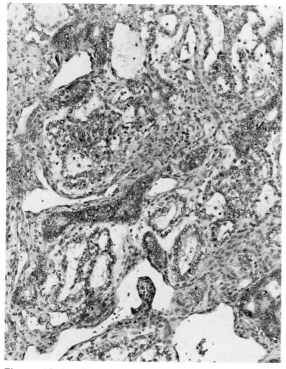

Figure 16–3. Embryonal carcinoma of the testis. An acinar, tubular and papillary pattern characterizes this neoplasm.

multitude of cell types reproducing normal adult tissues such as muscle bundles, bone, cartilage, squamous epithelium and even thyroid gland, intestinal wall or brain (Fig. 16–4). They represent about 25 per cent of testicular tumors.

On cut surface, these tumors present a characteristic variegated and cystic appearance. Teratocarcinomas are distinguished from teratomas by the overtly anaplastic nature of one or more of the tissue components, more often those of epithelial origin. Frequently, this anaplastic area resembles a seminoma or embryonal carcinoma and may show foci of choriocarcinoma. Despite the relatively benign appearance of the teratomas, many metastasize and hence are malignant. As a group, these tumors produce a degree of testicular enlargement intermediate between that produced by the seminoma and that produced by embryonal carcinoma, with an intermediate tendency toward local invasiveness.

Ten-year survival ranges from 50 to 75 per cent, depending on the degree of differentiation.

Choriocarcinoma accounts for only 1 per cent of testicular tumors.

The lesion may cause testicular enlargement, but more often the primary tumor is very small and cannot be palpated. Nonetheless, it is highly malignant, metastasizing early and widely. Histologically, these tumors reproduce the epithelial components of placental tissue, i.e., cytotrophoblast, composed of masses of cuboidal cells with central round nuclei, and syncytiotrophoblast, appearing as sheets of syncytial epithelium with an abundant pink vacuolated cytoplasm and large pleomorphic nuclei. These two cellular elements, however, are not arranged as in placental villi, but instead grow in disorderly array.

High levels of chorionic gonadotropins may be elaborated by choriocarcinomas. The appearance of such hormones in the male is virtually diagnostic of this form of cancer. Although chemotherapy in women with choriocarcinoma has proved very effective, in the male the tumor responds poorly and ten-year survival is only about 10 per cent.

A staging system for testicular tumors has been devised to aid in treatment planning and prognostication (Maier et al., 1969). Stage IA refers to tumor confined to one testis, without evidence of nodal or other metastases. When there is histologic evidence of involvement of the iliac or para-aortic nodes, the tumor is Stage IB. Clinical or radiologic evidence of lymph node metastases below the diaphragm indicates Stage II disease. Stage III disease implies involvement of nodes above the diaphragm or of other organs throughout the body.

ORCHITIS, EPIDIDYMITIS

In general, infections are more common in the epididymis than in the testis, but may ultimately reach the testis by direct or lymphatic spread. Most cases of epididymitis are nonspecific, secondary to urinary tract infection or to prostatitis. Rarely, epididymitis or orchitis results from hematogenous spread of distant infection.

With nonspecific infections the early changes are limited to the epididymis and comprise edema and a nonspecific leukocytic infiltration of the interstitial tissue. Later, the tubules are filled with exudate and there may be abscess formation or a generalized suppurative necrosis. Retrograde spread involves the testis. Any such nonspecific inflammation may become chronic. Pressure within the edematous testis or fibrous scarring of the tubules often leads to sterility. The hardier cells of Leydig usually are spared, so that endocrine function and libido remain intact.

The four major *specific* infections of the testis or epididymis are: gonorrhea, syphilis, tuberculosis and mumps. Gonorrhea and syphilis will be discussed in the section dealing with venereal diseases. Suffice it to say here that gonorrhea tends to affect primarily the epididymis, whereas syphilis first involves the testis. When tuberculosis involves the male external genitals, it almost invariably begins in the epididymis, from which it may spread to the testis. Tubercle formation is typical of that elsewhere in the body (p. 49).

In about 25 to 33 per cent of cases of *mumps* in adult males an acute interstitial orchitis, usually unilateral but occasionally bilateral, develops about one week following the swelling of the salivary glands. Rarely, cases of mumps orchitis have been described without significant involvement of the salivary glands.

The affected testis swells and, histologically, shows interstitial edema and a patchy mononuclear leukocytic infiltration. Although there is often some degree of atrophy on healing, the patchy nature of the process tends to permit preservation of fertility, even when the process is bilateral. However, when there has been especially intense generalized edema, compression of the blood supply may induce generalized atrophy and lead to sterility.

PROSTATE

There are three important lesions of the prostate: *inflammation*, usually as a result of nonspecific infection; *nodular hyperplasia*, commonly known as benign prostatic hypertrophy (BPH); and *carcinoma*. All three cause some degree of enlargement of the prostate. Because the prostate encircles the urethra any lesion that causes significant prostatic enlargement may easily encroach on the lumen of the urethra. Thus, diseases of the prostate commonly manifest themselves by urinary symptoms. These symptoms are variable but usually include such indications of partial obstruction as frequency of urination, nocturia and difficulty in initiating or maintaining the stream of urine.

PROSTATITIS

Although acute prostatitis is often caused by the gonococcus (p. 556), it may also be produced by a great variety of other organisms. Because of its location, the prostate is vulnerable to infection by organisms implanted anywhere along the urinary tract. Frequently, such nonspecific infections are iatrogenic, following catheterization, cystoscopy, urethral dilatation or partial resection of the prostate itself (Ghormley and Needham, 1953). Only occasionally is prostatitis caused by hematogenous seeding.

Acute prostatitis is characterized by suppuration, either in the form of minute, discrete abscesses or as large, coalescent areas of involvement. Diffuse involvement often leads to soft, boggy enlargement of the entire prostate. Histologically, the gland lumina may become virtually packed with a neutrophilic exudate, and the stroma characteristically contains a nonspecific leukocytic infiltrate.

Clinical findings vary. Symptoms may be limited to difficult urination, or there may be hematuria and perineal pain, with systemic indications of infection, such as fever, chills and malaise. Although healing is often fairly complete, with only slight residual scarring, the process sometimes becomes chronic.

Chronic prostatitis is most often a sequel to acute prostatitis, and thus represents the continued presence of a smoldering infection.

Because some degree of lymphocytic infiltration of the prostate is a normal accompaniment of aging, the diagnosis of chronic prostatitis should not be made unless other mononuclear leukocytes and neutrophils are also present, along with some evidence of tissue destruction and fibroblastic proliferation.

The development of granulomas without caseous centers may occur as a nonspecific inflammatory response to inspissated prostatic secretions. On the other hand, caseating granulomas represent tuberculous prostatitis, usually caused by direct spread of the tubercle bacillus from some other region of the genitourinary tract, such as the kidneys, bladder or epididymis.

There may be no clinical manifestations of chronic prostatitis, or it may be associated with various urinary disturbances, including nocturia, urgency and dysuria, along with a vague perineal discomfort. Because tuberculous prostatitis frequently leads to marked enlargement of the prostate, urinary obstruction may occur with this disease.

NODULAR HYPERPLASIA OF THE PROSTATE (BENIGN PROSTATIC HYPERTROPHY)

This is an extremely common disorder characterized by the development of large, fairly discrete nodules within the prostate. By long-standing tradition, this entity is known as "benign prostatic hypertrophy" or BPH. This, however, is a misnomer, since the basic process is hyperplasia rather than hypertrophy and, in either case, the qualification "benign" is redundant.

Beginning in the fifth decade of life, there is a progressive increase in incidence of nodular hyperplasia with age, until about 80 per cent of men beyond the age of 80 years are affected. Fortunately, not all who are affected are seriously inconvenienced. The cause of the lesion is unknown, but current opinion favors its somehow reflecting the relative hy-

perestrinism that occurs with age as testicular androgen output declines while adrenal estrogen secretion persists.

In the typical case, the prostatic nodules weigh between 60 and 100 gm.; aggregate weights of up to 200 gm. are seen. **The nodules are characteristically found in the median lobe and more central portions of the lateral lobes. This predilection is in striking contrast to that of prostatic carcinoma, which usually involves the posterior lobe** (Moore, 1943). Although the nodules do not have a true capsule, they are well demarcated on cross section because of the compression of the surrounding parenchyma. The urethra may be compressed to a slitlike orifice by the enlargement of the lateral lobes. The hyperplastic median lobe projects up into the floor of the urethra in a hemispheric mass, sometimes having the effect of a ball valve (Fig. 16–5).

In most cases, the hyperplasia is seen microscopically to result primarily from glandular proliferation. These new glands are variable in size, and their regular cuboidal to columnar epithelium is characteristically thrown into numerous papillary

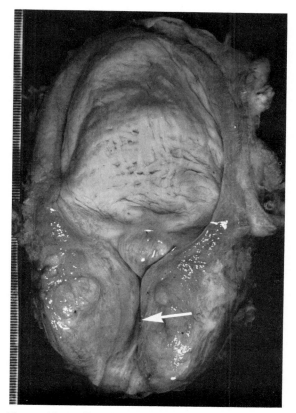

Figure 16–5. Nodular hyperplasia of the prostate. The urinary bladder and prostatic urethra have been opened. The enlargement of the prostate is seen as the two masses flanking the urethra (arrow). A median lobe projects under the floor of the bladder as a hemispheric mass.

buds and infoldings, which are more prominent than in the normal prostate. The gland formations are well developed and are separated from each other by stroma, however scant. Numerous small foci of hyaline concretions, termed corpora amylacea, are nested within these glands. Aggregates of lymphocytes are commonly found within the stroma. Sometimes the hyperplasia is predominantly fibromuscular, and in these cases the nodules may appear microscopically as almost solid masses of spindle cells. Whether glandular or fibromuscular, small areas of ischemic necrosis surrounded by margins of squamous metaplasia may be seen within the nodules or in the surrounding prostatic tissue. In addition, squamous metaplasia of the periurethral glands, which may be mistaken for carcinoma, is a common accompaniment of nodular hyperplasia.

The clinical significance of nodular hyperplasia lies entirely in its tendency to produce urinary tract obstruction by impinging upon the urethra. Despite the prevalence of this disorder, however, not more than 10 per cent of men over the age of 80 require surgical relief of the obstruction. Early symptoms include difficulty in starting, maintaining and stopping the stream of urine. There may also be frequency and nocturia, presumably because the raised level of the urethral floor leads to retention in the bladder of a large volume of residual urine after micturition. Hydronephrosis may ensue (see p. 455), as may infection, the all too frequent companion of obstruction.

Recently, the view that nodular hyperplasia and carcinoma of the prostate are unrelated has been challenged. In a long-term prospective study, the risk of developing carcinoma of the prostate was found to be 3.7 times higher among patients with nodular hyperplasia than among controls (Armenian et al. 1974). However, the methodology of this study has been questioned, and the conclusions remain unconfirmed (Williams and Blackard, 1974).

CARCINOMA OF THE PROSTATE

Carcinoma of the prostate is the most common cancer of men, occurring in from 14 to 46 per cent of males over the age of 50 years. This is a truly astounding incidence. Fortunately, however, most lesions are virtually microscopic in size, remain dormant and cause no clinical disease. These are discovered only as an incidental finding at autopsy or in glands removed because of concurrent nodular hyperplasia. Nevertheless, a small fraction of these cancers are lethal, invading contiguous structures and metastasizing widely. This fraction constitutes the third most frequent cause of death from cancer in the male, following cancer of the lung and of the colon and rectum. Moreover, its prevalence increases steeply in old age, so that by the age of 75 years it is the leading cause of death from cancer in males (Silverberg and Holleb, 1974). Thus, cancer of the prostate is recognized in two quite distinctive settings: as a small, dormant and localized lesion, and as an active, invasive and metastasizing one. Whether these two patterns represent two biological forms of cancer or are merely different stages of one disease is uncertain. Conceivably, the microscopic lesions may in some cases regress and in others eventually develop into clinically significant tumors. Except for their size, the so-called dormant and the aggressive forms are histologically indistinguishable.

The etiologic influences responsible for carcinoma of the prostate are not definitely known. Like nodular hyperplasia, its incidence increases with age, and it is speculated that the endocrine changes of old age, perhaps the augmented pituitary secretion of gonadotropins, are important predisposing factors (Strahan, 1963). Support for the general thesis lies in the inhibition of these tumors that can be achieved with orchiectomy or estrogen therapy. It has long been assumed that carcinoma of the prostate and nodular hyperplasia are unrelated. Their frequent concurrence was thought to be coincidental, since both are extremely common lesions in elderly men. However, the recent study showing that men with nodular hyperplasia were 3.7 times as likely to develop carcinoma of the prostate as were controls would seem to reopen the issue (Armenian, 1974).

Epidemiologic studies are of interest in seeking the causation of carcinoma of the prostate. There is a roughly fifteenfold geographic variation in the death rates from carcinoma of the prostate. The Scandinavian countries show a very high death rate from this form of cancer, whereas at the other extreme, the Japanese are relatively free of the disease. The United States occupies an intermediate position (Silverberg, 1973). The relative importance of hereditary and environmental factors in the genesis of carcinoma of the prostate is illuminated by other epidemiologic data. Immigrants from low-risk to high-risk geographic areas show an intermediate risk of developing this tumor. Within the United States there is some tendency toward familial aggregation. American blacks are affected somewhat more frequently than are whites (Cole 1974).

The morphologic diagnosis of carcinoma of the prostate is frequently difficult, both macroscopically and histologically. The tumor often blends imperceptibly into the background of the gland, al-

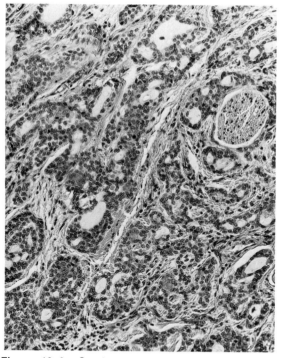

Figure 16–6. Carcinoma of the prostate. The neoplastic gland patterns are small and disorderly, and at the upper right, have encircled and permeated a perineurial lymphatic space.

though it may be apparent by its firm gritty texture or by a color somewhat yellower than the surrounding tissue. Histologically, most of these lesions are adenocarcinomas of varying degrees of differentiation. In general, the epithelial cells are surprisingly uniform, usually cuboidal or polygonal, with small central nuclei and scant cytoplasm. Usually they are arranged in recognizable glandular patterns, but occasionally they form cords or nests of cells (Fig. 16–6). When gland formation is orderly, it may be difficult histologically to distinguish carcinoma of the prostate from nodular hyperplasia. In these cases, the distinction may rest on the presence of invasion of blood vessels, perineurial and perivascular spaces or the prostatic capsule.

Usually carcinoma of the prostate is asymptomatic and does not spread, and the patient dies of other causes. Since the tumor most often arises in the posterior lobe, far removed from the urethra, it is unlikely to produce urinary symptoms so long as it remains small and localized. Those tumors that are aggressive and locally invasive, however, ultimately affect the urethra and bladder, producing such manifestations as frequency, dysuria and, sometimes, hematuria. Pain referred to the urethra, rectum and perineum reflects perineurial invasion. Often the first evidence of prostatic carcinoma is metastatic disease. A characteristic metastatic pattern is involvement, via the paravertebral venous

plexus, of the bones of the axial skeleton, which may produce either osteoclastic (destructive) or, more often, osteoblastic (stimulative) lesions.

Perhaps the most direct and fruitful diagnostic procedure is rectal palpation of the prostate, since the usual location of the lesion, in the posterior lobe, is closely applied to the rectal wall. Acid phosphatase, which is usually released into the blood by the prostate in small quantities, may be present in markedly increased quantities when there is widespread metastatic disease. However, this is not always the case, and normal levels do not rule out prostatic cancer with metastases. With osteoblastic lesions, there may also be elevated levels of alkaline phosphatase. A needle biopsy may confirm the diagnosis.

The survival statistics for men with the dormant form of prostatic carcinoma are similar to those of other men of comparable age. With clinically aggressive disease, however, there is a high mortality rate, depending on stage and grade. Overall five-year survival is about 33 per cent (Silverberg and Holleb, 1974).

Differences in the extent of spread at the time of diagnosis are the basis for a staging system using classifications from A to D. Stage A carcinoma of the prostate refers to the microscopic dormant form. A larger lesion still confined within the prostatic capsule is Stage B. Stage C implies local extracapsular extension, with or without involvement of pelvic nodes, or an elevated acid phosphatase. In Stage D disease, there is bony or extrapelvic involvement (Rubin, 1969). In addition, these tumors are graded from I to III on the basis of cellular differentiation. Grade I tumors are well differentiated, whereas Grade III tumors are extremely anaplastic. This grading system has been demonstrated to have prognostic value (Jewett et al., 1968).

VENEREAL DISEASE

The term "venereal disease" refers to disease which is sexually transmitted. Table 16–1 shows the more important venereal diseases and their causative organisms. In addition, there are many microbes known to be transmitted sexually but which are not proved to produce disease when so transmitted. These include some of the mycoplasma and diphtheroids, *Hemophilus vaginalis* and the cytomegalovirus. On the other hand, certain well-known diseases are suspected but not proved to be venereal, at least in some cases. These include carcinoma of the cervix (Beral, 1974; Nahmias and Roizman, 1973) and hepatitis B (Heathcote and Sherlock, 1973; Cameron and Dane, 1974). Although there are dif-

TABLE 16–1. SEXUALLY TRANSMITTED DISEASES IN MAN*

	ORGANISM	DISEASE
Spirochetes	T. pallidum	Syphilis
Bacteria	Gonococcus	Gonorrhea
	H. ducreyi	Chancroid
	Donovania	Granuloma inguinale
Viruses	Chlamydia	Nongonococcal urethritis
		Lymphogranuloma venereum
	Other viruses	Herpes simplex
		Molluscum contagiosum
		Condylomata acuminata
Protozoa	T. vaginalis	Trichomoniasis
Fungi	C. albicans	Moniliasis
	Epidermophyton inguinale	Tinea cruris
Parasites	Acarus scabiei	Scabies
	Phthirus pubis	Pediculosis

*From Wilcox, R. R.: A world look at the venereal diseases. Med. Clin. N. Amer., 56:1057, 1972.

ferences in epidemiology among the venereal diseases, it can be said in a general way that after a period of apparent control in the 1950's, they have in recent years reemerged as an explosive public health problem. The major venereal diseases—*gonorrhea, syphilis, chancroid, granuloma inguinale, lymphogranuloma inguinale* and *Herpes genitalis*—are discussed individually.

GONORRHEA

With the possible exception of nongonococcal urethritis, gonorrhea is the most frequent of the venereal diseases (Willcox, 1972). Its incidence is about 25 times that of syphilis (Lucas, 1972). Moreover, there has in recent years been an alarming worldwide resurgence in the frequency of this disease. In the United States the gonorrhea rate is now higher than at any time since the disease became reportable in 1919 (Lucas, 1972). The reasons for this resurgence will be discussed subsequently.

The organism which causes gonorrhea is *Neisseria gonorrhoeae*, a gram-negative diplococcus identical in appearance to the meningococcus, which is virulent by virtue of its rapid spread and its elaboration of an endotoxin. Infection with the gonococcus does not confer immunity, and reinfection may occur virtually as often as the individual is exposed. Like the other pyogenic cocci, this organism evokes a nonspecific, neutrophilic inflammatory reaction, manifested by the production of copious amounts of yellow pus.

Two to seven days after exposure, the anterior urethra and meatus of the male become hyperemic and edematous, and exude a mucopurulent material. In the female, the initial involvement is in Bartholin's and Skene's glands, as well as in the urethral meatus. The endocervix may also be primarily affected. Other potential sites of entry and initial involvement include the oropharynx and the anorectum (Lightfoot and Gotschlich, 1974). **Because stratified squamous epithelium is remarkably resistant to invasion by the gonococcus, lesions do not usually occur on the mucocutaneous surfaces of the external genitalia or in the vagina.** At this stage the major symptom in both sexes is dysuria owing to involvement of the urethra. **It is important to remember, however, that in perhaps 80 per cent of female cases and 40 per cent of male cases the disease is entirely asymptomatic** (Lucas, 1972; Handsfield et al., 1974). These people provide a huge reservoir from which the disease is spread.

Unless there is prompt and adequate therapy, gonorrhea tends to spread upward in the genital tract. In the male, the prostate, seminal vesicles and epididymides may become involved, producing marked perineal or scrotal pain and fever. With chronicity, abscess formation and tissue destruction occur in these organs. **The testes are relatively resistant to gonococcal infection.** Urethral strictures may develop, sometimes leading to hydronephrosis and serious secondary pyelonephritis. Gonococcal epididymitis frequently causes sterility.

In the female, untreated gonorrhea tends eventually to involve the oviducts, usually bilaterally but occasionally unilaterally. **For mysterious reasons, the endometrium is usually spared.** The lumina of the affected oviducts become filled with purulent exudate, creating a **pyosalpinx** (pus tube). At first, the exudate may leak out of the tubal fimbriae, but often the fimbriae eventually become sealed, sometimes against the ovary, producing a **salpingo-oophoritis.** As pus collects in these sealed tubes, they become distended, occasionally attaining a diameter of 10 cm. or more. A localized pelvic peritonitis commonly is present, with a tendency toward formation of extensive adhesions. This pattern of inflammatory involvement in the female is known as **pelvic inflammatory disease (PID).** Since gonococcal salpingitis is just one of a number of causes of PID, the general entity is discussed in more detail in Chapter 17. Permanent sterility almost always results when cases are neglected in either sex.

A transient gonococcal bacteremia sometimes results in metastatic dissemination of the infection, most often to the joints (*suppurative arthritis* or *tenosynovitis*), occasionally to the heart valves (*acute bacterial endocarditis*) and meninges (*suppurative meningitis*). Fortunately, these complications have become rare since the advent of effective chemotherapeutic measures. Advanced or disseminated disease is more likely in women than in men. This is because in women the initial stages are more often asymptomatic, so that they are less likely to seek treatment early in the course of the disease (Lightfoot and Gotschlich, 1974).

Another tragic complication of gonorrhea which has become rare is *gonococcal ophthalmia neonatorum*, caused by contamination of an infant's eyes as it passes through the birth canal of its infected mother. At one time this was an important cause of blindness, but has virtually been eliminated by the prophylactic instillation of silver nitrate or penicillin in the newborn's eyes.

Before leaving the subject of gonorrhea, a few words should be said about the reasons for its increasing incidence and about some other aspects of its epidemiology. After gonorrhea became a reportable disease in 1919, its incidence was fairly static (at about half its present rate) until World War II. Wartime presents ideal conditions for the resurgence of venereal disease—namely, an extended period of promiscuity in a large population of both men and women. Accordingly, the incidence of gonorrhea climbed steadily during World War II, reaching a peak in 1947. Then, with the return to peacetime conditions and the widespread use of penicillin, the gonorrhea rate declined rapidly. By 1957 the incidence had returned to prewar levels, and both gonorrhea and syphilis seemed under control. However, over the next several years the incidence again increased, at first gradually, then sharply in the mid-1960's, until it reached its present record levels. Why? There are several overlapping reasons, some more firmly established than others. The most obvious is the war in Vietnam, where venereal disease has become rampant. Vietnam, moreover, became a breeding ground for gonococcus strains that were increasingly resistant to penicillin as well as to other antibiotics. Thus, although very large dosages of penicillin remain effective, undertreatment is now frequent. Worldwide changes in attitudes and behavior are also tending to increase the risk of developing venereal disease. The advent of oral contraception has probably been of great importance, in part because it has permitted greater sexual freedom by removing the fear of pregnancy and in part because it has replaced the condom, which offered some protection against venereal disease. Greater population mobility has also been important. In addition, there is some evidence that the organisms responsible for both gonorrhea and syphilis are themselves undergoing changes. Apparently they are becoming less virulent, hence more likely to produce infections that are asymptomatic in the early stages (Willcox, 1972). Possibly this is due to the selective eradication of the more virulent organisms, which rapidly call attention to their presence.

At any rate, the effect of asymptomatic disease is to allow plenty of time for spread to other people before treatment.

What of the efforts to control gonorrhea? They are proving to be far less than adequate. The major thrust of such efforts is to locate and treat the sexual partners of each new case. Unfortunately, however, only about a third of new cases are reported (Lucas, 1972; Willcox, 1972). This under-reporting, along with the increasingly large asymptomatic reservoir and the absence of a simple serologic screening test (such as that for syphilis), makes the control of gonorrhea an exceedingly difficult challenge.

SYPHILIS (LUES)

Syphilis is far less frequent than gonorrhea, and efforts to control it have been much more successful. Like gonorrhea, its incidence increased dramatically during World War II; then, with the advent of penicillin and the return to peacetime conditions, it declined to a low point in 1957. Since then, there has been some resurgence in the incidence of syphilis, but, fortunately, it is still well below World War II levels. This reasonably good control of syphilis relative to gonorrhea probably reflects the remarkable success of the serologic screening tests (to be described) in finding new or latent cases. The result has been not only some containment of the rate of increase of early syphilis, but also—of far greater importance—an absolute decline in its tragic late sequelae and in congenital syphilis (Willcox, 1972).

Etiology and Pathogenesis. The causative organism is the spirochete *Treponema pallidum*, which is transmitted either by venereal contact or by an infected mother to the fetus in utero. The extreme vulnerability of *Treponema* to drying probably precludes any other mode of transmission. Although little is known of the toxicity or antigenicity of *Treponema pallidum*, its destructiveness is probably based on its invasiveness and on the elaboration of a weak endotoxin. Unlike the gonococcus, *T. pallidum* appears to have retained its original sensitivity to penicillin.

Immunity is conferred by a single syphilitic infection. Within one to four months after contraction of the disease, two distinct antibodies appear in the serum. One of these, *syphilitic reagin*, provides the basis for the complement fixation and flocculation diagnostic tests for syphilis. However these are not specific tests and there are a large number of *biologic false positive (BFP)* results with other disorders, such as infectious mononucleosis, primary atypical pneumonia, the "collagen" diseases and nearly any acute febrile disease. The second antibody, known as *treponemal immobilizing antibody (TPI)*, is technically more difficult to demonstrate, but it is quite specific. It is probable that the TPI antibody is responsible for the destruction of the spirochetes within the host and the development of active immunity.

Morphology. Syphilis may affect nearly any organ or tissue in the body. **In all sites, it evokes one of two morphologic patterns of tissue injury.** One of these is a type of vasculitis, termed obliterative endarteritis, which is characterized by a concentric endothelial and fibroblastic proliferative thickening of the small vessels in an involved area, with a surrounding mononuclear (principally plasma cell) inflammatory infiltrate, known as **perivascular cuffing.**

The second pattern of tissue injury is a granulomatous lesion known as a **gumma,** which, on occasion, may be difficult to distinguish from the lesions of tuberculosis or sarcoidosis. Gummas consist of a center of coagulative necrosis in which the native cells are barely discernible as shadowy outlines. This focus is surrounded by epithelioid cells infiltrated by mononuclear leukocytes (principally plasma cells) and enclosed by a fibroblastic wall. The small vessels in the enclosing inflammatory wall may show obliterative endarteritis and perivascular cuffing. With difficulty, treponemes may be demonstrated in the reactive inflammatory zone. Gummas may occur in any site in the body but most often are found in the liver, bones and testes. They vary in size from microscopic defects to grossly visible tumorous masses of necrotic material. Erosion of a cutaneous or mucosal gumma may yield a persistent, shaggy ulcer that shows a surprising resistance to local therapeutic measures.

Clinical Course. *Clinically, acquired syphilitic infection is characterized by three fairly distinct stages,* which will be discussed separately. The disease is infectious only in the first two stages. In addition, congenital syphilis may be looked upon as a fourth distinctive entity.

Primary Syphilis. This stage is marked by the development of a *chancre* at the site of inoculation, usually on the penis or on the vulva or cervix, within one week to three months following exposure. Usually there is an accompanying, somewhat tender, nonspecific regional lymphadenopathy. The primary chancre begins as a single indurated, button-like papule, up to several centimeters in diameter, which erodes to create a clean-based, shallow ulceration on an elevated base. The most distinctive histologic feature, deep within the base, is the obliterative endarteritis with perivascular plasma cell cuffing, so characteristic of lues. The more superficial reaction comprises a nonspecific diffuse mononuclear leukocytic infiltrate. With appropriate techniques, large numbers of treponemes can be demonstrated in the lesion. Although a systemic spirochetemia occurs within a day of infection and persists for weeks to years, the patient feels well at this stage, and serologic tests are usually negative. The primary chancre slowly heals spontaneously. Approximately 50 per cent of female patients and 30 per cent of males do not notice the primary lesion.

Secondary Syphilis. From one to three months following the development of the primary chancre, a *widespread patchy or diffuse mucocutaneous rash* ensues, accompanied by a generalized, nonspecific lymphadenopathy. This marks the second stage of syphilis. The lesions that constitute the rash are extremely variable. Most commonly, they are maculopapular, with each red-brown lesion being less than 5 mm. in diameter. In other cases, however, follicular, pustular, annular or scaling lesions predominate. Vesicular lesions do not occur. Histologically, the rash resembles the chancre, perhaps with a less marked mononuclear infiltrate, and spirochetes are present. In the region of the external genitals, the lesions may take the form of large, elevated plaques, designated *condylomata lata.* By this stage, serologic tests are usually positive. The patient continues to feel surprisingly well, and the striking absence of constitutional manifestations such as fever, chills or malaise is an important point in differentiating syphilis from other causes of generalized rash.

Tertiary Syphilis. The clinical importance of syphilis lies in the risk of developing the often seriously crippling or lethal lesions of tertiary syphilis. Only about one third of patients with untreated syphilis ever progress to this state, and, of these, about half remain asymptomatic. Another third of all untreated patients apparently achieve a spontaneous cure, with reversion to negative serologic tests. The remaining third continue to have positive serologic tests, but do not develop structural lesions.

Tertiary syphilis develops after a period of latency lasting from one to 30 years. It may affect any part of the body, but it shows a predilection for the cardiovascular system (80 to 85 per cent), and the central nervous system (5 to 10 per cent). Cardiovascular syphilis is discussed on page 280, and neurosyphilis on page 664. Other organs may be involved, singly or concurrently, giving rise to truly protean and often confusing clinical findings. In the liver, gummas may produce the coarsely nodular pattern of cirrhosis, termed *hepar lobatum* because of the simulation by the deep scars of multiple irregular lobes. Bone and joint gummas lead to areas of cortical and articular destruction. Pathologic fractures and joint immobilization may result. Testicular gummas often cause painless enlargement of the affected testis, thus simulating a tumor. In general, tertiary syphilis is a devastating disease, with a 15 to 30 per cent mortality rate. As mentioned, it is becoming increasingly rare.

Congenital Syphilis. Syphilis may be transmissible to the fetus by an infected mother for a variable period of months to years after she contracts the disease, presumably until the spirochetemia has abated. Transmission does not occur before the fifth month of gestation. Depending upon the magnitude of the infection, the fetus may die in utero or soon after birth, or it may survive. Surviving infants usually show a widespread, rather fulminant infection, with spirochetemia, that differs from any of the classic stages of acquired syphilis. The most striking lesions affect the mucocutaneous surfaces and the bones. A diffuse maculopapular rash develops, which differs from that of acquired syphilis by its tendency to cause extensive desquamation of the skin. A generalized osteochondritis and perichondritis are present. Destruction of the vomer of the nose produces the characteristic *saddle deformity;* inflammatory proliferation of the anterior surface of the tibiae causes the typical anterior bowing or *sabre shins;* and dental malformations create wedge shaped notched incisors (Hutchinsonian incisors) and "mulberry molars." A diffuse interstitial inflammatory reaction with prominent fibrosis may affect any organ of the body. In particular, the liver and lungs are frequently involved, with severe functional impairment. The eyes commonly show an interstitial keratitis or a choroiditis, and sometimes areas of abnormal pigmentation of the retinae.

Occasionally, congenital syphilis remains latent until early adulthood, then simulates tertiary syphilis in its manifestations, with the formation of gummas and the frequent development of neurosyphilis.

CHANCROID, GRANULOMA INGUINALE, LYMPHOGRANULOMA INGUINALE AND HERPES GENITALIS

These are four distinct venereal diseases, caused by four different infectious organisms. The diseases, however, are often confused because of their common tendency to produce ulcerative lesions of the external genitalia and tender inflammatory swelling *(buboes)* of the inguinal lymph nodes. The clinical and morphologic differences will be apparent in the following individual descriptions.

Chancroid (soft chancre) is an acute process caused by the gram-negative coccobacillus *Hemophilus ducreyi.* It is characterized by the development of a necrotic ulcer at the site of inoculation on the genitals and by suppurative inflammation in the regional lymph nodes.

Within two weeks following exposure, a small maculopapular lesion appears on the penis or vulva, followed over the next few days by rapid pustule formation and sloughing of the overlying skin, producing a painless ulcer between 1 and 3 cm. in diameter. This bears a superficial resemblance to the chancre of syphilis, but it does not have the characteristic induration of the syphilitic "hard" chancre. Histologically, the superficial necrotic debris covers a zone of granulation tissue and vasculitis, and this in turn overlies a zone of chronic inflammatory changes, with fibroblastic proliferation and mononuclear leukocytic infiltration. Often, autoinoculation produces multiple lesions. In about 50 per cent of cases, within two weeks after the appearance of the ulcer, the inguinal lymph nodes become enlarged and exquisitely tender. The histologic changes in the lymph nodes are essentially similar to those of the skin ulcer. There may be central abscess formation. Sometimes these abscesses drain to the surface.

Diagnosis is by culture or tissue biopsy. The course is usually self-limited, leaving only fibrous induration of the affected nodes and a scar at the site of the skin lesion.

Granuloma inguinale, in contrast to chancroid, is a chronic rather than an acute process, caused by the gram-negative coccobacillus *Donovania (Calymmatobacterium) granulomatis. It is distinctive in its tendency to form large, irregular keloid-like scars.* The extensive scarring may eventually produce lymphatic obstruction, which results in elephantiasis of the external genitalia. Although the sexual partners of patients are not always affected, it is thought to be a venereal disease, possibly of relatively low infectivity.

The initial lesion is a papule at the site of inoculation, usually on the external genitalia, which develops into a spreading, necrotic ulcer with a raised inflammatory border. Microabscesses form in the advancing margin of the lesion, and satellite papules and ulcers may appear along the course of lymphatic drainage. The lesion is characterized histologically by nonspecific acute and chronic inflammation, accompanied by an exuberant granulation tissue. The most distinctive finding is of large vacuolated macrophages containing many phagocytized organisms, termed Donovan bodies.

Diagnosis is by the demonstration of Donovan bodies, either in smears or in tissue biopsies. Rarely, the organism becomes widely disseminated, and may even cause death.

Lymphogranuloma inguinale (lymphogranuloma venereum, lymphopathia venereum) is very similar to granuloma inguinale in many ways, including its chronicity, but it is caused by a virus-like organism *Chlamydia trachomatis* (sometimes classified as rickettsiae).

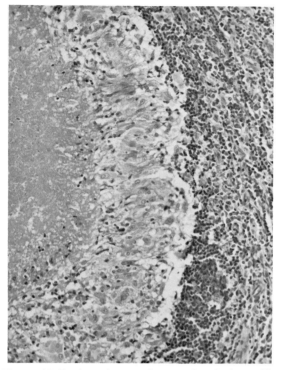

Figure 16–7. Lymphogranuloma inguinale. The margin of a characteristic "stellate" abscess rimmed by a granulomatous reaction. (From Robbins, S. L.: Pathologic Basis of Disease. Philadelphia, W. B. Saunders Co., 1974.)

Within a few days to three weeks following sexual contact, a tiny vesicle often, but not invariably, forms at the site of virus introduction. Usually this is on the glans penis or vulva, but the vaginal walls, cervix, urethra or anus may be primarily affected. The vesicle rapidly ulcerates, and a few weeks later, tender enlargement of the regional (usually inguinal) lymph nodes develops. Infrequently, the virus becomes widely disseminated. Histologically, the ulcer is characterized by a nonspecific mononuclear leukocytic infiltration, with fibroblastic proliferation and some vascular endothelial hyperplasia. The affected lymph nodes develop a granulomatous reaction surrounding a central area of suppuration, which may drain to the skin (Fig. 16–7). These lesions tend to coalesce, and contiguous lymph nodes become matted together. As with granuloma inguinale, obstruction of the lymphatic channels causes elephantiasis of the genitalia. More serious are the late sequelae in the female. Vaginal or posterior perineal lesions lead to involvement of the perirectal and deep pelvic nodes. Such involvement produces chronic fibrosis about the rectum, with resultant rectal strictures.

Lymphogranuloma inguinale, then, should be considered when evaluating rectal obstruction in the female. The *Frei skin test* indicates prior or present disease.

Herpes genitalis is caused by the Herpes simplex virus, antigenic type 2 (HSV-2). As such, it is the venereal counterpart of the oral "fever blisters" or gingivostomatitis produced by the closely related HSV-1. It is probably a very frequent infection. Evidence of its presence has been reported in approximately 1 of 500 Papanicolaou smears from the uterine cervix (Shelley, 1967; Nahmias et al., 1967). The infection may be primary, recurrent or chronic. In 90 per cent of cases, the *primary* infection is subclinical (Young, 1972). In the remaining cases, however, after an incubation period of about 6 days, painful focal lesions develop, often along with dysuria and systemic symptoms, such as fever, headache and malaise.

The lesions are single or multiple. In men, they occur on the inner surface of the prepuce, on the glans penis and on the nearby skin. In women, they most often involve the cervix, but also affect the vagina, vulva and labia. Grossly, the lesions appear as small vesicles, one or more millimeters in diameter, surrounded by marked erythema and edema. These rapidly rupture to form shallow ulcerations. Bilateral inguinal lymphadenopathy occurs, sometimes with exquisite tenderness. **Histologically, the hallmark of herpetic infection is the presence of multinuclear giant cells of epithelial origin containing intranuclear inclusions.** When such cells are found in Papanicolaou smears, they indicate herpetic cervicitis. The clinical manifestations of primary herpes genitalis last 3 to 6 weeks. **Recurrent** herpes genitalis is characterized by the periodic development of vesiculo-ulcerative lesions on an erythematous base. There is less edema and inflammatory response than with the primary disease, and the lesions disappear within a week to 10 days. They may recur several times a year. In some patients the lesions of herpes genitalis ulcerate and become **chronic,** particularly in those with diseases of the lymphoid tissue or those who are taking immunosuppressant drugs.

The major importance of herpes genitalis is twofold. Among pregnant women infected near the time of delivery, about 50 per cent of newborns delivered vaginally develop *neonatal herpes.* This is a severe, generalized disease which is often fatal. The second important effect of herpes genitalis is its possible contribution toward the development of *carcinoma of the cervix.* This subject will be more fully explored in Chapter 17. Suffice it to say here that prospective studies suggest that women with herpes genitalis have a higher risk of developing cervical cancer than women without HSV-2 neutralizing antibody (Nahmias and Roizman, 1973).

REFERENCES

Armenian, H. K., et al.: Relation between benign prostatic hyperplasia and cancer of the prostate. Lancet, 2:115, 1974.

Beral, V.: Cancer of the cervix: a sexually transmitted infection? Lancet, 1:1037, 1974.

Cameron, C. H., and Dane, D. S.: Hepatitis B antigen in saliva and semen. Lancet, 1:71, 1974.

Cole, P.: Personal communication 1974.

Dixon, F. J., and Moore, R. A.: Testicular tumors: clinicopathological study. Cancer, 6:427, 1953.

Dougall, A. G., et al.: Histology of the maldescended testis at operation. Lancet, 1:771, 1974.

Editorial: An epidemic of testicular cancer? Lancet, 2:164, 1968.

Editorial: Chlamydia and genital infection. Lancet, 2:264, 1974.

Eisenberg, H.: Cancer in Connecticut: Incidence and rates, 1935–1962. Hartford, Connecticut, State Department of Health, 1966.

Frank, I. N.: Urologic and male genital cancers. In Rubin, P. (ed.): Clinical Oncology for Medical Students and Physicians. 3rd ed. New York, American Cancer Society, 1970–71.

Franks, L. M.: Latent carcinoma of prostate. J. Path. Bact., 68:603, 1954.

Ghormley, K. O., and Needham, G. M.: Chronic prostatitis: a urologic quandary. J.A.M.A., 153:915, 1953.

Grumbach, M. M., et al.: Sex chromatin pattern in seminiferous tubule dysgenesis and other testicular disorders: relationship to true hermaphroditism and to Klinefelter's syndrome, with a review of gonadal ontogenesis. J. Clin. Endocr., 17:703, 1957.

Handsfield, H. H., et al.: Asymptomatic gonorrhea in men. New Eng. J. Med., 290:117, 1974.

Heathcote, J., and Sherlock, S.: Spread of acute type B hepatitis in London. Lancet, 1:1468, 1973.

Jewett, H. J., et al.: The palpable nodule of prostatic cancer. J.A.M.A., 203:115, 1968.

Lightfoot, R. W., and Gotschlich, E. C.: Gonococcal disease. Am. J. Med., 56:347, 1974.

Lucas, J. B.: The national venereal disease problem. Med. Clin. N. Amer., 56:1073, 1972.

Maier, J. G., et al.: An evaluation of lymphadenectomy in the treatment of malignant testicular germ cell neoplasms. J. Urol., 101:356, 1969.

Moore, R. A.: Benign hypertrophy of the prostate. A morphologic study. J. Urol., 50:68, 1943.

Nahmias, A. J., et al.: Genital herpes simplex infection: virologic and cytologic studies. Obstet. Gynec., 29:395, 1967.

Nahmias, A. J., and Roizman, B.: Infection with herpes-simplex viruses 1 and 2. New Eng. J. Med., 289:667, 719, 781, 1973.

National Advisory Council: Progress Against Cancer. Washington, D.C., U. S. Department of Health, Education and Welfare, Public Health Service, 1969.

Rubin, P.: Cancer of the urogenital tract: prostatic cancer. Introduction. J.A.M.A., 209:1695, 1969.

Shelley, W. B.: Herpes simplex virus as a cause of erythema multiforme. J.A.M.A., 201:153, 1967.

Silverberg, E.: Urologic Cancer. Statistical and Epidemiological Information. New York, American Cancer Society, Inc., 1973.

Silverberg, E., and Holleb, A. I.: Cancer statistics, 1974 — worldwide epidemiology. CA, 24:2, 1974.

Strahan, R. W.: Carcinoma of the prostate: incidence, origin, pathology. J. Urol., 89:875, 1963.

Wang, C.-I., et al.: Inguinal hernia, hydrocele and other genitourinary abnormalities. Am. J. Dis. Child., 119:236, 1970.

Willcox, R. R.: A world look at the venereal diseases. Med. Clin. N. Amer., 56:1057, 1972.

Williams, R. D., and Blackard, C. E.: Benign prostatic hyperplasia and cancer of the prostate. Lancet, 2:1265, 1974.

Young, A. W.: Herpes genitalis. Med. Clin. N. Amer., 56:1175, 1972.

CHAPTER 17

The Female Genital System and Breast

Each structure of the female genital tract—vulva, vagina, cervix, body of the uterus, oviducts and ovaries—tends to react to disease in a characteristic way. The clinical manifestations of disorders of the female genital tract, then, parallel anatomic divisions. This chapter will therefore be divided according to anatomic structure, with a short general statement as to the symptom complex produced by disease of each structure. Diseases of pregnancy and of the breast are described at the end of the chapter.

VULVA

Pathologic processes of the vulva tend to create visible epidermal lesions, which are vulnerable to secondary infection. The patient often complains of itching or pain, or of an exudative discharge.

Inflammatory lesions of the vulva in general parallel those of the penis. Reference should be made to Chapter 16 for consideration of these processes, which include gonorrhea, syphilis and the other venereal infections, since these diseases affect both the male and the female. In this section, we are concerned only with lesions specific to the female vulva, including *kraurosis vulvae* and *Bartholin's cyst,* as well as the more important *malignant neoplasms.*

KRAUROSIS VULVAE

Kraurosis vulvae refers to a marked exaggeration of the atrophy and fibrosis of the vulva which normally occur with advanced age. The skin loses its normal folds and becomes thin and parchment-like. Sometimes there is a glazed, reddened appearance. The labia atrophy and the introitus narrows. Histologically, the epidermis is thinned, with loss of the rete pegs, and the dermis is replaced by dense collagenous fibrous tissue.

The significance of kraurosis vulvae lies in the predisposition of the relatively avascular vulva to trauma and infection. On this basis, the disorder may cause considerable discomfort. Probably it does not significantly increase the risk of developing cancer of the vulva.

BARTHOLIN'S CYST

Obstruction of the excretory ducts of Bartholin's glands by inflammatory scarring, epithelial metaplasia or the accumulation of inspissated secretions may give rise to an exquisitely tender cystic dilatation of the ducts or the racemose glands, designated *Bartholin's cyst*. This lesion is quite common and may occur at any age. It should be differentiated from acute gonococcal infection of a Bartholin's gland.

The Bartholin's cyst is usually unilateral and appears as a tense, round mass in the labium minor, about 3 to 5 cm. in diameter, lined by columnar mucus secreting cells. When uncomplicated by infection, the cyst is filled with a mucinous secretion. Secondary infection is, however, frequent, and transforms the lesion into a pus-filled **Bartholin's abscess.**

TUMORS OF THE VULVA

Although a variety of nonspecific tumors, both benign and malignant, such as the fibroma, angioma and melanocarcinoma, may affect the vulva, only four are important enough to warrant description: the *papillomas, leukoplakia, squamous cell carcinoma* and *Paget's disease of the vulva.*

Papillomas of the vulva are entirely analogous to those of the penis, and reference should be made to Chapter 16 (page 547) for their description. The rather poorly defined, premalignant entity known as *leukoplakia* is also described in this earlier chapter. When leukoplakia affects the vulva, it appears as a patchy or diffuse, sharply circumscribed, whitish thickening. Its importance derives from the fact that roughly 25 per cent of these lesions progress through *carcinoma in situ (Bowen's disease)* to overt squamous cell carcinoma.

CARCINOMA OF THE VULVA

This uncommon squamous cell tumor is rare before old age. Roughly 50 per cent are preceded by leukoplakia.

The tumor begins as a small, grayish area of firm, elevated thickening which eventually becomes fissured and ulcerated. The ulcer is characteristically irregular and necrotic, with firm, elevated margins. On microscopic examination, these tumors are typical squamous cell carcinomas, ranging from well differentiated lesions with keratohyaline pearls and prickle cells to aggressive anaplastic tumors.

Not only is carcinoma of the vulva locally invasive, but it also tends to metastasize to regional lymph nodes at an early stage. Ultimately, widespread dissemination occurs to the lungs, liver and other organs.

Although carcinoma of the vulva is readily discernible by the patient and produces symptoms from secondary infection, such as pain, itching and exudation, it is often mistaken for dermatitis or leukoplakia, and the correct diagnosis is usually made late in the course. The five-year survival rate is about 30 per cent.

PAGET'S DISEASE OF THE VULVA

This is a rare tumor, analogous to *Paget's disease of the breast* (p. 590). It is thought to begin as a carcinoma of the mucous or sebaceous glands of the perineum which then grows along the excretory ducts to invade the epidermis.

Grossly, it appears as a red, crusted, map-like area, usually on the labia majora. On microscopic examination, characteristic large, anaplastic tumor cells, surrounded by a clear halo, are seen lying singly or in nests within the epidermis. Occasionally, these cells are seen in the apparent absence of an underlying glandular or ductal involvement. But, with sufficient investigation, a primary origin in one of the adnexal glands can generally be found as the source of the "Paget cells" lying within the epidermis.

VAGINA

The vagina of the adult is remarkably resistant to disease. The only primary disorders of the vagina that occur with any frequency are the more or less innocuous infectious disorders *trichomonal* and *monilial vaginitis.* Primary tumors are quite rare. Nearly always they are in the form of a typical *squamous cell carcinoma.*

Much less common are the *clear-cell adenocarcinomas.* Recently, these have received considerable attention because of an increased incidence in the teenaged daughters of women who had taken diethylstilbestrol during pregnancy (Herbst et al., 1971). From 1948 until about 1970 this drug was frequently given to pregnant women with threatened abortion in an attempt to maintain the pregnancy. The risk to their daughters of developing vaginal adenocarcinoma seems to be fairly small, about 0.4 to 0.9 per cent (Editorial, 1974a). More often these girls develop only a precursor lesion, *adenosis of the vagina*—the abnormal presence of glandular epithelium, either within the submucosa or replacing the normal surface squamous epithelium (Kurman and Scully, 1974). Those who do develop cancer are usually 15 to 20 years old.

A second very rare tumor of the vagina is a peculiar pleomorphic neoplasm of mesodermal origin termed *sarcoma botryoides.* This designation is descriptive of a soft, gray multilobate mass producing some vague resemblance to a cluster of grapes. Occasionally these masses may protrude through the introitus. Histologically, they have a loose, myxoid stroma, in which scattered anaplastic and bizarre mesenchymal tumor cells are found. Some of these cells reproduce features of striated muscle, indicating the true rhabdomyomatous nature of the tumors.

UTERUS

Diseases of the cervix and body of the uterus make up a large proportion of all of the illnesses afflicting the female, and represent the burden of disorders seen in gynecologic practice. Most fall into one of two large groups: disorders of the endometrium, and tumors of the uterine cervix and body. Thus, the wide range of lesions presents clinically in a fairly restricted number of ways, and the disorders therefore require careful appraisal to distinguish among them.

CERVIX UTERI

CERVICITIS

Cervicitis may be associated with such specific infections as gonorrhea, syphilis, chancroid and tuberculosis. These processes have been described elsewhere, and the cervical involvement does not significantly differ from the characteristic patterns of injury these infections impose on any tissue of the body.

Much more common is the relatively banal *nonspecific cervicitis,* present to some degree in virtually every multiparous woman. Although this somewhat baffling entity is known to be associated with a variety of organisms, including *E. coli,* alpha and beta hemolytic streptococci and a variety of staphylococci, the pathogenesis of the infection is poorly understood. Trauma of childbirth, instrumentation during gynecologic procedures, hyperestrinism, hypoestrinism, excessive secretion of the endocervical glands, alkalinity of the cervical mucus and congenital eversion of the endocervical mucosa have all been cited as predisposing influences.

Nonspecific cervicitis may be either *acute* or *chronic.* Excluding gonococcal infection, which causes a specific form of acute disease, the relatively uncommon *acute* nonspecific form is virtually limited to postpartum women and is usually caused by staphylococci or streptococci. The acute inflammatory infiltrate tends to remain largely limited to the exocervical os *(exocervicitis),* but, in severe cases, it may extend to the superficial endocervical mucosa and endocervical glands *(endocervicitis).*

The *chronic* form is the nearly ubiquitous entity usually referred to by the unqualified term "nonspecific cervicitis."

It begins as a slight reddening, swelling and granularity near the squamocolumnar junction, extending onto the external cervical os. With persistence of the inflammation, superficial irregular erosions or ulcerations develop. **Eventually, in severe cases, the continual inflammatory-reparative process results in distortion of the exocervix by irregular, friable nodules and ulcerations which may, on inspection, be confused with carcinoma of the cervix.** Histologically, a predominantly mononuclear inflammatory infiltrate, admixed with some polymorphonuclear leukocytes, is found subjacent to the endocervical mucosa, close to the squamocolumnar junction of the exocervical os. This infiltrate typically surrounds the endocervical mucous glands and fills their lumina. Usually the overlying epithelium undergoes some degree of inflammatory metaplastic change and, in severe cases, may show considerable dysplasia, with downward growth of epithelial pegs into the mouths of the endocervical glands, referred to as **epidermidization.** Such growth may completely envelop and compress the endocervical glands, a process **not** to be mistaken for invasion by a squamous cell carcinoma. Other morphologic features include cystic dilatation of the endocervical glands caused by inflammatory stenosis of their outlets **(nabothian cysts),** protrusion of the endocervical mucosa onto the external aspect of the cervix **(eversion)** and the development of lymphoid follicles **(follicular cervicitis).**

Nonspecific chronic cervicitis commonly comes to attention on routine examination or because of marked leukorrhea. When the lesion is severe, differentiation from carcinoma may be possible only by biopsy. *Clearly, cervicitis does not always lead to carcinoma, since the former is so much more frequent than the latter. However, it is believed to be an important predisposing influence (see page 565), and herein lies much of the clinical significance of the lesion.* In addition, severe cervicitis may lead to sterility through deformation of the cervical os.

TUMORS OF THE CERVIX

Although a wide variety of tumors may develop in the cervix uteri, all are rare except the squamous cell carcinoma and the relatively unimportant polyp.

Although *polyps* are quite common, occurring in 2 to 5 per cent of adult females, they are rather innocuous, being important principally as a cause of abnormal bleeding which must be differentiated from that due to more ominous causes.

These lesions typically arise within the endocervical canal. They may be sessile, hemispheric masses or pedunculated, spherical lesions up to 3 cm. in diameter. Those with long stalks may be seen on clinical examination, hanging down through the exocervical os and causing dilatation of the cervix. Characteristically, cervical polyps are soft, almost mucoid. Their histologic nature is that of a loose fibromyxomatous stroma containing cystically dilated endocervical glands. Although the covering epithelium is usually columnar and mucus secreting, superimposed chronic inflammation may lead to squamous metaplasia and ulcerations. Malignant transformation rarely, if ever, occurs.

CARCINOMA OF THE CERVIX

The story of carcinoma of the cervix is one of the most heartening in the annals of medicine. Once the second most important cause of cancer death in women (following cancer of the breast), it has now fallen to sixth place, and is responsible for only 5 per cent of female cancer mortality in the United States, or less than 8000 deaths per year (Silverberg and Holleb, 1974). This dramatic decline in the death rate from carcinoma of the cervix is largely attributable to the use of the Papanicolaou cytologic test ("Pap test") as a widespread screening device for the detection of cervical cancer (made possible, of course, by the fortuitous accessibility of the cervix). Very early diagnosis has permitted curative therapy in a remarkable percentage of patients. Thus, the price of liberation from cervical carcinoma, like that of liberty in general, is eternal vigilance.

The accessibility of the cervix to examination and biopsy has made possible another, more abstract, advance in medicine. By repeated observations over a period of years, it has been proved that carcinoma of the cervix arises in a series of stepwise progressions along a continuum of cell abnormalities ranging from hyperplasia to dysplasia to carcinoma-in-situ to invasive carcinoma (Fish, 1974; Rotkin, 1973). Indeed, it was through the study of this form of cancer that the concept of carcinoma-in-situ was developed. More will be said about this later. With early detection of cervical cancer, there has been a decline in the incidence of invasive carcinoma, with a reciprocal increase in that of carcinoma-in-situ (Kirk, 1974).

Incidence. Invasive cervical carcinoma now accounts for about 6 per cent of cancer in women. It reaches its peak incidence at about 50 years of age. However, the peak incidence of in-situ lesions is about 10 to 15 years earlier, and there is an impression in recent years that the disease has been showing a predilection for increasingly younger women.

Following is a list of epidemiologic associations with cancer of the cervix (Cole, 1974; Rotkin, 1973; Klein, 1973). One should, of course, be very cautious about ascribing a causative role to any of them. The incidence of cancer of the cervix is:

1. Higher in women who have an early first coitus.
2. Increased with the number of sexual partners.
3. Positively correlated with the incidence of antibodies to Herpes simplex virus, type 2.
4. Inversely correlated with socioeconomic status.
5. Higher in married women, increasing with the number of marriages.
6. Increased with the number of children.
7. Higher in prostitutes.
8. Higher in blacks than in whites.
9. Lower in Jews, Indian Muslims, Parsis, and nuns.
10. Lower in those using obstructive forms of contraception (condom, diaphragm).

Etiology and Pathogenesis. What clues about causation can be inferred from the incidence data? Obviously, the risk of developing this disease is strongly related to sexual practice. Reliable epidemiologic data on this subject are difficult to obtain. Nevertheless, attempts to evaluate each of these features separately indicate that a direct pathogenic role can be ascribed only to the first two: *early onset of coitus, and multiple sexual partners.* Most of the other factors, such as early and multiple marriage, early and multiple parity and low socioeconomic status, can be considered related to predisposing sexual practices (Rotkin, 1973). *Thus, it would seem that carcinoma of the cervix involves some initiating agent transmitted at an early age from male to female* — a one-way venereal disease, if you will. Multiple sexual partners would increase the likelihood of initially encountering this agent, as well as make possible repeated contact with it.

The very low incidence of this disease in Jewish women (0.25 that of controls), as well as in females of some other sects practicing male circumcision, led to the belief that the initiating agent was contained in the smegma which accumulates in the prepuce of the uncircumcised male. This hypothesis is made more attractive by the undoubted protection conferred by circumcision against carcinoma of the penis. Coitus only with circumcised males was thought similarly to protect against carcinoma of the cervix. Recently, however, this hypothesis has been challenged (Klein, 1973). It has been pointed out that studies tending to support this view have (a) dealt with select population groups in whom other variables may be operative, (b) focused on husbands rather than on all sexual partners, and/or (c) relied on the patient's own assessment as to whether her husband was indeed circumcised — a source which, strangely enough, appears to be unreliable. More recent studies in which an attempt was made to overcome these difficulties — by matching controls for ethnic groups, by attempting to include all sexual partners, and by verifying circumcision of husbands — have shown that patients with cancer of the cervix are no more likely to have uncircumcised sexual partners than are women in the control population (Terris et al., 1973; Rotkin, 1973; Aitken-Swan and Baird, 1965). As mentioned earlier, however, epidemiologic data concerning sexual practice are difficult to obtain, and the question of the role of circumcision remains unsettled.

The possible role of Herpes simplex virus, type 2 (HSV-2) in the causation of cervical cancer is also unsettled. It has been demonstrated that 80 to 98 per cent of patients with cervical carcinoma have neutralizing antibodies to this virus, as opposed to 20 to 55 per cent of controls (Plummer and Masterson, 1971). Moreover, immunofluorescent studies have revealed HSV-2 antigens within cells exfoliated from carcinomas of the cervix (Rapp and Buss, 1974). However, the significance of these findings is open to question, since both HSV-2 infection and carcinoma of the cervix may simply be independent covariables of sexual promiscuity. The fact that

antibody against HSV-1 (oral herpes) may cross-neutralize HSV-2 further complicates the issue (Plummer and Masterson, 1971). Still, attempts to match control populations for promiscuity do indicate some correlation between cervical cancer and the presence of antibodies against HSV-2 (Rawls et al., 1973).

Morphology. Carcinoma of the cervix usually begins at the squamocolumnar junction of the external cervical os. In most women this region is located somewhat outside the anatomic os. Before describing the appearance of these lesions, a few words should be said about their evolution. As mentioned, carcinoma of the cervix evolves as a sequential, multistep process in which there appears to be selection for increasingly autonomous cell forms. Thus, dysplastic cell forms may arise in a focus of basal cell hyperplasia. The dysplastic focus may then become increasingly atypical as less controlled cell forms are selected, until ultimately an anaplastic cell line emerges, still confined to the cervical epithelial mucosa. At this point the lesion is designated carcinoma-in-situ. The final step in the evolution of invasive carcinoma is penetration of the basement membrane with extension into the underlying stroma. **It is important to remember that this entire process is very slow, requiring years to decades. Moreover, progression of the disease from one step to the next is not inevitable** (Fish, 1974; Stern, 1973). At any point short of carcinoma-in-situ, the process may be reversed, sometimes spontaneously, sometimes by quite simple therapeutic measures to combat chronic inflammation. Even carcinoma-in-situ has been known to regress spontaneously, as well as to remain static for decades. This, however, is unusual. In general, the farther the process has evolved, the less likely is spontaneous regression.

In the in-situ stage, cancer of the cervix produces no gross changes. Histologically, one sees the changes characteristic of cellular anaplasia, con-

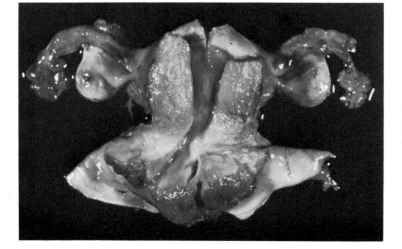

Figure 17–1. Carcinoma of the cervix. The uterus has been opened anteriorly. The cervix (below) is markedly enlarged by an invasive tumor that has fungated through the mucosal surface to produce the readily seen dark lobularity.

fined to the mucosa. Sometimes the anaplastic cells creep along the surface into the underlying endocervical glands, but such superficial spread should not be construed as invasion, since the basement membranes of these glands are not penetrated.

Invasive carcinoma takes one of three somewhat distinct macroscopic forms. The most frequent is a **fungating** tumor, which begins as a nodular thickening of the epithelium and eventually appears as a cauliflower mass projecting above the surrounding mucosa, sometimes completely encircling the external os (Fig. 17–1). The second is an **ulcerative** form, characterized by necrotic sloughing of the central surface of the tumor. The least frequent variety is the **infiltrative**, which tends to grow downward into the underlying stroma, rather than outward. Of course, with time these forms tend to merge as they infiltrate the underlying tissue, obliterate the external os, grow upward into the endocervical canal and lower uterine segment and eventually extend into and through the wall of the fundus into the broad ligaments. Advanced lesions may extend into the rectum or base of the urinary bladder. Only relatively late is there involvement of lymph nodes or distant metastases. The lymph nodes first affected are the external iliac and hypogastric chains, followed later by periaortic nodal involvement. Distant metastases, when present, usually affect the lungs, bones and liver.

The histology of 95 per cent of carcinomas of the cervix is that of a typical **squamous cell carcinoma** of varying differentiation (Fig. 17–2). The remaining 5 per cent are **adenocarcinomas**, presumably arising in the endocervical glands or mixed squamous and adeno- forms, termed **adenoacanthomas.**

Both a grading system, based on the degree of cellular differentiation, and a staging system, based on tumor spread, have been devised. Grades I through III refer to progressively undifferentiated lesions. The staging system is based only on the extent of the primary tumor, and does not address itself to nodal involvement or metastases. This reflects the relatively late dissemination of this form of cancer, along with the importance of the local effects of the primary lesion. The staging system is as follows:

Stage 0: Carcinoma-in-situ.

Stage I: Tumor confined to the cervix.

Stage II: Tumor extends beyond the cervix and involves the upper two-thirds of the vagina, but has not become fixed to the pelvic wall.

Stage III: Tumor has become fixed to the pelvic wall and involves the lower third of the vagina.

Stage IV: Tumor has extended beyond the true pelvis, or has involved the mucosa of the bladder or rectum.

Clinical Course. Carcinoma-in-situ of the cervix may be asymptomatic, or it may masquerade as chronic cervicitis. Usually it is detected on Pap smear. Although the smear calls attention to the possibility of cancer, it is not diagnostic. The Schiller test, also, is indicative but not diagnostic. This test is based on the fact that atypical cells become depleted of glycogen. The cervix is painted with a solution of iodine and potassium chloride; normal epithelium stains brown, whereas a cancerous focus remains unstained. However, lesser degrees of abnormality, such as hyperplasia or dysplasia, are also associated with a positive Schiller test (failure to stain). The final diagnosis, then, rests on a confirmatory biopsy. With advanced, invasive carcinoma, of course, the lesion may be immediately obvious on gross inspection. By this time there will usually have been clinical manifestations, most often leukorrhea, spotty irregular bleeding and post-coital bleeding. *The morbidity and mortality from this form of cancer are usually related to local effects rather than distant metastases.* The most common cause of death is renal disease from ureteral invasion by the tumor mass.

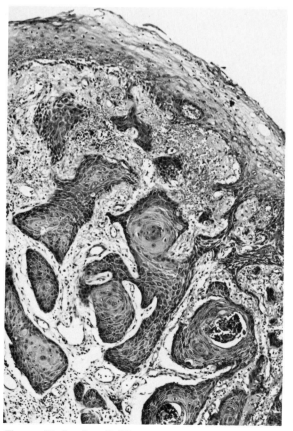

Figure 17–2. A well differentiated squamous cell carcinoma of the cervix, which has invaded below the normal mucosa (above).

The usual treatment for carcinoma-in-situ is total hysterectomy. Five-year survival approaches 100 per cent in these cases. In view of this prognosis and the slowness of these tumors to evolve, therapy can be postponed without risk to the patient if there is any doubt about the diagnosis and the physician desires to observe the lesion longer. Pregnancy may be an indication for postponement of therapy. Five-year survival with Stage I disease is 85 per cent; with Stage II disease, 75 per cent; Stage III disease, 55 per cent; and Stage IV disease, 15 per cent. It was mentioned earlier, as a medical triumph, that only 8000 women die of carcinoma of the cervix each year. In another sense, however, this is a great failure, since the efficacy of the Pap test, along with the nearly 100 per cent five-year survival with carcinoma-in-situ, indicates that theoretically all of these deaths are preventable.

CORPUS UTERI

ENDOMETRITIS

The endometrium is relatively resistant to infection. Occasionally, postpartal retention of placental fragments predisposes to an *acute,* nonspecific involvement of the uterine wall, usually caused by the hemolytic streptococci or staphylococci. Curettage permits prompt healing of the process.

Chronic endometritis may result from miliary spread of *tuberculosis,* as well as from a smoldering, *nonspecific* postpartal infection. Although the wall of the uterus is relatively resistant to invasion by the gonococcus, chronic endometritis is nevertheless in some cases a component of *gonococcal* PID (see p. 556). These three types of *secondary chronic endometritis* produce somewhat distinctive tissue reactions, which have been described elsewhere. In addition, the endometrial glands become irregular and the mucosa becomes infiltrated by plasma cells, the only type of leukocyte not normally present in the uterus late in the menstrual cycle. Occasionally, these histologic changes alone are found in patients who do not have tuberculosis or gonorrhea, and who have not been pregnant. In such cases, the diagnosis of *idiopathic* or *primary chronic endometritis* is probably justified. Sometimes, but not invariably, clinical complaints such as abnormal bleeding, discomfort, discharge or infertility accompany this histologic picture.

ENDOMETRIOSIS

The presence of endometrial glands or stroma, or both, in abnormal locations is termed *endometriosis.* When the aberrant tissue is contained within the myometrium, the condition is known as *internal endometriosis* or *adenomyosis.* Of greater clinical significance is the presence of foci of endometrial tissue outside the uterus, a disorder properly called *external endometriosis* or *pelvic endometriosis,* but often referred to by the unqualified term "endometriosis."

Internal endometriosis is found at postmortem examination in from 10 to 50 per cent of women. The etiology is unknown.

Grossly, the uterus is usually slightly enlarged, with irregular thickening of the wall to 2 to 2.5 cm. and a poorly defined endomyometrial junction. On histologic examination, penetration of the muscle bundles of the myometrium by nests of endometrial tissue is seen which, with serial sections, can be shown to represent downward extensions of the basal zone of the overlying endometrium. In most instances, these nests are composed of typical glands enclosed within a spindle cell stroma. Occasionally, however, only stroma is present, a picture sometimes designated **stromal endometriosis. In less than 10 per cent of cases of internal endometriosis, the buried endometrium is functional and menstruates.** Blood then accumulates within the endometrial foci, and considerable localized hemosiderosis may develop.

For obscure reasons, patients with internal endometriosis frequently have menorrhagia, colicky dysmenorrhea and premenstrual pelvic discomfort.

External endometriosis occurs in the following sites, in descending order of frequency: (1) ovaries, (2) uterine ligaments, (3) rectovaginal septum, (4) pelvic peritoneum, (5) umbilicus, (6) laparotomy scars and rarely, in other locations, such as the vagina, vulva, nasal mucosa and appendix (Groseclose, 1954). The disorder is of clinical importance during active reproductive life, between the ages of 20 and 40 years. Although it has been ascribed to relative or absolute hyperestrinism, a definite association between external endometriosis and elevated levels of estrogens has not been demonstrated.

As to pathogenesis, two theories are favored. One proposes that fragments of endometrium, which are regurgitated through the oviducts during menstruation, spill out of the fimbriated ends of the tubes to become implanted on serosal surfaces. The second theory suggests that the endometrial tissue arises through the abnormal differentiation of the coelomic epithelium which, after all, is the progenitor of the lining of the müllerian ducts. Conceivably, both pathogenetic mechanisms are operative in different cases. It is easy to explain the pelvic localizations by the former theory, but for endometrial implants

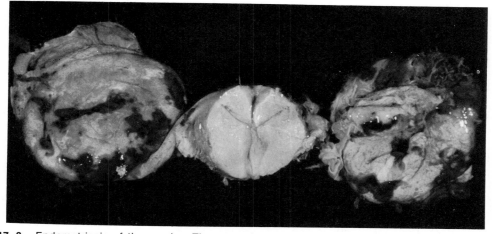

Figure 17–3. Endometriosis of the ovaries. The opened, subtotally removed uterus in the center is flanked by enlarged ovaries with marked endometriosis. The dark areas are masses of blood beneath the ovarian surface. The shagginess (seen best on the right) results from extensive adhesions to surrounding structures.

in the nose or umbilicus the theory of abnormal differentiation must be invoked.

In contrast to internal endometriosis, external endometriosis almost always contains functioning endometrium, which undergoes cyclic bleeding. Since blood collects in these aberrant foci, they usually appear grossly as red-blue to yellow-brown nodules or implants. They vary in size from microscopic to 1 to 2 cm. in diameter, and lie on or just under the affected serosal surface. Often, individual lesions coalesce to form larger masses. When the ovaries are involved, the large blood-filled cysts are transformed into so-called **chocolate cysts** as the blood ages. These cysts may become as large as 8 to 10 cm. in diameter, and are then referred to as **endometriomas.** With long-standing extensive disease, seepage and organization of the blood leads to widespread fibrosis, with adherence of pelvic structures (a "frozen" pelvis), obliteration of the pouch of Douglas, sealing of the tubal fimbriated ends and distortion of the oviducts and ovaries (Fig. 17–3). The histologic diagnosis depends on the finding within the lesions of two of the following three features: endometrial glands, stroma or hemosiderin pigment. When the disease is far advanced, with extensive scarring, both the gross and histologic diagnosis may be difficult because the characteristic features may largely be replaced by nonspecific fibrosis similar to that produced by, for example, PID (p. 573).

The clinical manifestations of external endometriosis depend upon the distribution of the lesions. Extensive scarring of the oviducts and ovaries eventually causes sterility. Pain on defecation reflects rectal wall involvement, and dyspareunia and dysuria reflect involvement of the uterine and bladder serosa. *In almost all cases, there is severe dysmenorrhea and pelvic pain as a result of intrapelvic bleeding and periuterine adhesions* (Meigs, 1942). Dys-

pareunia may be present on the same basis. For unclear reasons, menstrual irregularities are also common.

OTHER ENDOMETRIAL DERANGEMENTS

A variety of hormonal imbalances may result in derangements of the orderly cyclic proliferation and shedding of the endometrial mucosa. These endometrial abnormalities account for 15 to 20 per cent of gynecologic problems, and, next to leiomyomas of the uterus, are the most common causes of abnormal uterine bleeding. Four morphologic patterns are sufficiently well defined to merit individual discussion: cystic hyperplasia, adenomatous hyperplasia, atrophy of the endometrium, and out-of-phase cyclic changes in the endometrium known as chronic menstrual shedding.

Cystic hyperplasia, also sometimes known as *Swiss cheese endometrium,* is caused by a relative or absolute hyperestrinism. Most commonly, it develops shortly before menopause, and, in these instances, reflects the relative hyperestrinism resulting from the decline in progesterone levels with diminished ovulatory activity. Cystic hyperplasia is also seen when there are absolute increases in estrogen levels, as with persistence of follicle cysts in the ovary, such as may occur with the Stein-Leventhal syndrome, with functioning ovarian tumors, with excessive adrenocortical activity, and with exogenously administered estrogens, such as some of the contraceptive pills.

In all these situations, the endometrium is grossly thickened and velvety. Cystic dilatation of the glands produces a somewhat granular texture and a lacunar appearance on sectioning, which is

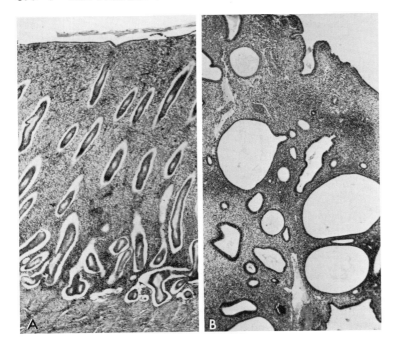

Figure 17–4. *A,* Normal proliferative endometrium. Compare with *B,* cystic hyperplasia of the endometrium.

somewhat reminiscent of Swiss cheese. On microscopic examination, cystic glands are seen interspersed with normal ones. In all glands, the tall columnar lining epithelial cells are regular, well-oriented and almost always nonsecretory. The intervening stroma often contains dilated, thin-walled vascular sinusoids, the source of the associated abnormal bleeding (Fig. 17–4).

Cystic hyperplasia usually manifests itself by excessive cyclic uterine bleeding (*menorrhagia*), and occasionally also by irregular spotty bleeding between menstrual periods (*metrorrhagia*). When encountered before puberty or after menopause, this form of hyperplasia strongly suggests either a functioning ovarian tumor or some adrenal cortical hyperfunction. Although some believe that there is an increased incidence of subsequent endometrial carcinoma in these patients, the risk is at worst only slightly augmented—probably to no more than 2 per cent of patients with this disorder.

In contrast, adenomatous hyperplasia clearly is associated with an increased risk of endometrial carcinoma. This form of endometrial hyperplasia occurs in women during active reproductive life. Although without doubt it is the result of some hormonal imbalance, the precise pathogenesis is unclear but probably involves hyperestrinism, perhaps having its origin in primary pituitary hyperfunction.

The endometrium in these cases may grossly resemble that of cystic hyperplasia, since it is markedly thickened, lush and velvety. Histologically, however, the difference is soon apparent.

The number of glands is markedly increased. These abnormal glands are rather unevenly distributed, so that focal aggregates of glands may be seen virtually back to back or separated only by a very scant stroma. Papillary inbuddings into the glands, as well as finger-like outpouchings into the adjacent stroma, are formed, The epithelial cells show a continuum of atypicality ranging from slight irregularity of the cellular and nuclear contours to more flagrant cytologic abnormalities with focal heaping and disarray of the epithelium. **Sometimes the atypism merits being called carcinoma-in-situ.**

Like cystic hyperplasia, adenomatous hyperplasia tends to produce menorrhagia, often with metrorrhagia. *Its principal clinical significance, however, lies in the fact that from 3 to 25 per cent of these patients eventually develop endometrial carcinoma.* Conversely, 19 of 32 patients with endometrial carcinoma were shown by retrospective studies of prior uterine scrapings to have once had adenomatous hyperplasia (Hertig and Sommers, 1949).

Atrophy of the endometrium is associated with hormonal changes which can be thought of as physiologically opposite to those which produce hyperplasia. It regularly occurs to some degree in postmenopausal women, but it may develop also in younger women if there is loss of ovarian or pituitary function.

The atrophic endometrium is thinned and glazed, consisting virtually only of the stratum basalis. Histologically, there is a compact endometrial stroma containing simple tubular nonproliferative and nonsecretory glands. Sometimes, in postmenopausal women, the glands are slightly dilated and the condition is then termed **senile cystic atrophy.**

Paradoxically, atrophy of the endometrium, like the hyperplastic disorders, may be responsible for menorrhagia or metrorrhagia.

Chronic menstrual shedding refers to abnormalities in the cyclic shedding and regrowth of the endometrium, in which some portion of the endometrium may progress normally into the secretory phase while residual areas remain in the proliferative phase.

This disorganized pattern is attributed to a peculiar resistance of some regions of the endometrium to the normal ovarian endocrine stimulation. When these endometrial changes develop, the menstrual shedding is incomplete, and persistent vaginal bleeding ensues.

TUMORS OF THE CORPUS UTERI

The most common uterine neoplasms are *endometrial polyps, leiomyomas* and *endometrial carcinomas* (comprising *adenocarcinomas* and *adenoacanthomas*). In addition, exotic mesodermal tumors are encountered, such as the *stromal sarcoma botryoides* (also encountered in the vagina and described on page 564). *All tend to produce bleeding from the uterus as the earliest manifestation.*

ENDOMETRIAL POLYP

These are sessile, usually hemispheric lesions, from 0.5 to 3 cm. in diameter, which project from the endometrial mucosa into the uterine cavity. On histologic examination, they are seen to be covered with columnar cells and to have an edematous stroma with cystically dilated glands similar to those seen with cystic hyperplasia.

Although endometrial polyps may occur at any age, they develop somewhat more commonly at the time of menopause. Probably their only clinical significance lies in the production of abnormal uterine bleeding that must be investigated to exclude more serious causes.

LEIOMYOMA

Benign tumors arising in the myometrium are properly termed "leiomyomas," although often they are referred to as "fibroids." *These are the most common benign tumors in females, developing in about 1 in 4 women during active reproductive life.* Although the etiology and pathogenesis are unknown, leiomyomas, once developed, seem to be estrogen dependent, as evidenced by their rapid growth during pregnancy and their tendency to regress following menopause. They have been shown to bind estradiol in greater amounts than does the normal endometrium (Farber et al., 1972). Whether or not hyperestrinism alone can ac-

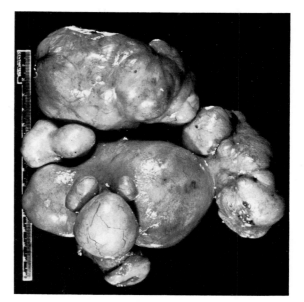

Figure 17–5. Leiomyomata of the uterus. The multiple subserosal, pedunculated, irregular tumors are viewed in the removed uterus. The uterine corpus is distorted beyond recognition. Only the cervix is identifiable as the lowermost projection.

tually initiate the formation of these tumors is, however, unclear.

Leiomyomas usually occur as multiple, sharply circumscribed but unencapsulated, firm, gray-white masses, with a characteristically whorled cut surface. The leiomyomas vary in size from barely visible seedings to massive tumors that may simulate a pregnant uterus. When these tumors are deeply embedded within the myometrium, they are termed **intramural.** Those located directly beneath the covering peritoneum of the uterine corpus are called **subserosal,** and those adjacent to the endometrium, **submucous.** Frequently, the subserosal and submucosal masses protrude either from the external surface of the uterus or into the endometrial cavity. Such lesions may be pedunculated (Fig. 17-5). Larger leiomyomas contain areas of yellow-brown to red softening, known as **necrobiosis** or **red carnaceous degeneration.** Proteolysis of these necrotic areas yields foci of cystic degeneration. Following menopause, as the tumors atrophy, they tend to become firmer and more collagenous, and sometimes they undergo partial or even complete calcification. Histologically, the tumors are characterized by whorling bundles of smooth muscle cells, duplicating the normal muscle bundles of the myometrium. Foci of fibrosis, calcification, ischemic necrosis with hemorrhage and more or less complete proteolytic digestion of dead cells may be present. After menopause, the smooth muscle cells tend to atrophy, eventually being replaced by fibrous tissue.

Leiomyomas of the uterus are often entirely asymptomatic and are discovered because of a palpably enlarged uterus. The most frequent manifestation is menorrhagia, with or without metrorrhagia. Large masses may produce a dragging sensation in the pelvic region. When situated in the lower uterine segment, they may create problems during childbirth.

Whether or not uterine leiomyomas ever undergo malignant transformation to become leiomyosarcomas is a controversial point. If they do, such transformation is indeed rare, since the benign tumors are commonplace, while their malignant counterparts are rare.

Grossly, **leiomyosarcomas** develop in several distinct patterns: as bulky masses infiltrating the uterine wall, as polypoid lesions projecting into the uterine cavity, or as structures with deceptively discrete margins that masquerade as large benign leiomyomas. Histologically, they show a wide range of differentiation, from well differentiated growths very similar to the leiomyomas to wildly anaplastic lesions approximating undifferentiated sarcomas.

The five-year survival rate with these lesions is about 20 to 40 per cent. After surgical removal, leiomyosarcomas show a striking tendency toward local recurrence, and some metastasize widely.

CARCINOMA OF THE ENDOMETRIUM

The most important cancer of the body of the uterus is endometrial carcinoma. This tumor is histopathologically distinct from cancer of the cervix. Almost certainly its causation is different as well. Perhaps the only similarity is the probability that carcinoma of the endometrium also arises over a period of years from a series of progressively abnormal cellular proliferations which eventually lead to in-situ carcinoma. The incidence of endometrial carcinoma has remained fairly static, while that of *invasive* cancer of the cervix has rapidly declined below it (Silverberg and Holleb, 1974). However, endometrial carcinoma remains less important as a cause of death than either cancer of the cervix or cancer of the ovary, and accounts for only 2 per cent of cancer deaths in women.

Etiology and Pathogenesis. Endometrial carcinoma is a disease of postmenopausal women, becoming more frequent with age. Like cancer of the breast and ovary, it shows a predilection for nulliparous women. Often there is a history of irregular menses and failure of ovulation. The similarity between this tumor and tumors of the breast and ovary goes deeper. *With all three, hormonal imbalances are thought to be important factors in their pathogenesis.* In the case of endometrial carcinoma, it has been suggested that this hormonal imbalance stems from abnormally low adrenal secretion of androgenic hormones, resulting in a relative, but not absolute, hyperestrinism (de Waard et al., 1968). Regardless of the origins of the estrogen excess, its effect is an abnormally intense proliferative stimulus to the endometrium. Normal endometrial cells contain specific receptor proteins which bind estradiol. Interestingly, cancerous endometrial cells also bind estradiol, indicating a continuing hormone dependence. It has already been mentioned that adenomatous hyperplasia, thought to be caused by hyperestrinism, is known to precede the development of endometrial carcinoma in many cases. In a manner similar to the stepwise development of cervical cancer from basal cell hyperplasia, it has been postulated that endometrial carcinoma develops from adenomatous hyperplasia, passing through an in-situ stage (Gusberg, 1973). Like cervical cancer, a developing endometrial carcinoma is probably reversible during much of its history. Certainly, adenomatous hyperplasia can usually be reversed by the administration of progestins.

The frequent association of ovarian cortical stromal hyperplasia with endometrial carcinoma raises the possibility in these cases that both may be the result of overstimulation of the ovaries by the pituitary. There is also a positive correlation between endometrial carcinoma on the one hand, and obesity and its common accompaniments, hypertension and diabetes mellitus, on the other (Garnet, 1958). It has been demonstrated that obese women tend to have higher estrogen levels than do their thinner sisters and, conceivably, this might be the basis for the increased incidence of endometrial carcinoma (de Waard et al., 1968).

Morphology. Endometrial carcinomas arise as in-situ lesions which, after a period of years, assume one of two macroscopic appearances (Gusberg et al., 1954). Either they infiltrate, causing diffuse thickening of the affected uterine wall, or they assume an exophytic form (Fig. 17–6). In both cases, they eventually fill the endometrial cavity with firm to soft, partially necrotic tumor tissue, and in time they extend through the myometrial wall to the serosa and thence by direct contiguity to periuterine structures. Late in the course, metastases to regional lymph nodes and later to distant organs occur. In about 85 per cent of these tumors, the histology is that of an **adenocarcinoma,** with well defined gland patterns lined with anaplastic cuboidal to columnar epithelial cells. Rarely, these cells have mucinous secretory activity, but most are nonsecretory and recapitulate the proliferative phase of the endometrial cycle. The remaining 15 per cent of endometrial carcinomas are **adenoacanthomas,** characterized by metaplastic transformation of the neoplastic columnar cells into

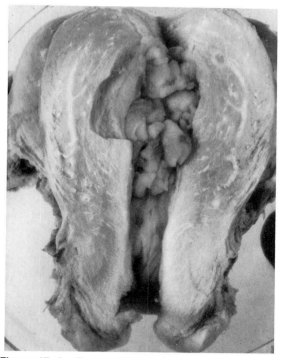

Figure 17—6. Endometrial carcinoma. The uterus has been opened anteriorly to disclose the fungating carcinoma in the endometrial cavity.

squamous cells along part of the circumference of the glands. Despite such curious aberrant differentiation, these tumors behave like adenocarcinomas.

Like most cancers, endometrial carcinoma is both graded according to cellular differentiation and staged according to the extent of the disease at diagnosis. The grades are I through III, from well differentiated to undifferentiated. The staging system incorporates a TNM evaluation as follows:

Stage O: Carcinoma-in-situ (TO NO MO).
Stage 1:   Tumor confined to the corpus uteri (T1 NO MO).

Stage II: Tumor extended to cervix (T2 NO MO).
Stage III: Tumor extended outside uterus but not outside true pelvis (T3 NO MO).
Stage IV--A: Tumor extended beyond true pelvis, e.g., to bladder and rectum (T4 NO MO).
Stage IV--B: Nodal involvement and metastases outside the pelvis (T1--4 N+M+).

Clinical Course. The first clinical indications of endometrial carcinoma are usually marked leukorrhea and irregular bleeding. This reflects erosion and ulceration of the endometrial surface. Even at this stage, the cervix may appear completely normal. Papanicolaou smears are of great value in the early detection of these lesions, particularly if the cytologic sample is aspirated from the uterine cavity itself, but the final diagnosis rests on histologic examination of curette scrapings. With radiotherapy and surgery, the prognosis is relatively good. Stage O endometrial carcinoma is entirely curable by hysterectomy. When Stage I and Stage II disease are treated by a combination of radiation and surgery, five-year survival is about 80 per cent. With more advanced disease, the prognosis is much poorer. Nevertheless, overall five-year survival for all stages of endometrial carcinoma is over 70 per cent (Cole, 1974).

OVIDUCTS

Except for tubal pregnancies, which will be considered later, the only lesion of importance to affect the oviducts is pelvic inflammatory disease. Cancers are extremely uncommon.

PELVIC INFLAMMATORY DISEASE (PID)

Although PID refers to an infection which involves more or less the entire female genital tract, salpingitis is its most prominent feature

Figure 17—7. Pelvic inflammatory disease. The uterus is flanked by bilateral large tubo-ovarian masses resulting from the accumulation of exudate within the sealed-off tubes and ovaries. Note the shaggy hemorrhagic surface responsible for pelvic adhesions.

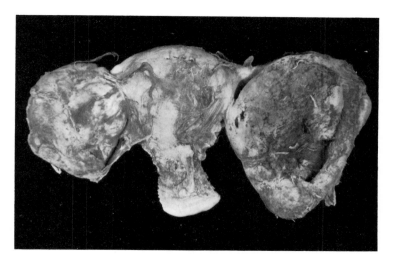

(Fig. 17–7). Pelvic inflammatory disease caused by the gonococcus was described in the discussion of gonorrhea in Chapter 16. Here we are concerned with the nonvenereal form, which, while very similar, differs in a few respects from the gonococcal disease.

With earlier diagnosis and more effective treatment of gonorrhea, other infections have assumed greater importance as causes of PID. Most of these follow childbirth, abortions or gynecologic instrumentation and are caused by the staphylococci, streptococci, coliforms or *Clostridium perfringens.*

Unlike the gonococcus, which spreads over the mucosal surfaces, nonspecific infections extend from their primary site through the lymphatic or venous channels. Accordingly, there is less superficial exudation but a correspondingly greater nonspecific inflammatory response within the deeper layers of the genital tract. The cervix, uterus, parametrium and oviducts commonly are involved. Eventually, the infection tends to spread through the wall of the affected structures to involve the peritoneum. Bacteremia is a more frequent complication of streptococcal or staphylococcal PID than of gonococcal PID, and it may lead to meningitis, endocarditis or suppurative arthritis.

The clinical presentation of well established PID gives little clue to etiology. Commonly, there is pelvic discomfort, dysmenorrhea and sometimes manifestations of an acute abdomen. Long-standing disease leads to fibrotic deformities of the oviducts with consequent sterility.

OVARIES

The ovaries are remarkably resistant to disease. Indeed, tumors are the only lesions important enough to warrant full discussion. Before proceeding to these, some of the frequent hyperplastic and cystic aberrations of the cyclic ovarian physiology deserve brief description.

BENIGN HYPERPLASTIC AND CYSTIC DISORDERS

Cortical stromal hyperplasia is found in a significant number of patients with endometrial hyperplasia or endometrial carcinoma.

The ovaries may be slightly enlarged or normal in size. The cortex is thickened by plump fibroblastic cells containing lipids, presumably steroids. Occasionally these cells create nodulation of the ovarian surface and, rarely, granulomatous foci appear in these nodules. The presence of lipid within the hyperplastic ovarian cells suggests that they are active in hormone production, and so it has been hypothesized that cortical stromal hyper-

plasia has a causative role in the development of the endometrial lesions.

Follicle and luteal cysts in the ovaries are so commonplace as to be virtually physiologic variants.

These innocuous lesions originate in unruptured graafian follicles or in follicles that have ruptured and have immediately been sealed. Such cysts are often multiple and develop immediately subjacent to the serosal covering of the ovary. Usually they are small—1 to 1.5 cm. in diameter—and are filled with clear serous fluid, but occasionally they accumulate enough fluid to achieve diameters of 4 to 5 cm. and may thus become palpable masses and indeed produce pelvic pain. They are lined by granulosal cells or luteal cells when small, but as the fluid accumulates under pressure it may cause atrophy of these cells. Thus the larger cysts often have only a compressed stromal enclosing wall. On occasion, these usually innocuous lesions rupture, producing intraperitoneal bleeding and acute abdominal symptoms.

The *Stein-Leventhal syndrome* is infrequent, but it is of great endocrinologic interest. It is characterized by multicystic ovaries, amenorrhea and sterility, often accompanied by obesity and hirsutism. Most often this poorly understood syndrome comes to attention when the patient is in her teens or early twenties.

The ovaries are usually, but not invariably, enlarged, contain multiple follicle cysts and sometimes have a thickened outer tunica, which gives rise to the terms "large white ovary" and "cortical stromal fibrosis."

TUMORS OF THE OVARY

Tumors of the ovaries, both benign and malignant, are a common form of neoplasia. Ovarian cancer is of particular importance. Although it is the least common of the three major forms of genital cancer in the female (cervical, endometrial and ovarian), it is the most lethal. Cancer of the ovary causes nearly 11,000 deaths per year, almost as many as cancer of the cervix and endometrium combined, and is the fourth most important cause of cancer death in women (Silverberg and Holleb, 1974). In part, its importance reflects the steady decline in the death rates from cervical and endometrial cancers in recent years, but it also reflects an absolute increase in the incidence and mortality of cancer of the ovary. Moreover, the prospect for a decrease in the death rate of ovarian cancer is not good because of the difficulty in making an early diagnosis. There is no simple screening technique, as for carcinoma of the cervix, nor are there dramatic early signs, such as the bleeding that often occurs with endometrial carcinoma. Thus, the clinician must rely on regular

TABLE 17-1. SIMPLIFIED CLASSIFICATION OF OVARIAN TUMORS

Type of Tumor	Frequency Among Ovarian Tumors	Age Group Affected

A. Of Surface (Germinal) Epithelial Origin
  1. Serous tumors
  2. Mucinous tumors
  3. Endometrioid tumors
  4. Clear cell tumors
  5. Brenner tumors
  6. Unclassifiable
	Over 50%	20–50 years

B. Of Germ Cell Origin
  1. Dysgerminoma
  2. Endodermal sinus tumors
  3. Teratoma-teratocarcinoma
  4. Choriocarcinoma
	Over 15%	Children and young adults

C. Of Ovarian Stromal Origin
  1. Fibroma—fibrosarcoma
  2. Granulosa-theca cell tumor
  3. Sertoli-Leydig tumor
	About 20%	20–50 years

D. Metastatic to the Ovary	About 6%	Variable

pelvic examinations and a high index of suspicion.

Within the ovary, any of the three basic cell types—the *surface* or *germinal epithelium,* the *germ cells* and the *stroma*—may give rise to neoplasms. It will be remembered that the ovary is covered by coelomic epithelium, which has the potential of differentiating into serous, ciliated columnar cells (such as are found in the oviducts) or mucous, nonciliated columnar cells (such as occur in the endometrium and endocervix). The stroma of the ovary is made up of connective tissue, which is capable of differentiating into theca, granulosa or luteal cells, and further contains ova that are totipotential. Because of this array of actual and possible cell types, ovarian tumors may take many forms and, therefore, their classification has long been a problem. In this chapter, a simplified approach is adopted and the tumors will be considered according to their presumed cell of origin, but it should be remembered that often the ancestry of a tumor is not clear. For a more complete and authoritative presentation, reference should be made to Scully (1970). Table 17–1 presents the tumors to be discussed, their classification and approximate incidences. Most of the tumors are either benign or malignant, but some tumors are intermediate, making it extremely difficult to be certain of their biologic behavior. *Table 17–2 is concerned only with the malignant forms of these tumors, and presents a breakdown of ovarian cancers by tumor type. Although the multiplicity of types of ovarian cancer is confusing, even to the pathologist, it may be comforting to remember that at least 75 per cent of these cancers are of only three types—serous, mucinous and endometrioid—and that all of the others are more or less rare.*

TUMORS OF SURFACE (GERMINAL) EPITHELIAL ORIGIN

Serous Tumors. These are the most common of the ovarian tumors. Although they may be solid, they are usually at least partially cystic, hence they are commonly known as *cystadenomas* or *cystadenocarcinomas. The ratio of benign cystadenomas to malignant cystadenocarcinomas is approximately 2 or 3 to 1.* However, the common existence of intergradations, characterized by epithelial anaplasia without invasion of the stroma, renders such a ratio only approximate.

Grossly, serous tumors tend to be large, ovoid, cystic structures, up to approximately 30 to 40 cm. in diameter. **About 33 per cent of the benign forms are bilateral, whereas 66 per cent of the more aggressive lesions are bilateral.** In the benign form, the serosal covering is smooth and glistening. In contrast, the covering of the cystadenocarcinoma shows rough irregularities, which represent penetration of the capsule by the invasive tumor. On transection, the cystic tumor may comprise a single cavity, but more often it is divided by multiple septa into a multiloculated

TABLE 17-2. FREQUENCIES OF MALIGNANT TUMORS

Type of Tumor	Proportion of Ovarian Cancers (Per Cent)
Serous tumors	35–50
Endometrioid tumors	16–22
Mucinous tumors	10–20
Unclassifiable	5–10
Granulosa-theca cell tumors	5–10
Metastatic	6
Clear cell tumors	4–6
Teratocarcinoma	2–4
Dysgerminoma	1–2

mass. The cystic spaces are usually filled with a clear serous fluid, although a considerable amount of mucus may also be present. Jutting into the cystic cavities are polypoid or papillary projections, which become more marked with increasing malignancy. **In general, the more malignant forms of this tumor tend to lose their cystic pattern and become at least partially solid.**

Histologically, the benign tumors are characterized by a single layer of tall columnar epithelium, which lines the cyst or cysts. The cells are in part ciliated and in part dome-shaped secretory cells. Microscopic papillae, consisting of a delicate fibrous core covered by a single layer of epithelium, may be present. Psammoma bodies are common. When there is an abundant stromal component, these lesions are often termed **cystadenofibromas.** With the development of frank carcinoma, microscopic examination discloses most importantly anaplasia of the lining cells. Invasion of the stroma is usually readily evident, and papillary formations are complex and multilayered and show invasion of the axial fibrous tissue by nests or totally undifferentiated sheets of malignant cells. Between these clearly benign and obviously malignant forms are intergradations in which slight epithelial anaplasia, as well as questionable invasion, is present. These are distinguished by the term "borderline tumors."

The prognosis with clearly invasive serous cystadenocarcinomas is poor, with a 10-year survival rate of only 13 per cent. In contrast, the borderline pattern seems to represent a distinct prognostic entity, with a 10-year survival of about 75 per cent.

Mucinous Tumors. Mucinous tumors are in most respects *entirely analogous to the serous tumors,* differing essentially in that the epithelial component consists of mucin secreting cells similar to those of the endocervical mucosa. These tumors are slightly less common than the serous tumors and are considerably less likely to be malignant, having a *benign-to-malignant ratio of about 7 to 1.* Like the serous tumors, the mucinous tumors are designated *cystadenoma* or *cystadenocarcinoma,* although here again intergradations occur. Again, when stromal proliferation is marked, the benign lesion may be termed a *cystadenofibroma.*

Mucinous tumors are bilateral in 10 per cent of patients. On gross examination, they may be indistinguishable from serous tumors except by the mucinous nature of the cystic contents (Fig. 17–8). However, they are somewhat more likely to be larger and multilocular, and papillary formations are less common.

Histologically, these mucinous tumors are identified by the apical vacuolation of the tall columnar epithelial cells and by the absence of cilia. Metastases or rupture of mucinous cystadenocarcinomas may give rise to the clinical condition

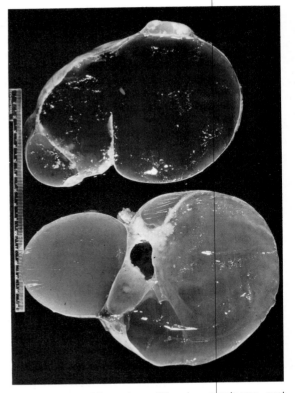

Figure 17–8. Bilateral multilocular mucinous cystadenomas of the ovaries, hemisected to reveal the gelatinous contents. The upper specimen has sustained some hemorrhage into the secretions, accounting for its darker color. Papillary projections are absent.

designated **pseudomyxoma peritonei.** The peritoneal cavity becomes filled with a glairy mucinous material resembling the cystic contents of the tumor. Multiple tumor implants are found on all the serosal surfaces, and the abdominal viscera become matted together. This form of pseudomyxoma peritonei is analogous to that encountered with rupture of a carcinomatous mucocele of the appendix (p. 505).

The prognosis with the mucinous cystadenocarcinoma is better than that with the serous counterpart. The 10-year survival rate is about 34 per cent. Borderline mucinous tumors are associated with a 68 per cent 10-year survival rate.

Endometrioid Tumors. *These tumors are characterized by the formation of tubular glands, similar to those of the endometrium, within the linings of cystic spaces. Although benign and borderline forms exist, endometrioid tumors are usually malignant. They are bilateral in about 10 per cent of patients. About 33 per cent of patients with these ovarian tumors have a concomitant endometrial carcinoma.* The relationship between the ovarian and the endometrial lesions is unclear, but it is likely that they represent separate primary tumors.

Grossly, the ovarian lesion may be solid or cystic. The cystic forms are usually indistinguishable on gross inspection from the serous and mucinous lesions just described. Sometimes these tumors develop as a mass projecting from the wall of an endometriotic cyst filled with chocolate-colored fluid. Microscopically, the cells lining the glandular formations are usually columnar, producing an **adenocarcinoma**. Sometimes, foci of metaplastic squamous cells are found, thus recapitulating the **adenoacanthoma** of the endometrium of the uterus. Varying degrees of anaplasia are present.

When these tumors are relatively well differentiated, there is a 62 per cent five-year survival rate. However, the more aggressive carcinomas permit only a 23 per cent five-year survival.

Miscellaneous and Unclassifiable Tumors.

Two frequent tumors of mysterious origin are considered here simply because they are more likely to be of surface epithelial origin than of germ cell or stromal derivation.

Clear cell tumors may exist in benign, borderline and malignant forms. All are characterized by large glycogen filled clear cells often arranged in tubular formations. Because of their resemblance to renal cell carcinomas, they have often been termed "**mesonephromas.**" Grossly, they may be solid or cystic or protrude as polypoid masses from the wall of a cyst that is filled with chocolate-colored fluid.

The five-year survival rate of the carcinomatous form is about 37 per cent.

The **Brenner tumor** is a solid, usually benign tumor consisting of an abundant stroma **containing nests or cysts of transitional epithelium resembling that of the urinary tract.** Occasionally, the nests contain columnar mucus secreting cells. Brenner tumors generally are smoothly encapsulated and gray-white on transection and range from a few centimeters to 8 to 10 cm. in diameter.

Possibly these tumors arise from the surface epithelium, but it is also hypothesized that they spring from rests of urogenital epithelium trapped within the germinal ridge.

In some instances, ovarian cancers are so undifferentiated as to be *unclassifiable*. Such tumors have been reported to be bilateral in over 50 per cent of cases. Ten-year survival is rare.

TUMORS OF GERM CELL ORIGIN

Dysgerminoma.

This infrequent tumor is the female counterpart of the seminoma (see p. 550), being identical to it both grossly and histologically. Like the seminoma, it is malignant and characteristically in the course of time invades and metastasizes widely. In about 10 per cent of cases, both ovaries are affected. The five-year survival rate is relatively high, about 70 to 90 per cent.

Endodermal Sinus Tumor.

This is a highly malignant tumor, roughly analogous to the embryonal carcinoma of the testis. It does, however, have a distinctive microscopic pattern which differs from that of the testicular tumor.

The endodermal sinus tumor consists of a network of tubular spaces lined with embryonal cells. Sometimes papillary structures containing blood vessels protrude into these spaces, in a pattern thought by some to recapitulate a yolk sac structure, hence the name "endodermal sinus tumor." Extracellular and intracellular hyaline bodies are common. These tumors may grow rapidly, and thus contain areas of hemorrhage and cystic necrosis. Widespread metastatic dissemination usually follows.

Five-year survival rarely, if ever, occurs.

Teratoma and Teratocarcinoma.

Ovarian teratomas and teratocarcinomas are similar to those of the testis, and reference should be made to the earlier description of these lesions (see p. 551). Like the testicular tumors, the ovarian neoplasms are characterized by the presence of multiple cell types and organoid patterns resembling normal adult tissues. Varying degrees of differentiation and malignancy are found. Some of these tumors are virtually solid, with only small cystic spaces, while others are almost entirely cystic.

The **solid teratomas** are composed of areas recapitulating adult tissues derived from more than one germ layer. Any of these patterns of differentiation may have anaplastic malignant changes. In addition, there may be microscopic areas resembling endodermal sinus tumors, testicular embryonal carcinomas or choriocarcinomas.

When malignant changes are present, the prognosis is correspondingly poor, with a two-year survival rate ranging from 13 to 50 per cent. Only rarely, when all the patterns of differentiation are mature and adult, are the solid teratomas benign.

Cystic teratomas result from largely ectodermal differentiation of totipotential germ cells, hence, these are called *dermoid cysts. They affect a slightly older age group than do the other tumors of germ cell origin, usually developing during reproductive life.* They apparently arise from a single germ cell after the first meiotic division (Linder et al., 1975).

Dermoid cysts are nearly always benign. Morphologically, these are fascinating tumors. They are bilateral in about 20 per cent of cases and are small compared to other ovarian neoplasms, usually being less than 10 cm. in diameter. Characteristically, they are enclosed by a smooth, glistening serosa. On sectioning, the thin cystic wall is seen to be lined by skin, with all its adnexal structures, including hair and sometimes even teeth. The cystic space is filled with a thick, yellowish,

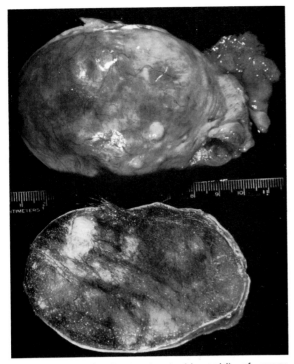

Figure 17–9. Cystic teratoma (dermoid) of ovary. The exterior is shown above and the cut surface below. The cystic space is jammed with sebaceous secretions and hairs.

sebaceous secretion, and matted strands of hair (Fig. 17–9). On microscopic examination, stratified squamous epithelium is seen, with underlying sebaceous glands and hair shafts. Usually, tissues from other germ layers are also present in these lesions, often including bone and cartilage. Sometimes dermoid cysts contain well developed thyroid acini, and occasionally this is the dominant tissue type in the tumor, which is then known as **struma ovarii.** In about 2 per cent of dermoid cysts, one of the tissue types present undergoes malignant transformation. In about 80 per cent of these cases the resultant cancer is a squamous cell carcinoma. Less frequently, melanomas, adenocarcinomas and sarcomas develop.

Choriocarcinoma. This rare tumor is exactly analogous to its counterpart in the testis (see p. 551). While it may arise as a primary lesion, presumably from germ cells, more often it is a component of one of the already mentioned tumors of germ cell origin. Choriocarcinoma arising in the placenta is described on page 581.

TUMORS OF OVARIAN STROMAL ORIGIN

This group of tumors includes fibromas and fibrosarcomas, as well as those tumors derived from specialized cells such as the granulosa-theca and luteal cells and their masculine counterparts, the Sertoli and Leydig cells (which may be present in the female in the hilus of the ovary).

Fibromas and Fibrosarcomas. The fibromas and fibrosarcomas of the ovary in no way differ anatomically from these kinds of connective tissue tumors occurring elsewhere in the body. In the ovary, the benign fibrous lesions are probably 100 times more common than the malignant forms. Ovarian fibromas are bilateral in about 10 per cent of cases. It is of interest that these benign tumors are frequently associated with ascites, and sometimes with right-sided hydrothorax, as well. *This triad of findings, i.e., ovarian tumor, ascites and hydrothorax, is designated "Meigs' syndrome."* Although Meigs' syndrome may also be caused by metastatic seeding of the serosal cavities, it is important to remember that ascites and hydrothorax are frequently associated with these benign fibromas of the ovary, hence these clinical findings do not of themselves connote malignancy.

Granulosa-Theca Cell Tumors. Tumors which arise from specialized elements of the ovarian stroma include the *granulosa-theca cell tumors* and the *Sertoli-Leydig cell tumors,* also known as *arrhenoblastomas.* While the granulosa-theca cell tumors are sometimes feminizing and the Sertoli-Leydig cell tumors may be masculinizing, in many instances these tumors do not elaborate hormones and have no endocrine effects.

Most important of these neoplasms are the granulosa-theca cell tumors, since they are not uncommon and those comprised primarily of granulosa cells frequently are malignant.

On external inspection, these lesions resemble fibromas, although often a yellow cast on the cut surface hints at their precise nature. The histologic picture is variable, depending on the dominant cell type. Granulosal cells predominate in about 17 per cent of these tumors, theca cells in 67 per cent and fairly equal mixtures of both in approximately 15 per cent. Scattered luteal cells may be present in all these tumors. Rarely, pure luteomas, composed largely of acidophilic, granular, apparent luteal cells are seen. The granulosa cell component of granulosa-theca cell tumors takes one of many histologic patterns. The small cuboidal to polygonal cells may grow in anastomosing cords or sheets, or, in occasional cases, may form small, abortive follicles filled with an acidophilic secretion (**Call-Exner bodies**). Theca cells are frequently indistinguishable from overly plump fibrocytes save by histochemical techniques which disclose a lipid content.

The granulosal cells probably do not elaborate hormones. It is the accompanying theca or luteal cells that are capable of secreting sex hormones. When hormonally active tumors develop in girls before puberty, they may cause sexual precocity. *Indeed, ovarian tumors are the most important pathologic cause of sexual precocity in females.* In the adult, the principal effects of the sustained hyperestrinism resulting from the hormone-elaborating tumors are endometrial hyperplasia, often with abnormal bleeding, endometrial carcinoma and fibrocystic disease of the breast.

Only the tumors composed predominantly of granulosa cells are malignant and, even in these cases, they are rather indolent lesions, with a five-year survival rate close to 90 per cent.

Sertoli-Leydig Cell Tumors. These are considerably less common than granulosa-theca cell tumors, but of somewhat greater malignancy. Most probably, these tumors originate from the remnants of the embryonic male mesonephric duct in the hilus of the ovary. Because they frequently are not masculinizing, the term *arrhenoblastoma* should not be used. The histologic pattern ranges from well differentiated recapitulation of testicular tubules to totally undifferentiated sheets of cells resembling a fibrosarcoma.

TUMORS METASTATIC TO THE OVARY

Metastases to the ovary most often arise from the gastrointestinal tract or nearby pelvic organs. The term *Krukenberg tumor* refers to those metastases characterized by mucin-secreting "signet ring" cells. Commonly, such lesions are primary in the stomach, but they may also be metastatic from the colon, breast or, indeed, any other organ containing mucous glands.

GRADING AND STAGING OF OVARIAN CANCER

In addition to classifying ovarian cancer according to its presumed cell of origin, as presented above, it is also graded according to cell differentiation, and staged according to the extent of involvement as determined by surgical exploration. The grading system is I through IV, from well differentiated to undifferentiated. The staging system is as follows:

Stage I: Growth limited to ovaries.
   I–A: Limited to one ovary; no ascites.
   I–B: Limited to both ovaries; no ascites.
   I–C: One or both ovaries; ascites present.
Stage II: Extension within the pelvis.
   II–A: Extension only to the uterus or tubes.
   II–B: Extension to other pelvic tissues.
Stage III: Widespread intraperitoneal metastases.
Stage IV: Metastases outside the peritoneal cavity.

Special category: Unexplored cases thought to be ovarian cancer.

CLINICAL COURSE OF OVARIAN CANCER

The clinical picture of most types of ovarian cancer is similar. In general, women most vulnerable are postmenopausal and nulliparous. Those with concomitant or past cancer of the breast or endometrium are also at increased risk. Obviously, in the individual case, this information is of value only insofar as it inspires the physician to consider the diagnosis. Unfortunately, there are usually no early symptoms. On palpation the ovary may seem large, and there may be some impression of thickening of the pelvic adnexa. Only late in the course are there symptoms referable to the expanding mass. These include vague gastrointestinal complaints, such as "gas" or constipation, sometimes along with distention and a sensation of heaviness. By this time, the lesion has usually metastasized. The pattern of dissemination is characteristic. Cancer of the ovary tends to seed the peritoneal and pleural cavities. The serosal surfaces become diffusely studded with 0.1 to 0.5 cm. nodules of tumor. Concomitant ascites, sometimes of massive proportions, is common. Visceral metastases occur in the liver, bones and lungs, as well as in the other ovary in half the cases. Survival rates for the specific types of tumor have already been given. Correlating these with grades and stages is difficult, since it would require data on a very large series of cases. Considering all tumor types combined, however, five-year survival is only 35 per cent. With Stage I disease, it is about 70 per cent; Stage II, 60 per cent; Stage III, 30 per cent; and Stage IV, 5 per cent (Rudolph, 1970–71).

DISEASES OF PREGNANCY

This discussion will concern itself only with those disorders having prominent morphologic lesions—i.e., ectopic pregnancy, hydatidiform mole and tumors of trophoblastic tissue. The toxemias of pregnancy often are associated with disseminated intravascular coagulation and are mentioned on page 365.

ECTOPIC PREGNANCY

Ectopic pregnancy refers to implantation of the fertilized ovum in any site other than the normal uterine position. The condition is not uncommon, occurring in up to 1 per cent of pregnancies. *In over 95 per cent of these cases, implantation is in the oviducts (tubal pregnancy); other sites include the ovaries, the abdominal cavity and the intrauterine portion of the oviducts (inter-*

stitial pregnancy). Any factor which retards passage of the ovum along its course through the oviducts to the uterus predisposes to an ectopic pregnancy. Most often such hindrance is based on chronic inflammatory changes within the oviduct, although intrauterine tumors and prior intratubal hemorrhage may also hamper passage of the ovum. Ovarian pregnancies probably result from those rare instances of fertilization and trapping of the ovum within its follicle just at the time of rupture. Gestation within the abdominal cavity occurs when the fertilized egg drops out of the fimbriated end of the oviduct and implants on the peritoneum.

In all sites, ectopic pregnancies are characterized by fairly normal **early** development of the embryo, with the formation of placental tissue, amniotic sac and decidual changes. An abdominal pregnancy is occasionally carried to full term. With tubal pregnancies, however, the invading placenta eventually burrows through the wall of the oviduct or so weakens it that tubal rupture, with intraperitoneal hemorrhage, usually ensues, typically about 2 to 6 weeks after the onset of pregnancy. In addition, the tube is usually locally distended up to 3 to 4 cm. by a contained mass of freshly clotted blood in which may be seen bits of gray placental tissue. The histologic diagnosis depends on the visualization of placental villi or, rarely, of the embryo. Less commonly, poor attachment of the placenta results in death of the embryo, with spontaneous proteolysis and absorption of the products of conception. Sometimes, in these cases, the embryo is not digested, but rather becomes calcified, forming a **lithopedion.**

Until rupture occurs, an ectopic pregnancy may be indistinguishable from a normal one, with cessation of menstruation and elevation of serum and urinary placental hormones. Under the influence of these hormones, the endometrium (in about 50 per cent of cases) undergoes the characteristic hypersecretory and decidual changes. *However, absence of elevated gonadotropin levels does not exclude this diagnosis, since poor attachment with necrosis of the placenta is common.* Rupture of an ectopic pregnancy is catastrophic, with the sudden onset of intense abdominal pain and signs of an acute abdomen, often followed by profound shock. Prompt surgical intervention is life-saving.

TROPHOBLASTIC DISEASE

Trophoblastic disease refers to three complications of uterine pregnancies which probably represent stages in progression from benign proliferation to malignant disease of the placenta. In order of increasing malignancy, they are *hydatidiform mole, chorioadenoma destruens* and *choriocarcinoma.* For completely obscure reasons, all are about 10 times as frequent in Asian as in Western countries. The monograph of Holland and Hreshchyshyn (1967) offers a detailed treatment of these interesting disorders.

HYDATIDIFORM MOLE

This disorder is characterized by failure of the embryo to develop, accompanied by a marked hydropic swelling of the chorionic villi. It is usually discovered in the fourth or fifth month of gestation. Hydatidiform mole occurs in about 1 in 200 pregnancies in Asia and 1 in 2000 pregnancies in the United States. The patient may be of any age of reproductive life, and may have borne normal infants.

The etiology and pathogenesis of this strange lesion are unknown. Two tentative theories have been suggested. The first considers the origin of the mole to be a "blighted" ovum or embryo. Because of the absence of a fetal circulation, fluid elaborated into the villi cannot be reabsorbed, hence it accumulates, with consequent progressive swelling and reactive hyperplasia of the chorionic epithelium of the villi. The second causative theory proposes that the primary defect is in the trophoblast, which subsequently causes death of the embryo. An interesting recent finding is that about 80 per cent of these moles are sex-chromatin positive, although no explanation exists for the greater vulnerability of the female conceptus.

At the time of discovery, the uterus is considerably larger than would be expected from the dura-

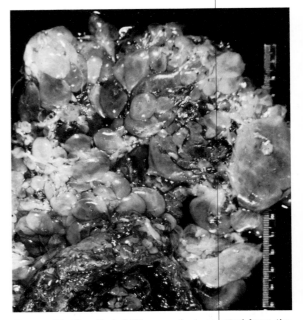

Figure 17–10. Hydatidiform mole evacuated from the uterus. The "bunch of grapes" appearance of the lesion is readily evident.

tion of pregnancy. **The mole appears grossly as a delicate mass of translucent cystic structures, not unlike a large bunch of grapes** (Fig. 17—10). The individual locules vary in size from microscopic to about 3 cm. in diameter. Although careful dissection may disclose a small amniotic sac, the sac contains no embryo. Microscopically, the hydatidiform mole is characterized by: (1) hydropic swelling of the chorionic villi. There is a loose edematous stroma covered by chorionic epithelium, both cytotrophoblast and syncytial trophoblast. (2) Inadequate vascularization of the villi, with only rudimentary or no capillary channels, rather than the normal vessels of the fetal circulation. (3) Variable degrees of hyperplasia of the covering chorionic epithelium, ranging from a single layer to masses of both cuboidal and syncytial cells. In some instances, the epithelium is entirely normal, and such moles are undoubtedly benign. However, variable degrees of atypicality leading to frank anaplasia are encountered, progressing until these lesions merge with the highly malignant choriocarcinomas, which will be described later.

Patients with hydatidiform moles usually have spotty bleeding from early pregnancy, often accompanied by passage of a watery fluid containing bits of tissue or individual locules. The diagnosis is established in the fourth or fifth month, when the uterus is noted to be abnormally large and there are no signs of the presence of a fetus. *An important diagnostic point is the presence of markedly elevated levels of serum and urine gonadotropins, which are usually at least 10 times higher than expected with a normal pregnancy.* After removal of the mole, usually accomplished readily in the benign forms by curettage, gonadotropin levels should return to normal within 4 to 8 weeks. A major morphologic criterion of the biologic behavior of these lesions is the extent of their invasion of the deeper levels of the endometrium and myometrium. Hence, it is standard practice to curet the lesions, first superficially and then deeply. The deep scrapings require greatest attention in order to discover evidence of invasion. Continuation of high levels of gonadotropins post-curettage strongly suggests that the lesion has progressed to the more malignant forms of trophoblastic disease. *Overall, from 4 to 17 per cent of hydatidiform moles are followed by the development of choriocarcinoma.* Among patients whose gonadotropin level is still elevated four weeks after removal of a hydatidiform mole, over 50 per cent develop choriocarcinoma unless prophylactic chemotherapy with folic acid antagonists is instituted.

CHORIOADENOMA DESTRUENS

When a hydatidiform mole is invasive, the lesion is termed *chorioadenoma destruens.*

After curettage of the mole, the well formed invasive villi remain and may even penetrate the uterine wall, causing rupture, sometimes with life-threatening hemorrhage. Local spread to adjacent pelvic structures may occur. Microscopically, the epithelium of the villi is seen to be markedly hyperplastic and somewhat atypical, with proliferation of both cuboidal and syncytial components.

While the marked invasiveness of this lesion makes removal technically difficult, metastases do not occur. In this sense, the significance of chorioadenoma destruens may be considered as intermediate between that of the hydatidiform mole and choriocarcinoma. Indeed, the recognition of well formed villi deep within the myometrium after passage of a mole augurs well for the patient in the sense that it indicates chorioadenoma destruens rather than choriocarcinoma.

CHORIOCARCINOMA

This highly aggressive malignant tumor arises either from the trophoblastic cells of pregnancy or, less frequently, from totipotential cells within the gonads. Choriocarcinomas are rare, occurring in approximately 1 in 1500 pregnancies in Asia and in fewer than 1 in 15,000 in the United States. In about 50 to 60 per cent of cases, it follows delivery of a hydatidiform mole; about 25 per cent arise in retained placental fragments following spontaneous abortion; and 10 to 22 per cent arise in a previously normal pregnancy. Stated in another way, the more abnormal the conception, the greater the hazard of developing choriocarcinoma. The latent period between termination of the pregnancy and diagnosis of choriocarcinoma varies remarkably, from 2 weeks to an extraordinary 7 years.

The tumor appears grossly as a soft, fleshy, yellow-white mass, invariably with foci of ischemic necrosis, cystic softening and hemorrhage. Often the mass is deceptively small. **In contrast to the hydatidiform mole and chorioadenoma destruens, chorionic villi are not formed; rather, the tumor is purely epithelial, with invasion of muscle and vessels by sheets and columns of anaplastic cuboidal and syncytial cells** (Fig. 17—11). The morphologic diagnosis of choriocarcinoma should not be made unless both types of epithelium can be seen. In as many as 45 per cent of cases (18 of 40 cases in one series), metastatic choriocarcinoma is discovered in the apparent absence of a primary lesion in either the uterus or the gonads. It is probable that this paradox reflects the marked tendency of the primary tumor to undergo necrosis, possibly with spontaneous regression, even though its distant seedings remain viable. By the time the tumor is discovered, widespread metastases are usually present, most often in the lungs (50 per cent), vagina (30 to 40 per cent), brain, liver and kidneys.

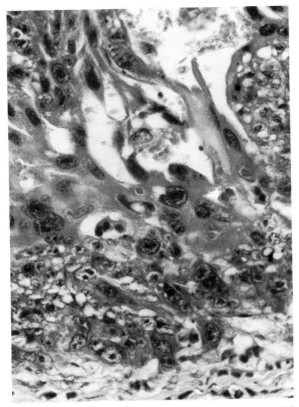

Figure 17–11. Choriocarcinoma. A nest of syncytial cells in the center field is surrounded by masses of cuboidal cells.

Most patients complain of a bloody, brownish discharge, beginning days to weeks after termination of pregnancy. Continued marked elevation of serum and urine gonadotropins for as much as eight weeks following termination of a pregnancy, whether abnormal or normal, indicates the likelihood of a choriocarcinoma. *In general, the hormone titers are at least 10 times higher than those associated with a hydatidiform mole and 100 times greater than those of a normal pregnancy.* With the higher titers, the prognosis is worse.

Until recently, this highly aggressive tumor was nearly uniformly fatal, usually within one year of discovery. Remarkable results, however, are achieved by treatment with folic acid antagonists, chiefly methotrexate, and the five-year survival rate, even if we include those patients with metastatic disease, is now at least 60 per cent.

Of interest is the possible synergistic role of a host immune response in the treatment of these tumors. Since the tumor tissue is derived from the embryo and is therefore "foreign" to the patient, such an immune response is theoretically possible. Support for this theory is drawn from the relatively poor response to chemotherapy of choriocarcin-omas which arise in the gonads and which therefore are "native" to the patient. It is possible, however, that other malignant components of these teratogenous tumors are responsible for the lack of success.

BREAST

Lesions of the breast are virtually limited to the female, with rare exceptions to be noted later. They usually take the form of palpable masses, sometimes painful, more often not. Some help in predicting the nature of a given mass can be had by knowing the likelihood of occurrence of the several possible lesions, and this varies with the age of the patient. The following table shows the most frequent causes of breast masses, ranked in order of frequency, in three age groups.

Under 35 Years:
   1. Fibrocystic disease (masses may be multifocal and bilateral)
   2. Fibroadenoma (solitary benign tumor)
   3. Mastitis (often during pregnancy or nursing, associated with pain and systemic signs)
   4. Carcinoma (infrequent in this group)
   5. Traumatic fat necrosis (rare; history of trauma in about 50 per cent of cases)

Between 35 and 50 Years:
   1. Fibrocystic disease
   2. Carcinoma (usually invasive scirrhous type)
   3. Fibroadenoma
   4. Mastitis
   5. Traumatic fat necrosis (rare)
   6. Papilloma (rare as cause of palpable mass)

Over 50 Years:
   1. Carcinoma
   2. Fibrocystic disease
   3. Traumatic fat necrosis
   4. Mastitis (rare in this group)

From this list it will be seen that, overall, the two most important entities are carcinoma and fibrocystic disease.

FIBROCYSTIC DISEASE (CYSTIC HYPERPLASIA, MAMMARY DYSPLASIA)

This is the most common disorder of the female breast. It is frequently but inappropriately called "chronic cystic mastitis." The many terms referring to this condition attest to the fact that its nature is still poorly understood. *Most probably it reflects some exaggeration of the normal repeated stimulation that occurs during the menstrual cycle, and thus is related to hyperestrinism, either absolute or relative.* It has been estimated that about 50 per cent of adult females have some degree of fibrocystic disease of the breast, but in many of these cases, of course, the changes are minimal (Frantz et al., 1951). Rarely does the disorder develop before adolescence or after menopause, although once developed, lesions may persist through old age. Not only does the severity of fibrocystic disease vary widely, but the morphologic lesions themselves also cover a broad spectrum, ranging from lesions that consist principally of overgrowth of the fibrous stroma to lesions characterized by cystic hyperplasia of the epithelium as well as stromal proliferation, to lesions marked almost entirely by epithelial proliferation (Foote and Stewart, 1945; Warren, 1946). Somewhat arbitrarily, then, three morphologic subdivisions are recognized—*fibrosis of the breast, cystic disease* and *adenosis*—which differ somewhat in the age group affected and in clinical significance. It should be remembered, however, that there is considerable overlap among them, and even in a single lesion, all patterns may be present.

FIBROSIS OF THE BREAST

This variant is characterized by overgrowth of the fibrous stromal tissue, unaccompanied by significant epithelial hyperplasia. It tends to affect somewhat younger women than the other patterns, being most frequent in women in their early thirties.

Usually the lesion is limited to the upper outer quadrant of one breast, but it may be bilateral. The mass is poorly defined, from 2 to 10 cm. in diameter, and of a rubbery consistency. On cut section, the appearance is of a tough, rubbery, gray-white homogeneous connective tissue, devoid of fat, within which tiny yellow-pink areas of glandular parenchyma may be barely visible. On histologic examination, the mass can be seen to consist of fibrous tissue which engulfs the epithelial structures and obliterates the loose periductal and lobular myxomatous stroma. Sometimes the ducts and buds are so compressed that they become markedly flattened or even atrophic.

CYSTIC DISEASE

This is the pattern which tends to affect the oldest age group, usually developing about the time of menopause. Both stromal and epithelial hyperplasia are present, along with the characteristic cystic dilatation of the ducts. These cysts are thought to develop because the periodic intense stimulatory changes of the menstrual cycle are not followed by the normal regression.

Unlike fibrosis, this disorder is usually multifocal and often bilateral, although occasionally it may take the form of an isolated cyst. The affected breast may have a diffuse nodular or shotty texture. On cut section, the cysts can be seen to vary

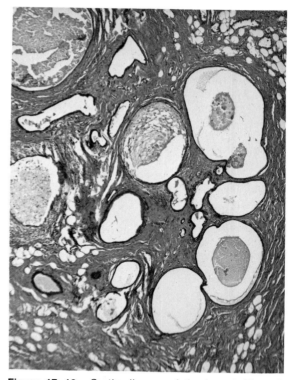

Figure 17–12. Cystic disease of the breast. The microscopic view shows numerous small cysts, some containing inspissated secretions. The epithelium is flattened and inactive.

in size from nearly microscopic to large lesions over 5 cm. in diameter. Some are filled with a thin, turbid fluid that imparts a blue cast to the unopened cyst, hence the surgical designation "blue dome cyst." When opened, the watery contents flow out readily, disclosing a smooth, glistening lining. Microscopic examination confirms varying degrees of cystic dilatation of the ducts. The smaller cysts are lined by cuboidal to columnar epithelium which is often multilayered in focal areas, sometimes with piled-up masses of proliferating cells or small papillary excrescences. Some cysts are lined with large cells having an abundant acidophilic cytoplasm, so-called apocrine gland epithelium. In most instances, a clearly defined basement membrane is present about these cysts, and the proliferating epithelium does not invade beyond its boundaries. The epithelium of larger cysts is typically compressed, and may even be totally atrophic, so that the lining consists only of collagenous fibrous tissue. The surrounding stroma tends to lose its loose myxomatous appearance and becomes densely fibrotic (Fig. 17–12).

ADENOSIS

Perhaps the variant of fibrocystic disease of greatest clinical import—because of its possible role as a precursor to cancer—is adenosis, also known as *benign epithelial hyperplasia*. This disorder affects an age range intermediate between those of fibrosis and cystic disease, roughly between ages 35 and 45 years.

Like fibrosis, adenosis is usually, but not invariably, unilateral and tends to affect the upper outer quadrant of the breast. Grossly, the lesion has a hard, cartilaginous consistency, similar to that of breast cancer (a point worthy of note by surgeons). Histologically, adenosis is characterized by the following four features: (1) Reduplication of the glands. Aggregated glands may be virtually back to back, with single or multiple layers of epithelial cells in contact with one another. Often the lumina are compressed, creating a double strand of cells. (2) Intraductal hyperplasia more marked than that seen with cystic disease, with multilayering of the epithelial cells. The larger ducts may be partially or completely plugged with cuboidal cells, which tend to produce closely packed gland patterns. The cells, nonetheless, are quite normal cytologically. The ductal basement membranes remain intact, and the proliferating epithelium does not invade the surrounding stroma. **Although some cystic dilatation of the ducts may be present, it is not a prominent feature of this variant of mammary dysplasia.** (3) The formation of small papillary protrusions into the ducts, known as intraductal papillomatosis, resulting from the piling-up of the epithelium. (4) Stromal thickening, which may compress and distort the proliferating epithelium. In some cases, this overgrowth of fibrous tissue completely compresses the lumina of the glands, so that they appear as solid cords of cells, a histologic pattern known as **sclerosing adenosis.** This pattern, especially, may be very difficult to distinguish histologically from an invasive carcinoma (Fig. 17–13).

The clinical presentation of all three variants of fibrocystic disease is of a mass or masses which become more pronounced, tender and slightly painful in the days immediately preceding each menstrual period, after which they become relatively quiescent. The significance of fibrocystic disease is twofold. First, when it is unilateral and unifocal, biopsy is necessary to distinguish it from a carcinoma (and even then, as has been pointed out, the distinction may be difficult). Although the presence of tenderness and of cyclic changes would militate against its being cancer, a purely clinical judgment is hazardous. Moreover, in such cases fibrocystic disease may mask a coexistent cancer. The second significant clinical aspect of fibrocystic disease is its possible role as a precursor to breast cancer. Although the issue is still being debated, it would seem that there is some relationship between the two diseases. One study has shown that the risk of developing breast cancer is 4.5 times greater for a woman with fibrocystic disease than for a normal control. Those with the mor-

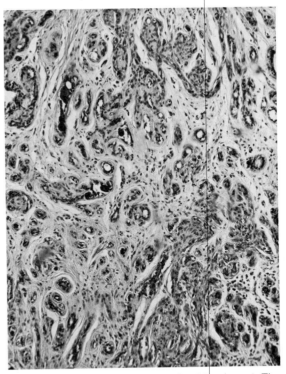

Figure 17–13. Sclerosing adenosis of the breast. The epithelial hyperplasia has produced the nests of cells, which appear quite disorderly. The overgrowth of fibrous tissue enmeshes and partially obliterates many of the epithelial nests, creating a pattern closely similar to the infiltrative growth of a cancer. Compare with Figure 17–16.

phologic variant adenosis are especially vulnerable. Conversely, among women who already have carcinoma of the breast, 60 to 90 per cent have concomitant fibrocystic disease. Clearly, then, the more florid instances of fibrocystic disease must be treated with great respect.

FIBROADENOMA

Fibroadenoma is the most common benign tumor of the female breast. While it may develop at any age, it is most frequent in the third decade. Some regard it as a variant of fibrocystic disease rather than as a true neoplasm, since it is thought to develop as the result of increased sensitivity of a focal area of the breast to estrogens. Moreover, the lesion may undergo slight increases in size during the late phase of each menstrual cycle. However, unlike fibrocystic disease, the fibroadenoma is a discrete, encapsulated, freely moveable nodule.

Usually this tumor occurs as a solitary lesion in the upper outer quadrant of the breast; rarely, multiple tumors are encountered. Differentiation lesions undergoes malignant transformation. Even then, however, their behavior is relatively innocent and while a few do metastasize to regional nodes, surgical excision effects a cure. To these tumors the designation **cystosarcoma phyllodes** has been given. For unknown reasons, the glandular component rarely becomes malignant.

MASTITIS

Bacteria may gain access to the breast tissue through fissures in the nipples which develop during the early weeks of nursing, or through eczema or other dermatologic conditions in non-nursing women. Most often the invading organisms are *Staphylococcus aureus* or the streptococci, which produce their characteristic patterns of tissue injury.

With the staphylococci, single or multiple abscesses may develop, whereas the streptococci cause a more diffuse, spreading infection that may eventually encompass the entire breast. In either case, the affected area is red, swollen and painful, as are the axillary nodes which drain the infection. Histologically, the ducts are filled with pus and the surrounding tissue is infiltrated with neutrophils.

When the suppurative necrosis is severe enough to destroy significant amounts of breast tissue, fibrous scarring ensues, which creates a localized area of firmness, often with retraction of the overlying skin or nipple. These findings may be confused with changes produced by cancer. Only rarely is sufficient breast tissue destroyed by mastitis to cause functional impairment.

"TRAUMATIC" FAT NECROSIS

This is an uncommon and innocuous lesion which is significant only because it produces a mass which must be differentiated from a cancer. Whether or not it is caused by trauma is controversial. Only about 50 per cent of these patients give a history of trauma, which even so may have been coincidental.

The lesion is small, often tender, rarely over 2 cm. in diameter and sharply localized. It consists of a central focus of necrotic fat cells surrounded by neutrophils and lipid filled macrophages, and, later, by an enclosing wall of fibrous tissue and mononuclear leukocytes. Eventually, the central debris is removed by the macrophages and giant cells and is replaced by scar tissue. A tendency for the fibrous tissue to adhere to the overlying skin sometimes results in dimpling or retraction, a picture which may also be caused by cancer.

PAPILLOMA AND PAPILLARY CARCINOMA

Papillary formations within ducts or cysts may occur as a single isolated neoplasm or as a diffuse hyperplastic process in the pattern termed *papillomatosis*, a component of fibro-

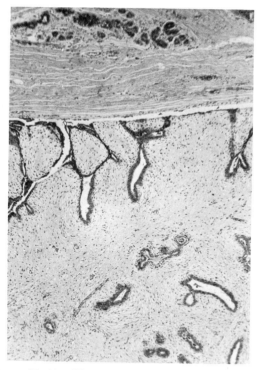

Figure 17–14. Fibroadenoma of breast. The margin of the nodule shows clear demarcation from the compressed breast substance above. The tumor is in part intracanalicular, particularly near the capsule. Toward the bottom, the pattern is pericanalicular.

from a solitary cyst is most difficult. The size of fibroadenomas varies remarkably. Typically, they are removed when about 3 cm. in diameter, but they may be considerably larger. **As the name implies, these tumors are composed of both fibrous and glandular tissue.** Grossly, they are firm, with a uniform gray-white color on cut section, punctuated by softer yellow-pink specks representing the glandular areas. Histologically, there is a loose fibroblastic stroma containing pleomorphic glandular and cystic spaces. Although in some lesions the glands are round to oval and fairly regular (the pericanalicular fibroadenoma), others are compressed by the stroma so that on cross section they appear as slits or irregular, star-shaped structures (the intracanalicular fibroadenoma). These glands are lined with single or multiple layers of cells that are regular and have a well-defined, intact basement membrane (Fig. 17–14).

Fibroadenomas that reach dimensions of 10 to 15 cm. in diameter are commonly termed **giant fibroadenomas.** These may markedly distort the breast and even cause pressure necrosis of the overlying skin, sometimes with rupture of the tumor through its capsule to the surface. Although such alarming behavior does not of itself imply malignancy, the stroma in a minority of these larger cystic disease (see p. 584). *In either case, these lesions are rarely large enough to be palpable and usually manifest themselves by a serous, turbid or bloody discharge from the nipple.* Both the solitary and multiple forms may be benign, malignant or borderline. Histologic differentiation may be difficult.

The neoplastic variant, the benign isolated papilloma, is a small lesion, usually less than 1 cm. in diameter, growing within a cyst or dilated duct, usually close to the nipple. It may be sessile or pedunculated. On microscopic examination, it can be seen to have a delicate central connective tissue framework covered by one to two layers of regular cuboidal epithelial cells. With progressive atypicality, the epithelium becomes anaplastic, growing in haphazard heaps and invading the stroma of the stalk or even the periductal tissue.

With diffuse hyperplastic papillomatosis, there is no well developed framework or stalk. Rather, the cells protrude into the lumina of the ducts or cysts in primitive papillary formation simply by virtue of the pressure from their proliferation. There is usually more distortion and disarray of the cells than with the solitary papillomas, even when the lesion is clinically benign. In some cases, the epithelium invades the basement membrane and extends into the periductal tissue, and is clearly malignant. When such occurs, the lesion takes on the significance of an infiltrative carcinoma.

CARCINOMA OF THE BREAST

In the United States carcinoma of the breast kills more women each year than any other cancer. It causes 20 per cent of all cancer deaths in women, or 32,500 deaths each year. Moreover, the incidence of this tumor is commensurately high. Excluding skin cancer and carcinoma-in-situ of the cervix, it accounts for 28 per cent of all cancer in women (Silverberg and Holleb, 1974). Moreover, it is an unusually cruel disease, often running a protracted course marked by extreme wasting and intense physical and psychological pain. It is not surprising, then, that a great deal of the effort to unravel the mysteries of cancer in general has been directed toward this particular form of carcinoma. A vast amount of experimental and epidemiologic data have been accumulated in an effort to find its cause or causes, and attempts have been made to arrive at a uniform grading and staging system in order to evaluate a wide variety of treatment modalities. It would seem that these efforts are finally yielding results. Where there was once ignorance, there is now emerging some cohesive picture of this disease and of those at highest risk of acquiring it, as well as exciting clues as to its etiology.

Incidence. Before considering what is known about the etiology and pathogenesis of breast cancer, we shall present a list of those factors known to affect the risk of developing breast cancer. Aside from the practical implications of being able to isolate high-risk individuals, the knowledge of these factors has been of great importance in suggesting possible etiologic influences. Breast cancer is more likely in women who:

1. Are older; the incidence increases sharply with age until menopause, then begins to plateau (Cole, 1974).

2. Live in North America or northern Europe (five to six times the risk in Asians or Africans) (MacMahon et al., 1973).

3. Have fibrocystic disease of the breast (three to four times the control rate) (MacMahon et al., 1973).

4. Have no children or who have their first child after age 30 (giving birth after age 35 three times the risk of giving birth before age 18) (MacMahon et al., 1973).

5. Have a history of breast cancer in their family (two to three times the control rate).

6. Are Jewish (two times other whites) (Cole, 1974).

7. Have an early menarche and a late menopause or both.

8. Have or have had cancer of the endometrium, ovary, colon or contralateral breast.

Etiology and Pathogenesis. The search for the cause of breast cancer has focused increasingly on three sets of influences: (1) viral, (2) hormonal, and (3) genetic. *The most exciting advances have centered on the question of a viral etiology.* This question was raised with the discovery that a virus, transmitted through the mother's milk, caused breast cancer in suckling mice (Bittner, 1936). This virus, called *mouse mammary tumor virus* or *MMTV*, was subsequently found to be an RNA B-type particle. Like other oncogenic RNA viruses, it contains RNA-dependent DNA polymerase (reverse transcriptase). In recent years, electron microscopic studies have revealed particles indistinguishable from the MMTV in the milk and breast tissue of humans. Such particles were described in the milk of 31 per cent of American women with a family history of breast cancer, in 39 per cent of Parsi women (an inbred religious sect in India with a high incidence of breast cancer) and in 12 per cent of American controls (Moore et al., 1971 *a*). They have also been described in the milk of 8 of 16 patients with this tumor as opposed to 1 in 43 controls (Feller and Chopra, 1971). Moreover, sera from women who have had breast cancer were more likely to neutralize the MMTV than those from controls. However, to confuse the issue studies have also revealed the presence of a number of other particles which may in some instances be difficult to distinguish from MMTV-like particles. These include particles similar to the RNA C-type virus which causes murine leukemia, as well as smaller viruses, mycoplasma and nonviral cellular fragments. In a recent study, C-type particles were seen even more often than MMTV-like forms, and both were found about as frequently in the milk of normal controls as in those with a family history of breast cancer (Sarkar and Moore, 1972).

Of great significance in further implicating a virus in breast cancer was the discovery of reverse transcriptase in some human milk samples containing virus-like particles (Schlom et al., 1971). This enzyme, *which is peculiar to oncogenic RNA viruses* (see p. 96) was found in four milk samples containing MMTV-like particles but in none of nine control samples. In another study, it was found in a number of milk samples both from women with and from those without a family history of breast cancer. Curiously, while it was present only in milk containing virus-like particles, the correlation was better for C-type particles than for the MMTV-like particles (Sarkar and Moore, 1972). Nevertheless, in a series of molecular hybridization experiments, *this RNA-dependent DNA polymerase was proved to synthesize DNA complementary to the RNA of the MMTV* (Schlom and Spiegelman, 1973). These important studies, then, show that the RNA in human breast cancer contains information identical (homologous) to that of the RNA of MMTV. Moreover, RNA from other human cancers and from normal breast tissue was not homologous to the MMTV. Interestingly, breast tissue from patients with fibrocystic disease also gave negative results. Of further significance in establishing the specificity of this particular MMTV agent was the fact that other viruses, including the Rauscher murine leukemia virus, were not homologous with the MMTV. These studies offer strong support for a role of MMTV-like viruses in the causation of breast cancer.

If a virus is indeed involved in the genesis of breast cancer, the question remains as to whether its presence is necessary in all cases. Conceivably, there are many causes of breast cancer. Even if a virus is *necessary*, epidemiologic data would indicate that its presence alone is not *sufficient* to produce a tumor, since these viruses seem to be so widespread. Thus, other promoting or co-carcinogenic influences may be necessary for the induction of breast cancer.

It has long been appreciated that hormonal influences play some role in the development of breast cancer. The evidence is largely epidemiologic, derived from the risk factors listed earlier. The common element in these risk factors, at least within a single geographic area, is a relatively long, uninterrupted period of cyclical ovarian function. Thus, the high-risk woman has an early menarche, a late menopause and no pregnancies to interrupt the repeated cycles. Moreover, women with other disorders thought related to hyperestrinism, such as fibrocystic disease of the breast and carcinoma of the endometrium and ovary, also show an increased vulnerability to breast cancer. Conversely, surgical removal of the ovaries is protective. Those who have their ovaries removed before the age of 35 have a 70 per cent reduction in the risk of breast cancer. This protective effect begins to be apparent about a decade after surgery, and persists throughout life. It has been suggested that the relevant factor is not the total level of estrogen, but rather the balance between the three estrogen fractions—estriol, estrone and estradiol. According to this theory, women with a low level of estriol relative to estrone plus estradiol have a greater risk of developing breast cancer (Lemon, 1969). Alternatively, other hormones have been implicated in the development of breast cancer. It has been postulated that low levels of thyroxin render breast epithelium abnormally sensitive to the proliferative effects of prolactin, and that the latter hormone then plays a role in promoting cancer (Editorial, 1974c). Others suggest an abnormality in adrenal function with a consequent hormone imbalance (DeWaard et al., 1968). Several reports have linked the antihypertensive agent reserpine with an increased vulnerability to breast cancer (Boston Collaborative Drug Program, 1974). The carcinogenic influence of reserpine might lie in its known effect of increasing prolactin secretion. Other studies, however, dispute any correlation between reserpine and breast cancer (Mack et al., 1975).

As was shown in the earlier list of risk factors, women who first become pregnant at an early age have a lower risk than those who first become pregnant later in life. The fact that an early first pregnancy offers protection, regardless of the number of subsequent pregnancies, is intriguing. It has been suggested that the first pregnancy "triggers" some favorable change in the breast tissue or in hormonal factors which confers protection against tumor development. The fact that the first pregnancy is protective only if it occurs before age 30 might indicate that tumor initiation occurs very early in life, within a decade after menarche. This would be followed by a long latent period, with overt tumor formation beginning in the fourth and fifth decades. In support of this view is a slightly increased risk with pregnancy *after* age 30.

This has been explained as a promoting effect of pregnancy *on already transformed cells.* There is some indication that women with breast cancer fall into two overlapping population groups. First, there are those discussed above whose tumor is initiated early in life and who develop overt cancer in middle age. The second group consists of those who develop breast cancer in old age, often after a late menopause. In both groups, the data are consistent with a long latent period.

In view of the likely influence of hormones on the development of breast cancer, two negative findings are of interest. The first is the failure to find any correlation between the use of oral contraceptives and breast cancer, despite some expectations to the contrary (Sartwell et al., 1973). However, it should be remembered that the "pill" has been in widespread use for only a decade, and the latent period for this form of cancer may be considerably longer. The second non-correlation is the lack of influence of lactation on the risk of developing breast cancer. For many years, it was thought that lactation offered protection, since breast cancer is relatively infrequent in Asia where prolonged breast-feeding is customary. However, recent data indicate that geographic differences cannot be ascribed to this factor, and that within a population group, there is no difference between the risks to those who breast-feed and those who do not (Yuasa and MacMahon, 1970).

Nevertheless, that there is some hormonal factor in the development of breast cancer seems clear. In many cases, this fact is used to advantage in the treatment of the disease. About 30 to 40 per cent of patients have a temporary remission after manipulation of hormone balance. This may be achieved through ovariectomy, adrenalectomy or hypophysectomy, as well as through the administration of exogenous estrogens or androgens. Tumors which respond to such treatment have been termed "estrogen-dependent." Recently, it has been shown that a number of breast cancers contain specific protein receptor molecules which bind estradiol. Patients with tumors binding estradiol were found to respond better to endocrine manipulations than those without such receptors. These receptors are not present in normal breast tissue, nor in tissue with fibrocystic disease (Editorial, 1974*b*).

Genetic influences involved in the development of breast cancer are very difficult to separate from viral and hormonal factors. Even in mice, in which high-risk strains have been bred for years, it would seem that the "inheritance" of a high risk can in most cases be traced to the presence of a virus. In humans, as shown in the list of risk factors, there is familial aggregation

of breast cancer. However, this is consistent with *either* genetic or environmental factors. All that can be said is that such familial aggregation probably cannot be ascribed to vertical transmission of a virus in milk, since an increased risk can be transmitted through paternal lines as well as maternal. The extreme geographic variation in the incidence of breast cancer is similarly difficult to analyze. As mentioned, it does not seem to be related to differences in breast-feeding customs. Probably it reflects primarily an environmental factor, since migrants from low-risk to high-risk areas develop an increasingly high risk. However, it requires two or three generations before the risk equals that of the host country (MacMahon et al., 1973).

In summary, then, the cause of breast cancer is still not definitely established. However, a number of breakthroughs in our understanding of this disease have occurred in recent years. Taking these together, it would seem that the most reasonable hypothesis is that an oncogenic RNA virus, perhaps identical to the MMTV, initiates the tumor. Tumor development is then promoted over a long latent period by hormonal influences. Whether genetic predisposition is necessary, perhaps as a determinant of immune response or of hormonal balance, is less clear.

Morphology. Cancer of the breast affects the left breast slightly more often than the right. In 4 to 10 per cent of patients there are bilateral primary tumors or a second primary tumor develops subsequently. The locations of the tumors within the breast are:

	Per Cent
Upper outer quadrant	50
Central portion	20
Lower outer quadrant	10
Upper inner quadrant	10
Lower inner quadrant	10

They may arise in the ductal epithelium (90 per cent) or within the lobular epithelium (10 per cent). Both ductal and lobular cancers are further divided into those which have not penetrated the limiting basement membranes (**noninfiltrating**) and those which have done so (**infiltrating**). Thus, carcinoma of the breast is classified as follows:

A. Arising in ducts
   1. Noninfiltrating — **intraductal carcinoma (comedocarcinoma)**
   2. Infiltrating
      a. **Scirrhous carcinoma**
      b. **Medullary carcinoma**
      c. **Colloid (mucinous) carcinoma**
      d. **Paget's disease**
B. Arising in lobules
   1. Noninfiltrating — **in-situ lobular carcinoma**
   2. Infiltrating — **lobular carcinoma**

Of these, the scirrhous carcinoma is by far the most

important. The morphology of each type will be discussed separately.

Intraductal carcinoma represents about 5 per cent of carcinomas of the breast. It takes the form of an anaplastic proliferation of the ductal epithelium which tends to grow within the ducts without invading the ductal basement membrane and underlying breast tissue. Eventually, the ducts become filled with cheesy necrotic tumor tissue, which can be extruded from the nipple with slight pressure (hence the name **comedocarcinoma**). This tumor remains difficult to palpate until late in its course, since there is no well-defined mass. Usually it manifests itself only by an ill-defined increase in consistency. Histologically, the neoplastic cells may initially assume a glandular or papillary pattern within the duct, but continued replication fills the ducts with compressed tumor cells until all architectural detail is lost. At this point they appear as solid cords of anaplastic cells. Eventually, intraductal carcinomas do invade the basement membrane, at which time they are considered infiltrative.

Scirrhous carcinoma, as mentioned, is the most common form of breast cancer, accounting for roughly 75 per cent of carcinomas of the breast. It grows as a deceptively delimited mass, rarely over 3 to 4 cm. in diameter, of stony hard consistency (Fig. 17–15). On cut section, the tumor is obviously infiltrative, retracted below the surrounding fibro-fatty tissue, and has a gritty texture which produces a grating sound when the tumor is scraped with a knife. Foci of chalky white necrosis and sometimes calcification are often evident on the cut

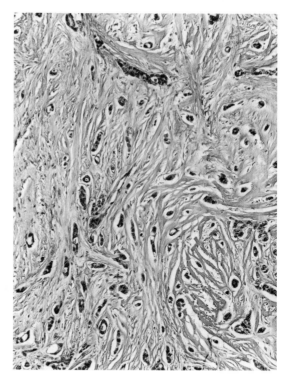

Figure 17–16. A high power detail of a scirrhous adenocarcinoma of the breast. The scattered islands of cancer cells are trapped in the striking desmoplastic stromal overgrowth.

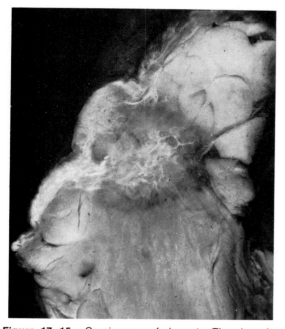

Figure 17–15. Carcinoma of breast. The invasive cancer is just below the skin. The chalky white lines are strands of the dense fibrous stroma so characteristic of these neoplasms.

surface. Histologically, the lesion is composed principally of dense fibrous stroma in which are found widely scattered nests or cords of tumor cells. These are round to polygonal, or compressed, and contain fairly uniform small dark nuclei with remarkably few mitotic figures (Fig. 17–16). At the margins of the tumor, the neoplastic cells can be seen infiltrating the surrounding tissue and frequently invading perivascular and perineurial spaces as well as blood vessels.

Medullary carcinoma represents about 5 to 10 per cent of breast carcinoma. The morphology of these tumors is in sharp contrast to that of scirrhous carcinoma. They tend to be soft and fleshy, rather than stony hard, and often become quite large (up to 10 cm. in diameter). On cut section, the tumor bulges above the surrounding tissue, rather than retracting below it. The reason for these differences is apparent on histologic examination. Unlike the scirrhous carcinoma, the medullary carcinoma has a very scant stroma. The tumor cells grow in large irregular sheets of undifferentiated polygonal to spindled cells, although occasionally well differentiated gland formations are present, meriting the designation medullary adenocarcinoma. There may be a marked lymphocytic infiltration in these tumors.

Colloid (mucinous) carcinoma is even more uncommon than the medullary carcinoma. It is characterized by the production of mucin, intracellularly and extracellularly. Grossly, these lesions are extremely soft, bulky gray-blue masses with the consistency of gelatin. There may be central cystic softening and hemorrhage. Histologically, one or more of three patterns is present. In the first pattern, the tumor cells are seen as small islands, or even isolated cells, floating in a large lake of basophilic mucin that flows into contiguous tissue spaces and planes of cleavage. At least some of the tumor cells have a vacuolated appearance because of the presence of intracellular mucin. In the second pattern, the neoplastic cells grow in well-defined glandular arrangements, the lumina of which contain mucinous secretions. Again, the neoplastic cells may be vacuolated. The third pattern consists of a disorganized mass of undifferentiated tumor cells, most of which are of the signet ring type, that is, they are distended with large vacuoles of mucin.

Paget's disease of the breast is an unusual form of ductal breast cancer which affects women in a slightly older age group than the other forms. It begins as a typical intraductal carcinoma, but involves the main excretory ducts from which it extends to infiltrate the skin of the nipple and areola. As a consequence, eczematoid changes in the nipple and areola antedate the formation of any palpable mass in the breast. The involved areolar and peri-areolar skin is frequently fissured, ulcerated and oozing. There is surrounding inflammatory hyperemia and edema, and superimposed bacterial infections are common. The histologic hallmark of this tumor is the invasion of the epidermis by pathognomonic neoplastic cells termed **Paget cells.** These are large hyperchromatic cells surrounded by a clear halo. In other respects the morphology of Paget's disease is similar to that of an intraductal carcinoma. The prognosis, however, is less favorable, since the diagnosis implies extension to the skin.

Lobular carcinoma, either **in-situ** or **infiltrating,** arises in the glandular epithelium rather than in the ducts. Although relatively infrequent, it is of some interest because of its peculiar tendency to be bilateral (about 20 per cent of cases) (Urban, 1967). Moreover, it is very frequently multicentric within the same breast. The in-situ form may be difficult to distinguish from fibrocystic disease, particularly the adenosis form, because of this tendency toward multicentricity. The diagnosis depends on the identification of anaplastic cells within the glandular spaces. With invasion, the in-situ form becomes infiltrative.

In all of the forms of breast cancer discussed above, progression of the disease leads to certain local morphologic features. These include a tendency to become adherent to the pectoral muscles or deep fascia of the chest wall, with consequent **fixation** of the lesion, as well as adherence to the overlying skin, with **retraction** or **dimpling** of the skin or nipple. The latter is an important sign, since it may be the first indication of a lesion, observed by the patient herself during self-examination. Involvement of the lymphatic pathways may cause localized lymphedema. In these cases the skin becomes thickened around exaggerated hair follicles, a change known as "orange peel." Sometimes, particularly in pregnancy, the tumor spreads so rapidly that it excites an acute inflammatory reaction, with swelling, redness and tenderness. This picture has been referred to as "inflammatory carcinoma." However, it is not a distinct morphologic pattern, but simply reflects rapid growth of any pattern.

Involvement of the lymph nodes is present in about two thirds of patients at the time of diagnosis. The particular chain involved depends on the location of the carcinoma within the breast, as shown by the chart below (Savlov, 1970–71).

As can be seen, involvement of the internal mammary chain, a relatively poor prognostic sign, is seen at diagnosis twice as frequently with lesions of the center or inner quadrants as with those of the outer quadrants. Favored sites for metastases, other than the lymph nodes, are the **lungs, bones, adrenals, brain, ovaries** and **liver.**

Grading and Staging of Breast Cancer. Breast cancer has been graded on the basis of histology in a number of ways. Perhaps the simplest system is the use of Grades I through III to indicate increasing degrees of anaplasia. Of greater importance has been the attempt to stage breast cancer on the basis of its spread at the time of diagnosis. This, of course, is not unrelated to histologic grade, since the more anaplastic lesions are likely to spread earlier and more widely. A staging system, if uniformly used, is of great value in comparing the efficacy of various treatment modalities. The system now in widespread use is based on the following TNM data:

Tumor

T1 — <2 cm. diameter, no fixation
T2 — 2 to 5 cm., skin involvement
T3 — 5 to 10 cm., pectoral fixation
T4 — > 10 cm., pectoral fixation

	Per Cent Outer Quadrant Lesions	Per Cent Center and Inner Quadrant Lesions
No nodal involvement	36	35
Axillary nodes only	46	25
Internal mammary nodes only	2	10
Both	16	30

Nodes

N0 — none
N1 — axillary, movable
N2 — axillary, fixed
N3 — supraclavicular nodes;
    edema of arm

Metastases

M0 — none
M1 — metastases

These data are applied to breast carcinoma as follows:

Stage I: A tumor less than 5 cm. in diameter without nodal involvement and no metastases (T1 N0 M0 or T2 N0 M0).

Stage II: A tumor less than 5 cm. in diameter with movable axillary nodes and no metastases (T1 N1 M0 or T2 N1 M0).

Stage III: All tumors of any size, with or without skin involvement or fixation, and with or without nodal involvement, but **without metastases (any combination of T and N plus M0).**

Stage IV: All tumors of any size, with or without skin involvement or fixation, and with or without nodal involvement, but **with metastases (any combination of T and N plus M1).**

Clinical Course. Breast cancer is usually discovered by the patient as a solitary, painless and movable mass. Less frequently, it is discovered by her physician. At this point, the lesion is typically less than 4 cm. in diameter, although, as mentioned, involvement of the lymph nodes is already present in about two thirds of patients. Obviously, the differential diagnosis includes fibrocystic disease, fibroadenoma, abscess and fat necrosis, as well as any other lesion producing a mass within the breast. The correct diagnosis almost always requires incisional or excisional biopsy. Signs of a poor prognosis include:

1. Edema of the overlying skin or arm.
2. Infiltration of the skin.
3. Fixation of the tumor or the axillary nodes.
4. Involvement of the internal mammary or supraclavicular nodes.
5. "Inflammatory carcinoma."

A great deal of controversy surrounds the appropriate treatment for breast cancer. The traditional approach in the United States has been radical mastectomy (removal of the breast, axillary nodes and pectoral muscles), but there are those who believe that less radical surgery, usually in conjunction with irradiation, gives equally good results. Thus, excision of the lesion ("lumpectomy") or simple mastectomy (removal of the breast alone) with

intensive prophylactic radiotherapy is gaining acceptance. In addition to surgery and radiation (the primary treatment modalities), a number of other measures may be taken secondarily, either as prophylaxis against recurrence or for palliation after recurrence. These usually involve manipulation of endocrine function, as described earlier, including ablative surgery and the administration of exogenous steroids. Chemotherapy may also be used. The possibility of a viral etiology suggests a role for immunotherapy, but this is still experimental.

Figures for overall five-year survival (including all forms and stages of the cancer) are difficult to ascertain, but range from 40 to 60 per cent. Of greater significance is the prognosis of treated patients when considered according to the stage at diagnosis. Thus, the five-year survival for treated Stage I and Stage II disease is 60 to 70 per cent; 10-year survival is 40 to 50 per cent (Anglem and Leber, 1973; Crile, 1973). The 10-year survival is probably of greater importance, since this disease is notorious for a protracted but inexorable course. At one time it was widely held that no form of therapy significantly altered the prognosis with breast cancer. This belief, of course, lent a sense of absurdity to efforts to establish the

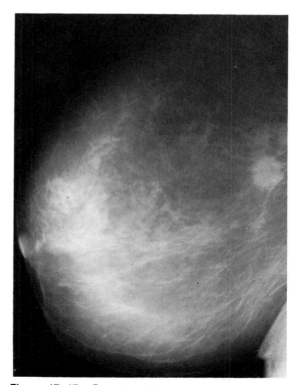

Figure 17–17. Breast carcinoma (mammogram). The nipple is seen on the left, and the deeply situated, deceptively discrete cancer on the far right, appearing as a somewhat radiopaque focus.

best treatment modality. However, it is now unmistakably clear that therapy does affect prognosis. Five-year survival with untreated disease is only about 20 per cent (Bloom, 1962). Moreover, the benefits of treatment are greatest in the early stages. Thus, it is important to detect breast cancer early in its course. Some promising new screening techniques are gaining acceptance, particularly for women at high risk. The one in most widespread use is mammography—x-rays of the breast which may disclose the increased density and spotty calcifications of breast cancer. With this technique, a tumor can be detected long before it is palpable (Fig. 17–17). Newer screening techniques include thermography, xerography and ultrasonic studies.

In summary, it can be said that rapid advances in the understanding of breast cancer are being translated into small gains for the victims of this disease. Nevertheless, it is not too optimistic to hope for an imminent breakthrough. Until then, breast cancer remains a particularly menacing threat to women.

MALE BREAST

The rudimentary male breast is relatively free from pathologic involvement. Only two disorders occur with sufficient frequency to merit consideration—*gynecomastia* and *carcinoma*.

GYNECOMASTIA

As in the female, the male breast is subject to hormonal influences, but is considerably less sensitive than the female breast. Nonetheless, enlargement of the male breast, or *gynecomastia*, may occur in response to absolute or relative estrogen excesses. *Gynecomastia, then, is the male analogue of fibrocystic disease in the female.* The most important cause of such hyperestrinism in the male is cirrhosis of the liver, with consequent inability of the liver to metabolize estrogens. Other causes include Klinefelter's syndrome, estrogen-secreting tumors, estrogen therapy and, occasionally, digitalis therapy. Physiologic gynecomastia often occurs in puberty and in extreme old age.

The morphologic features of gynecomastia are similar to those of intraductal dysplasia. Grossly, a button-like, subareolar swelling develops, usually in both breasts, but occasionally in only one.

CARCINOMA OF THE MALE BREAST

This is a rare occurrence, with a frequency ratio to breast cancer in the female of 1:125. It occurs in advanced age. Because of the scant amount of breast substance in the male, the tumor rapidly infiltrates the overlying skin and underlying thoracic wall. These tumors behave exactly as do the invasive scirrhous carcinomas in the female.

REFERENCES

Aitken-Swan, J., and Baird, D.: Circumcision and cancer of the cervix. Brit. J. Cancer, *19*:217, 1965.
Anglem, T. J., and Leber, R. E.: Operable breast cancer: the case against conservative surgery. CA, *23*:330, 1973.
Bittner, J. J.: Some possible effects of nursing on the mammary gland tumor incidence in mice. Science, *84*:162, 1936.
Bloom, H. J. G., et al.: Natural history of untreated breast cancer. Comparison of untreated and treated cases according to histological grade of malignancy. Brit. Med. J., *2*:213, 1962.
Boston Collaborative Drug Program: Reserpine and breast cancer. Lancet, *2*:699, 1974.
Cole, P.: Personal communication, 1974.
Crile, G., Jr.: Operable breast cancer: in defense of conservative surgery. CA, *23*:334, 1973.
Davis, H. H., et al.: Cystic disease of the breast: Relationship to carcinoma. Cancer, *17*:957, 1964.
deWaard, F., et al.: Steroid excretion pattern in women with endometrial carcinoma. Cancer, *22*:988, 1968.
Editorial: Vaginal adenocarcinomas and maternal estrogen ingestion. Lancet, *1*:250, 1974a.
Editorial: Estradiol receptors in human breast cancer. Lancet, *2*:631, 1974b.
Editorial: The thyroid, prolactin and breast cancer. Lancet, *1*:908, 1974c.
Farber, M., et al.: Estradiol binding by fibroid tumors and normal myometrium. Obstet. Gynec., *40*:479, 1972.
Feller, W. F., and Chopra, H. C.: Virus-like particles in human milk. Cancer, *28*:1425, 1971.
Fish, C. R.: Cervical intraepithelial neoplasia: rationale for investigation and management. Med. Clin. N. Amer., *58*:743, 1974.
Foote, F. W., and Stewart, H. E.: Comparative study of cancerous vs. noncancerous breasts. Ann. Surg., *121*:6, 197, 1945.
Frantz, V. K., et al.: Incidence of chronic cystic disease in so-called "normal breasts." A study based on 225 postmortem examinations. Cancer, *4*:762, 1951.
Garnet, J. E.: Constitutional stigmas associated with endometrial cancer. Am. J. Obstet. Gynec., *76*:11, 1958.
Gilbertsen, V. A.: Detection of breast cancer in a specialized cancer detection center. Cancer, *24*:1192, 1969.
Groseclose, E. S.: Clinical significance of endometriosis. Virginia Med. Monthly, *81*:253, 1954.
Gusberg, S. B.: An approach to the control of carcinoma of the endometrium. CA, *23*:99, 1973.
Gusberg, S. B., et al.: Precursors of corpus cancer. II. A clinical and pathological study of adenomatous hyperplasia. Am. J. Obstet. Gynec., *68*:1472, 1954.
Herbst, A. L., et al.: Adenocarcinoma of the vagina: association of maternal stilbestrol therapy with tumor appearance in young women. New Eng. J. Med., *284*:878, 1971.
Hertig, A. T., and Sommers, S. C.: Genesis of endometrial carcinoma. I. Study of prior biopsies. Cancer, *2*:946, 1949.
Holland, J. F., and Hreshchyshyn, M. M. (eds.): Choriocarcinoma. UICC Monograph Series, Vol. 3. Berlin, Springer-Verlag, 1967.
Jacobson, O.: Heredity in breast cancer: A genetic and clinical study of 200 probands as reported by Wynder, E. L., et al. Cancer, *13*:557, 1960.

Kirk, M. E.: Gynecology. Hum. Pathol., 5:253, 1974.

Klein, G.: Summary of papers delivered at the conference on herpesvirus and cervical cancer. Cancer Res., 33:1557, 1973.

Kurman, R. J., and Scully, R. E.: The incidence and histogenesis of vaginal adenosis. Hum. Pathol., 5:265, 1974.

Lemon, H. M.: Endocrine influences on human mammary cancer formation. A critique. Cancer, 23:781, 1969.

Linder, D., et al.: Parthenogenic origin of benign ovarian teratomas. New Eng. J. Med., 292:63, 1975.

Mack, T. M., et al.: Reserpine and breast cancer in a retirement community. New Eng. J. Med., 292:1366, 1975.

MacMahon, B., et al.: Etiology of human breast cancer. J. Nat. Cancer Inst., 50:21, 1973.

Meigs, J. V.: Endometriosis. New Eng. J. Med., 226:147, 1942.

Moore, D. H., et al.: Some aspects of a search for human mammary tumor virus. Cancer, 28:1415, 1971a.

Moore, D. H., et al.: Search for a human breast cancer virus. Nature, 229:611, 1971b.

Plummer, G., and Masterson, J. G.: Herpes simplex virus and cancer of the cervix. Amer. J. Obstet. Gynec., 11:81, 1971.

Rapp, F., and Buss, E. R.: Are viruses important in carcinogenesis? Am. J. Path., 77:85, 1974.

Rawls, W. E., et al: An analysis of seroepidemiological studies of herpesvirus type 2 and carcinoma of the cervix. Cancer Res., 33:1477, 1973.

Rotkin, I. D.: A comparison review of key epidemiological studies in cervical cancer related to current searches for transmissible agents. Cancer Res., 33:1353, 1973.

Rudolph, J.: Female genital tract cancer. In Rubin, P. (ed.): Clinical Oncology for Medical Students and Physicians. 3rd ed. New York, American Cancer Society, 1970–71.

Sarkar, N. H., and Moore, D. H.: On the possibility of a human breast cancer virus. Nature, 236:103, 1972.

Sartwell, P. E., et al.: Epidemiology of benign breast lesions: lack of association with oral contraceptive use. New Eng. J. Med., 288:551, 1973.

Savlov, E.: Breast cancer. In Rubin, P. (ed.): Clinical Oncology for Medical Students and Physicians. 3rd ed. New York, American Cancer Society, 1970–1971.

Schlom, J., and Spiegelman, S.: Evidence for viral involvement in murine and human mammary adenocarcinoma. Am. J. Clin. Path., 60:44, 1973.

Schlom, J., et al.: RNA dependent DNA polymerase activity in virus-like particles isolated from human milk. Nature, 231:97, 1971.

Scully, R. E.: Recent progress in ovarian cancer. Hum. Pathol., 1:73, 1970.

Silverberg, E., and Holleb, A. I.: Cancer statistics, 1974—worldwide epidemiology. CA, 24:2, 1974.

Stern, E.: Cytohistopathology of cervical cancer. Cancer Res., 33:1368, 1973.

Terris, M., et al.: Relation of circumcision to cancer of the cervix. Am. J. Obstet. Gynec., 117:1056, 1973.

Urban, J. A.: Bilaterality of cancer of the breast. Cancer, 20:1867, 1967.

Warren, S.: The prognosis of benign lesions of the female breast. Surgery, 19:32, 1946.

Yuasa, S., and MacMahon, B.: Lactation and reproductive histories of breast cancer patients in Tokyo, Japan. Bull. WHO, 42:195, 1970.

The Endocrine System

Hormones may be considered as blood-borne substances which, in very small amounts, regulate the activity of target cells without actually participating in energy-yielding reactions (Catt, 1970a). In the past 10 years several new hormones have been identified, and the total number by now is quite large. Some, such as histamine, are released by many cells throughout the body. Others, such as secretin, are released by the gut, which is not primarily an endocrine organ. Still others are elaborated by the pancreas, a dual exocrine and endocrine gland, which was considered in Chapter 15. The gonads, as is well known, are the sites of spermatogenesis and oogenesis, but they also secrete hormones. This chapter will be concerned only with those discrete organs whose principal function is the elaboration of hormones—the endocrine glands.

The diagnosis of endocrine disorders was at one time based largely on indirect assessments of glandular function. Sometimes rather crude bioassays were used. In other instances, if overactivity of an endocrine gland was suspected, clinical evaluation depended on attempts to suppress it and, conversely, suspected hypofunction was assessed by attempts to stimulate the gland. With the development of radioimmunoassay techniques, however, it has become possible in most cases to measure directly (Sutton's Law triumphant) the hormone levels.

THE PITUITARY

It will be remembered that the pituitary is composed of an anterior lobe, or *adenohypophysis*, and a posterior lobe, or *neurohypophysis*, which are separated by a rather rudimentary intermediate lobe. A narrow stalk connects the pituitary to the hypothalamus.

The adenohypophysis consists of three basic cell types—*acidophils* (30 to 40 per cent), *basophils* (5 to 10 per cent) and *chromophobes* (50 per cent)—classified according to the presence or absence of cytoplasmic granules and their staining properties. In addition, small numbers of transitional forms, known as *amphophils*, are recognized. It is thought that the chromophobes, as well as the transitional forms, represent acidophils or basophils that have become degranulated as a consequence of active hormone secretion (Catt, 1970*b*). At least seven hormones are synthesized and elaborated by the adenohypophysis. An eighth, termed lipotropic hormone, is postulated. All of these hormones appear to act through the stimulation of adenyl cyclase activity when bound to specific receptors in the cell membranes of target organs. For each of the seven hormones, corresponding peptide releasing factors from the hypothalamus have been isolated. In some cases, however, the releasing factor is relatively nonspecific and may affect the release of more than one pituitary hormone. For example, thyrotropin releasing factor (TRF) stimulates prolactin release as well as the release of thyroid stimulating hormone (TSH). The hypothalamus secretes in addition *inhibitory* factors for at least three hormones of the adenohypophysis—growth hormone, prolactin and melanocyte stimulating hormone (MSH). The neurohypophysis elaborates only two hormones, both of which are probably synthesized in the hypothalamus. The following list indicates the hormones of the pituitary and their probable cells of origin:

A. Adenohypophysis
  1. Growth hormone (GH) — Acidophils
  2. Prolactin (LTH) — ?Acidophils
  3. Adrenocortical stimulating hormone (ACTH) — Basophils
  4. Thyroid stimulating hormone (TSH) — Basophils
  5. Follicle stimulating hormone (FSH) — Basophils
  6. Luteinizing hormone (LH) — Basophils
  7. Melanocyte stimulating hormone (MSH) — ?Basophils
B. Neurohypophysis
  1. Antidiuretic hormone (ADH) — Supraoptic nucleus
  2. Oxytocin — Paraventricular nucleus

Lesions of the pituitary may express themselves by hyper- or hypofunction, or by local effects when an expanding mass impinges on surrounding structures.

HYPERPITUITARISM

Hyperfunction of the pituitary is usually caused by a functioning tumor. The majority

are benign adenomas. About 10 per cent of *clinically significant* pituitary adenomas are composed of acidophil cells; almost all the remainder are, in varying proportions, predominantly chromophobe. However, very small, *clinically insignificant* basophil tumors or foci of hyperplasia are discovered at autopsy in from 12.5 to 25 per cent of the population (Daughaday, 1968).

Both chromophobe and acidophil tumors tend to arise between the ages of 20 and 50 years, and they affect men more often than women. The chromophobe tumors are malignant in fewer than 20 per cent of cases, while the acidophilic tumors are almost never malignant. Because the chromophobe tumors tend to be larger, they are more likely to produce local manifestations.

Keeping in mind the above qualification, the gross morphology of all pituitary adenomas is similar. They range in size from microscopic to soft, spherical, red-brown masses over 10 cm. in diameter. They are usually well encapsulated and contained within the sella turcica. Progressive centrifugal growth may cause rupture of the capsule and the diaphragma sellae and extension of the tumor outside the sella, with apparent invasion of the cavernous sinuses, nasal sinuses and base of the brain. Occasionally, extension beyond the sella turcica may simulate the appearance of a malignant tumor. The cytologic detail of the typical pituitary adenoma is faithful to its cell of origin, although special stains may be necessary to identify the cell type. However, not infrequently, mixed cell populations are included within an adenoma composed predominantly of one cell type. The cells are regular, with little variability in size and shape, and mitoses are rare. They may simulate the glandular patterns sometimes seen in the normal adenohypophysis, or they may be arrayed in solid sheets or even in papillary formations. Often there are areas of ischemic necrosis resulting from the progressive development of pressure within these tumors.

The distinction between an adenoma and a carcinoma of the pituitary may be difficult. As was mentioned, benign tumors may rupture through their capsules to extend into the adjacent tissues, whereas malignant tumors may appear cytologically deceptively innocent. Perhaps the only certain criterion of malignancy is evidence of metastatic disease.

Chromophobe tumors (presumably representing degranulated chromophils) as well as acidophil tumors may be endocrinologically active. The histology does not provide any information about function. When there is hyperfunction, it may largely be limited to excess elaboration of growth hormone, or it may include hypersecretion of some of the other hormones as well. *It is probable that many of these tumors secrete ACTH as well as growth hormone. Thyroid and gonadal function may be decreased, increased or normal.* These variations in functional activity are not surprising when one remembers that acidophil tumors often contain some chromophobe cells, and these in turn may represent degranulated basophil cells. In those instances in which TSH and the gonadotropins are *not* elaborated, pressure from the expanding tumor may cause atrophy of the neighboring normal basophils and hence hypothyroidism and hypogonadism.

Hypersecretion of growth hormone in the adult leads to *acromegaly;* in children, the disorder takes a somewhat different form, termed *gigantism.*

ACROMEGALY

Acromegaly begins insidiously, usually between the ages of 20 and 40 years. The name of the disorder refers to one of its more striking features—a disproportionate overgrowth of the acral parts, caused by subperiosteal appositional bone growth, predominantly in the skull and small bones of the hands and feet. The patient develops a general coarsening of his facial features, with prominent cheek bones, prognathism and frontal bossing. The fingers and toes become broadened and spade-like. Often the patient is not aware of the gradually increasing size of his skull, hands and feet. The viscera also increase in size (visceromegaly). Some degree of hyperglycemia is seen in most acromegalics, sometimes with the development of overt diabetes mellitus. In addition, local indications of the intracranial mass are often present in these patients, including an enlarged sella turcica on x-ray, headache and, sometimes, bitemporal hemianopia from impingement of the tumor on the optic chiasm. Until recently, the diagnosis rested on clinical grounds and indirect laboratory procedures, but direct immunoassay of growth hormone is now possible.

GIGANTISM

Gigantism is considerably less common than acromegaly. It differs in that overgrowth is proportionate, since the epiphyses of these children have not closed, and there is a symmetrical increase in stature as well as in the size of the viscera. As with acromegaly, the thyroid, adrenal and gonads may be hyperplastic or atrophied. Sometimes these organs are hyperplastic initially, but eventually they may undergo exhaustion atrophy. Spontaneous infarction of the pituitary tumor may bring about a sudden, total reversal to panhypopituitarism.

HYPOPITUITARISM

The functional reserve of the pituitary is great, and about 75 per cent of the gland must be destroyed for symptoms to be pro-duced. Total obliteration of the pituitary is rare; it causes death from adrenal insufficiency within about two weeks. Causes of hypopituitarism include:

1. Sheehan's syndrome (postpartum pituitary necrosis).
2. Nonfunctioning pituitary tumors.
3. Congenital disorders.
4. Therapeutic ablation of the pituitary.

Usually there is a deficiency in all the hormones of the adenohypophysis (the neurohypophysis is only infrequently affected), but hypopituitarism may be unihormonal, for mysterious reasons.

SHEEHAN'S POSTPARTUM NECROSIS

Ischemic necrosis of the pituitary is believed to result from multiple pituitary thromboses incident to a sudden drop in blood pressure. Although theoretically it may follow hypotension from any cause, women who have severe hemorrhage during childbirth are most vulnerable. Perhaps the increased size of the pituitary during pregnancy renders it more susceptible to decreases in its blood supply. It has also been suggested that the minute thromboses may actually represent a generalized Shwartzman-type reaction based on sensitization of the patient to placental proteins. This would then represent a form of disseminated intravascular coagulation (DIC) (see p. 363).

Grossly, the gland may initially appear normal before the ischemic changes become evident, or it may appear hemorrhagic. As the necrotic cells are replaced by fibrous tissue, there is gradual, progressive shrinkage and scarring of the anterior lobe. Ultimately, the gland may be reduced to a fibrous nubbin weighing less than 0.1 gm. The histologic pattern is that of either ischemic or hemorrhagic infarction, depending on whether the vessels involved are predominantly arteries or veins. Fibrous replacement follows.

Symptoms of pituitary insufficiency may not appear for days, weeks, months or years after the causative hypotensive episode. In later developing cases, it is likely that progressive scarring slowly involves additional marginal cells, until the threshold of pituitary insufficiency is reached. In more severe, immediately developing cases, the patient fails to lactate after delivery and the breasts involute. Later, there is weakness and fatigability, loss of body hair, decreased pigmentation and failure of menses to resume. In general, the hormone deficiencies of partial hypopituitarism appear clinically in the following order: gonadotropins, growth hormone, TSH, ACTH.

NONFUNCTIONING PITUITARY TUMORS

The second most common cause of hypopituitarism is a pituitary tumor, either a *non-*

functioning chromophobe adenoma or a *craniopharyngioma.* The former does not differ significantly in appearance from its functioning counterpart.

The *craniopharyngioma* is, after the adenomas, the second most frequent type of pituitary tumor. It is probably derived from vestigial remnants of the craniopharyngeal anlage and is nonfunctional. Tumors of this type may arise in any position along the craniopharyngeal canal, and therefore some lie within the sella turcica, while others lie external to it.

Commonly, they are well encapsulated, up to 10 cm. in diameter, and either cystic or solid. **Of great diagnostic importance is the fact that over 75 per cent of craniopharyngiomas are sufficiently calcified to be apparent on x-ray.** The histologic pattern of these tumors is variable and often quite bizarre. Sometimes the architecture is similar to the enamel organ of the tooth, and these tumors are thus also known as **adamantinomas** or **ameloblastomas.** When solid, the tumors consist of nests or stands of the epithelial cells, interspersed within a loose fibrous myxoid stroma. The epithelial element closely resembles, at times, squamous epithelium (Fig. 18–1). The cystic forms may be lined with stratified squamous or columnar epithelium. Malignant transformation is rare.

These tumors produce hypopituitarism by their compression of the normal pituitary.

CONGENITAL HYPOPITUITARISM

This disorder may be transmitted as an autosomal recessive and be limited to a defi-

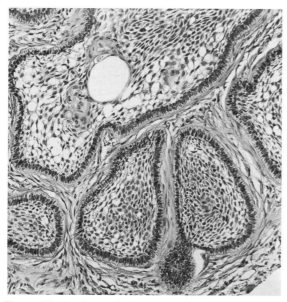

Figure 18–1. A craniopharyngioma of the pituitary growing as an adamantinoma. The epithelial nests have a peripheral palisade of columnar cells, which enclose loose squamoid cells.

ciency of growth hormone, or it may be sporadic, perhaps of hypothalamic origin, and sometimes include deficiencies of other pituitary hormones. In either case, the result of congenital growth hormone deficiency is *hypophyseal dwarfism.* Males are affected twice as often as females. These infants appear normal at birth, but sometime during the first year, their decreased growth rate is noted. Although growth takes place at less than one-half the normal rate, it continues until the fourth decade, so that a height of 4 to 5 feet may ultimately be reached. Intelligence is normal (Daughaday, 1968).

THERAPEUTIC ABLATION OF THE PITUITARY

Pituitary ablation is most often done for diabetic retinopathy and for palliation of metastatic breast cancer.

POSTERIOR PITUITARY

The neurohypophysis appears remarkably immune to disease. Loss of ADH results in diabetes insipidus, characterized by extreme polyuria. About one third of such cases are idiopathic, some familial. The remainder are attributable to tumors of the pituitary or midbrain, infiltrative processes such as eosinophilic granuloma, trauma and a variety of meningoencephalitides. There may be no histologic changes, or the changes may be confined to neuronal degeneration within the supraoptic nucleus.

Inappropriate hypersecretion of ADH is a functional disorder that is being recognized with increasing frequency. Although the underlying cause is often ectopic ADH secretion by a cancer, usually an oat-cell carcinoma of the lung, a large variety of intracranial and systemic disorders may, for rather obscure reasons, be associated with inappropriate ADH secretion.

THYROID

Disorders of the thyroid come to attention because of (1) *enlargement (goiter),* (2) *hyperfunction,* or (3) *hypofunction* of the gland, and are here classified in this way. With some diseases, however, such as the thyroiditides, the clinical presentation varies from patient to patient, rendering such an arrangement not always applicable.

ENLARGEMENT OF THE THYROID (GOITER)

Thyroid enlargement, either symmetric or asymmetric, may be caused by (1) inflammation (*thyroiditis*), (2) functional disorders (*diffuse* and *multinodular colloid goiters*), and (3) *tumors*. Congenital thyroid malformations (e.g., *thyroglossal cysts*) may produce an enlargement higher in the neck. In addition, hyperfunction of the thyroid may also be associated with goiter. The causes of hyperfunction are discussed in a later section.

THYROGLOSSAL CYSTS

These congenital lesions arise from partial persistence of the embryonic tract between the thyroid and the base of the tongue.

When this tract is not obliterated, cystic structures may arise which become filled with mucinous secretions, producing swellings up to several centimeters in diameter. These are palpable in the midline of the neck anterior to the trachea. The lining epithelium is stratified squamous when the cysts are high in the neck, i.e., near the tongue, but it is similar to that of the thyroid acini when the cysts are nearer the gland. Although these lesions are congenital, they slowly fill up with secretions and thus often become evident only in adult life.

Their major significance is as masses that must be differentiated from a tumor. In addition, they sometimes communicate as draining sinuses with either the skin or the base of the tongue.

THYROIDITIS

Acute and chronic nonspecific thyroiditis may be caused by a variety of viral and bacterial agents which secondarily affect the thyroid. In addition, there are two major specific forms of thyroid inflammatory disease.

Struma Lymphomatosa (Hashimoto's Disease). This is by far the most common form of thyroiditis. The classic case is characterized by: (1) modest symmetrical, rubbery enlargement of the thyroid gland, (2) mild hypothyroidism, (3) massive infiltration of the thyroid by lymphoid cells admixed with plasma cells, and (4) the presence of three thyroid-specific humoral antigen-antibody systems (Doniach and Roitt, 1968). Females have the manifest disease 30 times as commonly as males, and typically are most vulnerable about the time of menopause. It has become clear, however, that variations from this classic pattern abound and that this disorder may in most instances be asymptomatic, with little if any enlargement of the gland or functional impairment. In general practice in Great Britain, evidence for such subclinical thyroiditis was found in 4.6 per cent of women and 1.6 per cent of men (Hall, 1970). Variations in the expression of Hashimoto's disease are thought to be related in some manner to the innate regenerative capacity of the thyroid, which in turn may be dependent on the patient's age and sex. Whereas the fully developed lesion is commonly seen in menopausal females, males and older patients may instead show fibrous or atrophic changes, without regenerative goiter formation and with a correspondingly greater risk of functional impairment. In contrast, the goiter aspect may be dominant in young people. Indeed, a mild form of Hashimoto's disease has been cited as causing about 40 per cent of all nontoxic goiters in children and adolescents.

It is generally accepted that Hashimoto's disease, as well as primary myxedema and Graves' disease (two disorders to be discussed later), can all be considered as autoimmune in origin. Indeed, Hashimoto's disease was one of the earliest disorders recognized as having a probable autoimmune basis, and on this account remains dearly beloved among immunologists. This form of thyroid disease was of totally obscure nature until 1956, when Witebsky and Rose produced thyroid lesions in experimental animals immunized with homologous thyroid extract in Freund's adjuvant (Rose and Witebsky, 1956). At about the same time, Roitt and his associates (1956) identified precipitins to thyroid antigens in the serum of patients with Hashimoto's disease. Their observations set into motion the exciting era of the exploration of many other diseases of unknown etiology as possible additional instances of immune disorders. The precise nature of the immunologic disturbance with Hashimoto's disease is, however, still not clear. Whether it reflects a primary derangement in the immune system or, rather, represents a normal immune response to altered antigen or to abnormally high antigen levels in the circulation is controversial. It is possible that infection by an unknown virus, or some enzyme derangement of genetic origin, may cause alterations in thyroid proteins, rendering them antigenic. Most workers, however, favor the hypothesis that there is a primary derangement in the immune system. It has been suggested further that the effects may be widespread, often involving tissues other than the thyroid (DeGroot, 1970). Support for this view lies in the relatively high incidence in these patients of autoantibodies to a variety of other tissues, as well as in the concomitance of other possibly autoimmune disorders, such as pernicious anemia and Addison's disease.

The histologic features of Hashimoto's disease (as well as of primary myxedema and Graves' disease) suggest a cell mediated immune response. Indeed, Hashimoto's disease can be produced experimentally by the passive transfer of lymphocytes to a normal recipient from an animal in which the disease has been induced. In addition, circulating antibodies against (1) thyroglobulin, (2) a colloid antigen other than thyroglobulin, and (3) a microsomal antigen of the thyroid epithelial cells are present in various titers in almost all patients with Hashimoto's disease and in the majority of those with primary myxedema.

Despite the presence of these immunoglobulins, however, there are reasons for doubting that they cause the thyroid damage. Only the microsomal antibody, in the presence of complement, is cytotoxic for thyroid cells, and then only in tissue culture. Passive transfer of serum in experimental animals has failed to produce the disease in recipients. Although the microsomal antibody is in part IgG and might theoretically be expected to cross the placental barrier, it does not damage the thyroids of infants even when the mothers have active disease. Moreover, antithyroid antibodies, usually in low titer, have been demonstrated in a great many thyroid disorders involving very different morphologic changes. Perhaps, then, the autoantibodies are largely secondary to the destruction of thyroid tissue. Alternatively, it has been proposed that autoantibodies might first bind to cellular antigens in the thyroid. By coating the thyroid cells, these immune complexes render them vulnerable to Fc-bearing immunocompetent cells—so-called "antibody-dependent cellular cytotoxicity" (Sharp and Irvin, 1970). Obviously, the pathogenesis of Hashimoto's disease remains uncertain.

The gross morphologic change is usually a diffuse, rubbery enlargement of the thyroid, up to three to four times normal size, with no involvement of the capsule. At surgery, this lesion, which presents a pale gray, fleshy appearance on sectioning, is easily confused with a carcinoma. Some cases are characterized by marked fibrosis. Such fibrotic glands may be enlarged or they may be contracted and stony hard. Whether this fibrotic pattern is distinct from the rare disorder known as **Riedel's struma** is controversial. In the more typical form of Hashimoto's disease, there is a variable lymphocytic infiltrate, which, with increasing severity, tends to aggregate in focal areas and ultimately to organize into well developed lymphoid follicles surrounded by lymphoid pulp (Fig. 18–2). In these advanced cases, histologic sections of the thyroid may be confused with those of lymph nodes. In addition to the invading lymphocytes, there are intermingled plasma cells and a variable diffuse increase in interacinar connective tissue. All these changes occur at the expense of the normal thyroid architecture. The epithelial cells lining the remaining acini may become atrophic or, more commonly, may come to resemble **Hürthle cells**. These are large, granular, acidophilic cells which are found in certain thyroid adenomas.

When Hashimoto's disease is clinically

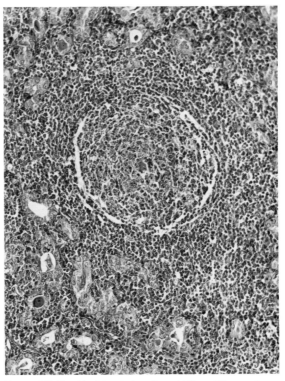

Figure 18–2. Hashimoto's thyroiditis. The microscopic field shows a prominent lymphoid follicle and a diffuse lymphocytic and plasma cell infiltrate interspersed among the somewhat atrophic thyroid acini.

overt, the patient usually seeks medical attention because of enlargement of the thyroid, occasionally with symptoms of pressure on the trachea or esophagus. *Thyroid function is normal or depressed.* The course is as variable as the expressions of the disease. Sometimes Hashimoto's disease remits spontaneously; in other cases, it remains more or less stable for years. Finally, there are those cases which from the beginning are dominated by manifestations of hypothyroidism, and those which only after a long course terminate in thyroid atrophy and primary myxedema (see p. 605). *It is now thought that primary myxedema represents an atrophic variant or end-stage of Hashimoto's disease.* The relationship of these disorders to Graves' disease, which is characterized by a different constellation of thyroid autoantibodies, is less clear. As mentioned, Hashimoto's thyroiditis frequently coexists with other disorders of presumed autoimmune origin, including SLE, Sjögren's syndrome, rheumatoid arthritis, Addison's disease and pernicious anemia. This would seem to indicate a genetic predisposition to autoimmune reactions. Woolner and his colleagues (1959) have called attention to the development of malignancy in 5 per cent of one series of patients with

Hashimoto's thyroiditis. Fifty per cent of these cancers were a form of lymphoma.

Subacute (de Quervain's, Granulomatous) Thyroiditis. This is a much less common form of specific thyroiditis. It is an acute to subacute inflammation, probably of viral origin, which manifests itself by painful swelling of the thyroid, often with malaise and other systemic reactions. In contrast to Hashimoto's disease, it is not considered to be an autoimmune disorder.

The morphologic changes consist of slight to moderate, often asymmetrical, enlargement of the thyroid. Early in the course, the histology shows patchy proliferation and necrosis of the thyroid acinar epithelium, surrounded by a nonspecific acute to subacute inflammatory infiltrate. **Prominent in this inflammatory infiltrate are large, foreign-body type giant cells which often contain phagocytized fragments of colloid.** With time, a granulomatous pattern may develop, with a predominantly mononuclear infiltrate and fibrotic reaction.

Thyroid function remains normal or only slightly increased. Almost invariably, spontaneous remission occurs within weeks to months.

DIFFUSE AND MULTINODULAR COLLOID GOITERS

In most cases, these goiters are caused by an absolute or relative lack of iodine, with consequent impairment of thyroxine formation (Zacharewicz, 1968). The pituitary then responds by an increased output of thyroid stimulating hormone (TSH), leading to diffuse hyperplasia of the thyroid gland. When this stimulus is subsequently removed, involution occurs, and the acini are left dilated and filled with colloid *(diffuse colloid or simple goiter)*. Sometimes this sequence of hyperplasia and involution occurs in cycles, or for some reason does not affect the gland uniformly. In these cases, areas of hyperplasia, involution and scarring all may coexist in the same gland, producing the *multinodular* or *multiple colloid adenomatous goiter.*

The prevalence of these goiters has been variously estimated as about 1 to 4 per cent of the population. A higher incidence is found in certain geographic areas, generally remote from the sea, where lack of iodine in the diet makes the thyroid disorder endemic. Women are affected four to eight times as commonly as men. Simple dietary deficiency is becoming less frequent as a cause of goiter because of the widespread practice of iodizing salt. Other causes of iodine deficiency include (1) the ingestion of goitrogenic foods, such as cabbage, cauliflower, turnips and soybeans, which contain a thiocarbamide that inhibits the oxidation of iodides; (2) inborn metabolic errors in the ability to utilize iodine, to deiodinate iodotyrosines, to couple iodotyrosines, or to liberate thyroxine; and (3) physiologic or pathologic stresses, such as puberty, pregnancy or infection, which increase thyroid demands and so may result in a relative iodine deficiency.

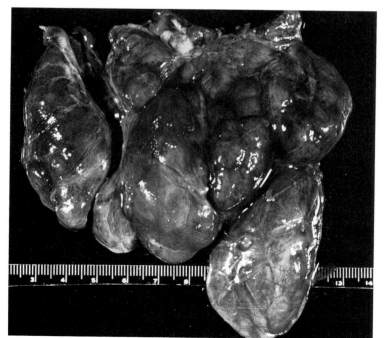

Figure 18–3. Multinodular colloid (multiple colloid adenomatous) goiter.

With **diffuse colloid goiter,** the thyroid is firm and symmetrically enlarged, up to 200 to 300 gm., which is 10 times its normal size. The capsule is usually uninvolved. The transected surface is pale, brown-gray, glistening, brittle and gelatinous. On histologic examination, large colloid-filled acini are seen, lined by flattened epithelial cells and separated by a scant stroma. Sometimes there is evidence of preexisting hyperplasia in the form of occasional small acini lined by cuboidal to tall columnar cells.

Multinodular colloid goiters may be truly enormous and, in general, are the largest type of goiter encountered, weighing up to 1000 gm. They may be markedly asymmetrical, consisting of masses of palpable nodules (Fig. 18–3). Expansion may occur downward behind the sternum to produce an **intrathoracic** or **plunging goiter.** Although the capsule is usually uninvolved, subcapsular hemorrhage sometimes causes adhesion to surrounding structures. Perhaps the most important histologic feature is the extreme variability of the tissue within these glands. Nodules of hyperplasia exist side-by-side with nodules composed of dilated, colloid-filled follicles. Grossly, this appears as meaty, red-brown parenchyma alternating with pale, gelatinous areas which are punctuated by small cysts, foci of red-brown hemorrhage and pale fibrotic reactions. Calcification is common in the scarred areas. **While the nodules may give the false impression of encapsulation on gross examination, they are actually merely surrounded by compressed stromal tissue.**

Both diffuse and multinodular colloid goiters usually come to attention because of progressive enlargement of the thyroid. When symptoms occur, they result from compression of the trachea or esophagus by the expanding mass. *In general, the increase in size of these glands is sufficient to keep the patient euthyroid.* Rarely, a focus within a multinodular goiter becomes hyperactive, producing a *toxic nodular goiter.* These will be mentioned further in the discussion of hyperthyroidism. The risk of malignant transformation of a multinodular colloid goiter is a subject of considerable debate. Some believe it to be quite small, less than 1 per cent, while others cite a hazard of about 6 per cent (Zacharewicz, 1968).

THYROID TUMORS

Benign adenomas and four kinds of malignant thyroid tumors are of clinical importance.

The *adenomas* are benign tumors having a range of histologic patterns which recapitulate the embryogenesis of the thyroid. Since all possess more or less well developed follicles, the entire range of lesions may be collectively termed *follicular adenoma.* They commonly occur in young adults, but may affect any age group. The lesion presents clinically as a solitary, discrete mass, usually up to 4 cm. in diameter.

Some tumors are composed of virtually solid cords of cuboidal epithelial cells, forming only occasional rudimentary acini (**embryonal adenoma**). At the other extreme are tumors consisting of well formed, dilated glands containing abundant colloid (**colloid adenoma**). An intermediate pattern, characterized by considerable variation in the size of the acini, as well as in the amount of intervening stroma, also occurs. When there is a very abundant loose stroma, with small, primitive acini, the designation of **fetal adenoma** is given. **Invariably, there is a well defined fibrous capsule.** Rarely, these tumors are made up of the large, granular, acidophilic **Hürthle cells** described on page 599. These cells are arranged in sheets and nests, as well as poorly defined glands. Because of the striking variation in size and shape of the cells, such tumors may be mistaken for cancers. In general, however, follicular adenomas clearly are benign on histologic examination.

Clinically, they frequently are confused with a nodule of a multinodular goiter. The incidence of malignant transformation varies from study to study, and has even been placed as high as 14 per cent, which is considerably higher than that of the multinodular goiter. However, this percentage is controversial (Zacharewicz, 1968). The evaluation of the significance of a thyroid nodule, i.e., determining whether it is benign or malignant, is one of the most difficult problems in clinical medicine. Well differentiated, functioning nodules will take up test doses of radioiodine (RaI) ("hot nodules") and are almost always benign. The less differentiated lesions of cancer are more likely to be "cold."

Thyroid cancer is infrequent and causes only about 0.5 per cent of all cancer deaths. Women are affected more often than men, in a ratio of 2:1. The peak incidence is between the ages of 40 and 60 years. Although the etiology and pathogenesis are buried in the mystery of all cancers, two important clinical associations are known. First, large amounts of radiation, particularly to the head and neck, seem to predispose to the later development of thyroid cancer (p. 98). Second, there is clinical and experimental evidence that prolonged TSH stimulation of the thyroid may eventually lead to malignant transformation.

The four principal types of thyroid cancer, all carcinomas, and their approximate relative frequencies are as follows (Woolner et al., 1961):

	Per Cent
Papillary carcinoma	61
Follicular carcinoma	18
Anaplastic carcinoma	15
Medullary (amyloidic) carcinoma	6

The *papillary carcinoma* tends to affect a somewhat younger age group than do the other thyroid cancers.

Grossly, they are usually solitary but may be multifocal lesions ranging from microscopic foci to areas up to 10 cm. in diameter. The cut surface varies from cystic to solid, often with a furry texture as a result of the myriads of tiny papillae. The pathognomonic histologic feature is a papillary axial stroma covered by epithelium, which varies markedly in its appearance from tumor to tumor and even from focus to focus within one lesion (Fig. 18–4). In some, the covering epithelium may be regular and cuboidal. These have erroneously been considered to be benign papillary adenomas. Others, however, may exhibit all degrees of anaplasia and disorientation of cells, with piling up of the epithelium and invasion of the stalk by sheets and masses of cells. Sometimes follicles filled with colloid are also present, but the diagnosis is based on the presence of papillae.

Usually these tumors become evident as palpable nodules within the thyroid which, if untreated, eventually extend via the lymphatics to the regional lymph nodes but seldom metastasize to distant organs. Others may remain undiscovered until removal of a lymph node bearing a metastatic deposit calls attention to the possibility of an occult primary lesion.

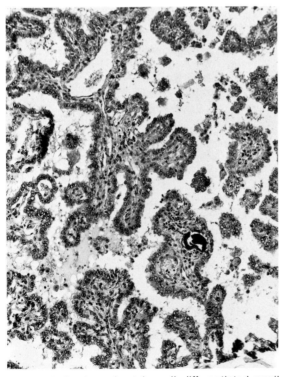

Figure 18–4. A moderately well differentiated papillary carcinoma of the thyroid. The epithelial cells display a slightly disordered array and show some variability in size.

Surgical resection and removal of involved nodes is almost always curative, particularly in younger patients. Because these tumors are TSH-dependent and because of their known indolence, some even advocate a trial of thyroxine chemotherapy to suppress the pituitary and therefore the tumor. Rarely do these cancers kill (Veith et al., 1964).

Follicular carcinomas are characterized by the formation of more or less well developed acini or follicles. They are seen in two different clinical settings. In the first, the tumor is discovered incidentally as a microscopic focus of anaplastic cells, which may be invading adjacent acini and blood vessels. Although it is possible that clinically overt disease does eventually develop from such lesions, they are of no significance at this stage.

More commonly, follicular carcinoma presents as a slowly enlarging irregular lump, often in an already nodular gland. The gray-white, firm tumor tissue tends to replace the thyroid parenchyma and eventually penetrates the capsule to become adherent to the trachea, muscles, skin and great vessels of the neck (Fig. 18–5). Often the recurrent laryngeal nerves are trapped in this process. The histologic pattern is of an adenocarcinoma with varying degrees of differentiation. Sometimes remarkably normal-appearing follicles filled with colloid are present; in other instances, the follicles are rudimentary at best and are surrounded by more anaplastic cells.

By their adherence to surrounding structures, these tumors produce pressure symptoms, such as dyspnea and dysphagia. Involvement of the recurrent laryngeal nerves leads to hoarseness and cough. *Most of these patients remain euthyroid.* However, a few become hypothyroid, owing to replacement of large amounts of thyroid tissue by the tumor, and still fewer are hyperthyroid because of an unusually well differentiated, functioning tumor. The prognosis with follicular carcinoma of the thyroid is variable, and depends largely on the extent of vascular invasion. When there is little or only equivocal vascular invasion, survival following thyroid excision is comparable to that of the control population. With vascular invasion, however, there may be distant metastases to bones and lungs. However, even in these cases, the disease may be remarkably indolent, with a mean life expectancy of six years.

Anaplastic carcinoma of the thyroid, in contrast to the preceding two types of thyroid cancer, is a highly malignant tumor which almost always causes death within a year. It affects older individuals, commonly between the ages of 60 and 80 years.

By the time it is brought to medical attention, the tumor is usually a bulky mass which has ob-

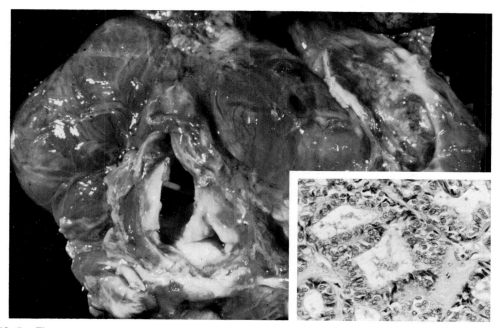

Figure 18–5. The gross appearance of a follicular carcinoma of the thyroid viewed from above. The gray-white tumor tissue has penetrated the capsule to produce the extrathyroidal mass seen on the right. The trachea is compressed and is held open by a prop. The insert on the lower right shows the tumor to be a moderately well differentiated carcinoma.

viously invaded beyond the thyroid capsule. The histologic pattern is totally undifferentiated. Sometimes the cells are small, round and fairly uniform, reminiscent of an undifferentiated sarcoma, while in other instances they are large, highly variable in size and shape, and often multinucleated.

Rapid advance in size, extension beyond the thyroid and widespread metastases, all occurring within one year, are characteristic of this aggressive neoplasm.

The *medullary carcinoma (amyloidic carcinoma)* is relatively uncommon, but it is of great interest on several accounts. *It arises from calcitonin-producing C cells* which lie deep within the lateral lobes of the thyroid. These cells are considered part of the APUD system (see p. 617). They neither take up iodine nor respond to TSH. You will recall that calcitonin tends to lower serum calcium by inhibiting bone resorption, as well as through effects on the kidney and gastrointestinal tract. Whether it plays a significant role in day-to-day calcium homeostasis in man, however, is unknown (Tashjian et al., 1974). Medullary carcinomas may elaborate very large amounts of calcitonin, as well as aberrant hormones, such as ACTH, serotonin and prostaglandins (Schimke et al., 1968). *Morphologically, the characteristic feature of these tumors is the presence of varying amounts of amyloid in the stroma.* This stroma separates sheets of small, round to spindle-shaped cells. It has been suggested that this "amyloid" may differ from that as-

sociated with immune reactions in that it contains or is composed of calcitonin (Tashjian et al., 1974). The generally nonaggressive behavior of these tumors belies their undifferentiated histologic appearance. In the absence of nodal metastases at the time of surgery, five-year survival is similar to that of normal controls. With positive cervical nodes, the 10-year survival rate is 42 per cent. With successful surgery, the serum calcitonin level falls; the reappearance of high levels may indicate recurrent or metastatic disease before any other manifestation appears (Goltzman et al., 1974).

Frequently, this tumor is seen together with pheochromocytomas, sometimes accompanied by cutaneous and mucosal neurofibromatosis and by adenomas or hyperplasia of the parathyroid glands. This concurrence of disorders is termed *multiple endocrine adenomatosis (MEA) II*, and is further discussed on p. 617.

HYPERTHYROIDISM

Hyperthyroidism is a state of hypermetabolism and hyperactivity of the cardiovascular and neuromuscular systems induced by abnormally high levels of circulating L-thyroxine or L-triiodothyronine, or both (Hall, 1970). The most common cause is *Graves' disease (exophthalmic goiter* or *diffuse primary hyperplasia of the thyroid)*, a syndrome characterized by the following three features, although any one patient may not necessarily have all: (1) goiter, caused by diffuse primary hyperplasia, (2) hyperthyroidism, and (3) eye signs, including exophthalmos, lid retraction and ophthalmoplegia (Hall, 1970). Much less frequently, hyperthyroidism, without the full syndrome of Graves' disease, is caused by a functioning (toxic) adenoma or an autonomously functioning focus within a multinodular colloid goiter. *Only very rarely is carcinoma of the thyroid gland associated with hyperfunction.* Excess pituitary secretion of TSH has been demonstrated as a cause of hyperthyroidism only in a few extraordinary cases of pituitary tumors.

Clinical manifestations of hyperthyroidism include elevations of body temperature, heart rate and systolic blood pressure; increased sensitivity to heat, with nearly continuous perspiration; marked irritability and "nervousness," with a fine tremor of the hands; weight loss despite increased appetite; fatigability; and muscle weakness. Sometimes, particularly in older patients, there are cardiac arrhythmias. Whether any of these manifestations is mediated by augmented catecholamine release is unclear (Cohen, 1975). Hyperthyroidism from any cause usually begins insidiously and tends to run a chronic course. However, physical or emotional stress may precipitate an acute crisis, termed "thyroid storm," characterized by extreme hyperpyrexia, delirium, dehydration, gastrointestinal disturbances and, ultimately, vasomotor collapse. Without prompt treatment, death may ensue.

GRAVES' DISEASE

As was mentioned on page 598, *Graves' disease*, like Hashimoto's disease and primary myxedema, is considered to be an autoimmune disorder. It affects females four times as commonly as males, tends to occur in young to middle-aged adults, and has a marked familial pattern (Werner, 1967). Whether these facts are indicative of a genetically determined disturbance of immune tolerance to which females are more vulnerable is speculative. Like Hashimoto's disease and primary myxedema, Graves' disease is characterized by a lymphocytic infiltration of the thyroid gland and the presence in most patients of circulating antibodies to various thyroid antigens. However, a unique feature of Graves' disease is the presence in 80 to 90 per cent of patients of a circulating thyroid stimulating agent known as LATS *(long acting thyroid stimulator).* This agent is an immunoglobulin of the IgG class which evidently acts on the TSH receptor to stimulate adenyl cyclase. It thus enhances the production of cyclic AMP and leads to increased synthesis of the thyroid hormones. It may also act as an antibody to

normal inhibitors of mitosis *(chalones)* within the cytoplasm of thyroid acinar cells. With the removal of normal inhibition of mitosis, the gland would then become both hyperplastic and hyperfunctioning (Garry and Hall, 1970). With the discovery of LATS, it seemed for a while that the etiology of Graves' disease was established. However, it has become increasingly difficult to ascribe either all the cases or all the changes of Graves' disease to this substance. The fundamental difficulty is that even with very sensitive assay techniques, about 20 per cent of patients with Graves' disease cannot be shown to have LATS in their sera. More recently, a second immunoglobulin has been identified in the sera of patients with Graves' disease, which also directly stimulates the thyroid gland (Adams and Kennedy, 1967). Evidently it competitively activates the same receptor as do LATS and TSH. Since it is thus capable of blocking the uptake of LATS, this new substance is known as *LATS-protector* (LATSP). Unlike LATS, LATS-protector is specific to humans. It is probably present in an even larger percentage of patients with Graves' disease than is LATS, and together these two immunoglobulins may account for the disorder in nearly all patients with Graves' disease (Adams et al., 1974). However, as the experience with LATS has demonstrated, we must not embrace such a conclusion without further evidence (Editorial, 1974a).

The pathogenesis of the eye signs is even more obscure. There is no indication that LATS or any of the other known thyroid autoantibodies is responsible for them. Conceivably, an as yet undiscovered antibody to other tissues occurs concurrently in many cases of Graves' disease. Certainly, one of the more distressing aspects of this disease is that treatment of the hyperthyroidism has little if any effect on the eye disorders. Once developed, the latter may have serious consequences. When exophthalmos becomes so severe that the lids cannot close completely, the eyes become vulnerable to trauma and infection, which may even terminate in destruction of the orbit.

The morphologic changes of Graves' disease include those of the thyroid and generalized changes related to the hypermetabolism. **The thyroid is symmetrically but only modestly enlarged** (no more than three times its normal size), up to 90 gm. Histologic changes comprise: (1) an increase in number and height of the acinar cells, causing them to pile up in papillary buds which project into the acini, (2) markedly diminished amounts of colloid, which, when present, is pale and thin, (3) interacinar infiltration by lymphoid tissue, which may form lymphoid follicles, and (4)

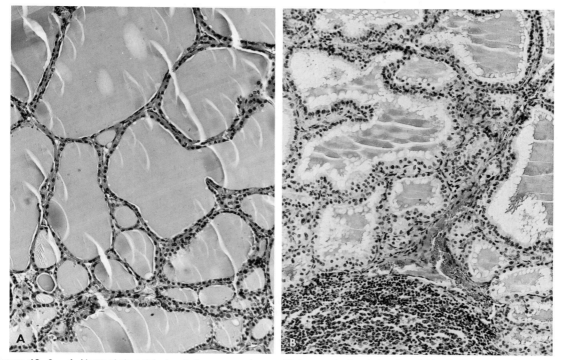

Figure 18–6. *A*, Normal thyroid gland, for comparison with hyperplasia of the thyroid in *B*. Note the resorption of colloid, producing the peripheral scalloping, and the lymphoid aggregate below.

increased vascularity of the gland (Fig. 18–6). Generalized lymphoid hyperplasia is seen throughout the body. Nonspecific degenerative changes may occur in the skeletal muscle, heart muscle and liver. Heart failure may be the cause of death in "thyroid storm." It should be remembered that the thyroid gland in most cases of Graves' disease is seen only after some form of preoperative medication has been given. This alters the histology of the gland in ways dependent on the medication. For example, iodine promotes colloid storage, devascularization and involution of the gland, while thiouracil tends to produce even more marked hyperplasia.

HYPOTHYROIDISM

This term refers to the hypometabolic, depressed state caused by a deficiency of one or both thyroid hormones. When severe and associated with generalized interstitial edema, it is known as *myxedema*. Causes include: (1) Hashimoto's disease, (2) iodine deficiency or inborn metabolic errors in its utilization, too severe to be compensated for by goiter formation, (3) pituitary insufficiency, and (4) surgical or chemical ablation of the thyroid in the treatment of Graves' disease.

MYXEDEMA

Hypothyroidism in the adult most often occurs as a variant or end-result of Hashi-

moto's disease (see p. 598). Usually the functional impairment is mild and even asymptomatic. Fully developed myxedema, however, produces a striking clinical picture, characterized by: (1) markedly slowed mentation, speech and movement, (2) deepened voice, (3) thick, dry, pale-yellow skin (color reflects carotenemia) and coarse, sparse hair, (4) thickened tongue, (5) generalized interstitial edema rich in proteins and mucopolysaccharides (the basis for the term *myxedema*), (6) intolerance to cold, and (7) fatigability and weakness. Sometimes there is massive pericardial and pleural effusion. The heart may show nonspecific degenerative changes and dilatation without hypertrophy (Hall and Nelson, 1968). These patients become hypercholesterolemic and show an accelerated development of atherosclerosis. Severe myxedema tends to occur in an older age group, often in the sixth decade. Although the female preponderance seen among patients with most thyroid diseases is present, it is less striking, with a female-male ratio of about 5:1. Circulating thyroid autoantibodies are present in about 98 per cent of patients whose disease is of recent onset and in 70 to 80 per cent of those with long-standing myxedema.

The histology has some resemblance to that of Hashimoto's disease (see p. 599), except for the lack of goiter formation and the prominence of such atrophic changes as flattening of the acinar epithelium and compression of the acini by fibrous tissue. The lymphocytic infiltrate of Hashimoto's disease becomes less prominent with progression to end-stage myxedema. In advanced stages, there may be virtually total fibrous replacement of the acini.

When the cause of hypothyroidism is pituitary insufficiency, the thyroid becomes involuted and atrophic. The histology may be indistinguishable from that of severe myxedema, but lymphocytes usually are not present.

CRETINISM

When severe hypothyroidism is present from birth, the syndrome, termed *cretinism*, is dramatic. These children become dwarfed, with ossification, epiphyseal union and dentition all being markedly delayed. Their tongues are enlarged and their abdomens protuberant. More important, if the condition is not treated promptly, the children suffer irreversible mental retardation. Although the principal cause of cretinism was once maternal iodine deficiency, congenital errors in thyroxine (and triiodothyronine) synthesis and release are becoming relatively more important as severe dietary deficiencies of iodine become less common.

ADRENAL CORTEX

Lesions of the adrenal cortex are usually expressed by hyperfunction or hypofunction of the gland. Exceptions to this rule include the nonfunctioning tumors which, when benign, tend to remain altogether asymptomatic and, when malignant, first manifest themselves late in their course by metastases or by the presence of a palpable mass. Endocrino-

logically functioning tumors, although they are less frequent than nonfunctioning neoplasms, are of greater clinical interest, and tumors in general will therefore be considered in the section dealing with adrenal hypercorticism.

HYPERCORTICISM

While a large number of steroids are elaborated by the adrenal cortex, only four are secreted in amounts sufficient to be of physiologic importance: the *glucocorticoids*, hydrocortisone (cortisol) and corticosterone; the *mineralocorticoid*, aldosterone; and the *androgenic steroid*, dehydroepiandrosterone (Ganong, 1965). *Hypercorticism usually involves the excess elaboration of only one of these three types of corticosteroids, and the resultant clinical syndrome varies accordingly.*

THE ADRENOGENITAL SYNDROME

This term refers to virilism resulting from secretion by the adrenal gland of abnormally large amounts of the androgenic steroids, particularly dehydroepiandrosterone. Usually, particularly in children, it is caused by a congenital deficiency of one of the enzymes necessary for the synthesis of the glucocorticoids and mineralocorticoids. Precursors then accumulate and are shunted through the unblocked pathways toward the synthesis of the androgenic steroids. *Moreover, since the glucocorticoids are required for negative feedback on the pituitary secretion of ACTH, their deficient synthesis leads to oversecretion of ACTH, with consequent hyperplasia of the adrenal.* The result, then, is excessive production of the androgenic steroids by default (Fig. 18–7). When the adrenogenital syndrome arises in adults, it is

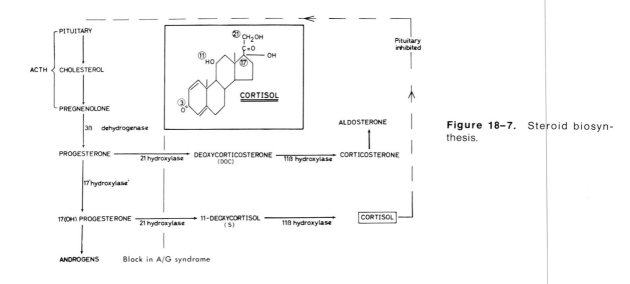

Figure 18-7. Steroid biosynthesis.

most often the result of an adrenal adenoma or carcinoma.

In children enzyme deficiencies are of principal importance in producing the adrenogenital syndrome. The most common is a more or less incomplete *deficiency of 21β-hydroxylase*. This biochemical defect is inherited as an autosomal recessive trait. Because of the incompleteness of the block, enough glucocorticoids and mineralocorticoids are synthesized to sustain life. In about one third of these cases, however, there is excessive *salt-wasting* as a result of the very low levels of aldosterone.

Less commonly, the adrenogenital syndrome is caused by *11β-hydroxylase deficiency*. Because this block occurs farther along the synthetic pathway, it permits the formation of excess amounts of a precursor of aldosterone called 11-deoxycorticosterone, which itself is an active mineralocorticoid. Hence, patients with this form of the adrenogenital syndrome show salt and water retention, with resultant *hypertension*.

A rapidly fatal, and fortunately rare, form of the adrenogenital syndrome is caused by a complete *deficiency of 3β-dehydrogenase*. No glucocorticoids or mineralocorticoids are formed, and death occurs in early infancy.

Virilism resulting from adrenocortical enzyme deficiencies usually becomes manifest in infancy or childhood, but mild cases may not be apparent until after puberty. When the adrenogenital syndrome is associated with a tumor, there are presumably enzyme deficiencies within functioning tumor cells.

Virilism in the female infant may take the form of *pseudohermaphroditism*, with a phalloid organ as well as uterus and ovaries. In older females, milder cases may appear as variable enlargement of the clitoris, with the later development of hirsutism, a male escutcheon, receding hairline and atrophy of the breasts. In the male child, the changes are not so striking. They consist chiefly of *macrogenitosomia* and sexual precocity, and may go unnoted unless the salt-losing or hypertensive features bring the syndrome to attention.

The **hyperplastic gland** most commonly associated with the adrenogenital syndrome varies in weight from about 2 to 12 gm. in the newborn up to about 30 gm. in the adult. Because of the rapid synthesis and turnover of the steroids, there is very little stored lipid within the cells, and the parenchyma consequently loses its yellowish color and becomes brown. Histologically, adrenal hyperplasia is characterized by the transformation of the clear cells of the zona fasciculata into compact cells indistinguishable from those of the zona reticularis. This transformation is presumed to result from the depletion of stored lipids in the hyperac-

tive cells. Sometimes a thin layer of clear cells remains just under the abnormally broad zona glomerulosa.

Those **benign adenomas** which cause the adrenogenital syndrome vary from small nodules of 10 gm. to bulky masses of 200 gm. All are well encapsulated. On sectioning, they are fleshy and red-brown. Their microscopic appearance is often similar to that of the normal zona reticularis, with compact cells arranged in alveoli. Occasionally, there are focal areas of clear cells.

Malignant tumors producing the adrenogenital syndrome are usually large carcinomas, which may weigh as much as 4000 gm. On sectioning, they are seen to consist of brown, friable tissue which, in accordance with their bulk, contains areas of necrosis and hemorrhage. The histologic pattern is variable. Usually the cells are compact, with ovoid vesicular nuclei, and are arranged in solid sheets around dilated vascular spaces lined with flattened epithelium. This picture may be modified by extreme degrees of anaplasia and the presence of large numbers of giant cells. Extension beyond the adrenal capsule, invasion of the kidney, metastasis to the opposite adrenal or widespread dissemination may occur with the more aggressive tumors. Adrenal cortical carcinoma, unfortunately, is usually discovered late in its course, and the five-year survival rate is only about 12 per cent.

It should be emphasized that there is very little correlation between the morphology of adrenal tumors, whether benign or malignant, and their function. When active, some or any constituents of the three groups of steroids may be produced. Thus, the morphologic description given applies to adrenal tumors in general and not just to those associated with virilism.

CUSHING'S SYNDROME

This clinical syndrome results from hypersecretion of the glucocorticoids. When fully developed, its components include: central obesity, with wasting of the distal limbs, moon facies, hypertension, hypokalemia, diabetes mellitus, osteoporosis, muscle weakness, acne, hirsutism and mental disturbances ranging from depression to euphoria to psychosis.

Cushing's syndrome may be caused either by adrenal tumors or, more often, by hypersecretion of ACTH. Both forms are most common between the ages of 20 and 40 years, and both affect females four times as often as males. The adrenal tumors are especially frequent during or just following pregnancy. Morphologic examination of the adrenals in a series of cases has shown functioning adrenal tumors in 30 per cent, bilateral adrenal hyperplasia in 60 per cent, and no evident pathology in the remaining 10 per cent (Forsham, 1968). The underlying causes can be further broken down as follows:

1. *Functioning adrenal tumor (primary Cushing's syndrome) — 30 per cent*
   a. Benign — over 15 per cent
   b. Malignant — less than 15 per cent
2. *Bilateral adrenal hyperplasia or hyperfunction (secondary Cushing's syndrome) — 60 per cent*
   a. Ectopic (nonpituitary) ACTH-secreting tumor — over 30 per cent
   b. Pituitary hypersecretion of ACTH — less than 30 per cent

Not included in this breakdown are the increasingly frequent instances of iatrogenic Cushing's syndrome in patients on long-term corticosteroid therapy.

Morphologically, adrenal tumors which produce Cushing's syndrome are not significantly different from those associated with the adrenogenital syndrome (Fig. 18–8). Perhaps the adenomas associated with Cushing's syndrome tend to be yellower, owing to larger numbers of lipid-laden cells scattered throughout the background of the predominantly compact cells. Secretion of glucocorticoids by these tumors, especially the malignant ones, is more or less independent of ACTH levels. Indeed, the high levels of circulating hydrocortisone suppress pituitary ACTH secretion, with consequent atrophy of the remaining normal adrenal tissue.

Only recently has it been appreciated that the most common single cause of Cushing's syndrome is ectopic secretion of ACTH by cancers of nonendocrine origin (Forsham, 1968). In about two thirds of these cases, the causative cancer is an oat-cell carcinoma of the lung. However, virtually every organ in the body has been known to give rise to ACTH-secreting tumors. Although ectopic ACTH-secreting tumors are being recognized with ever increasing frequency, it is probable that their incidence is still considerably underestimated. Examination of a series of 78 unselected visceral tumors showed that 6 (8 per cent) produced ACTH. The clinical diagnosis of Cushing's syndrome from this cause is, however, difficult. The cachexia of cancer and the short duration of the glucocorticoid excess in these often moribund patients tend to mask the features of Cushing's syndrome.

The original case of Cushing's syndrome described by Cushing was caused by pituitary hypersecretion of ACTH. Therefore, this form of the disorder is often designated "Cushing's *disease*." Although it was once thought that all patients with this disorder had basophilic pituitary tumors, it is now clear that perhaps no more than 10 per cent of cases of Cushing's syndrome are caused by pituitary tumors (Russfield, 1968). However, this issue remains controversial. It has been pointed out that pituitary tumors too small to be discernible on x-ray studies have subsequently been demonstrated on autopsy (Lagerquist et al., 1974). Among those discovered clinically, about half are small basophil tumors; the remainder are the larger chromophobe tumors having basophilic function. Although these lesions are usually benign adenomas, both types of lesions are malignant in about 25 per cent of cases. The pituitary tumors were described in the section on the hypophysis (p. 595).

The remainder, perhaps most, of those cases of Cushing's syndrome associated with pituitary hypersecretion of ACTH are of mysterious origin. There is no evidence of a pituitary tumor. It has been suggested that the "tumor" is actually a microscopic focus of autonomously functioning basophils, but this explanation is not entirely satisfactory. Alternatively, it has been postulated that the primary derangement is an increased elaboration of corticotropin-releasing factor (CRF) from the hypothalamus. However, this postulation leaves unexplained the basis for such a hypothalamic derangement.

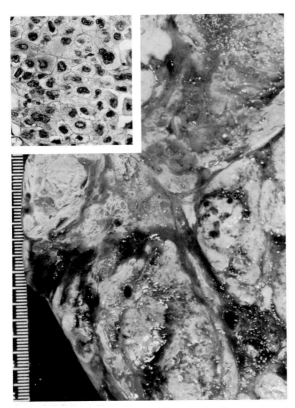

Figure 18–8. The transected surface of an adrenal carcinoma, showing obvious areas of necrosis and hemorrhage. The insert at upper left reveals some anaplasia, but there is still some resemblance to adrenal cortical cells.

Of interest in evaluating these theories is the recently appreciated finding that approximately 10 to 15 per cent of patients who undergo bilateral adrenalectomy for Cushing's syndrome later develop a clinically apparent, functioning pituitary tumor. These are diagnosed an average of three years after the hyperplastic adrenals have been removed. Whether the pituitary tumors result from the stimulation of a preexisting microscopic tumor by removal of the exaggerated feedback controls, or whether they represent the development of a new lesion, is unclear.

Regardless of ultimate cause, the result of either ectopic or pituitary hypersecretion of ACTH is bilateral hyperplasia of the adrenal glands. Although some degree of enlargement of these glands is usually grossly visible, it is in general not so marked as with the adrenogenital syndrome. Occasionally the adrenals appear grossly normal. Histologically, there is a prominent zona reticularis, which occupies the entire inner half of the cortex and extends in irregular tongues into a likewise thickened zona fasciculata. Sometimes there are fields of abnormally hypertrophied lipid laden or vacuolated cells, alternating with fields of apparently normal cortex. Some variation in nuclear size and shape may be present. Often the normal reticular pattern of the zona reticularis is lost. Typically the basophils in the pituitary undergo degeneration termed "Crooke's hyaline change."

While this text is not primarily concerned with clinical diagnosis, it might be of help in better understanding the causes of Cushing's syndrome to mention briefly the methods of diagnosis. Once it has been established that the patient indeed has pathologically elevated levels of circulating glucocorticoids (hence that he has Cushing's syndrome), usually an attempt is made to suppress adrenal function with moderately large doses of dexamethasone. This acts by inhibiting pituitary release of ACTH. If such suppression can be achieved, the diagnosis is likely to be pituitary hypersecretion of ACTH (Cushing's *disease*). If there is no suppression, then the diagnosis is either a primary tumor of the adrenal gland or an ectopic ACTH-secreting tumor. Determination of plasma ACTH will yield abnormally low levels in the former case and markedly elevated levels in the latter, as shown in the chart below.

PRIMARY HYPERALDOSTERONISM (CONN'S SYNDROME)

Primary hypersecretion of aldosterone is usually caused by a benign adrenal tumor. It leads to moderate *hypertension* and a constellation of findings attributable to *hypokalemia*, including polyuria (*hypokalemic nephropathy*), episodic muscle weakness and metabolic alkalosis, with a consequent drop in ionized calcium and a tendency toward tetany and paresthesias. Although there is some increase in extracellular fluid volume, overt edema is rare.

In contrast to the other corticosteroids, aldosterone release is not regulated solely by ACTH secretion. More important as control factors are the renin-angiotensin system (which responds to changes in position, extracellular fluid volume and osmolarity) and hyperkalemia, which probably has a direct stimulatory effect. It should not be surprising, then, that hyperaldosteronism may occur *secondary* to a number of disorders characterized by hemodynamic derangements, such as congestive heart failure, cirrhosis and other edematous states, as well as with intrinsic renal disease. *Primary hyperaldosteronism or Conn's syndrome, however, is usually caused by a benign adrenal tumor with or without accompanying cortical hyperplasia.* In a small minority of cases, it is caused by bilateral nodular hyperplasia of the zona glomerulosa, and only rarely by a malignant tumor (Forsham, 1968). *In contrast to secondary hyperaldosteronism, the primary disorder is associated with low levels of circulating renin.*

The incidence of primary hyperaldosteronism is controversial. Certainly aldosterone-secreting tumors are the most common of the functioning adrenal neoplasms. Perhaps as many as 4 per cent of individuals with hypertension harbor these tumors. The disorder is most common between the ages of 30 and 50 years, and affects women twice as often as men.

Although aldosterone-secreting adenomas may be multiple, they occur as single lesions in 90 per cent of cases. They appear as small, well encapsulated, yellow nodules, usually less than 3 cm. in diameter. Microscopically, the cells vary from large, lipid laden, clear cells similar to those of the zona fasciculata to smaller, darker cells characteristic of

Cause of Cushing's Syndrome	ACTH Levels	Dexamethasone Suppression
Pituitary hypersecretion of ACTH	High	Yes
Adrenal tumor	Low	No
Ectopic ACTH-secreting tumor	High	No

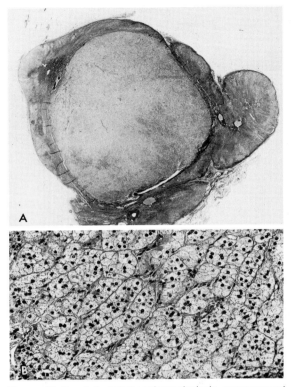

Figure 18–9. *A,* A slightly enlarged whole-organ mount of a section of an adrenal bearing an adenoma. The tumor has expanded into the medulla and is enclosed within a rim of adrenal cortex. The arrangement of the lipid laden cortical cells in nests is seen below in *B.*

the zona glomerulosa (Fig. 18–9). Most tumors contain a mixture of these cell types, although some may be composed exclusively of the glomerulosa type cell. Cellular arrangement tends to be in nests similar to those of the zona glomerulosa. Despite the appearance of the clear cells, histochemical studies have shown that they are capable of secreting aldosterone as well as corticosterone and hydrocortisone.

HYPOCORTICISM

Disorders which cause adrenal corticosteroid insufficiency are usually primary to the adrenal gland. Less frequently, hypocorticism is a part of panhypopituitarism, which was discussed in an earlier section, or it is caused by secondary involvement of the adrenal by disease that is primary elsewhere. Primary hypocorticism may appear insidiously and run a chronic course, or it may develop as a fulminant medical crisis.

CHRONIC PRIMARY HYPOCORTICISM (ADDISON'S DISEASE)

Clinically overt Addison's disease is uncommon, although it is likely that many undiagnosed borderline cases exist. Because of the

large functional reserve of the adrenal cortex, about 90 per cent of the parenchyma must be destroyed in order to produce symptoms of insufficiency. Most cases are seen in individuals between the ages of 20 and 50 years. Whereas in 1930 tuberculous destruction of the adrenal cortices was the cause of 70 per cent of Addison's disease, this lesion is now thought to cause less than 25 per cent of such cases. *Currently, most cases of Addison's disease are called idiopathic, but the condition may be an autoimmune disorder.* Less frequent causes include the deep fungi, amyloidosis and replacement of the adrenals by primary nonfunctioning tumors. Although metastatic disease to the adrenal glands is common, Addison's disease from this cause is relatively rare. Possibly the diagnosis tends to be overlooked in these cases because indications of adrenal insufficiency may be similar to those of widespread metastatic disease (Eisenstein, 1968).

Evidence for the autoimmune nature of *idiopathic Addison's disease* includes the following observations:

1. This disease is histologically similar to the "autoimmune" thyroid diseases (Hashimoto's thyroiditis, primary myxedema and Graves' disease), characterized by atrophy with a lymphocytic infiltrate.

2. From 50 to 67 per cent of these patients have circulating autoantibodies specific to adrenal tissue (Wuepper et al., 1969).

3. Other autoantibodies, especially against the thyroid gland and the gastric mucosa, are often present in these patients. Indeed, concurrent Addison's disease and Hashimoto's thyroiditis *(Schmidt's syndrome)* develop with more than chance frequency.

4. Lesions similar to those of idiopathic Addison's disease can be produced experimentally by injecting autologous adrenal tissue and Freund's adjuvant.

Morphologically, idiopathic Addison's disease results in small, irregularly contracted adrenal glands, with a combined weight as low as 2.5 gm. On sectioning, it can be seen that the cortex has collapsed around an otherwise normal medulla. The histology is of atrophy and destruction of the adrenal cells, with replacement by fibrous scarring. The few remaining viable cortical cells may be enlarged with an eosinophilic, lipid-poor cytoplasm (compact cells). A variable lymphocytic infiltrate is present.

Tuberculous adrenal glands, on the other hand, are enlarged, firm and nodular, with a thickened capsule. The histology is characteristic of tuberculosis in any site, with confluent areas of caseation necrosis and tubercle formation. Addison's disease caused by amyloidosis is also associated with enlargement of the adrenal glands, sometimes with a combined weight up to 40 gm. Grossly, these glands are firm and pale gray. On microscopic examination, it can be seen that most of the cortex is replaced by amyloid deposits.

An increasingly frequent cause of hypocorticism is chronic glucocorticoid therapy for some other disorder. This exerts a negative feedback effect on the hypothalamic-pituitary secretion of ACTH, leading to atrophy of the adrenal glands. Stress (as from surgery, trauma or infection) or sudden withdrawal of the medication then unmasks the adrenal insufficiency. Since such iatrogenic adrenal insufficiency usually manifests itself acutely, it is more fully described in the next section.

Addison's disease from any cause presents an insidious, rather ill defined clinical picture. The first indications are often a vague weakness and fatigability. *As the negative feedback on the hypothalamic-pituitary axis is abolished, ACTH (and perhaps MSH) levels rise, with a consequent increase in pigmentation of the skin, particularly of the mucous membranes, areolae and any surgical scars.* Most patients develop gastrointestinal disturbances, including anorexia with weight loss, nausea, vomiting and diarrhea. Blood sugar is low, and hypoglycemic symptoms may occasionally occur. Although some degree of hypotension is characteristic, actual syncope is uncommon. The heart becomes smaller, possibly because of its lightened work load as a result of chronic hypovolemia and hypotension.

Although patients with Addison's disease may continue indefinitely in their subactive precarious existence, any stress, such as surgery, infection or injury, may precipitate an acute crisis, characterized by a lag of about 12 hours, after which sudden, profound weakness, hyperpyrexia progressing to hypothermia, coma and vascular collapse occur. Without prompt therapy, death ensues.

ACUTE HYPOCORTICISM

Acute adrenal corticosteroid insufficiency may be caused by: (1) hemorrhagic destruc-

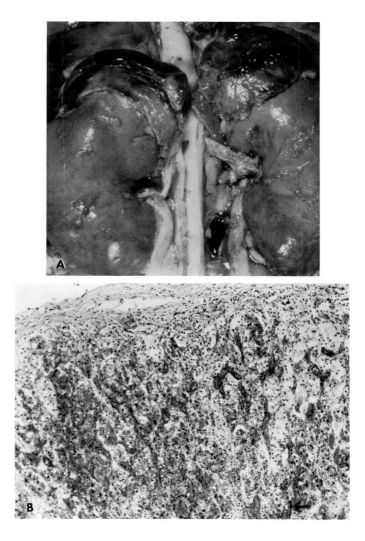

Figure 18–10. *A,* The kidneys and adrenals in situ in a child with the Waterhouse-Friderichsen syndrome. The dark adrenals are markedly hemorrhagic. *B,* Low power section. The cortical cells between the extravasated blood have undergone ischemic necrosis.

tion of the adrenal glands, including the Waterhouse-Friderichsen syndrome and hemorrhage due to local trauma, (2) adrenal vein thrombosis, (3) withdrawal of long-term steroid therapy (iatrogenic adrenal insufficiency), (4) stress in patients with Addison's disease (see previous discussion), and (5) in the neonate, congenital adrenal hypoplasia or lethal enzyme deficiencies in the synthesis of corticosteroids.

The *Waterhouse-Friderichsen syndrome* is classically produced by meningococcemia, although fulminant septicemia from other organisms, such as the pneumococci and hemolytic streptococci, may also be causative. These patients exhibit irritability, headache, abdominal pain, hyperpyrexia, with the later development of coma, hypothermia and vascular collapse. Often, however, the overwhelming infection causes death before indications of adrenal insufficiency ensue. *Characteristically, patients with the Waterhouse-Friderichsen syndrome develop widespread petechiae and purpura, as well as other manifestations of an underlying generalized bleeding diathesis.* Whether this bleeding tendency is based on direct or toxic damage to the vascular walls or, rather, represents a Shwartzman-type phenomenon is not clear. There is increasing evidence that it represents a form of disseminated intravascular coagulation (DIC) (see p. 363).

In any case, the adrenal gland shows hemorrhagic destruction, sometimes, but not invariably, with concomitant patchy thromboses. The hemorrhage begins in the zona reticularis and may remain localized to this area, compressing the medulla. Often the hemorrhage appears to have originated in the medulla. With peripheral extension, the hemorrhage treks outward toward the capsule, between the cords of the zona fasciculata, then spreads under the capsule. Lipid depletion and hemorrhagic necrosis of the cells are present (Fig. 18–10).

Similar morphologic changes are caused by hemorrhage resulting from trauma. Sometimes the trauma causes adrenal hemorrhage by inducing first adrenal vein thrombosis.

This mysterious vascular calamity is the most common cause of non-iatrogenic acute hypocorticism in adults (Forsham, 1968).

As mentioned, pharmacologic doses of corticosteroids suppress the hypothalamic-pituitary secretion of ACTH, with resultant *atrophy* of the adrenal glands.

The morphologic appearance is characteristic and is quite distinct from that of idiopathic Addison's disease. Although in both cases the glands are shrunken, iatrogenic hypocorticism is associated with lipid laden rather than lipid depleted glands. (It should be pointed out that the same picture is seen with primary pituitary hypofunction.)

When corticosteroid therapy is gradually discontinued, recovery of normal function is possible in most cases. In some patients, however, recovery is only partial, and stress may precipitate an acute adrenal crisis similar to that described with Addison's disease. Although these patients may show relatively little vascular collapse because of the preservation of aldosterone secretion, weakness, hyperpyrexia, nausea and vomiting may be extreme.

ADRENAL MEDULLA

The only significant disorders of the adrenal medulla are two tumors, the pheochromocytoma and the neuroblastoma.

PHEOCHROMOCYTOMA

This is a functioning, usually benign tumor composed of pheochromocytes, the cells which normally make up the adrenal medulla. It occurs chiefly in two age groups—in children and in adults between the ages of 30 and 50 years. Pheochromocytomas may occur sporadically or as a familial lesion, inherited through a dominant gene with a high degree of penetrance. In the latter case, they may occur concurrently with medullary carcinoma of the thyroid, sometimes along with multiple neurofibromatosis and hyperplasia or adenomas of the parathyroid glands. As mentioned in our discussion of medullary carcinoma of the thyroid, this constellation of lesions is known as *multiple endocrine adenomatosis (MEA) II.* It will be described more fully on page 617. Here we shall briefly mention the recent speculation that these lesions, along with carcinoid tumors, involve some widespread derangement in the so-called APUD system. This system refers to cells derived from neuroectoderm which ultimately migrate to various endocrine glands and the gastrointestinal tract. They have in common the capacity to take up and decarboxylate certain biogenic amines, hence the term APUD (*A*mine *P*recursor *U*ptake and *D*ecarboxylation). Certainly this hypothesis does much to explain the existence of multiple endocrinopathies (Pearse, 1969).

About 93 per cent of pheochromocytomas are located in the adrenal medulla; the remainder are usually found lying along the abdominal aorta, where collections of pheochromocytes may remain from their fetal wanderings. Although most pheochromocytomas are unilateral, about 9 per cent are bilateral. The bilateral tumors tend to be familial.

Pheochromocytomas vary markedly in size, ranging from 1 to 4000 gm., but averaging about 100 gm. Often remnants of the normal adrenal gland can be seen stretched over the surface or attached at one pole of the tumor. The cut surface is pale gray to brown, often with foci of necrosis and hemorrhage. Fibrous ingrowths from the capsule create a lobulated appearance. Microscopically, the tumors are composed of mature but pleomorphic pheochromocytes, i.e., large cells with central, single or sometimes double nuclei and abundant faint, granular, basophilic cytoplasm, in which granules can be demonstrated by the use of chrome salts (Fig. 18–11). The arrangements of these cells is variable. Sometimes they are arrayed in large trabeculae abutting on thin-walled sinusoids; in other instances, they may form small nests separated by fibrous trabeculae. Both patterns may be present in the same tumor. Cellular and nuclear pleomorphism is often noted, and giant and bizarre cells may be seen, even in clinically innocent lesions. About 10 per cent of pheochromocytomas are malignant. Differentiation of benign and malignant forms is extremely difficult on histologic grounds. Perhaps the only certain, if grim, criterion is the presence of metastases.

The clinical features of pheochromocy-tomas result from their elaboration of large amounts of catecholamines. In contrast to the normal tissue of the adrenal medulla, the tumors release predominantly norepinephrine. *Hypertension, either paroxysmal or sustained, is the classical presenting feature.* In addition, there are other indications of sympathetic overactivity, such as sweating, nervousness, pallor and tachycardia. Diagnosis depends primarily on the presence in the urine of high levels of catecholamines and their metabolites.

NEUROBLASTOMA

This highly malignant tumor is the fourth most common cause of death from cancer in children under the age of 15 years (Miller, 1969). Most neuroblastomas are found in the adrenal medulla, but a significant number arise in the cervical, thoracic and lower abdominal sympathetic chain. When these tumors develop in the retina, they are called *retinoblastomas.* Usually, neuroblastomas become apparent before the age of three years, and they affect males more often than females.

These tumors commonly weigh between 80 and 150 gm., and are lobular and soft, with a grayish cut surface. Often, areas of necrosis, hemorrhage and calcification are apparent. Histologically, the malignant cells are small and dark, resembling endothelial cells or lymphocytes, and tend to grow in haphazard masses. Careful searching near the periphery of the tumor, however, usually reveals the cells arranged in characteristic rosette formations, with the cells forming a glandlike pattern about young nerve fibrils growing into the center of each rosette.

Rapidly developing, widespread metastases, particularly to bone, are typical. Since these tumors secrete catecholamines, the combination, in a young child, of elevated urinary catecholamines and x-ray evidence of multiple bone metastases is virtually diagnostic (Editorial, 1975). Rarely, neuroblastomas undergo spontaneous maturation to the benign tumor called a *ganglioneuroma,* as was cited earlier (p. 109). Immune mechanisms may be responsible for such differentiation. With the rare exception of such happy transformations, the prognosis is poor. Children under the age of one year or those without bone metastases have a much better chance for survival (about a 60 per cent cure rate) (Putnam and Miller, 1970–71).

THE PARATHYROIDS

The pathology of the parathyroids may be divided into considerations of hyperfunction and hypofunction.

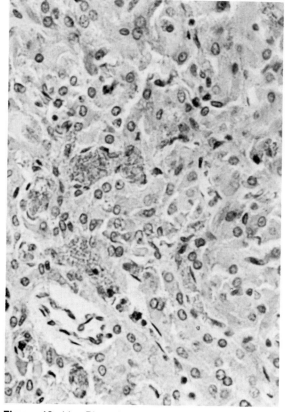

Figure 18–11. Pheochromocytoma. The plump neoplastic pheochromocytes have an abundant granular cytoplasm and small quite regular nuclei. Note the vascularity of the neoplasm.

HYPERPARATHYROIDISM

Hyperparathyroidism is defined as a sustained elevation in the secretion of parathyroid hormone (*parathormone* or *PTH*). As will be apparent, the condition may be associated with hypercalcemia, normocalcemia or even with hypocalcemia. In recent years our understanding of hyperparathyroidism has advanced rapidly. Widespread screening for hypercalcemia in hospital populations has contributed to this advance, as has the discovery that there is more than one immunoreactive form of PTH discernible by radioimmunoassay (Arnaud, 1973). Hyperparathyroidism is classified as primary when some parathyroid disorder produces hypercalcemia, or as secondary when hypocalcemia from any cause leads to a compensatory hyperfunction of the parathyroids. Yet another step removed in this chain of causation is a category of hyperparathyroidism sometimes termed "tertiary." This refers to the development of autonomous function or an adenoma in the hyperplastic parathyroid glands of secondary hyperparathyroidism. "Overcompensation" with hypercalcemia then ensues. Although some object to the rather grandiose and perhaps confusing term "tertiary," the concept remains valid. It has even been suggested that most cases of apparently primary hyperparathyroidism are in fact tertiary, that is, they were initiated by some unappreciated chronic stimulus to PTH secretion (Reiss and Canterbury, 1974).

PRIMARY HYPERPARATHYROIDISM

The causes of this disorder and their approximate frequencies are as follows:

	Per Cent
1. Single adenoma	80
2. Multiple adenomas	5
3. Multiple endocrine adenomatosis	5
4. Primary hyperplasia	9
5. Carcinoma	1

Not included in this analysis are the increasing number of cases of "hyperparathyroidism" based on cancer of nonendocrine tissue. Until recently it was thought that the hypercalcemia which occasionally accompanies cancer was caused by bone metastases. However, the discovery of several immunoreactive forms of active PTH has made it apparent that many, if not most, of these tumors elaborate ectopic PTH (Benson et al., 1974). Most often ectopic PTH-secreting tumors are oat-cell carcinomas of the lung or renal cell carcinomas.

Adenomas occur at all ages, with a slight male preponderance in the ratio of 1.5:1.0.

The lower glands are involved in about 75 per cent of cases. The usual adenoma appears grossly as a small, yellow-brown, soft, somewhat lobular mass, ranging in weight between 250 mg. and 5 gm. This soft yellowish tissue is usually readily distinguished from the firm red-brown substance of the thyroid. Sometimes these adenomas are found in aberrant locations within the neck or thorax, much to the distress of the surgeon. Histologically, all adenomas display a mixture of the three principal parathyroid cell types, with many transitional forms. The most common variant is composed principally of chief cells, but many wasserhelle ("clear as water") and oxyphil cells are also present. Others may comprise predominantly wasserhelle cells; rarely is the oxyphil the dominant cell. The cells commonly are arrayed in solid sheets, but occasionally they may produce cords, glandlike patterns or nodules separated by fibrous bands. **Adenomas may be extremely difficult to differentiate from foci of hyperplasia.** Of help in this regard is the greater likelihood that some variation in cell and nuclear size and shape will occur with the adenomas. Moreover, often a fragile capsule encloses the adenoma, outside of which the more normal residual parathyroid substance is visible.

Multiple adenomas may affect any or all of the parathyroid glands. A case has been reported of single adenomas in each of four parathyroid glands, all of differing cell types (Rubens et al., 1969).

Parathyroid hyperfunction is often a component of both forms of *multiple endocrine adenomatosis (MEA I and MEA II)*. These multiglandular derangements are discussed on page 617.

While *diffuse hyperplasia* of the parathyroids usually occurs secondary to hypocalcemia, it in some cases apparently develops as a primary disorder. *Nevertheless, the diagnosis of primary hyperplasia should not be made until the secondary form is ruled out.* Whether the cases of primary hyperplasia instead actually represent tertiary hyperparathyroidism is controversial. It has been suggested that conditions such as idiopathic hypercalciuria, a relatively common dysfunction, might present a continuing stimulus to PTH-secretion that eventually leads to autonomous and inappropriate hyperfunction of the parathyroid glands (Reiss and Canterbury, 1974).

There is considerable variation in the weight of hyperplastic parathyroids, even within the same patient. One gland may weigh as little as 100 mg. (normal weight is about 30 mg.), while another weighs as much as 20 gm. Irregular lobulation and pseudopod formations are sometimes present. Histologically, the principal cell is usually of the wasserhelle variety, but chief cells may predominate (Fig. 18–12). The cells are quite uniform in size. Occasionally foci of cystic necrosis simulate a glandular pattern. The normal fat content of the parathyroid is reduced.

Carcinoma of the parathyroids is uncommon. It is generally accepted that the diagnosis requires the demonstration of parathyroid hyperfunction, since nonfunctioning carcinomas of the parathyroid glands are so readily confused with some tumors arising in the thyroid. Moreover, because of the difficulty in distinguishing between the pleomorphism of some parathyroid adenomas and the minimal anaplasia of some carcinomas, it is further required that one of the following three features be present: (1) metastases, (2) capsular invasion, or (3) local recurrence following resection.

Most parathyroid carcinomas described have

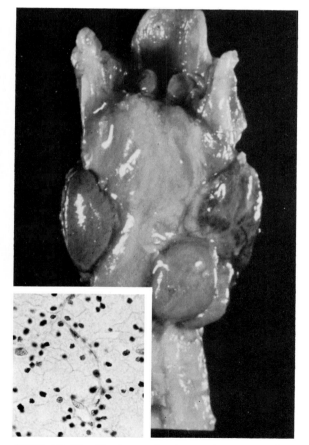

Figure 18–12. The larynx, trachea and upper esophagus viewed from the back. Two prominently enlarged parathyroids are readily evident, and a third is visible just anterior to the one on the lower right. The dark mass (upper right) is a portion of the thyroid lobe. Classical wasserhelle cells are seen in the insert.

been quite small, some even less than 1 gm. in weight. They tend to be irregular in shape and show lobulation and pseudopod formation, sometimes with adherence to surrounding structures. They are usually considerably more firm than adenomas. Most commonly, they consist of cords of cells in a trabecular arrangement, although some have gland patterns and others are composed of sheets of cells. **Hyperchromatism, pleomorphism and variation in nuclear size are all present, but not necessarily to a more marked degree than in some adenomas.** When these lesions metastasize, they usually affect only the regional nodes. Distant spread is uncommon, and death is more likely to result from the complications of hyperparathyroidism than from metastatic disease.

Clinically, the picture of primary hyperparathyroidism, whatever the underlying cause, is remarkably variable and often bizarre. Usually the condition is asymptomatic and is discovered only when hypercalcemia is found in routine laboratory testing. In one large series, primary hyperparathyroidism was found in 1 of every 834 patients screened, and 73 per cent of patients so discovered were asymptomatic (Keating, 1970). When symptoms do occur, they are usually related to the increased bone resorption and increased renal calcium resorption associated with excess PTH. Thus, a variety of bony changes may occur, including osteomalacia (see p. 251) and, in some cases, a lesion known as *osteitis fibrosa cystica*, which will be discussed below. Subperiosteal resorption of bone in the phalanges and distal clavicles, and loss of the lamina dura about the teeth are characteristic x-ray signs. *Osteitis fibrosa cystica generalista, also known as von Recklinghausen's disease of bone, develops in advanced hyperparathyroidism, whether primary or secondary, although it tends to be more severe with the primary form.* Its presence confirms the existence of hyperparathyroidism. More often, however, the nonspecific and less severe bony lesion *osteomalacia* is present. The reasons for the predominance of one bone lesion over another in the individual case of hyperparathyroidism are not clear. Certainly the variations cannot be entirely explained on the basis of severity. Other factors, such as the suddenness of onset, the amount of vitamin D in the diet and the amount of exposure to sunlight, have all been invoked to explain why osteomalacia predominates in some patients while osteitis fibrosa cystica develops in others.

The basic anatomic change with osteitis fibrosa cystica is osteoclastic resorption of bone, with fibrous replacement. Both microscopic and gross cysts form within the fibrous tissue. Frequently, the first manifestation of the well developed lesion is a cystic lesion in the jaw. In many instances, the radiographic cysts are in reality soft tissue masses referred to as "brown tumors." While these lesions conform to the general histologic characteristics of giant cell tumors of bone, they are more correctly considered as reparative giant cell granulomas. Although removal of the cause of parathyroid hyperfunction may be followed by amazingly rapid reversion of the bone to normal, cystic lesions persist in some cases.

The hypercalcemia itself gives rise to so-called "*metastatic calcifications.*" Calcifications within the renal tubules produce nephrolithiasis (see p. 453) and those in the renal parenchyma comprise nephrocalcinosis (see p. 454). Hyperparathyroidism underlies about 5 per cent of all urinary stones. *Metastatic calcifications* may also be found in the blood vessels, lungs and stomach. These calcifications, described on page 24, are not specific for primary hyperparathyroidism, but may occur when there is hypercalcemia from any cause. The increased levels of calcium produce virtual supersaturation of the serum, predisposing to precipitation of calcium salts in any site at which the circumstances are appropriate. Hypercalcemic calcification is particularly prone to occur in and about the renal tubules, in the alveolar walls of the lungs and in the gastric mucosa. This distribution is attributed to the fact that these sites excrete acids and are themselves relatively alkalotic. With increasing pH, calcium becomes less soluble.

Primary hyperparathyroidism must be distinguished not only from ectopic parathormone-secreting tumors, but also from other causes of hypercalcemia, including vitamin D intoxication, sarcoid, multiple myeloma, the milk-alkali syndrome and metastatic disease. The most direct method for making this distinction is by radioimmunoassay of PTH levels.

SECONDARY HYPERPARATHYROIDISM

The most common cause of secondary hyperparathyroidism is chronic renal insufficiency, with its attendant hypocalcemia and hyperphosphatemia. However, anything that causes a negative calcium balance may underlie this disorder. The anatomic changes in the parathyroid glands consist principally of hyperplasia of the chief cells. This usually affects all glands, but not infrequently, one, two or even three may be spared. Although the fat usually is largely replaced by hyperplastic cells, in general more fat remains than with primary hyperplasia. Despite the hypersecretion of PTH with secondary hyperparathyroidism, serum calcium levels remain normal or depressed, unless tertiary hyperparathyroidism supervenes.

HYPOPARATHYROIDISM

The most frequent cause of hypoparathyroidism is accidental removal of the parathyroid glands in the course of thyroidectomy.

Less often, hypoparathyroidism is *idiopathic.* This form of the disorder affects children nine times as often as adults, and females twice as often as males. There is some familial predisposition. Although the etiology and pathogenesis are unknown, there is speculation that idiopathic hypoparathyroidism, as with many cases of hypothyroidism and adrenal hypocorticism, is related to an autoimmune phenomenon. Evidence includes the following (Blizzard, 1969): (1) Idiopathic hypoparathyroidism frequently is associated with other disorders thought to have an autoimmune basis. In a study of 74 patients with this form of hypoparathyroidism, 18 were found to have concomitant Addison's disease and seven had pernicious anemia. (2) Parathyroid-specific circulating autoantibodies have been found in 38 per cent of patients with idiopathic hypoparathyroidism. (3) A lymphocytic infiltration of the parathyroids can be produced in experimental animals by injecting extracts of isologous parathyroid tissue.

The morphologic changes in the parathyroid glands of persons with idiopathic hypoparathyroidism have not been clearly defined. Fatty replacement of the parathyroid glands has been described. In some instances, there may be aplasia or severe atrophy of glands, or both, and cases are on record in which no parathyroid tissue could be found at postmortem (Golden and Canary, 1968).

Parathormone is necessary for life. With *total* parathyroidectomy, there is a rapid drop in the serum calcium, with a concomitant rise in inorganic phosphorus levels. Neuromuscular excitability appears, followed by frank tetany. Death usually results from laryngospasm, with resultant asphyxia.

Partial parathormone deficiency, on the other hand, may run a chronic course, characterized not only by increased neuromuscular excitability, sometimes with episodes of tetany, but also by cataracts, fragility of the fingernails, thickening of the skull, and, paradoxically, calcifications in the basal ganglia of the brain, sometimes with seizures.

Before closing our discussion, we shall mention briefly two recently recognized entities, rather awkwardly known as "pseudohypoparathyroidism" and "pseudopseudohypoparathyroidism." The former refers to a clinical and biochemical picture identical to idiopathic hypoparathyroidism with the exception that administration of PTH fails to correct the abnormality. Currently it is believed to be a familial disorder caused by an end organ inability to respond to PTH which, indeed, is secreted in increased amounts. Pseudopseudohypoparathyroidism refers to a similar clinical picture occurring in patients with normal calcium and phosphorus levels.

MULTIPLE ENDOCRINE ADENOMATOSIS

There are two recognized patterns of multiple endocrine adenomatosis, known as MEA I and MEA II. Both forms may occur apparently sporadically, but more often are inherited as autosomal dominants with incomplete penetrance. As shown in Table 18–1, MEA I consists of adenomas or hyperplasia of the pancreatic islets, parathyroids, adenohypophysis and adrenal cortex, often with peptic ulcer disease. Not all of these glands need be involved in any one patient. MEA II consists of pheochromocytomas and medullary carcinoma of the thyroid, often with cutaneous and mucosal neurofibromatosis and parathyroid adenomas or hyperplasia.

With neither pattern is the relationship among the endocrine derangements completely understood. There are two dominant theories concerning this issue. The first is that these multiglandular disorders stem from a derangement in cells derived from neuroectoderm. It is thought that many of the endocrine glands are normally populated by migrating cells of neuroectodermal origin which have the capacity to elaborate polypeptide hormones. This system of cells has come to be known as the APUD system because the cells have in common the capacity to take up and carboxylate certain biogenic amines (*Amine Precursor Uptake and Decarboxylation*) (Pearse, 1969). The system also includes certain cells of the gastrointestinal tract, in particular those that give rise to carcinoid tumors (p. 504). According to this theory, then, any congenital derangement in the growth potential of neuroectoderm might be reflected in multiple endocrine abnormalities.

The second theory concerning the relationship among the glandular dysfunctions postulates that only one of them is primary, that the others simply represent attempts to compensate for the basic disorder. For example, with MEA I, pancreatic islet cell lesions may secrete a variety of hormones, including insulin, glucagon and gastrin, as well as ectopic ACTH, MSH and serotonin. Many of these substances in turn are capable of causing hyperplasia, possibly with adenoma formation, in other endocrine organs. Gastrin secretion would, of course, lead to peptic ulcer formation. Most notably, glucagon has been shown to lower serum calcium, both by a direct effect on bone and by stimulating release of calcitonin from the thyroid (Avioli et al., 1969). The resultant chronic hypocalcemia may then cause reactive hyperplasia of the parathyroids, with adenoma formation. Similarly, with MEA II, it is possible that the parathyroid changes are secondary to the release of calcitonin by the medullary carcinoma of the thyroid (Schimke et al., 1968). It should be pointed out that these two theories are not mutually exclusive. More than one of the features of the MEA syndromes may indeed be caused by a derangement in the APUD system, whereas compensatory hyperfunction may be responsible for others. In particular, the frequent presence of hyperparathyroidism in both syndromes might be explained on the basis of compensatory hyperfunction, since it is doubtful whether parathyroid cells are part of the APUD system (Scully and McNeely, 1974).

It is impossible even to summarize all of the clinical presentations of MEA I and MEA II. In the individual patient, the effects of one or two of the functioning lesions usually overshadow those of the others. Among the more frequent presentations are: (1) intractable peptic ulcer disease, (2) hypercalcemia (evidence of hyperparathyroidism), (3) hypoglycemia (evidence of hyperinsulinism due to a pancreatic islet lesion), (4) Cushing's syndrome, and (5) hypertension related to pheochromocytomas.

THE THYMUS

Two pathologic entities of the thymus, *hyperplasia* and *tumors*, will be described here. These are of considerable interest because of their frequent association with a multitude of systemic disorders and also because of their possible relationship to each other.

HYPERPLASIA OF THE THYMUS

It will be remembered that there are no lymphoid follicles in the normal thymus. Under a variety of circumstances to be men-

TABLE 18–1. MULTIPLE ENDOCRINE ADENOMATOSIS SYNDROMES

LESIONS	MEA I	MEA II
Pituitary	++++	0
Medullary carcinoma of thyroid	++	++++
Parathyroid	++++	++
Adrenal cortex	++++	+
Pheochromocytoma	0	++++
Pancreas	++++	0
Peptic ulcer	++++	0
Neuromas	0	++++

tioned later, however, lymphoid follicles do develop within the thymus, chiefly in the medulla, along with a generalized proliferation of thymic lymphocytes and enlargement of the gland.

THYMIC TUMORS

All thymic tumors are known as thymomas. Because they span a range of patterns, they have been the subject of numerous classifications. The simplest divides most thymomas according to the principal cell types normally found in the thymus:

1. Small cell (lymphocytic) thymoma — about 15 per cent.
2. Epithelial thymoma, including a spindle cell variant — 20 per cent.
3. Mixed lymphoepithelial thymoma — 50 per cent.

In addition, a variety of nonspecific tumors, such as Hodgkin's disease, the lymphomas, and teratomas, may arise in the thymus. The older conception of a granulomatous thymoma probably represents Hodgkin's disease of this organ.

Histologically, the **small cell thymoma** consists of apparent lymphocytes dispersed in no distinct pattern. These cells may totally obliterate the underlying architecture, but occasionally leave small thymic corpuscles. Plump epithelial cells are usually scattered throughout this sea of lymphocytes. Hassall's corpuscles are infrequent to rare.

The **epithelial thymomas** are composed of large epithelial cells laid down in small islands and clusters throughout a lymphoid background. The epithelial cells have an abundant pale, acidophilic cytoplasm with a vesicular nucleus and appear much larger and paler than the surrounding lymphocytes. Cystic areas of softening are common. Hassall's corpuscles are more frequent than in the small cell type, but less frequent than in the spindle cell lesions to be described.

The **spindle cell variant** of the epithelial thymoma is one in which the cells assume elongated forms resembling fibroblasts. These may form broad bundles of cells or interlacing whorls that often form mature Hassall's corpuscles. In many cases these tumors are very vascular and produce strands of cells separated by vascular cords. In other cases they appear lymphangiomatous.

The **lymphoepithelial thymoma** is composed, as might be expected, of a mixture of well differentiated lymphocytes and scattered cords or clusters of epithelial cells. Which cell population predominates varies from one tumor to another. Hassall's corpuscles are usually rare and often poorly formed.

Grossly, all three patterns appear as sharply circumscribed, encapsulated, firm, gray-white masses, varying from several centimeters in diameter to massive lesions of 15 to 20 cm. in diameter. Approximately one third of thymomas penetrate the capsule to invade adjacent structures, and may therefore be considered malignant. However, even these more aggressive thymomas rarely spread outside the thorax.

As has been mentioned, thymic hyperplasia or tumors or both have been associated with many seemingly unrelated systemic disorders. These disorders can be classified as neuromuscular, hematologic, endocrinologic and immunologic.

Perhaps the best known association is with *myasthenia gravis* (see p. 634). About 75 per cent of patients with myasthenia gravis have hyperplasia of the thymus with lymphoid follicle formation, and 25 per cent have thymomas. Not surprisingly, these thymic lesions may coexist. Conversely, about 33 per cent of patients with thymomas have myasthenia gravis. The thymomas are usually of the epithelial type (Fisher, 1968). Frequently, these patients have circulating autoantibodies that are cross reactive to the thymus and to muscle tissue, but whether they play a role in the myoneural block that characterizes myasthenia gravis is unknown (Strauss, 1968). Thymectomy sometimes leads to dramatic improvement of myasthenia gravis. This supports a recent suggestion that the myoneural block is caused by thymopoietin itself, released systemically as a result of a thymic lesion (Goldstein and Schlesinger, 1975).

Anemia, granulocytopenia, thrombocytopenia and agammaglobulinemia all have been associated with thymic hyperplasia and, more often, with thymomas. Improvement or even remission has been known to follow thymectomy (Fisher, 1968).

Several endocrine disorders, including *Graves' disease, acromegaly* and *Addison's disease,* frequently are associated with thymic changes similar to those of myasthenia gravis. The basis for this association is unknown.

In view of the important immunologic role of the thymus, it is perhaps to be expected that thymic abnormalities are associated with many of the "collagen" or autoimmune diseases. Hyperplasia of the thymus with the development of lymphoid follicles has been described in patients with *SLE* and *rheumatoid arthritis,* among other collagen diseases. Whether the thymus in these cases is the site of forbidden clones, or instead is somehow involved in aberrations in cell-mediated immunity, is speculative. It seems clear, however, that elucidation of the part played by the thymus in these disorders will be of considerable importance in understanding the phenomenon of autoimmunity.

THE PINEAL

Because of the tendency of this gland to undergo calcification with age and because so little was known of its function, the pineal was largely relegated to a landmark on skull x-rays that enables the radiologist to determine whether there has been a shift of midline structures in the brain. Recently there has been renewed interest in its endocrine function. The pineal elaborates *melatonin*, a hormone derived from serotonin, which in lower animals antagonizes the effects of melanocyte-stimulating hormone (MSH), but in mammals has an inhibitory effect on gonad development and the estrus cycle. Thus, hyperfunction of the pineal is associated with delayed puberty, whereas hypofunction leads to precocious puberty. Melatonin secretion seems to be triggered by nerve responses to information about light received by the retina (Editorial, 1974*b*). The effect of light is inhibitory. Whether or not the activity of the gland continues unabated throughout life remains uncertain, as are the possible presence and nature of other pineal hormones.

The only lesions of importance in the pineal are tumors. They may be of three types: (1) **Pinealomas,** composed of nests of the large epithelial cells found in the adult pineal. These epithelial clusters are enclosed in a fibrous stroma containing an infiltrate of lymphocytes. This histologic appearance has a remarkable similarity to that of the seminoma of the testis (p. 550). (2) **Neuroglial tumors,** producing essentially gliomatous lesions resembling gliomas found in the central nervous system (p. 656). (3) **Teratomas,** derived from residual totipotential cells and similar to teratomas found anywhere in the body.

REFERENCES

Adams, D. D., and Kennedy, T. H.: Occurrence in thyrotoxicosis of a gamma globulin which protects LATS from neutralization by an extract of thyroid gland. J. Clin. Endocr., 27:173, 1967.

Adams, D. D., et al.: Correlation between long-acting thyroid stimulator protector level and thyroid ^{131}I uptake in thyrotoxicosis. Brit. Med. J., 2:199, 1974.

Arnaud, C. D.: Parathyroid hormone: coming of age in clinical medicine. Am. J. Med., 55:577, 1973.

Avioli, L. V., et al.: Role of the thyroid gland during glucagon-induced hypocalcemia in the dog. Am. J. Physiol., 216:939, 1969.

Benson, R. C., et al.: Radioimmunoassay of parathyroid hormone in hypercalcemic patients with malignant disease. Am. J. Med., 56:821, 1974.

Blizzard, R. M.: Idiopathic hypoparathyroidism. *In* Miescher, P. A., and Muller-Eberhard, H. J. (eds.): Textbook of Immunopathology. New York, Grune and Stratton, 1969, Vol. II, p. 547.

Catt, K. J.: Hormones in general. Lancet, 1:763, 1970*a*.

Catt, K. J.: ABC of endocrinology. II. Pituitary function. Lancet, 1:827, 1970*b*.

Cohen, J.: Beta-adrenergic blockade in hyperthyroidism. New Eng. J. Med., 292:645, 1975.

Daughaday, W. H.: The adenohypophysis. *In* Williams, R. H.: Textbook of Endocrinology. 5th Ed. Philadelphia, W. B. Saunders Co., 1974, p. 27.

De Groot, L. J.: Current concepts in management of thyroid disease. Med. Clin. N. Amer., 54:117, 1970.

Doniach, D., and Roitt, I.: Autoimmune thyroid disease. *In* Miescher, P. A., and Muller-Eberhard, H. J. (eds.): Textbook of Immunopathology. New York, Grune and Stratton, 1968, p. 516.

Editorial: The latest on L.A.T.S. Lancet, 2:433, 1974*a*.

Editorial: The pineal. Lancet, 2:1235, 1974*b*.

Editorial: Neuroblastoma. Lancet, 1:379, 1975.

Eisenstein, A. B.: Addison's disease: Etiology and relationship to other endocrine disorders. Med. Clin. N. Amer., 52:327, 1968.

Fisher, E. R.: The thymus. *In* Bloodworth, J. M. B.: Endocrine Pathology. Baltimore, Williams and Wilkins Co., 1968, p. 197.

Forsham, P.: The adrenal cortex. *In* Williams, R. H.: Textbook of Endocrinology. 5th Ed. Philadelphia, W. B. Saunders Co., 1974, p. 287.

Ganong, W. F.: Review of Medical Physiology. Los Altos, Calif., Lange Medical Publications, 1965, p. 294.

Ganong, W. F., et al.: ACTH and the regulation of adrenocortical secretion. New Eng. J. Med., 290:1006, 1974.

Garry, R., and Hall, R.: Stimulation of mitoses in rat thyroid by long-acting thyroid stimulation. Lancet, 1:693, 1970.

Golden, A., and Canary, J. J.: The parathyroid glands. *In* Bloodworth, J. M. B. (ed.): Endocrine Pathology. Baltimore, Williams and Wilkins Co., 1968, p. 181.

Goldstein, G., and Schlesinger, D. H.: Thymopoietin and myasthenia gravis: neostigmine-responsive neuromuscular block produced in mice by a synthetic peptide fragment of thymopoietin. Lancet, 2:256, 1975.

Goltzman, D., et al.: Calcitonin as a tumor marker. New Eng. J. Med., 290:1035, 1974.

Hall, R.: Hyperthyroidism—pathogenesis and diagnosis. Brit. Med. J., 1:743, 1970.

Hall, R. J., and Nelson, W. P.: Thyroid heart disease. Postgrad. Med., 44:127, 1968.

Hall, R., et al.: Ophthalmic Graves' disease—diagnosis and pathogenesis. Lancet, 1:375, 1970.

Keating, F. R.: The clinical problem of primary hyperparathyroidism. Med. Clin. N. Amer., 54:511, 1970.

Lagerquist, L. G., et al.: Cushing's disease with cure by resection of a pituitary adenoma. Am. J. Med., 57:826, 1974.

McKay, D. G., et al.: The pathologic anatomy of eclampsia, bilateral renal cortical necrosis, pituitary necrosis, and other acute fatal complications of pregnancy, and its possible relationship to the generalized Shwartzman phenomenon. Am. J. Obstet. Gynec., 66:507, 1953.

Miller, R. W.: Fifty-two forms of childhood cancer: United States mortality experience, 1960–1966. J. Ped., 75:685, 1969.

Nichols, J.: Adrenal cortex. *In* Bloodworth, J. M. B., Jr. (ed.): Endocrine Pathology. Baltimore, Williams and Wilkins, 1968, p. 224.

Pearse, A. G. E.: The cytochemistry and ultrastructure of polypeptide hormone-producing cells of the APUD series and the embryologic physiologic and pathologic implications of the concept. J. Histochem. Cytochem., 17:303, 1969.

Putnam, T. C., and Miller, D. R.: Pediatric solid tumors. *In* Rubin, P. (ed.): Clinical Oncology for Medical Students and Physicians. Rochester, N. Y., American Cancer Society, 1970–71, p. 375.

Reiss, E.: Primary hyperparathyroidism: A simplified approach to diagnosis. Med. Clin. N. Amer., 54:131, 1970.

Reiss, E., and Canterbury, J. M.: Spectrum of hyperparathyroidism. Am. J. Med., 56:794, 1974.

Roitt, J. M., et al.: Autoantibodies in Hashimoto's disease. Lancet, 2:820, 1956.

Rose, N. R., and Witebsky, E.: Studies on organ specificity. V. Changes in the thyroid glands of rabbits following active immunization with rabbit thyroid extract. J. Immunol., 76:417, 1956.

Rubens, R. D., et al.: Dissimilar adenomas in four parathyroids presenting as primary hyperparathyroidism. Lancet, 1:596, 1969.

Russfield, A. B.: Adenohypophysis. *In* Bloodworth, J. M. B., Jr. (ed.): Endocrine Pathology. Baltimore, Williams and Wilkins, 1968, p. 75.

Schimke, R. N., et al.: Syndrome of bilateral pheochromocytoma, medullary thyroid carcinomas and multiple neuromas. New Eng. J. Med., *279*:1, 1968.

Scully, R. E., and McNeely, B. U.: Case records of the Massachusetts General Hospital. New Eng. J. Med., *291*:1179, 1974.

Sharp, G. C., and Irvin, W. S.: Autoantibodies. Friend or foe? Am. J. Med. Sci., *259*:356, 1970.

Smith, B. R., and Hall, R.: Thyroid-stimulating immunoglobulins in Graves' disease. Lancet, *2*:427, 1974.

Strauss, A. J. L.: Myasthenia gravis, autoimmunity and the thymus. Adv. Int. Med., *14*:241, 1968.

Tashjian, A. H., Jr., et al.: Human calcitonin. Am. J. Med., *56*:840, 1974.

Veith, F. J., et al.: The nodular thyroid gland and cancer. New Eng. J. Med., *270*:431, 1964.

Werner, S. C.: Two panel discussions on hyperthyroidism. II. Etiology and treatment of hyperthyroidism in the adult. J. Clin. Endocrin. Metab., *27*:1763, 1967.

Woolner, L. B., et al.: Struma lymphomatosa (Hashimoto's thyroiditis) and related thyroidal disorders. J. Clin. Endocr., *19*:53, 1959.

Woolner, L. B., et al.: Classification and prognosis of thyroid carcinoma. A study of 885 cases observed in a thirty year period. Amer. J. Surg., *102*:354, 1961.

Wuepper, K. D., et al.: Immunologic aspects of adrenocortical insufficiency. Am. J. Med., *46*:206, 1969.

Zacharewicz, F. A.: Management of single and multinodular goiter. Med. Clin. N. Amer., *52*:409, 1968.

CHAPTER 19
The Musculoskeletal System

Diseases of the musculoskeletal system are here divided into those of bones, joints, and muscles. The hypothesis that the head bone is connected to the neck bone seems reasonably well established (although the etiology remains disputed). Beyond this, matters become more complicated. Because of the many cell types constituting bone, lesions affecting it are many and varied. Some of these have been described elsewhere in this book. The myeloproliferative disorders are discussed in Chapter 11. The healing of bone fractures is described on page 57. In addition, bone is a favored site for metastatic disease. Indeed, about two thirds of malignant lesions in bone are secondary rather than primary. Since these metastatic neoplasms do not differ significantly from their primary tumors, their description will not be repeated. Plasma cell myeloma, the most common of the *primary* tumors, is discussed on page 354. There remains for consideration in this chapter the very common metabolic diseases of bone and a large group of infrequently occurring primary bone tumors. In addition, a brief review of infection as it affects bone will be given. It should be pointed out that such osteomyelitis may represent extension of a septic arthritis, or vice versa.

The profusion of bone tumors may initially seem overwhelming and, unfortunately, differences in nomenclature add to the hardship. Sadly, this is one of those too frequent areas in medicine in which new ideas have simply fallen into step beside old ones rather than supplanting them. However, the problems *can* be sorted out, and that sinking feeling *will* pass. First, nearly all workers agree that the bone tumors fall into three groups, according to the dominant tissue type produced—whether bone, cartilage or soft tissue. In this chapter, we shall leave it at that, and consider the *osteogenic* and *chondroma* series of tumors separately from the remaining tumors, which produce neither bone nor cartilage. However, although in almost all cases these tumors arise within the skeletal system, rarely they may arise in extraskeletal metaplastic connective tissue. In recognition of this fact, some writers prefer to use the term "osteogenic tumors" broadly, to encompass all tumors which *arise* in bone, whether or not they *produce* bone. According to this system, even the chondroma and soft tissue tumors, when they arise in bone, are considered under this heading. For those osteogenic tumors which do produce bone, the term *osteosarcoma* is then used. So long as these differences in nomenclature are understood, they should present no problem. Beyond semantics, the study of bone tumors can be further simplified by remembering several characteristics which most of them have in common. First, primary bone tumors are usually malignant, in a ratio of roughly 3:1. Unlike most cancers, those of bone tend to manifest themselves first by producing pain. Also in contrast to the general pattern of malignant disease, they strike principally young people, often adolescents. This propensity, along with their almost uniformly poor prognosis (in common with other sarcomas), gives them importance beyond that indicated by their infrequency. Besides these characteristics, bone tumors have in common a tendency to arise in the region of the metaphyses of long bones, which are especially active areas of bone growth, as well as a tendency to form, extremely rapidly, large bulky masses with areas of necrosis and hemorrhage.

Discussion of joint diseases includes a presentation of the relatively common osteoarthritis and of the infrequently occurring synoviosarcoma. Septic arthritis is described briefly. Rheumatoid arthritis is discussed with other systemic disorders of immune pathogenesis in Chapter 6. Gout is considered with the genetic disorders in Chapter 5.

The muscles seem relatively resistant to disease. Only muscle atrophy, the progressive dystrophies, myasthenia gravis and trichinosis occur sufficiently frequently to warrant full description. Involvement of muscles by tumors, whether primary or secondary, is quite rare. The desmoid tumor and the rhabdomyosarcoma are briefly presented.

BONES

OSTEOPOROSIS

Osteoporosis refers to a generalized loss of cortical bone substance. Since it is an almost invariable accompaniment of aging, some would restrict its definition to those severe cases of bone loss characterized by pain and pathologic fractures, as well as by x-ray evidence of "thin" bones (Lutwak, 1969). However, others point out that the correlation between osteoporosis, with or without fractures, and clinical symptoms is so poor as to suggest that their concurrence may be coincidental (Morgan, 1968). In either case, osteoporosis is without doubt the most common of the metabolic bone diseases. Although both sexes are affected, osteoporosis occurs earlier and progresses more rapidly in females. It becomes evident soon after the menopause and results in the loss of 40 to 50 per cent of bone tissue between the fifth and ninth decades of life. In addition to aging, the disorder is seen in a variety of other circumstances, including: (1) malnutrition, (2) vitamin C deficiency, (3) prolonged immobilization, (4) various endocrinopathies, such as Cushing's syndrome and hyperthyroidism, as well as with the therapeutic administration of exogenous steroids, and (5) occasionally, as an idiopathic entity in otherwise healthy young men.

Etiology and Pathogenesis. The cause of osteoporosis is unknown. Most likely it represents a heterogeneous disorder, in which excessive bone resorption occurs through one of several possible mechanisms. It should be emphasized at the outset that after the age of 20 to 30 years all individuals undergo progressive loss of bone volume, at a rate estimated to be about 1 per cent per year (Harris and Heaney, 1969; Nordin, 1971; Baylink et al., 1964; Garn et al., 1967). Although both bone resorption and new bone formation take place continuously throughout life, there is a slight imbalance in favor of resorption. Osteoporosis, then, may be considered simply as an extreme form of a universal phenomenon. At one time it was thought that many if not all patients with osteoporosis suffered from inadequate calcium intake, either through a deficient diet or through malabsorption. However, recent studies have failed to show any general correlation between low calcium intake and osteoporosis, and this theory has been largely dismissed (Skosey, 1970). The known vulnerability of postmenopausal women naturally suggested some relation to ovarian function. It has been speculated that osteoporosis might in part be due to the loss of an opposing action of estrogen on the effects of parathormone (PTH) on bone (Editorial, 1969). Yet such a theory leaves unexplained the relative resistance of men of all ages. Alternatively, some workers believe that the increased frequency of osteoporosis in older women simply reflects more or less ordinary loss of bone volume in those who begin with a smaller skeletal frame. The fact that these patients are usually postmenopausal might be happenstance, and a not very surprising one at that (Newton-John and Morgan, 1970). Arguing against this theory of osteoporosis as a sort of physiologic accident is the finding that in some patients there is an absolute increase in the rate of bone resorption, to about 4 per cent per year. In this same study, an unexpected finding was a concomitant increase in the rate of bone *formation*. Thus, in this small group of patients there was an accelerated bone turnover, with absorption outpacing formation (Dudl et al., 1973).

These findings suggest some derangement in calcium homeostasis, possibly as a result of excessive PTH secretion or sensitivity, or perhaps because of decreased calcitonin secretion. However, all theories remain speculative, and there is as yet no universally accepted explanation for most cases of osteoporosis.

Morphology. Except when it is caused by immobilization of localized parts, osteoporosis is a systemic disorder affecting the entire skeleton. Nevertheless, it tends to be most marked in the spine and pelvis. Compression fractures of the vertebrae are likely to occur spontaneously, and there is also a vulnerability to fracture of other bones. The disorder may be characterized as "too little" bone. Cortical bone is thinned, with resorption of cancellous bone spicules and enlargement of the medullary cavity. Nevertheless, osteoporotic bone, although reduced in mass, has the same composition as normal bone, with no evidence of inadequate mineralization.

Clinical Course. As was mentioned, bone pain, especially backache, is a common complaint of patients with osteoporosis. However, whether the osteoporosis in these cases causes the pain or whether both simply represent two common conditions occurring coincidentally is debatable. X-rays show a generalized increased radiolucency of bone, frequently with compression fractures of vertebrae. *Serum alkaline phosphatase, calcium and phosphorus are characteristically within normal limits, and this is an important point in distinguishing osteoporosis from osteomalacia, to which it may be identical on x-ray* (see page 253). When there is an underlying predisposing influence that can be corrected, osteoporosis is reversible. In other cases, treatment seems to be of little avail, although calcitonin has been reported helpful in steroid-induced osteoporosis (Palmieri et al., 1974).

RICKETS AND OSTEOMALACIA

These disorders are caused by a lack of the active form of vitamin D — $1,25-(OH)_2D_3$. In childhood this deficiency produces *rickets; osteomalacia* is the adult counterpart. Both were described, along with vitamin D metabolism, in Chapter 8, and reference should be made to this earlier discussion. Suffice it to reiterate here that deficiency of the active form of vitamin D is a fairly common disorder, which may be seen in a number of clinical settings. The most important are: (1) simple dietary inadequacy of vitamin D, often combined with a lack of exposure to sunshine, (2) intestinal malabsorption from any cause, and (3) chronic renal insufficiency, in which osteomalacia appears as a component of renal osteodystrophy (p. 428).

OSTEITIS FIBROSA CYSTICA GENERALISATA (VON RECKLINGHAUSEN'S DISEASE)

This is the pattern of bone disease associated with severe hyperparathyroidism, whether primary or secondary. It is discussed in Chapter 18 on page 615. When secondary hyperparathyroidism results from chronic renal insufficiency, osteitis fibrosa cystica is a component of renal osteodystrophy (p. 428).

OSTEITIS DEFORMANS (PAGET'S DISEASE)

Osteitis deformans is a disorder of unknown etiology characterized by continuous destruction of bone and its simultaneous replacement by an abnormally soft, poorly mineralized material. This lesion is present in from 1 to 4 per cent of elderly individuals, although in most cases it is mild and asymptomatic. In some cases, however, it produces intense pain in the involved bones. The lesion is rarely present before middle age, and males are affected twice as often as females. A familial form exists, which seems to be transmitted as an autosomal dominant (Evens and Bartter, 1968). Some consider the disease to represent a benign neoplasia of bone mesenchymal cells, in which increased numbers of these cells differentiate first to osteoclasts and then to osteoblasts (Bordier et al., 1974).

Osteitis deformans may be polyostotic or monostotic. In the polyostotic form, usually the pelvis and sacrum are involved initially. The process may then extend to the skull, femur, spine, tibia, humerus and scapula, in decreasing order of frequency. The monostotic form most often affects the tibia.

As the normal bone is resorbed, it is replaced by a light, bulky, porous osteoid matrix with the consistency of dried bread. This material is highly vascular. Although the new defective "bone" is thicker than the normal bone, its softness leads to deformities under the stress of weight-bearing.

With the microscope, it can be seen that the haphazard destruction and reformation of bone destroys the original haversian lamellar pattern. **It is usually possible to identify narrow lines of cement substance between the original bone and the foci of new bone or osteoid tissue, and these create a characteristic tilelike or mosaic pattern.** Osteoblasts and osteoclasts are abundant. The former are usually found in apposition to new bone formation, and the latter in lacunar resorptive spaces. The marrow spaces between the cancellous spicules are filled with a loose fibroblastic connective tissue (Fig. 19–1).

X-rays show the affected bones to be enlarged and relatively radiolucent. In particular, the skull is often markedly thickened and the weight-bearing bones are bowed. "Burned out" cases occur, and in these, the bones may

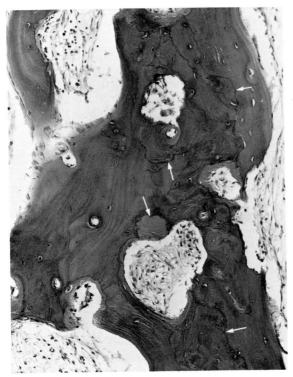

Figure 19–1. Paget's disease of bone. The thickened, irregular bony trabeculae show the classic mosaic pattern, outlined by the black lines traversing the bony trabeculae (arrows). These lines are produced by bone resorption and irregular patterns of new bone formation.

be abnormally dense. *Serum alkaline phosphatase is higher than in any other bone disorder, although serum calcium and phosphorus are characteristically normal.* Recently, it has been shown that the rapid turnover of bone may be suppressed by the administration of calcitonin, especially when supplemented by oral phosphates (Hamilton, 1974; Bordier et al., 1974).

Common complications of Paget's disease include pathologic fractures and impingement on the cranial nerves by the enlarging skull, often with consequent deafness or visual disturbances. In addition, the increased blood flow within the abnormal bone acts as multiple arteriovenous fistulae, which result in an increased work load for the heart and sometimes in high output heart failure. Most serious among the complications is the development of osteogenic sarcoma in bones affected by osteitis deformans. Such malignant transformation is reported in from 1 to 25 per cent of cases of Paget's disease, and carries with it a particularly grave prognosis, with a less than 1 per cent five-year survival rate (Boutouras and Goodsitt, 1963; Freydinger et al., 1963).

FIBROUS DYSPLASIA OF BONE

This disorder is characterized by focal areas of fibrous replacement of bone. Although the etiology is unknown, the anatomic changes suggest a derangement in the normal remodeling of bone, with the progressive replacement of resorbed bone by fibrous tissue and irregularly formed bone. Usually the lesion is monostotic, affects males slightly more often than females, and may appear at any time between infancy and middle age, with a median age in one series of 14 years (Firat and Stutzman, 1968).

Occasionally, fibrous dysplasia is polyostotic, and in a very small percentage of cases, the polyostotic form is associated with scattered areas of melanotic pigmentation of the skin (*cafe au lait spots*) and with sexual precocity. The concurrence of these disparate features is known as *Albright's syndrome.* In contrast to the monostotic form of fibrous dysplasia, Albright's syndrome occurs primarily in females. Although the multisystem involvement suggests some congenital defect, no hereditary or familial pattern has been established.

The monostotic form shows a predilection for the long bones of the extremities, the ribs and the bones of the skull and face. The lesion begins in the intramedullary cancellous bone and expands to involve the adjacent cortex. Although it is not encapsulated, it tends to remain enclosed within a shell of cortical bone. Histologically, there is a fibrous stroma containing nests of lipophages or islands of cartilage, but most important are trabeculae and masses of poorly formed membranous bone having no internal lamellar structure. This osteoid matrix is poorly delimited and projects into the fibrous stroma in irregular, tongue-like processes.

The clinical course is more or less unpredictable. Sometimes the lesion grows slowly and may even, apparently spontaneously, become stationary. In other patients, unless the lesion is cured by surgical excision, fibrous dysplasia progresses rapidly and inexorably, causing bone destruction and disfigurement. When the facial bones are involved, there may be severe distortions of the orbit, nose and jaw. Malignant transformation occurs rarely (Huvos et al., 1972).

HYPERTROPHIC (PULMONARY) OSTEOARTHROPATHY

This mysterious entity has three separate components, any of which may occur separately: (a) "clubbing" of the fingers, (b) periosteal proliferation of the distal ends of the long bones, and (c) swelling and tenderness of joints. These changes are seen in a multitude of diverse clinical settings. Clubbing is particularly common, and may be found with: (1) *Pulmonary diseases*, most importantly bronchogenic carcinoma and chronic lung sepsis—for example, lung abscess or bronchiectasis. An exception is pulmonary tuberculosis, which rarely if ever is associated with clubbing. (2) *Cardiovascular diseases*, particularly those associated with cyanosis, such as congenital heart disease with a right-to-left shunt. (3) *Hepatic disorders*, particularly biliary cirrhosis and liver abscesses. (4) A wide variety of *ulceroinflammatory gastrointestinal diseases*, including ulcerative colitis and Crohn's disease. (5) *Certain cancers*, including chronic myelogenous leukemia, carcinoma of the thymus and pleural mesothelioma.

The changes involved in clubbing of the fingers are edema, fibrous overgrowth at the tips of the fingers and an increased vascularization in the nail bed, with rounding or "watch glass" deformity of the nail. The normal inclination of the base of the nail toward the bone is lost. The tips of the digits become enlarged and often are dusky or cyanotic. These changes are more or less readily discernible on inspection, and therefore clubbing is a valuable diagnostic sign. Its presence may lead to the discovery of an unsuspected bronchogenic carcinoma.

Periosteal bone changes affect the distal radius, ulna, tibia, fibula, metacarpals and proximal phalanges. The amount of new bone formation varies from barely radiographically visible tufting to the formation of a complete enclosing layer about the metacarpals and first and second phalanges. Although any of the disorders leading to clubbing may produce periosteal proliferation, the most important underlying condition is bronchogenic carcinoma.

Hypertrophic osteoarthropathy is thought to involve increased blood flow to the bones, possibly as a result of some derangement in the autonomic nervous system (Editorial, 1975). Beyond this, the mechanism remains an enigma. With removal of the underlying disease, the bony changes promptly regress.

OSTEOGENIC TUMORS

As mentioned in the introductory material to this chapter, osteogenic tumors are here defined as those neoplasms that regularly produce bone. It will be remembered that some writers use this term differently, for all primary tumors which arise in bone, whether or not they produce bone. The three principal osteogenic tumors are the *osteoma*, the *osteoid osteoma* and the *osteogenic sarcoma* (sometimes referred to as *osteosarcoma*). By far the most important of these is the osteogenic sarcoma, which will be discussed here as a case history.

OSTEOMA

This is an infrequent and totally benign growth, found most often in the skull. Frequently it projects into the orbit or paranasal sinuses, and in such locations it is termed *hyperostosis frontalis interna*. Histologically, the growth is composed of dense normal bone. Because often little if any growth in these lesions is apparent, it has been suggested that they reflect reactive bone formation at sites of old injury rather than true neoplasms.

OSTEOID OSTEOMA

These, too, have been thought to represent reparative scarring in a focus of previous injury. However, most would consider these lesions to be small, benign, fibrous tumors. They are most likely to occur in persons under the age of 30 years, and they affect males twice as often as females. Although any bone may be involved, the femur and tibia are most commonly affected. The lesion typically arises within cortical bone, where it erodes the underlying normal bone, producing a discrete, red-brown nodule rarely over 1 cm. in diameter. Immediately surrounding it is a zone of delicate, porous bone and about this is a zone of dense, sclerotic bone. The tumor itself is composed of fibrous tissue containing patchy areas of osteoid matrix and poorly organized spicules of bone. On x-ray, the osteoid osteoma appears as a distinctive lytic lesion surrounded by a rim of densely hypertrophied bone. Despite its small size and benign nature, the lesion is extremely painful, and so it necessitates surgical removal.

OSTEOGENIC SARCOMA—A CASE HISTORY

The following case report is characteristic of one of the most malignant forms of cancer in man, the osteogenic sarcoma. Next to plasma cell myeloma, this is the most common of the primary malignant tumors of bone.

Present Illness. A 17 year old girl presented herself at the clinic with a painful mass located just above the left knee, of about four months' duration. Over this period it had gradually become worse, until a severe pain of a steady, boring nature developed, which was especially intense at night. Often it awakened her from sleep. At the time of consultation, she described the pain as "gnawing" and situated just over the left knee. She had also noted that the lower left thigh seemed to be somewhat more full than the right. She stated that she had lost about 7 pounds over the past month, which she thought was the result of fatigue and loss of appetite.

Physical Examination. The physical examination was entirely negative save for that relating to the left leg. There was a firm, tender mass in the distal thigh which had produced some overall enlargement. The circumference of the *right* thigh just above the knee was 37 cm. In contrast, the left thigh at the same level was 45 cm. The swelling was most prominent over the anterior aspect, and a firm mass was palpable in the soft tissues which was tender to moderate pressure. There was a peculiar dilatation of the veins in the subcutaneous area overlying the mass anteriorly. There was no evidence of increased heat or erythema, and no adenopathy was palpable in the inguinal region.

Alkaline phosphatase level was approximately 30 King-Armstrong units (normal range, 3 to 13 King-Armstrong units); serum calcium was 9.4 mg. per 100 ml.; phosphorus was 3.1 mg. per 100 ml. X-rays were taken of the left lower thigh and knee region. A large, soft tissue mass was seen circumferentially enveloping the distal femur, involving over 50 per cent of the diameter of the leg. It extended downward to just above the knee joint and proximally to the junction of the middle and lower thirds of the femur. The medullary cavity of the lower femur was irregularly filled with partially calcified material, which obscured cortical detail. This medullary calcification extended down to the articular cartilage of the distal end of the femur, and proximally into the middle third of the femur. There appeared to be an area of erosion of the anterior aspect of the cortex. The cortex was extremely thinned in the center of this area of erosion, but apparently it was not totally destroyed nor fractured. Radiating out from this region were a number of radiopaque streaks extending well into the surrounding soft tissue mass, creating a "sunburst" appearance. About 3 cm. proximal to the central focus of this sunburst, there was obvious elevation of the periosteum, with apparent delicate calcification interposed between the elevated periosteum and the preserved underlying cortex. Such an elevation produces an x-ray pattern referred to in orthopedic circles as *Codman's triangle;* this is considered to be indicative of a bone tumor, particularly an osteogenic sarcoma. The radiologic impression, then, was osteogenic sarcoma.

Comment. Many of the findings in this case pointed strongly and almost unmistakably to the diagnosis of osteogenic sarcoma. In a teen-ager, the occurrence of a tumor mass producing both radiolucent and radiopaque changes within the metaphyseal region of the femur, associated with a sunburst of calcification extending into an overlying soft tissue mass, is virtually pathognomonic of osteogenic sarcoma. The elevation of the periosteum to create Codman's triangle is not diagnostic of osteogenic sarcoma but is often associated with it. These radiologic changes represent lifting of the outer periosteum as the tumor penetrates from within, with reactive bone formation between the elevated periosteum and the underlying bony cortex. Presumably, the lesion first lifts the periosteum and then penetrates it, producing the sunburst, which extends well out into the soft tissues of the limb. The elevated alkaline phosphatase level in this setting is also highly suggestive of osteogenic sarcoma. Here again, the finding by itself is not diagnostic, since any form of reactive new bone formation, such as might be produced by osteomyelitis or a bone fracture, yields an elevation in the alkaline phosphatase level.

The location of the mass in this case, within the skeletal system, as well as within the bone involved, is typical of an osteogenic sarcoma. Approximately 70 per cent of these tumors arise in the femur or the tibia, usually in the metaphysis nearest the knee. Far less frequently, they involve the humerus (usually near the shoulder), the ilium, the mandible and the ribs. From the metaphysis of the long bones, they tend to extend in a broad front toward the epiphysis, which they may or may not penetrate, and in a conical form toward the diaphysis. Invasion through the metaphyseal cortex into the soft tissues is almost invariable. Osteogenic sarcomas present a wide range of histologic patterns. Some produce very little osteoid tissue and therefore have little calcification (*osteolytic osteogenic sarcoma*). These manifest themselves principally as soft tissue sarcomas causing destruction of bone without giving rise to areas of radiodensity within the tumor. Such lesions would not produce the sunburst appearance which was seen, for example, in the present case. At the other end of the spectrum are the tumors that produce abundant calcified osteoid tissue and are therefore densely radiopaque (*sclerosing osteogenic sarcoma*). The present case is intermediate between these extremes and on x-ray gave evidence of both bone destruction and neoplastic new bone formation.

Hospital Admission. The patient entered the hospital three days later for biopsy. Prior to biopsy, a chest x-ray disclosed multiple, rounded calcified shadows within both lung fields, up to 3 cm. in diameter, which were virtually diagnostic of metastatic osteogenic sarcoma. Despite the evidence of apparent metastatic disease, biopsy was performed, since it was deemed necessary to establish beyond doubt the nature of the primary le-

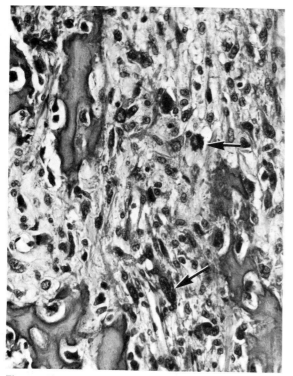

Figure 19–2. Osteogenic sarcoma. The high power detail illustrates the anaplastic fibrous tissue, with mitoses and giant cell formation (arrows). Osteoid trabeculae have been produced by the neoplastic cells, and anaplastic tumor cells are found lying within apparent bone lacunae.

sion. A 4 cm. incision was made in the anterior aspect of the left thigh, and immediately beneath the deep fascia, gritty, gray-white tumor tissue was encountered. A 1.5 × 1.0 × 1.0 cm. fragment was excised. On gross examination, definite gritty spicules of calcification were evident. Microscopic examination disclosed a highly anaplastic sarcoma (Fig. 19–2). It was composed of masses of spindle cells showing extreme pleomorphism, with large, deeply chromatic nuclei. Giant cells, some with huge, multilobate nuclei and others with multiple nuclei, were abundant. Mitoses were frequent and of extremely bizarre nature, some apparently having four or five tangled, atypical spindles. The preponderance of cells were of the fibroblastic, spindle cell variety. Scattered through this cellular background were islands and strands of pink amorphous, osteoid tissue in which tumor cells occupied the lacunar spaces. This osteoid tissue was well calcified in some areas. The diagnosis of osteogenic sarcoma was confirmed. Because of the apparent pulmonary metastases, surgery for the primary lesion was ruled out. The patient pursued a relentless, wasting, downhill course over three months to her death. The terminal event was an acute

respiratory infection, which lasted only two days.

Postmortem Examination. The body was that of a young, very emaciated female with skull-like facies and a skeletal system that appeared to be covered only by skin. There was extreme atrophy of the musculature of the entire body, particularly evident in the extremities. The tumor mass was plainly evident in the lower third of the left femur. At the level of maximal swelling, the left thigh had a circumference of 48 cm., in contrast to that of the wasted right thigh, which was 24 cm. On opening the chest, 560 ml. of serosanguinous fluid was found in the right pleural cavity and 400 ml. of similar fluid was found in the left pleural cavity. The lungs were voluminous and filled both pleural cavities, nearly hiding the heart from sight. The right lung weighed 1050 gm. (normal weight, 400 gm.). It was virtually solidified by bulky, gray-white tumor masses. The tumor extended in many places to the pleural surface, and at several points it appeared to have grown through the pleura. The left lung weighed 980 gm. and had a basically similar appearance. The trachea and main-stem bronchi were entirely free of significant findings, but within the second and third order bronchi and extending out into the terminal radicles was an abundant yellow mucinous secretion suggesting an inflammatory process. Multiple transections of both right and left lungs showed large, gray-white gritty tumor masses up to 10 cm. in diameter, replacing most of the lung substance. Only scant ribbons of pink crepitant lung parenchyma remained between the tumor masses. The abdominal cavity and its viscera were in general normal. The liver appeared somewhat more brown than usual and weighed about 200 gm. less than would be considered normal. Examination of the left thigh disclosed a large, gray-white tumor mass engulfing the lower third and most of the middle third of the femur. This tumor completely encircled the femur and extended virtually out to the skin. Incision into the tumor was performed with difficulty, since it contained a large amount of gritty, white, calcified tissue. Where it could be transected, the tumor had a gray-white, fish-flesh appearance, with minute flecks of white calcified deposits. Most of the tumor literally had to be sawed into sections. Its central portion was composed of a gray-white, bony mass that completely filled the medullary cavity of the femur from the distal articular cartilage up to the junction of the middle and upper third. The femoral cortex could be identified buried within the tumor, except for a 5 cm. area in the anterior metaphyseal region, where the cortex was completely destroyed or was indistinguishable from the bony mass that had encroached on it. The tumor that extended into the soft tissues about the bone was slightly less hard and contained more areas of soft, gray, gritty neoplasm. The joint space of the knee was not involved. The inguinal nodes apparently were normal. Examination of the vertebral bodies disclosed several 3 cm. foci of gray-white, apparent tumor tissue in the thoracic vertebrae.

Microscopic examination showed a variable histologic pattern throughout the many blocks of tumor tissue processed. In the central regions of the tumor taken from the medullary cavity, there was extensive bone formation. The bone was laid down in irregular, random masses and spicules having indistinct margins where it blended with the intervening spindle cell stroma. The cells occupying the lacunar spaces were atypical and anaplastic osteocytes. In the more peripheral regions of the tumor, where it had invaded the soft tissue, there was less bone formation and more of the fibroblastic spindle cell pattern already described in the biopsy. The anaplasia of the cellular element was extreme, as was the mitotic activity. As many as 10 mitoses could be found in a single high power field. Most of the cells were well preserved, but there were scattered foci of necrosis where the tumor had evidently outgrown its blood supply. The metastatic nodules within the lung contained slightly less osteoid tissue and consisted principally of extremely anaplastic spindle cells. The lesions within the vertebral bodies resembled the more ossified regions of the primary tumor in the left femur. Microscopic examination of the smaller bronchi disclosed many areas in which they were encircled by tumor but not invaded by it. However, there was an acute bronchitis, with an abundant outpouring of neutrophils within the bronchial and bronchiolar walls as well as within the lumina.

Anatomic Diagnoses. (1) Osteogenic sarcoma of lower third of left femur, with metastases to the lungs and to the thoracic vertebrae. (2) Acute suppurative bronchitis and bronchiolitis (staphylococcal). (3) Extreme cachexia. (4) Brown atrophy of liver (page 10).

Comment. This case history provides an all too clear demonstration of the fulminating, highly malignant nature of osteogenic sarcoma (and, indeed, of many anaplastic sarcomas). In particular, pulmonary metastases occur early, and it is probable that most patients have at least micrometastases in their lungs at the time of diagnosis. Overall five-year survival rates vary from study to study, but range between 5 and 20 per cent. Most patients are dead within 12 to 18 months of diagnosis. There is some indication, however, that aggressive chemotherapy at the time of surgical removal of the primary lesion may destroy pulmonary micrometastases and thereby improve the prognosis (Jaffe et al., 1974; Cortes et al., 1974). Improved results have also been reported following the use of vaccines made from lyophilized tumor cells (Marcove et al., 1973).

As this case exemplifies, osteogenic sarcoma tends to occur in young individuals whose skeleton is undergoing its most rapid phase of growth. Further support for the role of rapid bone growth comes from the evidence that taller adolescents are more vulnerable than are their shorter peers (Fraumeni, 1945). The peak incidence occurs by age 20. A second, smaller peak is encountered in patients over the age of 40. Many of these older patients have preexisting osteitis deformans (Paget's disease) with its extensive remodeling of bone (McKenna et al., 1964). Extreme anaplasia is a feature of virtually all osteogenic sarcomas. A few are better differentiated. Some of these may produce cartilage as well as bone.

All sarcomas tend to metastasize via the bloodstream. In the case under discussion, the massive metastatic dissemination was to the lungs, presumably through the bloodstream. The metastases to the vertebral bodies likewise presumably occurred through the bloodstream. Typically, osteogenic sarcomas metastasize to the lungs, to the liver and to other bones. It should be noted that in this case there was no lymph node involvement, even of the inguinal nodes draining the leg. However, spread via the lymphatics, with regional involvement, is sometimes seen. The cause of death, a terminal staphylococcal respiratory infection, is the common end point for many patients suffering from the advanced cachexia of malignant disease. It has been said that respiratory infection is the friend of those who are mortally ill with cancer.

CHONDROMA SERIES OF TUMORS

There are four important cartilaginous tumors: the *exostosis*, the *enchondroma*, the *chondrosarcoma* and the *chondromyxoid fibroma*.

EXOSTOSIS (EXOSTOSIS CARTILAGINEA)

This is a benign neoplasm which protrudes from the metaphyseal surface of long bones, most often the lower femur or upper tibia, and which is capped by growing cartilage. The cartilage produces endochondral bone. As an isolated defect, it develops commonly in children and adolescents and follows a very indolent course, sometimes with apparent cessation of growth followed by complete ossification. Multiple exostoses occur as a hereditary disorder (*hereditary multiple cartilaginous exostoses*). These appear earlier than the isolated lesions, usually in infancy, and typically cease to enlarge before adolescence is reached. The major clinical significance of these lesions, particularly in the hereditary form, lies in a reported potential for malignant transformation to a chondrosarcoma or an osteogenic sarcoma.

ENCHONDROMA

This is also a benign cartilaginous tumor, but, unlike the exostoses, it occurs deep within the bone, in the spongiosa. Most frequently involved are the small bones of the hands and feet. Young adults are principally affected. Multiple enchondromas, or *enchondromatosis*, may occur in childhood, a condition known as *Ollier's disease*. When this pattern is accompanied by hemangiomas of the skin, the involvement is termed *Maffucci's syndrome*.

Grossly, the enchondroma appears as a firm, slightly lobulated, glassy, gray-blue, translucent tissue which abuts on and erodes the overlying cortical bone. Usually reactive bone formation maintains a thin outer bony shell. With the light microscope, the tumor is seen to be composed of small masses of mature hyaline cartilage merging gradually through transitional cell forms with a scant fibrous stroma. Foci of calcification and even ossification may be present within the cartilage.

The erosive nature of these lesions may cause pain, swelling or pathologic fractures of the involved bone. On the other hand, the lesion may remain completely silent. As with the exostosis, malignant transformation is reported with the enchondroma, particularly the multiple pattern.

CHONDROSARCOMA

Although only about 10 per cent of malignant tumors arising in bone are chondrosarcomas, their clinical importance is greater than this figure would indicate, because adequate excision of this lesion permits an unusually good prognosis. This outlook is in sharp contrast to that afforded by the other malignant bone tumors. Five-year survival is 25 to 50 per cent (Stradford, 1970–71). Chondrosarcomas affect males three times as often as females, and tend to arise in adults somewhat older than those affected by most other bone tumors.

It is thought that they often result from malignant transformation of exostoses or enchondromas, and hence may have either a peripheral or a central location within the involved bone. With time, these tumors become quite bulky, destroying the native bone as they expand and frequently extending through the cortex into the surrounding soft tissues. The histologic appearance is similar to that of the enchondroma, with islands of mature hyaline cartilage in a fibrous stroma. However, the chondrosarcoma is differentiated by the presence of areas of poorly developed cartilaginous matrix containing overtly anaplastic cells. The stroma, too, may be sarcomatous. On the other hand, because foci of ossification may be present, this lesion is sometimes confused with a poorly os-

sified osteogenic sarcoma. In this case, the distinction rests on the pattern of bone formation. **The chondrosarcoma forms endochondral bone within cartilage, while the osteogenic sarcoma forms bone by direct osteoblastic production within a fibrous stroma.**

CHONDROMYXOID FIBROMA

A rare benign lesion, the chondromyxoid fibroma is important primarily because it is often misinterpreted as malignant. It usually arises within the marrow cavity of the upper metaphysis of the tibia or the lower metaphysis of the femur, and tends to erode the overlying cortex, producing pain. Grossly, it appears firm and gray-white, without sufficient myxoid tissue to produce sliminess. Histologically, the lesion consists of a loose myxomatous tissue containing spindled fibroblasts, stellate myxoma cells and collagenous hyaline fibrous tissue. Although some areas may differentiate into cartilage, osteoid or bone formation is uncommon. *The presence of apparently ominous, scattered multinucleated giant cells leads to the frequent misdiagnosis of these tumors as chondrosarcomas, or giant cell tumors.*

OTHER BONE TUMORS

GIANT CELL TUMOR (OSTEOCLASTOMA)

Giant cell tumors comprise a group of benign to malignant neoplasms characterized by the presence of numerous multinucleated, probably osteoclastic giant cells in a spindle cell stroma. Most patients are over the age of 20 years, and there is no sex preponderance.

As with many other bone lesions, the most frequently involved sites are the ends of long bones, particularly the lower femur, upper tibia and lower radius. Characteristically, giant cell tumors begin within the center of the marrow cavity and progressively expand outward, often reaching but not eroding the articular cartilage and producing a clublike deformity of the end of the bone (Fig. 19–3). Reactive new bone formation usually maintains a thin enclosing outer shell. The tumor itself is gray-brown, firm and friable, with scattered foci of hemorrhage and necrosis. With the light microscope, numerous irregularly scattered cells resembling osteoclasts or foreign body type giant cells are seen throughout a fibrous stroma composed of spindle cells which vary from well differentiated to frankly anaplastic (Fig. 19–4). From this stromal component, giant cell tumors are sometimes classified as Grades 1 to 3, from benign to malignant. **However, it is difficult to predict the clinical behavior of these tumors from their histology. Bone and cartilage formation typically do not occur in these tumors.**

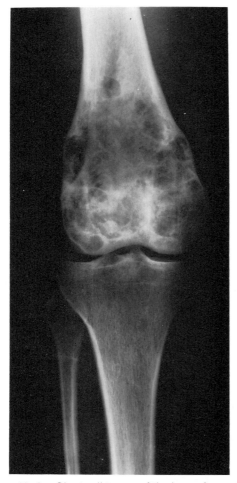

Figure 19–3. Giant cell tumor of the lower femur. The tumor has produced widening of the bone and multiple areas of cystic rarefaction. There is no apparent erosion of the bone cortex, nor extension into the surrounding tissues.

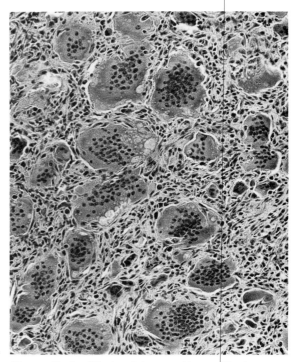

Figure 19–4. Giant cell tumor of bone. The large osteoclastic giant cells are separated by a scant fibroblastic stroma.

The clinical presentation of giant cell tumors is nonspecific, with pain, tenderness and occasionally pathologic fractures. Sometimes there is an externally palpable mass. X-rays may be virtually pathognomonic, showing a soap bubble appearance, consisting of large cystic areas of bone rarefaction traversed by strands of calcification and surrounded by a thin shell of bone. About 50 per cent of these tumors follow a benign course; another 35 per cent tend to recur after local excision, frequently in a more malignant form, and the remaining 15 per cent are aggressively malignant from the outset. Of those that are malignant, five-year survival is about 25 per cent (Stradford, 1970–71).

Often inflammatory or reparative lesions of bone contain giant cells, but these are called "tumors" only as misnomers. These lesions include the "brown tumors" of hyperparathy-roidism, the giant cell granuloma of the jaw bones in adolescents (also called *epulis*), and the giant cell tumor of synovial or tendon sheath origin. Histologically they may quite closely resemble giant cell tumors.

EWING'S SARCOMA (DIFFUSE ENDOTHELIOMA)

This rare and extremely malignant tumor arises within the marrow cavity of bone. Despite the unfortunate term "diffuse endothelioma," the presumed origin of this lesion from endothelial cells is not well substantiated. Alternatively, it has been suggested that the basic cell type is an undifferentiated mesenchymal tissue cell, perhaps closely related to the fibroblast. The uncertainty stems from the totally undifferentiated nature of the tumor. Like the osteogenic sarcoma, Ewing's sarcoma affects adolescents and young adults, with a slight male preponderance.

The two major sites of involvement are the metaphyses of the long tubular bones and the pelvis. Ewing's sarcomas grow rapidly and by the time the patient comes to medical attention, they may be large, fleshy gray masses, with areas of necrosis and hemorrhage, which have eroded the cortex and invaded the surrounding soft tissue. In about 50 per cent of cases, reactive new bone formation creates a concentric "onionskin" layering about the tumor. Histologically, these tumors consist of sheets of extremely undifferentiated small cells with rather uniform, prominent nuclei, often in mitosis, and scant cytoplasm. Giant cells are conspicuously absent. Because of the totally undifferentiated nature of the basic cells, these tumors may easily be confused with metastases from other undifferentiated cancers, particularly neuroblastomas.

Pain and tenderness are the dominant presenting clinical features of Ewing's sarcoma. Relatively early widespread dissemination occurs, and the prognosis is extremely poor, with a five-year survival rate variously reported as from 0 to 12 per cent (Stradford, 1970–71).

SEPTIC OSTEOMYELITIS

The two most important infections of bone are: (1) hematogenous pyogenic osteomyelitis caused principally by *Staphylococcus aureus*, followed in importance by the streptococci, pneumococci, gonococci, *H. influenzae* and the coliform bacilli, and (2) tuberculosis. Fortunately, both forms are becoming progressively less frequent.

Pyogenic osteomyelitis usually develops in children. In most cases, the primary focus of bacterial infection cannot be demonstrated, and a transient bacteremia from trivial causes is presumed. Occasionally, osteomyelitis results from direct contamination of a bone exposed by trauma or from spread of a neighboring soft tissue infection.

The bone involvement commonly begins in the metaphyseal marrow cavity and develops as a characteristic suppurative reaction. As the inflammatory pressure increases within the rigidly confined focus of infection, the vascular supply is often compromised, adding an element of ischemic necrosis to the suppurative damage. Eventually the inflammation may penetrate the cortex through the haversian system, often producing multiple sinus tracts. The suppuration and ischemic injury may then cause necrosis of a fragment of bone, known as a **sequestrum**. Extension into the joint is uncommon. In certain instances, the initial infection becomes walled off by inflammatory fibrous tissue, creating a localized abscess that may undergo spontaneous sterilization or become a chronic nidus of infection (**Brodie's abscess**). Intense reactive osteoblastic activity forms new bone that tends to enclose the inflammatory focus. This neo-osteogenesis, if continued for a sufficient period of time, gives rise to a densely sclerotic pattern of osteomyelitis, referred to as **Garré's sclerosing osteomyelitis.**

Hematogenous osteomyelitis usually manifests itself as an acute systemic febrile illness, accompanied by local pain, tenderness, redness and swelling. Blood cultures are usually positive during this stage. Necrosis of bone is typically not sufficiently advanced to be demonstrable on x-rays for the first seven to 10 days. Although spontaneous healing may occur, the usual course in the absence of adequate therapy is toward chronicity, with destruction of bone and the risk of metastatic dissemination of infection.

Tuberculous infection of bone occurs in approximately 1 per cent of patients with clinical tuberculosis. It often presents a diagnostic problem, since in about 50 per cent of these patients, concomitant pulmonary tuberculosis cannot be demonstrated (Davidson and Horowitz, 1970). Unlike pyogenic osteomyelitis, tuberculous osteomyelitis tends to arise insidiously and to extend into joint spaces. Often it is not noted until destruction is widespread. The long bones of the extremities and the spine (*Pott's disease*) are the favored sites of localization. Histologically, caseating tubercles develop which are entirely consonant with the disease wherever it occurs.

JOINTS

SEPTIC ARTHRITIS

Septic arthritis may be either pyogenic or tuberculous. *Pyogenic arthritis* usually represents hematogenous spread from a primary infection, often bacterial pneumonia, bacterial endocarditis or gonorrhea. Accordingly, the causative organisms are the staphylococci, streptococci, pneumococci and gonococci, and young adults are most often affected.

Characteristically, the infection is monoarticular and involves one of the large joints, such as the knee, hip, ankle, elbow, wrist or shoulder. The anatomic changes are typical of a suppurative infection. The synovial membranes become edematous and congested, and the joint space fills with purulent material. In severe cases, the inflammatory synovitis may ulcerate and involve the underlying articular cartilage, eventuating in destruction of the joint surfaces with scarring and, occasionally, calcification.

The clinical manifestations are those of an acute infection, with redness, swelling, tenderness and pain, often with accompanying constitutional symptoms. Because of the destructive tendencies of chronic suppurative arthritis, the acute phase requires prompt recognition and therapy for the preservation of normal joint function.

Tuberculous arthritis most frequently occurs in the spine and represents simply an aspect of tuberculous osteomyelitis (*Pott's disease*), with extension into the intervertebral discs. It may also occur as a monoarticular involvement in the large joints. Like tuberculous osteomyelitis, tuberculous arthritis is an extremely insidious destructive process, which tends to erode into the underlying articular surface and destroy the bone. Early diagnosis is imperative to prevent permanent damage.

OSTEOARTHRITIS (DEGENERATIVE ARTHRITIS)

Among the rewards of a long life is osteoarthritis, a chronic arthropathy which to some degree afflicts virtually everyone over the age of 50 years. In a general way, it can be ascribed to the inevitable trauma to the joints which accumulates over the course of many years. However, the precise etiology is unknown. It has been suggested that repeated trauma leads to increased thickness and decreased resiliency of subchondral bone, and that this impairs the joint's capacity to dampen stress (Radin et al., 1970). Moreover, there is some evidence of a tendency with age toward incongruity of articulating bone surfaces, which increases contact pressures acting over the joint (Editorial, 1973).

The spine and large joints of the body (i.e., those which are most subject to weight-bearing) are principally affected. The involvement may be either monoarticular or polyarticular. Unlike most arthritides, the basic anatomic change is degeneration of the articular cartilage, rather than inflammation of the synovia. This degeneration manifests itself as fissuring and irregularity of the cartilaginous surfaces, followed by fibrillation, microfractures and separation of small fragments. There is a very early decrease in the metachromatic staining capacity of the cartilage, which is thought to reflect depletion of proteoglycan (Mankin, 1974). With moderately advanced disease, the chondrocytes show proliferative activity, presumably reparative. Ultimately, however, nearly all the chondrocytes undergo degeneration (Weiss, 1973). The synovia may show some secondary inflammatory edema and thickening, but no significant leukocytic infiltrate and no pannus formation (see *Rheumatoid Arthritis*, p. 190). With destruction of the articular cartilage, the underlying bone is exposed. This becomes thickened, as a result of either compression or reactive new bone formation. Characteristic bony "spurs" project from the reactive bone at the margins of the joint space (Fig. 19–5). When large spurs project from opposing bones, they may come into contact with each other, causing pain and limiting motion. Either spurs or fragments of articular cartilage may break off, forming free intra-articular foreign bodies known as "joint mice."

Clinically, osteoarthritis appears insidiously as a slowly progressive joint stiffness. Pain and crepitus on motion, as well as occasional swelling of affected joints, may be present. Howev-

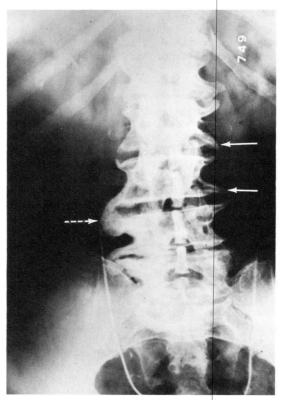

Figure 19–5. Osteoarthritis of the vertebral column. Prominent spur formation is seen along the intervertebral margins of the vertebral bodies (solid arrows). Fusion of spurs has created a bony bridge (dashed arrow).

er, there are no constitutional signs of an inflammatory disease. When osteoarthritis with spur formation affects the distal interphalangeal joints of the fingers, it appears clinically as firm, nodular enlargements of the joints, known as *Heberden's nodes.* These are extremely common in elderly individuals and constitute an important exception to the tendency of osteoarthritis to affect large, weight-bearing joints.

RHEUMATOID ARTHRITIS

This very important type of arthritis is discussed in Chapter 6 because of its probable autoimmune pathogenesis, as well as its systemic nature. Suffice it to say here that rheumatoid arthritis is a common disorder, which has been estimated to afflict about 2 per cent of the adult population of the United States. While its manifestations may remain largely restricted to the joints (usually taking the form of a remitting-relapsing symmetric polyarticular arthritis), in some cases the heart, lungs, blood vessels, muscles and skin are also involved.

SYNOVIOSARCOMA

As its name implies, the synoviosarcoma is a malignant tumor arising in synovial membranes, usually in joints but occasionally in tendon sheaths or bursae. It is the only tumor of joints that occurs with sufficient frequency to merit even a brief description. Often the misnomer "synovioma" is applied to it, despite its clearly malignant behavior. The tumor shows no sex preponderance, and most often it develops after middle age.

In 75 per cent of these patients, the lesion arises somewhere in the leg. It may grow rapidly, attaining a size of 15 cm. or more in diameter. On cross section, such bulky tumors typically show areas of hemorrhage and cystic necrosis, sometimes with spotty calcifications. Histologically, the synoviosarcoma is quite pleomorphic, with the various cell patterns tending to recapitulate the differentiation of cuboidal synovial cells from the more primitive spindle-shaped fibroblasts. Thus, there may be sheets of fusiform cells merging with cuboidal epithelium lining cleft-like spaces, which may contain serous or mucinous secretions similar to the fluid found within joint spaces. Papillary formations may project into these spaces. The individual tumor cells display all the characteristics of anaplasia, with variations in nuclear size and shape, hyperchromasia and mitotic activity. Five-year survival is about 30 per cent (Pories, 1970–71).

GANGLION

This is a small cystic swelling, up to 2 cm. in diameter, which arises from a joint capsule or tendon sheath, usually on the wrist but occasionally on the foot or knee. Anatomically, it consists of a collagenous fibrous wall, filled with mucoid fluid. The causation of these lesions is obscure.

MUSCLES

MUSCLE ATROPHY

Atrophic shrinkage, death and disappearance of muscle cells occur under a variety of circumstances, some generalized and some local. Among the systemic disorders are chronic malnutrition, panhypopituitarism, prolonged immobilization, SLE, dermatomyositis and advanced age, which presumably leads to muscle atrophy on the basis of diffuse ischemia. In these disorders, entire muscle masses are affected more or less uniformly.

Localized muscle atrophy results from interference with the innervation and may be caused by traumatic denervation or by neuromuscular disorders, such as polio, the peripheral neuritides and a variety of fortunately rare degenerative neuropathies. Obviously, the distribution of the muscle atrophy depends upon the pattern of involvement of the nerves. Whole muscles, bundles of cells or only a single neuromuscular unit may be affected.

When the process is generalized or when large bundles of myocytes are involved, the affected muscles become shrunken and flabby. On the other hand, minute focal involvements may produce no appreciable loss of muscle mass, since adjacent unaffected fibers undergo compensatory hypertrophy.

Within the affected area, no matter how small, the histologic changes are uniform. These consist initially of progressive shrinkage of the myocytes as a result of resorption of the sarcoplasm. Eventually, the striations are lost and the myocytes may be converted into virtually hollow tubes, encased by the sarcolemma and lined by the nuclei. Brown atrophy becomes apparent, in the form of a golden yellow perinuclear lipochrome pigment. In severe cases, cell death ensues, with fibrous replacement. At this time, a scant lymphocytic infiltrate develops, but this is usually minimal.

PROGRESSIVE MUSCULAR DYSTROPHY

This term includes a group of genetically determined myopathies characterized by progressive atrophy or degeneration of increasing numbers of individual muscle cells. With time, there is a tendency for virtually all muscles of the body to become involved, leading to profound weakness and often death, usually from complications resulting from involvement of the respiratory muscles.

Morphology. The involved muscles are shrunken, pale and flabby. With the light microscope, individual muscle fibers can be seen to be randomly affected, so that myocytes in various stages of degeneration may lie adjacent to abnormally large ones (**pseudohypertrophy**) (Fig. 19–6). This haphazard involvement is in contrast to the uniformity seen with muscle atrophy, as was discussed earlier. Degenerative changes include focal vacuolation, hyalinization, fragmentation of the cytoplasm and shrinking from the investing sarcolemmal sheath. The nuclei frequently proliferate and become pyknotic. An infiltration of fibrous and fatty tissue partially compensates for the loss of muscle mass. Probably about 50 per cent of the myocytes of a muscle must be affected before disease is clinically apparent.

Clinical Course. The muscular dystrophies are traditionally subdivided according to differing patterns of initial muscle involvement, which in turn correlate fairly well with the type of genetic transmission. Despite such dif-

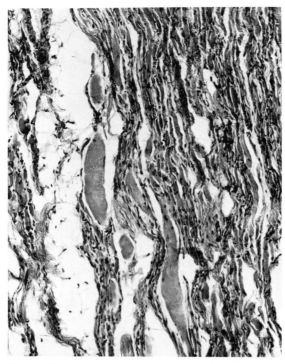

Figure 19–6. Muscular dystrophy, pseudohypertrophic pattern. The histologic detail of an involved muscle documents the extreme atrophy of some fibers with hypertrophy of other fibers. Strands of adipose tissue have appeared in the atrophic muscle on the left.

ferences, however, it should be remembered that the histologic changes are the same in all forms. The three major patterns are as follows:

A. Duchenne (pseudohypertrophic) muscular dystrophy
   1. Sex-linked recessive
      a. Aggressive
      b. Benign
   2. Autosomal recessive
B. Limb girdle muscular dystrophy: autosomal recessive (rarely dominant)
C. Facioscapulohumeral muscular dystrophy: autosomal dominant (rarely recessive)

The aggressive form of *Duchenne muscular dystrophy* is the most common, and certainly the most important of these disorders. Because it is transmitted as a sex-linked recessive, males are almost exclusively affected. The onset occurs soon after birth. Initially, the process involves the pelvic girdle, then extends to the shoulder girdle. *A characteristic feature is enlargement or "pseudohypertrophy" of the calf muscles.* As would be expected, increased serum levels of GOT, GPT, LDH, CPK, aldolase and myoglobin are present as reflections of leakage of these substances from the damaged muscle fibers. Complete paraly-

sis and death usually ensue within the first two decades of life.

A benign variant of the Duchenne type may begin as late as the fourth decade, and this form encroaches only slightly on the normal life span.

The *limb girdle pattern* of progressive muscular dystrophy usually begins in childhood. Since it is transmitted as an autosomal recessive, males and females are affected equally. In contrast to the situation with Duchenne muscular dystrophy, *pseudohypertrophy is not prominent.* The prognosis is variable; most patients survive for two to three decades with their disease.

Facioscapulohumeral muscular dystrophy, as the name implies, initially involves the muscles of the face and shoulder girdle. It usually begins in adolescence. It, too, affects males and females equally, since it is transmitted as an autosomal dominant. Here again, *pseudohypertrophy is not a regular feature.* Complete disability is rare and life expectancy is normal.

MYASTHENIA GRAVIS

This is a remitting-relapsing neuromuscular disorder characterized by paroxysmal weakness of skeletal muscles. Most likely there is a neuromuscular conduction block, since no consistent morphologic changes are seen within the involved muscles. However, there is a strong correlation with abnormalities of the thymus gland. Myasthenia gravis may be seen at any age in either sex but it is most prevalent among young women.

Etiology and Pathogenesis. It will be recalled from the discussion of the thymus on page 617 that about 75 per cent of patients with myasthenia gravis have hyperplasia of the thymus, characterized by the development of lymphoid follicles, and about 25 per cent have thymomas. Very often the two thymic lesions coexist. Because of the pivotal role of the thymus in the development of the immune system, it is not surprising that some immunologic derangement be sought as the cause of myasthenia gravis. Antibodies cross reactive to thymic tissue and striated muscle have been described in 30 to 75 per cent of patients with myasthenia gravis, particularly in those with thymomas. In addition, these patients often have a variety of other autoantibodies, such as antibodies against thyroglobulin, antinuclear antibodies and rheumatoid factor (White and Marshall, 1962). What is the basis for the cross reactivity of antibodies between thymic tissue and striated muscle? Electron microscopic studies have disclosed cells resembling striated muscle in the thymus glands of many species and in the fetal thymus in man (myoid cells). Accordingly, it has been proposed that an abnormal thymic reaction directed against myoid cells would also affect the muscles (Goldstein, 1971). It should be emphasized, however, that the mere existence of autoantibodies does not prove that they are of pathogenetic significance. Indeed, serum antibodies cross reactive with thymus and muscle are seen in patients who have thymomas but who do *not* have myasthenia gravis. This would argue against their role in any neuromuscular block (Strauss, 1968). Recently it has been reported that there is a serum factor (possibly distinct from the anti-muscle antibodies) in patients with myasthenia gravis which is capable of blocking the receptors for acetylcholine at the neuromuscular junction (Bender et al., 1975). Some workers believe that thymopoietin itself may be the serum factor which causes the neuromuscular block. They propose that abnormal amounts of this hormone may be liberated into the circulation as a result of a primary lesion of the thymus (Goldstein and Schlesinger, 1975).

We know even less of the etiology of myasthenia gravis than of its pathogenesis. There is some suggestion of an infectious etiology. It has been shown that thymocytes in patients with myasthenia gravis show new antigenic determinants on their surface. Moreover, an increased number of B cells was found within the cell population of these abnormal thymuses (Abdou et al., 1974). It has been speculated that these changes could result from a chronic nonlytic viral infection of the thymus, perhaps permitted by genetic factors (Datta and Schwartz, 1974). With regard to a genetic influence, it has been shown that there is a higher than expected frequency of the HL-A8 histocompatibility antigen in patients with myasthenia gravis, particularly in young women with thymic hyperplasia. Interestingly, among older men with thymomas, the increased risk is instead associated with the HL-A3 antigen (Fritze et al., 1974).

Morphology. In most cases, the muscles appear entirely normal, both grossly and microscopically. Occasionally, small interstitial accumulations of lymphocytes are found (**lymphorrhages**). The thymus usually shows hyperplasia, with the abnormal development of germinal follicles within the medulla. In addition, any of the three patterns of thymic tumors may be present (reference should be made to page 617 for a description of thymic hyperplasia and the thymomas).

Clinical Course. Myasthenia gravis manifests itself by rapid and profound fatigue of striated muscles. The muscles most severely involved are those in most active use: the extraocular muscles and those of the face, tongue and extremities. The primary danger to these patients is involvement of the respiratory muscles, which may lead to asphyxia. Usually the disease follows a long chronic course, interspersed with periods of spontaneous remission. The prognosis is highly variable and is not predictable in any one patient. Thymectomy produces dramatic improvement in some patients. In a large series of patients, 33 per cent died within six years of the onset of their illness, usually from respiratory involvement with superimposed pneumonia.

TRICHINOSIS

This common disorder is caused by infection with the larvae of *Trichinella spiralis.* Some degree of infection, often subclinical, has been found in up to 17 per cent of autopsies in the United States. Man contracts the disease by eating poorly cooked infected meat, usually pork. The larvae, which are encysted in the muscle of the meat, are released within the stomach and mature to adult worms within the duodenum. Here the female worm penetrates partially through the wall of the duodenum and her newly deposited larvae thus gain access to the bloodstream. They circulate throughout the pulmonic and systemic systems, ultimately emerging from capillaries to invade their preferred sites. The striated muscles provide the most suitable environment for their survival. The heaviest concentrations are usually found in the diaphragm and in the gluteus, pectoral, deltoid, gastrocnemius and intercostal muscles. The brain and the heart also are frequently involved. However, no tissue or organ is exempt.

In the striated muscles, the larva penetrates a muscle fiber, destroying it and evoking an inflammatory reaction characterized principally by lymphocytes and eosinophils. Later the focus becomes scarred, and a cystic wall is deposited about the coiled larva, which remains viable for many years (Fig. 19-7). Within two years, the cyst becomes calcified, and multiple foci can be demonstrated in the muscles on x-ray. In the heart, the larvae evoke a widespread interstitial myocarditis, undergo necrosis and do *not* become encysted. Invasion of the central nervous system is usually reflected by a diffuse mononuclear infiltration in the leptomeninges and by the development of focal gliosis in and about the small capillaries of the brain substance.

The clinical manifestations of trichinosis depend on the size of the infection and on the stage of the involvement. Since much of the meat in the United States is not inspected for trichina infection, it is likely that many, if not most, individuals have had some experience with the parasite. However, in most of these cases, the disease is mild or subclinical. It should be emphasized, nevertheless, that

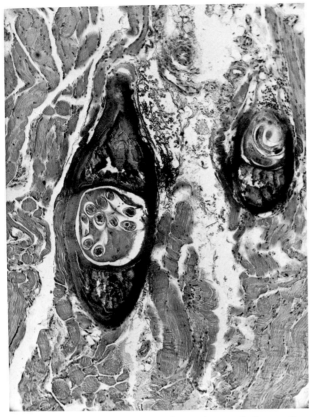

Figure 19-7. Trichinosis. Several encysted parasites are seen in striated muscle. The one on the right shows a coiled worm cut longitudinally. On the left, the parasite has been cut in numerous cross sections.

the only certain protection against serious trichinosis is adequate cooking of meat. With severe infection, the stage of invasion of the intestinal mucosa is usually marked by vomiting and diarrhea. During the hematogenous dissemination and muscular invasion, fever and widespread aches and pains appear. Muscle aches may persist. Often, invasion of the lungs evokes cough and dyspnea. The central nervous system involvement leads to headaches, disorientation, delirium and other neurologic impairments. Heart failure may ensue when the myocardial injury is severe. The mortality rate is, however, low.

After the third week of the disease, precipitin, complement fixation and flocculation tests are positive except in overwhelming disease. The diagnosis may be established by muscle biopsy. In addition, it is strongly supported by the presence of a peripheral eosinophilia, which may constitute up to 70 per cent of the circulating white cell count.

MYOSITIS OSSIFICANS CIRCUMSCRIPTA (TRAUMATIC MYOSITIS OSSIFICANS)

Occasionally, traumatic injury to muscle, usually accompanied by considerable hemorrhage, is followed by ossification at the site of damage. In the course of organization of the hemorrhage, cartilage may form and be followed by endochondral ossification, or calcification may occur en masse and be followed by ossification. The origin of the osteoblasts that lay down the bone is uncertain. Either they arise in situ from mesenchymal cells, or they are derived from adjacent periosteum, which is involved in the muscular injury. *Aside from the attendant pain, swelling and tenderness, the major significance of this lesion lies in the possibility of its being confused both clinically and histologically with a bone tumor.*

DESMOID TUMOR

This refers to a curious fibrous tumor which arises from the aponeuroses of muscles. Although histologically it appears quite benign and only rarely, if ever, does it metastasize, these lesions are locally invasive, hence they are best classified as very low-grade fibrosarcomas. About 70 per cent of desmoids occur in young women, frequently following pregnancy, and these usually affect the musculature of the anterior abdominal wall. However, men may also develop desmoids, and nearly any muscle of the body may be involved.

Desmoids appear grossly as firm, gray-white, poorly demarcated masses varying in size from small nodules 1 to 2 cm. in diameter to large masses up to 15 cm. in diameter. Microscopically, they resemble a somewhat cellular fibroma, with abundant collagenous fibrous tissue. The fibrocytes, which are uniform and innocent-appearing, insinuate themselves between muscle groups and individual muscle cells, frequently destroying the trapped myocytes.

The clinical presentation is of a slowly enlarging subcutaneous mass, sometimes but not usually producing pain.

RHABDOMYOSARCOMA

These are highly malignant, fortunately rare tumors of striated muscle. Three distinct histologic and clinical patterns are recognized: (1) adult pleomorphic (about 15 per cent), (2) embryonal alveolar (45 per cent), and (3) embryonal botryoid (40 per cent). Although the adult pattern is least common, it will be described first, since it is more likely to contain the specific features indicating its origin from striated muscles.

Adult pleomorphic rhabdomyosarcomas occur in either sex, usually between the ages of 30 and 60 years. The lower extremity is most often involved. The tumor mass grows extremely rapidly and may be as large as 25 cm. in diameter when the patient comes to medical attention. Grossly, these tumors are composed of soft, gray-red, fish-flesh tissue, with areas of necrosis and hemorrhage. Since the tumors are typically quite pleomorphic, the light microscope may show a variety of cell types—sometimes racket-shaped cells with single, long protoplasmic processes, occasionally ovoid giant cells with peripheral vacuoles separated by thin strands of cytoplasm (**spider-web cells**), but most often sheets of varying-sized, totally undifferentiated cells. With luck, persistent searching will usually disclose characteristic striated cells which resemble normal myocytes. **Only with the identification of such cells can the diagnosis of rhabdomyosarcoma be made with certainty.**

Embryonal alveolar rhabdomyosarcomas occur almost exclusively in children. They usually develop in a lower or upper extremity, but occasionally involve the trunk. Grossly, these tumors may be similar in appearance to the adult rhabdomyosarcoma, although they rarely achieve such massive dimensions. Microscopically, there are round to oval to occasionally elongated cell forms which show little resemblance to adult muscle cells. These are arranged in small nests or rosettes separated by an interlacing fibrous stroma. This scaffolding somewhat resembles the alveolar pattern of the lung, with the neoplastic cells filling the "alveolar" spaces; hence the name. Here and there racket-shaped cells and more differentiated striated cells can be identified.

Embryonal botryoid rhabdomyosarcomas occur most commonly in the genitourinary tract in adults of either sex and in the biliary tree, head and neck of children. Those of the vagina are often termed **sarcoma botryoides** and were described briefly on page 564. The term botryoid (grape-like) refers to the gross appearance of these cancers, which grow as large pendunculated, multilobate masses resembling a cluster of grapes. The predominant cell type within these tumors is an undifferentiated, small round cell having a large hyperchromatic central nucleus and scant cytoplasm. An abundant loose myxoid stroma may be present, simulating a myxosarcoma. With careful searching, racket shapes and elongated ribbon cells with cross striations can be found.

Rhabdomyosarcomas, especially the adult pattern, vary greatly in their growth rates and clinical behavior. In general, however, they are ugly tumors and widespread dissemination occurs early. Five-year survival is less than 10 per cent (Pories, 1970–71).

REFERENCES

Abdou, N. I., et al.: The thymus in myasthenia gravis. New Eng. J. Med., *291*:1271, 1974.

Baylink, D. J., et al.: Two new methods for the study of osteoporosis and other metabolic bone disease. II. Vertebral bone densitometry. Lahey Clin. Bull., *13*:217, 1964.

Bender, A. N., et al.: Myasthenia gravis: a serum factor blocking acetylcholine receptors of the human neuromuscular junction. Lancet, *1*:607, 1975.

Bordier, P., et al.: Effectiveness of parathyroid hormone, calcitonin and phosphate on bone cells in Paget's disease. Am. J. Med., *56*:850, 1974.

Boutouras, G. D., and Goodsitt, E. J.: Sarcoma arising in Paget's disease. Report of two cases and review of the literature. J. Internat. Coll. Surg., *40*:380, 1963.

Cortes, E. P., et al.: Amputation and adriamycin in primary osteosarcoma. New Eng. J. Med., *291*:998, 1974.

Datta, S. K., and Schwartz, R. S.: Infectious (?) myasthenia. New Eng. J. Med., *291*:1304, 1974.

Davidson, P. T., and Horowitz, I.: Skeletal tuberculosis. Am. J. Med., *48*:77, 1970.

Dudl, R. J., et al.: Evaluation of intravenous calcium as therapy for osteoporosis. Am. J. Med., *55*:631, 1973.

Editorial: Research into calcium metabolism. Brit. Med. J., *2*:528, 1969.

Editorial: Pathogenesis of osteoarthrosis. Lancet, *2*:1131, 1973.

Editorial: Finger clubbing. Lancet, *1*:1285, 1975.

Evens, R. G., and Bartter, F. C.: Hereditary aspects of Paget's disease (osteitis deformans). J.A.M.A., *205*:900, 1968.

Firat, D., and Stutzman, L.: Fibrous dysplasia of the bone. Review of twenty-four cases. Am. J. Med., *44*:421, 1968.

Fraumeni, J. F.: Stature and malignant tumors of bone in childhood and adolescence. Cancer, *20*:179, 1945.

Freydinger, J. E., et al.: Sarcoma complicating Paget's disease of bone. A study of seven cases with report of one long survival after surgery. Arch. Path., *75*:496, 1963.

Fritze, D., et al.: HL-A antigens in myasthenia gravis. Lancet, *1*:240, 1974.

Garn, S. M., et al.: Bone loss as a general phenomenon in man. Fed. Proc., *26*:1729, 1967.

Goldstein, G.: Myasthenia gravis and the thymus. Ann. Rev. Med., *22*:119, 1971.

Goldstein, G., and Schlesinger, D. H.: Thymopoietin and myasthenia gravis: neostigmine-responsive neuromuscular block produced in mice by a synthetic peptide fragment of thymopoietin. Lancet, *2*:256, 1975.

Hamilton, C. R., Jr.: Effects of synthetic salmon calcitonin in patients with Paget's disease of bone. Am. J. Med., *56*:315, 1974.

Harris, W. H., and Heaney, R. P.: Skeletal renewal and metabolic bone disease. New Eng. J. Med., *280*:303, 1969.

Huvos, A. G., et al.: Bone sarcomas arising in fibrous dysplasia. J. Bone Joint Surg., *54*:1047, 1972.

Jaffe, N., et al.: Adjuvant methotrexate and citrovorum-factor treatment of osteogenic sarcoma. New Eng. J. Med., *291*:994, 1974.

Lutwak, L.: Symposium on osteoporosis. Nutritional aspects of osteoporosis. J. Amer. Geriat. Soc., *17*:115, 1969.

Mankin, H. J.: The reaction of articular cartilage to injury and osteoarthritis. New Eng. J. Med., *291*:1335, 1974.

Marcove, R. C., et al.: Vaccine trials for osteogenic sarcoma. CA, *23*:74, 1973.

McKenna, R. J., et al.: Osteogenic sarcoma arising in Paget's disease. Cancer, *17*:42, 1964.

Morgan, D. E.: Osteomalacia and osteoporosis. Postgrad. Med. J., *44*:621, 1968.

Newton-John, H. F., and Morgan, D. B.: The loss of bone with age, osteoporosis and fractures. Clin. Orthop., *71*:229, 1970.

Nordin, B. E. D.: Clinical significance and pathogenesis of osteoporosis. Brit. Med. J., *1*:571, 1971.

Palmieri, G. M. A., et al.: Calcitonin in steroid-induced osteoporosis. New Eng. J. Med., *290*:1490, 1974.

Pories, W. J.: Soft tissue sarcomas. *In* Rubin, P. (ed.): Clinical Oncology for Medical Students and Physicians. 3rd ed. Rochester, N.Y., American Cancer Society, 1970–71, p. 299.

Radin, E. I., et al.: Subchondral bone changes in patients with early degenerative joint disease. Arth. Rheum., *13*:400, 1970.

Skosey, J. L.: Some basic aspects of bone metabolism in relation to osteoporosis. Med. Clin. N. Amer., *54*:141, 1970.

Stradford, H. T.: Bone tumors. *In* Rubin, P. (ed.): Clinical Oncology for Medical Students and Physicians. 3rd ed. Rochester, N.Y., American Cancer Society, 1970–71, p. 290.

Strauss, A. J. L.: Myasthenia gravis, autoimmunity and the thymus. Adv. Int. Med., *14*:241, 1968.

Weiss, C.: Ultrastructural characteristics of osteoarthritis. Fed. Proc., *32*:1459, 1973.

White, R. G., and Marshall, A. H. E.: The autoimmune response in myasthenia-gravis. Lancet, *2*:120, 1962.

CHAPTER 20
The Nervous System

It is difficult not to wax lyrical about the brain, perhaps because the brain not only controls the entire body but may be considered to do so for its own purposes—to perceive, feel and think; above all, to exist. The spinal cord and peripheral nerves may be considered intermediaries between brain and body.

Although the disease processes which afflict the nervous system are much the same as those which occur elsewhere in the body, three special features of the nervous system modify the expression of disease. These special features include: (1) the presence of unique cell types, i.e., the neurons and glia, (2) the correlation between function and loca-

tion in the nervous system, especially within the brain, and (3) the snug encasement of the brain by the skull. All three profoundly influence the response of the nervous system to a host of diseases and so will be discussed before going on to the presentation of individual disorders.

NEURONS AND GLIA—RESPONSE TO INJURY

The neurons and the glia (astrocytes, oligodendroglia and microglia) show limited and fairly stereotyped patterns of response to injury. Although some diseases attack one or more of these cell types selectively, their vulnerability to a nonselective influence, such as hypoxia, is in the following order (from most to least vulnerable): neurons, myelin sheaths, oligodendroglia, astrocytes, microglia, blood vessels. Although the glia may survive influences which destroy the neurons, any damage to neurons is almost invariably accompanied by some glial response.

NEURONS

The neuron reacts to disease in three ways. (1) Ischemia or an overwhelming acute toxic or infectious disorder may lead to **acute necrosis.** The neuron becomes shrunken and angular, with prominent processes (Fig. 20–1). The nucleus becomes pyknotic. The pigmented Nissl substance (endoplasmic reticulum) in the cytoplasm disappears **(chromatolysis),** and the cytoplasm assumes a homogeneous, brightly eosinophilic appearance. It should be remembered that by the time these changes are appreciated with the light microscope, the cell has been dead many hours. Thus, if the patient dies immediately after the neuronal injury, no morphologic changes whatever are apparent. If, however, the patient survives, at least for some hours, the above changes develop, followed ultimately by fragmentation of the cell processes, disruption of the membranes and autolysis or phagocytosis of the cell debris. An occasional dead cell is not removed, and can be seen to persist as a faint ghost. (2) A number of chronic disorders are associated with **degeneration** of neurons. Like acute necrosis, degeneration is characterized by contraction of the cell body. However, the cytoplasm becomes basophilic rather than eosinophilic, reflecting clumping and increased prominence of the Nissl substance. Lipofuscin pigment very commonly is seen within the cytoplasm of degenerating neurons. As long as the nucleus remains intact, these changes may be reversible. However, if the degenerative process continues, the nucleus ultimately becomes pyknotic and fragments. From this point on, the changes are basically the same as those of acute necrosis, with rupture of the cell membranes and autolysis or phagocytosis of the cell debris. Here, too, degenerated neurons sometimes remain intact, appearing as pallid ghosts. (3) When the axon is injured or severed, the cell body undergoes a series of alterations, termed the **axonal reaction.** Very similar changes may result from ischemia, which is not sufficiently intense or sudden to cause acute necrosis. They may also occur after many types of acute toxic or infectious injury. At first the neuron swells and loses its angularity, and the nucleus is displaced to the periphery opposite the axon hillock. The Nissl substance disappears, first near the center of the cell **(central chromatolysis).** Up to this point the neuron is still alive and the changes are reversible. Thus, the axonal reaction signifies a neuron in crisis. In the peripheral nervous system,

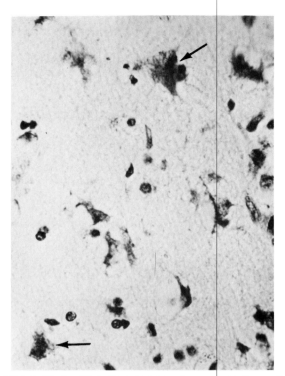

Figure 20–1. Shrunken and angular neurons (arrows) in the cerebral cortex, caused by ischemia.

the axon may regenerate following injury, in which case the cell body eventually resumes its normal appearance. Although axon regeneration cannot occur in the CNS, the cell body may be restored. Alternatively, the changes may progress to cell death. In the latter case, there is complete chromatolysis and the cytoplasm becomes vacuolated. With appropriate silver stains, it can be seen that the neurofibrils have disappeared. Ultimately, the cell processes and cell membranes fragment. These changes are irreversible and, as is the case with the other types of neuronal death, the neuron may disappear, or it may persist as a faint ghost.

MYELIN SHEATH

Death of the neuron or loss of the axon is always accompanied by degeneration of the **myelin sheath.** The converse is not true, however. A group of disorders is characterized by loss of myelin with preservation of the cell body and axon. The term **demyelinization** customarily refers to this selective phenomenon. The myelin progressively loses its affinity for myelin stains and ultimately appears as an unstained area surrounding the axon. However, the lipid breakdown products from the degenerating myelin stain black with sudan black and it can be seen with this stain that the myelin undergoes fragmentation and eventual phagocytosis.

OLIGODENDROGLIA

The most vulnerable of the glia are the oligodendroglia. These are normally found (1) streaming between the axons of the white matter, where they elaborate and maintain the myelin sheath, and (2) clustered about the neurons in the gray matter. In some of the demyelinating processes, the oligodendrocytes of the white matter degenerate. In the gray matter, the oligodendrocytes swell in response to nearly any type of injury to the neuron. They may also increase in number about a damaged neuron (**satellitosis**).

ASTROCYTES

The term **gliosis** refers to the proliferative response of the astrocyte to neuronal injury. These cells may be considered the CNS analogue of the fibroblast, although there are important differences. Nearly any degenerative or destructive process in the CNS is accompanied by proliferation of astrocytes. Initially the astrocytes enlarge, their cytoplasm becomes finely granular and the cell processes become longer, thicker and more numerous. Increased numbers of fibrils are formed within the cytoplasm and move outward into the cell processes. When the original insult is of a chronic degenerative nature, the astrocytes and their processes align themselves in parallel rows along the destroyed myelin sheaths (**isomorphous gliosis**). Acute destructive lesions, such as infarction, elicit a somewhat different astrocytic response. By the fourth day, hypertrophy and proliferation of astrocytes can be seen at the margin of the area of necrosis. Sometimes these cells become massively swollen with an eosinophilic cytoplasm (**gemistocytic astrocytes**). Multinucleated giant astrocytes may also be seen. The prominent glial processes assume an irregular tangled pattern (**anisomorphic gliosis**), and it is the intertwining of these fibrous processes that forms the typical glial scar. When the area of destruction is small, the defect may be completely filled by the glial scar. Often, however, shaggy cystic areas remain, sometimes criss-crossed by strings of glial processes. When the lesion is extensive, with violation of the blood-brain barrier, fibroblasts from the blood vessels or meninges enter the area and participate in scar formation. It should be remembered that severe insults may destroy the astrocytes themselves. In this case, the astrocyte swells, its processes fragment, the nucleus becomes pyknotic and the cell remnants ultimately undergo phagocytosis.

MICROGLIA

The microglia are part of the reticuloendothelial system—the histiocytes of the CNS. As the hardiest of the specialized cells of the CNS, they may remain alone in a focus of injury to remove the remnants of their fallen compatriots. This process is termed **neuronophagia** and begins about 48 hours after the onset of a destructive or demyelinating process. The microglia begin to evolve into **compound granular cells** (or **gitter cells**). Their cell processes are retracted, the cell assumes an enlarged, globoid appearance and the cytoplasm becomes finely granular. These scavengers increase in number in the injured focus over a period of days to weeks. A few may remain in the area for years. It is possible that monocytes from injured blood vessels contribute significantly to their numbers (Escourolle and Poirier, 1973). In more indolent pathologic processes, in many of the encephalitides and in paretic neurosyphilis (p. 664), the microglia assume a different form, termed **rod cells.** Here too the cell processes are retracted, but both the cytoplasm and nucleus become elongated or, as the name implies, rod-shaped. Especially in neurosyphilis, the rod cell cytoplasm may contain iron deposits.

CORRELATION BETWEEN FUNCTION AND LOCATION—CLINICAL IMPLICATIONS

Some organs, such as the liver, have a uniform population of parenchymal cells. One hepatocyte is much like another, and when the liver is injured or diseased the important consideration is the number of cells affected and not their location within the organ. It is true that in other organs, such as the kidney, there is more than one parenchymal cell type. But within each type the cells are homogeneous and the precise location of injury generally has little influence on functional impairment. In contrast, each locus within the nervous system corresponds to a different bodily process. Thus, the clinical effect of a lesion depends largely on its location within the nervous system. For example, injury in the precentral gyrus of the frontal cortex may produce a contralateral hemiparesis; the same injury in the posterior aspect of the superior temporal gyrus instead causes a receptive aphasia. Moreover, the location of a lesion may be far more important than its size. A small infarct of the prefrontal cortex may be of no apparent significance; in contrast, a lesion of the same size in the medulla oblongata may cause instant death. In general, as one proceeds caudally from the cerebral cortex (where there is dispersal of the neurons over a fairly large area) toward the medulla oblongata (where all the fibers and nuclei lie together in a relatively compact area), pathologic processes have increasingly dire consequences.

Before leaving the subject of the correlation between function and location in the nervous system, we should mention its importance to the clinician. Certain signs or symptom complexes enable the neurologist to infer the exact location of the causative lesion. Since many disorders tend to be selective for certain sites in the brain, this knowledge may in turn suggest the probable nature of the disease (diagnosis). Therapeutic and prognostic implications follow. Practical significance aside, deducing the location of a nervous system lesion from the pattern of functional impairment is an irresistible intellectual exercise for many neurologists.

ENCASEMENT OF THE BRAIN BY THE SKULL—EDEMA, HYDROCEPHALUS, INCREASED INTRACRANIAL PRESSURE AND HERNIATION

No other organ has so rigid an encasement as the brain. Although this provides great protection against injury, it becomes detrimental when there is any expansion of the intracranial contents. No matter what the mechanism, the rigid skull severely limits volume expansion and the result is a mounting intracranial pressure. This has grave implications for the patient, as will be described later. Such expansion results from: (1) space-occupying lesions, e.g., tumors; (2) edema of the brain; and (3) an abnormal accumulation of cerebrospinal fluid in the ventricles (hydrocephalus). Space-occupying lesions will be described later. Here we say a few words about edema and hydrocephalus.

EDEMA OF THE BRAIN

Edema as a cause of increased intracranial pressure is particularly important because it so frequently occurs as a response to a host of insults. In addition, it often accompanies and contributes to the increased intracranial pressure caused by a space-occupying lesion or by hydrocephalus.

The morphologic appearance of the edematous brain is striking. Grossly, it is heavy and boggy. The gyri are flattened and the sulci are obliterated. When there is no concomitant hydrocephalus, the ventricular system is compressed. Coronal sections show a blurred demarcation between white and gray matter, with the white matter relatively more voluminous than the gray. Microscopically, there is distention of the perivascular spaces and a loose appearance of the parenchyma. Myelin stains show pallor and splitting of the myelin lamellae. Electron microscopy has demonstrated that the increased fluid content is principally intracellular. In particular, there is usually swelling of the perivascular foot processes of the astrocytes, as well as of the neurons themselves. Two mechanisms of edema formation in the brain have been distinguished—vasogenic and cytotoxic—although there is much overlap. The vasogenic form is caused by damage to or alterations in the blood vessels. The edema fluid, which has a composition similar to plasma, is extracellular as well as intracellular. It accumulates chiefly in the white matter. The cytotoxic form reflects some cellular dysfunction. The fluid accumulation is almost entirely intracellular. The particular cell popula-

tion involved depends on the nature of the insult (Manz, 1974).

HYDROCEPHALUS

Hydrocephalus is another cause of increased intracranial pressure. It is almost always the result of some degree of obstruction of the third ventricle; the aqueduct of Sylvius (leading from the third to the fourth ventricle); the fourth ventricle; or the basal foramina (the foramen of Magendie and foramina of Luschka, leading from the fourth ventricle to the subarachnoid spaces). When there is no access between the ventricles and the subarachnoid spaces, the condition is termed **noncommunicating hydrocephalus.** When some access remains, the result is **communicating hydrocephalus.** In both there is increased cerebrospinal fluid (CSF) pressure somewhere in the system.

Whatever the cause, hydrocephalus is characterized by flattening of the gyri and obliteration of the sulci.

However, rather than the compression of the ventricles characteristic of simple edema, there is instead distention, sometimes to massive proportions. In extreme cases the cerebral cortex is converted to an atrophic shell surrounding an enormous bag of fluid. Usually there is some degree of secondary edema of the white matter immediately surrounding the ventricles.

The underlying causes of hydrocephalus are varied. Many cases result from congenital malformations near the base of the skull which interfere with the free flow of CSF. Others are due to tumors which obstruct the ventricular system or to scarring from infectious processes, usually tuberculous meningitis. Often there is no obvious cause. In some of these idiopathic cases it is assumed that there is overproduction of CSF by the choroid plexuses or, alternatively, under-resorption by the arachnoid villi. Rarely, hydrocephalus develops in middle age without any obvious anatomic abnormality and with no increase in CSF pressure ("*normal pressure hydrocephalus*"). Along with many other forms of hydrocephalus, it subsides when the CSF is surgically diverted by a ventriculojugular shunt. *Hydrocephalus ex vacuo* refers to a compensatory increase in CSF volume when there is primary atrophic disease of the brain. It, too, is associated with normal CSF pressure. The congenital malformations which lead to hydrocephalus are particularly important. They include the *Arnold-Chiari malformation* (Fig. 20–2), which involves herniation of the posterior cerebellum and the medulla through the foramen magnum, often accompanied by a meningomyelocele and platybasia (flattening of the base of the skull); the *Dandy-Walker-Taggart syndrome*, which involves occlusion of the foramina of Magendie and Luschka, oc-

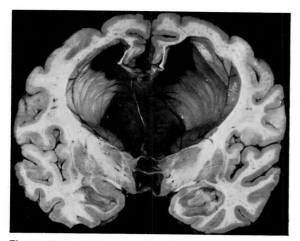

Figure 20–2. Hydrocephalus of moderate degree. This was associated with an Arnold-Chiari malformation. The basal ganglia have been displaced downward and laterally, and the overlying corpus callosum has been thinned.

cipital meningocele and hypoplasia of the cerebellar vermis; and *stenosis of the aqueduct of Sylvius*, which may or may not accompany the Arnold-Chiari malformation. The severity of these deformities varies. Some, such as complete obstruction of the aqueduct, are incompatible with life. Others may not become manifest until adulthood. When hydrocephalus develops in the fetus or in the infant before closure of the cranial sutures, considerable expansion of the skull is possible and the head may become grotesquely enlarged. Mental retardation often, but not always, results. When hydrocephalus develops after the sutures have closed, it is even more destructive to the brain since the skull can no longer yield to the pressure.

INCREASED INTRACRANIAL PRESSURE

Nearly any type of brain disorder may lead to increased intracranial pressure through one or more of three mechanisms (see p. 642). Hemorrhage and infarct, meningitis, encephalitis and brain abscesses, tumors, trauma and toxic encephalopathies—all may cause increased intracranial pressure. This in turn is the proximate cause of death of a great many patients with a variety of intracranial diseases. As such, it is analogous to CHF in heart disease or uremia in kidney disease.

In its early stages there are three clinical hallmarks of increased intracranial pressure: (1) headache, (2) vomiting, and (3) papilledema, or swelling of the optic discs. Later, drowsiness and coma, sometimes accompanied by generalized seizures, may follow. Headache is principally associated with an asymmetric rise in pressure, and is probably caused by distortion of the dura mater and blood ves-

sels. Although the headache may be ipsilateral to the lesion, it is more often diffuse or localized at the base of the skull. Typically, it is most severe upon awakening in the morning. Vomiting reflects increased pressure in the posterior fossa. Papilledema results from compression of the optic nerves and blood vessels by the surrounding columns of cerebrospinal fluid. Often there are associated retinal hemorrhages. Prolonged papilledema leads to atrophy of the optic nerves with progressive loss of vision.

HERNIATION OF THE BRAIN

The most feared consequence of increased intracranial pressure is herniation of a portion of the brain from one dural compartment to another. It will be remembered that the cranial cavity is divided into incomplete compartments by two reflections of the dura. The first is the *falx cerebri*, which descends from the vault of the skull along the midline and separates the cerebral hemispheres. The second is the *tentorium cerebelli*, a transverse septum which extends forward from the back of the skull and separates the occipital lobes above from the cerebellum below. The brain stem passes through the incisura of the tentorium. *Herniation usually reflects some asymmetry in the pressure increase.*

Three types of herniation are of particular importance. The most frequent is herniation of the medial portion of the temporal lobe through the incisura of the tentorium cerebelli, so that it comes to lie alongside the midbrain in the incisura (**tentorial pressure cone**). This has several consequences. Compression of the midbrain leads to loss of consciousness. The oculomotor nerve is also likely to be compressed, leading to transient ipsilateral pupillary constriction followed by fixed dilatation. Hemorrhages and infarcts appear in the midbrain and upper pons, as well as in the herniated portion of the temporal lobe. Compression of the aqueduct of Sylvius still further increases intracranial pressure, setting up a vicious circle. In the second type of herniation a pressure increase in the posterior fossa leads to herniation of the cerebellar tonsils through the foramen magnum (**foraminal** or **cerebellar pressure cone**). This compresses the medulla oblongata and usually results in instant death through failure of the cardiac and respiratory centers. In the third type, increased pressure in one cerebral hemisphere may cause the cingulate gyrus to herniate across the midline between the falx cerebri and the corpus callosum. This may cause obtundation, as well as shearing of the anterior cerebral arteries.

SUMMARY

Having discussed properties of the nervous system which are of particular importance in understanding neuropathology, we shall review them briefly before discussing individual diseases.

The first is the presence of cell types unique to the nervous system—namely, the neurons and glia. The neuron responds to a variety of insults in one of the three ways described—*acute necrosis*, *chronic degeneration* or *the axonal reaction*. The oligodendroglia may swell and cluster about the damaged neurons *(satellitosis)*, the astrocytes may proliferate and form a glial scar to replace dead neurons *(gliosis)* and the microglia may devour the debris as *compound granular cells* or become *rod cells*.

The second feature of the nervous system discussed was the correlation between location and function. Because of this correlation, the location of a pathologic process is often more important than its nature. Certainly the location determines the initial functional impairment.

Third, we discussed the implications of the encasement of the brain by the skull. Foremost among them is the ready development of *increased intracranial pressure* as a result of: (1) a space-occupying lesion, (2) edema from a variety of causes, or (3) hydrocephalus. The appearance of *edema of the brain* and the causes and morphology of *hydrocephalus* were described. Increased intracranial pressure may lead to *herniation of a portion of the brain*, the terminal event in a great many disorders of the brain.

In the discussions to follow, the many important diseases of the central nervous system (CNS) are presented first, followed by a much briefer presentation of disorders of the peripheral nerves. The diseases of the CNS are, in turn, classified according to etiology, where possible, and according to the dominant histopathologic process when the etiology is unknown. Thus we have: (1) trauma to the CNS, (2) vascular disease, (3) toxic, nutritional and metabolic disorders, (4) tumors, (5) infections, (6) the degenerative diseases, and (7) the demyelinating diseases. Classification by clinical presentation is, of course, impossible, since the clinical manifestations depend more on location than on the nature of the lesion.

TRAUMA TO THE CNS

In our era of violence, both accidental and otherwise, trauma to the CNS is an important cause of morbidity and mortality. Automobile accidents in particular contribute mightily to the incidence of CNS trauma. Either the brain or the spinal cord, or both, may be affected. Very often, of course, there are associated injuries elsewhere in the body.

TRAUMA TO THE BRAIN

Damage to the brain is rightly one of the most feared consequences of violence. Of 1000 consecutive head injuries studied, one in eight caused death within 2 days. Fully half resulted in prolonged morbidity. Frequent sequelae include hemiparesis, aphasia, hemianopsia, posttraumatic epilepsy, and the postconcussive syndrome, to be described later. Nearly three quarters of victims of head injury are males, tragically most between the ages of 10 and 40 years. The lesions produced are variable, depending on the location, type and force of the blow. The most important will be discussed separately. It should be remembered, however, that in most cases more than one of these lesions coexist. The pure form is relatively unusual.

Before describing the individual lesions, a few words should be said about the physics of blows to the head since this has an important bearing on the pathogenesis of brain injury. When the head sustains a blow, the skull, which is of lighter mass and first hit, accelerates and decelerates more rapidly than the brain. Thus the brain, with its greater inertia, is slammed against the walls of the skull. Moreover, unless the blow passes directly through the center of gravity, the head necessarily rotates to some degree. The skull rotates more than the brain and the outer layers of the brain rotate more than the deeper layers. This shearing force contributes importantly to the injury. It can be seen, then, that whereas the skull affords the brain a great deal of protection, it in some ways constitutes a liability.

CONCUSSION

This is defined as a transient impairment of consciousness without morphologic change. Its pathogenesis is poorly understood. It is of interest, however, that some degree of acceleration or deceleration seems to be necessary to produce concussion. If movement is prevented by holding the head immobile, a heavy blow may cause damage to the brain without loss of consciousness. In most cases of concussion, recovery of full consciousness occurs in, at most, 24 hours. However, a variety of troubling symptoms may persist for months. These include headache, irritability, unsteadiness, insomnia and personality changes.

CONTUSION

This refers to a bruise of the brain, that is, bleeding into brain tissue without disruption of its continuity. A blow to the head may cause a contusion in one of two ways. A relatively light sharp blow causes a contusion of the subjacent cortex by the instantaneous depression of the skull at the site of the blow. A heavier, blunter blow, however, accelerates the skull so that the brain is compressed against it at the site of the blow and torn away from it at the opposite side. Where the skull and brain separate there may be disruption of the leptomeninges with tearing of the blood vessels. When the skull decelerates, the brain continues to move and slams against the wall of the skull opposite the blow. When this happens, a *contrecoup lesion,* that is, a contusion on the side of the brain opposite the blow, is added to any damage at the site of the trauma. Thus, falls on the back of the head may produce contrecoup lesions in the tips of the frontal and temporal lobes; and falls on the front of the head may cause such lesions in the tips of the occipital lobes.

A contusion appears as a wedge-shaped area of hemorrhage with some degree of ischemic necrosis at the center. Eventually, large numbers of hemosiderin-filled scavengers appear, and there is scar formation by astrocytes and fibroblasts. As the scar retracts, the lesion appears as an orange-yellow depression on the surface of the brain. When the scarring is extensive, particularly if there has been disruption of the leptomeninges, the brain becomes plastered against the overlying dura to form a **meningocerebral cicatrix.**

Such scars are highly epileptogenic and frequently underlie the development of posttraumatic epilepsy.

LACERATION

Interruption of the continuity of brain tissue constitutes a laceration. By definition, penetrating injuries produce lacerations. In addition, lacerations are seen frequently with crushing injuries, and sometimes occur at the junction of gray and white matter in shearing injuries. A severe contrecoup lesion may take the form of a laceration rather than a contusion.

No matter what the cause, laceration of the brain implies some destruction of brain tissue and subsequent scarring. There is inevitably flooding of blood into the subarachnoid space. Even more than a contusion, a laceration tends to result in a meningocerebral cicatrix with possible posttraumatic epilepsy.

EPIDURAL HEMATOMA

Bleeding between the inner table of the skull and the dura produces an epidural hematoma. Usually this results from fracture of the skull with rupture of the middle meningeal artery or one of its branches. Because the blood cannot disseminate freely within this plane, it accumulates relatively slowly in a localized area.

Thus, after the injury these patients may be unconscious owing to a concussion, then regain consciousness (*lucid interval*), following which they may become progressively stuporous over the next several hours as the epidural hematoma slowly develops. It should be understood that not all patients exhibit a lucid interval, but when it is present it is of great diagnostic value. Unless evacuated, the hematoma progressively impinges on the underlying brain, causing a variety of neurologic deficits, convulsions, and eventual herniation and death.

SUBDURAL HEMATOMA

The formation of a hematoma between the dura and the leptomeninges may be acute or chronic. The acute form is often the result of a tear in the arachnoid and associated with a laceration or contusion.

Chronic subdural hematomas are of greater clinical interest because of their insidious behavior. They are usually caused by tearing of the bridging veins between the pia and the dura maters, usually as a result of a closed head injury (Fig. 20–3). Typically, they are seen in alcoholics and demented patients, that is, those who are especially vulnerable to falls. They may be bilateral owing to the contrecoup effect. The seepage of blood into the subdural space is very slow. It excites a fibroblastic response, and ultimately the

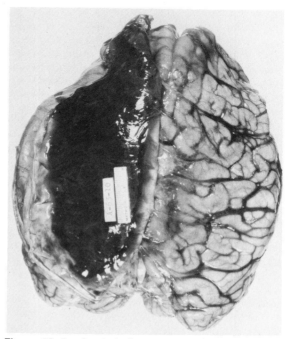

Figure 20–3. A relatively recent subdural hematoma revealed by folding back the covering dura mater.

hematoma becomes encapsulated in scar tissue. Sometimes the hematoma is resorbed, but usually it continues to expand as it accumulates fluid by osmosis.

Signs and symptoms develop weeks to months following the original trauma. Even then, manifestations are variable and may be quite subtle. Common indications include headache, increasing drowsiness, hemiparesis and seizures. In most cases an untreated chronic subdural hematoma eventually causes herniation and death. If the hematoma with its accumulated fluid is evacuated, recovery may be dramatic and complete. When the lesion is long-standing, however, there may be atrophy of the compressed hemisphere, with permanent neurologic deficits.

TRAUMA TO THE SPINAL CORD

Injury to the spinal cord is rarely lethal but may cause heart-rending disability. It is usually associated with fractures or dislocations of vertebrae. All of the types of trauma to the brain discussed earlier may be seen in the spinal cord.

Concussion of the spinal cord is extremely rare; it takes the form of loss of function for about 24 hours. **Contusion** results from a sudden blow, as from transient dislocation of a vertebra. **Laceration** may be caused by splintering of vertebrae; complete transection of the cord results from similar injuries. **Epidural** and **subdural hematomas** occur as complications of injury to the spinal cord just as they do with brain trauma. In addition, the anatomy of the vascular supply to the spinal cord is such that tearing of major blood vessels is especially likely with trauma (the vascular supply to the brain is less vulnerable). As a result, extensive areas of ischemic necrosis of the spinal cord (**myelomalacia**) may follow any form of injury. The nerve roots, too, may be stretched, bruised or compressed by trauma to the cord.

The signs and symptoms of spinal cord damage depend on the level and extent of injury. In general, paresthesias and weakness first develop distally, then extend upward toward the site of injury. As a contusion heals, there may be some recovery of function over a period of weeks. Lateral hemisection of the spinal cord produces the *Brown-Sequard syndrome*. This consists of ipsilateral loss of motor function and contralateral loss of sensation below the lesion.

VASCULAR DISEASE OF THE CNS

Vascular disease of the brain (especially "cerebrovascular accidents" or "strokes") is the third leading cause of death in the United States (Silverberg and Holleb, 1975). Spinal cord lesions resulting from vascular disease are very much less frequent and will not be discussed here. In the CNS, as elsewhere in the body, the significance of vascular disease lies primarily in the attendant ischemia of cells ordinarily served by the damaged vessels. The cells of the brain are especially vulnerable to such ischemia. This vulnerability in part reflects the enormous demands of nerve cells for oxygen. Although representing only about 2 per cent of the body's weight, the brain consumes 20 per cent of its oxygen. Moreover, this demand is invariable, since the brain cannot store energy nor temporarily exist by anaerobic metabolism. Hence, deprivation of oxygenated blood for even a few minutes leads to neuronal death. Not only is the brain extraordinarily vulnerable to ischemia, but also ischemic death of even a small area of brain tissue usually has clinical significance. There is virtually no functional reserve in the CNS.

Vascular disease of the CNS may produce either ischemic infarction or hemorrhage. Underlying causes are legion. *By far the most important etiologic factors are hypertension and atherosclerosis of the intracranial vessels.* Less important contributing disorders include the necrotizing arteritides, such as SLE (p. 184) and polyarteritis nodosa (p. 199); arteritis associated with certain chronic infections, such as meningovascular neurosyphilis (p. 664) and tuberculous meningitis (p. 664); and a variety of vascular anomalies, such as congenital aneurysms and arteriovenous malformations. In addition, some disorders lead to ischemia of the CNS without causing primary damage to the vessels. These include blood dyscrasias, such as leukemia and idiopathic thrombocytopenic purpura, which may lead to hemorrhage in the CNS with attendant ischemia; embolism to cerebral arteries from pathologic processes elsewhere in the body (to be discussed in a later section); and any cause of reduced delivery of oxygenated blood to the brain, such as hypotension, anemia or respiratory failure.

Vascular disease of the brain may be diffuse or localized. Any significant reduction in oxygen delivery to the brain as a whole (e.g., during shock) produces a diffuse morphologic pattern termed *anoxic encephalopathy.* This will be described in a later section. Suffice it to say here that all neurons are exposed to the same privations, although some are more vulnerable than others. Another form of diffuse vascular disease of the brain is *hypertensive encephalopathy,* considered in Chapter 13. Alternatively, vascular disease of the brain may be localized. An example is thrombosis complicating an atheromatous plaque in a cerebral artery. Hemorrhage or infarction resulting from such localized disease produces the clinical episode known as a *stroke* or *cerebrovascular accident (CVA)*. These terms have fallen into some disrepute; the first because it carries no information, the second because of concern about whether the disorder is actually "accidental." This concern would seem to represent a semantic problem at best and a knotty theologic dilemma at worst, and it may be desirable simply to find another name. Still the offending terms remain entrenched, albeit under siege, in the literature. It should be pointed out that sometimes a combination of diffuse and local factors operate together to bring about a CVA. For example, a congenital aneurysm may rupture only because of the stresses of hypertension. Or a slight drop in blood pressure may precipitate infarction only in the territory of an atheromatous vessel.

A few words should be said about the principal defenses of the brain against ischemic injury. These are twofold. *First, multiple homeostatic mechanisms, some of which are poorly understood, operate to maintain cerebral blood flow even in the face of profound hypotension.* An example of this defense is the powerful vasodilatation within the brain produced by low oxygen tension or high carbon dioxide tension in the blood. Thus, the brain, like the heart, is in this respect privileged. Even after other organs, such as the kidneys, are so deprived of blood that they can no longer function, blood flow within the brain may remain near normal levels. The second defense of the brain against ischemia is the existence of a rich network of collateral vessels. These include anastomoses between the external carotid artery and the ophthalmic artery, which can substitute for the internal carotid artery; the extensive anastomoses at the base of the brain where the internal carotid and vertebral-basilar systems join (circle of Willis); and the multitudinous superficial corticomeningeal anastomoses. If ischemic tissue can be perfused by collateral vessels within minutes after occlusion of the main channel, infarction may not occur. Even when the anastomotic network is not wholly adequate, it is usually sufficient to limit infarction to only a part of the area normally served by the occluded vessel.

In any given case of brain ischemia, whether diffuse or local, the adequacy of the brain's defense is itself modified by two factors. *The first is whether ischemia occurs suddenly or gradually.* Sudden hypotension is more likely to lead to anoxic encephalopathy than is a gradual lowering of the blood pressure. Likewise, sudden blockage of a vessel by an embolism may cause infarction, whereas gradual occlusion of the same vessel by an atheroma would not. *The second important factor modifying the defense of the brain against ischemia is the presence or absence of previous vascular disease.* A rather modest drop in blood pressure may cause anoxic encephalopathy in an elderly person with severe generalized atherosclerosis. By the same token, local infarction within the brain is more likely when a vessel is occluded if the potential collateral vessel is itself atherosclerotic. The latter situation may give rise to a *paradoxic infarct*, that is, infarction of an area outside that normally served by the involved vessel. For example, occlusion of the anterior cerebral artery may be adequately compensated by collateral vessels from the middle cerebral artery. Years later, stenosis of the middle cerebral artery might then produce infarction in the territory of the anterior cerebral artery.

It would be well to summarize our consideration of vascular disease of the CNS to this point. We have discussed reasons for the exceptional vulnerability of the CNS to ischemic injury. Such injury may be *diffuse* and take the form of *anoxic encephalopathy*, or it may be *local* and cause a *cerebrovascular accident (CVA)*, either through *hemorrhage* or through *infarction*. The most important *contributing factors* in cerebrovascular accidents are *hypertension* and *atherosclerosis*. The brain is defended against diffuse ischemic injury by systemic homeostatic mechanisms which augment cerebral blood flow during periods of hypoxia. The existence of multiple collateral networks offers further protection against local ischemic damage. The success of these defenses depends largely on whether the onset of ischemia is sudden or gradual and on whether there is preexisting vascular disease. With this recapitulation, we may turn our attention to the major morphologic patterns of ischemic injury: anoxic encephalopathy, hemorrhage and infarction.

ANOXIC ENCEPHALOPATHY

As indicated earlier, anoxic encephalopathy results from any process which diminishes the flow of oxygenated blood to the entire brain. As such, it may be caused by a multitude of conditions affecting either hemodynamics or the oxygen content of the blood. Foremost among such conditions are shock from any cause, respiratory failure, cardiac failure and profound anemia. Since lesions of the blood vessels are not the primary cause, anoxic encephalopathy may only loosely be considered a vascular disease. There is enormous variability in its severity. It ranges from a transient functional disorder to infarction of the entire brain. This is an extremely important entity, since it is the terminal event in a great many medical and surgical calamities. Indeed, if death be defined as irreversible loss of brain function, then anoxic encephalopathy may be considered our common end.

If the intensity or duration of hypoxia is slight, there may be no anatomic changes and the entire episode may be limited to euphoria followed by a period of drowsiness and impaired judgment. At the other extreme, oxygen deprivation which causes death within minutes likewise does not produce anatomic changes since such changes require hours to develop. Intermediate between these two extremes are the cases which can be discerned morphologically. In these cases, the brain is edematous and the demarcation between gray and white matter is blurred. Sometimes, for obscure reasons, the damage is more severe in some areas than in others, producing a patchy, muddy discoloration of the gray matter. Most vulnerable are the large cells of Sumner's sector of the hippocampus, the Purkinje cells of the cerebellum and the association centers of the cortex. The first microscopic changes are seen after 12 hours and consist of loss of staining properties. After 24 hours the affected neurons either swell or shrink. The swelling is similar to that of the axonal reaction (p. 640). More severely affected neurons undergo typical acute ischemic necrosis, becoming shrunken and angular (p. 640). Throughout the cortex, the injured or dying cells are interspersed with apparently unaffected ones. In severe cases, large areas of uniformly necrotic neurons are seen. If the patient survives, these are ultimately replaced by glial scars. In general, the resultant cortical atrophy is proportional to the number of neurons lost.

Clinically, severe hypoxia is manifested by unconsciousness, often with convulsions. The picture of decortication ensues. The head is retracted, the arms flexed and the legs extended. Secondary cerebral edema is common and may lead to herniation (p. 643). If the patient survives, severe neurologic sequelae may remain, including dementia, spasticity and recurrent seizures.

INTRACRANIAL HEMORRHAGE

Intracranial hemorrhage most often occurs either within the brain substance itself or within the subarachnoid space. Other locations are much less frequently involved. There is a strong association between hypertension and intracranial hemorrhage in either of these two locations. In addition, subarachnoid hemorrhage usually occurs at the site of a congenital saccular aneurysm (berry aneurysm). Other causes of intracranial hemorrhage include trauma, erosion of vessels by tumors, other vascular malformations and

blood dyscrasias which produce a hemorrhagic diathesis. Brain hemorrhage and subarachnoid hemorrhage will be discussed separately.

BRAIN HEMORRHAGE

Bleeding into the brain substance is a sudden, dramatic and highly lethal event. It usually occurs against a background of long-standing uncontrolled hypertension. Often there is concomitant atherosclerosis. In most cases the calamity is immediately preceded by some physical or emotional exertion which is thought to elevate the blood pressure still further. The incidence of brain hemorrhage is about the same in males and females; it increases with age until about age 65, when it reaches a plateau (Whisnant et al., 1971). In the early part of this century brain hemorrhage was by far the most frequent type of cerebrovascular accident. This predominance was in part artifactual, the result of a tendency to overdiagnose brain hemorrhage. However, there has no doubt been a real decline in its relative importance since 1920, probably due to several factors. These include a real increase in incidence of other forms of CVA, notably atherothrombotic infarction, and more recently, better control of hypertension. Various studies show that brain hemorrhage now constitutes from 7 to 17 per cent of

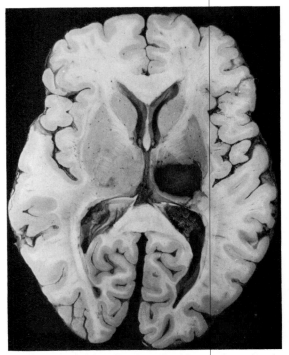

Figure 20–4. A localized cerebral hemorrhage involving the basal ganglia and the internal and external capsules.

CVA's (Kannel, 1971; Kuller et al., 1970; Whisnant et al., 1971). Despite its increasingly modest contribution to the incidence of CVA's, however, it remains the most lethal form.

In 80 per cent of cases the hemorrhage is in the cerebrum. Within the cerebrum, favored locations are the lateral basal ganglia, in particular the putamen and claustrum, and the external capsule (Fig. 20--4). In these sites the source of hemorrhage is often the lenticulostriate branch of the middle cerebral artery. Another 10 per cent occur in the midbrain or pons, and the remaining 10 per cent involve the cerebellum (Fig. 20—5). Regardless of the site of origin, brain hemorrhages tend to expand rapidly. Ultimately, they usually become massive lesions which may occupy most of an entire cerebral hemisphere. Very often rupture into the lateral ventricle occurs, causing massive intraventricular hemorrhage with sudden death. The gross appearance of these lesions is commensurate with their devastation. The hemorrhage appears as a large collection of blood with irregular margins which compresses and infiltrates the surrounding brain tissue. Small petechial hemorrhages are seen about its borders. The midline structures of the brain are distorted and the ipsilateral ventricle is all but obliterated. Cerebral edema is massive, in most cases leading to herniation of the brain (p.

643). Microscopically, it can be seen that at its center the hemorrhage completely destroys the normal architecture. In the surrounding tissue there is intense congestion of the blood vessels, with multiple small perivascular hemorrhages. In addition, the arterioles of the entire brain often show the changes of long-standing hypertension (p. 456). Polymorphonuclear exudation begins within hours. Compound granular cells begin to appear at two days and eventually become filled with hemosiderin. At about 10 days scar formation begins. Fibroblasts from the damaged blood vessels, as well as astrocytes, participate. If the patient survives, large lesions are ultimately converted into cystic scars with irregular orange-yellow borders. Smaller hemorrhages yield only pigmented areas of gliosis. Occasionally, multiple tiny scars of this type, termed "slit hemorrhages," are found on routine postmortem examination of the brains of hypertensive patients. These usually occur in the cerebrum at the junction of the white and gray matter. They indicate that tiny subclinical cerebral hemorrhages may occur.

The *classical* clinical picture of brain hemorrhage is, however, catastrophic. The onset is sudden and dramatic. Usually there is intense headache, sometimes accompanied by vomiting, and followed within minutes by loss of consciousness. Focal signs, of course, depend

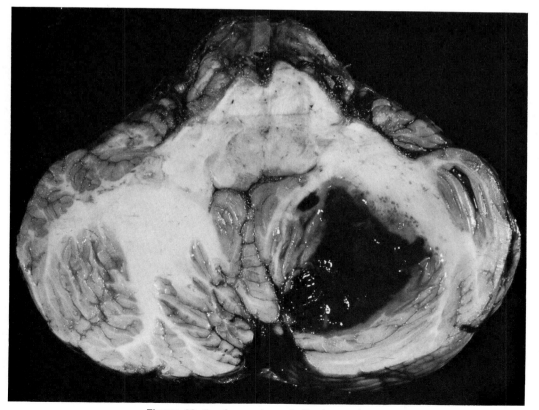

Figure 20—5. A recent cerebellar hemorrhage.

on the site of the hemorrhage. Cerebral hemorrhage usually produces a total contralateral hemiplegia, flaccid at the outset but later becoming spastic. Pontine hemorrhages are characterized by pinpoint pupils and hyperpyrexia. Cerebellar hemorrhages may produce intractable vomiting. In most but not all cases there is blood within the CSF. The prognosis is poor. Thirty day survival is only 17 per cent (Whisnant et al., 1971). The terminal event is usually intraventricular hemorrhage or herniation.

SUBARACHNOID HEMORRHAGE

Bleeding within the subarachnoid space accounts for 5 to 13 per cent of CVA's (Whisnant et al., 1971; Kuller et al., 1970; Kannel, 1971). There is a bimodal age distribution for this event, with peaks at age 40 and at age 70. Men and women are affected about equally. The most frequent cause of subarachnoid hemorrhage is rupture of a congenital saccular aneurysm (*berry aneurysm*). These aneurysms most often develop in the circle of Willis, usually at bifurcations. Favored sites are the junction of the anterior cerebral and anterior communicating arteries, the junction of the internal carotid and posterior communicating arteries and the first bifurcation of the middle cerebral artery (Fig. 20–6). The branches of the basilar artery are less frequently involved. Very often there are multiple aneurysms (Escourolle and Poirier, 1973). Although the defect in the wall of the artery which permits aneurysmal dilation is presumably present from birth, actual distention of the vessel occurs only later in life. Hypertension seems to contribute not only to the development of the aneurysm but also to its rupture. As with brain hemorrhage, there is very often a history of physical or emotional exertion immediately preceding the event.

The developmental defect in the affected artery consists of focal absence or hypoplasia of the muscular layer and internal elastic membrane, usually at a bifurcation. Thus, the wall of the vessel at this point may be formed of little more than a thin layer of fibrohyaline intima. Over the years this yields to form a small saccular dilatation, ranging from a few millimeters to several centimeters in diameter. It typically lies in the Y of the bifurcating vessel. The walls of the sac are often calcified and occasionally the aneurysm is filled with thrombus. Rupture is not inevitable and, indeed, these aneurysms are found incidentally in 1 to 2 per cent of routine autopsies. Sometimes they produce clinical signs and symptoms by impinging on adjacent structures rather than by rupturing. They may thus lead to palsies of cranial nerves which lie in the area, especially the third, but occasionally the fourth, fifth or sixth, as well as to vis-

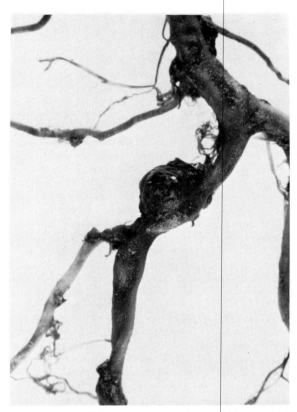

Figure 20–6. A berry aneurysm of the middle cerebral artery. The vessels have been dissected away from the brain.

ual defects referable to encroachment on the optic nerves or optic chiasm. Rupture, however, is the most calamitous consequence of a congenital saccular aneurysm. When this occurs, the entire subarachnoid space becomes flooded with blood, particularly about the site of the aneurysm. Sometimes the hemorrhage bursts into the brain substance itself and may even push through the parenchyma into the ventricle.

Sometimes frank rupture is preceded by a series of small leaks over a period of weeks to months, manifested clinically by transient headache and stiff neck. More often, however, rupture is unheralded and overwhelming. There is severe occipital headache, often with vomiting, followed rapidly by loss of consciousness. The CSF is always grossly bloody and under increased pressure. Signs of meningeal irritation (*meningeal signs*), including neck rigidity, Kernig's sign and Brudzinski's sign, are usually prominent. They, along with the frequent absence of focal signs, tend to distinguish subarachnoid hemorrhage from the other forms of CVA. However, exceptions occur, and the diagnosis cannot be made with certainty on a clinical basis. The prognosis with a subarachnoid hemorrhage is somewhat better than that with hemorrhage into the brain substance, but still is not good. Thirty-day survival has been reported as 35 per cent (Whisnant et al., 1971). About half those who die within the first month succumb to the initial hemorrhage. The others are victims of a recurrent hemorrhage which tends to occur within weeks of the initial bleed. After the first month the risk of recurrent hemorrhage in the survivors declines rapidly and by two months is less than 10 per cent.

INFARCTION OF THE BRAIN

Infarction of an area of the brain due to localized interference with its blood supply is by far the most frequent type of CVA. Almost any of the disorders mentioned earlier in the general discussion of vascular disease of the CNS may lead to an infarct. Even brain hemorrhage, paradoxically, results in an element of ischemic infarction of the nearby parenchyma. However, the most important causes of infarction of the brain are (1) thrombosis of an artery supplying the brain, usually as a complication of an atheroma, and (2) embolism to the brain from a thrombus elsewhere in the body. By common usage, then, infarction of the brain usually connotes thrombosis or embolism. Before discussing thrombosis

and embolism separately, as well as the clinical aspects of brain infarction, the histopathology will be presented.

Infarction of the brain may appear either anemic or hemorrhagic. The original insult is the same for each, that is, occlusion of a vessel. Ordinarily an anemic infarct results. Sometimes, however, blood flow is restored to the area (reflow) after the vessels have already been rendered abnormally permeable by ischemia. This permits a hemorrhagic diapedesis into the area, converting the lesion into a hemorrhagic infarct. Such reflow may result from opening of collateral vessels in the area or, more classically, it may occur when an embolus moves distally from the original site of occlusion.

In an anemic infarct, the first gross changes are apparent only after several hours. The affected gray matter becomes subtly duller and "opaque" and the demarcation between gray and white matter becomes indistinct. Within 2 to 3 days the infarct softens, becomes muddy in appearance and often looks mottled with tiny ecchymoses. There is intense edema of the surrounding tissue. Over the next week the necrotic tissue becomes friable, and the boundaries of the lesion stand out clearly. From 10 days onward, liquefaction with cavitation becomes increasingly evident, and scarring becomes apparent at the margins. The edema resolves. Eventually, the necrotic tissue is removed

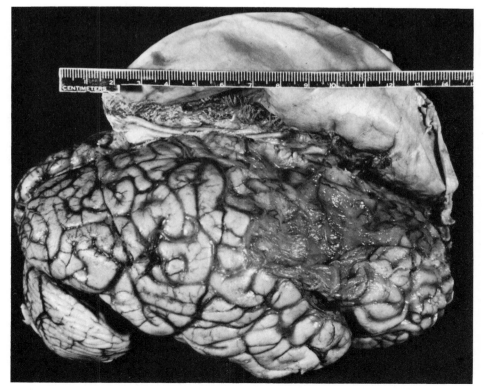

Figure 20–7. An old hemorrhagic infarct close to the temporoparietal sulcus. The gyri are atrophic; the area has undergone orange-brown discoloration and gliotic scarring.

and replaced by a ragged cystic scar. If the infarct is in contact with the leptomeninges, they become thickened and opaque to form the outer wall of the cyst. A hemorrhagic infarct produces the same gross changes, except that in the early stages there is blood in the area and later there is an orange-brown discoloration of the glial scar due to ingestion of hemosiderin by microglia and macrophages (Fig. 20–7).

The microscopic features and forms of ischemic injury of brain tissue were described in the general discussion of neuronal and glial response to injury beginning on page 639. Again, in the section dealing with anoxic encephalopathy (p. 647) ischemic damage to neurons was described. Here we will only briefly recapitulate. A reduction in staining capacity, principally of the neurons, is the first indication of ischemic injury and becomes apparent about 12 hours after the insult. At about 24 hours many neurons undergo changes similar to those of the axonal reaction, with swelling and rounding of the cell body, eccentricity of the nucleus and fading of the nuclear and cytoplasmic chromatin. At about the same time, congestion becomes marked. Cell death is confirmed by the appearance in most neurons of the more classical ischemic changes. The neurons become shrunken and increasingly angular, with pyknotic nuclei and strongly eosinophilic cytoplasm. At this point special stains of the myelin sheaths and of axis cylinders show these structures undergoing fragmentation and disintegration. Along with the myelin sheaths, the oligodendroglia within the area of infarction usually disappear. Within two days there is a marked polymorphonuclear exudation. Over the next few days these white cells are gradually replaced by histiocytes and compound granular cells which undertake removal of the necrotic debris. They become laden with fatty breakdown products, giving them a foamy appearance. These phagocytes attain maximum numbers at about two weeks, then gradually clear, although some may remain in the area for years. On the fourth day, gliosis becomes apparent at the margins of the infarct. Eventually, the typical cystic astroglial scar is formed. In hemorrhagic infarcts the basic changes are the same. However, large numbers of red blood cells can be seen within the parenchyma in the early stages, and later, red blood cells and hemosiderin are prominent within the phagocytic cells.

Having described the histopathology of brain infarcts we now turn our attention to the pathogenesis and clinical aspects. *The most important cause of infarction of the brain is thrombosis of an atheromatous artery supplying the brain. Indeed, this is the most important single cause of all CVA's, accounting for 44 to 75 per cent of them* (Kuller et al., 1970; Kannel, 1971; Whisnant et al., 1971). The likelihood of a CVA from this cause increases steeply with age. In a sense, then, age might be considered the most important risk factor. Males are slightly more vulnerable in the younger age groups, and females in the older. As mentioned, the thrombus usually forms on a pre-existing atherosclerotic lesion. A CVA from this cause is often termed an *atherothrombotic brain infarction (ABI)*. Thus, brain infarction joins myocardial infarction as a very serious complication of atherosclerosis. It might be assumed, then, that the risk factors are the same for brain infarction as for a myocardial infarction, and comprise those for atherosclerosis in general. Although this is largely true, there are some differences in emphasis. Some risk factors, such as hyperlipidemia, are more closely correlated with myocardial infarction, whereas others, most notably hypertension, are more closely associated with brain infarction. Nevertheless, glucose intolerance or diabetes, cigarette smoking and hyperlipidemia, as well as hypertension, are all to varying degrees correlated with atherothrombotic infarction of the brain.

Certain arteries supplying the brain are particularly prone to the development of atherosclerotic lesions. Most vulnerable are the carotid artery, especially in its cervical course, and the basilar artery. Within these vessels the lesions usually develop at bifurcations, at sites of curvature and where the vessels are fixed. Thus, frequently involved sites include the bifurcation of the common carotid artery, the carotid sinus, and the termination of the internal carotid artery where it gives rise to the anterior and middle cerebral and posterior communicating arteries. The basilar artery is most often involved at its origin from the vertebral arteries and at its termination, where it bifurcates to form the posterior cerebral arteries.

As elsewhere, atherosclerosis at these points leads to tortuosity and to gradual stenosis of the vessel. Complications, such as hemorrhage into the atheroma, and, most importantly, thrombosis, further interfere with blood flow. Although thrombosis is the usual precipitating event in brain infarction, uncomplicated atherosclerotic lesions themselves sometimes lead to infarction. This is most likely in elderly patients who experience a sudden adverse hemodynamic change, such as a cardiac arrhythmia or hypotension. In general, occlusion from thrombosis occurs relatively slowly, often permitting the development of an anastomotic collateral network. Indeed, total occlusion of the internal carotid may be entirely asymptomatic if the external carotid and ophthalmic arteries remain patent. If they do, the blood in the external carotid artery enters anastomoses with the ophthalmic artery whence by retrograde flow it reaches the internal carotid. When infarction does occur, it

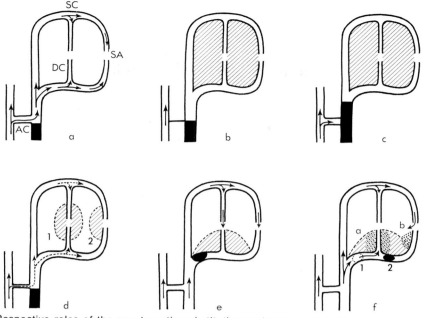

Figure 20–8. Respective roles of the anastomotic substitution pathways of circulatory supply and of the type of vascular occlusion in determining the occurrence and extent of cerebral lesions (*AC*, anastomotic vascular network; *SC*, superficial arterial circulation; *DC*, deep vascular territory; *SA*, superficial meningeal anastomoses).

a, Arterial occlusion, but with effective and adequate anastomotic substitution network of supply: no infarction.

b, Arterial occlusion without anatomically effective anastomotic network of supply (*AC*): massive infarction of the corresponding cerebral territory.

c, Arterial occlusion extending beyond the origin of the anastomotic network of supply. No anastomotic substitution byway of vascular supply: massive infarction.

d, Occlusion proximal to the anastomotic network of supply. Insufficient anastomotic substitution byway of arterial supply. Anemic infarct of variable extent in territory (2) distal to the junction of two vascular territories (last field of irrigation or watershed infarct) and in border zone between superficial and deep vascular territories (1).

e, Proximal occlusion of one dividing branch; anastomotic substitution byway of vascular supply provided by superficial meningeal anastomosis: limited proximal infarction.

f, Embolic occlusion. Mobilization of thrombus from 1 to 2. Sudden occlusion in 1, resulting in total ischemia of both deep and superficial vascular territories and in hemorrhages in the superficial territory when border zones are undergoing reirrigation (*b*); secondary mobilization of thrombus in 2, with hemorrhages due to secondary eruption of blood into the original ischemic deep vascular territory (*a*) (hemorrhagic infarct). (From Escourolle, R., and Poirier, J.: Manual of Basic Neuropathology. Philadelphia, W. B. Saunders Co., 1973.)

may be confined to the territory of the most distant branches of the internal carotid artery where the pressure drop is greatest and the collaterals least adequate. In this event, the infarcted area lies along the border between the territories of the anterior and middle cerebral arteries *(watershed infarct)*. In contrast, occlusion of an artery without major collaterals, such as the middle cerebral, usually produces extensive infarction, principally in its proximal territory, since there is *some* reirrigation distally from the superficial corticomeningeal vessels. Figure 20–8 shows schematically the relationships between the site of occlusion, the location of collateral vessels, and the area of consequent infarction, if any.

The clinical onset of an atherothrombotic brain infarction is usually more gradual and less devastating than that of the other forms of CVA. Symptoms may continue to develop over a period of hours or even days. Although the patient may be dazed or confused, actual loss of consciousness is unusual. Hemiplegia, confusion and aphasia are the most common signs and symptoms. The cerebrospinal fluid is often normal. Of course, the precise clinical syndrome depends on the location and size of the infarct. This in turn depends on: (1) the vessel occluded, (2) the site of occlusion within the vessel, (3) the competence of collateral channels, and (4) the speed of occlusion. The more important syndromes will be described subsequently. Although atherothrombotic brain infarction is the most frequent type of CVA, it is the least lethal. Thirty-day survival is 73 per cent, better than that with any of the other forms of CVA (Whisnant et al., 1971).

Brain infarction owing to embolism from sources

elsewhere in the body represents 3 to 14 per cent of CVA's. The source of the embolus is usually the heart. It may come from an atrial thrombus which forms during a cardiac arrhythmia, particularly atrial fibrillation; from a ventricular mural thrombus in myocardial infarction; or from valvular vegetations in endocarditis. Not to be overlooked as a possible source is a silent thrombus complicating an atheroma in one of the larger vessels supplying the brain, such as the carotid artery. Far less frequently, brain infarction is caused by fat emboli or air emboli. The incidence of embolic brain infarction increases with age, and both sexes are affected equally.

Although the distinction between atherothrombotic and embolic brain infarction is often difficult, certain features, when unequivocal, are helpful. Embolic occlusion is very sudden; hence the clinical onset is typically abrupt—the most abrupt of all forms of CVA. In contrast, as mentioned, atherothrombotic occlusion is usually gradual.

Emboli tend to travel to smaller vessels than those involved by thrombosis. The vessel most frequently occluded by an embolus is the middle cerebral artery. In this case the embolus has traversed the common carotid and internal carotid arteries before finally lodging in the middle cerebral artery. Because of the abruptness of occlusion and because the involved vessels may be functionally end arteries, collateral reirrigation is often inadequate. Infarction, then, is typically more extensive than that following thrombosis. Moreover, it is very often hemorrhagic because of the tendency of the embolus to dislodge and migrate farther along the affected vessel (Fig. 20–9). The blood that then rushes in behind the dislodged embolus leaks through the damaged vessel walls into the brain parenchyma.

Not surprisingly, the prognosis with embolic brain infarction is poorer than that with atherothrombotic infarction, although better than with either type of intracranial hemorrhage. Thirty-day survival is approximately 66 per cent (Whisnant et al., 1971).

In general, it is possible to infer from the clinical picture the specific artery involved by either thrombosis or embolism. The most important of the clinical syndromes result from stenosis or occlusion of the following arteries: the internal carotid, the middle cerebral and the vertebral and basilar arteries.

As mentioned earlier, gradual occlusion of the *internal carotid* artery may be entirely asymptomatic if the ophthalmic artery remains patent and the cardiovascular system is otherwise reasonably sound. Often, however, it results in intermittent transient episodes of dysfunction in any part of the vast territory ultimately supplied by the carotid artery. It

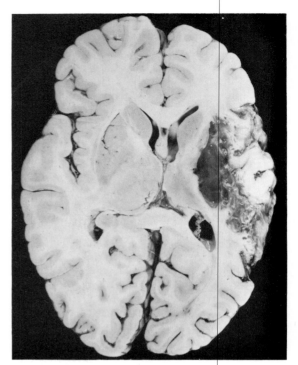

Figure 20–9. A large area of hemorrhagic infarction on the right.

should be remembered that this includes the territories of the anterior cerebral, middle cerebral and posterior communicating arteries, as well as of the ophthalmic artery. Thus there may be transient episodes of contralateral weakness (hemiparesis), of contralateral sensory deficits (hemiparesthesia) or of ipsilateral monocular blindness. These are known as *transient ischemic attacks (TIA's)*. They owe their transiency to the rapid development of collateral pathways. Auscultation of the carotid artery in the neck often reveals a bruit in these cases, a valuable diagnostic sign. When frank infarction does occur, it is often of the "watershed" type, involving the most distal ramifications of the carotid artery, particularly the boundary zone between the anterior and middle cerebral territories. In contrast to gradual occlusion, sudden total occlusion of the internal artery, as by a large embolus, or occlusion beyond the ophthalmic artery leads to massive infarction of the cerebral hemisphere. There is loss of consciousness, complete contralateral hemiplegia, and ultimately, in most cases, herniation of the edematous brain and death.

Infarction of the territory of the *middle cerebral artery* may reflect either occlusion of the internal carotid artery or of the middle cerebral artery itself. In the latter situation it is more frequently the result of an embolus than of thrombosis. With embolism to the middle cerebral artery, there is massive infarction, particularly in the proximal territory of supply. This results in contralateral hemiplegia, hemianesthesia and hemianopsia. If the dominant hemisphere is involved, aphasia, apraxia and agnosia also supervene. Often the patient does not survive. Less extensive infarction of the middle cerebral territory, owing to either gradual occlusion of the middle cerebral or of the internal carotid artery, is a very common cause of hemiplegia and aphasia.

Occlusion of the *anterior cerebral artery* is less frequent than that of the internal carotid or middle cerebral arteries. When it occurs, substitution through the contralateral anterior cerebral artery and the anterior communicating artery is possible.

Occlusion within the *vertebral or basilar arteries* may produce any of a variety of signs and symptoms. Transient ischemic attacks (TIA's) may occur since there are extensive anastomotic communications within this territory. In this sense, vertebral-basilar involvement is similar to that of the internal carotid artery. Common symptoms of vertebral-basilar TIA's are vertigo, deafness, diplopia, weakness, ataxia and cortical blindness. Again analogous to the internal carotid artery, the usual cause of vertebral-basilar occlusion is atherosclerosis with or without thrombosis. Emboli to these vessels are relatively rare. Sometimes the cause of ischemia is compression of a vertebral artery by osteoarthritic or spondylitic spurs where these arteries pass through the transverse foramina of the cervical vertebrae. Isolated involvement of the *posterior cerebral artery* is infrequent. Moreover, collateral chan-

nels from the internal carotid system offer additional protection to its territory.

The specific arterial syndromes just discussed stem from localized lesions and constitute typical CVA's. Less typical and more recently appreciated are multiple scattered infarcts termed *lacunar infarcts*. These are small cystic foci of ischemic necrosis surrounded by a zone of gliosis. They rarely exceed 1.5 cm. in diameter. Favored locations are the basal ganglia, the pons, thalamus and the internal capsule, although they may be found anywhere in the brain. Lacunar infarcts typically occur in elderly patients, particularly those with hypertension or diabetes. Sometimes these patients exhibit neurologic deficits, often pseudobulbar palsy (inappropriate crying or laughing), but frequently lacunar infarcts are unsuspected and found only on routine postmortem examination.

SUMMARY

To conclude our discussion of vascular disease of the CNS, the *three morphologic forms of ischemic injury to the brain* just described will be summarized briefly. *The first is anoxic encephalopathy*, which results from a generalized reduction in the supply of oxygenated blood received by the brain. It ranges from a transient functional disorder at one extreme, to sudden death at the other. In between are those cases in which morphologic changes develop. These consist of scattered areas of ischemic necrosis accompanied by marked edema of the entire brain. *The second form of ischemic injury to the brain is intracranial hemorrhage. The third is infarction of the brain. Together these two forms con-*

TABLE 20–1. FEATURES OF THE FOUR PRINCIPAL TYPES OF CVA

TYPE OF CVA	PROPORTION OF ALL CVA'S	AGE OF PEAK INCIDENCE	FAVORED LOCATIONS	CLINICAL ASPECTS	30-DAY SURVIVAL
Brain hemorrhage	12% (7% to 17%)	Increasing with age, plateau age 65	Cerebrum (80%)— putamen, claustrum, external capsule Pons or medulla (10%) Cerebellum (10%)	Sudden; headache; loss of consciousness; contra-lateral hemiplegia; CSF normal or bloody	17%
Subarachnoid hemorrhage	9% (5% to 13%)	Bimodal, ages 40 and 70	Congenital saccular aneurysm in anterior circle of Willis	Sudden; headache; loss of consciousness; meningeal signs; CSF bloody; ↑ pressure; ? preceding "leaks"	35%
Atherothrombotic infarction	60% (44% to 75%)	Increasing with age	Carotid bifurcation; carotid sinus, basilar bifurcation	Gradual; confusion; localizing deficits (hemi-plegia, aphasia, visual deficits); CSF normal; ? preceding TIA's	83%
Embolic infarction	8% (3% to 14%)	Increasing with age	Middle cerebral artery	Very sudden; confusion or loss of consciousness; localizing deficits; CSF normal or bloody	66%

stitute the entity known as cerebrovascular accident (CVA) or stroke. Intracranial hemorrhage is in turn subdivided into brain hemorrhage and subarachnoid hemorrhage. Brain hemorrhage is associated with long-standing uncontrolled hypertension. Most often the hemorrhage involves the cerebrum *(intracerebral hemorrhage)*, particularly the lateral basal ganglia and the external capsule. Subarachnoid hemorrhage usually results from rupture of a *congenital saccular aneurysm (berry aneurysm)* in the circle of Willis. At the site of the aneurysm there is absence or hypoplasia of the muscular layer and internal elastic membrane of the artery. Although this defect is presumably present from birth, rupture occurs in middle to old age and may be triggered by hypertension. *Infarction of the brain is usually caused by thrombosis complicating an atheromatous lesion in an artery supplying the brain (atherothrombotic brain infarction, or ABI). This is the most frequent type of CVA. Less often, infarction is caused by an embolus from a source elsewhere in the body, usually the heart.* Occasionally infarction seems to result from atheromatous narrowing of a vessel without superimposed thrombosis. Anatomically, the lesion in the brain may be *anemic* or *hemorrhagic.* In general, but by no means always, an atherothrombotic infarction is anemic whereas an embolic infarction is hemorrhagic. When collateral networks are present and rapidly utilized, there may be no infarction but rather a *transient ischemic attack (TIA).* These are particularly common with lesions in the internal carotid arteries and in the vertebral-basilar systems. Repeated TIA's may, however, eventually lead to a completed stroke. In some elderly patients, particularly those with hypertension or diabetes, multiple small infarcts known as lacunar infarcts are found scattered throughout the brain.

Table 20–1 shows some of the important features of the four principal types of CVA.

TOXIC, NUTRITIONAL AND METABOLIC DISORDERS OF THE NERVOUS SYSTEM

This category embraces a wide variety of insults which either primarily or secondarily affect the nervous system. Almost all of them are discussed elsewhere in this text. The metabolic encephalopathies associated with uremia (p. 429) and hepatic failure (p. 511) are two of the most important. Profound CNS disturbances are also characteristic of both severe hypoglycemia and of diabetic ketoacidosis (p. 127). Many of the intoxications which affect the nervous system, including those caused by alcohol, a variety of drugs, carbon monoxide and certain heavy metals, are discussed in

Chapter 8. Within this general category, only subacute combined degeneration of the spinal cord, associated with pernicious anemia, and Wilson's disease, caused by a defect in copper metabolism, are described in this chapter. Subacute combined degeneration of the spinal cord is considered with the demyelinating diseases on page 675, and Wilson's disease is briefly described with the degenerative diseases of the CNS on page 672.

TUMORS OF THE CNS

CNS tumors may be primary or they may represent metastatic deposits from cancer elsewhere in the body. Among the primary neoplasms, most are malignant. Their malignancy is by virtue of their histologic appearance and their relentless destructive growth. *They almost never metastasize.* Even the histologically benign tumors have a guarded prognosis since they may not be readily accessible to the surgeon and their location may cause serious disturbances, e.g., blockage of the flow of cerebrospinal fluid. Although primary cancer of the CNS accounts for only about two and a half per cent of all cancer deaths, it is unscrupulous in its destruction of children. Under the age of 15 years, cancer of the CNS represents fully 21 per cent of malignant lesions and is second only to leukemia as a cause of death from cancer (Silverberg and Holleb, 1975).

Any of the normal cell types present in the CNS may give rise to a specific type of neoplasm. Only the most important of these tumors will be presented here. By far the most frequent are those which originate in the glial cells, termed *gliomas.* Since all gliomas are to some degree malignant, the term is a misnomer. Most important among the gliomas are the *astrocytoma,* the *oligodendroglioma* and the *ependymoma.* The *medulloblastoma,* a particularly devastating tumor of children, although of uncertain origin, is often classified as a glioma. Among these four gliomas, the astrocytoma is the most common. It is further subdivided into Grades I through IV, in increasing order of malignancy. Grades III and IV are customarily lumped together as the highly malignant *glioblastoma multiforme.* Those primary tumors not of glial origin include the *meningioma,* which arises from cells of the arachnoid, and the *neurilemoma (Schwannoma),* which originates from the Schwann cells of the cranial nerves or spinal nerve roots. Both of these are usually benign, although malignant transformation may occur. Pituitary tumors, although intracranial, originate from endocrine rather than nervous tissue and are therefore discussed in Chapter 18. It is note-

TABLE 20-2. TUMORS OF THE CNS

```
BRAIN—80%
   Metastatic (most commonly from lung and breast)—30%
   Primary—70%
      Gliomas— ~35%
         Gioblastoma (astrocytoma III and IV)—17%
         Astrocytoma I and II—8%
         Oligodendroglioma—2%
         Ependymoma—3%
         Medulloblastoma—5%
      Meningioma— ~15%
      Pituitary—12%
      Neurilemoma—8%

SPINAL CORD—20%
   Meningioma and Schwannoma—56%
   Ependymoma—16%
   Glioma—7%
```

TABLE 20-3. CNS TUMORS OF CHILDREN

Tumor	Per Cent
Medulloblastoma	30
Astrocytoma I and II	30
Ependymoma	12
Other	28

worthy that, with the possible exception of the medulloblastoma, none of the important primary CNS tumors arise from the neurons themselves.

Exact relative incidences of the various CNS tumors are difficult to ascertain. Most large studies are weighted in some fashion—by age, by survival time, by availability of tissue for histologic diagnosis. However, some statistics are reasonably well established, and approximations to which most would agree can be given for others. These are presented in Table

20-2. As can be seen, brain tumors outnumber those of the spinal cord by about 4:1; moreover, they are far more likely to be malignant. Among the brain tumors, about a third are metastatic. Of the primary tumors, about half are gliomas and, in turn, half of these are astrocytomas Grades III and IV (glioblastomas). However, as Table 20–3 shows, in children these incidences are quite different. Before discussing in a general way the clinical features of CNS tumors, the histology and some of the distinguishing features of each of the major ones will be presented individually. After reading this material, reference should be made to Table 20–4 for an overview (p. 661).

ASTROCYTOMA, GRADES I AND II

These tumors are seen principally in young adults, although they may occur at any age.

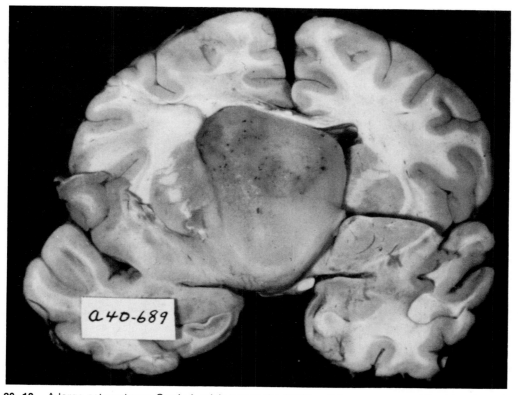

Figure 20–10. A large astrocytoma, Grade I, arising near the midline; it has compressed the lateral ventricle and distorted the opposite hemisphere.

In adults they usually involve the cerebrum; in children they show a predilection for the posterior fossa. Their appearance is variable. Grossly, they are often white, gray or pink, moderately firm, irregular masses (Fig. 20—10). Within the tumor there are frequently cysts containing clear to yellowish fluid, as well as occasional foci of calcification. The microscopic appearance is of sheets of fairly innocent appearing astrocytes. Although the nuclei may be slightly larger and the chromatin more dense than normal, pleomorphism is minimal and there are no mitoses and no giant cells. Grade II astrocytomas differ from the Grade I lesions only in degree. The nuclei show somewhat greater variation in size and shape, they stain more darkly and the cell processes are thicker. In addition, there is some noticeable angiomatoid proliferation of small blood vessels within the tumor.

Despite the innocence of their appearance, astrocytomas of Grades I and II are slowly invasive, and often recur after removal. With treatment, five-year survival with Grade I astrocytoma is about 60 per cent. With Grade II it is 38 per cent (Bouchard, 1966).

ASTROCYTOMA, GRADES III and IV (GLIOBLASTOMA MULTIFORME)

These highly malignant tumors affect a slightly older age group than do the better differentiated astrocytomas. The average age is about 50 years, and there is a slightly greater risk in men. Unfortunately, the higher grade astrocytomas are the most common single type of primary brain tumor.

Although they may occur anywhere in the CNS, they show a predilection for the white matter of the cerebrum. Their appearance is even more variable than the astrocytomas of Grades I and II. They range in size from quite small lesions, only a few centimeters across, to enormous masses virtually replacing an entire hemisphere. Grossly, the tumor appears as a soft yellow-gray to pink-gray infiltrative mass. The pinkish color reflects the intense vascularity of these lesions and many assume a mottled pattern. Often the cut section presents creamy yellow areas of necrosis, red-brown foci of hemorrhage and occasional cysts containing clear fluid (Fig. 20—11). The histology of these lesions is also variable. The tumor cells themselves are highly pleomorphic. They may be polygonal, fusiform or unipolar, and have bizarre hyperchromatic nuclei (Fig. 20—12). Mitoses and multinucleated giant cells are seen in virtually every microscopic field. In addition, tangled angiomatoid knots of blood vessels typically are prominent. The new vessels are unusually convoluted, with thickened cellular walls. Mitotic figures may be seen within the endothelial cells. As mentioned, foci of necrosis and hemorrhage are almost always apparent.

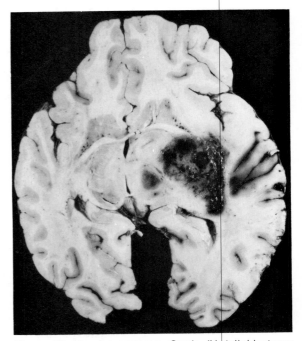

Figure 20–11. Astrocytoma, Grade IV (glioblastoma multiforme), showing prominent hemorrhage and areas of cystic softening. The neoplasm and the surrounding edema have produced considerable expansion of the hemisphere.

The behavior of these tumors is as ugly as their appearance. They grow rapidly, almost always recur after treatment and usually lead to death within a few months. Even with treatment, two-year survival with Grades III and IV astrocytoma is only 20 per cent (Bouchard, 1966).

OLIGODENDROGLIOMA

Like the higher grade astrocytomas, oligodendrogliomas most frequently occur in middle age and are usually located in the cerebral white matter. They differ in their relatively benign course, although they, too, are technically malignant and in many cases ultimately cause death.

Typically, they are solid grayish lesions, often containing gritty areas of calcification and sometimes cystic areas and foci of hemorrhage. The unusual tendency of these tumors to produce concentric lamellated calcifications permits their identification by x-ray in about half the cases. Histologically, the tumors consist of sheets of oligodendrocytes within a scant vascular connective stroma. Although the cell membranes and the small regular nuclei of the oligodendrocytes take the H&E stain, the abundant cytoplasm does not, and the effect is of a field of small dark spheres lying in the center of sharply circumscribed empty spaces.

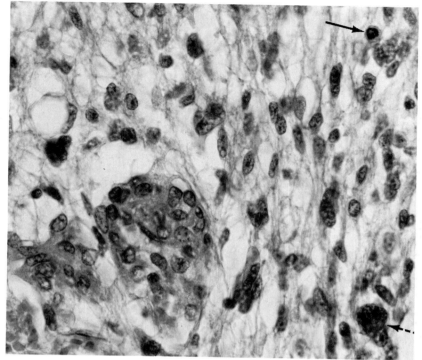

Figure 20–12. Microscopic detail of an astrocytoma, Grade IV. A mitotic figure (solid arrow), giant cell (dashed arrow) and a cluster of endothelial cells are evident.

These tumors are in general slowly growing. Often they are present for years before diagnosis, and permit survival for years afterwards. Occasionally, however, they behave in a more malignant fashion and rapidly cause death. There appears to be no very good correlation between the histologic appearance and their clinical course. Five-year survival is about 50 per cent (Bouchard, 1966; Weir and Elvidge, 1968).

EPENDYMOMA

These tumors arise from the cells lining the ventricular system of the brain and the central canal of the spinal cord. Their most frequent locations are the fourth ventricle, the lumbosacral enlargement of the cord and the filum terminale. Young adults and children are primarily affected.

The appearance of these tumors is variable. They range from moderately firm, gritty lesions to soft, gray, fleshy ones. Cystic cavities and foci of calcification may be present. The histologic pattern also varies, not only from tumor to tumor but also within the same tumor. However, three broad architectural types are usually distinguished — the **cellular**, the **epithelial** and the **papillary**. **Cellular ependymomas** are composed of sheets of polygonal cells in a scant stroma. Within these sheets may be **perivascular pseudorosettes.** These consist of ependymal cells arrayed around blood vessels with their pale tapered processes abutting on the vessel wall. This creates the appearance of a pale

halo around the vessel which separates it from the surrounding circle of ependymal nuclei. The **epithelial ependymoma** contains true **rosettes**, consisting of circular arrangements of elongated ciliated ependymal cells surrounding a central canal. Pseudorosettes may also be seen. The **papillary ependymoma** occurs primarily in the spinal cord and filum terminale. As its name suggests, it is composed of a branching fibroglial stroma covered by a single layer of cuboidal ependymal cells. In the filum terminale the stroma may be myxomatous. Despite the variability of the ependymomas, two histologic hallmarks may be present and aid in their diagnosis — the rosettes, described above, and small basophilic granules termed **blepharoplasts,** which may sometimes be seen in the cytoplasm of the tumor cells.

The clinical course of ependymomas is as variable as their appearance. They have been graded from I to IV in a manner similar to the astrocytomas but with less success in prognostication. Usually they are slowly growing. However, their location along ventricular pathways leads to obstruction of the CSF at a very early stage, with serious consequences. Removal is difficult and recurrences are typical. Lesions of the filum terminale are more easily resected and may be cured.

MEDULLOBLASTOMA

These are highly malignant tumors of the cerebellum. About two thirds of their victims are children under the age of 15 years, most often boys. The cell of origin is controversial, and they are only loosely classified as gliomas. The favored theory is that they arise from remnants of the superficial granular layer of the cerebellum—primitive cells normally present in fetal life and early infancy, from which the neuronal and glial cells of the cerebellum may differentiate.

The tumor most often arises from the vermis of the cerebellum and characteristically grows as a gray fleshy mass hanging down into the fourth ventricle, which it rapidly obstructs. Occasionally the lateral lobes of the cerebellum are involved. Microscopically, the medulloblastoma is densely cellular, with very little stroma and few blood vessels. The cells are small, often tapered at one pole (carrot-shaped), with dark round or oval nuclei. They may be arranged in sheets or parallel rows. Typically, they are arrayed around vessels to form pseudorosettes. Mitoses are abundant. Although metastasis outside the nervous system is rare, medulloblastomas frequently spread throughout the subarachnoid-ventricular system, giving the brain and spinal cord a frosted appearance.

As mentioned, the medulloblastoma is a particularly unpleasant cancer, and children with this tumor do not usually survive more than a year. Recently, however, aggressive radiotherapy has brightened the picture somewhat. With this modality, in conjunction with surgery, five-year survival has been reported as high as 40 to 75 per cent (Bloom et al., 1969; Paterson, 1963; Hope-Stone, 1970).

MENINGIOMA

The most important benign tumor of the CNS is the meningioma. Malignant transformation does sometimes occur and, at best, even the benign form is difficult to extirpate, but so bleak is the outlook with CNS tumors in general that the meningioma is the patient's best hope. They usually occur in middle age and affect women more often than men. Probably they arise from the arachnoidal villi, since their cells are of arachnoidal origin, but they are always attached to the dura mater.

Favored locations are near the superior sagittal sinus and on the sphenoid ridges. Other important sites include the lateral convexities of the skull, the vicinity of the sella turcica and of the olfactory groove, and the cerebellopontine angle. In addition, the meningioma is one of the most frequent spinal cord tumors; the usual location is the thoracic segment. Occasionally they are multiple. Grossly, these are usually nodular, grayish-white, rubbery lesions, although they are occasionally soft and fleshy. A variation is the **meningioma en plaque**, which, as its name suggests, is a flattened,

spread-out lesion seen particularly at the convexities of the skull. As benign tumors, meningiomas are encapsulated and compress but do not invade the brain substance. Calcification of meningiomas is common, often giving them a gritty texture on sectioning, and this may be intense enough to permit x-ray visualization of the tumor. Moreover, these lesions characteristically excite an osteoblastic reaction from nearby bone, a valuable diagnostic feature when localized thickening of a portion of the skull is seen on x-ray. The histology of meningiomas falls into three patterns. The **meningotheliomatous** tumor is composed of sheets of large polygonal cells with prominent oval, vesicular nuclei and a pale, finely granular cytoplasm. On ordinary stains the cell boundaries are indistinct. The stroma tends to be hyalinized and quite vascular. In the **psammomatous** meningioma the cells assume a whorling pattern (Fig. 20–13). The centers of these whorls are occupied by "psammoma bodies"—small foci of hyalinization and calcification lying at the center of a whorl of tumor cells. They probably result from degeneration of the central cells within a whorl. The third pattern is the **fibroblastic** meningioma. This is composed of bundles of streaming spindle cells separated by thick collagenous bands. Small areas of the meningotheliomatous pattern also usually can be found. Many intergrades among these three patterns occur. Psammoma bodies, although most abundant

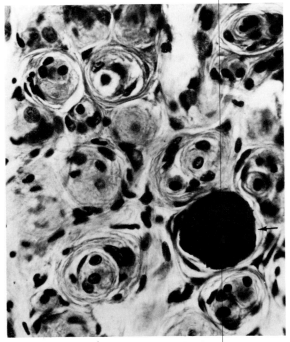

Figure 20–13. Microscopic detail of a psammomatous meningioma, showing numerous concentric whorls and a large psammoma body (arrow).

TABLE 20–4. PRIMARY INTRACRANIAL NEOPLASMS

Neoplasm	Age and Sex	Cell of Origin	Favored Locations	Gross Appearance	Histology	Malignancy
Astrocytoma Grades I and II	Young adults	Astrocyte	Cerebrum	Variable; irregular, gray-pink, cystic	Sheets of well differentiated astrocytes, ± proliferation of blood vessels	+
Astrocytoma Grades III and IV	Middle age M > F	Astrocyte	Cerebrum, white matter	Variable; soft, yellow-gray-pink, necrosis, hemorrhage, cysts	Variable; pleomorphism, mitoses, giant cells, marked proliferation of blood vessels	+++
Oligodendroglioma	Middle age	Oligodendrocyte	Cerebrum, white matter	Solid gray; foci of calcification, sometimes cysts	Masses of enlarged oligodendrocytes, scant vascular stroma	+
Ependymoma	Young adults, children	Cells lining ventricular system	Fourth ventricle, distal spinal cord	Variable; soft–firm, fleshy, gritty, foci of calcification, sometimes cystic	Variable; *cellular or epithelial or papillary,* rosettes, blepharoplasts	+
Medulloblastoma	Children M > F	? Primitive bipotential cells	Vermis of cerebellum	Soft, gray, fleshy, in fourth ventricle, frequent seeding of subarachnoid space	Sheets of small cells, dark nuclei, scant stroma, mitoses, pseudorosettes	++
Meningioma	Middle age F > M	Arachnoid cells	Parasagittal, sphenoid ridge; lateral convexities, thoracic spinal cord	Nodular gray-white, rubbery encapsulated, calcification, sometimes meningioma en plaque	*Meningotheliomatous*— sheets of polygonal cells *psammomatous*— whorls (psammoma bodies) *fibroblastic*—spindle cells	Usually benign
Neurilemoma	Middle age	Schwann cells of cranial nerves or spinal nerve roots	CN VIII in cerebellopontine angle, thoracic spinal cord	Variable, irregular, nodular, cystic, encapsulated	Bundles long bipolar cells, palisading nuclei	Usually benign

in the psammomatous type, are also seen in the other two.

As mentioned, some meningiomas, despite their apparent benign cytology, behave as malignant neoplasms and invade the adjacent bony structures.

NEURILEMOMA (SCHWANNOMA)

Like the meningioma, the neurilemoma is classically benign, although malignant behavior sometimes develops and recurrence after removal is frequent. It arises from cells of the neural sheath (Schwann cells) of cranial nerve or spinal nerve roots as they exit from the CNS. Typically, the neurilemoma develops during middle age.

The most frequent and the classical location is in the cerebellopontine angle, at the root of the vestibular portion of the eighth cranial nerve where it emerges from the brain stem (**acoustic neuroma**). In von Recklinghausen's neurofibromatosis, multiple acoustic neuromas may be present. Only occasionally does the neurilemoma arise from other cranial nerves. In the spinal cord, it is a relatively important tumor. Here they are subdural lesions, most frequently involving the dorsal nerve roots in the thoracic segment of the cord. Neurilemomas have a variable gross appearance. Often they are irregularly nodular lesions containing multiple small cysts and foci of hemorrhage or yellowish degeneration. They are encapsulated and, like meningiomas, compress rather than invade surrounding structures. Microscopically, the neurilemoma consists of interlacing dense bundles of spindled cells, often with rod-shaped nuclei. Classically, there is palisading of the nuclei, i.e., the nuclei appear regimented into parallel rows. Although this appearance certainly points to the diagnosis, it is often not present. Moreover, the typical bundles of long slender cells are sometimes replaced by a looser structure of more rounded cells in no apparent pattern. Although collagenous and reticulin fibers are abundant, there are no nerve fibers within the tumor.

The usual location of neurilemomas within the cerebellopontine angle produces a characteristic constellation of clinical findings. Involvement of the eighth nerve itself leads to tinnitus and some degree of deafness. Later, the tumor impinges on the fifth and seventh cranial nerves, which also lie in the cerebellopontine angle, and palsies of these nerves develop. More serious are indications of direct compression of the brain stem or of obstruction of the fourth ventricle, with resultant hydrocephalus. While cures are theoretically possible, in practice extirpation is difficult and recurrences are frequent.

An overview of tumors of the CNS is presented in Table 20–4.

METASTATIC TUMORS OF THE CNS

As mentioned earlier, at least 30 per cent of CNS tumors are metastatic from sites elsewhere in the body. Most probably this figure actually understates the true proportion of the CNS tumors that are metastatic, since these are probably often clinically overshadowed by the primary process and diagnostic tissue is less avidly sought from these than from primary tumors. The most common sources of metastatic lesions to the CNS are carcinomas of the lung and of the breast. Other important sources include carcinoma of the GI tract, renal cell carcinoma and melanoma. Remarkably often, symptoms of brain metastases are the first indication of the primary lesion.

The metastatic deposits are usually multiple and present a characteristic gross appearance regardless of their source. They tend to be spherical, seemingly well demarcated and often straddle the junction of white and gray matter. Histologically, of course, they duplicate the primary tumor.

CLINICAL COURSE WITH CNS TUMORS

The clinical picture of the CNS tumors is related more to the location of the lesion than to the type of neoplasm. However, it should be remembered that location and tumor type are themselves not unrelated. The medulloblastoma, for example, is virtually always located in the cerebellum. Bearing this in mind, a few general comments can be made about the clinical course of CNS tumors. Signs and symptoms are of two kinds: (1) those due to compression or destruction of nearby normal tissue (local effects), and (2) those arising from an increase in intracranial pressure (general effects). Since the CNS is the control center of the body, it should not be surprising that the local effects include a multitude of far-flung, disparate abnormalities depending entirely on the location of the lesion. Examples include Jacksonian seizures when the precentral gyrus is involved, contralateral homonymous hemianopsia when the optic tracts are affected, staggering and loss of balance with cerebellar tumors, and subtle impairment of judgment with prefrontal lesions. The onset of seizures in an adult should always cause concern. In about 35 per cent of such cases, an intracranial neoplasm is discovered. Meningiomas are especially likely to cause seizures, and do so in about two thirds of cases (McDonald and Lapham, 1970–71). Increased intracranial pressure (discussed on p. 643) may be caused by the volume of the tumor mass itself, by obstruction of the ventricular system or by hemorrhages and edema. The ability of a relatively small lesion to produce marked edema is a poorly understood attribute of CNS tumors. Probably it is related to increased vascular permeability. With rapidly growing tumors the edema accumulation may be massive. Not surprisingly, then, headache is the most common single presenting symptom of a brain tumor (Walker, 1975).

Although some of the indications of CNS tumors may be episodic, e.g., seizures, the usual untreated course is of inexorable progression of CNS signs and symptoms. A remarkable peculiarity of CNS tumors is the fact that distant metastases rarely occur, even when there is extensive seeding of the leptomeninges. Diagnosis usually requires a constellation of tests. Skull x-rays are abnormal in about 30 per cent of cases. Meningiomas and oligodendrogliomas may be calcified, or the calvarium or sphenoidal ridge may be thickened at the point of attachment of a meningioma. Increased intracranial pressure may cause erosion of the posterior clinoidal processes of the sella turcica. A calcified pineal body is often shifted away from the midline. Lumbar puncture in the face of probable increased intracranial pressure is risky, since it may shift the pressure gradient between brain and cord enough to hasten herniation. Good diagnostic sensitivity is obtained with the electroencephalogram (EEG) (positive in 75 per cent of cases, although not precise in localization), brain scan (positive in 75 to 85 per cent of cases) and selective angiography of the carotid or vertebral vessels. Pneumoencephalography, a highly unpleasant procedure for the patient, can diagnose and localize lesions with 95 per cent reliability. Computer assisted tomography (CAT-scan), a recently developed noninvasive radiographic technique, promises to become the diagnostic tool of first choice. The general outlook for all CNS cancers is poor. Five-year survival is about 25 per cent for males and 35 per cent for females (Silverberg and Holleb, 1975).

INFECTIONS

Infections of the nervous system are often limited to the coverings of the brain or the spinal cord (*meningitis*). In other cases, however, they involve the parenchyma of the brain (*encephalitis*) or of the spinal cord (*myelitis*) or both (*encephalomyelitis*). Sharply circumscribed *brain abscesses* also occur. A host of infectious agents may be involved, including flukes and round worms. Most important are the pyogenic bacteria, the viruses and the tubercle bacillus. Table 20–5 at the end of this section shows the salient features of the more important infections. Meningitis, encephalomyelitis

and brain abscesses will be discussed separately.

MENINGITIS

Meningitis may be pyogenic, granulomatous or lymphocytic (viral or syphilitic). In all three it most often conforms to the distribution of the cerebrospinal fluid (CSF) and thus involves the arachnoid and pia maters (*leptomeningitis*), and the subarachnoid space, including the Virchow-Robin spaces and the ventricles.

PYOGENIC MENINGITIS

This is commonly caused by the pneumococcus in infants and the elderly, by the meningococcus in previously healthy adults, by *H. influenzae* in young children and by gram-negative bacilli in newborns (Seligman, 1973). Other causes include the streptococci, *Staphylococcus aureus* and a variety of opportunistic infectious agents in patients who are debilitated or receiving immunosuppressive drugs. The meninges are usually invaded during the course of a septicemia. The primary involvement is often pneumonia, endocarditis or osteomyelitis. Infections of the face (e.g., paranasal sinusitis) or of the ear (e.g., otitis media and mastoiditis) may also lead to meningitis. Penetrating injuries may implant organisms directly.

Grossly, a cloudy, purulent exudate develops in the subarachnoid space, principally over the vertex and at the base (Fig. 20–14). The leptomeninges

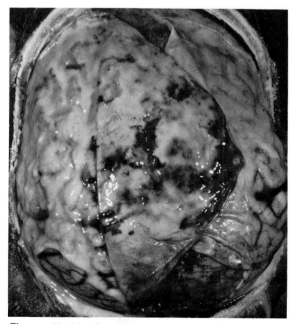

Figure 20–14. Pyogenic meningitis. A heavy layer of suppurative exudate is disclosed by folding back the dural covering.

become opaque and congested. At the beginning the inflammatory cells are almost entirely neutrophils. Later, the exudate becomes fibrinous and contains mononuclear inflammatory cells as well. Thrombophlebitis of the dural sinuses or bridging veins is frequent and may lead to a venous infarct of the subjacent cortex. Ultimately, fibrosis with thickening of the meninges ensues. Sometimes adhesions between the meninges and the brain impinge on cranial nerves or block the outflow of CSF from the ventricles. Such strategic scarring leads to cranial nerve palsies or to hydrocephalus.

The clinical onset of pyogenic meningitis is sudden and dramatic, with severe headache, fever and chills, progressing rapidly to delirium and coma. In all forms of meningitis, *meningeal signs,* i.e., Kernig's sign, Brudzinski's sign and neck stiffness, are present. With prompt treatment, most patients survive, but approximately 20 per cent suffer permanent neurologic impairments (Zacks, 1971). These may be severe, and include hydrocephalus, blindness, deafness, cranial nerve palsies, seizures, mental retardation and the subsequent development of brain abscesses.

GRANULOMATOUS MENINGITIS

This form of meningitis may be caused by the tubercle bacillus or by a variety of fungi, most notably *Cryptococcus neoformans.*

It differs from pyogenic meningitis clinically by a less stormy onset, and histologically in producing a mononuclear exudate with granuloma formation entirely typical of the organism. Usually the leptomeninges and subjacent superficial cortex are involved. Arteritis of the bridging vessels is common. The process is most pronounced at the base of the brain, where a shaggy fibrous and necrotic exudate may compress the overlying brain and cord. Characteristic granulomatous nodules may be scattered throughout the meninges.

Tuberculous meningitis is usually metastatic from the lung or occurs in association with miliary tuberculosis. Cryptococcal meningitis, too, is usually metastatic from the lung and represents the most important extrapulmonary site of this infection. Very often, fungal meningitis attacks patients who are already debilitated, as for example by a lymphoma or Hodgkin's disease. The clinical picture of granulomatous meningitis is of a somewhat gradual onset of nonspecific symptoms, such as malaise, headache and low-grade fever, along with the development of meningeal signs. Occasionally, however, the onset may be quite abrupt and mimic that of pyogenic meningitis. Infrequently, a mass of confluent tuberculous granulomas, called a *tuberculoma,* may develop in the brain parenchyma and clinically simulate a tumor.

Without treatment, granulomatous meningitis is fatal within weeks to months. Prompt therapy of tuberculous meningitis permits recovery, although residua may remain. The management of fungal meningitis is more difficult and the prognosis is therefore guarded. Differentiation among the various causes of granulomatous meningitis is important, and may be accomplished by finding the causative organisms in the CSF on smear or appropriate cultures.

LYMPHOCYTIC MENINGITIS

This is typically caused by viruses (*aseptic meningitis*). An exception is neurosyphilis, caused by *Treponema pallidum,* included here because of a similar tissue reaction. Neurosyphilis, however, differs from viral meningitis in many, largely clinical respects. Viruses which cause lymphocytic meningitis include many ECHO and Coxsackie viruses, the mumps virus and that of lymphocytic choriomeningitis. Most of these are enteric viruses and reach the nervous system from the GI tract via the blood.

The tissue reaction is characteristic. Grossly, the meninges may appear entirely normal or may be somewhat opaque. Although early in the course of the disease the leptomeningeal infiltrate may include many neutrophils, it subsequently is composed almost entirely of lymphocytes and plasma cells. In particular, these mononuclear cells form a cuff around blood vessels (**perivascular cuffing**).

The onset of viral meningitis is sudden, with headache, fever and meningeal signs. In most cases the disease is self-limited, with ultimate full recovery, although fatalities do occur.

In contrast, neurosyphilis is insidious in onset, with protean, often puzzling symptoms. It represents a form of tertiary syphilis which affects only a few of those who contract primary syphilis. Those who do develop neurosyphilis always pass through a stage of asymptomatic syphilitic meningitis within two to three years of manifesting the primary lesion. This stage is recognizable by the appearance of increased numbers of lymphocytes and a positive serologic reaction in the CSF.

Ultimately, symptomatic neurosyphilis may take one of three forms: (1) **Meningovascular neurosyphilis**—characterized by a mononuclear infiltration of the leptomeninges, particularly about the optic chiasm and brain stem, along with typical syphilitic endarteritis and, occasionally, gummatous formations (p. 558). (2) **Paretic neurosyphilis**—characterized by atrophy of the entire brain owing to loss of nerve cells, with perivascular cuffing and transformation of the microglia into rod cells. (3) **Tabes dorsalis (locomotor ataxia)**—characterized by atrophy of the posterior roots of the lumbar region, sometimes accompanied by optic nerve atrophy.

As one might surmise, clinical presentations with neurosyphilis are diverse. Meningovascular syphilis may produce hydrocephalus with its signs and symptoms, or palsy of the second, third and eighth cranial nerves. Paretic neurosyphilis begins with subtle mental changes and progresses to abject dementia. Tabes dorsalis is characterized by sudden lightning pains and paresthesias of the legs or trunk, accompanied by loss of normal pain sensation, vibration sense and deep reflexes. The Argyll-Robertson pupil is almost always present.

BRAIN ABSCESS

Abscesses within the parenchyma of the brain may be single or multiple. They are caused by pyogenic bacteria which reach the brain by the same routes which may also lead to meningitis, i.e., septicemia, nearby infections of the ear or paranasal sinuses, and direct implantation from trauma or during surgery. Occasionally they occur as a late complication of meningitis. The location of the abscess within the brain varies with the route of infection.

Those resulting from septicemia tend to be multiple and often are situated at the junction of the white and gray matters. Infections of the mastoid may lead to a brain abscess within the cerebellum, and those of the middle ear may result in a temporal lobe abscess.

The histology of a brain abscess is characteristic of abscesses elsewhere. There is a central cavity containing pus surrounded by neutrophils. Rimming this is a layer of granulation tissue (composed of mononuclear cells as well as neutrophils, small blood vessels and a scaffolding of connective tissue). A dense outer capsule is formed by a combination of fibrosis and gliosis. Adhesions of the meninges often seal off a point of entry from the rest of the subarachnoid space.

The clinical evolution of a brain abscess tends to be insidious, although at times it may mimic a rather acute encephalitis. In its more chronic presentation it may be entirely quiescent for many weeks to months, often long after the primary source of infection has been forgotten. When symptoms do appear, they are of two types: (1) those referable to a general increase in intracranial pressure, including headache, vomiting and eye signs, and (2) local indications of a space-occupying lesion, such as hemiparesis, hemianopsia, difficulties in coordination and seizures. Unless the abscess is surgically drained, the patient eventually dies, usually of herniation of the brain due to increased intracranial pressure. Sometimes the abscess ruptures into a ventricle, producing a *ventricular empyema*, which is rapidly fatal.

ENCEPHALITIS, MYELITIS, ENCEPHALOMYELITIS

More or less generalized infection of the brain or spinal cord parenchyma is almost always caused by viruses. These viral infections take one of three forms: (1) acute viral encephalitis, (2) "slow" viral encephalitis, characterized by a prolonged incubation period and chronic course, and (3) postinfectious encephalomyelitis, probably an allergic response to a viral infection elsewhere in the body.

ACUTE VIRAL ENCEPHALITIS

A great many viruses may cause encephalitis or encephalomyelitis. Some of these, such as the arboviruses, poliovirus and the rabies virus, show a special predilection for damaging nervous tissue (*neurotropic viruses*). Others, such as the mumps virus, are capable of attacking many tissues. The mode of exposure, of course, varies with the etiologic agent. The arboviruses, which cause Eastern equine encephalitis, Western equine encephalitis, Venezuelan equine encephalitis, St. Louis encephalitis and Japanese B encephalitis, among others, are transmitted by the bite of a mosquito or tick. Rabies, of course, is transmitted by the bite of rabid animals, chiefly dogs. Poliomyelitis is caused by an enteric virus. Perhaps the most common single cause of encephalitis within the United States is the Herpes simplex virus. There is some evidence that it remains latent within the trigeminal ganglia from which it may occasionally migrate to the brain.

Acute viral encephalitis produces fairly uniform histologic changes. Gross alterations are minimal, consisting only of slight edema and sometimes petechiae. Microscopically, the basic process involves chiefly the gray matter. There is progressive degeneration and destruction of the nerve cell bodies. Inclusion bodies have been identified in some of the encephalitides. These include the intranuclear inclusion bodies of rabies (Negri bodies) and cytomegalovirus encephalitis. In all cases there is proliferation of the microglial cells, with the formation of rod cells. The blood vessels are surrounded by lymphocytes and plasma cells (perivascular cuffing) (Fig. 20–15). Some reactive mononuclear inflammation of the leptomeninges almost always occurs. Despite the general uniformity of the histologic picture of encephalitis, there are variations in this pattern which are specific for certain viruses. Thus, the poliovirus selectively destroys the cells of the anterior horn of the spinal cord and of the motor nuclei of the cranial nerves, and the Betz cells of the motor cortex.

The clinical picture of viral encephalitis varies with the causative agent. Infections with the arboviruses, for example, are frequently

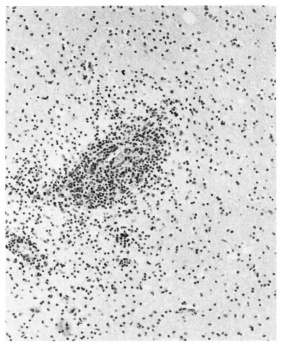

Figure 20–15. Microscopic detail of the cerebral white matter with viral encephalitis. There is striking perivascular cuffing by lymphocytes.

subclinical. In other cases, however, they cause severe disease which, after an incubation period of a few days to three weeks, explodes suddenly in a manner similar to that of pyogenic meningitis. Headache, chills and fever, vomiting and often meningeal signs are present. Marked drowsiness progresses to stupor and coma within a few days. Infection with poliovirus also may be inapparent. When overt it begins after an incubation period of 7 to 14 days with headache, fever and meningeal signs. It may then progress to include a lower motor neuron type of paralysis. Respiratory embarrassment occurs when there is involvement of the respiratory center of the medulla or of the spinal anterior horn cells which give rise to the phrenic or intercostal nerves. The onset of rabies is nonspecific, with headache, fever and malaise, following an incubation period of one to three months. Concomitantly, there are paresthesias near the wound caused by the bite of the rabid animal. Exquisite central nervous system sensitivity ensues. Uncontrollable muscle spasms and even seizures follow nearly any stimulus, including the sight of food or water (hence the popular name, *hydrophobia*) and intense pain results from the slightest touch. Within a week, total flaccid paralysis ensues.

The prognosis with acute viral encephalitis is variable. Rabies is nearly always fatal. At the other extreme, mumps encephalitis is almost always benign. Eastern equine encephalitis carries a mortality of up to 80 per cent, and survivors often suffer severe residua. The other arthropod-borne encephalitides tend to be milder.

"SLOW" VIRAL ENCEPHALITIS

One of the more intriguing recent discoveries in the field of neuropathology is the apparent existence of "slow" viral infections of the central nervous system. These have very long incubation periods, measured in months to decades. Possibly they develop only in conjunction with an altered or abnormal immune status. Such "slow" viral infections have been demonstrated in the following more or less rare but lethal disorders: subacute sclerosing panencephalitis (SSPE), progressive multifocal leukoencephalopathy (PML), Creutzfeldt-Jakob disease, and kuru, a disease of New Guinea cannibals transmitted by eating diseased brain tissue. With far less certainty, "slow" viruses are suspected in certain other degenerating and demyelinating diseases. These include motor neuron disease, Schilder's disease and, most importantly, multiple sclerosis (p. 673) (Zacks, 1971).

Subacute sclerosing panencephalitis (SSPE) begins insidiously in childhood or adolescence. Subtle intellectual deterioration is followed by progressive dementia, myoclonic jerks, seizures and decerebration. Death follows within months to years.

As the name suggests, SSPE affects the gray matter of the entire brain and often the white matter as well. There is shrinkage and loss of neurons (**chronic degeneration,** p. 640), accompanied by marked gliosis. Demyelination may be spotty or diffuse. There is a meningeal and perivascular mononuclear inflammatory infiltrate. Intranuclear acidophilic inclusions can be seen within the neurons and glia.

In 1965 paramyxovirus-like particles were reported in these inclusions (Bouteille et al., 1965). Subsequently, measles antigen was demonstrated in brain sections from some of these patients, as well as high levels of antibodies to measles virus in the serum and CSF (Connolly et al., 1967). By serial subculture and cocultivation with other cell types, a measles-like virus was finally recovered (Payne et al., 1969; Horta-Barbosa et al., 1969), but the difficulty in isolating it suggests that *complete* infectious units (virions) are not present within the brain. Rather, SSPE appears to represent an occult infection involving only the viral nucleocapsids, with limited expression of the viral genes.

Progressive multifocal leukoencephalopathy (PML) is a rare disease which develops almost exclusively in patients with other chronic disease, especially lymphoproliferative disorders, or in those undergoing immunosuppressive therapy. Like SSPE it begins insidiously with subtle changes in mentation, then progresses inexorably through gross hemispheric neurologic deficits, such as hemiplegia or hemianopsia, to death within a few months of onset.

The lesions are characterized histologically by multifocal demyelination of white matter with loss of the oligodendrocytes which maintain the myelin sheath. The axons are spared. Nearby surviving oligodendrocytes are enlarged and contain intranuclear inclusions. There is a proliferation of astrocytes and these may be quite bizarre, containing abnormal mitotic figures and multiple nuclei. A minimal mononuclear inflammatory response may occur.

Intranuclear inclusions within the oligodendrocytes were reported in 1965 to be virtually packed with papovaviruses (ZuRhein and Chou, 1965; ZuRhein, 1969). Two specific viruses were subsequently identified—one called the JC-virus and another closely related or identical to simian-virus 40 (SV-40) (Narayan et al., 1973). Both are members of the polyoma subgroup of papovaviruses. This is especially interesting for two reasons. First, PML becomes the first disease in man found to be related to the simian-virus 40 (or indeed to any of the polyoma viruses). Second, these viruses are oncogenic in their natural hosts as well as in experimental animals and transform cells in culture. Recent seroepidemiologic studies show that *asymptomatic* infection with JC-virus is quite common. Antibody against JC-virus was found in 69 per cent of adults tested (Padgett and Walker, 1973). Moreover, within the last 20 years, millions of people have been inoculated with SV-40 virus inadvertently as a contaminant of polio vaccine produced in monkey kidney tissue cultures.

Creutzfeldt-Jakob disease and *kuru* are two diseases less certainly associated with viruses. They are known as *spongiform encephalopathies* because of the swollen, vacuolated appearance of the neurons, with displacement of the nucleus. There is an accompanying astrocytosis but no inflammation. Two spontaneously appearing diseases of lower animals—mink encephalopathy and scrapie of sheep and goats—involve similar pathologic changes and are included with the spongiform encephalopathies (Zlotnik et al., 1974). In both Creutzfeldt-Jakob disease and kuru, an infectious agent is indicated by the fact that they can be transmitted to chimpanzees by the intracerebral inoculation of diseased brain suspensions. However, specific organisms have not yet been recovered (Editorial, 1974c). Creutzfeldt-Jakob disease occurs in middle age and produces dementia and myoclonus, leading to death within a year. Kuru, as mentioned, is a disease of New Guinea cannibals. It begins as cerebellar ataxia, progressing to generalized decortication and death within six months.

Despite the fairly clear association of measles virus with SSPE and of certain papova viruses with PML, the basic nature of these "slow" virus infections remains a fascinating mystery, with implications beyond the importance of these two uncommon diseases. Why do viruses which are known to be very common in man, producing conventional measles in one case and almost always no known disease in the other, go on to cause progressive neurologic disease in only a small minority of their hosts? Does this minority necessarily have a defective immune capacity? Although a concomitant immunologic derangement can be strongly argued in the case of PML, which is associated with disorders such as Hodgkin's disease or chronic lymphocytic leukemia, it is not an obvious factor in SSPE. In the case of SSPE, an autoimmune component has been suggested. Measles virus is known to alter cell membranes, and it may thus introduce new antigens into the membrane and trigger an immunologic response to the host as well as to the invading viruses (Weiner et al., 1973). However, this does not explain why only a small number of measles victims go on to develop SSPE. Recently a two-virus theory has been proposed (Baguley and Glasgow, 1973). This theory is based on the extraordinarily high incidence of SSPE which occurred in the 13 years following vaccination of a group of schoolchildren with SV-40 contaminated Salk vaccine. *Both* measles virus and a papovavirus were subsequently recovered from the brain tissue of three of these patients. Perhaps the measles virus, by causing cell fusion, in some way facilitates the spread of the papovavirus, or perhaps they interact at a molecular level. If subsequent studies do show that both are in fact necessary to produce SSPE, a papovavirus, oncogenic in animals, emerges as the common element in two chronic neurologic diseases of man.

POSTINFECTIOUS ENCEPHALOMYELITIS

This disorder occurs as a complication of various viral infections elsewhere in the body, especially the exanthems, such as measles, varicella and rubella. It may also develop following inoculation against smallpox. Although it is thought to represent an allergic phenomenon rather than actual invasion by the virus of the CNS, inclusion bodies have been reported in the brain and the issue therefore remains unsettled.

Histologically, the lesions are quite specific.

TABLE 20–5. INFECTIONS OF THE NERVOUS SYSTEM

Type	Entity	Entry of Organism	Distribution	Histopathology	Cerebrospinal Fluid (CSF)	Clinical Features	Prognosis	Other
Pyogenic meningitis	Pneumococcus, meningococcus, streptococcus, H. influenzae, staphylococcus	Septicemia, otitis, paranasal sinusitis, mastoiditis, penetrating wounds	Subarachnoid, occasionally subdural or spinal epidural	Acute polymorphonuclear fibrinopurulent exudate	Turbid, ↑pressure, many PMN's, ↑protein, ↓sugar, organisms on smear or culture	Sudden onset, headache, fever, chills, meningeal signs, agitation, coma	Good with therapy, may be permanent neurologic impairment	
Granulomatous meningitis	Tubercle bacillus, Cryptococcus neoformans, Coccidioides immitis	Metastatic from lung	Subarachnoid, occasionally spinal epidural	Granuloma formation typical of organism	↑pressure, lymphocytes, ↑protein, ↓sugar, organisms on smear or culture	Subacute to chronic, malaise, headache, meningeal signs	Variable, may be permanent impairment	
Lymphocytic meningitis	Viral ECHO 4, 6, 9, 11, 14, 16; Coxsackie B and A 7, 9; mumps; lymphocytic choriomeningitis; neurosyphilis	Usually contaminated food or water Blood-borne with neurosyphilis	Subarachnoid	Chronic inflammatory infiltrate (lymphocytes and plasma cells), perivascular cuffing	↑pressure, lymphocytes, slight ↑protein, normal sugar	Sudden onset, headache, fever, meningeal signs; neurosyphilis—often slow onset with protean signs	Good, may be residua with neurosyphilis	Argyll-Robertson pupil in syphilis

MENINGITIS

Brain abscess	Staphylococcus, pneumococcus, streptococcus	Same as pyogenic meningitis; may follow meningitis	Brain, often junction of white and gray matter	Focus of liquefaction surrounded by granulation tissue and fibrous capsule	↑ pressure, lymphocytes, ↑ protein, normal sugar, sterile	Variable, may mimic encephalitis, brain tumor or chronic infection (malaise, fever, headache)	Fair, often residua	
Acute viral encephalitis	Arthropod-borne viruses (equine encephalitis, St. Louis, Japanese B); rabies; poliomyelitis; Herpes simplex; Herpes zoster; cytomegalovirus	Bite of mosquito or tick for arboviruses, others variable	Brain and occasionally spinal cord, typically gray matter, varies with disease	Degeneration of nerve cells, microglial proliferation and formation of "rod cells," perivascular cuffing, often inclusion bodies	↑ pressure, lymphocytes, slight ↑ protein, normal sugar, sterile	Vary with disease, usually sudden onset, headache, fever, drowsiness	Variable, often residua	Negri bodies with rabies
"Slow" viral encephalitis	Subacute sclerosing panencephalitis (SSPE), progressive multifocal leukoencephalopathy, ?? multiple sclerosis	?	Brain, often diffuse	Degeneration of nerve cells in SSPE, demyelination white matter, gliosis, inclusion bodies	May be normal, occasionally lymphocytes	Variable in SSPE and PML, chronic onset, subtle mental changes, dementia, myoclonus, decortication	Fatal in months to years (MS may remit)	? Caused by persistent measles and/or papovaviruses
Postinfectious encephalomyelitis	May follow: measles, varicella, rubella, vaccinia, smallpox, influenza	—	Brain and cord, diffuse	Demyelination of white matter (scattered), perivenular lymphocytes and plasma cells	May be normal, occasionally ↑ lymphocytes	About 1 week after infection, headache, fever, delirium	Good, occasionally fatal or residua	Probable autoimmune basis

ENCEPHALITIS, ENCEPHALOMYELITIS

They consist of scattered foci of demyelination throughout the brain and spinal cord, without loss of axons, accompanied by an infiltrate of lymphocytes and plasma cells about the venules of the CNS ("perivenular encephalomyelitis"). This histologic pattern closely resembles that of experimental allergic encephalomyelitis, which can be induced by the injection into experimental animals of a protein component of myelin, termed basic encephalitogen (Webb et al., 1974).

The disorder has an abrupt clinical onset, usually during the week after the exanthem appears, or within 3 weeks of smallpox inoculation. There is headache and fever, which may be followed by stupor, convulsions and severe neurologic impairment. Fortunately, the disorder is usually transient and clears within days to weeks. However, with measles, which it complicates in 1 of 1000 cases, the mortality rate may be up to 20 per cent (Weiner et al., 1973).

DEGENERATIVE DISEASES OF THE CNS

The degenerative diseases of the CNS are characterized by slowly progressive loss of neurons without known cause. The definition is rather arbitrary, and implies that enlightenment about the etiology of a disorder removes it from the group. Thus, Wilson's disease (hepatolenticular degeneration) is now considered a metabolic derangement rather than a degenerative disease. Nonetheless, the concept of degenerative diseases of the CNS is useful, if only because the label can be remembered as encompassing perhaps the cruelest group of disorders in neurology.

To some extent the degenerative process tends to be selective for certain levels of the nervous system. Thus, one set of disorders predominantly involves the cerebral cortex; another, the basal ganglia; and a third, the cerebellum and spinal cord. Degeneration of the peripheral nerves may also occur; this is considered in the discussion of the peripheral neuropathies (p. 675). Each of these sets of disorders produces a fairly distinct symptom complex. For this reason, they are discussed separately in the following sections. However, it should be remembered that some of the individual disease entities may affect more than one anatomic level and thus produce mixed pictures.

CORTICAL DEGENERATION

Degeneration of the cerebral cortex produces the symptom complex known as *dementia*. In the early stages the demented individual may exhibit little more than anxiety or depression as he experiences increasing difficulty with memory and comprehension. Thus, the disorder may go unrecognized, or masquerade as a psychogenic disturbance. Later, as the full-blown syndrome develops, there is the gradual onset of obvious memory impairment, particularly for recent events; defective comprehension and judgment; labile affect; and some degree of disorientation. This is the picture the layman terms "senility." Aphasia, apraxia and agnosia may supervene, as well as locomotor impairment corresponding to the degree of mental deterioration. In advanced stages there may be pathologic reflexes, including the grasp and sucking reflexes and bilateral extensor plantar responses, exaggerated normal reflexes and resistance to passive movement (gegenhalten). Paroxysms of affectless crying or uncontrollable laughter with dysarthria and dysphagia (*pseudobulbar palsy*) may also occur. Eventually, the patient may become little more than a vegetable—totally withdrawn, mute and motionless.

There has been an unfortunate tendency on the part of clinicians to attribute dementia rather indiscriminantly to atherosclerotic changes in the cerebral vessels. Whereas it is true that dementia may be a sequela of a cerebrovascular accident, and that stepwise mental deterioration may result from lacunar infarcts (p. 655), there is no very good evidence that *slowly progressive* dementia results from atherosclerosis (Hachinski et al., 1974). Both cortical degeneration and atherosclerosis affect the same age groups, however, and it is not surprising that they often are seen together. *Probably the most important causes of cortical degeneration are pre-senile dementia (which includes both Alzheimer's disease and Pick's disease) and senile dementia.* Although these will be considered separately, there is some reason to believe that Alzheimer's disease and senile dementia represent extremes of a spectrum, with the former occurring earlier in life and progressing more rapidly (Barrett, 1972). Before continuing, it should be emphasized that disorders other than cortical degeneration may produce dementia and that some of these are treatable. Such disorders include subdural hematoma, meningioma, a variety of metabolic derangements and normal pressure hydrocephalus. It is important to exclude treatable lesions before attributing dementia to a degenerative process.

ALZHEIMER'S DISEASE

This degenerative process is characterized by progressive severe atrophy of the entire brain, particularly the frontal cortex. It has its onset relatively early, between the ages of 40 and 60 years, and progresses steadily from subtle emotional lability and intellectual impairment through total dementia to death by inanition, dehydration or respiratory infection within 5 to 15 years (Haase, 1971; Heston et al., 1966). There is some tendency to familial occurrence.

The gross changes consist of shrinkage of the brain, with narrowing of the gyri and widening of the sulci, and dilatation of the ventricles (**hydrocephalus ex vacuo**). Microscopically, there is loss of many neurons, particularly in the cortex, and replacment by astrocytes and microglia. In addition, there are three histologic hallmarks of this disease. The first is the **senile plaque**. This consists of a core of amorphous material, identified by histochemical studies as amyloid, surrounded by a fibrillar ring, consisting of degenerated neuronal and glial processes (Barrett, 1972). It varies in size from 20 to 150 μm. in diameter, and is found in variable numbers only in the gray matter. The second histologic hallmark is the **neurofibrillary tangle** present within some affected neurons. With silver impregnation this is seen as a prominent, flame-shaped skein of intracytoplasmic fibrils which probably results from some alteration of the neurofilaments. The third hallmark is **intraneuronal granulovacuolar degeneration**. This appears as small, clear, intracytoplasmic vacuoles, up to 5 μm. in diameter, which contain an argyrophilic granule. **None of these features is specific to Alzheimer's disease.** Any of them may be seen in other degenerative processes and, in small numbers, in the brains of elderly individuals with no known disease. **It is their concurrence and abundance, in association with widespread loss of neurons, that permits the histologic diagnosis of Alzheimer's disease.**

PICK'S DISEASE

This is clinically indistinguishable from Alzheimer's disease. It is far less frequent, and affects women more often than men. In the individual case, the distinction between Alzheimer's disease and Pick's disease is on anatomic grounds.

In Pick's disease, the atrophy is highly selective. Only the frontal and temporal lobes are involved, and in these areas there is sparing of the precentral gyrus, the hippocampus and the auditory area of the superior temporal gyrus. Histologically, there is loss of neurons in the affected areas, with glial replacement. **Senile plaques and neurofibrillary tangles are not present, except incidentally.** Round homogeneous argyrophilic inclusions may be seen within the cytoplasm of neurons. These are termed **Pick's neuronal inclusions.** Although they are specific for the disease, they are present in only a minority of cases (Escourolle and Poirier, 1973).

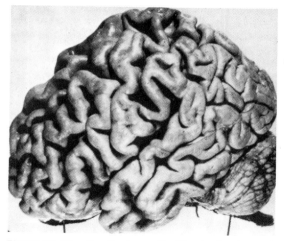

Figure 20–16. Senile dementia. The brain shows diffuse cortical atrophy, particularly marked in the frontal, parietal and superior temporal lobes, with narrowing of the gyri and widening of the sulci. (Courtesy of Dr. Robert D. Terry.)

SENILE DEMENTIA

This form of cortical degeneration occurs in an older age group, usually over the age of 60 years. Often there is concomitant atherosclerotic disease of the cerebral vessels, and it is difficult to say how much, if any, this contributes to the process. The clinical picture is much the same as with presenile dementia, although it tends to progress more slowly.

Anatomically, too, senile dementia is very similar to Alzheimer's disease. There is diffuse cerebral atrophy with dilatation of the ventricles (Fig. 20–16). Microscopically, senile plaques and neurofibrillary tangles may be present, although they are not so abundant as with Alzheimer's disease. As mentioned earlier, it is possible that senile dementia is simply a milder form of Alzheimer's disease with a later onset.

DEGENERATION OF THE BASAL GANGLIA

Degenerative processes which affect the basal ganglia give rise to a variety of clinical signs based on interference with the extrapyramidal motor system. Broadly speaking, these include: (1) the presence of certain stereotyped involuntary movements—namely, tremor, choreiform movements, athetosis or dystonia, (2) a disturbance of voluntary movements, which usually takes the form of slowness to initiate movement and loss of spontaneous gestures, and (3) a disturbance of muscle tone, which may be either increased or decreased. The precise clinical syndrome varies with the specific disease and the area most affected. By far the most important cause of degeneration of the basal ganglia is Parkinson's disease, to be discussed later. Other important causes include Wilson's disease and Huntington's chorea. Both of these are familial.

Wilson's disease (hepatolenticular degeneration), as mentioned earlier, is caused by a defect in copper metabolism which is inherited as an autosomal recessive characteristic. There is a deficiency of ceruloplasmin, the serum copper-transporting protein, and copper is deposited in large amounts within the tissues. The disease becomes manifest in adolescence, and is characterized by corneal discoloration (*Kayser-Fleischer ring*) and cirrhosis of the liver, as well as degenerative lesions of the putamen and, to a lesser extent, the globus pallidus, the thalamus and the cerebral cortex. The manifestations of the liver involvement usually precede those of the nervous system. The pattern of cirrhosis ranges from a delicate scarring reminiscent of posthepatitic cirrhosis to coarse irregular lesions similar to those of postnecrotic cirrhosis. Special studies disclose abnormal deposits of copper within the liver.

Huntington's chorea is inherited as an autosomal dominant disorder which becomes manifest in middle age. The degeneration affects chiefly the head of the caudate nucleus, which may be almost totally atrophied, and the putamen. In addition, there is some degeneration of the frontal and parietal cortex. The lesions take the form of loss of neurons, with marked replacement gliosis. A deficiency of the neurotransmitter γ-aminobutyric acid (GABA), has been demonstrated in the affected areas (Perry et al., 1973). The onset of choreiform movements is the first clinical indication of Huntington's chorea. This is eventually followed by dementia, and both progress over a period of 10 to 15 years until the patient is completely incapacitated.

PARKINSON'S DISEASE (PARALYSIS AGITANS)

This is a disorder of unknown etiology characterized clinically by (1) a coarse rhythmic tremor of the hands, face and tongue, (2) akinesia, with loss of spontaneous movements, masked facies and poverty of voluntary movements, and (3) intermittent or "cogwheel" rigidity. An identical clinical picture may result from a variety of other processes, including lacunar infarcts (arteriosclerotic Parkinsonism), encephalitis (postencephalitic Parkinsonism), poisoning with manganese or carbon monoxide and, in a small number of cases, therapy with reserpine or phenothiazines. *It is proper, then, to speak of a Parkinsonian syndrome, of which the most frequent cause is Parkinson's disease.* It would seem that in all cases the

syndrome is associated biochemically with a deficiency of dopamine in the dopaminergic neurons of the caudate, putamen, globus pallidus and substantia nigra. According to neurochemical studies, the severity of the manifestations of Parkinsonism is directly pro portional to the deficiency (Hornykiewicz, 1973). Thus, the dramatic effect of treatment with L-dopa (the immediate precursor of dopamine, which, unlike dopamine, crosses the blood-brain barrier) is due simply to replacement. Recognizing the biochemical abnormality, however, tells us little about the pathogenesis or the basis of the lesions in Parkinson's disease proper.

The most striking anatomic changes of Parkinson's disease are seen in the substantia nigra. Grossly, this area of the brain appears pale. With the light microscope it can be seen that most of the neurons have disappeared and are replaced by glial cells. Phagocytes contain the displaced pigment. Within the residual neurons are spherical, eosinophilic, intracytoplasmic inclusions termed **Lewy bodies**. Less dramatic changes are seen within the globus pallidus and, to a lesser extent, within the caudate and putamen. These consist of nonspecific degenerative changes.

Parkinson's disease has its clinical onset in middle to old age. It usually begins with tremor in one hand, which eventually spreads to both arms, the face and tongue. Akinesia and rigidity follow. Although the disease is not in itself life-threatening, it is to a variable extent incapacitating and the characteristic immobility may lead to problems of malnutrition, infection and thromboembolism.

CEREBELLAR AND SPINAL DEGENERATION

There exist a large number of degenerative processes which affect the cerebellum or the spinal cord. In some cases the lesions are localized to one of these structures; in others, the involvements are spinocerebellar or corticospinal. Many of these disorders are hereditary. Fortunately, most are rare. Degeneration of the cerebellar cortex with resultant ataxia may occur as a distant effect of *carcinoma*. The pathogenesis is unknown. *Alcoholism* may also lead to degeneration of the cerebellar cortex, again for mysterious reasons.

Friedreich's ataxia is the most important of the hereditary spinocerebellar disorders. It is characterized by atrophy with demyelination of the spinocerebellar, the corticospinal and the posterior columns of the spinal cord. In addition, there is an associated foot deformity (pes cavus), some degree of kyphoscoliosis and, sometimes, an interstitial myocarditis. The clinical onset is in adolescence, and it leads to complete disability within a few years.

Motor neuron disease refers to a group of disorders which involve degeneration of motor neurons anywhere within the CNS. It includes *spinal muscular atrophy*, characterized by degeneration of the anterior horn cells; *amyotrophic lateral sclerosis*, in which the pyramidal tracts as well as the anterior horn cells are involved; and *progressive bulbar palsy*, which involves the cranial nerve nuclei. The pathogenesis of these disorders is unknown. Their onset is usually in early middle age, with progressive weakness and atrophy of the denervated muscles. All lead to death within a few years. The bulbar form is particularly lethal, since it interferes with swallowing and breathing and easily leads to aspiration pneumonitis.

THE DEMYELINATING DISEASES

A great many pathologic processes result in secondary demyelination. These include any sizable lesion located in the white matter, such as a tumor or infarct, as well as the degenerative diseases. Here, however, we are concerned only with those disorders in which the *primary* lesion is loss of myelin, with relative sparing of the axon. By this strict definition, there are not a large number of demyelinating diseases. By far the most important among them is *multiple sclerosis.* This is one of the most frequent of nonvascular nervous system diseases. It will be discussed in some detail below. A closely related disease, *Schilder's disease,* will also be described briefly. Another important demyelinating process to be described is *subacute combined degeneration of the spinal cord,* the neuropathy associated with pernicious anemia (p. 336). *Progressive multifocal leukoencephalopathy, subacute sclerosing panencephalitis* and *postinfectious encephalomyelitis* may also be considered demyelinating diseases. They are discussed in the section dealing with "slow" viral infections of the CNS (p. 666). Relatively rare causes of demyelination are the *leukodystrophies,* a group of familial disorders characterized by the formation of abnormal myelin (rather than the loss of normal myelin), probably on the basis of an inherited enzymatic defect (Escourolle and Poirier, 1973).

MULTIPLE SCLEROSIS (DISSEMINATED SCLEROSIS)

This is a relatively frequent, relapsing and remitting disorder, characterized by the unpredictable appearance of circumscribed patches of demyelination throughout the CNS. It most often has its onset in young adulthood, and affects men and women equally. The etiology and pathogenesis are unknown. Recently, the possibility that multiple sclerosis is caused by a virus, in particular measles or another paramyxovirus, has gained considerable support. The evidence is epidemiologic, pathologic and immunologic (Editorial, 1974a). The epidemiologic indications of an infectious etiology have been appreciated for some time. The disease is very much more frequent in the higher latitudes of both the northern and southern hemispheres. Those who move from a low-risk to a high-risk area before adolescence develop a high risk of acquiring multiple sclerosis; however, those who make the same move after adolescence sustain a low risk. Thus, it would seem that the initial event in the development of the disease occurs in early life. In addition, there appears to be a familial tendency toward the disease which is independent of any heritable factor. On the basis of migration and family studies, a latent period of 3 to 23 years between the initial event and the clinical onset can be inferred (Weiner et al., 1973). These data are all consistent with exposure in childhood to a virus which later in some way leads to multiple sclerosis. The presence of perivascular mononuclear inflammatory infiltrates in the lesions of multiple sclerosis offers some pathologic support for a possible viral causation. The first bit of immunologic evidence for a viral causation was the report in 1962 of higher than average titers of measles antibodies in the serum and CSF of patients with multiple sclerosis (Adams and Imagawa, 1962). Since then it has been demonstrated that some of these antibodies are produced in the brain. The anti-measles antibodies within the serum include IgM as well as IgG, which suggests a continuing infection by the virus somewhere within the body (Editorial, 1974). Finally, there have been recent reports of the presence and recovery of paramyxovirus-like particles from the brain tissue of patients with multiple sclerosis (ter Meulen et al., 1972; Field et al., 1972; Prineas, 1972). If multiple sclerosis is indeed caused by a paramyxovirus, it is certainly not a classical infection. Conceivably, the viruses persist as defective particles in the nervous systems of hosts with some subtle immunologic impairment. Multiple sclerosis would then represent a "slow" virus infection. The concept of an immunologic impairment is supported by the fact that certain histocompatibility antigens are significantly more common in multiple sclerosis patients than in controls; possibly these are associated with some immunologic deficiency. It has been suggested that a T-cell derangement

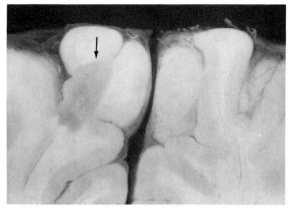

Figure 20–17. A plaque of multiple sclerosis virtually replacing the central white matter of a cerebral gyrus (arrow).

may permit persistence of the virus and also lead to increased B-cell activity, with the production of antibodies against components of both the virus and the host (Editorial, 1974a). Some autoimmune contribution is supported by several aspects of the disease, including its similarities to experimental allergic encephalitis and to postinfectious encephalomyelitis, as well as a reported response to intensive immunosuppressive therapy (Ring et al., 1974). It has been hypothesized that the relapsing-remitting character of the disease may reflect an interplay between a slow virus infection of the oligodendrocytes and an intermittent autoimmune response whenever critical levels of virus production are reached (Adams and Dickinson, 1974). The answers to some of these questions seem tantalizingly close.

The morphologic hallmark of multiple sclerosis is the plaque of demyelination. Grossly, these plaques appear as rather sharply circumscribed areas, from 1 mm. to several centimeters in diameter, scattered throughout the white matter of the CNS (Fig. 20–17). Favored locations are the optic nerves, the periventricular areas of the cerebrum, the cerebellar peduncles, the brain stem and the dorsal spinal cord. New plaques tend to be pinkish, owing to vascular congestion, and edematous. Older ones have a grayish translucency and are retracted. Microscopically, the plaques are characterized by demyelination, with loss of the oligodendrocytes (Fig. 20–18). Usually the axons are preserved, although in severe, long-standing multiple sclerosis there may be some axonal degeneration. In active lesions, compound granular cells, which engulf the degenerating myelin, are very prominent. In addition, as mentioned, there is a perivascular cuff of lymphocytes and plasma cells. Reactive gliosis follows, especially around the perimeter of the plaque. In the older lesions, the

gliosis is increasingly marked and the inflammatory aspect becomes muted.

The clinical picture of multiple sclerosis is highly variable, as the widespread anatomic distribution of the lesions would suggest. The onset is usually rather sudden, and may take the form of visual disturbances, ataxia, weakness or paresthesias of a limb, or one of a multitude of other, less frequent symptoms. In any case the initial manifestation usually disappears within a few days to weeks. The subsequent course of the disease is variable. After the initial attack, there may be an interval of months to years before relapse. Relapse may be heralded by the return of the original symptom or by the development of an entirely different one. This tendency to remit and the varied symptomatology are the most important clinical clues to the nature of the disease. In general, the longer the interval between the initial attack and the first relapse the better the prognosis. Occasionally, remission may be apparently permanent. At the opposite extreme, in unfortunate patients the course is progressive from the outset. Most patients fall in between these two extremes. With each attack there is some permanent neurologic

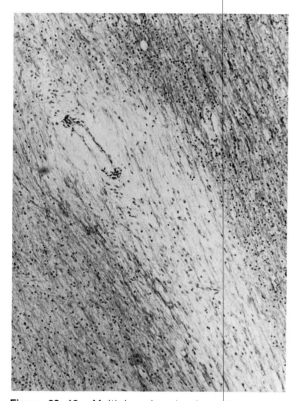

Figure 20–18. Multiple sclerosis. A myelin stain to reveal a focus of demyelination virtually enclosing a small vessel.

damage and they become more or less incapacitated, but only after many years.

SCHILDER'S DISEASE

This disease is similar to multiple sclerosis in many respects. It differs in that it evolves without remissions, and it tends to affect children. The lesions are nearly identical to those of multiple sclerosis, although they tend to be larger and more often involve secondary degeneration of the axons. Children with this disease follow a tragic course, developing blindness, deafness, aphasia, hemiplegia, anesthesia and mental deficiency. Some regard this disease as a severe variant of multiple sclerosis; others consider it a leukodystrophy (Zacks, 1971).

SUBACUTE COMBINED DEGENERATION OF THE SPINAL CORD (COMBINED SYSTEMS DISEASE)

This is the neuropathy that accompanies pernicious anemia and is presumed to result from vitamin B_{12} deficiency. In most cases it develops only after long-standing overt pernicious anemia, although occasionally its clinical onset precedes the discovery of anemia. Only rarely does it accompany other forms of vitamin B_{12} deficiency, such as that resulting from malabsorption.

The lesions are found in the dorsal and lateral columns of the spinal cord. Grossly, these areas of the cord appear shrunken and grayish-white. The first alteration seen with the microscope is swelling of the myelin followed by demyelination of the dorsal columns, particularly in the lower cervical and upper thoracic regions. Only later does degeneration of the axons take place. The lesions extend rostrally and caudally, as well as to the lateral columns. In severe cases the other long tracts are also involved. The gray matter is spared. In a few cases the brain stem, optic nerves and cerebral cortex contain foci of demyelination.

Clinically, subacute combined degeneration is heralded by paresthesias of the hands and feet. Neurologic examination at this point usually reveals loss of vibration sense and diminution of the knee and ankle jerks. Because of the loss of proprioception, the patient becomes ataxic. When the corticospinal tracts become involved, spasticity and extensor plantar responses ensue. In severe cases, a spastic paraplegia may develop.

DISORDERS OF PERIPHERAL NERVES (PERIPHERAL NEUROPATHY)

Peripheral neuropathy may accompany a variety of metabolic, nutritional, toxic and neoplastic disorders, or it may occur as an isolated disorder. Whether isolated or a part of a well-defined disease entity, the precise pathogenesis of the neurologic involvement is in most cases unknown. Following is a general description of the distribution, histology and clinical features of the peripheral neuropathies. Some of the more important individual neuropathies are then presented.

Peripheral neuropathy may affect only one nerve trunk *(mononeuropathy)* or two or more nerve trunks in isolation *(mononeuropathy multiplex)*, or it may diffusely involve all nerves of a certain type *(polyneuropathy)*. In the latter case, the longest neurons are most severely affected; hence the feet are usually the earliest sites affected. When polyneuropathy is progressive, the signs and symptoms later have a "glove and stocking" distribution, then spread proximally.

The histological manifestations of peripheral nerve disorders, regardless of cause, are limited. There are two principal lesions. The first is **Wallerian degeneration.** This reflects injury to the neuron or axon and takes the form of fragmentation and loss of the distal portion of an axon, with secondary breakdown of the myelin sheath. In its most well-defined form, it is seen distal to the point of section of a peripheral nerve, in which case the cell

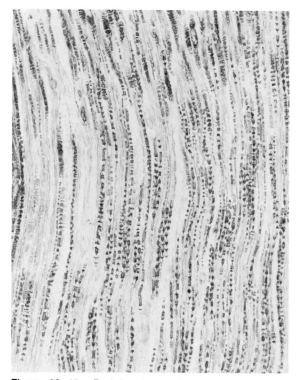

Figure 20–19. Peripheral neuritis. A myelin stain which discloses foci of total loss of myelin and fragmentation of the residual myelin.

body simultaneously undergoes the changes described as an **axonal reaction** (p. 640). However, Wallerian degeneration also occurs in the distal axon of a neuron undergoing a generalized insult—for example, in certain metabolic derangements. It is thought that this vulnerability of the distal axon reflects its greater distance from its source of nutrients and protein synthesis (Sibley, 1972). In progressive disease, Wallerian degeneration may then spread proximally ("dying-back phenomenon"). The second important lesion in peripheral neuropathy is **segmental demyelination (segmental degeneration of Gombault).** This appears as patchy dissolution of the myelin sheath with anatomic preservation of the axon (Fig. 20–19). It is thought to result from focal derangements of the Schwann cells from infectious agents or toxic or metabolic injury. Usually this is accompanied by transient functional impairment of the axon. Remyelination with complete restoration of function may follow and requires about two weeks (Zacks, 1971). This form of injury is thought to represent a relatively early indication of neuronal distress, which in many cases precedes the development of Wallerian degeneration. Thus, they may be seen together. In addition to these two forms of primary neuronal injury, the peripheral nerves may undergo infarction from vascular disease, such as diabetes mellitus or polyarteritis nodosa, or be directly destroyed by localized proliferative processes, such as tumors.

Clinically, peripheral neuropathy is characterized by motor weakness, sensory loss and pain. The predominant symptom varies markedly from case to case and among the various neuropathies. Tendon reflexes are diminished or absent in the affected limbs, and nerve conduction velocities are variably reduced.

Table 20–6 shows the more important peripheral neuropathies and some of their salient features. Those that are secondary to another pathologic process are in most cases presented along with the parent disorder, as will be indicated.

Acute idiopathic polyneuritis (Guillain-Barré syndrome) is thought to be the peripheral nervous system equivalent of postinfectious encephalomyelitis, that is, an immunoallergic phenomenon. A variety of viral and bacterial infections are reported to have preceded it by days to weeks. Most often, the antecedent illness is a nonspecific respiratory or enteric infection, but it may be one of the childhood exanthemata, vaccinia, typhoid-paratyphoid immunization or infectious mononucleosis (Sibley, 1972). Histologically there is widespread segmental demyelination accompanied by a perineurial lymphocytic inflammatory infiltrate. It has been suggested that the myelin is specifically attacked by sensitized lympho-

TABLE 20–6. PERIPHERAL NEUROPATHIES

Idiopathic:
  Acute idiopathic polyneuritis (Guillain-Barré syndrome): Polyneuropathy, demyelination, affects mainly proximal muscles, may affect muscles of respiration.
  Acute brachial neuritis: Mononeuropathy multiplex, demyelination, affects muscles of the brachial plexus.
  Bell's palsy: Paralysis of seventh cranial nerve.

Nutritional:
  Alcoholic polyneuropathy (p. 241): Wallerian degeneration and segmental demyelination; chiefly sensory; ? toxic rather than nutritional.

Metabolic:
  Diabetic neruopathy (p. 137): Polyneuropathy, segmental demyelination, chiefly sensory; or mononeuropathy or mononeuropathy multiplex, probably of vascular origin, chiefly motor.
  Uremic neuropathy (p. 429): Polyneuropathy, Wallerian degeneration and segmental demyelination, reversible with transplantation, sometimes with hemodialysis. (editorial, 1971).
  Acute porphyric polyneuropathy: Acute, similar to Guillain.Barré, chiefly motor, may affect muscles of respiration.

Toxic (arsenic, lead, mercury, gold, INH): Variable effects.

Carcinomatous Neuropathy: Sensorimotor, Wallerian degeneration and segmental demyelination.

Neuropathy of Dysproteinoses (p. 354): Variable, usually polyneuropathy, demyelination with multiple myeloma, improves with treatment of tumor (Davis and Drachman, 1972).

Traumatic: Mononeuropathy or mononeuropathy multiplex.

Infectious:
  Leprosy: Mononeuropathy multiplex.
  Diphtheria: Segmental demyelination.
  Herpes zoster: Primarily dorsal root ganglion, may be inflammation or Wallerian degeneration of corresponding peripheral nerve.

Heredofamilial:
  Charcot-Marie-Tooth disease (peroneal muscular atrophy): Polyneuropathy, degeneration.
  Dejerine-Sottas disease (hypertrophic interstitial polyneuritis): Whorling proliferation of Schwann cells around axons, with compression.
  Refsum's disease (heredopathia atactica polyneuritiformis): polyneuropathy, proliferation of Schwann cells.

cytes. The onset is typically heralded by weakness of the legs, followed within hours by numbness and paresthesias of the hands and feet. Paralysis of all extremities usually ensues. In contrast to most other peripheral neuropathies, this is typically most profound in the proximal muscles. Involvement of the cranial nerves may also occur, particularly diplegia of the facial nerve. *The most important feature of acute idiopathic polyneuritis is its tendency to affect the muscles of respiration.* Respiratory insufficiency develops in 10 to 20 per cent of cases, often suddenly. Prompt mechanical respiration in these cases is necessary to prevent death. Usually, the disease reaches its peak within a week, remains stationary for another two weeks, then gradually subsides. CSF protein is elevated, often between 100 and 400 mg. per 100 ml. Although about 10 per cent of patients suffer some neurologic deficit, recovery is usually complete.

Acute brachial neuritis (neuralgic amyotrophy) is a degenerative process which affects one or more roots of the brachial plexus (Editorial, 1974*b*). Usually it is unilateral. Sometimes it occurs as a part of a serum sickness syndrome, in particular following the administration of tetanus antitoxin; in other instances it represents a familial recurrent disorder; most often it is idiopathic. Intense pain in the arm and shoulder is the first symptom, followed in a few days by weakness. Although the pain subsides within days, muscle weakness may persist for months. In about 20 per cent of cases, there is some permanent weakness and muscle atrophy (Bardenwerper, 1962).

Trauma is the most common cause of mononeuropathy. Although the trauma may produce disruption of the nerve, most commonly it acts by acute or repetitive compression or stretching. Thus, an alcoholic who falls asleep on a park bench with his arm draped over the back may awake with a radial nerve palsy as well as a hangover. In the carpal tunnel syndrome, the median nerve is compressed. Other nerves vulnerable to compression or stretching include the ulnar nerve at the elbow, the lateral femoral cutaneous nerve and the peroneal nerve at the fibular head.

In concluding this book with a presentation of neuropathology, we have perhaps lent support to the view that when the nervous system is finished, so are you. Be that as it may, this relatively brief tour through the basics of pathology is now completed.

REFERENCES

Adams, D. H., and Dickinson, J. P.: Etiology of multiple sclerosis. Lancet, *1*:1196, 1974.

Adams, J. N., and Imagawa, D. T.: Proc. Soc. Exp. Biol. Med., *3*:562, 1962.

Baguley, D. M., and Glasgow, G. L.: Subacute sclerosing panencephalitis and Salk vaccine. Lancet, *2*:763, 1973.

Bardenwerper, H. W.: Serum neuritis from tetanus antitoxin. J.A.M.A., *179*:763, 1962.

Barrett, R. E.: Dementia in adults. Med. Clin. N. Amer., *56*:1405, 1972.

Bloom, H. J. G., et al.: The treatment and prognosis of medulloblastoma in children. Am. J. Roentgenol., *105*:43, 1969.

Bouchard, J.: Radiation Therapy of Tumors and Disease of the Nervous System. Philadelphia, Lea & Febiger, 1966.

Bouteille, M., et al.: Sur un cas d'encéphalite subaigue à inclusions. Etude anatomo-clinique et ultrastructurale. Rev. Neurol., *113*:454, 1965.

Connolly, J. H., et al.: Measles-virus antibody and antigen in subacute sclerosing panencephalitis. Lancet, *1*:542, 1967.

Davis, L. E., and Drachman, D. B.: Myeloma neuropathy. Arch. Neurol., *27*:507, 1972.

Editorial: Uremic neuropathy and renal transplantation. Lancet, *2*:418, 1971.

Editorial: Measles and multiple sclerosis. Lancet, *1*:247, 1974*a*.

Editorial: Neuralgic amyotrophy. Lancet, *2*:878, 1974*b*.

Editorial: Kuru, Creutzfeldt-Jakob, and scrapie. Lancet, *2*:1551, 1974*c*.

Escourolle, R., and Poirier, J.: Manual of Basic Neuropathology. Philadelphia, W. B. Saunders Co., 1973.

Field, E. J., et al.: Viruses in multiple sclerosis? Lancet, *2*:280, 1972.

Haase, G. R.: Disease presenting as dementia. *In* Wells, C. E. (ed.) Dementia. Philadelphia, F. A. Davis Company, 1971.

Hachinski, V. C., et al.: Multi-infarct dementia. Lancet, *2*:207, 1974.

Heston, L. L., et al.: Alzheimer's disease. Arch. Neurol., *15*:225, 1966.

Hope-Stone, H. F.: Results of treatment of medulloblastomas. J. Neurosurg., *32*:83, 1970.

Hornykiewicz, O.: Parkinson's disease: from brain homogenate to treatment. Fed. Proc., *32*:183, 1973.

Horta-Barbosa, L., et al.: Isolation of measles virus from brain cell cultures of two patients with subacute sclerosing panencephalitis. Proc. Soc. Exp. Biol. Med., *132*:272, 1969.

Kannel, W. B.: Current status of the epidemiology of brain infarction associated with occlusive arterial disease. Stroke, *2*:295, 1971.

Kuller, L., et al.: Nationwide cerebrovascular disease morbidity study. Stroke, *1*:86, 1970.

Manz, H. J.: The pathology of cerebral edema. Hum. Pathol., *5*:291, 1974.

McDonald, J., and Lapham, L.: Central nervous system tumors. *In* Rubin, P., ed.: Clinical Oncology for Medical Students and Physicians. 3rd ed. Rochester, N.Y., American Cancer Society, 1970–71.

Narayan, O., et al.: Etiology of progressive multifocal leukoencephalopathy. New Eng. J. Med., *289*:1278, 1973.

Padgett, B. L., and Walker, D. L.: Prevalence of antibodies in human sera against JC-virus, an isolate from a case of progressive multifocal leukoencephalopathy. J. Infect. Dis., *127*:467, 1973.

Paterson, R.: The Treatment of Malignant Disease by Radiotherapy. Baltimore, Williams & Wilkins Company, 1963.

Payne, F. E., et al.: Isolation of measles virus from cell cultures of brain from a patient with subacute sclerosing panencephalitis. New Eng. J. Med., *281*:585, 1969.

Perry, T. L., et al.: Huntington's chorea. New Eng. J. Med., *288*:337, 1973.

Prineas, J.: Paramyxovirus-like particles associated with acute demyelination in chronic relapsing multiple sclerosis. Science, *178*:760, 1972.

Ring, J., et al.: Intensive immunosuppression in the treatment of multiple sclerosis. Lancet, *2*:1093, 1974.

Seligman, S. J.: The rapid differential diagnosis of meningitis. Med. Clin. N. Amer., *57*:1417, 1973.

Sibley, W. A.: Polyneuritis. Med. Clin. N. Amer., *56*:1299, 1972.

Silverberg, E., and Holleb, A. I.: Cancer statistics, 1975. CA, *25*:8, 1975.

ter Meulen, V., et al.: Fusion of cultured multiple sclerosis brain cells with indicator cells: presence of nucleocapsids and virions and isolation of parainfluenza-type virus. Lancet, *2*:1, 1972.

Walker, M. D.: Malignant brain tumors—a synopsis. CA, *25*:114, 1975.

Webb, C., et al.: Lymphocytes sensitised to basic encephalitogen in patients with multiple sclerosis unresponsive to steroid therapy. Lancet, 2:66, 1974.

Weiner, L. P., et al.: Viral infections in demyelinating diseases. New Eng. J. Med., 288:1103, 1973.

Weir, B., and Elvidge, A. R.: Oligodendrogliomas, an analysis of 63 cases. J. Neurosurg., 29:500, 1968.

Whisnant, J. P., et al.: Natural history of stroke in Rochester, Minnesota, 1945 through 1954. Stroke, 2:11, 1971.

Zacks, S. I.: Atlas of Neuropathology. New York, Harper & Row, 1971.

Zlotnik, I., et al.: Transmission of Creutzfeldt-Jakob disease from man to squirrel monkey. Lancet, 2:435, 1974.

ZuRhein, G. M., and Chou, S. M.: Particles resembling papova viruses in human cerebral demyelinating disease. Science, 148:1477, 1965.

ZuRhein, G. M.: Association of papova virions with a human demyelinating disease (progressive multifocal leukoencephalopathy). Progr. Med. Virol., 11:185, 1969.

Index